Maternity Nursing

Sharon J. Reeder, R.N., Ph.D.

Associate Professor of Nursing, School of Nursing,
University of California, Los Angeles

Luigi Mastroianni, Jr., M.D., F.A.C.S., F.A.C.O.G

William Goodell Professor and Chairman, Department of Obstetrics and Gynecology,
University of Pennsylvania School of Medicine

Leonide L. Martin, R.N., M.S., M.P.H.

Family Nurse Practitioner, Lecturer, Department of Nursing
California State College, Sonoma

Maternity Nursing

fourteenth edition

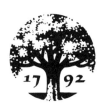

J. B. Lippincott Company

Philadelphia • Toronto

Fourteenth Edition

Copyright © 1980, 1976, 1971, 1966, 1960, 1952, 1948, 1943, 1940, 1937, 1934, 1933, 1931, 1929 by J. B. Lippincott Company

ISBN 0-397-54253-4

Library of Congress Catalog Card Number 79-22993

Printed in the United States of America

5 7 9 8 6 4

Library of Congress Cataloging in Publication Data
Main entry under title:
Maternity nursing.
   Includes index.
   1. Obstetrical nursing. I. Reeder, Sharon J.
RG951.Z3   1980   618.2   79-22993
ISBN 0-397-54253-4

To

Leo G. Reeder

March 13, 1921–September 25, 1978

The authors wish to dedicate the fourteenth edition of *Maternity Nursing* to the memory of Leo G. Reeder who was killed in an aircrash tragedy on September 25, 1978. Leo had been a contributor to several editions of *Maternity Nursing*.

He was a pioneer in the field of medical sociology. His interest and work in the fields of population, social epidemiology and utilization of health services had far-reaching implications for the areas of reproductive health and maternal-child health. His contribution to the health field in general is well recognized by his colleagues and his presence and encouragement are deeply missed by his wife and many friends.

S.J.R.

L.M., Jr.

L.L.M.

Contributors

CLAUDIA J. ANDERSON, PH.D., R.N.
Chairperson
Department of Obstetrics and Gynecological Nursing
Rush-Presbyterian-St. Lukes Medical Center
Chicago, Illinois
Emotional Reactions to Pregnancy *in Chapter 17:*
Psychosocial Aspects of Normal Pregnancy

IDA STANLEY BIRD, R.N., M.N.
Assistant Clinical Professor
Childbirth Educator
Center for the Health Sciences
U.C.L.A.
Los Angeles, California
Chapters 18 and 19: **Parent Education; Nutrition in Pregnancy**

ROBERTA GERDS, R.N., M.N.
Assistant Clinical Professor
School of Nursing
U.C.L.A.
Los Angeles, California
Chapters 29 and 30: **Care of the Newborn Infant; Infant Nutrition**

BRETT B. GUTSCHE, M.D.
Professor of Obstetrics and Gynecology
Professor of Anesthesia
University of Pennsylvania School of Medicine
Chapter 25: **Analgesia and Anesthesia for Childbirth**

MARGO MCCAFFERY, R.N., M.S.
Consultant in the Nursing Care of People with Pain
Santa Monica, California
Chapter 24: **The Nurse's Contribution to Pain Relief During Labor**

ANN MCDONNELL, R.N.
Nurse Coordinator, Genetics Counselor
Department of Obstetrics and Gynecology
University of Pennsylvania School of Medicine
Co-author, *Chapter 15:* **Genetic Counseling and Diagnosis During Pregnancy**

MICHAEL T. MENNUTI, M.D.
Assistant Professor
Department of Obstetrics and Gynecology
University of Pennsylvania School of Medicine
Chapter 37: **Electronic Fetal Monitoring and Fetal Intensive Care**
Co-author, *Chapter 15:* **Genetic Counseling and Diagnosis During Pregnancy**

RICHARD SCHWARZ, M.D.
Chairman, Department of Obstetrics and Gynecology
Downstate Medical Center, Brooklyn, N.Y.
Chapter 36: **Fetal Diagnosis and Treatment**

MAUREEN SHANNON-BABITZ, R.N.
Chapter 40: **Alternatives in Maternity Care**

Preface

The 14th edition of *Maternity Nursing* again reflects extensive revision. Several new chapters have been added, most of the chapters have been rewritten and the remainder have been completely updated.

In the past five years, society has continued to change at a phenomenal pace and the institutions within society continue their reorganization, particularly the family and the educational and health systems. As society changes, so must those who occupy roles in society. Thus, as clients change their orientations, values and behavior, health providers must change in order to maintain a synchrony in their roles.

The family system continues with innovation and experimentation with many lifestyles becoming more apparent. With these various lifestyles come a melange of attitudes and behaviors regarding reproduction, family planning, sexuality, birthing and childrearing. Of necessity, these broaden the scope of maternal care. Moreover, the continuing innovation occurring in the health care delivery system, especially in nursing, has an additional impact on the specialty. These current issues are examined in depth to enable students to gain a better insight into their importance so that this knowledge can be incorporated into their care of families during the reproductive process.

Unit 1 has been reorganized to provide a variety of fundamental concepts regarding the structure and function of the modern family and health systems, emerging multiple life styles, and various social factors relating to health. These concepts are explored in depth as a basis for discussion of the current thinking regarding changing role relationships in the family, nursing and parenting, reproductive behavior and utilization of maternity services. This information provides a broad conceptual base which the student must have in order to deliver high quality nursing care to families.

Unit 2 has been rewritten to elaborate on information regarding sexual and reproductive anatomy and physiology, as well as conception and ovum development. Sections on development and physiology of the embryo and fetus have been revised to reflect current data and thinking. This unit supplies the basic anatomy and physiology upon which students can base their nursing care.

Unit 3 is a new unit. Areas of sexuality and various facets of reproduction are examined in depth. Common concerns that individuals have regarding sexuality are addressed and the chapters dealing with contraception, pregnancy termination, infertility and genetic counseling provide additional necessary information for the delivery of quality maternity care.

Units 4 through 6 deal with the normal reproductive cycle from conception through the post-partal period. Several new chapters have been added which include psychosocial aspects of pregnancy and the postpartum period, nutrition in pregnancy and infant nutrition. These chapters will enable the student to gain a knowledge of the total normal reproductive cycle and its management. Throughout these and the other chapters in the book, dimensions of effective nursing care for each phase of the reproductive cycle have been expanded, based on recent research and conceptual developments in nursing practice and related disciplines.

Units 7 and 8 reflect current research and practice regarding the assessment and management of maternal and infant disorders. A full chapter has been devoted to electronic monitoring and its appropriate use. Fetal diagnosis and the management of the high risk infant has been extensively updated to reflect current thinking and management. The information in these chapters is essential as the field of perinatal medicine and nursing continue to evolve.

Unit 9 examines several special considerations in maternity nursing. The current issue of alternatives in childbirth is addressed and the topics of home deliveries, birth centers, lay midwives and nurse midwives are discussed to enable the student to see the place of these important events and the contribution of these providers in the total maternity spectrum. The section on the evolution of maternity nursing has been rewritten to reflect current trends. Health care is not carried out in a vacuum, nor did present-day maternity care spring from nothing. It was shaped and nurtured by a variety of economic and social factors. Thus, a good understanding of the history of the field will enable the student to appreciate current practice and predict future care patterns.

Many new photographs, drawings, illustrations and figures have been added to this edition. All of the suggested readings have been updated with references from current professional literature.

Sharon R. Reeder, R.N., Ph.D.

Luigi Mastroianni, Jr., M.D.

Leonide L. Martin, R.N., M.S.

Acknowledgments

With the preparation of the fourteenth edition of this book, we wish to thank our contributors who have given a special dimension to the book with their varied expertise. We wish also to express our gratitude for the help and encouragement of our many colleagues and friends in the revision of this volume. We would like to thank Ms. Teresa Seeman for her assistance in researching the literature and Mrs. Trudy Krohn and Mrs. Pat Quist for their expert typing and editorial services.

We are also indebted to Mrs. Ruth Lubic, General Director of Maternity Center Association of New York, for permission to publish the exercises taught by the Maternity Center Association in its prepared childbirth program. The authors would also like to express their appreciation to colleagues, publishers, and organizations for the use of illustrations, assessment tools, and other forms that are found in the text. We wish to express our gratitude also to the many parents, nursing students, and staff members who granted permission for photographs to appear in this book.

Finally, we take this opportunity to thank the J. B. Lippincott Company, particularly Mr. David T. Miller and Ms. Dorothy Hoffman for their interest and cooperation. Most particularly, we wish to thank Ms. Diana Intenzo, our editor, whose steadfast monitoring and assistance helped make this edition possible.

Contents

Philosophy of Family-Centered Care

Of all the phenomena that the human species experiences, birth is perhaps the most awe-inspiring, emotional, and dramatic episode of one's lifetime. It is, indeed, a family affair, and the reproductive health of the total family is the cornerstone upon which a healthy society rests. Thus, the study of obstetrics and the nursing care of women and their families during the various phases of childbearing includes not only the study of anatomical and physiological adaptations to human reproduction, but also the study of human growth and development and the many complex, interdependent relationships to the total society that are inextricably bound to this growth.

Knowledge of the anatomy and physiology of the reproductive organs and of the development of the unborn child from conception to birth is basic to the understanding required by everyone who participates in maternity care. The physiological mechanism by which conception takes place and the new human being develops is not only a fascinating story in itself, but also one that has far-reaching implications for the mother, the child, and the family. All that a person becomes depends on many factors: his or her heritage, the prenatal environment, the care at birth, and the care thereafter throughout infancy and childhood. Thus, it becomes apparent

that the health, well-being, and safety of each mother, father, and infant must be protected, and simultaneously that the highest level of wellness possible for every childbearing family be achieved in the broadest sense of physical, emotional, and social well-being. Moreover, it is also important to understand the extent to which the structure and function of the family, as it relates to the larger society, influence the reproductive behavior and health of the childbearing family.

This chapter is planned to orient the student to maternity nursing. The philosophy and assumptions underlying care for the family during reproduction will be given and basic concepts of care will be examined. Basic and new evolving terminology will be defined. In the remainder of the unit, information and concepts relating to childbearing families and their intermeshing with society will be explored.

THE EVOLUTION OF THE CONCEPT OF MATERNITY CARE

All definitions and modes of health care have a history. Maternity care is no exception. The student is referred to Chapter 41 for an in-depth presentation of the history of the field. For the moment, we will concern ourselves with a brief overview of some terms and the concepts of care that have become associated with them.

Obstetrics

Obstetrics is defined as that branch of medicine which deals with parturition, its antecedents and its sequels. Thus, it is concerned principally with the phenomena and the management of pregnancy, labor, and the puerperium under both normal and abnormal circumstances.[1]

The etymology of "obstetrics" is mentioned here to serve as basic information. Briefly, the word obstetrics is derived from the Latin *obstetricia* or *obstetrix,* meaning *midwife.* The verb form *obsto (ob,* before, plus *sto,* stand) means to stand by. Thus, in ancient Rome a person who cared for women at childbirth was known as an *obstetrix,* or a person who *stood by* the woman in labor. In both the United States and Great Britain, this branch of medicine was called *midwifery* until the latter part of the 19th century. The term obstetrics really came into usage little more than a century ago, although reference to a variety of words of common derivation can be found occasionally in earlier writings.

The post-World War II era brought dramatic changes in the care of childbearing women and concomitant changes in terminology relating to them. In the then-current frame of reference, it seemed, and continues to seem, more appropriate to use the term *maternity* care since this term focuses on the *recipient* of care rather than on the *provider.* Moreover, it has come to imply a broader meaning of the care of the mother and her offspring; it emphasizes the importance of interpersonal relationships that are significant in the family and takes into consideration all the factors that are crucial in promoting the general health and well-being of the entire expanding family group.

The World Health Organization Expert Committee on Maternity Care has defined maternity care as follows:

The object of maternity care is to ensure that every expectant and nursing mother maintains good health, learns the art of child care, has a normal delivery, and bears healthy children. Maternity care in the narrower sense consists in the care of the pregnant woman, her safe delivery, her postnatal examination, the care of her newly born infant, and the maintenance of lactation. In the wider sense it begins much earlier in measures aimed to promote the health and well-being of the young people who are potential parents, and to help them develop the right approach to family life and to the place of the family in the community. It should also include guidance in parent-craft and in problems associated with infertility and family planning.[2]

Thus, from the rather narrow definition that focused primarily on the provider of care, we have come to expand our concept of obstetrics to include not only the childbearing woman herself, but all those in her social network who are significant to her.

Maternal Child Health

Despite the fact that the use of the term *maternal and child health* seems to imply a relatively new concept of care, it was in usage more than 50 years ago. In 1912 the U.S. Children's Bureau was created by an act of Congress for the purpose of promoting maternal and child health "among all classes of people." It was said to be a community health nurse who first conceived the idea of a federal bureau of this kind and originally suggested the plan to President Theodore Roosevelt in 1905. The Children's Bureau has continually stressed the importance of community health nursing in maternal and child welfare. Between the years 1921 and 1929, community health nursing consultants were employed by the Bureau, and their services were offered to the states for maternal and infant hygiene. In rural areas throughout the United States, community health nursing services were greatly extended, and 2,978 centers for prenatal and child health work were established.

Since these early beginnings, the Children's Bureau has continued to make significant contributions to the promotion of maternal and child health in this country.

Trends in Maternal-Child Care

Trends in U.S. maternal and child health services were assessed in a report by the late Dr. Edward Schlesinger of the University of Pittsburgh, who had long been active in efforts to upgrade such programs. Writing in *Health and Society,* Dr. Schlesinger cited current and past developments to explain why those in the maternal–child health field feel that they are in the throes of a profound "identity crisis."[3]

These developments are germane to maternity care because they exemplify a broad spectrum of thinking about delivery of health services in general. New systems of personal health services are being developed to serve entire populations regardless of age or categorical needs. Thus, expanding "special purpose" programs in early childhood and adolescence that tend to include their own independent health services have called into question the more traditional types of health services for mothers and children. The latter have tended to be separate and clearly identifiable programs in maternity and newborn care; in health supervisory services for infants, preschoolers, and school-age children; and in rehabilitative services for handicapped children. The new special purpose programs, because of their breadth, often lose specific aspects of care that are badly needed.

However, there have been certain reasons for the development of these newer programs, the most important of which is the unprecedented decline in the U.S. birth and fertility rates. Therefore, further expansion of maternal and child health services can no longer be justified *solely* by the argument of a continuing increase in the number of mothers and children to be served. Moreover, the U.S. infant mortality rate, although poor in relation to the rates of other industrialized nations, has also reached record lows, thus making arguments for broadened services on this point no longer as compelling as they were. Hence, with a much smaller population to serve and a slightly better infant survival rate, what can be the rationale for continued expansion of maternal–child health services? It appears that the argument must be shifted to the need to provide adequate services in order to maintain and expand the gains of recent years, *especially for those segments of the population that have not shared equally in these gains.*

One other reason for the newer programs deserves mention because it is concerned with basic funding for maternal–child health services. In 1973, there was a drastic reorganization of the federal child development and child health services under the Health Services Administration. While necessary, this reorganization fragmented services and diminished the visibility of mothers' and children's health needs within the federal government. There is no longer a single, clear focus for the expression of concerns for those involved with the health of mothers and children. Before the reorganization, there was firm federal-local cooperation in the provision of special project grants for specific purposes in geographic areas of need—primarily inner-city neighborhoods. However, since the reorganization, the concept of revenue sharing has threatened to reverse this and other salubrious trends that had been growing since 1935 with Title V funding. Inherent in all of this is the hazard that the health needs of the inner-city and other special need populations will receive less emphasis.

Toward Better Maternal-Child Health

In view of these current outside forces and trends, we will summarize in the form of recommendations the major areas of concern in maternal–child health:

1. First, it is necessary to have integration of high-quality maternal–child health services within evolving comprehensive systems of prepaid group health care plans. Moreover, services should include prevention, detection, and maintenance.
2. Second, adequate funding of preventive and ambulatory services, especially during the newborn period, must be included in all the mechanisms for financing maternal–child health services.
3. Third, the present services and special projects must be extended to meet the needs of specific high-risk and disadvantaged groups.
4. Fourth, there is a need to resolve the dilemma of providing health services in settings which do not focus primarily on health, that is, schools.
5. Fifth, there must be a focus on concern for maternal and child health within the federal government and for mechanisms for child advocacy both within and without the federal government. The recent fragmentation has left the federal government without a clear point of entry for those interested in maternal–child health services.
6. Finally, there is a need for continuing, critical evaluative research to explore innovations and alternative methods of delivery of care. For instance, it is necessary to have a much clearer idea about whether increased technology really results in higher quality of care.

PHILOSOPHY AND ASSUMPTIONS ABOUT MATERNITY CARE

Philosophy

Health providers' responses to their clients' needs in both health maintenance and illness management must take into consideration current attitudinal, social, and cultural changes. Health care is not delivered in a vacuum; it takes place in a larger social context and is greatly influenced by current thinking and change manifested by the host society. From this thinking and change philosophies of care evolve.

The authors of this text believe maternity care to be a philosophy of patient care rather than a special area of medical services or nursing. We believe that begetting children is a family affair; thus, the medical and nursing care of maternity patients is properly a family-centered activity. In most situations today the childbearing woman is a healthy individual in the normal physiological process of childbearing. However, like all individuals facing any other new experience in the family life cycle, the woman and her partner may begin the experience at various stages of preparation for pregnancy and childbirth, with various kinds of stress and different levels of contentment.

It is safe to say that in almost no other normal physiological process does one find such individual extremes of reactions within a normal context. For both the woman and her partner, these reactions may be based on events going back to childhood, as well as to those experienced as an adolescent and adult. Certainly, they are influenced by the immediate home environment from which the couple comes and to which they will soon return with their newborn. Moreover, the level of satisfaction with which the expectant parents leave the provider's presence, or the level of contentment with which the newly delivered mother and infant leave the hospital environment will be modified by the interpersonal relationships of those most significant to them in that environment.

Assumptions

Therefore, underlying the above philosophy are the following assumptions.

1. All individuals have the right to be born healthy, and to ensure this right, every pregnant woman and every fetus has the right to quality health care.
2. Individuals' sexuality is inextricably bound to reproduction but not subordinate to it; changing societal attitudes toward sexuality, role relationships, and childbearing, together with technological advances in fertility control, have combined to make parenthood increasingly a voluntary state.
3. Reproduction is not experienced alone; whatever the circumstances, it involves one or more individuals.
4. Reproduction is part of a normal psychophysiological process and can be physically and emotionally rewarding for the individuals involved.
5. The childbearing experience is a developmental opportunity; it can also be a situational crisis during which family members benefit from the solidarity of the family unit.
6. The profound physiological changes and adjustment that both the mother and her offspring experience during the childbearing process make them particularly vulnerable to changeable and noxious environments and situations that would ordinarily not prove hazardous.
7. Each individual's attitudes, values, and health behavior are influenced by the culture and society from which he or she comes; thus, each individual's reproductive outcomes and childbearing experience will be influenced by his or her cultural heritage.

Having stated our guiding philosophy and the assumptions underlying that philosophy, we will next examine our view of nursing's role in this philosophy of care.

MATERNITY NURSING / FAMILY-CENTERED CARE

Definition

Maternity nursing can be defined as the delivery of professional quality health care while recognizing, focusing on, and adapting to the physical and psychosocial needs of the childbearing woman, the family, and the newly born offspring. The emphasis is on the provision of professional, quality care that fosters family unity while maintaining physical safety of the childbearing unit.

Implicit in this definition is the notion of a family-centered approach. This notion, in turn, assumes that the family is the basic unit of society and, as such, is to be viewed as a total unit within which each member is a distinct individual entitled to consideration. It is further assumed that childbearing and the rearing and socialization of children are unique and important functions of the family. Therefore, the experience of childbearing is appropriate and beneficial to share as a unit.

It is important to note that, when we speak of the "family," we do not necessarily mean the traditional nuclear family composed of a married pair and their children. A family may be any constellation of interacting individuals who are considered to be "significant others" to the individuals involved. In Chapters 3 and 4 we will examine, in more detail, the various definitions and family forms that are emerging today.

Maternity nursing involves direct, personal ministrations to the childbearing woman and her infant, as well as the related activities of teaching, counseling, and supervision, during the various phases of the childbearing experience. A cornerstone of care is patient/consumer education with respect to health maintenance and reproductive health. It differs from the practice of nursing in other areas in that the clinical focus involves primarily the care of the childbearing unit—the mother, father, and infant (in contrast, for example, to the care of surgical patients or psychiatric patients). It is unique in that the nurse is called upon to attend, educate, and counsel all age groups, from the fetus through childhood, adolescence, and adulthood, since the childbearing unit may span all those stages in the life cycle.

How the maternity nurse meets the needs of mothers, fathers, and their infants cannot be spelled out in stereotyped activities any more than it can in any other situation in which individualized care is the underlying objective. She will intervene to relieve or reduce her clients' problems caused by physiological, psychological, or social stress. In addition, she will consult with her clients and their families to make them aware of the principles of health maintenance so that they may incorporate these into their preventive health behavior patterns.

A significant aspect of maternity nursing on the professional level is that the nursing care involves purposeful, sustained interaction between the nurse and her client(s). During this encounter, the nurse makes an assessment of the client(s)' problems and resources, and then takes action to relieve the problem and support the strengths with appropriate nursing measures. If the condition requires additional services from the other members of the health team, referral and/or consultation is given.

Implementation

The successful implementation of family-centered nursing care includes recognition that the provision of high caliber care requires a team effort by the woman and her family, the health care providers, and the community. The composition of the team may vary from setting to setting and includes obstetricians, pediatricians, family physicians, certified nurse-midwives, nurse practitioners, and maternity clinical nurse specialists. While physicians are responsible for providing direction for medical management, other team members share appropriately in managing the health care of the family, and each team member must be individually accountable for the performance of his or her facet of care. The team concept includes the cooperative interrelationships of hospitals, providers, and the community in an organized care system so as to provide for the total spectrum of maternity/newborn care within a particular geographical region.[4]

Expanding Roles

Expanded roles in maternity nursing is not a new concept and, in fact, predates the expanded role concept now prevalent in nursing in general. Prior to the 19th century there was little interest by anyone in providing quality maternity care to mothers and families. Care was generally delivered by untrained women who had achieved a modicum of expertise by an apprenticeship/doer method. In the mid-1900s physicians became more interested in obstetrics. In Britain nurse-midwifery educational programs were implemented. In 1925, Mary Breckinridge, who had trained in England as a midwife, spearheaded the organization of the Frontier Nursing Service in Kentucky. In 1925, the Frontier Graduate School of Midwifery opened its doors and for many years was the premier school of midwifery in the United States. Today there are numerous educational programs throughout the United States that are undertaking the preparation of nurses for various expanded roles in the field.

A brief overview of the main categories of personnel in the expanded role will be useful to the student. At the time of this writing, several additional subspecialties are emerging. However, the following will provide a basis for later comparisons.

Nurse-midwife. Certified nurse-midwives are registered nurses who have completed a specified program of study and clinical experience recognized by the American College of Nurse Midwives. They must also pass a certification test before beginning practice. They are qualified to take complete health histories and perform complete physical examinations for their patients. They can provide complete antepartal care, including teaching and counseling. They are qualified to give comprehensive care during the intrapartal period, including delivery of the infant. They are able to deliver care to the mother and infant in the postpartal period, including family-planning information and devices. Thus, they attend both the mother and infant throughout the maternity cycle as long as the mother's progress is considered normal and uncomplicated. The student is directed to Chapter 41 for a more detailed examination of the role and functions of this practitioner.

Obstetrical-gynecological Nurse Practitioner. These individuals are registered nurses who have completed an additional formal educational program that meets criteria specified for state licensure and certification. These programs may be at the master's level. These practitioners work in collaboration with physicians and may have varying degrees of supervision from their physician colleagues. They function in somewhat the same way that nurse midwives do; however, they do not deliver infants.

Obstetrical-gynecological nurse practitioners provide immediate and continuing assessment of the newborn and its mother and aid the family in assuming the new parental role. Their focus of practice is on providing primary health care to normal pregnant and nonpregnant women with an emphasis on health maintenance. They can also diagnose and treat certain common abnormalities,

such as uncomplicated cystitis or vaginitis, under the aegis of the collaborating physician's standing and contingency protocols.

Women's Health Care Specialist. This level of practitioner may be a registered nurse or a licensed vocational nurse, or may have experience in another ancillary medical role. The length of training is variable, usually around three to six months, depending upon the entry level of professional education of the applicant. These programs do not have the in-depth preparation that the longer midwifery or Masters degree programs do. Women health care specialists can screen for physical abnormalities in their patients; they then refer any person with suspected pathology to a physician. They can perform routine gynecological examinations, and provide family-planning counseling; they can also insert and remove intrauterine devices. Like the ob-gyn practitioner, they can, under physician's orders, treat simple gynecological problems. Their focus of care is primarily on women as their name implies, but many of these practitioners expand their focus to include a more family-centered approach in their patient teaching and counseling.

Maternity Clinical Specialist. This specialist is a registered nurse who has completed a university-based, Masters degree program of graduate courses designed to provide in-depth knowledge of the reproductive process and development of clinical expertise in the actual delivery of complex nursing care to the childbearing unit. Her functions include health education, counseling, dissemination of family-planning information and assisting the family with their parenting role. These professionals may not have physical assessment (diagnosis) skills and hence would not do complete physical examinations or medically treat common disorders. Patient and family education, counseling, and delivery of complex, expert nursing care is the focus of practice. They also are resource persons for staff education and patient care coordination.

New Directions—Perinatal Nursing

As knowledge continues to burgeon in the field of reproductive health, there has been an effort in the last decade to provide an umbrella of conceptualization about maternal-fetal health care in the form of *perinatal medicine* which would serve to decrease the segmentation and fragmentation of health care for the mother and her child. Perinatal nursing, in turn, is emerging as a new specialty of professional maternity nursing. It is evolving in response to a need that arises from past gaps, failures, and successes in the delivery of quality nursing care during the reproductive process. It encompasses many of the best features of the above roles, and the knowledge base is not significantly different from the midwife or Masters-prepared maternity nurse/practitioner. It would seem that this specialty ought to continue to flourish since professional nurses are capable of assuming new roles that are appropriate for new responsibilities and conceptions of nursing and for the health care of the childbearing unit in general.

THE NURSING PROCESS IN MATERNITY CARE

Implicit in the delivery of effective, professional nursing care is the ability to utilize a method that helps the nurse arrive at informed judgments about clients that have a sound data base. With the data base and these appropriate clinical judgments, nursing care can be planned and implemented so as to enable clients to maintain or return to a state of high-level wellness. This method has been conceptualized as *nursing process* by a variety of authors in an effort to describe a lucid, organized, scientifically based problem-solving approach to professional nursing practice.[5-7]

Nursing process is the organizing conceptual framework used throughout this text to help the student learn to make nursing judgments appropriate to her nursing care. It supplies a mechanism which enables the nurse to arrive at a responsible valid judgment about clients from which to plan, implement, and evaluate nursing care that is responsive to the clients' varied needs.

Components of the Process

The nursing process is composed of such phases as assessment, planning, implementation or intervention, and evaluation. Other authors have conceptualized the process as including observation, infer-

ence, validation, assessment, action, and evaluation.[8] Over the years, new terminology has evolved, and as nursing science develops, other terminology no doubt will be employed. Thus, we have in the literature such terms as nursing diagnosis, clinical judgment, assessment, nursing prescriptions, and so on. All of these terms refer in some way to the components of the nursing process and constitute the anatomy of nursing practice. Figure 1-1 presents a model for a contextual scheme of some current terms used in the conceptualization of nursing process.

It is important to point out that, in the midst of the press and crush of everyday practice, where human lives may be at stake, calm fact-finding and judicial deliberation become increasingly difficult. Some of our most crucial nursing problems arise from conflicts between principle and expediency. Hence, we need to have a method so internalized as to be second nature so that we can arrive quickly at appropriate decisions and conclusions about our patients.

The components of the process also can help the student understand how nursing practice can be made operational. The various operations have been classified under headings derived from Bloch.[9] One is not to assume that these categories are mutually exclusive or stand alone. Rather, there are constant feedback loops in the process (see Fig. 1-1). Many authors might consider the data collection part of the nursing diagnosis stage. We present this interpretation as one means of conceptualizing more clearly the nursing process (see Fig. 1-2).

Figure 1-2 also illustrates the similarity of the nursing process to the scientific method. The scientific method is utilized by other disciplines to provide a way of problem-solving for their members and as a basis from which to formulate research that will expand the theoretical base of the discipline. Since nursing also has the concern of expanding its theoretical knowledge to provide a sound basis for its practice, it becomes very important that the nursing process be scientifically grounded.

Assessment

As we review the process, it can be seen that components 1 and 2 constitute a reconnoitering stage in which information is gathered and the diagnosis begun. Resources such as the chart, the

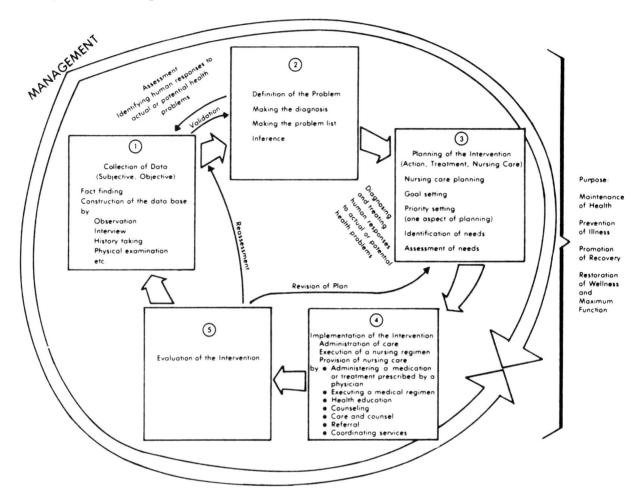

Figure 1-1. Contextual scheme for some currently used terms in the conceptualization of nursing practice. (Block, D.: Some crucial terms in nursing: what do they really mean? Copyright © 1974, American Journal of Nursing Company. Reproduced with permission from Nursing Outlook, 22:4, Nov. 1974)

family, the patient, members of the health team, and elements in the environment can be utilized. The nurse also may utilize the ability to "role take" to speed up the data collection.★ This term refers to the ability to project oneself into the place of the patient in order to imaginatively construct the role of the patient, so as to provide appropriate cues for predicting and understanding the meaning of the patient's behavior, and thus, for determining appropriate behavior on the part of the nurse. The process by which the role of each particular patient is inferred stems from basic knowledge about the patient role in general, prior experience with the individual or others like her, and/or a specific bit of

★For a detailed definition and explanation of the concept of "role taking" and its application in maternity nursing, see the Reeder article in the Suggested Reading.

behavior that is being manifested. As the student gains more experience with various individuals involved in the patient role who are confronted with different kinds of health-illness conditions (including maternity patients), this role-taking ability will be facilitated.

Nursing Diagnosis

As we acquire our data, we become able to decide the existence and extent of a problem. We can say in the most general terms that a problem does exist when there is a health goal to be obtained, but the individual (patient) sees no well-defined, well-established means of attaining it. For instance, she may be too ill or weak to help herself. Again, the goal may be so vaguely defined or unclear that the

patient cannot determine relevant means of achieving it. Thus, the patient may not understand or
know how to accept conditions and instruction for
achieving the goal of health.

A decision about the existence and extent of the
problem initiates the diagnosis. There are many
definitions of this term. For our purposes we shall
regard a nursing diagnosis as a conclusion based on
a systematic and scientific appraisal of an individual's
health-illness condition, resulting from critical anal-

ysis of his or her behavior (alone and with others),
the nature of the condition and the numerous other
factors, environmental, social, or psychological,
that may affect the client's general state. This conclusion serves as a guide for our nursing care.

It is well to remember also that the statement of
the diagnosis may be several words and be more
descriptive than etiological. As we find additional
information about our patients, we may move from
descriptive to more etiological statements. More-

Figure 1-2. Relationship of scientific method to nursing process.

Components of the Nursing Process

1. Collection of Data (subjective, objective)
   a. Gathering of information on the physical, social and
      psychological aspects of the health status of the indi-
      vidual and family
   b. Construction of the data base by: observation, inter-
      view, history taking, physical examination, role tak-
      ing, etc.
   c. Develop impressions

2. Definition of the Problem
   a. Making decisions regarding deficit(s) or potential
      deficit(s) in health status of the individual and family
      assigning resources
   b. Making these nursing diagnoses based on clinical
      judgment and inference, and review of related
      information; i.e., theoretical formulations, research

3. Planning the Intervention
   a. Making decision(s) regarding the action(s) believed to
      be appropriate to effect a solution of defined
      problem(s)
   b. Decision(s) include goal setting, priority setting, nurs-
      ing prescriptions

4. Implementation of the Intervention
   a. Execution of a nursing regimen by: administering a
      prescribed medication or treatment, executing a med-
      ical regimen, providing comfort measures and
      physical care, providing counseling, providing referral
      services, coordinating services for the patient, pro-
      viding health education

5. Evaluation of the Intervention—this in turn may lead to
   further reassessments.
   a. Determining the degree of effectiveness of the
      action(s) taken in solving the defined problems by: ob-
      servation, interview of patient status and conditions,
      physical examination, reading of current records, etc.
   b. Prediction of future nursing action and patient poten-
      tial for change

6. Terminate or modify relationship

Scientific Method

1. Recognize general problem area
   a. Survey pertinent information (liter-
      ature, past experience, observation)
   b. Construct data base (organize,
      select)
   c. Develop "hunches"

2. Define specific problem
   a. Make decisions about relevance

   b. Review related information (re-
      search already done, theoretical
      formulations)

3. Propose hypotheses

4. Test hypotheses
   a. Establish base-line data
   b. State criteria for acceptance or re-
      jection
   c. Collect data

5. Analysis data—interpret results

6. Terminate or modify study
   a. Recommendations/predictions for
      future research

Assessment — Intervention — Evaluation & reassessment

over, there may be several diagnoses relating to a constellation of interrelated problems the patient has; for instance, if the nurse were to write diagnoses regarding a labor patient, they might be as follows: "anxiety regarding process of labor"; "elevated temperature"; "inefficient but painful contractions."

Finally, one can have the same nursing diagnosis but have different pathological conditions that give rise to it. In the case of a newly delivered infant, for instance, the diagnosis might be "inadequate oxygenation"; the cause for one infant might be a congenital heart defect; for another infant, immature lungs associated with prematurity. Thus, the total interrelationship of all the influencing factors is to be considered as it gives direction to our care plan.

Intervention

Components 3 and 4 are concerned with the planning and implementation of knowledgeable intervention in the form of nursing activities that encompass everything from the administration of comfort measures to counseling and health education. These activities are directed at moving the patient toward increased positive adaptation to the environment and a high level of wellness.

Here nursing prescriptions are given. These are directions and suggestions that are incorporated into the nursing regimen or care plan. They constitute mutually agreed upon directives to the client that have bearing in furthering the well-being of the patient. They function much the same way as medical prescriptions, but are often more elaborate and are formulated in consultation with the client and family.

It is well to remember that the implementation phase is fluid since it is based upon the diagnosis or diagnoses which may be reassessed at any point in the process. Moreover, as we administer care, the patient's condition will be expected to change, which, upon evaluation, will necessitate possible new diagnoses and modification of care. Therefore, continuous feedback loops are built into the process.

In this phase, the nurse has the responsibility to disseminate her plan of care to her medical and nursing colleagues so that comprehensive care for the patient can be attained. This can be done by means of the Kardex, verbal reporting, charting, and nursing assessment care plans. Most hospitals have instituted these care plan forms, and they

provide a thorough but brief summary of pertinent patient data together with space to write and record nursing prescriptions, interventions, evaluations, and patient response to care.

Evaluation and Reassessment

Component 5 includes both evaluation and prediction facets. A worthwhile evaluation includes an estimation of the results of our past nursing care activities to help us predict the validity of our care for the future. Any statement of the effectiveness and reliability of our actions is best made with qualifications indicating the degree or amount of effectiveness and reliability claimed.

1. What is the present state of the client?
2. Were all symptoms relieved?
3. What was the extent of the results?
4. On what evidence (observation of self, others, verbal response, cessation of symptoms)?
5. Who was involved (nurse, patient, others)?
6. In what contexts (what else was happening when the action was performed)?

When these points are established, we can begin to build categories of nursing action that are effective under certain circumstances for certain patients given certain conditions. As we ascertain the extent of our effectiveness we are then in a better position to predict the patient's potential for change toward stability and/or a wellness condition. Thus, we arrive at the nursing prognosis.★

THE SOCIAL CONTEXT OF MATERNITY CARE

We mentioned earlier that maternity care is practiced in the context of the total society and, as such, is influenced by the values, attitudes, and practices of that society. Of late, society is adopting a new stance, particularly with regard to women. Since at least half of the maternity nurse's clientele will be women, attitudes and practices regarding them have great relevance for nursing practice. In concluding this chapter, we would like to leave the student

★The student is encouraged to utilize the Suggested Reading for the articles on the nursing process and clinical judgment for a thorough and varied treatment of the subject.

with some information which we hope will be doubly thought-provoking for him or her.

Martin has pointed out in her recent book that the maelstrom of social change this country has experienced, particularly in the last 25 years, has greatly expanded the options open to women. At one time women had to make a choice between a family or a career; now women are increasingly combining the two—as men have always been privileged to do. Moreover, many types of occupations and professions formerly closed to women are becoming more accessible. Federal legislation now supports equal treatment of working women, and more mechanisms to challenge discrimination and unfair employment practices against women are being developed at the state level. Antidiscrimination laws have also had an impact on educational institutions. This is forcing a gradual change in the social biases toward a male privilege, perpetuated through values taught in primary and secondary schools, and culminating in the sex-linked admissions practices and career choices fostered by colleges and universities.[10]

Growing numbers of women and men no longer accept the traditional definitions of "feminine" and "masculine" identities and roles. They are seeking more individualized definitions of self that offer wider ranges of expression of their unique characteristics as *persons* rather than simply *woman* or *man*. Indeed, the common qualities shared by both women and men are felt to far outweigh their sex-related differences. Hence, social roles are developing that provide each sex with a much broader repertoire of behaviors. Women, in particular, expect more choices of lifestyle to be open to them. They may choose to marry or not, to have children or not, or to pursue any career or employment that is suited to their particular talent or interest. They expect to have a voice in the determination of their lives and well-being. And, increasingly, they are demanding a large decision-making role regarding economic and social policies that affect their lives and the larger society in which they live.

Women who choose to rear families spend significantly less of their lifetime in childbearing and childrearing. This fact, of course, has a direct impact on the structure and function of the family. Today's families are smaller and the last child is often born in the mid- to late 20s. Thus, the woman in her late 30s finds that childrearing activities no longer consume the great majority of her time. Moreover, the high degree of technology in the majority of American households has freed her from hours of household chores; thus, homemaking does not provide the fulltime occupation that it once did. With her lifespan lengthened and her health improved, the 35- to 40-year-old woman can be healthy and vigorous and can look ahead to another 25 years or so of productivity in a sphere outside the home.[11]

It has been said that roles are differentiated in pairs—that is, every role has its complementary role. Thus, as women's roles change and broaden, so too must men's. Slowly more egalitarian relationships are developing between the two sexes. Increasingly, men are assuming more responsibility in childrearing and running the household, just as their partners are forging ahead with careers. When both parties are pursuing a career, there is a growing tendency for household management, chores, and child-related activities to be shared equally. Thus, social power is very slowly being equalized and sex-linked exploitation is very gradually being diminished. However, there is still a long way to go before true equality can be achieved.

The authors hope that students would ponder these societal changes and the relevance that they have for nursing practice and themselves as persons.

In the following chapters, we will examine in more depth some of the above ideas as we look at the various aspects of American families and the influence of a variety of social factors in the delivery of care.

REFERENCES

1. Pritchard, J. A. and P. McDonald. *Williams Obstetrics,* ed. 15. New York, Appleton-Century-Crofts, 1976, p. 1.

2. World Health Organization Technical Report Series, No. 51. Geneva, Switzerland, World Health Organization, 1952.

3. Schlesinger, E. *Health and Society* 23:16–20, 1974.

4. Committee on Perinatal Health, The National Foundation—March of Dimes. *Toward Improving the Outcome of Pregnancy: Recommendations for the Regional Development of Maternal and Perinatal Health Services,* 1976.

5. Orem, D. E. *Nursing Concepts of Practice.* New York, McGraw-Hill, 1971.

6. Riehl, J. and Callista Roy. *Conceptual*

Models for Nursing Practice. New York, Appleton-Century-Crofts, 1974.

7. Little, D. and D. Carnevali. *Nursing Care Planning,* ed. 2. Philadelphia, J. B. Lippincott, 1976.

8. Carrieri, V. K. and J. Sitzman. Components of the nursing process. *Nurs. Clin. North Am.* 6: 115–121, Mar. 1971.

9. Bloch, D. Some crucial terms in nursing: What do they really mean? *Nurs. Outlook* 22: 689–694, Nov. 1974.

10. Martin, L. *Health Care of Women.* Philadelphia, J. B. Lippincott, 1978, pp. xiii–xiv.

11. *Ibid.*

SUGGESTED READING

Aspinall, M. J., et al. The why and how of nursing diagnosis. *MCN* 2, 6:355–58, Nov./Dec. 1977.

Curtin, L. and J. A. Petrick. Reproductive manipulation: Technical advances, options and ethical ramifications. *Nurs. Forum* 16, 1:6–25, 1977.

Durand, M. and R. Prince. Nursing diagnosis: Process and decision. *Nurs. Forum* 5, 4:50–64, 1966.

Levine, N. A conceptual model for obstetric nursing. *JOGN Nsg.* 5, 2:9–15, 1976.

Mundinger, M. O. and G. Johnson. Developing a nursing diagnosis. *Nurs. Outlook* 23: 94–98, Feb. 1975.

Reeder, S. Becoming a mother, nursing implications in a problem of role transition. A.N.A. Regional Clinical Conferences, 204–210. New York, Appleton-Century-Crofts, 1968.

Reiter, F. K. The clinical nursing approach. *Nurs. Forum* 5, 4:39–44, 1966.

Roy, Callista. A diagnostic classification system for nursing. *Nurs. Outlook* 23:90–93, Feb. 1975.

Two

Statistical Profiles

Vital Statistics | Natality | Population | Mortality

In the following paragraphs, we shall discuss several types of statistics that are relevant to the care of mothers and their infants and families. Statistical profiles are useful since they summarize a large amount of data about various populations and therefore supply health providers and policymakers with a valuable overview of needs and gaps in care.

VITAL STATISTICS

Vital statistics reports give us quantitative data that have been systematically gathered and collated. Definitions relating to these data are presented here because they relate to statistical changes in the large body of people with whom we are concerned.

In this country these vital statistics reports are published officially by the U.S. Public Health Service, National Center for Health Statistics, Vital Statistics Division. The following terms have been defined by the National Center for Health Statistics. Mortality and morbidity terminology is classified according to the World Health Organization's Manual of International Classification of Diseases, Injuries and Causes of Death. This volume is known by the shortened title, ICD. The ICD is periodically revised and its ninth revision is scheduled for publication in 1979. Some of the definitions below are expected to be changed as a result of the revision.

BIRTHRATE.   The number of births per 1,000 population. Also known as the crude birthrate.

MARRIAGE RATE.   The number of marriages per 1,000 total population.

FERTILITY RATE.   The number of births per 1,000 women aged 15 through 44 years.

NEONATAL.   The period from birth through the 28th day of life.

NEONATAL DEATH RATE.   The number of neonatal deaths per 1,000 live births.

STILLBIRTH OR FETAL DEATH.   A death in which the infant of 20 weeks or more gestational age dies in utero prior to birth.

PERINATAL MORTALITY.   The current definition approved by WHO includes all stillborn infants whose gestational age is 28 weeks or more, plus all neonatal deaths under seven days per 1,000 births. The 1979 revision of the ICD, however, uses birth weight as a criterion rather than gestational age. It also recommends two different categories of reporting. For national data collection, the recommendation is that 500 gm. be used as the minimum weight of stillborn and live-born infants. For international comparisons, however, the weight should be 1,000 gm. or more. When weight is unknown, either gestational age (28 weeks) or body length corresponding to 1,000 gm. may be used. Obviously, these different criteria will make comparisons with previous data impossible and will also make national and international statistical comparisons difficult. There is current debate as to the efficacy of using the newly developed criteria.

INFANT MORTALITY RATE. The number of deaths before the first birthday per 1,000 live births.

MATERNAL MORTALITY RATE. The number of maternal deaths resulting from the reproductive process per *100,000* live births.

RACE AND COLOR. Births in the United States are classified for vital statistics according to the race of the parents in the categories of white, black, American Indian, Chinese, Japanese, Aleut and Eskimo combined, Hawaiian and part-Hawaiian combined, and "other nonwhite." In most tables a less detailed classification of "white" and "nonwhite" is used.

The category white includes births to parents classified as white, Mexican, Puerto Rican, or "not stated." If one parent is Hawaiian and the other is not, the birth is classified as part-Hawaiian. If one parent is black, and the other is not Hawaiian, the birth is classified as black. In other cases of mixed parentage in which both parents are nonwhite, the child is assigned the father's race; if the father is white, the child is assigned the mother's race.

NATALITY

Overall the number of registered births in the United States has decreased in the last three decades from over 4 million live births in 1957 to 3.5 million in 1968 and 3.15 million in 1975. However, provisional data from the National Center for Health Statistics indicates a slight (about 1 percent) rise in the number in 1976 as compared to the previous year. At the same time, both the overall birthrate and the fertility rate continue to decline.

Birth Rates

The increase in the number of births is the result of the increase in the number of women in the childbearing ages (15 to 44). This number has risen rapidly due to the high birthrates of the 1940s and the 1950s—the so-called baby boom of the post-World War II era. Although the fertility rate reached a record low in 1976 for the fifth consecutive year, the decline was not enough to offset the 2 percent increase in the number of women of childbearing age.

Thus, as can be seen, an important consideration which influences the number of children being born annually is the size and the age composition of the female population of childbearing age. Although the fertility rate is computed on the basis of births per 1,000 women between ages 15 and 44, most of the childbearing is concentrated among women in their 20s. In 1973, for example, three out of five births were to women who were in the 20- to 29-age interval.

Another factor that influences the number of births is the number of marriages. In general, there has been a slight rise in the rate of marriages since 1968. However, more married couples are electing not to have children, and there are children being born more often now from social contract and other nonlegal unions. Thus, marriage is not as accurate a predictor as it was formerly.

Multiple Births

Over the years, there has been a decline in the frequency of multiple births in the United States. The frequency of these births is another factor that bears on the natality rate. The rate at present is about ten per 1,000 deliveries. Changes in age and the racial composition of the population, as well as the use of certain ovulation-producing drugs for infertility, contribute to fluctuations in the rate over time. There are differences, for instance, in the occurrence of twins, depending on the number of births the mother has had before delivery of the multiple birth. It should also be mentioned that

H105.142 Rev 5 78

COMMONWEALTH OF PENNSYLVANIA
DEPARTMENT OF HEALTH
VITAL STATISTICS
CERTIFICATE OF LIVE BIRTH

TYPE OR PRINT IN PERMANENT INK

PRIMARY DIST. NO. _____

STATE FILE NO. _____

A. _____

B. _____

C. _____

D. _____

E. _____

F. _____

G. _____

H. _____

I. _____

CHILD—NAME	FIRST	MIDDLE	LAST	SEX	DATE OF BIRTH (Mo. Day Year)	HOUR
1.				2.	3a.	3b. ___ AM PM

HOSPITAL NAME (If not in Hospital, Give Street and Number)	City, Boro, or Twp. of Birth	COUNTY OF BIRTH
4a.	4b.	4c.

I CERTIFY THAT THE STATED INFORMATION CONCERNING THIS CHILD IS TRUE TO THE BEST OF MY KNOWLEDGE AND BELIEF	DATE SIGNED (Mo, Day, Year)	CERTIFIER—NAME AND TITLE (Type or Print)
5a. (Signature) ▶	5b.	5c.

	CERTIFIER'S MAILING ADDRESS (Street or R.F.D. No., City or Town, State, Zip)
Name and Title of Attendant at Birth if other than Certifier (Type or Print) 5d.	5e.

MOTHER—MAIDEN NAME	FIRST	MIDDLE	LAST	AGE (At time of this Birth)	STATE OF BIRTH (If not in U.S.A., Name Country)
6a.				6b.	6c.

MAILING ADDRESS 7.	STREET AND NUMBER	CITY AND STATE	ZIP CODE

WHERE DOES MOTHER ACTUALLY LIVE? 8.	STATE	COUNTY	CITY, BORO, TWP. (Specify)

FATHER—NAME	FIRST	MIDDLE	LAST	AGE (At time of this Birth)	STATE OF BIRTH (If not in U.S.A., Name Country)
9a.				9b.	9c.

INFORMANT 10a.	Relation to Child 10b.	REGISTRAR'S SIGNATURE AND DATE RECEIVED 11.

CONFIDENTIAL INFORMATION FOR MEDICAL AND HEALTH USE ONLY

Death Under One Year Of Age —
Number of Death Certificate For This Child

Multiple Births
Enter State File Number for Mate(s)

Live Birth(s)

Fetal Death(s)

RACE—MOTHER (e.g., White, Black, American Indian, etc. — Specify)	RACE—FATHER (e.g., White, Black, American Indian, etc. — Specify)	EDUCATION—MOTHER (Specify only highest grade completed)		EDUCATION—FATHER (Specify only highest grade completed)		IS MOTHER MARRIED TO FATHER?
12.	13.	ELEMENTARY OR SECONDARY (0-12) 14.	COLLEGE (1-4 or 5+)	ELEMENTARY OR SECONDARY (0 12) 15.	COLLEGE (1-4 or 5+)	☐ Yes ☐ No 16.

PREGNANCY HISTORY (Complete each section)

LIVE BIRTHS (Do not include this child)		OTHER TERMINATIONS (Spontaneous and Induced)		Date Last Normal Menses Began (Mo. Day, Year) 18.	Month of Pregnancy Pre Natal Care Began (1st, 2nd, etc.) (Specify) 19a.	Pre-Natal Visits — Total (If none, so state) 19b.	Length of Pregnancy in weeks. 20.
17a. Now living	17b. Now dead	17d. Before 16 wks.	17e. After 16 wks.	BIRTH WEIGHT 21.	THIS BIRTH—Single, Twin, Triplet, etc. (Specify) 22a.	If NOT Single Birth — Born First, Second, Third etc. (Specify) 22b.	APGAR SCORE
Number ___ None ☐	Number ___ None ☐	Number ___ None ☐	Number ___ None ☐				1 Min. 23a. / 5 Min. 23b.
17c. Date of Last Live Birth (Mo. Year)		17f. Date of Last Other Termination (Mo. Year)		Method of Delivery 24.	COMPLICATIONS OF PREGNANCY (Describe or write "none") 25.		

CONCURRENT ILLNESSES OR CONDITIONS AFFECTING THE PREGNANCY (Describe or write "none") 26.	COMPLICATIONS OF LABOR AND/OR DELIVERY (Describe or write "none") 27.
BIRTH INJURIES OF CHILD (Describe or write "none") 28.	CONGENITAL MALFORMATIONS OR ANOMALIES OF CHILD (Describe or write "none") 29.

Figure 2-1. Certificate of live birth used by Pennsylvania Department of Health. Similar forms are used by other cities and states.

there are differences between the rate of monozygotic, or identical twins, and dizygotic, or fraternal twins. The relative proportions of monozygotic and dizygotic twins are not the same for all races. The incidence of dizygotic twins is white 60 percent, black 70 percent, Japanese 40 percent. In the United States the twinning rate varies slightly from one region to another; the region with the highest rate of 10.5 is the Northeast; the lowest rate, 9.4, is in the West.

The Birth Certificate

In 1915 the federal government began to collect data on registered births and organized birth registration. At first only ten states and the District of Columbia were included in this method of reporting births, but it gradually expanded so that by 1933 the entire country was included. At the present time all 50 states and the District of Columbia demand that a birth certificate be filled out on every birth, and that it be submitted promptly to the local registrar. After the birth has been registered, the local registrar sends a notification to the parents of the child. Also, a complete report is forwarded from the local registrar to the state authorities, and then to the National Office of Vital Statistics in Washington.

Complete and accurate registration of births is a legal responsibility (Fig. 2-1). The birth certificate gives evidence of age, citizenship, and family relationships and as such is often required for military service, passports, and to collect benefits on retirement and insurance. On the basis of birth certificates, information that is essential to agencies concerned with human reproduction is compiled by the National Office of Vital Statistics.

POPULATION

The population of the United States more than doubled during the first half of this century and has continued to grow in tremendous proportions as was predicted. Between the time of the 1950 census and 1970, the population of the United States grew from 151 million to over 200 million. The predominant growth factor resulted from natural increases rather than international migration. This growth has required huge public and private expenditures for such basic facilities as shelter, schools, and highways. The high birthrates of the 1940s and the early 1950s first produced pressures for expansion of elementary education, then for the expansion of secondary education facilities, and, as we are aware now, for college facilities and jobs.

Three vital factors determine the rate at which population grows: births, deaths, and migration. The decline in the death rate that was so apparent in the first half of this century has fluctuated near the same relatively low level (9.7 deaths per 1,000 population) for the last decade. Control of immigration began in this country about a half century ago. However, recent modifications will undoubtedly exert an influence on this factor in our population growth.

One should not be deceived by the falling birthrate, which at first glance gives the impression that there is no need to have any concern about a "population problem" in the United States. The impression left by the tabulation of birthrates is that the number of live births has been relatively stable. However, it must be remembered that the birthrate is related to the number of births *per 1,000 population.*

The decline in the annual number of births is partly related to the age and sex structure of the population. The majority of Americans are young. More than half are under 28 years of age, but the proportion is shifting because of the fluctuating birthrates. The young adult group, composed of persons between ages 18 and 34, is now the fastest growing portion of the population, reflecting the high birthrates that followed World War II. This group, now 22 percent of the total, will increase to 28.5 percent of the total by 1980. The 40-to-50-year-old segment of the population is not expected to increase proportionately, but moderately large increases are anticipated in the older age groups, that is, persons 65 years and over.

According to population projections made by the Bureau of the Census, during the next ten years the number of women of childbearing age will probably rise in this country.

The uncertainty as to how much the population will grow rises from the unpredictable number of children who will be born to contemporary young couples. Though their fertility potential is huge, much will depend upon whether they choose to increase or decrease their family size.

MORTALITY

Maternal Mortality

Maternal mortality refers to deaths that result from childbearing; that is, the underlying cause of the woman's death is the result of complications of pregnancy, childbirth, or the puerperium.

In 1968 there were 950 maternal deaths registered in the United States. Over the past decade, there has been a decline so that now complications from pregnancy and childbirth account for about .03 of all the deaths per 1,000. The maternal mortality rate in 1974 was about 15 per 100,000 and provisional data from 1976 indicate a maternal mortality rate of 14.5 per 100,000 live births.

The reduction in maternal mortality rates has been rather consistent since 1951 (Fig. 2-2). The dramatic decline in these rates began about the mid-30s and continued until 1956. During the succeeding five years, the maternal mortality rate declined more slowly, reaching an all-time low in 1962. In 1963 the rate rose slightly to 35.8 per 100,000 live births, but resumed its decline the following year and reached a record low in 1976.

The risk of maternal death for all mothers is lowest at ages 20 to 24 (15 per 100,000 in 1970). It is slightly higher under age 20, and from age 25 on. Increasing age is associated with a steep rise in maternal mortality. At 40 to 44 years of age, the mortality rate is six times greater than at 20 to 24. At the oldest age in the reproductive age span, 45 years or older, the mortality is about 12 times greater than the low figure.

Causes of Maternal Mortality

The reduction in maternal mortality from the hypertensive disorders of pregnancy was the largest single factor responsible for the reduction in the

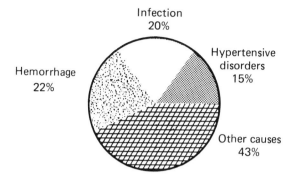

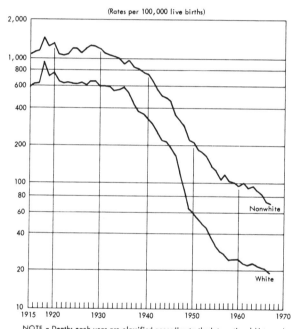

MATERNAL MORTALITY RATES BY COLOR:
BIRTH-REGISTRATION STATES, 1915-1975

(Rates per 100,000 live births)

NOTE – Deaths each year are classified according to the International Lists used at that time; for discussion of comparability, see Technical Appendix.

Figure 2-2. (Top) Causes of maternal mortality, percentage distribution by cause, 1975. (Data from Vital Statistics of the United States, 1975, Vol. II—Mortality, Part A, Table 1-15, U.S. Department of Health, Education, and Welfare, Public Health Service, 1975) *(Bottom)* Maternal mortality by color: birth registration states, 1915-1975. Deaths from complications of pregnancy, childbirth, and the puerperium per 100,000 live births in the specified groups. (Data from Vital Statistics of the United States, 1975, Vol. II—Mortality, Part A, Table 1-16, U.S. Department of Health, Education, and Welfare, Public Health Service, 1975)

total maternal mortality rate (from 82.7 per 100,000 live births in 1949–51 to 14.5 in 1976). Hemorrhage and sepsis (cases other than abortion) were next in importance as conditions affecting the mortality rate. Subsequently, these three conditions will be

discussed in detail, but it is important to stress the fact that deaths from these causes are for the most part preventable. Substantial achievements in maternity care have caused the death rate from puerperal infection and hypertension of pregnancy to fall more dramatically than that from hemorrhage.

Consequently, *hemorrhage* remains a predominant cause of death in childbirth. According to the official classification, only the direct cause of death is considered, even though the predisposing cause may be an important factor. For example, in a case in which the mother has a massive hemorrhage and then (in her weakened condition) develops a puerperal infection that eventually causes her death, the death is classified as due to puerperal infection. Hemorrhage is often a predisposing factor, and in this manner its toll in maternal mortality probably exceeds all other causes combined.

Puerperal infection is a wound infection of the birth canal after childbirth, which sometimes extends to cause phlebitis or peritonitis. The nurse can play an important role in helping to prevent such infections by maintaining flawless technique in performing nursing procedures.

The *hypertensive disorders of pregnancy* are certain disturbances peculiar to gravid women, characterized mainly by hypertension, edema, albuminuria, and in some severe cases by convulsions and coma. Antepartal care is an important part of prevention or early detection of symptoms, and with suitable treatment the disturbance often can be allayed.

Reduction in Maternal Mortality

Many factors are responsible for achieving the overall reduction in maternal mortality in this country during the past 25 years.

Medical management has improved. The widespread use of blood and plasma transfusions and antibiotics, together with careful maintenance of fluid and electrolyte balance and sophisticated anesthesia management, has changed obstetrical practice substantially. Legalized abortion has also helped reduce the number of maternal deaths associated with abortion.

Perhaps more important is the development of widespread *training and educational programs* in obstetrics and maternity which have provided more and better qualified specialists, professional nurses, and other personnel to deliver care in this area. Better hospital facilities and the increase in hospital deliveries have also helped reduce maternal mortality. The development of alternate hospital facilities to meet consumer demands for a more homelike setting for parturition may also prove to be a helpful factor.

The distinct *change in attitudes* of physicians, nurses, and parents also has contributed to this progressive saving of mothers. Childbirth is no longer an event to be awaited helplessly by the expectant mother with what fortitude she is able to muster; instead, it is the climax of a period of preparation—a true state of preparedness attained through the cooperation of the physician, the nurse, and the expectant parents. As indicated before, this preparation for childbirth, based on careful medical and nursing supervision throughout pregnancy, is called antepartal, or prenatal care.

Antepartal care has been an important achievement in maternity care during the present century. It will be of interest to the nurse to know that this salutary contribution to the mother's welfare was initiated by the nursing profession. It had its beginning in 1901, when the Instructive Nursing Association in Boston began to pay antepartal visits to some of the expectant mothers who were to be delivered at the Boston Lying-In Hospital. This work gradually spread until, in 1906, all of these women prior to confinement were paid at least one visit by a nurse from the association. By 1912, this association was making about three antepartal visits to each patient. In 1907, another pioneer effort in prenatal work was instituted when George H. F. Schrader gave the Association for Improving the Condition of the Poor, New York City, funds to pay the salary of two nurses to do this work. In 1909, the Committee on Infant Social Service of the Women's Municipal League in Boston organized an experiment of antepartal work. The pregnant women were visited every ten days—oftener if necessary. Blood pressure readings and urine tests were made at each visit. This important work was limited because of the effort to make it as nearly self-supporting as possible; therefore, only mothers under the care of physicians and hospitals were accepted. Thus began the movement for antepartal care that has been extremely important in promoting the health and well-being of many pregnant women.

Another important factor in the reduction of maternal mortality has been the development of *maternal and child health programs* in State Departments of Public Health, particularly the work of community health nurses. These nurses visit a large number of the mothers who otherwise would re-

ceive little or no medical care, bringing them much-needed aid in pregnancy, labor, and the puerperium. This service fills a great need not only in rural areas, but also in metropolitan centers.

Perinatal Mortality

The two groups of problems in infant mortality that are of chief concern in maternity are (1) those in which the fetus dies in the uterus prior to birth, and (2) those in which it dies within a short time after birth (neonatal death). The term perinatal mortality is used to designate the deaths in these two categories.

Fetal Death

In an effort to end confusion arising from usage of a variety of terms, such as stillbirth, abortion, miscarriage, and so on, the World Health Organization recommended the adoption of the following definition of fetal death:

Fetal death is a death prior to complete expulsion or extraction from its mother of a product of conception, irrespective of duration of pregnancy; the death is indicated by the fact that after such separation the fetus does not breathe or show any other evidence of life such as beating of the heart, pulsation of the umbilical cord, or definite movement of voluntary muscles.[1]

WHO further defined fetal death by indicating four subgroups, according to gestational age in weeks.

Infant Mortality

Two decades ago, there was reported a total of 103,390 infant deaths before the first birthday. By 1970, the infant mortality rate was 20.0 per 1,000 live births, the lowest in U.S. history, and provisional data for 1976 suggest that rate has declined further to 15.1.[2] A falling fertility rate, better contraceptive practices, increasing availability of safe abortion, together with a higher standard of living in the general population, have been suggested as factors in this decline in infant mortality.

However, it has been pointed out that this national figure does not accurately reflect trends in the large urban areas and the southern states where the rate has declined less.

Many causes are responsible for infant mortality. The vast number of infant deaths is the result of several main causes: respiratory distress syndrome, preterm birth, asphyxia and atelectasis, congenital malformations, and birth injuries.

During the first four weeks of life early gestational age and low birth weight are the chief causes of death. Birth injuries, another of the main causes of infant loss, accounted for almost 7,000 infant deaths in 1970. Almost one-third of these deaths were due to intracranial and spinal injury at birth. In the vast majority of these cases, death occurred in less than seven days of life. These conditions will be discussed in detail later. It suffices to say that one of the first and most important of them, immaturity, is largely a nursing management problem. Indeed, in all the wide range of nursing care there is no area that offers such a challenge to the nurse or such lifesaving possibilities as that of caring for the preterm infant.

The welfare of some 4,000,000 babies born annually in the United States is very much the concern of maternity nurses and obstetricians and one of the main objectives of the entire field of maternity care. To reduce the enormous loss of newborn lives, to protect the infant not only at birth, but also in the prenatal period and during the early days of life, to lay a solid foundation for his health throughout life—these are the problems and the challenge.

Reproductive Wastage

The vast number of infants lost by spontaneous abortion is a matter of grave importance. The abortion rate in this country exceeds stillbirths and neonatal deaths in fetal wastage. About 10 percent of all pregnancies terminate in spontaneous abortion because of such factors as faulty germ plasm, unsatisfactory environmental conditions, hormonal and *otherwise* many unknown etiological causes.

As our knowledge of determining and diagnosing these factors becomes greater, it is hoped that more definitive inroads will be made in this area.

Today, the concerns for the United States stemming from the overall problem of maternal and fetal reproductive wastage reflects a symptom of far-reaching social change. The tremendous reduction in maternal and infant mortality rates presents concrete evidence of the noteworthy progress that has been achieved in maternity care in this country. Nevertheless, the current major concern is that a large segment of our population is not receiving maternity care.

The needs resulting from problems of maternal and child health in rural areas continue today, but what is alarming is that now there is a parallel situation in the larger cities.

Since World War II, major shifts in population have occurred; urban middle-class families have migrated to suburban areas, whereas large numbers of families from rural areas have moved to the large urban industrial areas. Despite the increase in employment and in income generally, the population still includes a large segment of disadvantaged, low-income families who recently have concentrated in the major cities. With the increased cost of health services in general and the cost of hospital care in particular, these low-income families are straining the local resources of the communities in which they reside. Also, the number of maternity patients in these areas has greatly increased as a result of migration, producing overcrowding of clinics and hospital maternity in-service divisions. To accommodate such large numbers of patients, many of the hospitals with large maternity services have had to resort to limiting the mother's hospital stay, some women being discharged 24 hours after delivery. The most serious problem by far is that many of these women are receiving poor or, often, no antepartal care, due in part to dissatisfaction with the kind of care provided. Inadequate care during pregnancy has been demonstrated to bear a direct relationship to the rate of immaturity.

Moreover, with spiraling inflation, it has been pointed out that middle-class couples are feeling the impact of not being able to afford adequate health care. They are not eligible for welfare coverage, yet not affluent enough to seek the kind of care that is appropriate.

It has been mentioned previously that social factors play a role in morbidity and mortality and, in fact, influence the reproduction efficiency of childbearing women.

Much of the difficulty in providing adequate care is due to a shortage of professional personnel in the maternity field. The rapid growth of the population has not been accompanied by a proportionate increase in physicians and nurses who are attracted to this area of specialization. Student nurses might well investigate the reason for this apathy and in good time provide some solution to this problem. These factors will be explored in greater detail in subsequent chapters.

REFERENCES

1. National summaries: fetal deaths, U.S., 1954. National Office of Vital Statistics 44:11, Aug. 1956.

2. National Center for Health Statistics, Annual Summary for the United States, 1976. *Monthly Vital Statistics Reports* 12:13, Dec. 12, 1977. DHEW Publication No (PAS) 78–1120.

SUGGESTED READING

Aubry, R., and J. Pennington. Identification and evaluation of high-risk pregnancy: The perinatal concept. *Am. J. Ob.-Gyn.* 16:3–27, Mar. 1973.

Hickey, Louise A., et al. Maternity day care program offers economical, family-oriented care. *Hospitals, JAHA* 51, 23:85–89, Dec. 1, 1977.

Lawson, J. Avoidable factors in maternal deaths. *Nurs. Mirror* 139, 11:48, Sept. 12, 1974.

Osofsky, H. and N. Kendall. Poverty as a criterion of risk. *Clin. Ob. and Gyn.* 16:103–119, Mar. 1973.

Schneider: Changing concepts of prenatal care. *Post-grad. Med.* 53:91–97, June 1973.

Three

The Family in a Changing World

WHAT IS THE FAMILY?

Most people know intuitively what they mean by "the family." They have known families throughout their lifetime and intuitive definitions are sufficient for everyday conversation and action. However, when we begin to define what constitutes a family, or analyze this unit as a social institution, or attempt to deliver comprehensive care to it, it becomes apparent that what we have considered as *the* family is inappropriate for systematic treatment. The characteristics of the families of our own personal experience often do not fit "families" of other segments of society. Family life in different cultures exhibits even greater contrasts.

The family has been defined in a variety of ways. Torbett refers to it as "a group of two or more persons who are united by blood, marriage, or adoption residing in a common household wherein they create and maintain a common culture and interact with each other by way of familial roles."[1] Other authors have defined the family as a unit of interacting personalities or as a system of roles.[2,3] Common to all of these definitions is the fact that the members—whether they be a married dyad or a single parent and child, have anonymous role relationships, or belong to a union unsanctioned by law—relate to each other in some way; that is, they

interact with specified patterns of behavior, and in so doing differentiate or structure roles for themselves.

THE RELATIONSHIP OF FAMILY THEORY TO NURSING PRACTICE

Since nurses in their interaction with families will come into a situation in which there is a set of ongoing role relationships, it is important that they consider a number of factors when providing care for their clients. The structure and functioning of the family determines their use of health services. Hence, all members of the health team need to be aware of a variety of theories regarding human behavior and how families develop their various patterns of behavior. This awareness necessitates using knowledge from other specific disciplines where it is appropriate, in order to deliver optimum health care.

Family-centered Care

The concept of family-centered care and its logical extension, family nursing, has always been a part of nursing. Some areas of practice, notably that of community health, have traditionally claimed more interest, expertise, and responsibility for total family care than others. Delivering care in the client's home has allowed the nurse more insights into the family and its workings and the implications its structure and function have for the health of its members. Moreover, it has allowed the nurse to assess as a whole the problems and progress of the family members.

However, other nursing specialists, notably those in maternal-child health, have also demonstrated interest in family care, focusing initially on the mother-child dyad and later on parenting. In addition, midwifery has used a family-centered approach to home delivery services by utilizing family resources to prepare for care of the mother-infant couple in the home setting.[4] Parents' classes under the auspices of the Maternity Center Association and the Child Study Association in conjunction with the Children's Bureau have also promoted the development, over time, of nursing care of the total family.[5] The philosophy behind this approach has been to meet expressed needs and concerns of parents through the nurse's group leadership role, not necessarily through a course of preplanned instruction. Thus, as nursing has evolved to keep pace with today's health needs, it has become apparent that concepts from other disciplines are badly needed in order to supply a total picture of the family unit for which high-quality care is to be provided.

Probably no force has been so potent or recent in supplying these valuable concepts as the theorists and researchers in the social and behavioral sciences. Efforts to theorize and to conduct research about the family as a social phenomenon have brought together many disciplines and encouraged cooperation and collaboration in the study of that complex social entity. These multidisciplinary contributions have stimulated many teachers and students of nursing to seek advanced preparation and to conduct research about families that have implications for their practice.

The comprehensive overview of family study by Christensen in his *Handbook of Marriage and the Family*,[6] as well as the identification and classification of conceptual frameworks relating to the family unit done by Hill and Hansen, and Nye and Berardo,[7,8] have been invaluable resources for helping to delineate content in clinical nursing courses and providing conceptual frameworks for the develop-

ment of assessment tools and the testing of nursing intervention techniques.

Perhaps most significant, nursing is now joining with other related disciplines whose basic interests and expertise in the family may someday ensure team approaches to research in clinical matters, multidisciplinary educational programs, and, most important, team effort in family care.[9] Society's demands, needs, and aspirations are causing rapid changes in all health fields, including nursing practice and educational programs. Tired of fragmentation in service, high costs, barriers to the entry into health services, and the inertia and unresponsiveness of the health care system in general, consumers are taking action in what amounts to a social movement.[10,11]

As a result, health professionals find themselves in the center of a revolution in the health care system. Only by multidisciplinary collaboration will they be able to rise to the occasion and provide adequate health services.

ROLES, ROLE THEORY, AND IMPLICATIONS FOR NURSING PRACTICE

As background for understanding the family, we must deal with another concept that permeates both lay and professional language today. That concept is role, and it is an integral part of the structure and function of the family.

As with the concept of family, we have an intuitive sense of what a "role" is, but when attempts are made to systematically study the construct, we find a broad latitude in definitions and understandings of it. Psychological and sociological approaches to role are closely interrelated, since an individual's personality develops within a social system which, in our culture, is the family. Hence, roles may be viewed from a psychosocial viewpoint that enables us to focus on the individual and how he integrates his role relationships, and also from a sociological viewpoint which guides us in focusing on group or social relationships, primarily those within the family. We must also deal with culture, for the "self" can be viewed as the unit of personality, an individual's "status" or position as the unit of society, and "role" as the unit of culture.[12]

Definition of Role and Status. Basic to any discussion of role are the definitions of *role* and *status*. Status, or position, generally refers to a person's location in a system of interaction. On the other hand, role applies to *behavior* that reflects the goals, values, and sentiments operating in a given situation. A further clarification of these definitions can be made by contrasting role as defined by two major theorists, Ralph Linton and George Herbert Mead. According to Linton, roles tend to be defined as constellations of rules or expectations for behavior associated with a given status or position.[13] In the Meadian, or interactionist tradition, however, roles are defined, created, stabilized, or modified as a consequence of interaction between the self and others.[14]

Role vs. Interaction. From an interactionist frame of reference, then, role is more than a series of do's and don'ts for the behavior expected of a person occupying a given position. Rather, it is a constellation of behaviors that emerges from interaction between the self and others, that constitutes a meaningful unit, and that is an expression of the values, goals, and/or sentiments that provide direction for that interaction. It is true that these constellations of behaviors become patterned over time and that the actors proceed "as if" there were prescriptions for performance.

However, there is much more latitude in the Meadian conception of role, since it allows for innovative, individualistic designing of a person's role performance on the basis of assignment of some sentiment or goal to the behavior of relevant others.

This conception of role is particularly salient for nursing practice, since it allows for a broader interpretation of the behavior of all actors than do more traditional concepts. Moreover, it does not limit either the interpretation of the behavior or the nurse's response to the behavior to a prescribed set of do's and don'ts. Hence, it permits creativity and innovation in interaction with clients.

Complementary Roles. Another basic concept in role theory is that of the *complementarity* of roles or the fact that all roles are learned in pairs. Thus, a role does not exist in isolation but is patterned to mesh with that of a role partner. For instance, the nurse's role meshes with the patient's role, the husband's with the wife's, the child's with the parent's, and so on. Some of these roles that are basic in society, such as husband, wife, child, and so on, have become more patterned in the various cultures than others, and thus firmer expectations have come about. But we need only look at the innovative variation in recent family lifestyles to appreciate how traditional role prescriptions and expectations can, and often must, be modified.

Whether there be firm or loose expectations, this pairing or complementarity of roles provides for reciprocal arrangements in interaction and therefore allows social interaction to proceed in an orderly fashion, since there emerges a predictability in interaction. The actors "know" what they are to do. Without this complementarity, it would be difficult to maintain stable interaction networks such as exist in the family system. Indeed, the family's equilibrium depends on this role pairing.

Socialization of Roles and Role Models. Roles are learned through the process of socialization. In socialization, individuals learn the ways of social groups so that they can function within these groups. Socialization takes place through both intentional and incidental instruction, that is, by providing specific instruction regarding a certain facet of behavior and by providing examples of desired behavior—in other words, role modeling. All of the various socialization agencies—the family in the beginning and later the church and schools—teach the child certain role behaviors through intentional programs of learning and study.

However, operating conjointly may be incidental learning in which the child adopts the ways of others in his environment through play acting, peer group relations, and observations of adult and peer role models.

Thus, the significant others in the child's world teach him, both by defining the world for him and by serving as models for his attitudes and behavior. The child learns through a system of rewards and punishment and, if he behaves as the significant others desire, he receives positive attention and invitations to continue his participation and interaction. If, on the other hand, he behaves otherwise, he is refused attention, reprimanded, or physically punished.

It is important to remember that much of the role learning that takes place in the family is indirect. The child learns by observing and participating in the interpersonal relations patterns established by the family, the examples set by the other family members, and the role that he develops for himself within the family. Hence, he learns and *adopts* basic role skills from family members and concurrently *adapts* to the roles of the other family members.

Emotional Basis of Role Learning.   Another important aspect of role learning is that it is not merely a cognitive process. It comes to be associated with multiple emotional or affective ties that the individual makes with others. These attachments begin with the mother and gradually include increasing numbers of persons with whom the child interacts and comes to identify with. As these attachments grow, the child develops a sense of "self" in that he can take a position from the outside and view his own thoughts, feelings, and actions. In this way, he gradually internalizes the behavior that is expected of him as he figuratively stands back and looks at himself and guides, judges, and reflects on his own behavior according to his perceptions of others' expectations for his behavior.

It has been noted that, while individuals learn role behavior in much the same way, there are differences in respective role performances. This differential role performance may be due to differences in the ways persons respond in interpersonal situations, their knowledge of the role in general, their motivation to perform specific roles, their attitude toward themselves, and finally, their response to the behavior of other persons in the interaction.[15]

Tension in Role Relations.   Another aspect to be considered when considering the concept of role is that of tension and/or discontinuities in role relations. Many terms have been used to illustrate the idea of tension or interruptions in a smooth process of interaction. Terms such as role conflict, role strain, role change, role transition, and the like have been used to convey the various aspects of tension that can occur in a role system.

We have made the point that role interaction is dynamic. As theories of the development of human nature change, so do socialization patterns. As these latter change, variant family life systems evolve, which in turn redefine reciprocal role relationships. Tensions and disruptions in smooth and rewarding role interaction may occur at any point.

Summary.   The major determinants of the degree of adjustment an individual makes to a role can be summarized as follows: (1) the clarity with which a specific role and its complementarity is defined and demonstrated; (2) the clarity or definiteness of the transitional procedures in the acquisition of a new role; (3) how well the role is learned and enacted—this is partly dependent on 1 and 2 and the strength of the socialization process to the new role; (4) the consistency of the responses a role evokes; (5) a role's compatibility with the other roles in the individual's set of roles; (6) a role's congruity with the emotional needs of the individual; and (7) the degree of complementarity that exists between reciprocal roles.

When there is a high degree of adjustment, the enactment of an individual's set of roles can be rewarding in that they define for him his niche, his self-concept anchorage, a sense of belongingness and purpose. They give him social recognition and support which, in turn, allow him to buy or earn desired conditions or things in the world and to view himself as a worthwhile, contributing member of society.[16]

FAMILY ROLES AND THE NURSE

Concepts from role theory encompass a body of knowledge that is vital for the nurse who works with families or individual family members. The application of these concepts can greatly increase the nurse's understanding of the role strains and changes inherent in the phenomenon of family stress that can be precipitated by childbearing, chronic or acute illness in the family, or death of any of the family members.

For example, consider the change in the interaction patterns that must be accomplished when a new infant is incorporated into the household— restructuring of all of the members' roles is necessitated, and this is doubly complicated when there are other children present. Sibling rivalry is only one aspect of the impact of a new infant on the family.

Or, consider the situational crisis when parents bear a mentally retarded or otherwise defective child. Following the grief reaction and concomitant frustration, conflict, and high anxiety, the family equilibrium can be regained only when parents restructure their roles to either encompass or reject the afflicted member and learn to cope with the situation.

Finally, consider acute catastrophic illness in the father of a family with several children. When such an illness occurs, the man is thrust into the role of patient which is, in essence, a dependent role. This necessitates a reorganization of the role behaviors of the other family members. The wife must become more dominant, the children generally must assume more responsibility, and hence, their positions change vis-à-vis other family members. These few examples point up the necessity for the nurse to consider family role relations if she is to intervene in a holistic way.

The Role of Mother

Each society provides many cues and signals that tell individuals how it defines a role and identifies appropriate behavior for the role. These cues may be overt or covert and may be perceived in a subliminal way. In our culture, the ideal mother has been traditionally the nurturer, the one who gave sustenance and unconditional love.

A woman's concept of the mother role is based on the norms of the culture, the social class and ethnic group to which she belongs, and the type of socialization she has received from her immediate family.

Motherliness.   It is important to remember that there is a difference between the role of mother and feelings of motherliness. In a sense, both are learned, but mothering, the enactment of the role of mother, involves skills and a certain understanding of the developmental process of the child. Thus, *motherliness* can be thought of as an emotional feeling that develops over time as the mother has increasing contact with her infant (see Chapter 1). It is a feeling that the child is emotionally hers, and there is a need to identify the infant with the rewarding values and qualities that she considers part of herself and her life.

This development of motherliness begins with the maternal claiming process and is evident in the initial and early mother-newborn contact when the mother touches (at first timidly) and later enfolds her infant and exclaims, "Oh, he is finally here! How did I ever produce that?"

Our hospital procedures militate against this early claiming behavior, but fortunately we are now beginning to relax many of the restrictions that tend to disrupt the reality testing of this ownership process.

Anxieties and Conflicts in Motherhood.   All mothers need reassurance that they are now, indeed, mothers—and adequate if not excellent ones. The disappointment the mother feels when the infant sleeps at the breast instead of nursing is very familiar to everyone. Mothers excoriate themselves with criticism when they are awkward in handling their first-born. They try desperately to "pull themselves together," to assume care of the infant only hours after delivery. Although seemingly small and unimportant, these initial anxieties are the basis of the future relationship between mother and child. Moreover, they are complicated by the many conflicts in modern society where the role of mother has come into increasing competition with other social roles a woman may enact. Paramount among these conflicts are (1) fantasies of idealized motherhood versus feelings of inadequacy in actual role performance; (2) the need for dependency versus the adult goal of independence and responsibility; (3) love versus resentment for the baby due to fatigue and increased responsibility for such a dependent being; (4) feelings for the baby versus feelings for the husband; and (5) self-actualization versus the demands of motherhood.[17]

If the mother has had problematic relations with her own mother during the early socialization years, these, too, may affect her role enactment. She may project many of these negative feelings onto her own child or, conversely, bend over backwards to avoid socialization techniques her mother used, thereby limiting or missing important features that she might have kept and used. Also, if the normal and increasing dependency needs of pregnancy and the early postpartum are not met, she may not be able to care easily for and give love to her dependent child.

One final point deserves mention. For many, children of one age are more appealing than those of another. A mother may be able to respond to the needs of a dependent infant but not adapt readily to the four-year-old's search and insistence on autonomy.

Thus, the role of mother and its enactment is shaped by many interacting factors and therefore will have a wide range of behavioral manifestations.

The Role of Father

It has been said that, if the 20th century is proclaimed the "Century of the Child," it certainly will not be remembered as the "Century of the Father."[18] Research on the dynamics of the father role or the development of fatherliness has received much less attention than that of motherhood. Recently, there has been some impetus in research, but it will be some time before there is solid empirical evidence regarding this topic.

Fatherliness. As with the mother role and motherliness, there is a difference between the father role or fatherhood and feelings of *fatherliness*. The role of father is learned as is the role of mother—but feeling tones are not initiated physiologically as with the mother. And this may be a very important difference. Moreover, the admission and enactment of fatherliness in our culture is still wrought with conflicts stirred up by discontinuities in cultural conditioning. This is gradually changing with the more modern attitudes toward relaxed sex role structuring. However, we still have a long way to go. By and large, the image of the virile male is still not compatible with the demonstration of tender feelings that have usually been attributed to the female domain.

Traditionally, the male-father in our society was supposed to be a leader, hero, disciplinarian, mentor, an authority figure, and the family bulwark against the outside, reality-oriented world. Yet fatherliness must involve feelings of tenderness and gentleness, empathic capacity, the ability to respond emotionally, the valuing of a love object more than the self and, finally, the finding of a gratifying living experience in the experiences of others. Obviously, these feelings are quite different from the simple pride of a man in his child as a symbol of his virility, or his feelings that the child represents a challenge to his own adequacy.[19]

It becomes apparent that, as long as women have an emotional investment in men, they will not be free to express their motherliness wholeheartedly until their relationships with their mates are integrated into the men's fatherliness. It would seem that the coordination of the feelings of motherliness and fatherliness in those who choose to be parents is essential to the mature, creative psychosexual development of both parents and eventually their children's.

Conflicts in Fatherhood. It may be that the same basic problems that confront a woman in delineating her role as mother also face the man in defining his father role. Interviews with young fathers indicate that they are immersed in many instrumental problems, such as rearranging work or study schedules, finding or preparing adequate housing, taking on extra jobs to ease the finances, and the like. They also have basic questions and fears about their preparation for the parenting role, as well as changes in their wives during pregnancy and the postpartum periods. In some, the prospect of fatherhood also rekindles thoughts of the less happy aspects of their childhood and their relations with their parents. Their fears and concerns about their rest, quiet, and privacy, their sexual relationships, and their wives' increasing demands for attention all become realities with the advent of childbirth.

We can speculate that these developments and problems may be due, at least partly, to our current lack of systematic obstetrical care of the father. It is true that we invite him to childbirth classes (and this has been a big step), and that we are allowing him greater participation in the actual birthing process. However, there is still no systematic attempt (or even acknowledgment of the necessity) to prepare him for his father role. All of these problems are the common components of severe role conflict and how they are resolved becomes the key to ultimate appropriate role transition.[20]

Creative Fatherhood. Josselyn has delineated several functions that a father can *creatively* undertake to enrich and maintain a healthy family life. First, a father can be a *true* companion, help-mate, and inspiration for the mother. Second, he can be an awakener of emotional potential for his child as well as a beloved friend and teacher. Third, he can present a role model for masculine love, ethics, and morality. Fourth, he can be a stabilizing influence as the child proceeds through his maturational stages. Fifth, he can be a model and mentor for social and occupational behavior. Sixth, he can provide a model, as mentor and protector for children in general, and finally, he can be a counselor for and friend of the adolescent.[21] While each of these activities will be modified to meet the needs of a rapidly changing society, it is apparent that they provide more of a basis for sound family interaction than does the traditional role of father as sire, disciplinarian, and breadwinner.

The Role of Child

Of all the family roles, the child's role is perhaps the most dynamic, since it is constantly evolving through techniques of socialization. These techniques are essentially future-oriented, since they focus on and emphasize what the child is to become rather than what he or she is. Helping the child learn appropriate social roles requires that the parents be emotionally healthy and stable enough to keep the anxiety level at a point that will allow the child's self-esteem to be in relative equilibrium with the environmental demands that are made. This does not mean that there will be no demand or no anxiety—without these, no learning takes place. However, they must not be excessive or incompatible with reality.

Socialization of the Child.   There are many techniques of socialization, and the evidence indicates that no one technique is better than another. Rather, each set of parents must choose and modify what is best for them, and this will depend on the many factors that we have previously alluded to. Spiegel has attempted to delineate the various steps in the maintenance of role complementarity so that the family can balance the demands society's expectations place on it, the family's attitudes, and the child's needs and eventually arrive at a progressively healthier family role equilibrium. He conceives of these steps along the torturous route of socialization as comprising two major groups of five steps each linked by a sixth, or middle step.

Role Induction Procedures.   The first group consists of *role induction procedures* by which compliance of the child is elicited. These are primarily manipulative and ensure that the child gradually realizes that he or she must learn and that his or her parents are the chief source of learning.

The first and second steps are *coercion* and *coaxing* in which punishment and rewards are used respectively to focus the child's attention on the fact that there are rules that must be observed and that the parents are the enactors of these rules.

The third step is *evaluation* in which a value judgment of good or bad is placed on the behavior and implies or directly gives praise or blame to ensure appropriate behavior.

The fourth step is *masking*, or withholding correct information or giving wrong information for the sake of settling a conflict. This can be pernicious and a crisis may occur if the child uncovers the truth—trust can be lost and reality is distorted.

Fifth is the technique of *postponing* which can be useful because it puts off dealing with a conflict until a fresher look can be taken at the situation. Of course, if this maneuver is over-utilized, it will intensify and prolong the difficulty.

The sixth is the transitional step and has been called *role reversal* or *role taking*—that is, putting oneself in the role or position of the other and looking at the situation from the point of view of another. Some call this empathic ability. It is the first glimmer of adult thinking and requires a rather well-developed understanding of self and reality. The ability to perform this maneuver early and successfully depends on the degree of masking that goes on in the family. The less the extent of masking, the better the success of role taking.

Role Modification.   The second group of procedures have been called *role modification* maneuvers. The basic characteristic here is *communication* and how individuals learn to complement each other in role change.

Role modification begins with the seventh step of *joking, or humor,* in which individuals develop the ability to laugh at themselves and each other (but affectionately). It is felt to be an outgrowth of role taking and the first of several tension-relieving mechanisms that families employ.

The eighth step employs the *intervention of a third party* (not necessarily a professional) who brings to the situation certain skills, a point of view, or knowledge that is not available to the parents or child within the family unit.

Mutual exploration is the ninth step, in which each person probes the capacity of the other to come to a solution regarding a conflict or problem. Here, trust and regard are expressed and invested in all members, including the children (to the extent of their capacity).

The tenth step, *compromising goals* is an extension of mutual exploration. Here, goals are altered but to no single person's detriment.

Similarly, the last step, *consolidation,* is the refined, integrated effort of learning to compromise successfully. It is associated with adjustment, redistribution of rewards, and role clarification.

Needless to say, the evolution through these various steps does not necessarily proceed smoothly, nor at times are all accomplished, especially steps 8 through 10. However, the more frequently they can be utilized, the easier each subsequent role adaptation and transition will become.[22]

The Role of the Nurse

The understanding and application of role theory in nursing practice provides a conceptual base for understanding the populations that we serve and gives some anchorage to our therapeutic method. It increases our capacity to view the forces of personality, family interaction, social systems, the health condition, and nursing intervention as a unit. It provides a needed framework for studying motivations for childbearing, reproductive behavior, childrearing techniques, and cultural goals. In addition, it provides a basis for understanding ourselves and our colleagues who provide health care.

Nursing is an applied science. The broad implications of its scientific nature challenge its practitioners to document this aspect with intellectual experimentation, innovations in practice, and constant research. If, indeed, we in maternity nursing, define the family as the unit to be served, we must have a thorough knowledge of its dynamics—and that includes much more than the physiological and psychological stages the *mother* passes through during pregnancy, labor, delivery, and the postpartum. The utilization of role theory provides a vehicle to tie all of these disparate aspects of childbearing into related units amenable for study and, hence, practice.

Aspects of the Nurse's Role.   There are multiple facets or aspects of the nurse's role. First, the nurse is a practitioner—she assesses, prescribes, and implements nursing regimens for her patients and assists the physician in implementing his medical regimen for his patients. Another facet of her role is that of role model or mother surrogate. Maternity nurses and community health nurses have long been experimenting with providing role models for mothers who are inexperienced or exhibit maladaptive behavior in childrearing and child care. Again, in high-risk situations of child neglect or rejection, techniques of mothering the mother are implemented. Basically, the nurse meets the dependency needs of the mother, and in so doing, allows her to move on to mothering her own children. The nurse

may also provide a role model for her peers and other professional colleagues as she initiates newcomers into the institutional or agency routines and practices and demonstrates an interest in delivering high-quality care.

Another facet of the nurse's role is that of teacher and, more recently, that of counselor. Nurses are becoming increasingly involved in parent education on all levels in order to socialize groups of parents expeditiously, thus avoiding the role strain and conflicts that can occur with the assumption of new roles. The counselor aspect has come into the fore with family-planning services and abortion and genetic counseling. Similarly, this aspect has become apparent in parental counseling with regard to health problems of the school child, management of sibling rivalry, childhood and maternal nutrition, and the like.

Finally, in her "expanded role" she may bring new physical diagnosis-clinician skills to her basic role. She finds in many instances that her work in an ambulatory care setting provides the bridge between the family in the community and the institution to which they must go from time to time for more severe conditions.

The potential for developing these multiple facets of the nursing role is unlimited and will only be fully realized when nursing recognizes its own unique and independent contribution to health.

When delivering care to individuals and families, nurses must observe and analyze the role behaviors of the persons involved, including their own. Cognizance must be taken of the various dimensions of the roles: the behaviors, values, expectations, and attitudes of the actors, as well as their underlying motivations and emotions. Role conflict and perceptions of inadequacy in role performance have the potential to undermine emotional and physical well-being. On the other hand, satisfactory role performance is a vital self-concept enhancing experience and can promote growth and emotional well-being.[23]

THEORETICAL APPROACHES TO THE STUDY OF THE FAMILY

In attempting to systematically study and delineate patterns of interaction in the family, scholars of the family, primarily sociologists, have developed several interpretive approaches to variations in family life, each one generating unique understanding about family organization while at the same time emphasizing a different aspect. These variations in emphasis result in slightly modified definitions of the family in each approach. For instance, some students of the family try to define the family in terms of a set of ends; others in terms of a kind of social structure organized to gain more general ends in societies; and still others in terms of structure and ends emerging in the unique history of each society.[24]

Conceptual Frameworks in Family Study

Five different conceptual frameworks have been designated that can be useful to nurses who deal with families. These have been summarized by Hill and Hansen as follows.[25]

1. *The interactional approach* views the family as a unity of interacting personalities. Each person has a position in the family in which he perceives the norms or role expectations held by the other individuals (or by the family as a whole) as the basis for his attitudes and behavior. The individual will define his role expectations primarily in light of their source and his own self-conception. The family is studied through analyzing the interactions of the role-playing members. The primary focus is on the internal structure of the family; this framework, however, neglects the family's relation to the community.

2. *The structural functional approach* views the family as a social system and one of the components of the complete social system—or society. It analyzes the functions which the family performs for society as a whole. The emphasis in this approach has been upon the statics of structure with a concomitant neglect of change and dynamics.

3. *The situational approach* is based on the assumption that all behavior is purposive in relation to the situation that triggered it. The situation itself, or the individual's behavior in the situation, is the focus for the study of families by means of the situational approach.

4. *The institutional approach* takes the perspective that the family must be considered a social unit in which individual and cultural values are the prime concern. The individual's values and learned needs are transmitted from one generation to the next within the family system.

5. *The developmental approach* focuses upon the study of the developmental phases of the family from the wedding to old age, and finally the dissolution of the family through death. The changing developmental tasks and role expectations of parents and children as they go through the family life cycle, as well as the developmental tasks of the family as a whole, are the basis for this approach.

As previously stated, any of these frameworks can be used depending upon the problem under study. It is important to remember that these frameworks are helpful tools and are not to be considered "right" or "wrong." In choosing a framework, an individual must consider the assumptions he makes about human behavior, how he views people in relation to the environment, and the problem that he is trying to solve.

The Interactional Approach

One of the most useful of the above frameworks for those who must deal with the family as a unit is the interactional framework. This conceptual scheme provides a system for viewing the personal relationships between the man and woman and parents and children, as well as the impact of various health conditions on the family unit. The family is conceived of as a unit of interacting personalities and, as such, is a living, changing, growing thing. This conceptualization, then, does not view the family in a legalistic way or in a family contract sense, but rather as it exists by virtue of the interaction of its members. Thus, a single parent with a child would be a family unit, a household with several monogamous couples with children would constitute a family unit, as would an unmarried couple with or without children.

Within the family, each member occupies a position or positions to which a number of roles are assigned or allocated. Through socialization and role differentiation (structuring a role) the individual perceives certain norms (rules) or role expectations that the other members of his family have for his behavior in his role performance. The response of the others in the family reinforces or challenges this conception that he is developing. Thus, a person defines his role expectations in a given situation in terms of a reference group (others who are important to him) and also by means of his own self-concept.

Implicit in this formulation is the fact that human beings interpret or define one another's actions instead of merely reacting to them. For instance, a woman's response to her mate is not made merely on the basis of his actions; it also depends upon the meaning which both partners attach to such actions. Thus, the family members act and react by using symbols, and the key concept involved in the use of symbols is *communication*.

Interpersonal relations among family members based on communication is one of the major distinguishing aspects of the interactional approach. Foote and Cottrell have pointed out that the emphasis in this framework is on the development of competence in interpersonal relations and as such describes a *process* rather than a *state*.[26]

Family Interaction and Crisis.   Several problems for investigation have grown out of these concerns and emphases on family unity, communication, and interpersonal competence. The one that is particularly important for health practitioners is that of the study of discontinuities in family life, particularly family crises or stress. This includes the impact of the reproductive process and parenthood on the family, stress created by acute or chronic illness of the various family members at any time during the life cycle, and the crisis brought about by death of a family member, particularly during the reproductive years.

Using this approach to the family, a practitioner can get inside the family group and analyze its coping as far as it involves interaction among members. Each family member, therefore, can be viewed as a developing member in a changing group. This approach can be particularly useful to the helping professions not only because it provides a practical way of inspecting the family, but also because it allows the professional to isolate and specify the potential sources of difficulty as family members relate to one another and to their society.[27]

Pregnancy as Crisis.   Much of the "pregnancy as crisis" literature has developed from this orientation. LeMasters, Dyer, and Hobbs have been contributors in this vein. The extent to which parenthood is a crisis is likely to vary according to definitions (i.e.,

crisis as a crisis or a critical event), measurements, and the amount of time between the birth of a child and the undertaking of the particular research study.

There is little doubt that, when a dyad of a man and woman becomes a triad of a mother, father, and child, a major reorganization of positions, roles, and interaction patterns takes place. The effect of the birth of a child and the preschool years of children on the adjustment of the parents seems fairly well-established. General marital satisfaction of couples tends to decrease after the birth of their children through the preschool and school years, until the children are getting ready to leave the nest. Thus, the experiences of childbearing and childrearing appear to have a rather profound and negative effect on marital satisfaction, particularly for the mother, who may even feel her basic self-worth is affected.[28]

All of this has grave implication for maternity health professionals with respect to our family-planning counseling, assistance during the reproductive process, and especially in delineating those successful aspects in the parents' coping behavior that can be useful in lessening this "critical" event.

Summary

In summary, there are several conceptual frameworks for the study of the family. Of particular use to practitioners is the interactional approach which strives to interpret family phenomena in terms of internal processes. These processes consist of role enactment (role playing) status or position relations, communication problems, decision making, stress reactions, and socialization processes. Little attempt is made to view the overall institutional or cross-cultural relationship of family structure and function, and this has been one of the criticisms of this approach. However, this framework can be used to study the relationship of the family unit to the community, but it is more difficult since one must move from the microlevel of the small cluster of interacting persons to the larger macrolevel sweep of the community. However, where the interface of these units occurs is important for health practitioners.

Other critics feel that the interactional approach fails to recognize the biogenic and psychogenic influences on family behavior. This criticism seems destined to be short-lived since these influences are recognized by the interactionist as factors that indeed set limits but are not determinants with respect to family interaction patterns. The focus is on the family in process, irrespective of the biological or personal makeup of its members, not on a static entity. What appears to be needed at this point for this framework to reach its greatest utility is better agreement and more precise definitions of its assumptions and concepts as well as extension of the framework through application and research. In this way, the interactional approach will function for the study of the family and eventually will mesh with other frameworks into what could be called a general family theory.[29]

REFERENCES

1. Torbett, D. The single-parent family. In J. P. Clausen, et al., *Maternity Nursing Today*. New York, McGraw-Hill, 1973.

2. Schvaneveldt, J. The interactional framework in the study of the family. In A. Reinhardt and M. Quinn, *Family Centered Community Nursing*. St. Louis, C. V. Mosby, 1973, pp. 119–138.

3. Turner, R. H. *Family Interaction*. New York, John Wiley & Sons, 1966.

4. Ford, L. The development of family nursing. In R. D. Hymovich and M. Barnard (eds.), *Family Health Care*. New York, McGraw-Hill, 1973, pp. 3–17.

5. Corbin, H. Development of parent classes in the United States. *The Bulletin for Maternal and Child Health, A Symposium: Education for Parenthood*. American Assoc. Mat. and Infant Health, Inc., 1960.

6. Christensen, H. T. *Handbook of Marriage and the Family*. Chicago, Rand McNally, 1964.

7. Hill, R. and D. Hansen. *Marriage and Family Living*, 22:299–311, 1960.

8. Nye, I. and F. Berardo. *Conceptual Frameworks for the Study of the Family*. New York, Macmillan, 1966.

9. Ford, *op. cit.*, p. 9.

10. *Ibid.*

11. Reeder, L. G. The patient-client as a consumer: some observations on the changing professional-client relationship. *J. Health and Soc. Behav.* 13:400–12, Dec. 1972.

12. Robischon, P and D. Scott. Role theory and its application in family nursing. *Nurs. Outlook* 17:52–57, July 1969.

13. Linton, R. *The Cultural Background of Personality*, New York, Appleton-Century Co., 1945.

14. Mead, G. H. *Mind, Self and Society from the Standpoint of a Social Behaviorist*. Chicago, U. of Chicago Press, 1934.

15. Robischon and Scott, *op. cit.*, p. 53.

16. *Ibid.*

17. *Ibid.*

18. Hines, J. D. Father—the forgotten man. *Nurs. Forum* 10:177–200, 1971.

19. Josselyn, I. Cultural forces, motherliness and fatherliness. *Am. J. Orthopsychiat.* 26:264–271, Apr. 1956.

20. Robischon and Scott, *op. cit.*, p. 55.

21. Josselyn, *op. cit.*

22. Spiegel, J. P. Resolution of role conflict within the family. *Psychiat.* 20:1–16, Feb. 1957.

23. Robischon and Scott, *op. city.*, p. 56.

24. Farber, B. *Kinship and Family Organization*. New York, John Wiley & Sons, 1966.

25. Hill and Hansen, *op. cit.*

26. Foote, N. and L. S. Cottrell. *Identity and Interpersonal Competence*. Chicago, U. of Chicago Press, 1955.

27. Schvaneveldt, *op. cit.*, pp. 119–138.

28. Eshleman, J. H. *The Family: An Introduction*. Boston, Allyn & Bacon, 1974.

29. Schvaneveldt, *op. cit.*, pp. 120–123.

Four

Emerging Family Forms

Family Forms of the Seventies and Eighties / General Considerations in Working with Parents / Ethnic, Social Class, and Cultural Variations

FAMILY FORMS OF THE SEVENTIES AND EIGHTIES

Ethnic historians and scholars of race relations and the family have emphasized the pluralistic character of American society. Over the years there has been a good deal of discussion as to whether this society was a melting pot cooking an amalgam of ethnic and cultural distillates called "American," or a salad bowl with a variety of shapes, hues, and various ethnic, religious and racial identities. The argument continues, but the salad bowl concept appears to be winning.

It is interesting to note that the acceptance of pluralism and especially variability and differences has never been strong among those with an interest in the family, including health practitioners. This may be because the family, the bulwark of society, is a sensitive area surrounded by many judgmental and normative statements about what "ought to be." So often the family is still thought of as having some "ideal" form, which is preordained, often religiously sanctioned, and adhering to an ideal set of values. Thus, forms that vary from the traditional nuclear family of husband, wife, and children living in their separate residence with the male as bread-winner and female as homemaker have been viewed as deviant. Research in the 1950s and 1960s on single-parent families, working mothers, or dual-work families was, for the most part, concerned with the deleterious effects of the absence of spouses or the effect of gainful employment on the children. The implication was, of course, that the woman should be in the home "where God intended her to be" and if a spouse was alone for any reason, he or she had the obligation to remarry (not just live with someone) as soon as possible.[1]

Several factors have been identified as responsible for the changes that we now are seeing in the structure and function of the modern family. A number of social indicators suggest that changes in the roles of both women and men have come about extremely rapidly in the 1960s and the 1970s. The changes in women's roles particularly have been caused primarily by three interrelated factors: changes in the economy affecting labor-force participation; changes in the age structure of our society; and finally, changes in values.[2] Thus, there are more younger women who may delay marriage, and who, after commitment to a partner, work outside the home and choose to do so out of desire to realize themselves as individuals. Moreover, there is a restructuring of values and roles within the home toward a more egalitarian or democratic orientation.

Pickett has noted that the control base in families has shifted from patriarchal domination to egalitarianism and sometimes women-centeredness. He points out that a new "ideal type" of democratic family has emerged which he calls "romantic monogamy" where partners are expected to be dutiful parents, dual wage earners, restrained but fascinating lovers, and finally, and most important, providers of unqualified emotional support. Since the goals of this relationship are incredibly demanding, a highly flexible divorce system has arisen as if in response. Partners may shift, but the *monogamous ideal* remains.[3]

Obviously, some have used divorce as a safety valve quite readily, but others have tried to modify the new ideal-type model from within or have attempted to build or select a model that better suits their needs. Thus, we see the phenomenon of a pluralism in family forms existing side by side, with members of each of these forms having different problems to solve and issues to face.

It is important to remember that not many persons remain in one type of family structure throughout their lifetime, although most have some experience in the more traditional nuclear family.[4] Thus, we see, along with the traditional family structures, emerging experimental structures that can have an effect on the socialization and health of their members and, hence, on their reproductive motivation and performance.

Traditional Family Structures

There are a variety of forms in traditional family structures. The most prominent among these are:

1. The nuclear family in which husband, wife, and children live in a common household. A single or a dual career may be pursued, and, in the case of the wife, her career may be continuous or interrupted as the children are born.
2. The nuclear dyad in which a husband and wife live alone. They may be childless or not have children living at home. Again, there may be a single or dual career or a "second career" where the wife enters the labor force after the children have left home.
3. The single-parent family in which there is one head as a consequence of death, divorce, abandonment, or separation. Here there are usually preschool or school-age children. There may or may not be a career; when financial aid is not forthcoming from the absent spouse, there is usually some form of occupation pursued by the parenting spouse.
4. The single adult living alone.
5. The three-generation family or extended family. These may be characterized by any variant of forms 1, 2, or 3.
6. The kin network in which nuclear households or unmarried members live in close geographical proximity and operate within a reciprocal system of exchange of goods and services.[5]

Each of these will have its problems and resources with respect to health needs and utilization of services. Generally, traditional households are looked upon more favorably by society because they are considered stable and provide a legitimating anchorage for the children born of these unions.

It has been said that nuclear families suffer from isolation and cannot cope with illness (or repeated pregnancy, reproductive wastage, and the like); hence, they must turn to professionals for sustenance and care. However, current research indicates that the nuclear family probably has less isolation and better coping ability than formerly was thought.[6] This is due to the fact that there appears to be great role adaptability and flexibility in time of stress as well as a greater utilization of kin and other social networks for advice and sustenance during childbearing as well as for other health conditions.

It is apparent that extended family forms can be helpful to counter isolation and to provide help during periods of stress. It must be remembered, however, that kin and friends can also deter family members from appropriately defining themselves in need of care as well as prohibiting or deterring them from prompt and continued utilization of health services.

Emerging Experimental Structures

1. The commune family. This form can be further divided into:
   a. A household of more than one monogamous couple with children, sharing common facilities, resources, and experiences; socialization of the child is a group activity. Each member is a responsibility of the other members, and there is mutual con-

cern for the various aspects of the members' lives including health matters.

   b. A household of adults and children in which there is "group marriage"; that is, all the individuals are "married" to each other and all parent the children. A status system usually develops with the leader(s) believed to have charisma. These are very small in number.

2. The unmarried parent and child family, often a mother and child for whom marriage is not desired or possible. Children can be natural offspring of the parent or adopted.

3. Unmarried couple and child family. Again, these may be of two varieties:

   a. A social contract marriage in which there is an ideologic commitment to a relationship not sanctioned by law, which must be constantly worked at in order to maintain its vitality and meaningfulness. Common value systems are shared that strongly emphasize humanism and personal relationships. A great deal of time is spent by the members, including the children, in sharing mutual emotional experiences and ideas. The father plays a prominent role in the caretaking and socialization of the children and both parents have intimate, continued, and sustained contact with their children.

   b. The second type of unmarried couple and child family is that usually referred to as common-law marriage with the children either born to the partners or informally adopted. These unions are often found among the poorer strata of society who experience exceptional problems and constraints associated with legal marriage.[7]

It is with the emerging experimental forms of family styles that today's nurse may have the least experience. Therefore, we will discuss some basic principles of care that have special relevance for these families. It is worth noting that as little as five years ago these families were known as "alternate" lifestyle families. However, their ethic and philosophy have become so much a part of the mainstream of society that they no longer can be so classified. While we still use the term alternate or alternative from time to time in reference to them, it is more appropriate to consider their lifestyle as evolving rather than alternative.

Social Contract Families or the Unmarried Marrieds

As stated previously, social contract families are composed of two partners whose structure exists as a social rather than a legal contract. We in maternity nursing become acquainted with these patients when giving family planning counseling and services during pregnancy and childbirth. The literature and current research suggests that in many ways, this group shares the philosophy of the "turned-off" middle-class countercultures. Living together in this form, however, has little similarity to the "shacking-up" of previous generations, or with the large number of common-law marriages found among some of the poor who experience constraints and problems associated with legal marriage, such as no finances to obtain a divorce or inability to manage the bureaucracy to facilitate legal severance. Rather, this form of marriage involves an ideologic commitment to a relationship instead of joint living by virtue of a legal status. Basic to this rejection of a legal marriage is the conviction that the bond of love and trust that binds the partners is more important and stronger than the legal bond authorized by church or state.

In the family setting, parents spend long periods of time with one another and share emotional exchanges of closeness and rejection, desire and repulsion, and all of the certainties and uncertainties involved in living together and bearing and raising children. There is, for the most part, a great deal of frankness and openness about these statuses which include the children. There is little secretiveness about their approach to life, and both names may be displayed on the mailboxes, in financial arrangements, and the like. There are no hang-ups on their part regarding the legitimacy of the children.

Since the possible instability of the relationship can be critical to pregnancy outcomes and the children's development, researchers have explored these facets of alternate family forms. Motivations for this lifestyle are very important. Some partners do not accept the civil contract per se; others do not accept the relevance of the civil marriage contract to their relationship as it exists for them at the moment, wanting no civil constraints on their "splitting" if things change between them. Others seek to avoid the obvious unhappiness in their own family life and unbringing. In general, from the participants' point of view, living together in this family structure is seen as representing true maturity and an acceptance of the faith placed in one another.

The women's liberation movement and the raising of women's consciousness have played a strong philosophical role in determining reproductive behavior and childrearing activities. The choice of having a child appears even more determined than in the traditional nuclear family. Contraception services appear to be utilized and the option of termination of pregnancy is freely available and utilized without the apparent guilt associated with such termination in some of the traditional families. From this point of view, and because of the close interaction and caretaking when the children are born, this family style has been considered a very motivated form of parenting.[8]

The Single Parent

The single or unmarried mother is far from a new phenomenon in our society. However, there has been a significant change reflecting this alternative way of bearing and raising children in today's society. Available and effective birth control measures have reduced the population for adoption and, more important, there has arisen a new perspective on the part of many single parents to keep their children and raise them without the stigma that has previously been associated with unwed pregnancy. There has been a gradual institutionalized acceptance of single parenting. The women's movement and the early counterculture movement among middle-class students were forceful agents in making parenthood a viable option for the woman whether she is married or not. Young women from middle-class families, in increasing numbers, are allowing their pregnancies to continue to term and are electing to keep their children. Older single women are becoming pregnant by choice and keeping their babies or are adopting one or more children. Single men also have chosen adoption as a means of experiencing parenthood without the responsibility of marriage.

Under such conditions, a variety of styles of parenting have emerged since different supports are needed by these parents who are alone. The single mother, particularly, must enlarge her social support networks if she is to become economically independent and socially involved.

Family Style Dwelling. Among the family styles that have been encountered among the single mother group are small group homes or boarding homes where a small number (four to ten) live together with their children; foster homes for mother and child; and apartment complexes where each family lives in its own unit.[9] The actual physical arrangements for the child differ among residences, but, in general, there are separate sleeping quarters for the parent and child with common dining and living facilities. The opportunity for the children to eat and play together, share toys, and have a shared caretaker is considered one of the advantages for children in groups such as these.

Community Support Programs. Many communities have developed programs that facilitate a young mother's return to school or work so that she can gain skills that will enable her to be independent. These programs are still in the early stages and are largely experimental but do indicate that society recognizes the complex needs of women who rear children alone. Child care facilities, caretaking arrangements and infant caretakers in the home reflect the kinds of assistance the community has developed, which means that most children of single parents are exposed to multiple caretaking as early as six weeks of life.

Organizational Support. Societal recognition has also encouraged single parents to move toward developing organizations and social networks that provide them with tangible supportive contacts. The expansion of such organizations as Parents Without Partners, the Momma League, LaLeche League, and the like into activity programs, information and training centers, and consciousness-raising efforts suggest that the middle-class parent has become more sensitive to his/her needs as a person as well as a parent.

The Single Male Parent. While voluntary single male parents are still much in the minority, they are becoming more numerous. Their living arrangements include group living as well as living alone with the child. Because the male's economic status is generally better than the female's, he has more options for child care and living quarters. Thus, caretakers in the home are found more frequently, although ample use is made of child care centers and children programs. This particular population provides an opportunity for observing an alternative in family style that has voluntarily and proudly rejected the traditional nuclear family.[10]

Communes

The creation of a communal alternate to the isolated nuclear family is not new in this country. Generations have sought a new start and protested the status quo. Causes of their dissent and the ways in which they chose to organize their new communal existence varied in the past as they do with today's communards. Some were based upon religious conviction, some on economic idealism, some on rebellion against authority. Some attempted to establish a model of government based upon an absence of central authority; others sought a strict line of hierarchical authority with the rejection of those members who did not adhere to the authority prescribed. Some had relatively long histories, such as the Bruderhof, while others, such as "Brook Farm," an intellectual community in Massachusetts, dissolved rapidly.

Current Communal Lifestyle.   Lifestyles displayed by the current commune movement are perhaps even more varied than those of the historical models. This makes attempts to define this alternate lifestyle difficult. Communes vary today in type of membership, organizational structure, and general purpose. Some are involved in agricultural subsistence seeking a closeness to the land characterized by the early close-knit communities reported to have existed in history, while others are composed of middle-class young professionals who do not wish to disengage from the urban scene and its various technological comforts. Size also varies from 12 or less to hundreds.

A significant number of present-day communes is based upon religious commitments of various persuasions. Eastern philosophy is often a guiding force in many of these religiously oriented communes. In others, the "Jesus movement" is central, with the members searching for a new way to live out the traditional Judeo-Christian convictions. Of late there have been some tragic happenings in some of these communal group living arrangements. It remains to be seen what effect these events will have on the total commune movement.

Communes are often formed around common interests, crafts, or some unifying goal. They start with people who like each other and share similar value systems, orientations, and convictions. This aspect is extremely important in these intentional communities, and some see their alternate family arrangement as the beginning of a social revolution that will bring about radical change in society.

Family Structure within the Commune.   Some communes are reported to be group-marriage oriented, but they are in the minority. One such group lives in Taos, New Mexico, and another exists nationally with a sizable base in Los Angeles. Children are shared with the group and there is little concern about knowing or caring which individuals have been biologically responsible for the conception of the child. The rearing of the child is considered more important than who the parents are.

Other groups are oriented as extended families, with couples remaining essentially monogamous in their own private quarters, although partners may change from time to time. Still others live together under a community concept rather than a family unit, sharing resources that are more effectively achieved in multiple family cooperatives, such as expenses, household chores, and child care responsibilities. The women's consciousness movement has given particular impetus to these groups.

As we stated previously, the life span of the current communes varies. Such issues as organization of work and other aspects of living, interpersonal relationships, mutual values, economic feasibility, and ability to cope with outside community harassment have been suggested as important to the stability of communal arrangements.

Parent-child Relationships.   Living arrangements largely determine parent-child relationships. Great ingenuity is shown—tents, lean-tos, and cabins in the rural areas; apartment houses, motels, and sometimes "single family" dwellings in the city.

The number of children varies from commune to commune. In general, the adults are conscious of the population explosion, and few parents with more than three biological children are in evidence; however, there are some "families" who have eight to ten children. Birth, pregnancy, and children are esteemed and joyously regarded as an expression of a natural and ecologically appropriate experience. Adult-child relations are often determined by proximity of living and sleeping quarters. Relations with biological parents may be infrequent, with children being physically separated from them and assigned to caretakers, as is the case in some instances. In addition, the child's relationship with other adults is related to the extent of the existence of a hierarchical structure. In a family, multiple dwelling arrangements can permit a child to move among households, as when he is in conflict with other members, lonely for playmates or when his family is "splitting" for a time.

Childrearing Practices.   Investigators have found a wide range of childrearing practices among the communards. Some of the attitudes and value systems that are likely to affect the child's development and, hence, have relevance for health professionals are summarized here:[11,12]

1. Breast-feeding appears routine and there is usually close tactile contact between mother and child in the first year. Strapped to the mother's back, the baby goes everywhere with her, and is touched frequently.

2. There is often a clear break in the intense mother-infant relationship at around two-and-one-half years, when there is a push in the direction of independence and self-reliance. The mother begins to think of her own needs and returns gradually to activities.

3. Good health, together with a desire for wholesomeness, are reversed. Natural foods are stressed and "junk" foods are restricted. Institutional medical and dental care may be limited to emergencies with self-help medical and pharmacological expertise encouraged. Few preventive measures are sought from organized medicine except prenatal care. The emphasis is on prevention through healthful, natural living.

4. Nonviolence is generally espoused among the counterculture groups, although assertiveness among the children, especially the girls, is sanctioned. Children are often left to work out peer relationships and direct interrelations are fostered. Only the demands of safety take precedence. Children are disciplined, however, and a broad spectrum of this exists from verbal admonition to physical punishment.

5. Humanistic and interpersonal relationships and the direct expression of affectional needs are valued. Artificial repression of sexuality and intimacy are eschewed. Thus, exposure to nudity and observation of adult sexual activity may be permitted.

6. Children socialize each other, since, when the child gets into his own groups, he is dependent upon his peers' support. There is a great deal of age specific role peer modeling.

7. Early decision making is encouraged in the child. This is related to the philosophy that the child has individual rights and thus has a role in participatory democracy. This group decision making by parents is often modeled by children as an important mode for solving problems even though their decisions are by necessity immature.

8. The parents experience some difficulty with serving as role models for their children. They appear to be quite reluctant to "lay their trip" on the child. Yet, they admit to value and lifestyle preferences that are consonant with their attitudes, and, because of their verbal admonishings and role modeling, reinforce those behaviors of the child that are consonant with their attitudes. Another problem is that the parents may not be willing to serve as sex role models because of their general acceptance of an antisexist philosophy. Yet many of the males are out and out sexists. There is also ambivalence about having the girls identify with the not completely emancipated women.

9. Competency to handle daily life is stressed, while competition and achievement striving are played down; thus, individual potential and creativity are felt to be promoted. Sensory impressions, intuition, and the occult, as opposed to the rational, are data that are considered an enhancement of creativity. Children, because of their competency, are expected to distinguish between what is appropriate behavior within the "family" and the "outside world."

10. The materialistic values are seen as tied in with technological advances and nonhumanistic goals; thus, dependence on material possessions is minimized whenever possible. Shared objects, toys, and utensils are far in the majority. Some of the children see the adults "ripping off" the outside society and ignoring the social contracts involved in per-

sonal ownership (i.e., stealing). There is such great variability in these groups that it is evident that follow-up is indicated to see what the impact is of these childrearing practices.

One of the other findings of the studies that have been done indicates that many of the practices within these lifestyles and relating to childrearing are also practiced in the present-day nuclear family. Much of what appears in the mass media—TV, newspapers, and so on—logically finds expression in many of these evolving lifestyle families.[13]

GENERAL CONSIDERATIONS IN WORKING WITH PARENTS

There are several principles that health professionals will want to remember when delivering services to any couple, particularly those who may be experimenting with a variant lifestyle. A general rejection of so-called traditional values pervades our culture with more and more emphasis placed on the right of each individual to find values and a philosophy that is meaningful to him or her. Thus, couples experimenting with varient lifestyles may assume a questioning attitude which may prove disconcerting to some health providers.

Evaluating Health Information

Health professionals often expect patients to accept their information as true because it is drawn from a scientific body of knowledge. However, thoughtful patients may not necessarily accept Western scientific knowledge. They may, indeed, regard modern science as attempting to bring forth more and more "laws" aimed at finding absolute truth in a relative world and, hence, having little to do with health and, more important, happiness.

On the other hand, information from other sources, including health information, is also subjected to scrutiny and evaluation before acceptance. Thus, many practices that could be potentially harmful are often rejected. If patients have any kind of a relationship with a professional to whom they can turn for criteria against which to compare advice, they will usually make appropriate choices.

The tendency to evaluate medical information

given by the health professional on an experiential rather than a scientific basis does not preclude an interest in what the health professional has to say. In our experience, particularly in the free clinics, we find that the nurse is respected as a person who has knowledge in her field and *who shares some of the patient's concerns and feelings.* Expectant parents will have many questions and, when the nurse responds to their inquiries, they may go on to relate information that they have gathered from other sources. It becomes important to discuss this information seriously and with respect since it is valuable to the parent. Health teaching documented with rational explanation and practical experiences is much more readily accepted. The advice and teaching must be practical also. To insist that a vegetarian eat meat, even if she may have anemia, is simply too impractical, especially if there are others in the family to consider.

Moreover patients who follow evolving lifestyles are, for the most part, well educated and, because of this and their value system, expect a fuller and more complete explanation than many other patients. If a mother prefers a vegetarian diet and wants to know the food values of the foods she wishes to include in her diet, she will not be satisfied with only a suggested menu. Exchanges and equivalents must be discussed. It is not sufficient to tell a mother in an antepartal clinic to return in so many weeks for another blood test without telling her the reason for returning and the purpose of the procedure. If patients reject some of the advice, this, too, is to be treated with respect.[14]

Choosing Antepartal Services

The factors that affect the couple experimenting with a family lifestyle also affect the traditional lifestyle couple. These include past experience with health personnel, geographic location, feelings about the pregnancy, the influence of significant others, and the parents' physical condition. Increasingly, there is a high priority placed on ambience and interpersonal relations during the pregnancy and at the time of delivery. Modern up-to-date equipment and technological expertise may be much less important than an environment that simulates the home. The rise of alternative birth centers which provide a homelike atmosphere and indeed, the rise in the number of home births attest to this value.

Selection of services is made on the basis of consultation with friends, referrals from professionals and past experience with health providers. In general, couples are taking a more militant stand regarding participation in the planning and execution of their care and tend to seek out health professionals who allow them this right. It becomes important then to be sure that the patients be duly informed about the nature of their care, including their right to sign themselves out of the hospital. This information together with a genuine indication of regard for the couple is usually sufficient to lessen the apprehension about having a hospital delivery or seeking antenatal care from a "traditional" establishment provider.

Choosing the Place and Method of Delivery

Selecting a hospital for delivery or choosing between a hospital and home delivery involves many of the same factors as those considered in the selection of antepartal services. For most couples today, childbirth is regarded as a natural process; thus, prepared childbirth classes and the Le Boyer method of delivery are very popular. Today, parents come to their deliveries much more knowledgeable than previously. This is due, in part, to the large variety of books now available dealing with nutrition in pregnancy, the physiology of pregnancy, labor and delivery, and even "how-to" books on home delivery. Parents therefore expect their requests to be considered. Hospitals that have the reputation for having a great deal of restrictions and "hassle" are avoided, regardless of the quality of technological expertise offered.

The need for control over one's own life may also be a strong motivating factor in the choice of a home delivery.[15] These types of deliveries still remain controversial due to a variety of factors. Safety of the mother and infant continues to be a grave concern for the health professionals, and there are data that indicate that this concern is well founded. However, birth carries a strong symbolic meaning and the home typifies this meaning. The traditional hospital setting is seen by many couples as a sterile place with little room for intimacy and family integration.[16] Many hospitals are now instituting birthing rooms or birth centers which simulate a homelike atmosphere that is free from many of the restrictions and rigidities imposed by the traditional delivery suite. It is hoped that this alternative will encompass both the symbolic atmosphere that is desired and adequate safety features for the mother and infant.

ETHNIC, SOCIAL CLASS, AND CULTURAL VARIATIONS

The recent emphasis on cultural pluralism and ethnic heritage in America seems to contradict the contention that ethnic groups tend to shed their distinctive family patterns as they become socially mobile. It can be seen, however, that the move toward the celebration of national origins represents an extolling of distinctive ethnic art, language, dress, and food patterns for the purpose of promoting a positive identity and ancestral pride in those who have had little of either.

If we examine the contemporary family roles of various ethnic groups, we see that the process of acculturation has been accelerated or delayed by several factors including opportunity available in the new environment, the extent of discrimination, and the degree of cultural and physical similarity or difference between the acculturating group and the dominant society. There are many groups that comprise the "salad bowl" of America and, unfortunately, we cannot include all of them here. However, we will highlight some of the groups to give an indication of the current state of thought on contemporary family roles.

We would like to make clear at the outset that the variations among the different ethnic groups in family styles, health beliefs and practices, utilization of health services, and the like are a function of the socioeconomic status of the individuals far more than their particular ethnicity. Since minority groups in general are often poorer than their white counterparts and because more individuals within each group tend to be poorer than the same proportion of whites, there has been an inability to gain access to education and other resources that money can buy. Thus, behavior and beliefs which differ from the mainstream white middle-class dominant society have come about or been retained. Thus, misconceptions have arisen attributing these behaviors to ethnicity.

Native American Families

Of all of the ethnic groups that abound in this country, the American Indian has perhaps the most remarkable history—one that reflects severe exploitation, astounding endurance, and incredible capability for adaptation. The name "Indian" itself was a European appellation and was applied indiscriminately to the several thousand tribes that inhabited the North American continent at the time of its discovery by Columbus. From that time onward, the native American's history has been marred by disease, starvation, deliberate attempts at genocide, and blatantly inconsistent treatment by governmental agencies.

Even today, there is no single accepted definition of American Indian or native American. Governmental agencies and the Census Bureau rely on the individual to define himself or herself as Indian; some require proof of at least one quarter Indian blood. Hence, even enumerating the number of tribes and individuals is difficult. In 1976 it was estimated that this population was increasing so that now there may be around one million Indians in the country who are associated into over 300 tribes.

Approximately one half of the Indian population lives on reservations whose development was a result of a racist governmental policy of "exclusion." Reservation lands were much less acceptable than the lands originally inhabited by the various tribes. Life on the reservation, even today, is fraught with the twin plagues of poverty and substandard housing which, in turn, gives rise to myriad health problems.[18,19]

An urban resettlement program was attempted in 1952 which was supposed to aid the assimilation of the Indian into the mainstream American culture. Participants were given job training and limited aid in finding jobs and housing. The program is generally regarded as a failure. Because of bureaucratic red tape and disinterest, financial and other aid was so meager that it did not begin to achieve the goals originally outlined. Those who did leave the reservation often found themselves separated from their families since the housing allowance was inadequate to accommodate an entire family. Moreover, the traditional social supports found on the reservation disappeared in the city. Thus, the urban Indian became a true "marginal" man. He was distrusted by his own people and unable to participate in traditional tribal life. Moreover, he was stigmatized and ignored by those with whom he was supposed to assimilate. It is estimated that about half of those who attempted the urban move have returned to the reservation.[20]

An attempt is being made through the use of Urban Indian Centers to meet some of the needs of these urban migrants. These centers supply health services, educational services, job counseling, and the like. It is still too early to comment on the success of this innovation, but it would seem that these programs are achieving at least a modicum of success.[21]

The cultural background of the native American will vary according to tribal affiliation. Thus, generalizations about the American Indian family must be made with caution. In the main, however, family life is influenced by tribal beliefs and there is a great deal of variation among the tribes with respect to holding to traditional values and customs. This variability occurs in both the reservation and urban Indian communities.

For the most part, the family remains the basic unit of native American society. The Indian idea of family is the extended family that includes grandparents, aunts, uncles, and even close friends. Children are valued and admired and all members participate in the childrearing. Each has certain things that must be taught to the child and the responsibility is taken seriously.

In many tribes, the lineage is matriarchal and the child automatically becomes a member of the mother's clan at birth. Indian women have traditionally worked very hard, but they have also been very influential in tribal affairs. Indeed, they have been "the heart of the home" and several have also been leaders of their tribes.[22,23]

Health beliefs also vary according to tribal identity and religion is a powerful force in giving direction to childbearing, childbirth, and childrearing. Again it is difficult to make generalizations, but a few principles will be attempted here. For the most part, pregnancy is thought of as a natural process in the normal cycle of life and death. In general, a harmonious prenatal period is stressed with an attempt to help the mother be content, keep away from ill or evil persons and things and think good thoughts. When facilities permit, prenatal care and hospital delivery is sought from obstetricians or other physicians. Tribal midwives are also utilized. The tribal medicine man is relied upon also to provide special foods and beverages that are believed to be helpful in increasing strength and preventing illness. He also supplies charms and amulets to aid in a healthy delivery.[24]

In spite of the fact that the majority of native American women deliver in hospitals, their maternal mortality rate is nearly 2 percent higher than the overall maternal mortality rate for the United States.[25] It is becoming glaringly apparent that health providers who work with these clients must make more of an effort to become familiar with the customs and needs of these patients if they are to provide adequate services. A recent positive development has been a rapprochement between traditional western medicine and the native healers. Programs have been developed which permit sharing of each's beliefs and techniques. Thus, the best of each tradition can be incorporated into the care of patients, which results in an upgrading in the quality of care delivered.

Black Families

One of the most significant factors affecting the family roles of the black population of the United States has been the concentration of a majority of these families at income levels that are grossly inadequate. This has been due largely to discrimination which is more severe for blacks than for other less visible groups. New opportunities have opened up for the black community in recent years; however, these have benefitted mainly upper-working-class and middle-class families. The poorest strata have not gained proportionally.

Another factor that has been woven into the fabric of what some have called mythology about the black community has been the lack of a strong patriarchal tradition among the black family. The mother is seen as the head of the household and provider, while the father is seen as mostly absent, a nonprovider, and a powerless parent. However, research has indicated that, among the middle-class and upper-working-class families, there is no significant difference from whites with respect to family role differentiation and the acceptance of a middle-class value system.

In a thoughtful review and evaluation of the empirical research findings regarding lower-class black families, TenHouten concluded that the bulk of the findings do *not* show these fathers and husbands to be powerless in either their conjugal or parental roles. Black wives do appear to be powerful in their parental roles, but there is no indication that this emasculates the black father.[26] Indeed, there is a healthy effect in that fathers tend to be more expressive in their marital and parental roles and are helpful and willing to share in childrearing and homemaking chores. Moreover, this freedom from patriarchy has enabled the black woman to be more pragmatic, resourceful, and flexible than her counterparts from other cultures in which the tradition of authoritarianism and patriarchy is strong.

Since they typically do not have authoritarian fathers, black children do not experience one of the psychological stresses of low-achievement motivations. The increased economic opportunities that will allow black fathers to become economic role models for their children, combined with an early emphasis on independence typical among black families, and confident setting of standards by black mothers should result in higher levels of achievement motivation among black children than those among children whose fathers play a more repressive role. There is already evidence that middle-class black children have higher levels of motivation and aspiration than do their white counterparts.

Blacks in the lower socioeconomic strata, especially when confined to the ghetto and/or rural areas and deprived of educational and other acculturating opportunities, tend to hold a traditional value system that includes a strong sense of family (or familism), superstition, religiosity, and fatalism. This is in contrast to the "middle-class" value system generally held by highly industrialized urban societies. These values—rationalism, pragmatism, individualism, equalitarianism, secularism, and achievement—have also become known as the dominant American values.

Whether the individual's value system is traditional or middle-class urban, it becomes part of his belief system and is incorporated into the roles of husband, wife, parent, and child.[27] Thus, when dealing with these patients, health professionals often find their values competing with those of the patients. When the basic values are examined, it becomes clearer why there occur certain health beliefs, differential utilization of health services, delay in seeking care and often nonadherence to prescribed regimens.

Mexican-American Families

Mexican-Americans have been the forgotten minority in the United States, possibly because the Southwest has been somewhat neglected by both academicians and writers with the exception of John Steinbeck. There are more than 5 million Mexican-Americans, who are mainly second-generation offspring of peasant immigrants from Mexico. They are concentrated in the border states of Texas, Arizona, New Mexico, and California, and comprise the second largest minority group in the United States.

Since World War II, the isolation of the Mexican-American has been declining; this has been due to the fact that many participated in the war and gradually new perspectives and opportunities have come about which have had an impact on family roles and traditional value and belief systems. Neighborhood enclaves (barrios) still exist, of course, and in some small rural or isolated urban areas, even the middle-class Mexican-American tends to reside in them.

Familism appears to be the strongest surviving traditional value within the older Mexican-American community, along with patriarchalism and machismo—the cultural ideal of masculinity which equates maleness with sexual prowess.[28] These traditional values and certain folk beliefs persist, particularly because of the isolation of the barrios and the persistence of these values and beliefs make difficult the acceptance of modern health knowledge and practice.

Mexican-Americans in the barrios who are educated and have had a positive experience with health services, have accepted the ideas of scientific medicine and health care, allow their children to be immunized, attend clinics and, in some cases, have accepted some kind of family planning. However, there are many others who have their own set of folk beliefs about illness and its treatment which they practice in conjunction with medical care or before seeking scientific health care. These beliefs about diseases and their cures are derived from experience and experimentation and are handed down from generation to generation. Two or more cures may be recognized for one disorder and disorders generally fall into two categories—those of emotional origin and those of magical origin. Folk healers (primarily curanderas [women], or curanderos [men]) are often utilized and some have

an important and respected standing in the community. It is felt by the majority of the uneducated that physicians do not know how to treat folk disorders because they lack either faith, knowledge, or understanding of them.

Among those with little education, there is no distinction between the natural and supernatural and many illnesses can be a result of evil forces, witches, spells cast by other persons, or punishment for some sin committed either knowingly or unknowingly. One common condition that health professionals should be aware of is the following: *mal aire* or bad air, especially night air. It can enter through any of the body cavities under certain circumstances and results in illness of both mother and child. *Mal ojo,* or the evil eye, is a culturally defined disease, primarily of children. It is caused when someone looks admiringly or covetously on the child or adult. Its symptoms are restlessness, crying, and headache as well as other nonspecific symptoms. *Susto* or fright can be caused by a frightening experience that can result in excessive nervousness, loss of appetite, and loss of sleep. *Mollera calda* or fallen fontanel is a common disorder among infants. It is believed to be due to a fall or from taking the nipple out of the baby's mouth too suddenly, thus causing the fontanel to be sucked in. Symptoms include irritability, crying, diarrhea, sunken eyes, and vomiting. There are other afflictions as well as their home remedies that it is wise for the nurse to know if she will be dealing with these patients. The reader is referred to the books by Hymovich and Barnard, and Reinhardt and Quinn for excellent presentations of these conditions and specific nursing intervention.[29,30]

Japanese-American Families

The modernization of the Japanese family in America has proceeded more slowly in some respects than in Japan because the isolation of the Japanese-American from the effects of technological development and rapid social change has been more pronounced here. However, in California, where the largest concentration of Japanese ancestry occurs, this segment of the population has the highest median levels of income and education of any minority group. Japanese-Americans also have very low rates of crime and delinquency, indicating at the same time the greater persistence of the traditional values of obedience and conformity to parental values and norms. The generational pattern of increasing acculturation is very clearly illustrated in the contemporary Japanese-American community, since other factors such as urban-rural residence do not vary significantly.

A majority of the Issei or first-generation immigrants who were born in Japan arrived here some time between the end of the 19th century and 1924, when immigration from the Orient and Eastern Europe was sharply restricted by the Johnson Act. While the Issei came largely from rural agricultural areas and occupations, they were unusual in that they were relatively literate, compared with peasant immigrants from Europe, and they valued education even before their arrival in this country.

Second-generation Japanese-Americans—the Nisei—born largely before 1940, experienced an unusual push into modernity not only by the parents' preexisting emphasis on education, but by the West Coast evacuation of Japanese-Americans during World War II. Familistic values were weakened by the loss of confiscated family homes and businesses, which removed an important source of Issei control over their second-generation offspring. Thus, after the war, the Issei, who were forced to seek out independent, nonfamily occupational opportunities, were thereby more speedily acculturated into the modern values of individualism and equalitarianism in family relationships, although a cultural lag in this respect is still quite pronounced among many Japanese-Americans.

The third generation—the Sansei—born largely since World War II and now in high school, college, or in the adult occupational world, are the most totally acculturated of all. However, certain subcultural differences remain in family role conceptions, even within the third generation, that are traceable to the survival of traditional ethnic values in marital roles and in childrearing practices.

In the Orient, the patriarchal tradition has been much more crystalized than in the West. The deference and obedience of wife and children toward husband and father, and of the younger generations toward elders, was more intense and more formalized in ritual, ceremony, religion, and law in the Orient than in Western society.

The extended family form, the ancestral clan or house as the basic family unit, was far more salient in the Orient as reality and as cultural ideal, for all social strata. Arranged marriages and emphasis on lineage, important indicators of the value of familism, were common even among the poor in Japan. The values of obedience, deference, duty, and responsibility were constantly reinforced by pervasive mechanisms of control that elicited shame and guilt for the slightest deviation from established convention.[31]

Frequent sources of role conflict, in the Sansei generation especially, are found in the greater prevalence of strict disciplinary measures in childrearing, the greater emphasis on conformity and unconditional obedience, on humility and emotional reserve (particularly the suppression of anger), the continued extensive use of shame and guilt as mechanisms of control, the greater submissiveness of women, even within the higher strata, and the greater strength of extended family pride and intergenerational emotional dependence. These are the residual of traditional values of the parents.

Male dominance is stronger in Oriental homes, at all class levels, than in any other ethnic group in this country. While the emphasis within Japanese-American homes on achievement and competitiveness has promoted educational and occupational success, the continuing stress of familism and authoritarian values has retarded the flexibility, independence, and the self-reliance that are important attributes of individualistic achievement in highly industrialized society.

While recent studies of the Sansei generation have indicated a shift toward greater independence in this generation, both males and females remain, typically, less assertive, more deferent and conforming, and more emotionally reserved than their Anglo peers. The rigid conformity, status distinctions, and authority relations of traditional Japan that continue to affect family roles of Japanese-Americans in this country are likely to disappear with time, but more quickly in the occupational world than in the world of the family, where they appear less immediately dysfunctional.[32]

There are few folk beliefs and, in general, scientific medicine is accepted especially by the second- and third-generation Japanese-American. Preventive medicine is solicited and, because of the high educational levels as well as high achievement aspirations, health and medical regimens are usually followed. Among the older generation there may be some reliance on herbal medicine and interest in acupuncture.

REFERENCES

1. Sussman, M. Family systems in the 1970's: Analysis, policies, and programs. *Annals Am. Academy* 396, July 1970.

2. Lewis, G. L. Changes in women's role participation. In I. Frieze, et al. (eds.), *Women and Sex Roles, A Social Psychological Perspective.* New York: W. W. Norton, 1978, pp. 137–8.

3. Pickett, R. S. Monogamy on trial part II, the modern era. *Alternate Lifestyles* 1, 3:281–301, Aug. 1978.

4. Sussman, *op. cit.*

5. *Ibid.*

6. Reeder, S. J. The Impact of Disabling Health Conditions on Family Interaction. Unpublished Doctoral Dissertation, 1974.

7. Sussman, *op. cit.*

8. Eiduson B. J., et al. Alternatives in childrearing in the 1970's. *Am. J. Orthopsychiat.* 43: 720–31, Oct. 1973.

9. *Ibid.*

10. *Ibid.*

11. *Ibid.*

12. Johnston, C. and R. Deisher. Contemporary communal childrearing. *Pediat.* 52:326, Sept. 1973.

13. Eiduson, *op. cit.*

14. Bancroft, A. V. Pregnancy and the counterculture. *Nurs. Clin. N. Am.* 8:67–76, Mar. 1973.

15. Maralee. *Our Babies, Our Lives, Our Right to Decide.* Chicago, Chicago Seed, 1972.

16. Bancroft, *op. cit.*

17. Taylor, T. W. *The States and Their Indian Citizens.* Washington, D.C., U.S. Government Printing Office, 1972.

18. Levitan, S. and B. Hetrick. *Big Brother's Indian Programs; With Reservations.* New York, McGraw-Hill, 1971.

19. Billard, J. B. (ed.). *The World of the American Indian.* Washington, D.C., National Geographic Society, 1974, pp. 311–382.

20. Clark, A. L. *Culture Childbearing Health Professionals.* Philadelphia: F. A. Davis, 1978, Chap. 2.

21. *Ibid.*

22. Foreman, C. T. *Indian Women Chiefs.* Muskogee, Oklahoma, Hoffman Printing Co., 1954.

23. Billard, *op. cit.*

24. Vogel, G. *American Indian Medicine.* New York, Ballantine Books, 1973.

25. U.S. Department of Health, Education and Welfare. Report of a Regional Task Force: Health of the American Indian. Washington, D.C., U.S. Government Printing Office, 1973.

26. TenHouten, W. The black family: Myth and reality. *Psychiat.* 33:145–173, 1970.

27. Yorburg, B. *The Changing Family.* New York, Columbia U. Press, 1973, pp. 141–49.

28. *Ibid.*

29. Hymovich, D. P., and M. Barnard. *Family Health Care.* New York, McGraw-Hill, 1973, pp. 128–137.

30. Reinhardt, A. and M. Quinn. *Family Centered Community Nsg.* St. Louis, Mosby, 1973, pp. 72–77.

31. Benedict, R. *The Chrysanthemum and the Sword.* Boston, Houghton-Mifflin, 1946.

32. Yorburg, *op. cit.*, pp. 145–149.

Five

Culture, Society and Maternal Care

The Social and Cultural Meaning of Childbearing / The Sick Role, Illness and Pregnancy / Childbearing Motivations / Sociocultural Factors Affecting Childbearing / Additional Factors in the Use of Maternity Services

In most societies, conceptions of health and well-being reflect the orientations of the person's social class or group membership. Values, attitudes, perspectives, and the behavior that we engage in are formed and conditioned by the social groups in which we participate from earliest childhood. Consequently, there are differing orientations to health and health care reflecting memberships in differing ethnic, racial, religious, and social class groups. These varying health orientations become manifest both in the behavior of individuals and the institutions that are organized to deliver health services.

In recent years, there has been a heightened awareness of the importance of social and cultural factors in health status, specifically maternal care. Although Americans are accustomed to thinking of their health status as being the best and highest in the world, their health care is still far short of its potential. Large segments of the population either do not have access to adequate medical care or are deprived of quality care in the services that they do receive. There has been a great stimulus to improve the prenatal care system, in particular, in order to improve the delivery of maternal care services and thus reduce preterm, low-birth weight, and infant deaths. Essentially, there has been an expansion and elaboration of the existing system of maternity

services. Whether such an approach to maternity problems will have the desired effects depends on a variety of factors, not the least of which are those concerning the health values, beliefs, orientations, and ultimately behaviors of the target populations.

In the present chapter the focus is upon those forces and features in society that influence the field of maternity services. First, it is important to examine the social and cultural meaning of pregnancy: what are the current social, cultural, and economic forces that influence motivations for childbearing? Second, we will discuss some of the critical issues in access and use of maternal services and finally present some aspects of the nurse's role in these matters.

THE SOCIAL AND CULTURAL MEANING OF CHILDBEARING

For nurses to function appropriately, to use their talents more creatively than in the past, they must have an understanding of the social and cultural meaning of pregnancy. As discussed in Chapter 1 pregnancy itself needs to be considered in terms of the social context in which it occurs, namely, the family and the larger society. Moreover, pregnancy and childbearing in general have different meanings in various societies and even within any given society.

In Western society the expectations and the prescriptions for behavior surrounding pregnancy are relatively ill-defined, and in some situations they do not exist. Consequently women are often uncertain when and how often they ought to visit the physician, whether they can continue employment, and what is expected of them by significant others. Part of the reasons for these loose definitions is related to the lifestyles of population subcultures and part of the answer lies in factors related to the social structure of society.

THE SICK ROLE, ILLNESS, AND PREGNANCY

How a society or groups within a society define pregnancy and cope with pregnancy tends to vary considerably. In some societies, pregnancy is regarded as a "normal" situation—a kind of status passage through which most women, at some time or other, will pass. In other societies, pregnancy may be regarded as an illness and is reacted to as other illnesses are. Moreover, there is considerable variation, even within societies, in the way health and illness are perceived by different social classes, ethnic groups, and age categories.

The Sick Role Concept.   The sick role has been developed as a concept by sociologists to study the role behavior of persons who are considered to be sick or to have an illness. In brief, the sick role concept refers to the process by which every society ensures that an adequate level of health and normative conformity exists among the majority of its members most of the time. Society has various mechanisms for accomplishing this purpose. It accommodates individuals or groups who are ill by placing them in a special position or status. The term "social role" refers to both the regular way of acting expected of persons occupying a given position and the social position itself. Typically there are certain rights or privileges, as well as expectations, associated with given social positions. Parsons has presented an insightful and systematic analysis of the expectations associated with occupancy of the sick role.[1] There are two main rights:

1. The sick person is allowed exemption from the performance of normal social role obligations.
2. The sick person is allowed exemption from the responsibility for his own state.

In addition there are two main obligations:

3. The sick person must be motivated to get well as soon as possible.
4. The sick person should seek technically competent help and cooperate with medical experts.

The sick role is generally thought of as only a theoretical model for the purposes of understanding the processes contributing to and the various conditions to be fulfilled in the legitimation of illness conditions. In reality, the concept is not universally applicable to all who claim to be ill; it varies depending on the unique background of the person, the particular illness involved, and the social context within which legitimation is sought.

Behavioral scientists have made a number of criticisms of the sick role, including the fact that Parsons has left open the problem of the chronically ill, as well as some illness that is not considered serious enough to warrant more than a slight reduction in normal activities. Furthermore, much illness never reaches the stage of formal consultation with a qualified physician. Individuals who are ill may receive what they consider to be competent help from other than professional medical personnel. Furthermore, Parsons has suggested that his sick role formulation is especially applicable to psychiatric or emotional illnesses. Finally, Parsons's formulation may not be relevant to all societies, and various studies have demonstrated that there are both intercultural and intracultural variations in the definitions of the conditions to which the sick role is thought to be applicable.

The Sick Role and Pregnancy. The state of pregnancy in its usual or normal situation, where there are no resultant obstetrical or delivery complications, must be considered in the discussion of the applicability of the sick role concept. If a woman is experiencing complications of pregnancy, certainly this would make her eligible for the sick role as discussed above. The question that arises is whether pregnancy is in fact a "normal" state.

One may conceivably take the position that illness, or sickness, is statistically normal in most members of the population at some point in their lives; similarly, pregnancy can likewise be considered statistically normal in that most of the population of possible conceivers at some time are in this state. Pregnancy can also be considered "normal" in the sense that it is a necessary biological function for the species. Indeed, it can even be considered a desirable state of affairs. In this latter sense, it is not similar to illness at all. McKinlay has noted that pregnancy differs from illness by "calling forth in both the woman and her significant others a set of responses which are in many ways different from those elicited with the onset of an illness."[2] Considering whether the four sick role expectations noted above apply to pregnancy, McKinlay suggests that for a variety of reasons the state of pregnancy is in some ways different from illness and cannot be analyzed in terms of any of the four expectations associated with the sick role.

There is a tendency in the more advanced societies to consider some point during pregnancy as illness and to treat it in a manner similar to that in which illness is handled. For example, women are discouraged from home deliveries and are hospitalized for delivery. Blood pressure, height, weight, and so on are usually taken at several points during the pregnancy. Treating women "as if" they are ill may perhaps encourage the adoption of certain behaviors because the women perceive this type of treatment as being similar to that for an illness. In sum, the state of pregnancy and the expectations covering it differ from routine illness behavior and the situation is relatively unstructured. This relatively unstructured situation may produce a sense of role ambiguity in pregnant women. Women may take matters into their own hands and reduce the strain from ambiguity by structuring the situation in particular ways, including adopting the sick role.

For women who are at greater risk, particularly, and who react excessively or unfavorably under the strain of pregnancy, the sick role becomes meaningful and relevant.

Thus, both in the "normal" circumstances of pregnancy and in pathological conditions, the sick role plays an important part in maternal care.

CHILDBEARING MOTIVATIONS

One of the most important factors in human reproduction that is determined and influenced by culture and society is the *motivation* for childbearing. In the

past 15 years, numerous studies have appeared concerned with factors influencing the number of children desired by and born to married couples. Most of these studies have focused on the *number* of children desired rather than on the attitudes held by women regarding *why* they want children. A brief consideration of some of the social and psychological aspects motivating childbearing will be discussed.

No biological event has greater significance for society than reproduction and its outcome. Reproduction is important in family dynamics and population dynamics, which, in turn, have a heavy impact on individual and national welfare. Women begin their preparation for childbearing early in life. In a sense, they begin it at the time of their own conception.

As mentioned previously, society is primarily organized for families with children and the argument for having children can be very persuasive. Couples without children are still generally made to feel "out of place," especially if they have been married very long. Research has indicated that the value of having children remains generally accepted by the vast majority of Americans.[3]

In this context it is understandable that all levels of society should be organized in favor of children. As Rossi has noted, the cultural pressure to become parents is great enough that a couple may plan to bear children in spite of a latent desire to the contrary. For the female, the pressure to become a mother may be the equivalent of the cultural insistence that the male assume a productive occupational role.[4]

The availability of acceptable means for preventing conception permits a good deal of childbearing today to be a consequence of motivated human action rather than a mere biological result of sexual behavior. Regardless of when pregnancies occur or if they are planned, the number of children a couple has and the time at which it has them are partially a function of the nature of the couple's childbearing motivations.[5]

Present Societal Trends Affecting Childbearing Motivation

Fertility Control. Elsewhere in this book we discuss techniques of contraception and family planning from a more technical perspective. Here we wish to highlight certain social implications of fertility control. A number of important trends occurring in the United States have already resulted in low fertility. Indeed, the U.S. birthrate in 1974 reached an all-time low. At the current level, American families are having just enough children to replace themselves. In the opinion of many demographers, a revolution in the fertility regime of American women is taking place that has profound implications for society, including maternity services. At the core of the fertility changes is the apparent change in values associated with fertility control. The widespread use of the pill resulted not only in a more effective means of controlling fertility, but also in a change in the rules under which fertility decisions are made.

First, it must be recognized that the extensive use of oral contraceptives, not only vastly improved contraceptive protection, but also separated contraception from sexual activity. Now childbearing can be voluntary in a radically different sense than ever before. Under the previous fertility regimen, women could not confidently plan a lifetime of childlessness nor the prevention of unwanted pregnancy. Not surprisingly, under this regimen the role expectations of women were structured around motherhood. In fact, cultural values with respect to fertility were, in part, rationalizations of the inevitable. For example, in the early 1960s about one-half of all births were accidental: one-fifth were reported by their mothers as unwanted.[6]

The widespread use of the pill has facilitated the adoption of other effective means of preventing unwanted births (the IUD, sterilization, and abortion) and has led to reductions in the number of children intended by U.S. women. Contraceptive sterilization had been a relatively infrequent occurrence in the population prior to the introduction of the pill. In recent years there has been a dramatic reversal of this pattern with majority approval and greater use of this procedure. By 1970, for example, among women older than 30, sterilization was the most prevalent contraceptive method.[7]

Competing Social Roles. All of the foregoing processes in contraceptive practice indicate a drastic realignment of values in fertility. These new fertility control values have given more support to the equal opportunity concept by making nonfamilial roles a realistic and viable option for women. Thus the potential for complete fertility control makes child-

bearing a matter of choice in a sense never before realized. Motherhood itself now becomes a matter of rational evaluation. The costs as well as the virtues can now be weighed. This is, of course, not a new discovery. There has always been a large literature on the psychological and emotional costs of motherhood. They have, however, become more relevant and prominent particularly in the context of increased concern with equality of opportunity for women.

Thus, as other social roles become more feasible, the opportunity costs of childbearing are increased. One of the consequences is to place motherhood more directly in competition with these alternative, socially desirable roles. As fertility becomes more a matter for *decision,* greater emphasis is placed on planning. Among the factors that must be taken into account in the decision are the direct social, psychological, and economic costs of children themselves, and also the loss of the wife's earnings and intrinsic satisfaction with her occupation.

This is no small matter. Modern lifestyles are significantly dependent on the wife's earnings. In a majority of the families in which both the husband and wife have incomes, the wife's income represents over one-fifth of the total family income.[8]

Impact on Maternity Services

The implications of all this are enormous, for fertility statistics influence almost every facet of our lives. Consider the following as examples: (1) elementary school enrollment has been dropping since 1970 and this is now being seen in high schools; (2) a slowdown in the birthrate affects the Social Security system of the country; (3) there will be changes in the consumption patterns that may influence smaller cars and even smaller houses; (4) last, but not least, there is an impact upon maternity services.

Two trends in particular are worth mentioning; first, not only are some hospitals closing their maternity units, but perhaps more important, hospitals are merging their obstetrical units. This will hopefully improve the quality of obstetrical care for mothers and newborns, in addition to controlling costs and avoiding duplication of services. In addition, the experience of fertility control may make women more sensitive and aware of the need for better maternal care during pregnancy. Indeed, the increased availability of safe abortion after 1970 has been temporarily associated with a reduction in pregnancy-associated maternal mortality.[9,10] There is also good reason to connect the trends in fertility control to the recent rapid decline in infant mortality.

It should be recognized that no one knows for certain that the current pattern of fertility control will continue indefinitely. Nevertheless, it is important to note that the "baby boom" children of the 50s are now forming their own families. Consequently, within the next few years, there will be an increase of approximately 20 percent in the number of women in the childbearing age groups of 15 to 44 years. Thus, the absolute number of births may rise even if the *birthrate* does not. This occurred in 1974 for the first time in four years, and will have relevance for continued, high-quality maternity services.

SOCIOCULTURAL FACTORS AFFECTING CHILDBEARING

Sociodemographic Factors and the Use of Maternity Health Services

Social Class. Social class is an important determinant of maternal reproductive behavior and maternal use of services. Since socioeconomic status or social class has such a pervasive influence upon health and health care, it is well to briefly describe the central features of this concept.

Social class, or socioeconomic status, is a complex concept referring to a theoretical formulation of relationships between subgroups in our society. It is a term frequently used by sociologists and epidemiologists in medical research as an effort to subdivide populations into a few descriptive categories that differ in a variety of social and economic characteristics, background, and behavior.

Typically, in determining socioeconomic status, the usual procedure is to select as indicators of social differences one or several characteristics, each of which are closely related to income, education, occupation, housing and place of residence, social values, and the general lifestyle of population subgroups. By far the most widely used indicator of socioeconomic status or social class is occupation. It is the best indicator of a person's income, edu-

cation, standard of living, social values, and a variety of other attributes.

However, not all social differences stem from socioeconomic status. Dividing a population along one social dimension does not automatically provide categories that are socially meaningful in other respects. It can be demonstrated that such social variables as age, geographic region, height, parity, and ethnicity each contribute independently to the total picture of social variation in pregnancy outcome. The same may be said of other more complex social influences.

It is generally accepted that adequate medical care during pregnancy, particularly in the early stages of pregnancy, reduces the incidence of neonatal mortality, congenital malformations or other birth defects, maternal mortality, prematurity, and so on. The relationship between low socioeconomic status and failure to receive adequate antenatal care has been well documented. The data appear to be similar in the United States, Great Britain, and in various other Western nations. Not only do the lower-class women typically comprise the highest proportion of those who have not received antenatal care, they are also the women, as a group, who contribute to the highest proportion of underutilizers of antenatal care.[11]

According to the latest sources of data for the United States, the average white mother had 60 percent more visits for medical care than the average nonwhite mother. This is undoubtedly related less to the ethnicity of the mother than to the influence of socioeconomic status. According to these data, as family income increased, the number of visits for medical care also increased. Women living in families below the poverty level made, on the average, 9.3 visits for medical care; women from middle-income families averaged 13.7 visits. Most of the women in the lowest income group visited medical facilities (clinics, hospitals) for their care as contrasted to the women in the highest income group where the majority visited physicians for medical care.

Thus, income appears to be a major factor in the number of visits for prenatal care. There is a large jump in number of visits when the income goes over the poverty line (i.e., $5,000 and over).

Medical Organization and Social Class. Before discussing how the characteristics of lower-income persons influence their behavior in connection with the issues of health, illness, and the utilization of medical services, it is appropriate to briefly discuss some aspects of medical organization and care for lower-income groups. The national commitment for equality of medical care for all citizens has led to a variety of important legislative acts. The emphasis is on extending and improving the system of medical organization so that medical care can be offered more rapidly, more effectively, and more efficiently to the poor as well as to those more economically advantaged. For example, the maternal and infant care projects (MIC) supported by the U.S. Children's Bureau has had an important impact on maternity care throughout the United States. These projects are supposed to help reduce the incidence of mental retardation and other handicapping conditions caused by complications associated with childbearing and to help reduce infant and maternal mortality. The projects are concentrated in low-income areas of large and small cities, and the emphasis is on early, comprehensive prenatal care for all patients in the geographic area served. As with most of these new programs, there are many problems that have yet to be resolved before they can be called truly successful.

However, there is a serious question as to whether the inequities in the medical care system can be overcome unless changes are made reflecting greater understanding of lower socioeconomic lifestyles. It is well known that when medical facilities are set up in convenient proximity to lower-income housing, they do not automatically draw clientele.

There are two factors that contribute to inequities of medical care. The first of these relates to the way in which medical organization facilities are structured; the second is concerned with the characteristic lifestyles of lower-income groups.

What are the features of medical care organization that tend to blunt the effectiveness of medical care for lower-income patients? These negative features of medical organization include the following: first, there is the massiveness of medical organization itself. As noted earlier, most of the lower-income women tend to visit medical facilities such as hospitals and clinics. These are often large and complex organizations, characterized by great specialization and a fair degree of impersonality. Lower-class patients are ill-equipped by lack of education and experience to cope with complex bureaucratic organization.[12]

Professionalization.   A second feature of medical organization that tends to decrease the quality of care for lower-income patients is that of professionalization with its resultant characteristic set of goals, its perspectives toward work and patients which results in a gap between the patients and the professionals. Lower-income people are less skilled in obtaining information from professionals. They tend to be less aggressive in demanding explanations. On the other hand, higher-income patients have greater aggressive and interactional skills and can cope more effectively with the professionals' failure to communicate.

There are other, more subtle, disadvantages stemming from professional stances, from which lower-income patients suffer. These have been discussed by a number of investigators in the field of mental disorders. That is, middle-class patients are preferred by most providers, and are seen as more treatable. In other words, there may be a distinct bias expressed against the lower-income patient, based honestly on professional conceptions. Also, many regimens are impossible for low-income patients to carry out. The simple order that medication is to be taken "with each meal" may not recognize that many lower-income families eat irregularly and may not have three meals a day.

Middle-class Bias.   Another characteristic of medical organization that influences the quality of medical care is the middle-class bias of most professional health workers. The staff members, typically, do not understand the perspectives, attitudes, customs, and lifestyles of the patients. They simply take for granted that the patients have the same attitudes about health as they do. Hence, they tend to issue orders that are not understood or cannot be easily followed by lower-income patients. Furthermore, there is a tendency to think of lower-income people in stereotyped terms, "they cannot keep appointments; they have little sense of time or responsibility, and so on." Lower-income patients may perceive these class biases and this may affect the underutilization of medical services.

The many hours of waiting, the impersonal routines of institutional care in large hospitals or clinics, particularly in the municipal and county hospitals, the real or imagined perceptions of racial and class bias all tend to maximize dissatisfactions of lower-income patients and reduce the possibility of utilization of health facilities. Furthermore, the distances that patients must travel to the medical facilities and the cost of transportation are realistic matters. Customarily, poor people organize their lives so as not to go far for the necessities of living. This is one of the factors in the relative success of the MIC program that reached into the lower-income communities and brought the clinic facilities into the neighborhood. Similarly, the neighborhood health centers have been relatively successful for this reason.

Lifestyles and Social Class. It is important to take into account the characteristic lifestyles of the poor. The lower-income person's experience of himself or herself and his or her world is highly distinctive in our country. It is also distinctive for its problems and crisis-dominated character. As S. M. Miller has commented about these people, their "life is a crisis-life constantly trying to make do with string where rope is needed." In other words, health concerns are minor to those who feel they confront much more pressing troubles. Health problems are just one crisis among many that they must try to cope with, control, or just live with.

Indeed, the value orientations of the medical system reflect the values of the middle- and upper-middle classes. These have been characterized as activistic, rational mastery, future-time orientation to life. A large body of empirical research data suggests that the values of the middle class tend to result in a specific outlook on life that gets reflected in health beliefs and behavior. Thus, the lower classes, whose position in the social structure does not support a belief in the rational mastery of the world, tend to have a quite different orientation of the world. There is a feeling of lack of control over events; occurrences are viewed as "luck" or fate rather than as planned by rational design. Planning, education, and involvement in organized activity are less important in this framework; they seek help from those in their social network rather than from "experts" or professionals.[13,14]

Another problem is that many lower-income households are often much more understaffed than those of higher income. This understaffing of households means that each individual's health receives relatively little attention as far as preventive measures are concerned, and when someone is sick it is more difficult to care for him or her at home. When the main family member is sick, he or she will be in a disadvantaged position in caring properly for himself or herself. There is a necessity for poor people to learn to live with illness rather than to use their limited financial and psychological resources to do something about illness.

Lower-income people also do not conform to the expectations of how "good" and "considerate" patients should behave in medical settings. Their behavior is often frustrating and annoying to medical and nursing personnel for a variety of reasons.

In short, the cultural values and health beliefs tend to shape the maternal behavior of pregnant women just as they influence other types of health practices. These values are not easily mutable; thus, in the absence of either powerful attempts to change behavior or the system itself, it is well to recognize the differences in assumptions, values, beliefs and behaviors, and attempt to adjust the structure of the maternal health service delivery system.

Ethnicity and Geographic Area

The evidence we have to date indicates that white mothers receive care earlier in pregnancy than non-white mothers. There is a consistent difference between white and nonwhite mothers in the receipt of medical care during each of the trimesters of pregnancy. There is evidence that women living in metropolitan areas receive care earlier than those outside metropolitan areas; this holds true for both white and nonwhite women. Furthermore, more of the nonwhite women in metropolitan areas are known to have received care than nonwhite women residing outside metropolitan areas. It is worth noting, though, that for any given income or educational group the differences between metropolitan and nonmetropolitan areas are insignificant with respect to the time when mothers first receive medical care.

Age and Parity

Furthermore, there is a differential by age and parity; women in the younger age group tend to come later than women in the other age groups. This is maybe due to the fact that the highest rates of illegitimacy are in the youngest age groups. Both the young mother and the unwed mother tend to be late-comers to prenatal care. Multiparas who have had little trouble with previous pregnancies also tend to come later and be more lax in keeping appointments.

ADDITIONAL FACTORS IN THE USE OF MATERNITY SERVICES

The issues discussed here are also related to the *changing relationships between the client-patient and the providers of maternity services,* physicians and nurses. Walker has succinctly summarized the changes in maternity nursing caused by changing social factors and consumer demands.[15] She notes, as we have, the use of different terminology in the profession from "obstetrical nursing" to "maternity nursing" to "family-centered maternity care." Consumers complain that it is becoming more and more difficult to find a primary care physician who will give them the personal attention they want. Regardless of the social class level of the woman, it is very difficult for her to receive continuity of care from the personnel who provide maternity services. Regardless of its other merits, group practice sometimes disrupts the relationship between patient and physician; hospital structure requires nursing personnel to change with shift changes; patients have difficulty determining the status of the person in the medical office to whom they are speaking on the telephone. Patients feel that the obstetrician seems to relinquish his responsibility for the neonate during the postpartum period. Similarly, in this period, the pediatrician (from the mother's perspective) does not appear to be centrally involved with the needs of the mother. All of these features of the medical care system are reflected in the concept of "fragmented health care," and consumer dissatisfaction.

Consumer Satisfaction. *Consumer satisfaction,* that is, the satisfaction of pregnant women, refers to the attitudes toward the medical care system of those who have experienced a contact with the system. It is different from the medical and health beliefs of the patient in that it is concerned with the satisfaction of the patient with the quantity or quality of care actually received. There are several dimensions to this concept. These include: (1) accessibility-convenience of services (convenience of care, and emer-

gency care); (2) availability (family physicians, hospitals, specialists, complete facilities); (3) continuity (regular family physician, same physician); (4) physician conduct (consideration for feelings, explanations, prudent risks, quality, regular checkup); (5) financial aspects (cost of services, insurance coverage, payment mechanisms). However, little is known about the relationship of these features of patient satisfaction to other social-psychological dimensions such as perceived health, values, psychological well-being, and general sentiments about life.

Communication. A crucial feature of this aspect of maternity care is the quality and quantity of patient-provider *communication*. Here we refer not only to the physician, but also to the nurse in communicating with the patient and her needs. One of the more important transactions that occurs in the provider-patient relationship is effective communication from the provider to the patient concerning the nature of the patient's condition and the actions to be taken. The degree to which the patient has understood the physician and can verbalize the physician's advice and instructions depends on the quality of the relationship.[16] Similarly, good medical care results in communication from the patient to the physician. In particular, the degree to which the patient's concerns, worries, and fears about her condition have been perceived by the physician are equally important.

Commentators on the physician-patient relationship frequently have discussed the social class and value differences between providers and patients as one barrier to communication, and ultimately to utilization of medical services. Numerous studies have demonstrated that working-class patients tend to be diffident in questioning physicians, especially about their health or illness condition. These studies indicate that middle-class patients tend to obtain most of their information about illness by asking their physicians and nurses direct questions. In contrast, working-class patients receive their information from a "passive process in which they were given information without asking; they also tended to receive less information."[17]

Despite their reluctance to request information, working-class maternity patients are not much different from upper-class patients in their *desire* for information.[18] Although upper-class patients may desire more technical details about their health condition, there is no general social class difference in patients' desires for as much information as possible presented in nontechnical language.

Part of the issue of better communication between physician and patient results from a reflection of a general social class difference in language use which was alluded to previously. Working-class patients sense that physicians do not expect them to ask questions; they tend to hold the physicians in awe; and there is social distance. But even middle-class patients hesitate to freely communicate with their physician about troublesome problems or symptoms. A virtual legend has been created by the media about the hard-working, busy physician. It has become generally accepted throughout our society that all physicians are extremely busy professionals. Thus, although there may be some apparent social class differences in the quantity and quality of communication with physicians, it is a matter of degree of communication.

The Role of the Nurse as Communicator. Given this situation, the maternity nurse has a crucial role to play. By and large the nurse is not perceived by the patient in the same manner as the physician. Patients perceive the nurse as filling a substantially different role with accompanying differences in expectations. Thus, the nurse has an opportunity to fill a much-needed role in the delivery of health care by seizing the initiative and closing the communications gap in the patient-provider relationship. Such action would be congruent with patient expectations; moreover, several studies have indicated that the nurse can perform roles involving the receiving and giving of information to patients far more effectively than physicians.[19]

These problems of communication have been emphasized here because, among other things, the patient's perceived difficulties in communicating with medical providers has a direct influence upon the use of health services.

REFERENCES

1. Parsons, T. Definitions of health and illness in the light of American values and social structure. In *Social Structure and Personality.* Glencoe, Ill., The Free Press, 1964, pp. 257–291, 436–347.

2. McKinlay, J. B. The new latecomers for antenatal care. *Brit. J. Prev. Soc. Med.* 24:52, Feb. 1970.

3. Blood, R. O. and D. M. Wolfe. *Husbands and Wives.* Glencoe, Ill., The Free Press, 1960.

4. Rossi, A. Transition to parenthood. *J. Marriage and Fam.* 30:33, Feb. 1968.

5. Flapan, M. A paradigm for the analysis of childbearing motivations of married women prior to birth of the first child. *Am. J. Orthopsychiat.* 39:402–417, Apr. 1969.

6. Bumpass, L. L. and C. F. Westoff. The 'perfect contraceptive' population. *Sci.* 1969: 1177, 1970.

7. Lipman-Blumen, J. Demographic trends and issues in women's health. In V. Olesen (ed.), *Women and Their Health: Research Implications for a New Era.* Washington, D.C., HEW, #HRA 77-3138, 1977.

8. *Ibid.*

9. Pakter, J., et al. Impact of the liberalized abortion law in New York City on pregnancy associated deaths: A two-year experience. *Bull. N.Y. Academy Med.* 49:804–818, 1972.

10. Wright, N. H. Family planning and infant mortality rate death decline in the United States. *Am. J. Epidemiology* 101:182–187, Mar. 1975.

11. McKinlay, *op. cit.*

12. Strauss, A. L. Medical organization, medical care in lower-income groups. *Soc. Sci. Med.* 3:143–177, 1969.

13. Hyman, H. The value systems of different classes. In R. Bendix and S. Lipset (eds.), *Class, Status, and Power.* Glencoe, Ill., The Free Press, 1953, pp. 426–442.

14. Milio, N. Values, social class and community health services. *Nurs. Research* 16, 1, Winter 1967.

15. Walker, L. Providing more relevant maternity services. *JOGN, Nursing* 34–36, Mar./Apr. 1974.

16. Waitzkin, H., and Stoeckle, J. D. The communication of information about illness. *Adv. Psychosom. Med.* 8:180–215, 1972.

17. Pratt, L., et al. Physicians' views on the level of medical information among patients. *Am. J. Public Health* 47:1277–1283, 1975.

18. Milio, op. cit.

19. Walker, op. cit.

Six

Social Risk Factors and Reproductive Outcomes

Sociodemographic Risk Factors / Behavioral Risk Factors / Life Events and Life Crises as Risks

In this chapter the focus is upon selected risk factors that are associated with such reproductive outcomes as infant and maternal mortality, low-birth weight, and other complications of pregnancy.

SOCIODEMOGRAPHIC RISK FACTORS

Maternal Age

In one of its earliest studies, the U.S. Children's Bureau demonstrated a relationship between age of mother and infant mortality. This relationship has been observed many times in the past—that is, high mortality rates among infants of the youngest mothers and also among those of older mothers. Moreover, there is a strong correlation between socioeconomic status and age of mother; births to parents with more education and/or higher family income tend to occur to substantially older mothers. The lower the socioeconomic status, the greater the tendency for the mother to be younger. Of course, women age 35 and over account for only about 5 percent of all U.S. births.

First births to older women are of particular interest because they have been viewed as "high risk" and attention has usually been focused on the maternal rather than the fetal results. More recently, however, given careful prenatal care, the emphasis has shifted to fetal risk.

On the other hand, older *multiparous* women are also at increased risk for neonatal mortality and spontaneous abortion.[1]

Age and parity are two biological categories that have specific social significance. They are associated with perinatal mortality, stillbirths, and more complications of pregnancy and possible risk of brain damage to the baby. The role of the maternity nurse is to counsel women with respect to the problems associated with pregnancy. Thus, patient education is particularly important for this type of patient.

Teenage Pregnancy

Associated with maternal age is the problem of adolescent pregnancy. Notable among the social and health costs of these pregnancies are the following: (1) About one-half of school-age mothers will have a subsequent unwanted pregnancy within two years of the birth of the first child; (2) evidence indicates that approximately 60 percent of those who had their first baby at school-age become welfare recipients; (3) young mothers have a disproportionate number of babies of low-birth weight, which is associated with mental retardation and other handicapping conditions; (4) problems associated with pregnancy are particularly acute in mothers age 15 and younger.[2]

We cannot consider this issue systematically without placing it within a broader social context. The so-called teenage sexual revolution is related to a number of concurrent trends. For example, there is an increased number and proportion of births to women under age 20. One-third of all births are to girls 17 or younger and about two-fifths of these births are out-of-wedlock. Thus, we shall consider out-of-wedlock births jointly with the problems of teenage or adolescent pregnancy.

Out-of-Wedlock Births. Out-of-wedlock birthrates have been increasing since 1940 for girls age 19 and younger. Among nonwhite individuals the rates for girls age 14 increased between 1940 and 1950 but have been rather stable since then. Similarly, there are variations for both white and nonwhites in the period 1940 to 1976; the rate for nonwhites seems to be declining recently, but the rate for whites appears to have risen steadily since 1940. The fact that the rate continues to increase is considered prima facie proof of increased sexual activity of revolutionary proportions. In a definitive study of the problem, however, Cutright casts doubt on this conclusion.[3]

There are alternative explanations for rising out-of-wedlock births than the simple one of a sexual revolution. In an examination of this issue, Cutright suggests that recent health status changes may explain a great deal of the recent increase in teenage out-of-wedlock births. He presents evidence of two health status changes: those that affect the ability of young girls to conceive (fecundity) and those that affect their capacity to avoid spontaneous abortion.

In addition, Cutright examined the interrelationships of customs, laws, and mean age of menarche. Data indicate that the mean age of menarche has decreased in the United States and western Europe. There is general agreement that one major factor responsible for the decline is improved nutrition and health during preadolescent years. Recent research suggests that improved nutrition increases the rate of physical growth, which in turn, decreases the age at menarche.[4]

Problems in Teenage Pregnancies. Childbearing at any age is a momentous event. For the teenager, however, it is often accompanied by a different set of problems from those experienced by older mothers. For very young mothers, at least those under age 15, risks that the baby will be stillborn, die soon after birth, or be born with a low-birth weight, are much higher than those for women in their 20s.

The relationship of *infant mortality* to maternal age has been noted earlier. In a recently published study matching infants' death certificates to infants' birth certificates, the National Center for Health Statistics reported that, at all ages, the infant mortality rate is considerably higher among nonwhites than among whites.[5] Moreover, neonatal mortality in infants of young mothers is much higher than that for infants of older mothers in both color groups.

The increased risk of *low-birth weight* may be the most important medical aspect of teenage pregnancy. Increased mortality risk is only one of the dangers facing infants of low-birth weight. There are apparent linkages to epilepsy, cerebral palsy and mental retardation, and to higher risks of deafness and blindness.

Various studies are not conclusive about the relationship of age of the mother to the intelligence of the child or physical and mental handicaps. Despite this inconclusiveness, these data document that the infant born to a teenage mother has a much higher risk of suffering *severe handicaps* than infants of older mothers.

For the mother there are increased *risks of complications* of pregnancy, including toxemia, prolonged labor, and iron-deficiency anemia. Poor diets, inadequate prenatal care, and immaturity are probably all contributing factors. The primary concern would appear to be with social rather than biological factors.

The Role of the Nurse. What is the role of the nurse in preventing early childbearing? Any action must start with the assumption that these are not inevitable consequences. Many women want to become mothers, but there are data to indicate that a substantial proportion wish that their first child had come later.[6] Organized family-planning programs and self-help clinics can be important factors in the future in preventing early unintended motherhood.

We cannot close this discussion of early childbearing without recognition of the fact that knowledge, accessibility, and contraceptive technology are not the only problems. More than one study has documented that a substantial proportion of young mothers say that they had not used contraception because they did not care whether they became pregnant or not.[7] Some of these women are simply not motivated to take advantage of the opportunities to control their fertility. Altering their motivation would be a major undertaking in society.

Socioeconomic and Ethnic Indicators of Risk

Certain indicators of socioeconomic status—such as family income, education of mother and father and ethnicity—can be risk factors in pregnancy. Low-income individuals are considerably more predisposed to lowered health status and obstetrical complications during pregnancy. Low-birth weight is particularly prevalent in the lowest socioeconomic status groups, especially the black population. The role of ethnicity becomes readily apparent when one analyzes data which have accrued since 1935 on racial background. Throughout this period marked differences have occurred on the basis of racial background, with nonwhites faring much worse than whites. Indeed, the relative differential has actually risen during this period. The racially related differentials in mortality have also been noted beyond the first year of life. It should be stressed that virtually all of the racially related differentials in mortality are socioeconomically related.

Undernutrition

One of the most important sequelae of low-socioeconomic status is undernutrition. Government studies have revealed that, compared to more affluent persons, the poor are twice as deficient in four essential diet ingredients. Most striking, poor persons had about four times as much clear-cut iron deficiency anemia and twice as many borderline cases as had the nonpoor. In three categories of essential diet ingredients—vitamin A, vitamin C, and riboflavin—the poor were found to have about twice as much of clear-cut deficiency as the nonpoor. The survey also found a greater percentage of low height and weight measurements for children living below the poverty line than for those who were more affluent.[8]

Obviously, there is a complex interaction between undernutrition, poverty, and other environmental or genetic factors.

Effects on Fetal Brain Development. Studies have shown that deficiencies in the diet of a pregnant woman can have profound effects on a number of pregnancy outcomes. For example, it has been shown that nutritional and genetic factors may interact during prenatal development with consequent irreversible results on the development of the baby's brain. This is one of the most important recent discoveries in the field of mental retardation. It is estimated that one-tenth of the children born today are seriously affected as a consequence of malnutrition. Recent work at the National Institute of Health suggests that there is a correlation between the level of the amino acids in the blood of a pregnant woman and the subsequent intelligence of her baby.

Low Birth Weight. Undernutrition has been identified as one of the causes of low-birth weight in infants born to poor urban mothers.[9] Extremely low-birth weights have been reported among poorly fed groups in Asia and Africa. The relationship between low-birth weight and malnourished populations may be more complex than a simple nutritional explanation. Rather than dietary deficiency in pregnancy, one specific factor, the small size of the baby, may reflect long-term maternal undernutrition dating back to the early childhood of the woman. Conceivably, malnutrition over many generations in underdeveloped societies may have favored the emergence of genetically different kinds of women with lower dietary requirements. This, however, is highly speculative and needs much carefully designed research to confirm such a possibility.

Hypertensive disorders (toxemias). The effect of socioenvironmental influences was most dramatically illustrated in World War II in Great Britain. During this period, the mortality from the pregnancy hypertensive disorders (toxemias) fell dramatically. The underlying reason for the drop in mortality resulting from this condition in England and Wales was that large numbers of women were evacuated from their homes in the cities into the country. The antenatal clinics were understaffed and improvisational. The major advantage brought about by this change of social environment was that the rationing system benefited expectant and nursing mothers and children. For the first time, women of the lower socioeconomic groups were fed as well as other population groups and better than previously. Suffice to say that eclampsia as a syndrome is most commonly seen in poor and badly nourished populations and that there is some evidence that the incidence has been profoundly modified by environmental changes, either situational or behavioral.

Role of the Nurse. What can be done to improve the nutritional and other risk factors associated with socioeconomic status and ethnic or racial groups? Clearly, the role of the maternity nurse is relatively limited, but not inactive. The nurse can be a force both in the community and in the clinic setting to help improve preventive services to those at highest risk because of situational factors. Better ways can be devised to use the nurse and other health personnel to provide health education to the individuals at risk. This assumes that the nurse herself is equipped with the knowledge concerning nutrition and other precursors of problems of pregnancy to provide the appropriate knowledge to the patient. Moreover, the nurse can be a positive force in the community to exert influence on other institutions such as the schools, health departments, government agencies, and voluntary agencies to provide preventive measures to the population at greatest risk.

BEHAVIORAL RISK FACTORS

Up to now, the discussion has been concerned primarily with factors not easily controllable by the nurse or other health personnel. An individual's social position in society cannot be influenced easily by nursing interventions. As the present section will show, however, the risk factors of smoking and substance abuse are mutable, and hence, the nurse can have some degree of influence on the patient.

Smoking

In recent years the literature has grown substantially, reflecting a heightened awareness of the important and substantial effects of smoking on pregnancy outcome. The earlier studies demonstrated that mothers who smoked cigarettes had smaller babies than nonsmoking mothers and subscribed this finding to the direct effect of smoking.

Recent evidence, based on prospective studies and other well-designed research, has partly substantiated the fact that fetal size, growth, and mortality are related to smoking of cigarettes by the mother. According to the U.S. Public Health Service, some 4,600 stillbirths each year in the United States probably can be attributed to women's smoking habits. Research indicates that women who smoke have a 30 percent higher rate of stillbirths than those who do not. These women also have a 26 percent higher rate of perinatal mortality.

A positive association between maternal cigarette smoking and reduced infant birth weight emerges from every study of these two characteristics. The hypothesis that the relationship between smoking and weight reduction in the infant is one of cause and effect is supported by several types of evidence. This relationship has been consistently observed in a wide variety of populations differing by geographical location, race, and social and economic circumstances. Furthermore, there is an inverse relationship between mean birth weights and the number of cigarettes smoked during pregnancy, an evident dose-response effect.

However, there have been a few studies that have not confirmed these findings. Since smoking is a preventable behavior, the focus of concern is to determine whether babies who would otherwise be alive and healthy might die, before or after birth, because their mothers smoked.

Meyer and her colleagues found that mothers who are young, reasonably healthy, having their first or second child, and smoking *less than a pack of cigarettes* a day have an increased risk of perinatal loss of *less* than 10 percent. "At the other extreme, heavy smokers who are high parity, public patients, those who have had previous premature births or whose hemoglobin is under 11 Gm. have an increased risk of perinatal loss of over 70 percent. Other groups are intermediate . . . perinatal mortality increased with maternal smoking, with the magnitude of increase ranging from 4 percent to 97 percent."[10] Thus, their data suggest that maternal smoking may *interact* with other factors in its influence on perinatal mortality.

Meyer and her associates have examined further the contrary evidence from other studies and suggest that these studies selected study populations that were, in one way or another, not typical of the general population and/or did not impose appropriate statistical controls on the study population.[11]

Thus, in conclusion, the weight of evidence indicates that maternal smoking during pregnancy increases the infant's perinatal morbidity and mortality risk. This risk increases directly with the number of cigarettes smoked. The presence or absence of other risk factors alters the risk.

Role of the Nurse.   Thus, the implications for prevention are clear. Counseling the patient at the first visit, particularly in the case of mothers with other risk factors, can be done by the maternity nurse. Health education, although it needs to begin early in life, must be an essential part of prenatal care and smoking is one behavior that is preventable. Moreover, the nurse by her own behavior can provide an appropriate role model for the mother and father.

Drugs

There has been considerable interest in the potential genetic and teratogenic effects of a variety of foods and drugs for the mother and her offspring. Teenagers and young adults now comprise the majority of the population for whom this interest applies. Many of these patients will admit to use of drugs or else give some evidence of drug use. Detection of maternal addiction is based on history or physical evidence of administration, particularly puncture marks.

The true prevalence of drug-addicted mothers is unknown. But the indications are that, in large urban centers at least, the ratio of drug-addicted mothers to total deliveries has increased in the past 20 years. This is particularly true for those deliveries that take place in public hospitals.

Use of Services.   Most drug-addicted patients are latecomers for prenatal care. Indeed, most patients delay until they feel that they are ready for delivery in order to avoid a long labor without drugs and in order to satisfy their need for a last "fix" before submitting to "authority." As a result, there is evidence that a substantial proportion of deliveries to this population occurs at home, in the ambulance, or on the stretcher.[12] This is especially true of the

heroin addict. Also, addicts make considerable efforts to nourish their addiction during enforced periods of confinement in a hospital. Such patients will either hide the drug or obtain it from others in or outside the hospital. A portion of these patients supplement their supply with barbiturates or tranquilizers.

Effect on Mother and Infant.   As far as heroin addicts are concerned, there is some difficulty in evaluating the data on total length of labor, but available evidence indicates that labor is not prolonged. Greatest difficulties tend to occur after delivery when withdrawal in the infant and mother is a risk factor. Symptoms of withdrawal in the mother include nausea, tremors, sweats, abdominal pain, cramps, and yawning. (Chapter 39 discusses withdrawal symptoms in the infant.)

The attitude of the medical and nursing staff becomes a critical factor at this stage. The pregnancy outcomes of heroin-addicted mothers are typical of any nutritionally deprived groups of low-socioeconomic status receiving inadequate prenatal care, with one important exception, congenital addiction of the baby.

There is some suggestion in the literature that narcotic use by the mother may lead to intrauterine growth retardation. The long-term effects on growth and development are now being observed and evaluated in at least one prospective study. As of today, the effects of narcotic addiction on the reproductive process are not clearly reflected in our standard measures of maternal and perinatal mortality rates. Available evidence indicates that the addicted individual, even after withdrawal, detoxification, or rehabilitation remains at risk in that subsequent intake, even years later, may result in the immediate urge for more drugs.

Thus, a pregnant woman who is a user of narcotic drugs of unknown potency and amount is carrying a potentially addicted fetus, and while detoxification of the newborn infant seems to be initially successful, a detoxified baby is still a problem infant. Even with use of methadone in the management of the pregnant addict, it is possible to magnify the effects on the fetus.

It is important to note that the problem of drug *usage,* as distinct from drug addiction, is of considerable magnitude. Although the former is seen more often in private and community hospitals, the addictive patient is a growing problem there also. It is increasingly apparent that our *drug-using* population is encompassing greater numbers of individuals from the middle- and upper-socioeconomic segments of our society. For these reasons, all maternal service personnel need to be familiar with both the maternal and neonatal aspects of drug use.

Alcohol

Women cannot assume that it is safe to drink even small amounts of alcohol during their pregnancies. Research in recent years is indicating that there is no "safe" level for alcohol consumption during this time. The Department of Health, Education and Welfare has warned that an alcoholic intake of six drinks a day (3 ounces of absolute alcohol) can lead to birth defects in the infant.[13]

Drs. Kenneth Jones and David Smith coined the term "fetal alcohol syndrome" to describe the pattern of birth defects found in infants whose mothers consumed moderate to large amounts of alcohol during their pregnancies. This syndrome has become the third most commonly recognized cause of mental retardation in the United States, exceeded only by Down's syndrome and an incompletely enclosed spinal cord. It is estimated that the incidence is two to three per 1,000 live births. It is characterized by mental retardation, low-birth weight (2,500 gm. or less), short stature, small heads and a variety of joint and heart defects, as well as fine motor dysfunctions.

It is important to note that a woman does not necessarily have to be an alcoholic to place her infant at risk for this condition. However, women who are chronic alcoholics run a much higher risk of having defective infants. Jones and Hansen found that women who drink 2 to 4 ounces of hard liquor per day run a 10 percent risk of having an abnormal child. Women who drink 4 ounces or more have a 19 percent risk. If the average daily consumption is less than 2 ounces, the apparent risk is low but still present.[14]

Heavy alcohol consumption is most likely to affect fetal structure during the first trimester when organogenesis is taking place. Frequently abortion will take place. During the second trimester the infant's weight is most likely to be affected when there is mostly an increase in cell size rather than cell volume.

The Role of the Nurse. If the nurse suspects her patient has a drinking problem or even drinks moderately but consistently, it is important that she explore her reasons for drinking and refer the mother for counseling if necessary. Often patients' lifestyles are such that "social drinking" is expected, and the mother may not realize the impact of her behavior on her fetus. The hazards of the syndrome can be clearly explained and various counseling and assistance avenues utilized.[15]

LIFE EVENTS AND LIFE CRISES AS RISKS

Life events and life crises in the sense used here refer to such events as divorce, illness, death of a significant other, such as a family member, job loss, and the like, rather than to the occurrence of the actual pregnancy itself, although this too may be a factor in pregnancy outcome. Appropriate intervention by nursing staff can be especially effective in meeting the needs and reducing the risks associated with such life crises. The interest in the relationship between the psychological and social world of the individual and human disorders and disease have a long history. But even the findings of carefully designed and conducted investigations have not always yielded clear-cut and unambiguous results concerning this relationship. This is in sharp contrast to the dramatic results that have been obtained with animal experiments in which the various elements in the social environment have been correlated. Nevertheless, there is accumulating evidence of the intimate interaction between the social environment, physiological reactions and pathological outcome in the individual. This is particularly true for certain of the chronic diseases, such as heart disease and cancer.[16]

Data on the relationship between disorders of pregnancy and life changes and experiences that may be stressful are relatively scanty.

It should be clear that an outcome such as low-birth weight is the result of multiple interactions between the human organism and the environment. In a paper published in 1963, Gunter focused on the psychological and stressful environmental factors operative in the mother *before* conception and during pregnancy. Almost ten years elapsed before another study appeared that was related to the Gunter study, although the importance of the variables had long been recognized and applied in research directed toward other problems.[17] The emphasis in Gunter's research was on critical life events that occurred *before* the onset of pregnancy, such as (1) death within the immediate family of orientation or procreation; (2) desertion by husband or by one or both parents of the subject; (3) economic need; (4) interpersonal problems, such as difficulties with husband (including divorce), difficulties with in-laws, family, or neighbors; and (5) physical disability including illness, accident, and bodily harm incidents. She also had obtained data on events that occurred *during* the gestation period.

Gunter found that the "social and life situation of the mother are related to and may, in part, determine the outcome of pregnancy in terms of the birth weight of the infant." A decade later, Nuckolls and her associates at North Carolina went beyond an attempt to assess only the effects of life experiences on pregnancy outcome. They included, in addition, the supportive or protective psychological or social elements of the patient, which was termed the adaptive potential for pregnancy (TAPPS). In short, Nuckolls and her group were attempting to assess the "balance" between the protective and the deleterious social and psychologic processes and the relationship of this balance to various health parameters of pregnancy and the puerperium.[18]

The results showed that considering the multiple life changes and the psychosocial assets separately, they were not related to complications of pregnancy. When taken together, however, Nuckolls found that in the presence of mounting life changes, women with high psychosocial assets had only one-third the complication rate of women whose psychosocial assets were low. In the absence of such life changes, particularly for the period before pregnancy, the level of psychosocial assets was irrelevant.

As these investigators point out, additional research is needed, but their data help to explain some of the discrepant results in the literature. In short, the research and the approach casts serious doubt on the utility of specificity (as far as current clinical syndromes are concerned) in research concerned with psychosocial factors in disease etiology. Similar psychosocial factors may be related to different disease syndromes. At the present, this research approach is very promising and additional work needs to be done using the approach.

Attitudes and Emotions. Much has been written in recent years on the role of emotional and attitudinal factors and psychological stress *during* the pregnancy as these may be related to pregnancy outcomes. The evidence is inconclusive, but more important, much of it is based on poorly designed research and inadequate samples of the population at risk. Despite this poor state of affairs, there is a general consensus in medical science that psychological factors are in some way associated with various aspects of the maternity cycle. Indeed, some investigators have asserted that early psychological assessment of pregnant women holds promise of being predictive of the course and outcome of pregnancy. Most of the literature makes an attempt to measure the attitudes of the woman toward her pregnancy and to measure other psychosocial factors as these may influence the outcome.[19]

Surely there are attitudinal differences among women toward their individual pregnancies. There is also an intimate interaction between the psychological stress experienced by the person and psychological reactions, as Heinstien has noted.[20] Complications of pregnancy, labor, and delivery are obscured by this interaction. Thus, physiological changes and discomfort may trigger psychologically negative attitudes toward the pregnancy and, conversely, life stress may precipitate somatic problems.

There is no doubt that many, perhaps a majority, of women experience some psychological stress and anxiety during pregnancy. However, the literature in medical and nursing journals alike tends *to assume* some of these conditions are psychosomatic or emotional in origin. In a paper critical of the cloudy thinking that has characterized such conditions as menstrual pain, nausea of pregnancy, and pain in labor, as caused or aggravated by psychogenic factors, Lennane and Lennane suggest sexual prejudice as the basis for such thinking. Such scientific evidence as exists clearly suggests organic causes for these conditions.[21]

The point here is that nurses must not unwittingly and uncritically accept long-established attitudes that are rooted in prejudice rather than in scientific evidence. Stereotypic thinking is not only poor in scientific terms, but, equally important, it tends to influence the course and quality of treatment of women patients.

The Role of the Nurse. Nursing staff has an important role to play in assisting the pregnant woman to utilize her psychosocial assets to the fullest in coping with the fears, anxieties, somatic complaints, and other problems associated with the pregnancy in the prenatal and intrapartal periods. Emotional and social support during and following the pregnancy cannot only be a comfort to the patient, but may also assist in reducing problematic outcomes.

REFERENCES

1. Jolly, C., et al. Research in the delivery of female health care: The recipients' reaction. *Am. J. Ob.-Gyn.* 110, 3:291–294, June 1, 1971.
2. Card, J. J. and L. L. Wise. Teenage mothers and fathers: The impact of early childbearing on the parents' personal and professional lives. *Family Plan. Perspect.* 10, 4:199–205, July/Aug. 1978.
3. Cutright, P. Illegitimacy in the United States: 1920–1968. Final Report to the Commission on Population Growth and the American Future. Washington, D.C., U.S. Government Printing Office, 1972.
4. Tietze, C. Teenage pregnancies: Looking ahead to 1984. *Family Plan. Perspect.* 10, 4: 205–207, July/Aug. 1978.
5. Infant Mortality Rates: Socioeconomic Factors, United States, Series 22, No. 14, Vital and Health Statistics. Washington, D.C., Department of Health, Education and Welfare, 1972.
6. Presser, H. Early motherhood; ignorance or bliss. *Family Plan. Perspect.* 6, 1:8–14, Winter 1974.
7. Lindemann, C. *Birth Control and Unmarried Young Women.* New York, Springer, 1974.
8. Ten-State Nutrition Survey in the United States, 1968–1970. Washington, D.C., Department of Health, Education and Welfare, Pub. No. (HSM) 72-8129 through 72-8134, 1972.
9. Ibid.
10. Lipman-Blumen, J., Meyer, M. B., and Comstock, G. W. Maternal cigarette smoking and perinatal mortality. *Am. J. Epidemiology* 96: 1–10, July 1972.
11. Meyer, M. B., et al. The interrelationship of maternal smoking and increased perinatal mortality with other risk factors: Further analysis of the Ontario perinatal mortality study, 1960–1961. *Am. J. Epidemiol.* 100:443–452, Dec. 1974.
12. Stone, M. L., et al. Narcotic addiction in pregnancy. *Am. J. Ob.-Gyn.* 109:716–723, Mar. 1971.
13. Alarm Sounded on Alcohol, Pregnancy. *OCOG Newsletter,* 21:3, Aug. 1977.
14. Jones, K. L., et al. Pattern of malformation in offspring of chronic alcoholic mothers. *Lancet* 1:1267–1271, June 9, 1973.
15. Luke, B. Maternal alcoholism and fetal alcohol syndrome. *AJN* 12, 12:1924–1926, Dec. 1977.
16. Syme, S. L. and L. G. Reeder (eds). Social stress and cardiovascular disease. *The Milbank Memorial Fund Quarterly,* Apr. 1967.
17. Gunter, L. M. Psychopathology and stress in the life experience of mothers of premature infants. *Am. J. Ob.-Gyn.* 109:716–723, Mar. 1971.
18. Nuckolls, K. B., et al. Psychosocial assets, life crisis and the prognosis of pregnancy. *Am. J. Epidemiol.* 95:431–441, 1972.
19. Heinstien, M. I. Expressed attitudes and feelings of pregnant women and their relations to physical complications of pregnancy. *Merril-Palmer Quarterly* 1:217–236, Jan. 1967.
20. *Ibid.*
21. Lennane, K. J. and R. J. Lennane. Alleged psychogenic disorders in women—a possible manifestation of sexual prejudice. *New Eng. J. Med.* 288, 6:288–292, Feb. 8, 1973.

UNIT 2

Biophysical Aspects of Human Reproduction

Sexual and Reproductive Anatomy

Sexual and Reproductive Physiology

Conception and Ovum Development

Development and Physiology of the Embryo and Fetus

Seven

Sexual and Reproductive Anatomy

Pelvis / Female Organs of Reproduction / Mammary Glands / Male Organs of Reproduction

PELVIS

The pelvis, so called from its resemblance to a basin (*pelvis*, a basin), is a bony ring interposed between the trunk and the thighs. The vertebral column, or backbone, passes into it from above, transmitting to it the weight of the upper part of the body, which the pelvis in turn transmits to the lower limbs. From an obstetrical point of view, however, we must consider it as the cavity that contains the generative organs and, particularly, as the canal through which the fetus must pass during birth— the birth canal.

Bony Structure

The pelvis is made up of four united bones: the two hipbones (*os coxae* or innominate) situated laterally and in front, and the sacrum and the coccyx behind (Fig. 7-1).

Anatomically, the hipbones are divided into three parts: the ilium, the ischium, and the pubis. These bones become firmly joined into one by the time the growth of the body is completed (i.e., at about ages 20 to 25), so that when the pelvis is examined no trace of the original edges or divisions of these

three bones can be discovered. Each of these bones may be roughly described as follows.

The *ilium,* which is the largest portion of the bones, forms the upper and back part of the pelvis. Its upper flaring border forms the prominence of the hip, or crest of the ilium (hipbone).

The *ischium* is the lower part below the hip joint; from it projects the tuberosity of the ischium on which the body rests when in a sitting posture.

The *pubis* is the front part of the hipbone; it extends from the hip joint to the joint in front between the two hipbones, the symphysis pubis, and then turns down toward the ischial tuberosity, thus forming, with the bone of the opposite side, the arch below the symphysis, the pubic or subpubic arch. This articulation of the two pubic bones encloses the cavity of the pelvic anteriorly.

The *sacrum* and the *coccyx* form the lowest portions of the spinal column. The former is a triangular wedge-shaped bone, consisting of five vertebrae fused together; it serves as the back part of the pelvis. The coccyx forms a tail end to the spine. In the child the coccyx consists of four or five very small, separate vertebrae; in the adult these bones are fused into one. The coccyx is usually movable at its attachment to the sacrum, the sacrococcygeal joint, and may become pressed back during labor

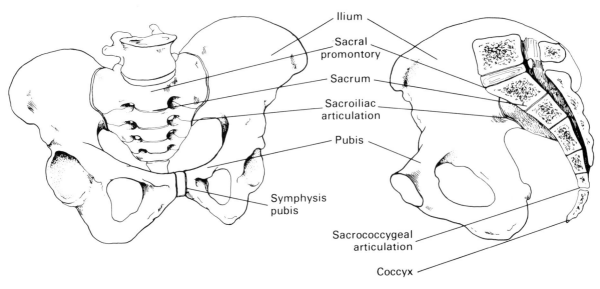

Figure 7-1. Front and lateral view of the pelvis showing major bones and articulations.

to allow more room for the passage of the fetal head.

Of special importance is the marked projection formed by the junction of the last lumbar vertebra with the sacrum; this is the *sacral promontory* and is one of the most important landmarks in obstetrical anatomy.

Articulation and Surfaces

The *articulations,* or joints of the pelvis, which have obstetrical importance, are four in number. Two are behind, between the sacrum and the ilia on either side, and are termed the *sacroiliac articulations;* one is in front between the two pubic bones and is called the *symphysis pubis,* and the fourth, of little consequence, is between the sacrum and coccyx, the *sacrococcygeal articulation.*

All of these articular surfaces are lined with fibrocartilage, which becomes thickened and softened during pregnancy; likewise, the ligaments that bind the pelvic joints together become softened, and as a result greater mobility of the pelvic bones develops. A certain definite though very limited motion in the joints is desirable for a normal labor; however, there is no change in the actual size of the pelvis. From a practical standpoint, the increased mobility that these joints develop in pregnancy produces a slight "wobbliness" in the pelvis and throws greater strain on the surrounding muscles and ligaments. This accounts in large part for the

frequency of backache and legache in the latter months of pregnancy.

The pelvis is lined with muscular tissue that provides a smooth, somewhat cushioned surface over which the fetus passes during labor; these muscles also help to support the abdominal contents.

Divisions: True and False Pelves

Regarded as a whole, the pelvis may be described as a two-storied, bony basin that is divided by a natural line of division, the *inlet* or *brim,* into two parts. The upper part is called the false pelvis and the lower part is called the true pelvis (Fig. 7-2A).

The *false pelvis,* or upper flaring part, is much less concerned with the problems of labor than is the true pelvis. It supports the uterus during late pregnancy and directs the fetus into the true pelvis at the proper time.

The *true pelvis,* or lower part, forms the bony canal through which the fetus must pass during parturition; for descriptive purposes it is divided into three parts: an inlet or brim, a cavity, and an outlet.

Pelvic Inlet

Continuous with the sacral promontory and extending along the ilium on each side in circular fashion is a ridge called the *linea terminalis,* or brim (Fig. 7-2A). This bounds an area or plane, the *inlet,* so named because it is the entryway or inlet through which the fetal head must pass in order to enter the true pelvis.

The pelvic inlet, sometimes called the pelvic brim or superior strait, divides the false from the true pelvis. It is roughly heart-shaped, the promontory of the sacrum forming a slight projection into it from behind (Fig. 7-2B). Generally it is widest from side to side, and narrowest from back to front (i.e., from the sacral promontory to the symphysis). It should be noted that the fetal head enters the inlet of the average pelvis with its longest diameter (anteroposterior) in the transverse diameter of the pelvis (Fig. 7-3A). In other words, as shown in Figure 7-3B, the greatest diameter of the head accommodates itself to the greatest diameter of the inlet.

As the inlet is entirely surrounded by bone, it cannot be measured directly with the examining fingers in a living woman. However, the measurements of its anteroposterior diameter can be estimated on the basis of the diagonal conjugate diameter (see Fig. 7-8). The measurements of these diameters are very important, since variations from the normal (e.g., smaller in size or flattened) may cause grave difficulty at the time of labor (see Chapter 25).

Pelvic Outlet

When viewed from below, the *pelvic outlet* is a space bounded in front by the symphysis pubis and the pubic arch, at the sides by the ischial tuberosities, and behind by the coccyx and the greater sacrosciatic ligaments (Fig. 7-3C). It requires only a little imagination to see that the front half of the outlet resembles a triangle, the base of which is the distance between the ischial tuberosities, and the other two sides of which are represented by the pubic arch. From an obstetrical point of view, this triangle is of great importance, since the fetal head must utilize this space to gain exit from the pelvis and the mother's body (Fig. 7-3D). Nature has provided a wide pubic arch in females, whereas in males it is narrow (see Fig. 7-6). If the pubic arch in women were as narrow as it is in men, vaginal delivery would be extremely difficult since the fetal head, unable to traverse the narrow anterior triangle of the outlet, would be forced backward against the coccyx and the sacrum, where its progress would be impeded.

In the typical female pelvis, the greatest diameter of the inlet is the transverse (from side to side), whereas the greatest diameter of the outlet is the anteroposterior (from front to back) (Fig. 7-3 A/C). Moreover, the fetal head, as it emerges from the pelvis, passes through the outlet in the anteroposterior position, again accommodating its greatest diameter to the greatest diameter of the passage. Since the fetal head enters the pelvis in the transverse position and emerges in the anteroposterior, it is obvious that it must rotate some 90° as it passes through the pelvis. This process of rotation is one of the most important phases of the mechanism of labor and will be discussed in more detail in a later chapter.

Figure 7-2. (Left) Side view of true and false pelvis. (Right) Front view showing linea terminalis (pelvic brim).

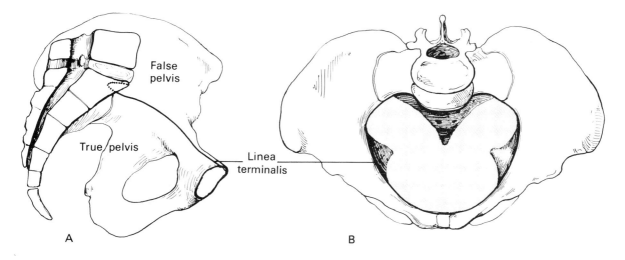

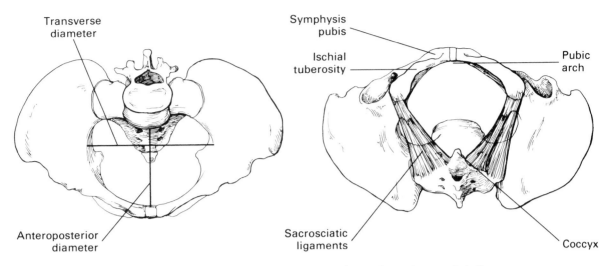

A. Inlet of normal female pelvis showing transverse and anteroposterior diameters.

C. Pelvic outlet and sacrosciatic ligaments.

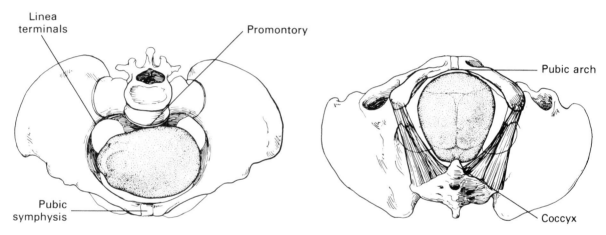

B. Largest diameter of the fetal head passing through the largest diameter of inlet. Therefore it enters transversely.

D. Largest diameter of the fetal head passing through the largest diameter of the outlet. Therefore, it passes through anteroposteriorly.

Figure 7-3. Views of pelvic inlet and outlet with fetal head in place.

Pelvic Cavity

The *pelvic cavity* is the space between the inlet above, the outlet below and the anterior, the posterior, and the lateral walls of the pelvis. The pelvic canal is practically cylindric in shape in its upper portion and curved only in its lower half. It is important to note the axis of the cavity when viewed from the side (Fig. 7-4). It is apparent that during delivery the head must descend along the downward prolongation of the axis until it nearly reaches the level of the ischial spines and then begins to curve forward. The axis of the cavity determines the direction which the fetus takes through the pelvis in the process of delivery. As might be expected, labor is made more complicated by this curvature in the pelvic canal, because the fetus has to accommodate itself to the curved path as well as to the variations in the size of the cavity at different levels.

Pelvic Variations

The pelvis presents great individual variations—no two pelves are exactly alike. Even patients with normal measurements may present differences in contour and muscular development that influence the actual size of the pelvis. These differences are due in part to heredity, disease, injury, and development. Heredity may be responsible for passing on many racial and sexual differences. Such diseases as tuberculosis and rickets cause malformations. Accidents and injuries during childhood or at maturity result in deformities of the pelvis or other parts of the body that affect the pelvis. Adequate nutrition and well-formed habits related to posture and exercise have a very definite influence on the development of the pelvis.

It must be remembered also that the pelvis does not reach the final stages of maturity until the age of 20 to 25 when ossification is completed.

There are several *types of pelves*. Even pelves whose measurements are normal differ greatly in the shape of the inlet, in the proximity of the greatest transverse diameter of the inlet to the sacral promontory, in the size of the sacrosciatic notch, and in their general architecture. These characteristics have been used in establishing a classification of pelves which has been of great interest and value to obstetricians. The four main types according to this classification are shown in Figure 7-5. The manner in which the fetus passes through the birth canal and, consequently, the type of labor vary considerably in these pelvic types.

In addition, of course, there are many pelvic types which result from abnormal narrowing of one or the other diameters. These contracted pelves will be described in Chapter 25.

In comparing male and female pelves, several differences are observed (Fig. 7-6). The most con-

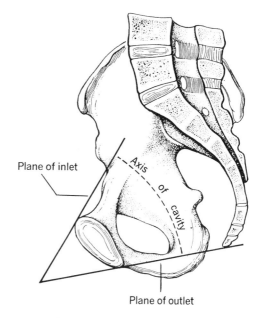

Figure 7-4. Pelvic cavity showing plane of inlet and outlet. The direction the fetus takes through the pelvis is determined by the axis of the cavity. (From: Chaffee, E. E., and Lytle, I. M.: *Basic Physiology and Anatomy*, ed. 4. Philadelphia, J. B. Lippincott, 1980.)

spicuous difference is in the pubic arch, which has a much wider angle in women. The symphysis is shorter in women, and the border of the arch probably is more everted. Although the female pelvis is more shallow, it is more capacious, much lighter in structure, and smoother. The male pelvis is deep, compact, conical, and rougher in texture, particularly at the site of muscle attachments. Both males and females start life with pelves that are

Figure 7-5. The four types of female pelves. (From Brunner, L. S., and Suddarth, D. S.: *The Lippincott Manual of Nursing Practice,* ed. 2. Philadelphia, J. B. Lippincott, 1978, p. 1168.)

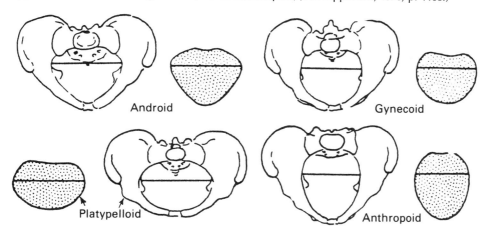

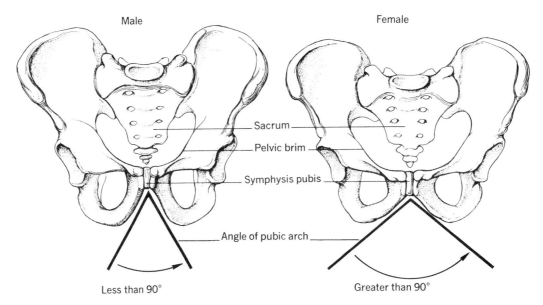

Male

Female

Sacrum
Pelvic brim
Symphysis pubis
Angle of pubic arch
Less than 90°
Greater than 90°

Figure 7-6. Comparison of male and female pelves. (Left) male pelvis, narrow and compact; pelvic arch less than right angle. (Right) female pelvis, broad and capacious, pubic arch greater than right angle. (From Chaffee, E. E., and Lytle, I. M.: *Basic Physiology and Anatomy,* ed. 4. Philadelphia, J. B. Lippincott, 1980.)

identical in type; the major differences do not appear until puberty and are therefore due to the influence of the sex hormones. (For the definition and description of the sex hormones, see Chapter 6.)

Pelvic Measurements

The entire childbirth process centers on the safe passage of the fully developed fetus through the pelvis. Slight irregularities in the structure of the pelvis may delay the progress of labor, while any marked deformity may render delivery by the natural passages impossible.

The pelvis of every pregnant woman should be measured accurately in the antepartal period to determine before labor begins whether or not there is anything in the condition of the mother's pelvis that may complicate the delivery. This examination is a part of the antepartal evaluation.

Types of Pelvic Measurements

Internal pelvic measurements, made manually, are an important means of estimating the size of the pelvis. In the past, a number of external pelvic measurements were recorded. Except for measurement of the outlet, these are of dubious value in evaluating the true pelvis; thus they are no longer used. In the majority of abnormal pelves, the most marked deformity affects the anteroposterior diameter of the inlet.

Diagonal Conjugate. Internal pelvic measurements are made to determine the actual diameters of the inlet. The chief internal measurement taken is the *diagonal conjugate,* or the distance between the sacral promontory and the lower margin of the symphysis pubis. The patient should be placed on her back on the examining table, with her knees drawn up and her feet supported by stirrups. Two fingers are introduced into the vagina, and, before the diagonal conjugate is measured, the contour of the pelvis is evaluated by palpation. Included in this evaluation are the height of the symphysis pubis and the shape of the pubic arch, the motility of the coccyx, the inclination of the anterior wall of the sacrum and the side walls of the pelvis, and the prominence of the ischial spines.

To obtain the length of the diagonal conjugate, the two fingers passed into the vagina are pressed inward and upward as far as possible until the middle finger rests on the sacral promontory. The point on the back of the hand just under the symphysis is then marked by putting the index finger of the other hand on the exact point (Fig. 7-7A), after which the fingers are withdrawn and measured. The distance from the tip of the middle finger to the point marked represents the *diagonal conjugate measurement*. This distance may be measured with a rigid measuring scale attached to the wall or with a pelvimeter (Fig. 7-7B). If the measurement is greater than 11.5 cm., it is justifiable to assume that the pelvic inlet is of adequate size for childbirth.

True Conjugate. An extremely important internal diameter is the *true conjugate* or, in Latin, the conjugata vera (C.V.), which is the distance between the posterior aspect of the symphysis pubis and the promontory of the sacrum. However, direct measurement of this diameter cannot be made except by means of an x-ray study; consequently, it has to be estimated from the diagonal conjugate measurement. It is believed that if 1.5 to 2.0 cm., according to the height and the inclination of the symphysis pubis, is deducted from the length of the diagonal conjugate, the true conjugate is obtained. For example, if the diagonal conjugate measures 12.5 cm., and the symphysis pubis is considered to be "average," the conjugata vera may be estimated as about 11.0 cm. In this method, the problem consists of estimating the length of one side of a triangle, the conjugata vera; the other two sides, the diagonal conjugate and the height of the symphysis pubis, are known. If the symphysis pubis is high and has a marked inclination, the examiner takes this into consideration and may deduct 2.0 cm.

The length of the conjugata vera is of utmost importance, since it is about the smallest diameter of the inlet through which the fetal head must pass. Indeed, the main purpose in measuring the diagonal conjugate is to give an estimate of the size of the conjugata vera.

Obstetrical Conjugate. Students sometimes are confused when they are confronted with the term *obstetrical conjugate*. This term identifies a diameter that begins at the sacral promontory and terminates just below the conjugata vera on the inner surface of the symphysis pubis a few millimeters below its upper margin. The obstetrical conjugate is in reality the shortest diameter through which the fetal head must pass as it descends into the true pelvis. A distinction is rarely made between the conjugata vera and the obstetrical conjugate, except in x-ray pelvimetry (see below).

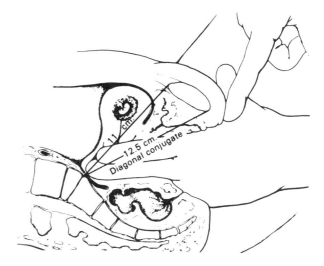

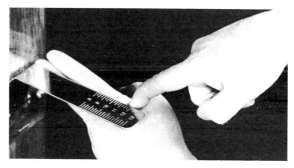

Figure 7-7. Method of obtaining diagonal conjugate diameter (12.5 cm.).

Tuberischii Diameter. Next to the diagonal conjugate, the most important clinical dimension of the pelvis is the transverse diameter of the outlet, the diameter between the ischial tuberosities. This is sometimes called the *tuberischii diameter* (often abbreviated T.I.), or biischial diameter, or intertuberous diameter (see Fig. 7-3C). This measurement is taken with the patient in the lithotomy position, well down on the table and with the legs widely separated. The measurement is taken from the innermost and lowermost aspect of the ischial tuberosities, on a level with the lower border of the anus. The instruments usually employed are the Williams's pelvimeter (Fig. 7-8) or the Thoms's pelvimeter. The intertuberous diameter may also be estimated by inserting the closed fist between the tuberosities. The known diameter of the hand can then be used as a reference. A diameter in excess of 8.0 cm. is considered adequate.

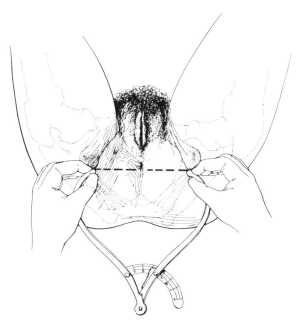

Figure 7-8. Method of measuring tuberischii, or intertuberous diameter of outlet.

X-ray Pelvimetry

The most accurate means of determining pelvic size is x-ray pelvimetry. This subjects the maternal ovaries and the fetal gonads to a certain amount of irradiation. Although the amount involved is minimal, exposure of pregnant women to irradiation should be avoided unless this procedure is really necessary. Hence, x-ray pelvimetry is used prior to labor only in cases in which there are sound reasons for suspecting pelvic contraction, such as small manual measurements or a history of difficult labor in the past.

Pelvimetry is also indicated when there has been failure to progress normally in labor, to rule out previously unsuspected cephalopelvic disproportion. It is also important to evaluate pelvic size in term breech presentations, since the head is the largest part of the fetus and the adequacy of the pelvis is not really tested until the body has already been delivered. For this reason, many examiners evaluate pelvic size with pelvimetry routinely in the primigravida at term with a breech presentation.

A variety of pelvimetry techniques have been developed. One that has stood the test of time, with minor modifications, is that devised by Dr. Herbert Thoms, a pioneer in this field. For a complete study, two x-ray films are made as follows:

1. The patient is placed on the x-ray table in a semirecumbent position so that her pelvic inlet is horizontal and as nearly parallel as possible with the plate beneath her (Fig. 7-9). The exact plane in which the patient's inlet lies, both front and back, is now determined and recorded. After an exposure of the film has been made, the patient is removed from the table, and a lead plate or grid containing perforations a centimeter apart is placed in the plane previously occupied by the inlet of the patient. Another exposure is now made on the same film. When the latter is developed, the outline of the inlet is shown, as are the dots produced by the perforations in the lead plate. Since the projected dots on the film represent centimeters in the plane of the inlet, the diameters of the inlet can be read off directly as centimeters.

2. A somewhat similar procedure is carried out with the patient standing and from the lateral view (Fig. 7-10). Here, however, an upright lead and iron rod, with a centimeter scale notched on its edge, is placed posterior to the patient and close to the gluteal fold. After an

Figure 7-9. Pelvic inlet roentgenogram. The scale represents corrected centimeters for various levels of the pelvic canal. The top line is used for measuring the diameters of the inlet. The other levels are established on the lateral roentgenogram. Pelvic morphology is readily established by viewing both lateral and inlet views. Thoms's technique.

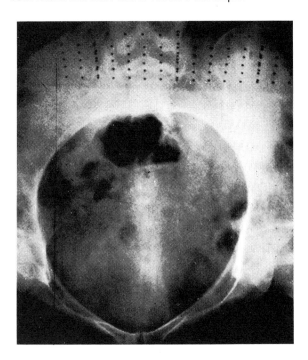

exposure has been made, the developed film will show a lateral view of the symphysis pubis, the sacral promontory, other bony landmarks, as well as, of course, the notched centimeter scale for establishing the distance between important points.

Diameters which may be measured by x-ray pelvimetry are the obstetrical conjugate, posterior sagittal at the inlet, midpelvis and outlet, and the anteroposterior diameter at the midpelvis and outlet.

Other techniques use stereoscopic procedures that allow for three-dimensional vision of the film, thereby giving a clear image of all pelvic relationships.

When x-ray films are made late in pregnancy by any of these methods, it is possible to secure also an impression of the size of the fetal head. When this is considered in relation to the pelvic picture, helpful information may be obtained in forecasting whether or not this particular pelvis is large enough to allow this particular fetus to pass through.

Preventive Care Based on Pelvimetry

The importance of the knowledge gained through skillful performance of internal pelvimetry cannot be overestimated. It should never be neglected in the case of a woman pregnant for the first time, or in any case in which the patient has suffered previously from difficult or prolonged labors.

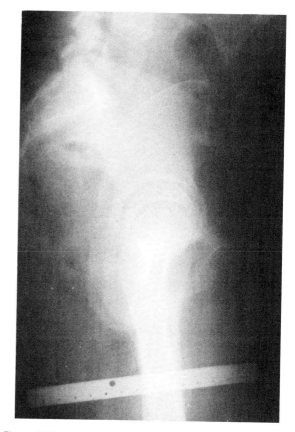

Figure 7-10. Lateral roentgenogram. The scale represents corrected centimeters in the midplane of the body. The various diameters may be measured with calipers. The lateral morphologic aspects are readily visualized.

FEMALE ORGANS OF REPRODUCTION

The female organs of reproduction are divided into two groups—the external and the internal.

External Organs

The external female reproductive organs are called the *vulva,* from the Latin word meaning *covering.* This includes everything that is visible externally from the lower margin of the pubis to the perineum, namely, the mons veneris, the labia majora and minora, the clitoris, the vestibule, the hymen, the urethral opening and various glandular and vascular structures (Fig. 7-11). The term vulva often has

been used to refer simply to the labia majora and minora.

The *mons veneris* is a firm, cushion-like formation over the symphysis pubis and is covered with crinkly hair.

The *labia majora* are two prominent longitudinal folds of adipose tissue covered with skin that extend downward and backward from the mons veneris and disappear in forming the anterior border of the perineal body. These two thick folds of skin are covered with hair on their outer surfaces after the age of puberty, but are smooth and moist on their inner surfaces. At the bottom they fade away into the perineum posteriorly, joining together to form a transverse fold, the posterior commissure, situated directly in front of the fourchette. This fatty tissue is supplied with an abundant plexus of veins that may rupture as the result of injury sustained during labor and give rise to an extravasation of blood, or hematoma.

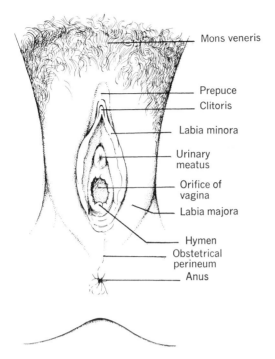

Figure 7-11. External genitalia of female. (From Chaffee, E. E., and Lytle, I. M.: *Basic Physiology and Anatomy,* ed. 4. Philadelphia, J. B. Lippincott, 1980.)

The *labia minora* are two thin folds covered entirely with thin membrane and situated between the labia majora, with their outer surfaces in contact with the inner surfaces of the labia majora; the labia minora extend from the clitoris downward and backward on either side of the orifice of the vagina. In the upper extremity each labium minus separates into two branches which, when united with those of the opposite side, enclose the clitoris. The upper fold forms the prepuce and the lower the frenum of the clitoris. At the bottom, the labia minora pass almost imperceptibly into the labia majora or blend together as a thin fold of skin, the fourchette, which forms the anterior edge of the perineum or perineal body.

The *clitoris* is a small, highly sensitive projection composed of erectile tissue, nerves, and blood vessels and is covered with a thin epidermis. It is analogous to the penis in the male and is regarded as the chief seat of voluptuous sensation. The clitoris is so situated that it is partially hidden between the anterior ends of the labia minora.

The *vestibule* is the almond-shaped area that is enclosed by the labia minora and extends from the clitoris to the fourchette. It is perforated by four openings: the urethra, the vaginal opening, the ducts of Bartholin's glands and the ducts of Skene's glands. *Bartholin's glands* are two small glands situated beneath the vestibule on either side of the vaginal opening. *Skene's glands* open upon the vestibule on either side of the urethra.

The *hymen* marks the division between the internal and the external organs. It is a thin sheaf of mucous membrane situated at the orifice of the vagina. It may be entirely absent, or it may form a complete septum across the lower end of the vagina.

The hymen presents marked differences in shape and consistency (Fig. 7-12). In the newborn child it projects beyond the surrounding parts. In adult virgins it is a membrane of varying thickness which presents an aperture that varies in size from a small opening to one that readily admits one or even two fingers. The opening is circular or crescent-shaped. In rare instances, the hymen may be imperforate and cause retention of menstrual discharge if it occludes the vaginal orifice completely.

The *perineum* consists of muscles and fascia of the urogenital diaphragm, which lies across the pubic arch, and the pelvic diaphragm, which consists of the coccygeus and the levator ani muscles. The levator ani is the larger and consists of three portions which form a slinglike support for the pelvic structure, and between them pass the urethra, the vagina, and the rectum (Fig. 7-13). Between the anus and the vagina the levator ani is reinforced by a central tendon of the perineum to which three pairs of muscles converge: the bulbocavernosus, the superficial transverse muscles of the perineum, and the external sphincter ani. These structures constitute

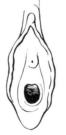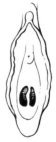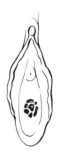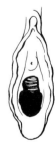

Figure 7-12. Variations of the hymen. From left to right: virginal, nondilated; septate, septum may or may not stretch; cribriform; parous, at least one full-term delivery. (From Pierson, E. C., and D'Antonio, W. V.: *Female and Male.* Philadelphia, J. B. Lippincott, 1974, p. 39.)

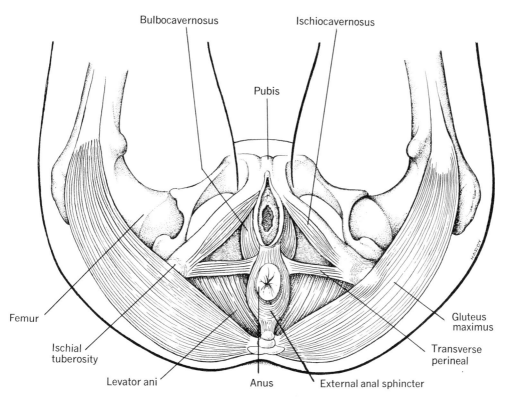

Figure 7-13. Muscles of the pelvic floor (female perineum). (From Chaffee, E. E., and Lytle, I. M.: *Basic Physiology and Anatomy,* ed. 4. Philadelphia, J. B. Lippincott, 1980.)

the perineal body and form the main support of the perineal floor. They are often lacerated during delivery.

Internal Organs

The internal organs of reproduction are the vagina, the uterus, the fallopian or uterine tubes, and the ovaries (Figs. 7-14, 7-15, and 7-16).

Ovaries

The *ovaries* are two almond-shaped organs situated in the upper part of the pelvic cavity on either side of the uterus. Their chief functions are the development and the expulsion of ova and the provision of certain internal secretions, or hormones. These organs correspond to the testes in the male. They lie embedded in the posterior fold of the broad ligament of the uterus and are supported by the suspensory, the ovarian, and the mesovarium ligaments (Fig. 7-16).

Each ovary contains in its substance at birth a large number of germ cells, or primordial ova. This huge store of primordial follicles present at birth more than suffices the woman for life. It is usually believed that no more are formed, and that this large initial store is gradually exhausted during the period of sexual maturity. Beginning at about the time of puberty, one, or possibly two, of the follicles that contain the ova enlarges each month, gradually approaches the surface of the ovary, and ruptures. The ovum and the fluid content of the follicle are liberated on the exterior of the ovary; then they are swept into the tube. The development and the maturation of the follicles containing the ova continue from puberty to menopause.

The arteries that supply the ovary are four or five branches that arise from the anastomosis of the ovarian artery with the ovarian branch of the uterine artery (see Fig. 7-16). The veins draining the ovary become tributaries to both the uterine and the ovarian plexus. Superiorly the ovarian vein drains into the inferior vena cava on the right and into the renal vein on the left.

The nerves supplying the ovaries are derived (*Text continues on p. 80*)

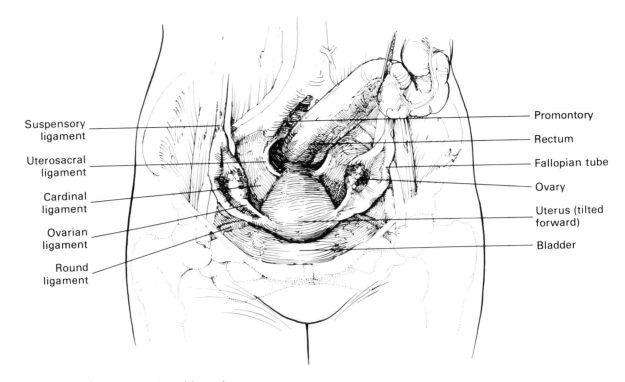

Figure 7-14. Pelvic contents viewed from above.

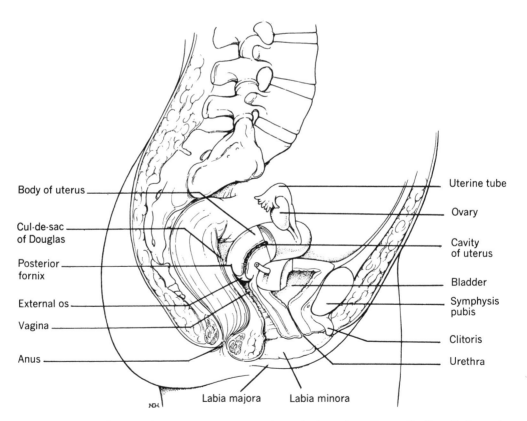

Figure 7-15. Female reproductive organs as seen in sagittal section. (From Chaffee, E. E., and Lytle, I. M.: *Basic Physiology and Anatomy,* ed. 4. Philadelphia, J. B. Lippincott, 1980.)

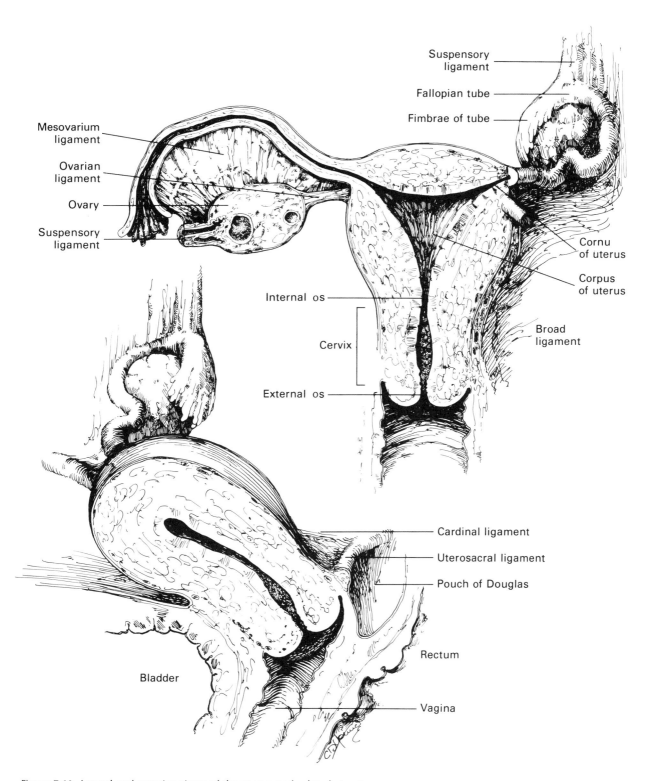

Suspensory
ligament

Fallopian tube

Fimbrae of tube

Mesovarium
ligament

Ovarian
ligament

Ovary

Suspensory
ligament

Cornu
of uterus

Corpus
of uterus

Internal os

Cervix

Broad
ligament

External os

Cardinal ligament

Uterosacral ligament

Pouch of Douglas

Rectum

Bladder

Vagina

Figure 7-16. Lateral and anterior views of the uterus and related structures.

from the craniosacral and the thoracolumbar sympathetic systems. The postganglionic and visceral afferent fibers form a plexus surrounding the ovarian artery, which in turn is formed by contributions from the renal and the aortic plexuses and corresponds to the spermatic plexus in the male.

Fallopian or Uterine Tubes

The fallopian or uterine tubes are two trumpet-shaped, thin, flexible, muscular tubes, about 12.0 cm. long. They extend from the upper angles of the uterus, the cornua, in the upper margin of the broad ligament, toward the sides of the pelvis. They have two openings: one into the uterine cavity and the other into the abdominal cavity.

The opening into the uterine cavity is minute and will admit only a fine bristle. The abdominal opening is larger and is surrounded by a large number of fine fringes; hence the term *fimbriated end.* The fimbriated extremity lies near the ovary, but it is not necessarily in direct contact with it. It is generally believed that the cilia upon the fimbriated end of the tube create a current in the capillary layer of fluid lying between the various pelvic organs.

The tubes convey the discharged ovum by peristaltic action from the ovaries to the cavity of the uterus; by their tentacle-like processes the fimbriated ends of the tube draw the escaped ovum into the tube.

The tubes are lined with mucous membrane containing ciliated epithelium. The muscular layer is made up of longitudinal and circular fibers which provide peristaltic action. The serous membrane covering the tubes is a continuation of the peritoneum, which lines the whole abdominal cavity.

The fallopian or uterine tubes receive their blood supply from the ovarian and the uterine arteries (see Fig. 7-17). The veins of the tubes follow the course of these arteries and empty into the uterine and the ovarian trunks. The nerves which supply the uterus also innervate the tubes.

Uterus

The uterus is a hollow thick-walled, muscular organ (Fig. 7-16). It serves two important functions: 1) it is the organ of menstruation, and 2) during pregnancy it receives the fertilized ovum and retains and nourishes it until it expels the products of conception at the time of labor.

The uterus varies in size and shape according to the age of the individual and whether or not she has borne children. The uterus of the adult nullipara weighs approximately 60 gm. and measures 5.5 to 8.0 cm. in length. It resembles a flattened pear in appearance and has two divisions: the upper triangular portion, the *corpus,* and the lower constricted cylindric portion, the *cervix,* which projects into the vagina. The fallopian or uterine tubes extend from the *cornu* (the Latin word meaning *horn*) of the uterus at the upper outer margin on either side. The upper rounded portion of the uterus between the points of insertion of the tubes is the fundus (Fig. 7-16).

The nonpregnant uterus is situated in the pelvic cavity between the bladder and the rectum. Almost the entire posterior wall and the upper portion of the anterior wall is covered by peritoneum. The lower portion of the anterior wall is united to the bladder wall by a layer of loose connective tissue. The lower posterior wall of the uterus and the upper portion of the vagina are separated from the rectum by an area called Douglas's cul-de-sac, or pouch of Douglas.

Due to its muscular composition, the uterus is capable of enlarging to accommodate a growing pregnancy; at the termination of pregnancy it weighs about 1 Kg. or 2 pounds. It is made up of involuntary muscle fibers arranged in all directions, making expansion possible in every direction to accommodate the products of conception. Due to the nature of this arrangement of the muscle, the uterus is able to expel its contents at the termination of normal labor. Arranged between these muscular layers are many blood vessels, lymphatics, and nerves.

The cavity of the uterus is somewhat triangular in shape, being widest at the fundus, between the small openings into the fallopian or uterine tubes, and narrowest below at the opening into the cervix. The anterior and posterior walls lie almost in contact, so that if a cross-section of the uterus could be examined, the cavity between them would appear as a mere slit.

The uterus is lined with mucous membrane, the endometrium, and is divided into two parts: the cavity of the body of the uterus and the cavity of the cervix.

Cervix. The *cervix* is less freely movable than is the body of the uterus. Its muscular wall is not so

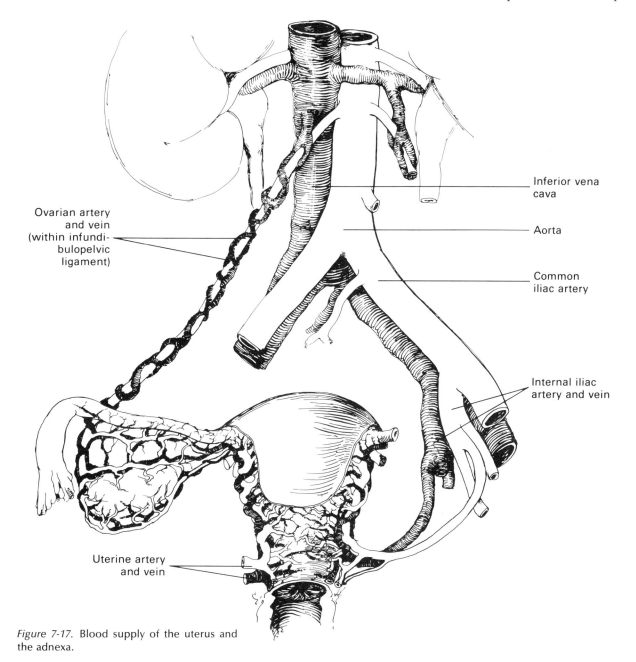

Figure 7-17. Blood supply of the uterus and the adnexa.

Ovarian artery and vein (within infundibulopelvic ligament)

Inferior vena cava

Aorta

Common iliac artery

Internal iliac artery and vein

Uterine artery and vein

thick, and its lining is different in that it is much folded and contains crypts, which produce mucus and are the chief source of the mucous secretion during pregnancy. The cervix has an upper opening, the *internal os,* leading from the cavity of the uterine body into the cervical canal, and a lower opening, the *external os,* opening into the vagina. The cervical canal is small in the nonpregnant woman, barely admitting a probe, but at the time of labor it dilates to a size sufficient to permit the passage of the fetus.

Ligaments. The uterus is supported in two ways: by ligaments extending from either side of the uterus and by the muscles of the pelvic floor. The ligaments that support the uterus in the pelvic cavity are the broad ligaments, the round ligaments, and the uterosacral ligaments (Fig. 7-16).

The *broad ligaments* are two winglike structures that extend from the lateral margins of the uterus to the pelvic walls and serve to divide the pelvic cavity into an anterior and a posterior compartment.

Each consists of folds of peritoneum which envelop the fallopian or uterine tubes, the ovaries, and the round and the ovarian ligaments. Its lower portion, the *cardinal ligament* is composed of dense connective tissue that is firmly united to the supravaginal portion of the cervix. The median margin is connected with the lateral margin of the uterus and encloses the uterine vessels.

The *round ligaments* are two fibrous cords which are attached on either side of the fundus just below the fallopian or uterine tubes. They extend forward through the inguinal canal and terminate in the upper portion of the labia majora. These ligaments aid in holding the fundus forward.

The *uterosacral ligaments* are two cordlike structures which extend from the posterior cervical portion of the uterus to the sacrum. These help to support the cervix. The uterovesical ligament is merely a fold of the peritoneum which passes over the fundus and extends over the bladder. The rectovaginal ligament is a fold of the peritoneum which passes over the posterior surface of the uterus and is reflected upon the rectum.

Uterine Blood Supply.   The uterus receives its blood supply from the ovarian and the uterine arteries (Fig. 7-17). The uterine artery, the principal source, is the main branch of the hypogastric, which enters the base of the broad ligament and makes its way to the side of the uterus. The ovarian artery is a branch of the aorta. It enters the broad ligament and on reaching the ovary breaks up into smaller branches that enter that organ, while its main stem makes its way to the upper margin of the uterus, where it anastomoses with the ovarian branch of the uterine artery.

The uterovaginal plexus returns the blood from the uterus and the vagina. These veins form a plexus of thin-walled vessels that are embedded in the layers of the uterine muscle. Emerging from this plexus, the trunks join the uterine vein, which is a double vein. These veins follow on either side of the uterine artery and eventually form one trunk, emptying into the hypogastric vein, which makes its way into the internal iliac.

Uterine Nerve Supply.   The uterus possesses an abundant nerve supply derived principally from the sympathetic nervous system but partly from the cerebrospinal and parasympathetic system. Both the sympathetic and the parasympathetic nerve supplies contain motor and a few sensory fibers. The functions of the nerve supply of the two systems are in great part antagonistic. The sympathetic causes muscular contraction and vasoconstriction; the parasympathetic inhibits contraction and leads to vasodilatation.

Position of Uterus.   Since the uterus is a freely movable organ suspended in the pelvic cavity between the bladder and the rectum, the position of the uterus may be influenced by a full bladder or rectum, which pushes it backward or forward. The uterus also changes its position when the patient stands, lies flat, or turns on her side. Also, there are variations in position such as anteflexion, in which the fundus is tipped far forward; retroversion, in which it is tipped far backward (Fig. 7-18); and prolapse, due to the relaxation of the muscles of the pelvic floor and the uterine ligaments.

Lymphatic Vessels.   The lymphatic vessels drain into the lumbar lymph nodes.

Vagina

The *vagina* is a dilatable passage lined with mucous membrane situated between the bladder and the rectum. The vaginal opening occupies the lower portion of the vestibule. The vagina is from 8.0 to 12.0 cm. long, and at the upper end is a blind vault, commonly called the *fornix,* into which the lower portion of the cervix projects.

The fornices (plural of fornix) are divided into four parts for convenience of description. The lateral fornices are the spaces between the vaginal wall on either side and the cervix; the anterior fornix is between the anterior vaginal wall and the cervix; the posterior fornix is between the posterior vaginal wall and the cervix. The posterior fornix is considerably deeper than the anterior since the vagina is attached higher up on the posterior than the anterior wall of the cervix. The fornices are important because the examiner is usually able to palpate the internal pelvic organs through their thin walls.

The vagina serves three important functions: 1) it represents the excretory duct of the uterus through which its secretion and the menstrual flow escape; 2) it is the female organ of copulation; and 3) it forms part of the birth canal during labor. Its walls are arranged into thick folds, the columns of the vagina, and in women who have not borne children,

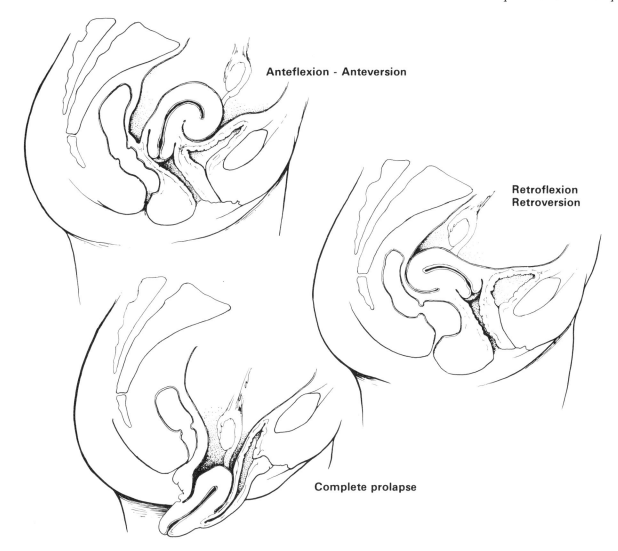

Anteflexion - Anteversion

Retroflexion Retroversion

Complete prolapse

Figure 7-18. Positions of the uterus, showing anteflexion-anteversion, retroflexion-retroversion and complete prolapse.

numerous ridges, or *rugae,* extend outward and almost at right angles to the vaginal columns and give the surface a corrugated appearance. Normally, the anterior and the posterior walls of the vagina lie in contact, but they are capable of stretching to allow marked distention of the passage, as in the process of childbirth.

The vagina receives its abundant blood supply from branches of the uterine, the inferior vesical, the median hemorrhoidal, and the internal pudendal arteries. The passage is surrounded by a venous plexus; the vessels follow the course of the arteries and eventually empty into the hypogastric veins. The lymphatics empty into the inguinal, the hypogastric, and the iliac glands.

Related Pelvic Organs (See Fig. 7-15)

Bladder. The *bladder* is a muscular sac that serves as a reservoir for urine. It is situated in front of the uterus and behind the symphysis pubis. When empty or only moderately distended, it remains entirely in the pelvis, but if it becomes greatly distended, it rises into the abdomen. Urine is conducted into the bladder by the ureters, two tubes that extend down from the basin of the kidneys over the brim of the pelvis beneath the uterine vessels to open into the bladder at about the level of the cervix. The bladder is emptied through the urethra, a short tube which terminates in the urethral meatus. Lying on either side of the urethra and almost parallel with it are two small glands, less than 2.5 cm. long, known as Skene's glands. Their ducts empty into the urethra just above the meatus. Often in cases of gonorrhea, Skene's glands and ducts are involved.

Anus. The *anus* is the entrance to the rectal canal. The rectal canal is surrounded at the opening or anus by its sphincter muscle, which binds it to the coccyx behind and to the perineum in front. It is supported by the muscles passing into it.

The muscles involved are those that aid in supporting the pelvic floor. The rectum is considered here because of the proximity to the field of delivery.

MAMMARY GLANDS

The *breasts,* or mammary glands, are two highly specialized cutaneous glands located on either side of the anterior wall of the chest between the third and the seventh ribs (Fig. 7-19). They are abundantly supplied with nerves. The breasts contain tissue which responds to hormones. Thus breast devel-

opment at puberty and lactation during pregnancy occur as a result of endocrine influences.

The internal mammary and the intercostal arteries supply the breast glands, and the mammary veins follow these arteries. Also, there are many cutaneous veins that become dilated during lactation. The lymphatics are abundant, especially toward the axilla. These breast glands are present in the male, but exist only in the rudimentary state.

Internal Structure

The breasts of a woman who never has borne a child are, in general, conic or hemispheric in form, but they vary in size and shape at different ages and in different individuals. In women who have nursed one or more babies they tend to become pendulous. At the termination of lactation, certain exercises aid in restoring the tone of the breast tissue.

The breasts are made up of glandular tissue and fat. Each organ is divided into 15 or 20 lobes, which are separated from each other by fibrous and fatty walls. Each lobe is subdivided into many lobules, which contain numerous acini cells. The *acini* are

Figure 7-19. Glandular tissue and ducts of the mammary gland. (From Chaffee, E.E., and Lytle, I. M.: *Basic Physiology and Anatomy,* ed. 4. Philadelphia, J. B. Lippincott, 1980.)

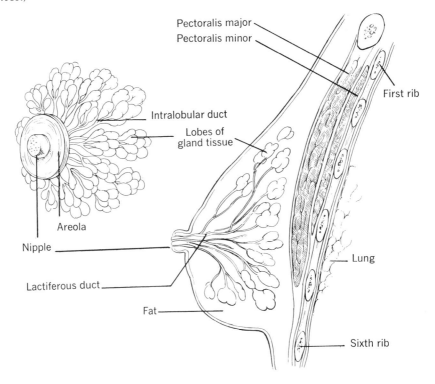

Pectoralis major
Pectoralis minor
First rib
Intralobular duct
Lobes of gland tissue
Areola
Nipple
Lactiferous duct
Fat
Lung
Sixth rib

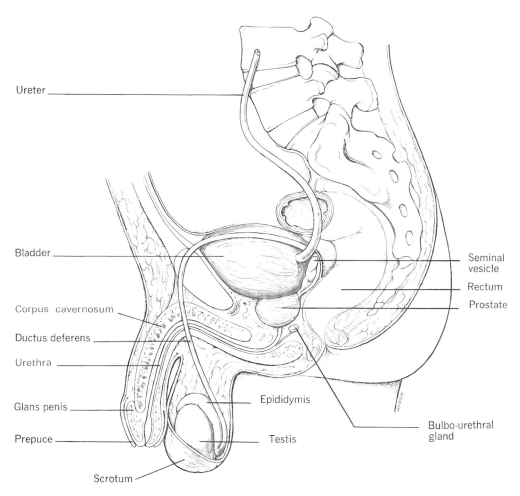

Ureter

Bladder

Corpus cavernosum

Ductus deferens

Urethra

Glans penis

Prepuce

Scrotum

Seminal vesicle

Rectum

Prostate

Epididymis

Testis

Bulbo-urethral gland

Figure 7-20. Organs of the male reproductive system. (From Chaffee, E. E., and Lytle, I. M.: *Basic Physiology and Anatomy,* ed. 4. Philadelphia, J. B. Lippincott, 1980.)

composed of a single layer of epithelium, beneath which is a small amount of connective tissue richly supplied with capillaries. By the process of osmosis the products necessary for the milk are filtered from the blood, but the secretion of the milk really begins in the acini cells. As the ducts leading from the lobules to the lobes and from the lobes approach the nipple, they are dilated to form little reservoirs in which the milk is stored; they narrow again as they pass into the nipple. The size of the breast depends on the amount of fatty tissue present and in no way denotes the amount of lactation possible.

External Structure

The external surface of the breasts is divided into three portions. The first is the smooth and soft area of skin extending from the circumference of the gland to the areola.

The second is the *areola,* which surrounds the nipple and is of a delicate pinkish hue in blondes and a darker rose color in brunettes. The surface of the areola is more or less roughened by small fine lumps of papillae, known as the glands of Montgomery. These enlarged sebaceous glands, white in color and scattered over the areola, become more marked during pregnancy. Under the influence of gestation, the areola becomes darker, and this pigmentation in many cases constitutes a helpful sign of pregnancy.

The *nipple* or third portion is largely composed of sensitive, erectile tissue and forms a large conic papilla projecting from the center of the areola and having at its summit the openings of the milk ducts. These openings may be from 3 to 20 in number.

The care of the breasts (see Chaps. 20 and 28) constitutes one of the important phases of the nursing care of the maternity patient throughout pregnancy and the puerperium.

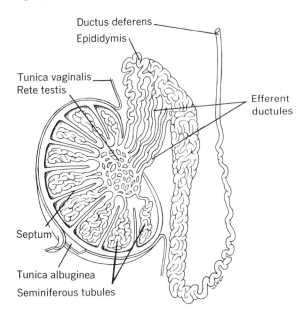

Figure 7-21. Diagram of structural features of the testis and epididymis. (From Chaffee, E. E., and Lytle, I. M.: *Basic Physiology and Anatomy*, ed. 4. Philadelphia, J. B. Lippincott, 1980.)

MALE ORGANS OF REPRODUCTION

The male reproductive system consists of the penis, the testes, and a system of excretory ducts with their accessory structures (Fig. 7-20).

Penis. The *penis,* the male organ of copulation, consists of the cavernous bodies (erectile parts) and a urethra through which the seminal fluid passes during ejaculation. The cavernous bodies contain blood spaces which are usually quite empty, and the organ is flaccid. When these spaces fill with blood, the organ becomes turgid. The flow of blood is controlled by the autonomic nervous system (vasodilator fibers) and varies with sexual arousal. The enlarged conic structure at the free end of the penis which contains the external orifice of the urethra is called the glans penis. Unless it has been removed by circumcision, the glans is covered by a fold of retractable skin, the foreskin or prepuce.

Testes. Not unlike the ovaries, the testes have a dual function—hormone production and the formation and release of gametes, in this case, spermatozoa. Unlike the ovaries, the testes are located outside the abdominal cavity in the scrotum (meaning bag). During early fetal life, the testes are abdominal. With growth of the fetus, they move

downward, entering the scrotum via the inguinal canal shortly before birth. The testes are approximately 5.0 cm. long and are contained in a fibrous protective covering, the tunica albuginia, which subdivides the testes into lobules (Fig. 7-21). Each lobule contains seminiferous tubules, coiled ducts in the walls of which spermatogenesis occurs. The testes also contain testosterone-producing cells, the interstitial cells of Leydig, as well as larger supporting cells, the Sertoli cells, which are important for sperm transport within the seminiferous tubules.

Spermatogenesis is a heat sensitive process. The 2 to 3° difference between scrotal and abdominal temperatures allows spermatogenesis to proceed normally in the cooler environment. Testosterone production is not affected by temperature. When there has been failure of the testes to descend, spermatogenesis is severely impaired, but testosterone production remains unaffected.

The *canal system* consists of the epididymis, which is made up of numerous seminiferous tubules, the vas deferens, which passes from the epididymis to the ejaculatory duct, the ejaculatory duct (formed by the union of the vas deferens and the duct of the seminal vesicle), and the urethra, which is surrounded by the prostate gland and traverses the penis (Figs. 7-20 and 7-21).

The accessory structures consist of the seminal vesicles (sacculated structures located behind the bladder and in front of the rectum), the prostate gland, which surrounds the base of the urethra and the ejaculatory duct, and the bulbourethral glands or Cowper's glands, which lie at the base of the prostate and on either side of the membranous urethra. Cowper's glands produce a mucinous substance that lubricates the urethra and coats its surface.

Transport of Spermatozoa. When spermatozoa are released into the seminiferous tubules, although endowed with tails, they are not yet capable of motility. They acquire motility as they pass along the epididymis in which they are stored. The ducts of the epididymis lead to the vas deferens, which provides the transporting passage along which spermatozoa traverse to the base of the penis. The ductus deferens or vas deferens has contractile power that allows it to propel the spermatozoa upward to the base of the penis. Seminal plasma, the fluid in which spermatozoa are transported during the ejaculatory process, is made up of the secretions of the accessory glands of the male reproductive tract. These include the seminal vesicles which empty into the ejaculatory duct, which in turn empties into the urethra, the prostate gland which surrounds the urethra, the ejaculatory ducts at the base of the penis, and the bulbourethral glands. During ejaculation, the seminal vesicles discharge their contents and propel spermatozoa that are already in the vas deferens along the urethra. The seminal plasma also receives a contribution from the prostate gland which expels a thin alkaline secretion into the base of the urethra. The function of the secretions of the accessory glands is to facilitate transportation of spermatozoa along the urethra during the ejaculatory process, and provide a temporary milieu in which the spermatozoa can survive. On intravaginal ejaculation, spermatozoa almost immediately begin to traverse the cervical mucus and within a matter of minutes some are on their way to the site of fertilization.

SUGGESTED READING

Chaffee, E. E., and Lytle, I. M.: *Basic Physiology and Anatomy*, ed. 4. Philadelphia, J. B. Lippincott, 1980.)

Goss, C. M., ed. *Gray's Anatomy of the Human Body*, ed. 29. Philadelphia, Lea & Febiger, 1973.

Eight

Sexual and Reproductive Physiology

Sexual Maturity / Menstrual Cycle / Menopause / Female and Male Reproductive Capacity / Human Sexual Response

A general review of reproductive physiology is included here to serve as background for the more practical aspects of maternity nursing. An understanding of physiology is essential, so that the nurse may recognize the special relation of physiology to problems in obstetrics.

SEXUAL MATURITY

Female. Evidence of sexual maturity in the female begins at the time of puberty, with the onset of dramatic bodily changes. Early in the course of puberty, axillary and pubic hair appears. Shortly thereafter, there is a gradual change in the contour of the labia. The breasts also begin to mature at this time and there is a sudden increase in bodily growth.

These changes usually precede the onset of the first menstruation—the *menarche*. Establishment of the menstrual cycle is the most clearly identifiable sign of puberty and serves as an indication that the internal sex organs are approaching maturity. These physical changes are accompanied by emotional changes, as the young girl recognizes these outward signs that she is now approaching womanhood. The whole process of puberty spans about three years and is completed with the menarche.

The time sequence of changes that culminates in the attainment of reproductive potential varies considerably among individuals (Fig. 8-1). Bodily manifestations of puberty, such as the beginning of breast development, the appearance of pubic hair, and a spurt of growth, precede the actual onset of menstruation by a variable amount of time.

Throughout puberty there is an interplay of physiological and sociocultural forces, and often the nurse is called upon to explain the bodily and psychological changes in puberty to mothers who have daughters approaching their teens. There is often anxiety about the onset of pubertal changes that are thought to be occurring too early or too late. Therefore, it is important to recognize the wide variability from one young woman to the next.

Male. Changes associated with puberty in the male occur somewhat later, on the average, than in the female and span an interval of about four years. These include development of axillary, pubic, and body hair, and maturation and growth of the testes and penis over a two-to-three-year period, accompanied by growth spurt and general muscular development.

Development of internal glands (prostate, bulbourethral, seminal vesicles) occurs in concert with penile and testicular growth. These provide the

88

seminal fluid in which spermatozoa are delivered during ejaculation. Ejaculation of fluid with penile erection may occur as soon as a year after the beginning of growth of the penis, even before it is of mature size. Generally, the ability to grow a full beard signals the completion of sexual maturity in the male.

Menarche

Menarche usually occurs between the ages of 12 and 16, although heredity, race, state of nutrition, climate, and environment may influence its early or late appearance; for example, maturity tends to occur earlier in warm climates and later in cold regions. The reproductive period spans about 35 years, from some point after the beginning of menstruation until its cessation during the menopause between ages 45 and 50.

Throughout childhood the *gonadotropins*, hormones produced by the pituitary gland which stimulate the ovaries, appear in very low concentrations. Estrogen, produced by the ovaries in the adult, remains undetectable. Puberty is ushered in when there is a rise in the release of gonadotropins from the pituitary gland. These stimulate the ovary to secrete increasing amounts of *estrogen*, the hormone responsible for many of the bodily changes of puberty.

An orderly sequence of endocrinological events resulting in ovulation may not occur initially. The first few menstrual cycles following the menarche may not, in fact, be associated with ovulation. However, once menstruation has occurred, it must be assumed that there is ovulation and, therefore, fertility and the potential for pregnancy.

Ovulation and Menstruation

Each month, with considerable regularity, a blister-like structure about 1.0 cm. in diameter develops on the surface of one or the other ovary. Within this bubble, almost lost in the fluid and cells about it, lies a tiny speck, scarcely visible to the naked eye; a thimble would hold 3 million of these specks. This speck is the human ovum—a truly amazing structure. It not only possesses within its diminutive compass the potential of developing into a human being, but also embodies the mental as well as

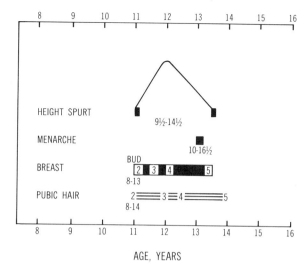

Figure 8-1. Sequence of events at adolescence in girls. An average girl is represented; the range of ages within which some of the events may occur is noted. Breast development progresses from the development of the breast bud (2) through full development (5). There is progression from downy pubic hair (2) through complete development of hair over the mons (5). (Modified for Tanner, J. M.: *Growth at Adolescence*, ed. 2. Oxford, England, Blackwell Science Publication, 1969. Pierson, E. C., and D'Antonio, W. V.: *Female and Male: Dimensions of Human Sexuality*. Philadelphia, J. B. Lippincott, 1974.)

physical traits of the woman and her forebears: perhaps her own brown eyes or her father's tall stature; possibly her mother's genius at mathematics or her grandfather's love of music. These and a million other potentials are contained in the ovum, which is so small that it is about one-fourth the size of the period at the end of this sentence.

In the process of ovulation, one blister on one ovary ruptures at a given time each month and discharges an ovum. The precise day on which ovulation occurs is a matter of no small importance. For instance, since the ovum can only be fertilized (impregnated by the spermatozoon, or male germ cell) within hours after its escape from the ovary, the day after ovulation a woman is no longer fertile. However, a person is potentially fertile for a number of days preceding the actual time of ovulation, since spermatozoa survive in the female reproductive tract for hours, even days, awaiting the arrival of the ovum.

In a given cycle, the time of ovulation is unpredictable. Even the person who consistently has regular menstrual periods could experience a delayed ovulation, or early ovulation in any one cycle. This possibility of irregularity, combined with the potential for fertility any time prior to ovulation due to the fact that spermatozoa retain their ability for fertilization, makes it difficult to identify accurately the fertile phase of a given cycle.

It should be remembered that the only really infertile interval is after ovulation has occurred. The time between ovulation and menstruation is relatively constant (14 ± 2 days); the time between menstruation and ovulation is variable enough that ovulation cannot be accurately predicted from one cycle to the next. It should be assumed that intercourse will result in conception unless some means of contraception is used, or the patient is assured, by the use of the temperature chart described later, that she is past ovulation.

Graafian Follicle.   In delving further into the process of ovulation, we find that at birth each ovary contains a huge number of undeveloped ova, probably more than 400,000. These are rather large, round cells with clear cytoplasm and a good-sized nucleus occupying the center. Each ovum is surrounded by a layer of a few small, flattened or spindle-shaped cells. The whole structure—ovum and surrounding cells—is a *follicle,* while in its underdeveloped state at birth it is a *primordial follicle.*

The formation of primordial follicles ceases at birth or shortly after, and the large number contained in the ovaries of the newborn represents a lifetime supply. The majority have disappeared before puberty, so that there are then perhaps 30,000 left. This disintegration of follicles continues throughout reproductive life, with the result that usually none is found after the menopause.

Meanwhile, from birth to the menopause a few of these primordial follicles show signs of development. The surrounding granular layers of cells begin to multiply rapidly until they are several layers deep, and at the same time become cuboidal in shape. As this proliferation of cells continues, a very important fluid develops between them—the *follicular fluid.*

After puberty, the cells within the developing follicles produce estrogenic hormones which in turn act on the reproductive organs and bring about cyclic bodily changes. During each menstrual cycle, several follicles develop further. One of these is finally selected by a process not as yet completely understood for complete maturation and ovulation.

Follicular fluid accumulates in such quantities that the multiplying follicle cells are pushed toward the margin; the ovum itself is almost surrounded by fluid and is suspended from the periphery of the follicle by only a small neck of cells. The structure is now known as the *graafian follicle,* after Von Graaf, the Dutch physician who, in 1672, first described it.

As it increases in size so enormously, the graafian follicle naturally pushes aside other follicles, forming each month, and a very noticeable, blister-like projection appears on the surface of the ovary. At one point the follicular capsule becomes thin, and as the ovum reaches full maturity, it breaks free from the few cells attaching it to the periphery and floats in the follicular fluid. The thinned area of the capsule now ruptures, and the ovum is expelled from the ovary in the process of ovulation (Fig. 8-2).

Changes in the Corpus Luteum.   After the discharge of the ovum, the ruptured follicle undergoes a change. It becomes filled with large cells containing a special yellow-colored matter. The follicle then is known as the *corpus luteum,* or yellow body. If pregnancy does not occur, the corpus luteum reaches full development in about eight days, then retrogresses and is gradually replaced by fibrous tissue, the *corpus albicans.*

If pregnancy occurs, the corpus luteum enlarges somewhat and persists throughout the period of gestation, reaching its maximum size about the fourth or fifth month and retrogressing slowly thereafter. The corpus luteum secretes an extremely important substance, progesterone, which will be discussed later in this chapter.

In the absence of pregnancy, the corpus luteum remains active for about two weeks. The constancy of progesterone production by the corpus luteum accounts for the relatively standard duration of the postovulatory phase of the menstrual cycle, 14 ± 2 days.

MENSTRUAL CYCLE

Menstruation in Relation to Pregnancy

Menstruation is the periodic discharge of blood, mucus, and epithelial cells from the uterus. It usually occurs at monthly intervals throughout the repro-

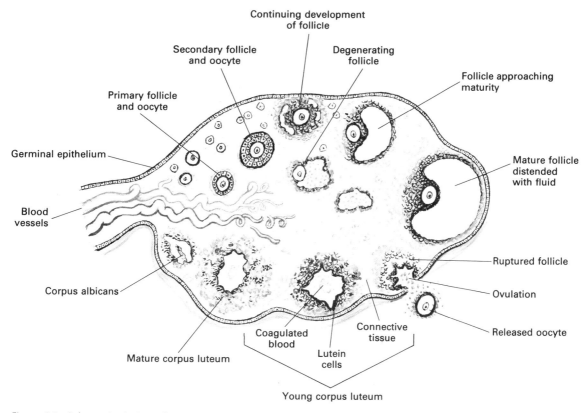

Figure 8-2. Schematic design of an ovary, showing the sequence of events in the origin, growth, and rupture of an ovarian follicle, and the formation and retrogression of a corpus luteum. Atretic follicles are those that show signs of degeneration and death. For proper sequence, follow clockwise around the ovary, starting at the mesovarium. (From Patten, B. M.: *Human Embryology,* ed. 3. New York, Blakiston, McGraw-Hill, 1968.)

ductive period, except during pregnancy and lactation, when it is usually suppressed. Accordingly, the span of years during which childbearing is possible—that is, from about ages 12 to 45—corresponds to the period during which ovulation and, therefore, menstruation occur. In general, a woman who menstruates is able to conceive, whereas one who does not is probably infertile. Ovulation and menstruation are closely interlinked, and since no process of nature is purposeless, menstruation must play some vital and indispensable role in childbearing. What is this role?

If day by day we were privileged to watch the *endometrium,* the lining membrane of the uterus, we would observe some remarkable alterations. Immediately following the termination of a menstrual period, this membrane is very thin, measuring a few millimeters in depth. Each day thereafter it becomes a trifle thicker and harbors an increasing content of blood, while its glands become more and more active, secreting a rich nutritive substance.

About a week before the onset of the next expected period, this process reaches its height; the endometrium is now of the thickness of heavy, downy velvet and has become soft and succulent with blood and glandular secretions. At this time the ovum, if it has been fertilized, is embedded into this luxuriant lining.

All these changes have only one purpose: to provide a suitable bed in which the fertilized ovum may rest, secure nourishment, and grow. If an ovum is not fertilized, these alterations serve no useful function. Accordingly, through a mechanism that even today is obscure, the swollen endometrium disintegrates, and the encased blood and glandular secretions escape into the uterine cavity. Passing through the cervix, they flow out through the vagina, carrying the tiny unfertilized ovum with them. In other words, menstruation represents the abrupt termination of a process designed to prepare board and lodging, as it were, for a fertilized ovum. It forecasts the breakdown of a bed that was not needed because the "boarder" did not materialize. Thus, its purpose is to clear away the old bed so that a new and fresh one may be created the next month.

Hormonal Control of Menstruation

The menstrual cycle is regulated primarily through the highly coordinated function of the brain, the hypothalamus, the pituitary, the ovaries, and the uterus. If, while watching the changes in the endometrium during the menstrual cycle it were possible to inspect the ovaries from day to day, it would be noted that the uterine alterations are directly related to certain changes that take place in the ovary. If it were possible to look further, it might be seen that the alterations that occur regularly in the ovarian cycle are directly related to certain phenomena that take place in the anterior pituitary gland and the hypothalamus, a portion of the brain that lies above the pituitary. Thus, the whole sequence represents the harmonious, integrated reactions of several processes within the human organism, all of which are necessary to maintain proper relationships in the menstrual cycle.

Phases of the Menstrual Cycle

Proliferative Phase. Immediately following menstruation, it will be recalled, the endometrium is very thin. During the subsequent week or so it proliferates markedly. The cells on the surface become taller, while the glands that dip into the endometrium become longer and wider. As the result of these changes, the thickness of the endometrium increases six- or eightfold.

Each month during this phase of the menstrual cycle (from approximately the fifth to the fourteenth days), a graafian follicle is approaching its greatest development and is manufacturing increasing amounts of follicular fluid. This fluid contains a most important substance, the estrogenic hormone *estrogen.* The word *hormone* comes from a Greek word that means *I bring about,* and in the case of estrogen, it brings about (among other things) the thickening of the endometrium described.

Each month, then, after the cessation of menstruation, the cells in and around the developing graafian follicle produce estrogen which acts on the endometrium to cause it to grow (proliferate). For this reason this phase of the menstrual cycle is commonly called the *proliferative phase,* although it is sometimes referred to as the *follicular,* or *estrogenic* phase.

Secretory Phase. Following the release of the ovum from the graafian follicle (ovulation), the cells which form the corpus luteum begin to secrete, in addition to estrogen, another important hormone, *progesterone.* This supplements the action of estrogen on the endometrium in such a way that the glands become very tortuous or corkscrew in appearance and are greatly dilated. This change occurs because the glands are swollen with a secretion.

Meanwhile, the blood supply of the endometrium is increased; it becomes vascular and succulent. Since these effects are directed at providing a bed for the fertilized ovum, it is easy to understand why the hormone that brings them about is called progesterone, meaning *for gestation.* It is also clear why this phase of the cycle, occupying the last 14 ± 2 days, is commonly called the *secretory phase* and why occasionally it is referred to as the *progestational, luteal,* or *premenstrual phase.*

Menstrual Phase. Unless the ovum is fertilized, the corpus luteum is short-lived. Since corpus luteum cells secrete both progesterone and estrogen, cessation of corpus luteum activity means a withdrawal of both of these hormones. As a result, the endometrium degenerates. This is associated with rupture of countless small blood vessels in the endometrium with innumerable minute hemorrhages. Along with the blood, superficial fragments of the endometrium, together with mucin from the glands, are cast away, all of which constitutes the menstrual discharge (Fig. 8-3). Naturally, this phase of the cycle (from approximately the first to the fifth days) is called the *menstrual phase.*

Role of the Pituitary Gland

The pituitary gland is of considerable importance in the function of the reproductive system.★ The anterior lobe of the pituitary, the "master clock," releases, among other hormones, the gonadotropins, whose function is to stimulate the ovary.

★The posterior lobe of the pituitary gland produces oxytocin, a hormone that has an important role in obstetrics, but one that differs altogether from the purpose of the present discussion.

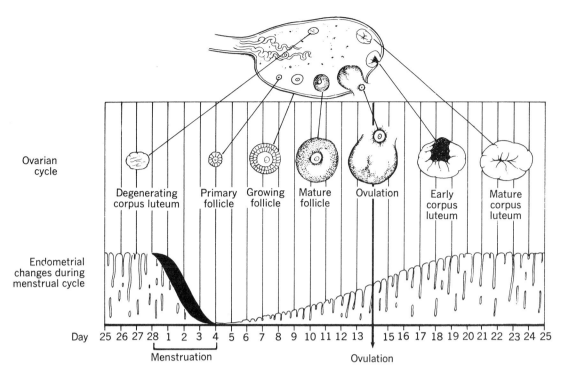

Ovarian
cycle

Degenerating
corpus luteum | Primary
follicle | Growing
follicle | Mature
follicle | Ovulation | Early
corpus
luteum | Mature
corpus
luteum

Endometrial
changes during
menstrual cycle

Day 25 26 27 28 1 2 3 4 5 6 7 8 9 10 11 12 13 15 16 17 18 19 20 21 22 23 24 25

Menstruation

Ovulation

Times approximate

Figure 8-3. Schematic representation of one ovarian cycle and the corresponding changes in thickness of the endometrium. It is thickest just before the onset of menstruation and thinnest just as it ceases. (From Chaffee, E. E., and Lytle, I. M.: *Basic Physiology and Anatomy,* ed. 4. Philadelphia, J. B. Lippincott, 1980.)

These hormones produce the ovarian alterations associated with ovulation. There are two principal gonadotropins. One is *follicle-stimulating hormone* (FSH). As its name implies, FSH stimulates the development of the follicle. The other is *luteinizing hormone (LH),* which has its principal activity during ovulation and the luteal phase of the cycle.

The release of the gonadotropic hormones by the pituitary is regulated by the *hypothalamus*—a specialized structure within the brain located just above the pituitary. The hypothalamus has a vascular connection to the pituitary gland, as well as nervous connections with the central nervous system. Indeed, its function can be modified by influences within the central nervous system. Thus, the function of the pituitary gland may be affected by the brain. The cyclic release of gonadotropin is brought about through the influence on the pituitary gland by a hormonal agent released by the hypothalamus. This is called gonadotropin-releasing hormone or LH/FSH-releasing hormone (GnRH or LH/FSH-RH), since it directly affects the release of both FSH and LH from the pituitary gland.

Other Functions of Estrogen and Progesterone

In addition to their role in controlling menstruation, estrogen and progesterone have other far-reaching and important functions. Estrogen is responsible for the development of the secondary sex characteristics, that is, all those distinctive sex manifestations that are not directly concerned with the process of reproduction. Thus, the growth of the breasts at puberty, the distribution of body fat, the size of the larynx and its resulting influence on the quality of the voice, as well as mating instincts, are all the results of estrogenic action. Thus, it may almost be said that a woman is a woman because of estrogen.

Aside from its action on the endometrium, progesterone also has a relaxing action on the uterine muscle. Thus, it plays an important role in preserving the life of the embryo in early pregnancy, both by preventing its expulsion from the uterus and by preparing the endometrium to receive and nourish it.

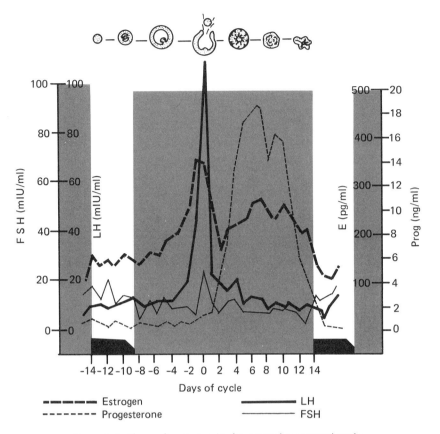

Figure 8-4. Plasma hormones in the normal menstrual cycle.

Sensitive laboratory methods now allow accurate measurement of day-to-day changes in circulating pituitary and ovarian hormones (Fig. 8-4). The interplay between pituitary and ovary, influenced in turn by the central nervous system through the hypothalamus, brings about orderly development of the follicle and ovulation.

At the end of a given cycle and at the beginning of the subsequent cycle (Fig. 8-4) the pituitary gland releases increased amounts of FSH. With the help of small amounts of LH, FSH stimulates maturation of several ovarian follicles. These produce modest amounts of the estrogen, estradiol. The levels of estradiol in the bloodstream begin to rise and estradiol in turn acts negatively at the central nervous system-hypothalamic-pituitary level, inhibiting the release of additional amounts of FSH. Consequently, the level of FSH in the circulating blood begins to fall. FSH also acts on the follicle to make it more sensitive to the second pituitary hormone, LH.

About two days before ovulation, all but the one follicle that is destined to ovulate begin to regress, in a process called atresia. That one follicle undergoes rapid growth, and estrogen production rises sharply. The increased amount of estrogen produced at this point then acts positively at the central nervous system-hypothalamic-pituitary level, stimulating a rapid increase in gonadotropin-releasing hormone (GnRH) levels. In turn, GnRH causes release from the pituitary gland of large amounts of LH, as well as additional FSH. This dramatic rise in LH stimulates the completion of maturation of the follicle and within 24 hours after the LH surge, ovulation takes place.

The increased levels of preovulatory estrogen prepare the genital tract for sperm migration. The secretions of the cervix, scanty and viscous early in the cycle, become thin and watery and more receptive to spermatozoa. The vaginal wall also reflects the effect of estrogen. A vaginal smear taken at this time reveals a large percentage of mature or "cornified" cells. The endometrium displays maximal proliferation (see Fig. 8-3).

Following ovulation the cyclic pattern continues. The ruptured follicle is transformed into a corpus luteum. The second function of LH is maintenance of the corpus luteum. These endocrine events are associated with further modifications in the cervical mucus, vagina, and endometrium. The mucus becomes thick, "tacky," and viscous, and is no longer as receptive to spermatozoa. The vaginal smear reflects the influence of progesterone with a decreasing "maturation index." The endometrium takes on secretory changes preparatory to implantation.

Progesterone secretion by the corpus luteum reaches its maximum about five to seven days after ovulation (Fig. 8-4). This is the time when the fertilized egg, now a *blastocyst,* is ready to implant. If pregnancy has occurred, another hormone, *human chorionic gonadotropin (hCG),* appears within two to three days of implantation. This hormone acts on the corpus luteum, maintaining its progesterone-providing function, and transforms it into a corpus luteum of pregnancy. If pregnancy has not intervened, the corpus luteum begins its demise at this time. Approximately ten to eleven days after ovulation, progesterone levels decline precipitously, and on about the fourteenth postovulatory day, no longer the beneficiary of hormonal support, the endometrium begins to shed in the process of menstruation.

BODILY MANIFESTATIONS OF OVARIAN FUNCTION

From what has been said concerning the underlying mechanism of menstruation, it is clear that the monthly flow of blood is only one phase of a marvelous cyclic process that not only makes childbearing possible, but also profoundly influences both body and mind. For this reason the time of the onset of menstruation is a critical period in the life of a young woman.

The average age at which the onset of menstruation occurs is between 12 and 14 years. It may be as early as the ninth year or as late as the eighteenth year and still be within normal limits. Although the interval of the menstrual cycle, counting from the beginning of one period to the onset of the next, averages 28 days, there are wide variations even in the same woman. Indeed, there is scarcely a woman who menstruates exactly every 28 or 30 days each month. This question has been the subject of several studies on normal young women, chiefly nursing students who have conscientiously recorded the time and the nature of each period. These investigations show that the majority of women (almost 60 percent) experience variations of at least five days in the length of their menstrual cycles; differences in the same woman of even ten days are not uncommon and may occur without explanation or apparent detriment to health.

The degree and intensity of the outward manifestations of the ovulatory cycle vary from one individual to the next. Some women consistently experience pelvic discomfort during ovulation, or "mittelschmerz," so named because it typically appears in the middle of a 28-day menstrual cycle. Slight staining or occasional bleeding may occur in association with ovulation. In the postovulatory interval there may be breast tenderness and fullness which typically reaches a nadir just before menstruation. Premenstrual "tension" characterized by increased irritability may also occur after ovulation.

Cyclic changes in the quality of the cervical mucus may be observed and are often easily detected by the patient when she is made aware of this possibility. In some cases, a clear translucent mucus appears at the labia or may be wiped from the cervix to provide suggestive evidence of impending ovulation. In the postovulatory phase of the cycle, the mucus becomes sticky and less abundant. Daily observations of cervical mucus changes have been suggested as a useful parameter in utilizing the "rhythm" method of contraception.

Normal menstruation should not be accompanied by pain, although there may be some general malaise, together with a feeling of weight and discomfort in the pelvis. Painful menstruation is known as *dysmenorrhea.* If there is a great irregularity or extremely profuse flow or marked pain, a pathologic condition may be present. Absence of menses is known as *amenorrhea.* The most common cause of amenorrhea is pregnancy, but sometimes it is brought about by emotional disturbances, such as fear, worry, or fatigue, which work through the central nervous system and hypothalamus, or by debilitating disease (anemia, tuberculosis).

Variations in Basal Body Temperature

Beginning about the first year of life, slight daily variations in body temperature occur normally in all human beings. These temperature variations have relation to the time of the day and the nature of the circumstances surrounding the individual. For example, the body temperature is lowest in the morning before breakfast, after a good night's rest, and prior to assuming activity. Then after a day of normal activity the body temperature is usually highest toward afternoon and early evening. The fact that physiological variations in basal body temperature also occur in relation to the menstrual cycle is important here, because it can be useful in estimating the time of ovulation. Such an index becomes extremely important in studies of fertility and sterility.

In the woman who is ovulating, there is normally a rhythmic variation in the basal body temperature curve during the course of the menstrual cycle (Fig. 8-5). The basal temperature is lower during the first part of the menstrual cycle, the proliferative phase. It rises in association with ovulation and remains relatively higher during the luteal phase of the cycle. The rise in the basal temperature occurs as a result of the influence of progesterone, produced by the corpus luteum following ovulation. Progesterone causes this thermogenic effect through its influence on the central nervous system. The basal temperature rises as much as 0.5 of a degree, and a relatively higher temperature is sustained until just before the onset of the menstrual period. This interval occupies the 14 ± 2 terminal days in the cycle.

If pregnancy occurs, the levels of progesterone are maintained, and under its influence the basal temperature remains high past the expected time of the period. In the absence of pregnancy, the basal temperature usually drops a day or so before the menstrual period.

The Use of the Basal Temperature Graph

The basal body temperature is one of the most practical means for the diagnosis of ovulation. It is the relative difference in basal body temperature during the course of the cycle which is the important diagnostic criterion for ovulation. It is only useful in the timing of ovulation retrospectively. Thus, when there is infertility, efforts to time intercourse to coincide with changes in the temperature chart have not proved worthwhile. In fact, such regulation of coital habits is not recommended. However, for the diagnosis of ovulation, the temperature chart

has proved valuable. The temperature chart is also useful as an adjunct to the rhythm method of family planning (see Chapter 12).

Directions

1. The first day of menses is considered to be the first day of the menstrual cycle. The duration of menstrual flow is recorded, beginning on cycle day 1, with X's on the chart (Fig. 8-5). The date of onset of flow is recorded, and each subsequent date is recorded in the spaces provided. Following cessation of flow, the morning temperature is taken. Oral temperatures are as satisfactory as rectal recordings and are certainly more convenient. The temperature should be taken immediately after waking and before getting out of bed, talking, eating, drinking, or smoking. Ideally, it should be taken at about the same time every morning.

2. The thermometer is read to within 0.1 of a degree, and the reading is recorded on the chart.

3. Any known cause for temperature variation should be noted on the chart, for example, interrupted or shortened sleep, a cold, indigestion, emotional disturbance. If intercourse has occurred, that fact should be recorded with a circle around the recording the following morning.

4. Some women can recognize ovulation by mittelschmerz; others have vaginal bleeding or clear preovulatory vaginal discharge. Such manifestations should be recorded on the chart.

MENOPAUSE

The term *menopause* means the cessation of menstruation. In about 50 percent of women this usually occurs during the middle years, between the ages of 45 and 50. About 25 percent will reach menopause before the age of 45 and 25 percent after the age of 50. In common usage, the term menopause generally means cessation of *regular* menstruation. Since this is a normal process of aging and takes place gradually, the periods may become scanty or irregular, or intermittantly heavy before ceasing altogether. The commonly used term "menopausal female" really refers to the perimenopausal woman.

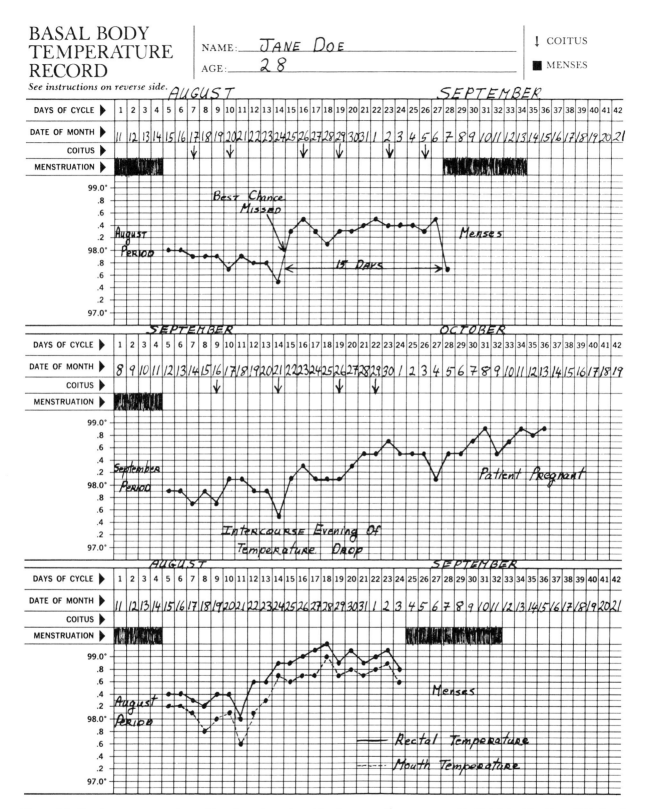

Figure 8-5. Basal temperature chart. Directions for using this chart are given on page 96. (Published by Merrell-National Laboratories, Division of Richardson-Merrell Inc., Cincinnati, Ohio 45215.)

The cause of natural menopause is cessation of ovarian activity, that is, estrogen production and ovulation. Often the terms menopause and climacteric are used synonymously, but the usage is not accurate. The latter encompasses the total syndrome of endocrine, somatic, and psychic changes occurring at the termination of the reproductive period in the female. It is derived from the Greek meaning *rung of the ladder,* or critical point in human life. The withdrawal of estrogen production associated with the cessation of ovarian function is evidenced by decreasing size of the ovary, the uterus, and the breasts. The external genitals become flattened and the vaginal walls lose their folds, elasticity, and lubrication, becoming shiny and smooth. The decrease in estrogen levels may also produce intermittent "hot flashes" and some emotional instability—for example, irritability and sudden outbursts of tears much like the emotional lability associated with premenstrual tension. Increasing dryness of hair and skin are also associated with the perimenopausal years.

Each individual reacts somewhat differently to this withdrawal of estrogen. These reactions are unpredictable, vary from woman to woman, and depend to some extent on her previous emotional history, her present support systems within the family, and to a very real extent, on the fact that the menopausal reproductive-endocrine system may be quite labile during this interval which may last as long as eight or nine years.

Hot flashes are not an old wives tale; they are real and a result of vasomotor instability. This instability also results in sweating and brief sensations of cold "all over." There may be redness and perspiration that is visible to onlookers, or the sensations may be equally intense on another occasion but with no visible signs. Their daily frequency may vary and there can be long intervals, sometimes weeks with no symptoms at all.

The menopause may result from other than the natural physiological alterations of the climacteric. The term *artificial menopause* describes the cessation of menstruation produced by some artificial means, such as an irradiation of the ovaries or surgical operation for the removal of the ovaries (oophorectomy) or the uterus (hysterectomy). Each of these brings about one manifestation in common (i.e., the woman will no longer menstruate), but beyond this the manifestations in the patient are not identical.

Certain misunderstandings based on incorrect interpretation of terminology are rather widespread and should be clarified. The fact that a woman has had a hysterectomy and ceases to menstruate does not mean that her healthy ovaries will now cease to function. Hysterectomy involves only the removal of the uterus. On the other hand, if the ovaries are also removed surgically or are treated by irradiation, the source of estrogen is withdrawn abruptly and thus the symptoms caused by the sudden withdrawal of this hormone will occur. Because there is much misinformation among the lay public on this point, sometimes intensive preoperative and postoperative counseling is required. Abrupt interruption of ovarian function in a woman who is still having regular periods may create more withdrawal symptoms than in a woman who is in her perimenopausal years. In the younger woman, estrogen replacement to alleviate signs and symptoms of estrogen withdrawal may be imperative for a time. The need for estrogen replacement in the older woman after surgical removal of ovaries will vary from patient to patient.

Physiology of the Menopause

When one considers that the menopause is experienced by all middle-aged women, it may seem surprising that the endocrine and metabolic events associated with it are still incompletely understood. This lack of information is due, in part, to difficulties associated with long-term, longitudinal studies spanning many years. In addition, the sensitive endocrine assays which would allow study of the endocrinological events associated with the menopause have only recently become available. Because of this, estrogen replacement therapy with its possible short- or long-term effects has created much controversy in both the lay and scientific literature.

It is now known that several years before the menopause there is an increase in *circulating levels of both FSH and LH.* The actual levels of estrogen and progesterone produced by the ovaries are decreased. These are only slight changes, and in spite of them, ovulation and menstruation continue to occur. The decreasing production of estradiol and progesterone is the factor that undoubtedly allows release of increased amounts of gonadotropins from the pituitary, resulting in higher circulating levels of FSH and LH.

In normal postmenopausal women, FSH and LH levels are consistently high. The ratio of FSH and LH is always greater than one. Both of the gonadotropins are released in a pulsating fashion, similar to that seen in younger women but much more pronounced, with bursts occurring every 10 to 20 minutes. There is also periodic fluctuation in gonadotropin levels which occurs about every two hours. After removal of the ovaries in regularly menstruating women, gonadotropin levels begin to rise within two days. The rise in the FSH is more dramatic than that of LH.

Estrogen production by the postmenopausal ovary is miniscule. Surgical removal of the ovary after the menopause does not affect circulating estrogens in any significant way. However, the postmenopausal ovary does continue to produce androgens, and in increased amounts, evidenced in some women who begin to notice the appearance of dark hair on the upper lip and chin. Since varying amounts of circulating estrogen are found in the postmenopausal women, it has been suggested that the estrogen may be produced elsewhere in the body and also that other tissues are able to convert the circulating androgen (testosterone) to estrogen. Fat, the liver, and some areas of the hypothalamus are capable of this conversion. Such estrogen production varies from one postmenopausal woman to the next, and this variability may account for some of the variations in menopausal symptoms.

The mechanism responsible for *vasomotor symptoms* is not known. Obviously, neuroendocrinological factors are at work. It has been suggested that catecholamines that act as neurotransmitters in the brain—they transfer information from one neuron to another—may respond to fluctuating gonadotropin or ovarian hormone levels. Catecholamines are responsible for modulating behavior and motor activity as well as the function of the hypothalamus and pituitary. Disturbance in catecholamine activity produces vasodilatation in the brain which could bring about hot flashes. Many other environmental influences are operating in the life of a postmenopausal woman and it is difficult to separate these from the physiological events associated with decreased ovarian function. While it is clear that emotional and physical stress can be related to increased frequency of vasomotor symptoms and signs, this relationship does not always occur in a predictable fashion. Hot flashes are the result of vasomotor instability and are clearly related to the estrogen deficiency associated with the cessation of ovarian function.

The *changes in the vaginal mucosa* also vary among menopausal women. Even minimal changes may result in painful intercourse (dyspareunia). Thinning of the vaginal lining and the decrease in lubrication can be corrected with estrogens administered orally or locally with vaginal suppositories or cream. Dyspareunia is a common symptom that should not be overlooked in the management of the postmenopausal woman.

Osteoporosis, demineralization of the bones, commonly occurs following menopause. Decreasing levels of estrogens are known to be associated with loss of bone calcium which is evidenced by high levels of circulating calcium in the plasma. This circulating calcium is excreted by the kidneys leaving the body in a negative calcium balance. Osteoporosis is a serious medical condition in elderly women as hip fractures in this age group are common. Healing is poor when there is osteoporosis, leading to long hospitalization and the morbidity associated with a nonambulatory status. Unfortunately, osteoporosis is seldom discovered in its beginning stages; often it is not until a fracture occurs that its existence is noted. Evidence of osteoporosis in the postmenopausal woman is generally felt to be an indication for estrogen therapy.

Estrogen Replacement

A good case could be made for routine use of estrogen in all postmenopausal women were it not for some of its side effects. The most serious of these is a greater incidence of endometrial carcinoma among estrogen-treated women than in the nontreated. Such factors must be carefully weighed and a risk-benefit ratio established for each individual patient.

One must consider the severity of the symptoms against the potential hazards of estrogen treatment and the quality of life. Signs and symptoms that interfere with working outside or inside the home or with a good sexual life are clear indications for treatment. Absolute contraindications to estrogen treatment include liver disease, cerebrovascular disease, venous thrombosis and embolism, and an estrogen-dependent malignancy of the breast or uterus. The use of estrogen in the menopausal years requires a carefully considered medical decision and, if instituted, careful monitoring during the course of treatment.

FEMALE AND MALE REPRODUCTIVE CAPACITY

Women have a limited reproductive life span, beginning soon after menarche, declining somewhat in the late reproductive years, and finally terminating at the menopause. At most, there is an opportunity to release no more than 500 ova during the course of reproductive life. In the male, spermatogenesis is initiated at the time of puberty and sperm production continues well into senescence. The number of mature spermatozoa produced by the testes during this very long interval are in the billions, and the reproductive capacity of a given fertile male is nothing short of phenomenal.

Another important difference is that in the male the capacity to reproduce is necessarily associated with sexual excitement, erection of the penis and ejaculation. As a requisite for procreation, the male must have had an erection and the associated stimulation required to produce it. In contrast, the capacity of the female to reproduce may be disassociated from sexual excitement and receptivity. Consider that conception can occur by mechanical placement of the ejaculate through artificial insemination. The capacity of the woman for sexual pleasure, however, is extremely important. There is no doubt that the physical aspects of a relationship play a critical role in the communication process that brings a couple closer together.

HUMAN SEXUAL RESPONSE

Female Sexual Response

Sexual excitation in the female which culminates in orgasm or "climax" is a complex process that has only recently been studied. Interest in coitus, culminating in penetration, is initiated through levels of communication which traditionally are not looked upon as sexual. How it is that a given female is sexually attracted to a given male or vice versa is not completely understood. The aspect of this process which is better understood is the physiology of female sexual excitement leading to orgasm.

Sexual arousal is brought about by touching and caressing. Some areas of the body are more sensitive to sexual stimulation than others, and the sexual organs—the breasts and external genitals, predominantly the clitoris—are the most responsive areas in this regard. During the course of sexual communication there is a rising awareness of sexual function, which, during continued sexual stimulation, is maintained at a plateau (Fig. 8-6). In the "plateau phase" a number of bodily changes occur. The most identifiable of these is the appearance of a fluid that traverses the vagina and provides lubrication so that penetration can occur easily. This vaginal transudate occurs as a result of vascular engorgement in the vaginal area. The labia become engorged and increase somewhat in size and the

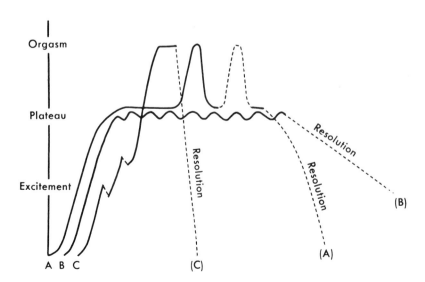

Figure 8-6. Female sexual response cycle. (From Masters, W., and Johnson, V.: *Human Sexual Response.* Boston, Little, Brown, 1966.)

clitoris becomes erect. Concomitantly, the nipples become erect and there are skin changes—the sexual flush. At the height of sexual excitement, the contour of the vagina changes and there is a deepening of the vaginal vault behind the cervix.

The clitoris plays the most important role in sexual excitation. Stimulation of the area in and around the clitoris produces the most dramatic physiological changes. If there has been penetration, the movement of the penis in the vagina stimulates the labia and indirectly stimulates the clitoris through motion of the clitoral hood. Just prior to orgasm, the clitoris retracts behind the clitoral hood. The orgasm itself is associated with a sense of pleasure and release. Additional orgasms can occur following the initial orgasm. A period of resolution follows during which the various bodily changes subside.

Male Sexual Response

During sexual excitation, the most dramatic bodily change in the male is penile erection. This can occur in response to visual or mental influences, whereas the ejaculatory process itself usually occurs as a result of direct stimulation. Ejaculation may occur spontaneously, as a result of nocturnal emission, but always with erection. It is usually brought about by direct stimulation of the penis manually or vaginally. Erection occurs through central nervous system influences that result in accumulation of blood within the erectile tissue of the penis. There is an increase in penile size and the normally flaccid organ becomes erect and turgid. Valves located in the blood vessels at the base of the penis close, preventing the egress of blood and maintaining erection. Immediately prior to ejaculation, a small amount of secretion appears at the opening of the urethra. This is the product of the bulbourethral

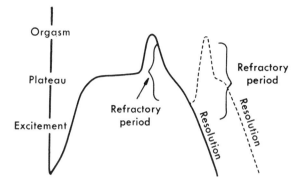

Figure 8-7. Male sexual response cycle. (From Masters, W., and Johnson, V.: *Human Sexual Response*. Boston, Little, Brown, 1966.)

glands and may contain some spermatozoa. At the height of sexual excitement, the urethra closes at the neck of the bladder, preventing discharge of urine at the time of ejaculation. Muscular elements within the penis contract spasmodically, ushering the semen containing spermatozoa along the urethra beyond the glans penis. On culmination of the ejaculatory process, which occupies a matter of seconds, there is a gradual deturgescence of the penis, followed by a refractory period (Fig. 8-7). The refractory period usually lasts from 15 to 20 minutes during which time an additional erection and ejaculation will not occur in spite of intensive stimulation. Knowledge of the refractory period has been useful in sexual counseling when the problem is premature ejaculation. After the first ejaculation the total reservoir of spermatozoa is not, in fact, depleted. In the second, and occasionally third ejaculation, semen may still contain active fertile spermatozoa and is capable of successful impregnation. The normal ejaculate contains between 1.5 and 4.0 ml. of fluid and there are some 60 to 150 million spermatozoa per ml. of which 60 to 70 percent are motile and presumed to be capable of fertilization.

SUGGESTED READING

Greep, R. O., Koblinsky, M. A.: *Frontiers in Reproduction and Fertility Control*. Cambridge, Mass., The MIT Press, 1977.

Greep, R. O., Koblinsky, M. A., and Jaffe, F. S.: *Reproduction and Human Welfare: A Chal-lenge to Research*. Cambridge, Mass., The MIT Press, 1977.

Gwatkin, R. B. L.: *Fertilization Mechanisms in Man and Mammals*. New York, Plenum Press, 1977.

Masters, W. H., and Johnson, V. E.: *Human Sexual Response*. Boston, Little, Brown, 1966.

Masters, W. H., and Johnson, V. E.: *Human Sexual Inadequacy*. Boston, Little, Brown, 1970.

Pierson, E. P.: *Sex Is Never an Emergency*, ed. 2. Philadelphia, J. B. Lippincott, 1975.

Speroff, L., Glass, R. H., and Kase, H. G.: *Clinical Gynecologic Endocrinology and Infertility*, ed. 2. Baltimore, Williams & Wilkins, 1979.

Yen, S. S., and Jaffe, R. B.: *Reproductive Endocrinology: Physiology, Pathophysiology and Clinical Management*. Philadelphia, W. B. Saunders, 1978.

Nine

Conception and Ovum Development

Maturation of Ovum and Sperm Cells / Fertilization and Changes Following Fertilization / Implantation of the Ovum

In all of Nature's wide universe, there is no process more wondrous, no mechanism more fantastic, than the one by which a tiny speck of tissue, the human egg, develops into a 7-pound baby. So miraculous did primitive peoples consider this phenomenon that they frequently ascribed it to superhuman intervention and even overlooked the fact that sexual intercourse was a necessary precursor. Throughout unremembered ages, our own primitive ancestors doubtless held similar beliefs, but now we know that pregnancy comes about in only one way: from the union of a female germ cell, the egg, or ovum, with a male germ cell, the spermatozoon. These two germ cells, or *gametes* become fused into one cell, or *zygote,* which contains the characteristics of both the female and the male from which these gametes originated.

MATURATION OF OVUM AND SPERM CELLS

Until about two days before ovulation, the ovum remains in a resting stage of development. Its nucleus is large and round and has been described as vesicular, because it resembles a bleb or vesicle.

While still in the follicle, the ovum undergoes the process of *meiosis,* the special method for cell division, through which it is matured and its genetic material (chromosomes) is prepared for fertilization.

The spermatozoon is fully matured when it is discharged in the ejaculate. It has undergone a meiotic process preparatory to fertilization before it leaves the testis.

In all human cells, with the exception of the mature sex cells, there are normally 46 chromosomes (chroma, color; soma, body). Normally, the chromosomes within each somatic cell are paired. Thus, each cell contains 22 pairs of autosomes (auto, self) and one pair of sex chromosomes. Female cells normally contain two X chromosomes; male cells normally contain one X and one Y chromosome. The sex chromosome of the mature ovum is always of the X type. The mature spermatozoon may have either an X chromosome or a Y chromosome (Fig. 9-1). When fertilization occurs with a spermatozoon containing the X chromosome, the resulting product is genetically female. When an ovum is fertilized by a spermatozoon containing a Y chromosome, the resulting product is genetically male.

Thus, in the human being, age, state of health, and natural physical strength have nothing to do with the determination of the sex of the offspring.

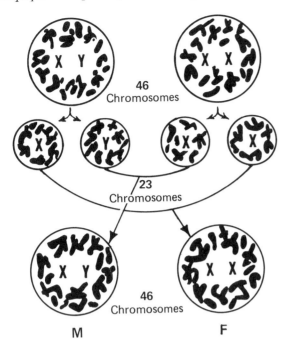

Figure 9-1. The sex of the offspring is determined at the time of fertilization by the combination of the sex chromosomes of the spermatozoon (either X or Y) and that of the ovum (X). The ovum fertilized by a sperm cell containing the X chromosome produces a female (44 regular chromosomes + 2 X chromosomes). If it is fertilized by a spermatozoon containing the Y chromosome, the union produces a male (44 regular chromosomes + X + Y).

Note: The structures depicted as chromosomes are diagrammatic only. In this illustration it was not possible to include the total correct number.

The sex is determined at the time of fertilization by the spermatozoon—not by the ovum. At the completion of the fertilization process, the fertilized ovum contains 46 chromosomes, the number normally present in all somatic cells.

Prior to fertilization, each gamete undergoes a reduction in its total number of chromosomes to one-half the usual number, the *haploid number.* This reduction occurs through the process of meiosis (Fig. 9-1). In the meiotic process, each gamete normally receives only one chromosome of each pair. Thus, each mature spermatozoon has 23 chromosomes in its nucleus, and each mature ovum also contains 23 chromosomes, the haploid number.

The cells that will eventually produce mature spermatozoa within the seminiferous tubules are called spermatogonia. These are located at the periphery of the seminiferous tubules (Fig. 9-2). They divide by mitosis, forming a new generation of germ cells, the primary spermatocytes. These cells, in time, undergo a reduction division through the process of meiosis (Fig. 9-2). Although their cytoplasm divides, the chromosomes do not split; instead, they are divided between each of two new cells, each now containing 23 chromosomes, the haploid number. These new haploid cells are called secondary spermatocytes. One contains 22 regular chromosomes (autosomes) and an X chromosome. In the other, there are 22 autosomal chromosomes and a Y chromosome. These cells divide again forming four spermatids, each with 22 autosomal chromosomes, two with X and two with Y sex chromosomes. Each spermatid develops a tail and eventually will become a mature spermatozoon.

The reduction division of the oocyte begins as the follicle is being prepared for ovulation (Fig. 9-2). While still within the follicle, the primary oocyte through the process of meiosis divides into two cells, a secondary oocyte and a first polar body, so called because it is observed at one pole of the developing ovum. Upon penetration by the spermatozoon a second polar body is released and, as a result of its release, the number of chromosomes is halved. The final product, the fertilized ovum, once again contains a set of 46 chromosomes, 23 from one ovum and 23 from the spermatozoon. Thus, the chromosomes of the fertilized ovum are derived from both germ cells (i.e., one half from the ovum and one half from the spermatozoon that fertilized the ovum).

The individual chromosomes differ in form and size, ranging from small, spherical masses to long rods. By the use of cell culture techniques, it is possible to photograph the individual chromosomes in a given cell. (Techniques for chromosomanalysis are considered in Chapter 15).

The Ovum

As described in Chapter 8, ova normally are discharged from the human ovary at the rate of one a month. Under the influence of the gonadotropins, the graafian follicle that is destined to release an ovum has matured. The ovum itself has been pushed to one side of the fluid-filled cavity of the follicle. It is surrounded by a translucent coat, the *zona pellucida.* Immediately adjacent to the zona pellucida, and connected to it, is a layer of follicular cells, the *corona radiata,* so named because the cells are arranged

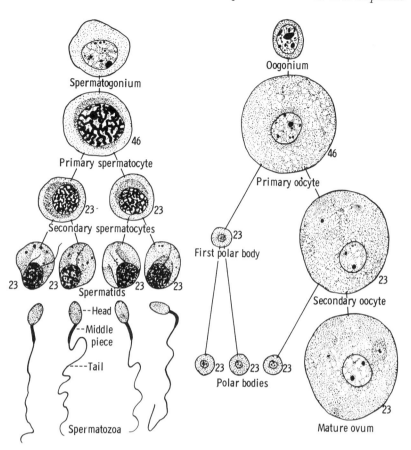

Figure 9-2. Diagram of gametogenesis. The various stages of spermatogenesis are indicated on the left; one spermatogonium gives rise to four spermatozoa. On the right, oogenesis is indicated; from each oogonium, one mature ovum and three abortive cells are produced. The chromosomes are reduced to one-half the number characteristic for the general body cells of the species. In man, the number in the body cells is 46, and that in the mature spermatozoon and secondary oocyte is 23. (From Chaffee, E. E., and Lytle, I. M.: *Basic Physiology and Anatomy*, ed. 4. Philadelphia, J. B. Lippincott, 1980.)

in a radial pattern. Peripheral to this is a more loosely arranged layer of cells, the *cumulus oophorus*. The ovum, surrounded by this entourage of cells, having matured through release of its first polar body, is released through the process of ovulation. Transfer of the ovum within its sticky cumulus mass into the fallopian or uterine tube, the site of fertilization, occurs relatively rapidly and with great efficiency. At this time, the ovum is a relatively large cell, measuring about 0.2 mm. (1/25 of an inch) and is barely visible to the naked eye.

Transport Through the Fallopian Tube

The fallopian or uterine tube is an important structure which serves a number of functions in reproduction (Fig. 9-3). It is responsible for the transfer of the ovum into its lumen from the rupturing follicle, and for providing a temporary environment for the ovum and the spermatozoon. It also provides the environment in which the fertilization process occurs, and in which the ovum passes through many cell divisions during the early stages of human life. Finally, the tube is responsible for transport of the fertilized, cleaving ovum into the uterus after a three-day interval.

The tube is uniquely designed anatomically for its various functions. At its ovarian end, it is endowed with specialized structures, the *fimbriae.* These are arranged in fronds and are lined with hairlike projections, the *cilia,* which beat in such a manner as to direct any overlying fluid—as well as any particles that float thereon—in the direction of the uterine cavity. The remainder of the fallopian or uterine tube is also lined with cilia, and these are important in the transportation of the newly released ovum along the tube (Fig. 9-4). The cilia create a current which courses along the tube, and which is partially responsible for the transportation of particles through it.

The anatomical arrangement at the fimbriated end of the tube is important in ovum pickup mechanisms. A separate strand of fimbria, the *fimbria ovarica,* extends from the tube to the ovary to which it is attached. This contains a separate bundle of smooth muscle. At the time of ovulation

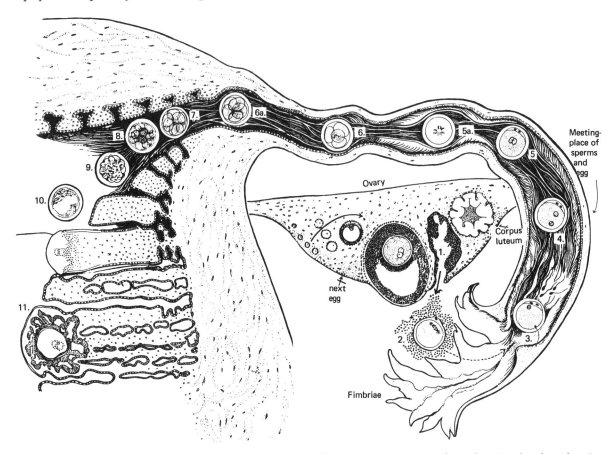

Figure 9-3. Travel of egg from ovary through implantation, with alterations en route: three days in tube, four days in uterus before implantation which occurs midway on rear wall or front of uterus. (1) Follicle ruptures. (2) Ovum with adhering granulosa cells; first polar body; second maturation spindle. (3) Sperm enters egg; second maturation division. (4) Male and female pronuclei. (5) Pronuclei fusing; fertilization accomplished. (5a) First cleavage division. (6–7) Early cleavage. (8) Morula. (9–10) Early and later gastrula. (11) Implanted growing embryo. (R. L. Dickinson, M.D., New York, adapted from Sellheim, with suggestions from Streeters, Frank, Hartman, and Miller)

this muscle contracts, pulling the ovary in the direction of the tubal opening. The remainder of the fimbria are thought to embrace the ovary near the point of ovulation, or over it, and they exercise muscular movement which moves them to and fro over the rupturing follicle. Thus, the cilia lining the fimbriae soon come into contact with the cumulus oophorus surrounding the ovum and as they beat in the direction of the tubal lumen, they carry the sticky cumulus mass past the tubal ostium to a point well within the fallopian or uterine tube. Through these mechanisms an efficient process of ovum transfer is arranged, and ovum pickup is practically assured, despite the fact that the ovum itself is miniscule in size.

Once the ovum is safely past the tubal ostium, it is transported rapidly to a point well within the fallopian or uterine tube. There, fertilization occurs. The fertilizing spermatozoon has previously been conditioned in the female reproductive tract so that it has acquired the ability to fertilize an ovum.

After fertilization, the ovum passes through several cell divisions, during which it is retained in the fallopian or uterine tube for approximately three days. Eventually it develops into a solid mass of cells, a *morula,* so called because it resembles a mulberry. It is finally transferred into the uterus at the 8 to 16 cell stage.

In the human, the mechanism by which the ovum is retained in the tube is not as yet clear. However, the importance of the three-day residence within the tube can be extrapolated from experiments in other mammals. In the rabbit, for example, if the ovum is removed from the tube and placed in the uterus prematurely, it degenerates and fails to implant. Although for obvious reasons the actual experiment has not been carried out in the human, it is generally accepted that the three-day residence within the human tube is important. Premature expulsion of the ovum from the tube could result in failure of implantation. Prolonged retention could result in ectopic pregnancy, with implantation into the tube itself and consequent tubal rupture and hemorrhage. The latter condition constitutes a serious obstetrical emergency. The importance of the fallopian or uterine tube, a once-neglected organ that bridges the space between the ovary and the uterus, is now quite evident.

Spermatozoa

The minute, wriggling *spermatozoa* are in some respects even more remarkable than the ova which they fertilize. In appearance they resemble microscopic tadpoles, with oval heads and long, lashing tails about ten times the length of the head. The human spermatozoon consists of three parts: the head, the middle-piece (or neck) and the tail (Fig. 9-5). The head of the spermatozoon is covered by a specialized structure, the acrosome. This acrosomal cap is an envelope in which enzymes that play an important role in sperm penetration are contained. The nucleus, and consequently the chromatin material, is in the head; the tail serves for propulsion.

Spermatozoa are much smaller than ova, their overall length measuring about one quarter the diameter of the egg, and it has been estimated that the heads of 2 billion of them—enough to regenerate the entire population of the world—could be placed, with room to spare, in the hull of a grain of rice.

As a result of the wriggling motion of the tails, spermatozoa swim with a quick vibratory motion and have been "timed" under the microscope at rates as fast as 3 mm. a minute. To ascend the uterus and the fallopian or uterine tube, they must swim against the same currents that waft the ovum downward; in their ascent, they are assisted by the muscular action of the uterus, which propels them upward in the direction of the tube. Spermatozoa have been observed in the fallopian or uterine tube within minutes of insemination.

The most amazing feature of spermatozoa is their huge number. At each ejaculation, during inter-

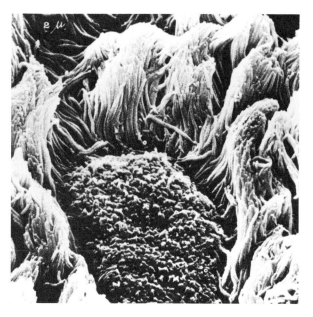

Figure 9-4. Scanning electron micrograph of the human fallopian tube showing ciliated cells surrounding a nonciliated cell in the midproliferative phase of the menstrual cycle. (From Patek, E., Nilsson, L., and Johannison, E.: *Fertil. steril.* 23:459, 1972)

course, about 300 million are discharged into the vagina. If each of these could be united with an ovum, the babies that would be created would exceed the total number born in the United States during the past 100 years—all from a single ejaculation.

Of the millions of spermatozoa deposited in the vagina during coitus, many are expelled immediately; some remain in the vagina for an interval and are later extruded. Those retained in the vagina lose their motility at the end of about an hour because

Figure 9-5. Spermatozoa.

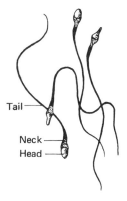

of the rather hostile acid environment provided by the vagina.

Some spermatozoa reach the cervix almost immediately after ejaculation. Those transferred into the secretions of the cervix find a more favorable environment there and may remain motile for as long as several days, especially in the preovulatory phase of the cycle.

Thousands of spermatozoa find their way into the cavity of the uterus; fewer still reach the lumen of the fallopian or uterine tube. Only one is afforded the privilege of continued biological life through fertilization and, at that, only occasionally. The remainder are disposed of in the reproductive tract, and as they degenerate they are phagocytized by the white blood cells in that region. However, it should be remembered, that once the spermatozoon is in the female reproductive tract it may retain its motility and, therefore, its potential ability to fertilize for hours, and even for days. Spermatozoa are conditioned to fertilize an ovum after they are exposed to the female reproductive tract, a process called *capacitation*. Within the female reproductive tract they "lie in wait" for the ovum.

FERTILIZATION AND CHANGES FOLLOWING FERTILIZATION

After the ovum is well within the fallopian or uterine tube, dispersion of the cumulus oophorus occurs. These cells begin to separate, partly as a result of the influence of the enzyme hyaluronidase contained in the acrosome surrounding the head of the spermatozoon. The spermatozoon makes its way through this peripheral layer of cells; meanwhile the densely packed corona radiata has undergone certain changes. These cells become looser under the influence of tubal fluid, and the spermatozoon then finds its way through this layer to the zona pellucida. It is now thought that the zona pellucida is penetrated by the spermatozoon because of a trypsin-like enzyme that is present in the sperm acrosome. Prior to penetration, openings are created in the outer membrane of the acrosome through which the enzyme-rich contents of the acrosome escape. This process, called the *acrosome reaction,* leads to a loss of the membrane over the anterior half of the sperm head. The spermatozoon makes a channel through the zona pellucida as the trypsen-like enzyme desolves the protein containing zona

with which it comes into contact. Having traversed the zona pellucida, the spermatozoon is then in a position to penetrate the membrane of the ovum itself. As the spermatozoon penetrates the ovum, it brings its tail with it.

Once penetration is complete, a physiological barrier occurs, and penetration of the ovum by other spermatozoa is prevented. Soon after penetration, the nucleus of the spermatozoon and the nucleus of the ovum undergo characteristic changes. They become pronuclei—distinct, clearly identifiable bodies of chromatin, each contained in a membrane. The male pronucleus and the female pronucleus then fuse, and the process of fertilization is now biologically complete. The new cell presents the full complement, or *diploid number* of chromosomes, one half from the spermatozoon and one half from the ovum. Soon thereafter, the first cell division occurs. In this process, the male and female chromosomes and their genes are mingled and finally split, forming two sets of 46 chromosomes, one set of 46 going to each of the two new cells. This process is repeated again and again until masses containing 8, 16, 32, and 64 cells are produced successively. These early cell divisions produce a morula. At the 8 to 16 cell stage, the dividing ovum is delivered into the uterus.

Retention in the fallopian or uterine tube occupies about three days. The fertilized ovum then spends some four days in the uterine cavity before actual embedding takes place. Thus, a total interval of some seven days elapses between ovulation and implantation.

Meanwhile, important changes are taking place in the internal structure of the fertilized ovum. Fluid appears in the center of the mulberry mass which pushes cells to the periphery of the sphere. At the same time it becomes apparent that this external envelope of cells is actually made up of two different layers, an inner and an outer. A specialized portion of the inner layer, after some 260 days, will develop into the long-awaited baby. The outer layer is a sort of foraging unit, called the trophoblast which means "feeding" layer; it is the principal function of these cells to secure food for the embryo (Fig. 9-6).

While the ovum is undergoing these changes, the lining of the uterus, it will be recalled, is making preparations for its reception. Considering that ovulation took place on the fourteenth day of the menstrual cycle and that the tubal journey and the

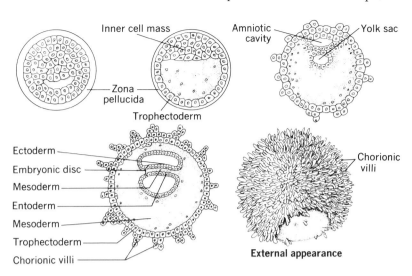

Figure 9-6. Early stages of development. (*Top, left and center*) The cells are separated into a peripheral layer and an inner cell mass; the peripheral layer is called the trophoblast, or trophectoderm; the entire structure is called a blastodermic vesicle. (*Top, right*) The formation of the amniotic cavity and yolk sac is indicated. The former is lined with ectoderm, the latter with entoderm. (*Bottom, left*) The location of the embryonic disk and the three germ layers is shown, together with the beginning of the chorionic villi. (*Bottom, right*) The external appearance of the developing mass is shown; the chorionic villi are abundant. (From Chaffee, E. E., and Lytle, I. M.: *Basic Physiology and Anatomy*, ed. 4. Philadelphia, J. B. Lippincott, 1980.)

uterine sojourn required 7 days, 21 days of the cycle will have passed before the ovum has developed its trophoblastic layer of cells. This is the period when the lining of the uterus has reached its greatest thickness and succulence. In other words, the timing has been precisely correct; the bed is prepared, and the ovum has so developed that it is now ready to embed itself.

IMPLANTATION OF THE OVUM

The embedding of the ovum is the work of the outer foraging layer of cells, the *trophoblast,* which possesses the peculiar property of being able to digest or liquefy the tissues with which it comes into contact. This process is carried out by means of enzymes. In this manner these cells not only burrow into the uterine lining and eat out a nest for the ovum, but also digest the walls of the many small blood vessels that they encounter beneath the

surface. The mother's bloodstream is thus tapped, and presently the ovum finds itself deeply sunk in the lining epithelium of the uterus, with tiny pools of blood around it. Sprouting out from the trophoblastic layer, finger-like projections now develop and extend greedily into the blood-filled spaces. Another name for the trophoblast, and one more commonly employed as pregnancy progresses, is the *chorion;* the finger-like projections are *chorionic villi.* These chorionic villi contain blood vessels connected with the fetus and are extremely important, because they are the sole means by which oxygen and nourishment are received from the mother. The entire ovum becomes covered with villi, which grow out radially and convert the chorion into a shaggy sac.

The cells of the chorionic villi begin to produce HCG. This hormone maintains progesterone production by the corpus luteum. In turn, progesterone stimulates and supports endometrial growth, providing suitable environment for continued development of the conceptus.

SUGGESTED READING

Greep, R. O., Koblinsky, M. A.: *Frontiers in Reproduction and Fertility Control.* Cambridge, Mass., The MIT Press, 1977.

Greep, R. O., Koblinsky, M. A., and Jaffe, F.: *Reproduction and Human Welfare: A Challenge to Research.* Cambridge, Mass., The MIT Press, 1977.

Gwatkin, R. B. L., *Fertilization Mechanisms in Man and Mammals.* New York, Plenum Press, 1977.

Seitz, H. M., B. G. Brackett, and L. Mastroianni, Jr. Fertilization. *In* Hafez, E. S. E. and Evans, T. N.: *Human Reproduction: Conception and Contraception.* Hagerstown, Md., Harper and Row, 1973, pp. 119–131.

Ten

Development and Physiology of the Embryo and Fetus

Physiologic Overview / Size and Development of the Fetus / Duration of Pregnancy / Calculation of the Expected Data of Confinement (EDC) / Physiology of the Fetus and Placenta / Fetal Circulation / Periods of Development

PHYSIOLOGIC OVERVIEW

With completion of implantation, the fertilized ovum has survived a series of delicately programmed events. It has been released from its follicle within the ovary, the meiotic process having been initiated. Following ovulation the ovum has been transported successfully into the lumen of the fallopian tube. There a single, properly conditioned spermatozoon has traversed the barriers surrounding the ovum to initiate the fertilization process. Ovum meiosis is completed, and there is fusion of the male and female genetic components, followed by a series of mitotic divisions. Three days later the ovum, now multicellular, is ushered out of the fallopian tube into the uterus. It lingers free in the uterine cavity, bathed in uterine fluid while it develops further into a blastocyst. Implantation occurs on about the seventh postfertilization day and the conceptus begins to derive its nourishment from the blood and tissue juices of the endometrium.

As development continues, the conceptus begins to produce human chorionic gonadotropin (hCG) which maintains production of progesterone by the corpus luteum. Thus, the newly formed pregnancy is now essentially self-sufficient and is in control of its own environment. Support of the corpus luteum by hCG results in continued maintenance of the endometrium by progesterone, and the next expected menstrual period is missed. At this point the conceptus is traditionally referred to as an embryo.

Throughout this two-week interval, there is a substantial incidence of pregnancy loss. It is estimated that 35 percent of fertilized ova develop abnormally and fail to progress beyond two weeks. Such a pregnancy loss is not surprising when one considers the complicated series of events which culminate in a successfully implanted pregnancy.

From the second week on, development occurs relatively rapidly. The mechanisms which support pregnancy, as the now nearly self-sufficient embryo develops, will be considered in this chapter.

The Decidua

The thickening of the uterine endometrium, which occurs during the premenstrual phase of menstruation, was described in Chapter 8. If pregnancy ensues, this endometrium becomes even more thickened, the cells enlarge, and the structure becomes known as the *decidua*. It is simply a direct continuation in exaggerated form of the already modified premenstrual endometrium.

For purposes of description, the decidua is divided into three portions. The part which lies directly under the embedded ovum is the *decidua basalis* (Fig. 10-1). The portion which is pushed out by the embedded and growing ovum is the *decidua capsularis*. The remaining portion, which is not in immediate contact with the ovum, is the *decidua vera*. As pregnancy advances, the decidua capsularis expands rapidly over the growing embryo and at about the fourth month lies in intimate contact with the decidua vera.

Amnion, Chorion and Placenta (Fig. 10-1)

Amnion. Even before the above noted structures become evident, a fluid–filled space develops about the embryo, a space which is lined with a smooth, slippery, glistening membrane, the *amnion.* The space is the amniotic cavity. Because it is filled with fluid, it is often called the bag of waters; in this the fetus floats and moves. At full term this cavity normally contains from 500 to 1,000 ml. of liquor amnii, or the "waters."

The amniotic fluid has a number of important functions: it keeps the fetus at an even temperature, cushions it against possible injury, and provides a medium in which it can move easily; furthermore, it is known that the fetus drinks this fluid.

At the end of the fourth month of pregnancy, the amniotic cavity has enlarged to the size of a large orange and, with the fetus, occupies the entire interior of the uterus. At this point, the amniotic fluid, which contains viable cells which are cast off by the fetus, can be sampled by amniocentesis and the chromosomal make-up of the fetal cells evaluated in culture for prenatal diagnosis of genetic abnormalities (see Chap. 36).

Chorion. As explained in Chapter 9, the early ovum is covered on all sides by shaggy chorionic villi, but very shortly those villi which invade the decidua basalis enlarge and multiply rapidly. This portion of the trophoblast is the *chorion frondosum* (leafy chorion). Conversely, the chorionic villi covering the remainder of the fetal envelope degenerate and almost disappear, leaving only a slightly roughened membrane, the *chorion laeve* (bald chorion). The chorion laeve, of course, lies outside the amnion with which it is in contact on its inner surface, while

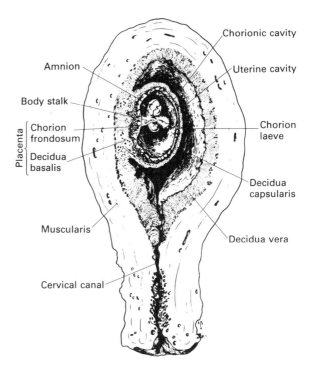

Figure 10-1. Pregnant uterus shown in sagittal section, The embryo is about one month of age. (From Chaffee, E. E., and Lytle, I. M.: *Basic Physiology and Anatomy*, ed. 4. Philadelphia, J. B. Lippincott, 1980.)

its outer surface lies against the decidua vera. The fetus is thus surrounded by two membranes, the amnion and the chorion, and in ordinary clinical discussions these are usually referred to simply as "the membranes."

Placenta. By the third month, another important structure, the placenta, has formed. This is a fleshy, disklike organ; late in pregnancy it measures about 20 cm. in diameter and 2 cm. in thickness. It receives its name from the Latin word meaning flat cake.

The placenta is formed by the union of the chorionic villi and the decidua basalis (Fig. 10-1). An analogous situation is seen when a tree or a plant sends down its roots into a bed of earth for nourishment; when the plant is removed, a certain amount of the earthy bed clings to the interlocking roots. Similarly, a thin layer of the uterine bed clings to the branching projections of chorionic villi, and together they make up this organ which supplies food to the fetus, as the roots and the earth provide nourishment for a plant.

At term the placenta weighs about 500 gm., or 1 pound. Its fetal surface is smooth and glistening,

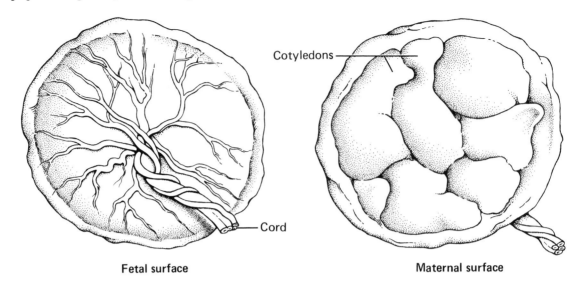

Cotyledons

Cord

Fetal surface   Maternal surface

Figure 10-2. The human placenta.

being covered by amnion, and beneath this membrane may be seen a number of large blood vessels. The maternal surface is red and fleshlike in character and is divided into a number of segments, or *cotyledons,* about 2.54 cm. in diameter (Fig. 10-2).

The placenta and the fetus are connected by the *umbilical cord,* which is usually about 45 cm. in length and about 1.5 cm. in diameter. The cord usually leaves the placenta near the center and enters the abdominal wall of the fetus at the umbilicus, a trifle below the middle of the median line in front. It contains two arteries and one large vein, which are twisted upon each other and are protected from pressure by a transparent, bluish-white, gelatinous substance called *Wharton's jelly.*

The Three Germ Layers

With nutritional facilities provided, the cells which are destined to form the baby grow rapidly. At first they all look alike, but soon after embedding, certain groups of cells assume distinctive characteristics and differentiate into three main groups: an outer covering layer (ectoderm), a middle layer (mesoderm), and an internal layer (entoderm).

From the *ectoderm* the following structures are derived the epithelium of the skin, hair, nails, sebaceous glands and sweat glands; the epithelium of the nasal and oral passages; salivary glands and

mucous membranes of the mouth and nose; the enamel of the teeth; and the nervous system.

From the *mesoderm* are derived muscles, bone, cartilage, the dentin of the teeth, ligaments, tendons, areolar tissue, kidneys, ureters, ovaries, testes, the heart, blood, lymph and blood vessels, and the lining of the pericardial, pleural, and peritoneal cavities.

From the *entoderm* arise the epithelium of the digestive tract, and the glands which pour their secretion into this tract; the epithelium of the respiratory tract (except for the nose) and of the bladder; the urethra, the thyroid, and the thymus.

SIZE AND DEVELOPMENT OF THE FETUS

Size at Various Months

The physician, as well as the nurse, is sometimes called upon to estimate the intrauterine age of a fetus which has been expelled prematurely.

In general, length affords a more accurate criterion of the age of the fetus than weight. Hasse's rule suggests that, for clinical purposes, the length of the embryo in centimeters may be approximated during the first five months by squaring the number of the month to which the pregnancy has advanced;

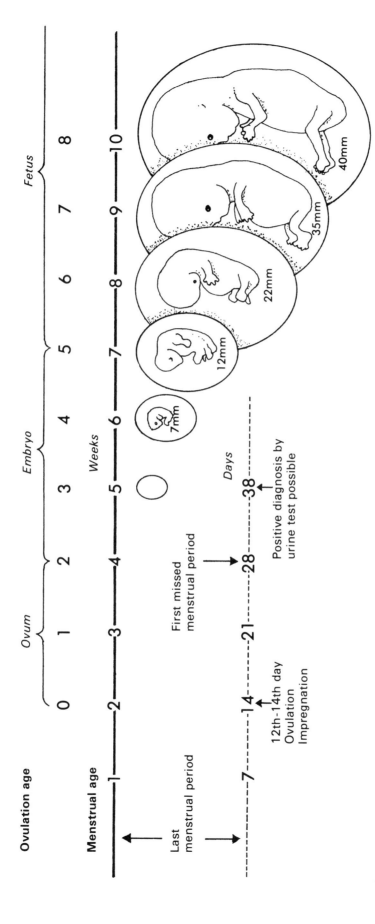

Figure 10-3. Growth of ovum, embryo, and fetus during the early weeks of pregnancy.

113

Fetal Development

1st Lunar Month
1. *Length* 0.75–1 cm. (0.3–0.4 inch)
2. Trophoblasts imbed in decidua.
3. Chorionic villi form.
4. Foundations formed for nervous system, genitourinary system, skin, bones, and lungs.
5. Buds of arms and legs begin to form.
6. Rudiments of eyes, ears, and nose appear.

4 weeks

2nd Lunar Month
1. *Length* 2.5 cm. (1 inch)
   Weight 4 gm.
2. Fetus is markedly bent.
3. Head is disproportionately large, owing to brain development.
4. Sex differentiation begins.
5. Centers of bone begin to ossify.

8 weeks

3rd Lunar Month
1. *Length* 7–9 cm. (2.8–3.6 inches)
   Weight 5.20 gm.
2. Fingers and toes are distinct.
3. Placenta is complete.
4. Fetal circulation is complete.

3 months

4th Lunar Month
1. *Length* 10–17 cm. (4–6.7 inches)
   Weight 55–120 gm. (1.9–4.2 oz.)
2. Sex is differentiated.
3. Rudimentary kidneys secrete urine.
4. Heart beat is present.
5. Nasal septum and palate close.

4th month

5th Lunar Month
1. *Length* 30 cm. (12 inches)
   Weight 280–300 gm. (9.9–10.6 oz.)
2. Lanugo covers entire body.
3. Fetal movements are felt by mother.
4. Heart sounds are perceptible with fetoscope.

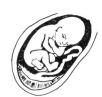

5th month

Fetal Growth by Month

in the second half of pregnancy, the month may be multiplied by five. Conversely, the approximate age of the fetus may be obtained by taking the square root of its length in centimeters during the first five months, and thereafter by dividing its length in centimeters by five. For instance, a fetus 16 cm. long is about four months old; a 35-cm. fetus is about seven months old.

Development Month by Month

Most women consider themselves one month pregnant at the time of the first missed menstrual period, two months pregnant at the second missed period, and so on. Since conception does not take place until ovulation, 14 days after the onset of menstruation in a 28-day cycle, it is obvious that an embryo

6th Lunar Month
1. *Length* 28–34 cm. (11.2–13.4 inches)
   Weight 650 gm. (1.4 lb.)
2. Skin appears wrinkled.
3. Vernix caseosa appears.
4. Eyebrows and fingernails develop.

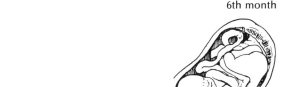

6th month

7th Lunar Month
1. *Length* 35–38 cm. (13.8–15 inches)
   Weight 1200 gm. (2.6 lb.)
2. Skin is red.
3. Pupillary membrane disappears from eyes.
4. If born, infant cries, breathes, but usually expires.

7th month

8th Lunar Month
1. *Length* 38–43 cm. (15–17 inches)
   Weight 2000 gm. (3.5–4.2 lb.)
2. Fetus is viable.
3. Eyelids open.
4. Fingerprints are set.
5. Vigorous fetal movement occurs.

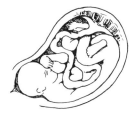

8th month

9th Lunar Month
1. *Length* 42–49 cm. (16.5–19.3 inches)
   Weight 1700–2600 gm. (3.7–5.7 lb.)
2. Face and body have loose wrinkled appearance due to subcutaneous fat deposit.
3. Lanugo disappears.
4. Amniotic fluid decreases somewhat.

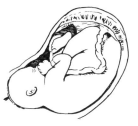

9th month

10th Lunar Month
1. *Length* 48–52 cm. (18.9–20.5 inches)
   Weight 3000–3600 gm. (6.6–7.9 lb.)
2. Skin is smooth.
3. Eyes are uniformly slate-colored.
4. Bones of skull are ossified and nearly together at sutures.

Fetal Growth by Month (continued)

does not attain the age of one month until about a fortnight after the first missed period (assuming a 28-day cycle), and its "birthday" by months regularly falls two weeks or so after any numerically specified missed period (Fig. 10-3). If the cycle is longer than 28 days, or if ovulation was delayed in the conceptive cycle, the duration of actual pregnancy, relative to the last menstrual period, will be shorter. This should be remembered in evaluating the month-by-month development of the fetus.

In speaking of the age of a pregnancy in months, physicians use the term *lunar months,* that is, periods of four weeks. Since a lunar month corresponds to the usual length of the menstrual cycle, it's easier to "figure" in this way (Fig. 10-3).

Month by month, the fetus develops as follows:

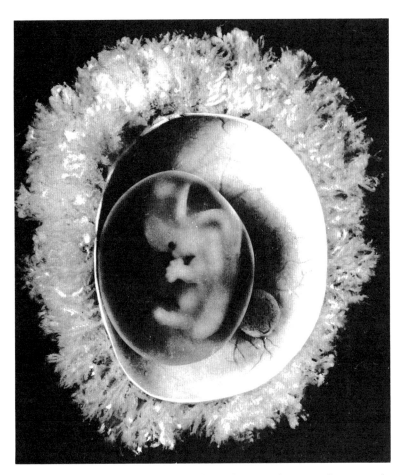

Figure 10-4. Human embryo photographed by Chester F. Reather. This specimen represents about 40 days' development and is shown in the opened chorion. It is reproduced at a magnification of 1.7. (Carnegie Institution, Washington, D.C.)

END OF FIRST LUNAR MONTH. The embryo is about 7 mm. long if measured in a straight line from head to tail—for it does have a tail at this early stage—and recognizable traces of all organs have become differentiated. The backbone is apparent but is so bent upon itself that the head almost touches the tip of the tail. At one end of the backbone, the head is extremely prominent, representing almost one-third of the entire embryo. (Throughout intrauterine life, the head is always very large in proportion to the body, a relationship which is still present, although to a lesser degree, at birth.)

The rudiments of the eyes, the ears, and the nose now make their appearance. The tube which will form the future heart has been formed, producing a large, rounded bulge on the body wall; even at this early age this structure is pulsating regularly and propelling blood through microscopic arteries. The rudiments of the future digestive tract are also discernible—a long, slender tube leading from the mouth to an expansion in the same tube which will become the stomach; connected with the latter the beginnings of the intestines may be seen. The incipient arms and legs are represented by small nubbins that resemble buds.

END OF SECOND LUNAR MONTH. The fetus, the term used for the product of conception after the fifth week of gestation, now begins to assume human form (Fig. 10-4). Due to the development of the brain, the head becomes disproportionately large so that the nose, the mouth, and the ears become relatively less prominent. It has an unmistakably human face and also arms and legs, with fingers, toes, elbows, and knees. During the past four weeks it has quadrupled in length and measures about 2.2 cm. from head to buttocks.

The external genitalia become apparent, but it is difficult to distinguish between male and female. During the second month, the human tail reaches its greatest development, but by the end of the month it is less prominent and then undergoes retrogression.

END OF THIRD LUNAR MONTH. The fetus is somewhat over 7.5 cm. long and weighs almost 28 gm. The sex can now be distinguished because the external genitalia are beginning to show definite signs of sex. Centers of ossification have appeared in most bones; the fingers and the toes have become differentiated, and the fingernails and the toenails appear as fine membranes. Early in this month, buds for all the temporary "baby" teeth are present, and sockets for these develop in the jawbone. Rudimentary kidneys have developed and secrete small amounts of urine into the bladder, which probably escape later into the amniotic fluid. Movements of the fetus are known to occur at this time, but they are too weak to be felt by the mother.

END OF FOURTH LUNAR MONTH. The fetus from head to toe is now 16 cm. long and weighs about 113 gm. The sex, as evidenced by the external genital organs, is now quite obvious.

END OF FIFTH LUNAR MONTH. The length of the fetus now approximates 25 cm., while its weight is about 227 gm. A fine downy growth of hair, *lanugo,* appears on the skin over the entire body. Usually, about this time the mother becomes conscious of slight fluttering movements in her abdomen, which are due to movements of the fetus. Their first appearance is called *quickening,* or the perception of life. At this period the physician often is able to hear the fetal heart for the first time. If a fetus is born now, it may make a few efforts to breathe, but its lungs are insufficiently developed to cope with conditions outside the uterus, and it invariably succumbs within a few hours at most.

END OF SIXTH LUNAR MONTH. The length of the fetus is 36 cm., and its weight is 680 gm. It now resembles a miniature baby, with the exception of the skin, which is wrinkled and red with practically no fat beneath it. At this time, however, the skin begins to develop a protective covering, *vernix caseosa,* which means cheesy varnish. This fatty, cheesy substance adheres to the skin of the fetus and at term may be .3 cm. thick. Although a few fetuses of this size have survived, the outlook must be regarded as extremely grave.

END OF SEVENTH LUNAR MONTH. The fetus measures about 37 cm. in length and weighs approximately 1 kg. If born at this time, it has some chance of survival.

END OF EIGHTH LUNAR MONTH. The fetus measures about 40 cm. and weighs approximately 1.8 kg. Its skin is still red and wrinkled, and vernix caseosa and lanugo are still present. In appearance it resembles a little old man. With proper incubator and good nursing care, infants born at the end of the eighth month have better than even chances of survival, possibly as high as three chances in four.

END OF NINTH LUNAR MONTH. For all practical purposes the fetus is now a mature infant, measures some 47 cm. and weighs approximately 2.7 kg. Due to the deposition of subcutaneous fat, the body has become more rotund and the skin less wrinkled and red. As though to improve its appearance before making its debut into the world, the fetus devotes the last two months in the uterus to putting on weight; and during this period gains 220 gm. a week. Its chances of survival are now as good as though born at full term.

MIDDLE OF TENTH LUNAR MONTH. Full term has now been reached and the fetus weighs on an average about 3 kg. if a girl and 3.4 kg. if a boy; its length approximates 50 cm. Its skin is now white or pink and thickly coated with the cheesy vernix. The fine, downy hair which previously covered its body has largely disappeared. The fingernails are firm and protrude beyond the end of the fingers.

DURATION OF PREGNANCY

The length of pregnancy varies greatly; it may range, indeed, between such wide extremes as 240 days and 300 days and yet be entirely normal in every respect. The average duration from the time of conception is 9½ lunar months, that is, 38 weeks or 266 days. From the first day of the last menstrual period its average length is 10 lunar months, that is, 40 weeks or 280 days. That these average figures mean very little, however, is shown by the following facts. Scarcely one pregnancy in ten terminates exactly 280 days after the beginning of the last period. Less than one-half terminate within one week of day 280. In 10 percent of cases, birth occurs a week or more before the theoretical end of pregnancy, and in another 10 percent, it takes place more than two weeks later than we would expect from the average figures cited above. Indeed, it would appear that some fetuses require a longer time, others a shorter time, in the uterus for full development.

TABLE 10-1
DEVIATION FROM CALCULATED DATE OF CONFINEMENT, ACCORDING TO NAEGELE'S RULE, OF 4,656 BIRTHS OF MATURE INFANTS

Deviation in days	Early Delivery	Delivery on Calculated Date	Late Delivery
0		189(4.1)*	—
1–5	860(18.5)*	—	773(16.6)*
6–10	610(13.1)	—	570(12.2)
11–20	733(15.7)	—	459(9.9)
21–30	211(4.5)	—	134(2.9)
31 and over	75(1.6)		42(0.9)

The menstrual cycles of the mothers were 28 ± 5 days. The infants were at least 47 cm. in length and 2,600 gm. in weight (Burger and Korompai).

* Numbers in parentheses represent percent of cases considered.

Source: Eastman, N. J., and Hellman, L. H.: *Williams Obstetrics*, ed. 13. New York, Appleton-Century Crofts.

CALCULATION OF THE EXPECTED DATE OF CONFINEMENT (EDC)

In view of the wide variation in the length of pregnancy, it is obviously impossible to predict the expected day of confinement (often abbreviated EDC) with any degree of precision. The time-honored method, based on the above "average figures," is simple. Count back three calendar months from the first day of the last menstrual period and add seven days (Naegele's rule). For instance, if the last menstrual period began on June 10, we would count back three months to March and, adding seven days, arrive at the date of March 17. An easier way to calculate this is to substitute numbers for months. Then, this example becomes: 6/10 − 3 months = 3/10 + 7 days = 3/17. Although it may be satisfying to the curiosity to have this date in mind, it must be understood that less than 5 percent of all pregnant women go into labor on the estimated date of confinement, and in 35 percent a deviation of from one to five days before or after this date may be expected (Table 10-1).

Yet, whether pregnancy terminates one week before or two weeks later than the day calculated, the outlook for mother and baby is usually as good as though it had ended at "high noon" on the due date.

Actually, women seldom go overterm; in most of these cases it is the system of calculation and not nature which has erred. For example, ovulation and, hence, conception may have occured some

days later than calculated; this error would make the beginning and the end of pregnancy that many days later. If, in addition to this circumstance, we were dealing with a fetus which required a slightly longer stay in the uterus for complete development, it would be clear that the apparent delay was quite normal and for the best.

PHYSIOLOGY OF THE FETUS AND PLACENTA

During the period when the ovum lies unattached in the uterine cavity, its nutriment is provided by an endometrial secretion, often called *uterine milk,* which is rich in glycogen. When burrowing into the endometrium, the ovum lies in a lake of fluid representing the broken-down product of endometrial cells and obtains nourishment from this source.

Very early in pregnancy, certainly by the third or the fourth week, the chorionic villi have blood vessels within them (connected with the fetal bloodstream), and since these villi have already opened up the maternal blood vessels, nourishment is available from the maternal blood via the placenta.

Placental Function

The human placenta is a truly versatile organ. It functions as a lung in the transfer of gases, as a gastrointestinal tract in the transport of nutrients, as a kidney in the excretion of wastes, as skin in the transport of heat, much like a liver in its conjugation of drugs and hormones, and as an endocrine gland through production of various protein and steroid hormones. The normal human term placenta weighs approximately 500 gm. and covers about one-quarter of the uterine wall. During the course of pregnancy its weight and mass increase in proportion with that of the fetus. The normal fetal to placental weight ratio at term is 6:1.

The structure and function of the placenta differs among mammalian species. Homo sapiens has a villous hemochorial placenta. It is villous because the fetal vessels are contained within fingerlike villi which extend into an intervillous space (Fig. 10-5). There they are bathed by maternal blood (hemo) which transfers nutrients from across the chorionic

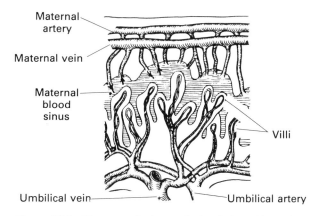

membrane (chorial) which constitutes the outer surface of the villi. Nutrient-rich and well-oxygenated blood enters the intervillous space via the maternal spiral arteries. This blood surrounds the villi which themselves contain fetal blood that has been delivered to them by the umbilical arteries, and therefore has been depleted of both nutrients and oxygen. An exchange occurs, during which oxygen and nutrients from the blood in the intervillous space are delivered into the blood contained in the villous capillaries. The newly restored blood is then returned to the fetus along the veins contained within the villi, which converge into the umbilical vein.

Figure 10-5. Diagram of placental circulation. Note that maternal and fetal circulations are completely separate. (From Chaffee, E. E., and Lytle, I. M.: *Basic Physiology and Anatomy*, ed. 4. Philadelphia, J. B. Lippincott, 1980.)

Fetoplacental Oxygen Exchange

The partial pressure of oxygen (PO_2) in the intervillous space is approximately 40 mm. of mercury. This is the highest oxygen tension to which the fetal circulation is exposed. At any given time the oxygen which is contained in the intervillous space is capable of satisfying fetal oxygen consumption for approximately one and a half minutes. On their way to the intervillous space, the spiral arteries traverse the muscular wall of the myometrium. With each uterine contraction the spiral arteries are compressed by the myometrium and blood flow through these vessels is interrupted. Thus delivery of oxygen to the intervillous space is interrupted. The normal fetus can tolerate this brief period of oxygen deprivation without damage. In certain cases of abnormal labor, when the contractions are unusually prolonged, the resulting anoxia could in time cause fetal damage.

The umbilical cord is the other vulnerable link in the system for maternal-fetal exchange of oxygen. Under certain conditions of labor the umbilical cord can be compressed, for example, between the fetal head and the pelvis, or entangled above the fetus. Prolonged interference with cord circulation can seriously affect fetal oxygenation.

On gross examination of the maternal side of the placenta, one can usually see approximately 20 cotyledons or lobes. These are further divided into approximately 200 lobules, each of which is a circulatory unit containing a single spiral artery. When a spiral artery becomes obstructed, as when there has been a thrombosis or organization of a clot within its lumen, the blood supply to that circulatory unit is interfered with, and the net result is tissue destruction or infarction of the area. Many term placentas contain an area of infarction. Fortunately, the placenta is endowed with a substantial reserve. It has been estimated that only half of the placental surface is required for maintaining a normal maternal-fetal exchange.

At the microscopic level, three layers of tissue separate the fetal circulation from the maternal blood. A molecule passing from the fetus to the mother must traverse these tissues. The outermost layer is that of the fetal trophoblast, which contains the outer syncytiotrophoblast and the inner cytotrophoblast. Immediately beneath is a connective tissue layer. The innermost layer is the endothelial layer of the fetal capillary itself. As pregnancy progresses, the fetal capillaries are brought closer and closer to the surface of the villi and thus exchange is facilitated. At term, the diffusion distance for a molecule is approximately 3.5 microns as compared to 0.5 microns in the adult lung.

Nutrition Placental Transmission

There are six well documented mechanisms for the transport of nutrients from the mother to the fetus: diffusion, facilitated diffusion, active transport, bulk flow, pinocytosis, and defects in placental membrane.

1. *Diffusion,* is the passage of a substance from one area to another on the basis of its concen-

tration gradient. Materials which are transported by diffusion include the respiratory gases, oxygen and carbon dioxide, the electrolytes, sodium and chloride, and some lipid soluble vitamins. The transport of gases is dependent on their partial pressures. The mechanism of diffusion is important because clinically evident placental failure is generally the result of a limitation in substances exchanged by diffusion.

2. *Facilitated diffusion,* the second important mechanism of transfer, involves passage along a concentration gradient that occurs when the concentration of material on the maternal side is greater than that on the fetal side. This kind of transfer occurs without the use of energy, but at a faster rate than can be explained on the basis of the concentration gradient alone, and is carrier mediated, that is, it is transferred by cellular elements which carry it into and through the membrane. Glucose, a most important fetal fuel, is transported by the mechanism of facilitated diffusion.

3. *Active transport,* the third mechanism, requires the passage of substances from one area to another against a concentration gradient, and it is energy dependent. This mechanism requires the expenditure of energy by the cells. Amino acids are transported against a 2 to 1 concentration gradient from mother to fetus. Iron, calcium, iodine, and water soluble vitamins are transported by the mechanism of active transport.

4. *Bulk flow,* the fourth mechanism, involves the transfer of substances by hydrostatic or osmotic gradients through micropores in the membrane. This mechanism is important in maintaining maternal–fetal exchange of water.

5. *Pinocytosis,* the fifth mechanism of transport, involves the transfer across a cell of materials contained in small vessels located at or near the cell membrane. Microdrops of plasma are taken up by the trophoblast and, in this way, immunoglobulins may reach the fetus.

6. *Breaks in the placental membrane* is the final mechanism by which substances are transported from mother to fetus. Defects in the placental membrane can allow the transfer of very large materials, such as red blood cells. This process is responsible for sensitization of the Rh negative woman carrying an Rh positive fetus. Rh positive fetal red blood cells are carried into the maternal circulation and produce antibodies. This occurs with greatest frequency at the time of delivery, when the incidence of breaks in the placental membrane is greatest.

Placental Permeability

Diffusion is the most important mechanism regulating the transfer of substances between mother and fetus, for impaired diffusion is often the cause of clinically evident placental dysfunction. Diffusion depends upon the characteristics of the placental membrane. It is purely a physical process and requires no energy. The process is governed by certain principles, which, in combination, are described in Fick's law. Fick's law states that the rate of transfer of materials is directly proportional to the permeability of the membrane and to the actual area of the membrane, but inversely proportional to the thickness of the membrane. This means that the more permeable the membrane and the greater the area presented by the membrane, the greater the rate of transfer. Conversely, the thicker the membrane, the slower the rate of transfer.

Other determinants of permeability for any molecule include the size of the molecule, as well as its molecular charge and lipid solubility properties. In general, molecules with a molecular weight greater than 1,000 do not cross the placental membrane. For example, the anticoagulant heparin is a large molecule which, because of its size, will not traverse the placental membrane, hence, heparin treatment can be used safely in pregnancy. In contrast, the anticoagulant Coumadin is a much smaller molecule which readily crosses the placenta and, when used in pregnancy, may affect the fetus.

Lipid solubility is an extremely important characteristic in the transport of drugs from mother to fetus, as is the electrostatic charge on the molecules themselves. Many of the narcotic agents and analgesics used in labor and delivery are designed to reach the maternal brain quickly in order to provide rapid pain relief. The characteristics which allow this rapid transport to the brain also allow them to cross the placental membrane rapidly, and thus they can equally quickly affect the fetal central nervous system.

Factors Influencing Placental Exchange

Blood Flow to Uteroplacental Circulation

In general, impaired exchange of carbon dioxide and oxygen is not usually related to problems of diffusion. There is little, if any, resistance to the diffusion of these molecules. Their transfer is most often affected by interference with blood flow into the intervillous space and back to the fetus. Oxygen is brought to the intervillous space by the maternal uterine circulation. Uterine blood flow at term is approximately 600 to 700 ml. per minute, representing 10 percent of the total maternal cardiac output. Almost 90 percent of the total uterine blood flow goes into the intervillous space, while 10 percent supplies the myometrium. The amount of blood which flows into the intervillous space is directly affected by the perfusion pressure within the uterine arteries themselves. Under resting conditions, uteroplacental circulation is widely dilated, and therefore has little capacity to expand further. This circulation is, however, capable of marked vasoconstriction, which occurs through hormonal or neural mechanisms. Hence uterine blood flow during pregnancy can be increased significantly by only one mechanism—maternal bedrest. At rest, blood flow to other organs and tissues, such as muscle and fat, is diminished and the supply of blood to the placenta and fetus is enhanced.

Many mechanisms exist by which blood flow to the uteroplacental circulation may be diminished. Each uterine contraction interrupts the supply of blood into the intervillous space. A contraction lasting 45 seconds stops the blood flow for approximately 30 seconds. During this interval, the fetus must exist on stored nutrients or on those present in the stagnant blood of the intervillous space. This stress is well tolerated by the normal fetus. Abnormally prolonged uterine contractions, or a decrease in maternal blood pressure can diminish blood flow to the uteroplacental circulation. For example, the large term uterus may compress the inferior vena cava, interfering with the return of blood to the right heart. Cardiac output and, therefore, delivery of blood to the uteroplacental unit are decreased. Diminished uterine blood flow can also result from chronic hypertension and pregnancy-induced hypertension due to vasoconstriction. Various pharmacologic agents such as vasopressers may also

cause constriction of these vessels. Finally, vigorous maternal exercise will increase blood flow to the muscles and may divert blood from the uteroplacental circulation.

Fetal Blood, Fetal Hemoglobin, Bohr Effect

Several other important determinants of oxygen transfer from mother to fetus should be considered. These include the actual affinity of fetal blood for oxygen, the concentration of fetal hemoglobin within the fetal blood, and the Bohr effect (to be discussed). *Fetal hemoglobin,* because of its special characteristics, has a greater affinity for oxygen than does maternal blood. By virtue of certain biochemical constituents, maternal hemoglobin has a greater capacity to unload oxygen, while fetal hemoglobin is endowed with a greater ability to accept oxygen. The actual concentration of hemoglobin in fetal blood is also greater than in maternal blood. Fetal blood contains 15 gm. of hemoglobin per 100 ml., in contrast to approximately 12 gm. per 100 ml. in the adult. Since hemoglobin is the agent which actually carries the oxygen, and since the fetus has more hemoglobin, a given unit of fetal blood can carry much more oxygen than can maternal blood.

The Bohr effect is the effect of pH on the ability of hemoglobin to accept or unload oxygen. A more acid pH is associated with an increased ability of hemoglobin to unload oxygen, while a more alkaline pH will increase the ability to accept oxygen. Blood returning from the fetal circulation in the umbilical artery is more acid, and therefore endowed with a greater capacity to unload oxygen. It reaches the intervillous space, where it gives up its hydrogen ions and carbon dioxide, and its pH rises. Concomitantly, these hydrogen ions and carbon dioxide are accepted by the maternal circulation, and the pH of the maternal blood decreases. The increased fetal pH results in a greater capacity to accept oxygen, and the decreased maternal blood pH results in a greater capacity to deliver oxygen. This is the Bohr effect.

Adjustments in Fetal Blood Flow

During periods of oxygen deprivation, fetal blood flow is redistributed. Increased amounts of blood are supplied to the fetal brain and heart, while blood flow to the fetal gastrointestinal tract is diminished. This helps to ensure survival of the most vital fetal organs during a time of temporary oxygen lack. Nature has endowed the fetoplacental unit with a unique system of checks and balances whose purpose is preservation of fetal well-being throughout pregnancy.

The Placenta as an Endocrine Organ

From very early pregnancy the cells which eventually form the placenta are hormonally active. Even before the skipped menstrual period the trophoblastic cells which have been responsible for allowing the embryo to invade into the endometrium have begun to secrete the hormone, human chorionic gonadotropin (hCG).

Human Chorionic Gonadotropin (hCG). This hormone (hCG) is produced by the syncytial cells of the trophoblast. It is a glycoprotein with a very large molecular weight of 36,000 to 40,000. It is similar to pituitary LH in both structure and activity, but it differs physiologically in that its levels are maintained in the circulation for longer periods of time. It is composed of two subunits: an alpha subunit, which is similar to the alpha subunit of pituitary glycoprotein hormones, and a beta subunit which is specific and unique to human chorionic gonadotropin. The beta subunit has recently been isolated and has been used to make antibodies for a pregnancy test, a test which is specific for human chorionic gonadotropin levels.

HCG appears in maternal blood by the eighth day after ovulation in the fertile cycle. Its levels increase steadily in early pregnancy, reaching a maximum in 60 to 90 days, and then the levels in the blood begin to fall. Very little hCG is secreted into the fetal compartment in comparison to the large quantities that are released in the maternal circulation. It is the circulating hCG that has served as the basis for all of the commonly used pregnancy tests.

Human Placental Lactogen (hPL)/Human Chorionic Somatomamotropin (hCS). The placenta produces a second protein hormone, human placental lactogen (hPL), also called human chorionic somatomamotropin (hCS). This hormone is also formed in syncytial cells within the trophoblast of the placenta. Its production increases progressively during pregnancy, with a very marked increase after the twentieth week. Very little hCS reaches fetal circulation. There is a distinct correlation between hCS levels and placental weight. For example, maternal hCS levels are higher in multiple gestations. This hormone has an action similar to human growth hormone, and its purpose is to regulate maternal metabolism so as to maintain a supply of nutrients for the fetus. Specifically, hCS facilitates transport of glucose across the placenta by the process of facilitated diffusion. As its name implies, hCS also has a mammotropic effect.

Progesterone and Estrogen. The placenta also produces the steroid hormones progesterone and estrogen. During the course of pregnancy there is a steady increase in *progesterone* levels which reach maximum just prior to delivery. This progesterone maintains the endometrium and endometrial blood supply, brings about uterine growth, inhibits the activity of the uterine muscle, and stimulates alveolar development in the maternal breast. It also has significant effects on the mother's metabolism.

The estrogens, estriol, 17B-estradiol, and estrone, are products of the placenta. Estriol is biologically the weakest of the three major estrogens, but it is produced in greatest quantity. Its production by the placenta involves a unique interplay between the fetal adrenals, fetal liver, and placenta. The raw material from which it is derived is produced by the fetal adrenal gland. This precursor to estriol is a weak androgen, dehydroepiandrosterone (DHA) sulfate. Ninety percent of all the estriol which is seen in pregnancy is derived from fetal adrenal DHA-sulfate. The fetal liver modifies DHA-sulfate further and converts it to a hormone, which the placenta can then use in estriol production. Thus, the requisites for the placenta to produce significant quantities of estriol are an intact fetal adrenal gland and a normally functioning fetal liver.

The placenta itself converts the modified DHA-sulfate into estriol. The estriol levels in the blood rise steadily during pregnancy. There is a positive correlation between urinary estriol excretion and fetal weight. The levels of the other two hormones, estradiol and estrone, parallel those of estriol in maternal blood.

The physiologic functions of the estrogens during pregnancy are multifold. They include stimulation of growth of the uterus and uterine placental blood flow, stimulation of contractile activity of the myometrium, and growth of mammary tissue. The

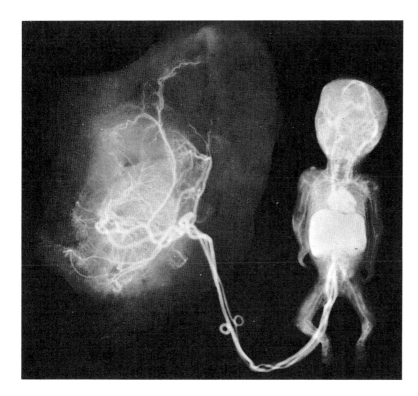

Figure 10-6. Roentgenogram showing fetal and placental circulation at 11 weeks gestation, injected with Thorotrast (a contrast medium) by Charles H. Hendricks, M.D., and Frederick P. Zuspan, M.D. (Department of Obstetrics and Gynecology, Western Reserve University)

estrogens also have significant effects on maternal metabolism.

Clinically it is important to understand the mechanism behind estrogen production by the placenta because estrogen levels can be used to detect certain deficiencies in the fetoplacental unit. If, for example, the placenta is not functioning properly (as in diabetes) the estrogens are not produced in normal amounts. Periodic determination of estrogen levels, either in the urine or in the blood, can be useful clinically in assessing the progress of such affected pregnancies.

EFFECTS ON THE NEWBORN. Maternal estrogen is transmitted to the fetus and produces certain effects in the newborn which may be very striking. First, as the result of the action of this hormone, the breasts of both boy and girl babies may become markedly enlarged during the first few days of life and even secrete milk—the so-called witch's milk (see Chapter 29, Breast Engorgement). Second, estrogen causes the endometrium of the female fetus to hypertrophy, as it does that of an adult woman. After birth, when this hormone is suddenly withdrawn, the endometrium breaks down, and bleeding sometimes occurs. For this reason, perhaps one girl baby in every fifteen manifests a little spotting on the diaper during the first week of life. This is entirely normal and clears up by itself within a few days.

FETAL CIRCULATION

Since the placenta acts as the intermediary organ of transfer between mother and fetus, the fetal circulation differs from that required for extrauterine existence. The fetus receives oxygen through the placenta, since the lungs do not function as organs of respiration in utero. To meet this situation, the fetal circulation contains certain special vessels ("bypasses" or "detours") which shunt the blood around the lungs, with only a small amount circulating through them for nutrition.

The oxygenated blood flows up the cord through the umbilical vein and passes into the inferior vena cava; on the way to the inferior vena cava, part of the oxygenated blood has gone through the liver, but most of it has passed through a special fetal structure, the *ductus venosus,* which connects the umbilical vein and the inferior vena cava (Fig. 10-6). The liver is proportionately large in a newborn infant because it receives a considerable supply of

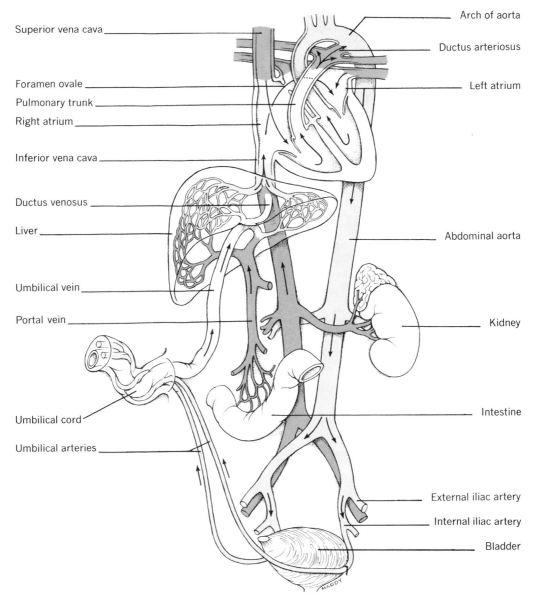

Figure 10-7. Diagram of the fetal circulation shortly before birth; course of blood is indicated by arrows. (From Chaffee, E. E., and Lytle, I. M.: *Basic Physiology and Anatomy*, ed. 4. Philadelphia, J. B. Lippincott, 1980.)

freshly vitalized blood directly from the umbilical vein.

From the inferior vena cava, the current flows into the right auricle and goes directly on to the left auricle through a special fetal structure, the *foramen ovale*, passing thence into the left ventricle and out through the aorta. The blood which circulates up the arms and the head returns through the superior vena cava to the right auricle again, but instead of passing through the foramen ovale, as before, the current is deflected downward into the right ventricle and out through the pulmonary arteries, partly to the lungs (for purposes of nutrition only), but mainly into the aorta through the special fetal structure, the *ductus arteriosus*.

The blood in the aorta, with the exception of that which goes to the head and the upper extremities (this blood has been accounted for), passes downward to supply the trunk and the lower extremities (Fig. 10-7). The greater part of this blood finds its

TABLE 10-2
CHANGES IN FETAL CIRCULATION AFTER BIRTH

Structure	Before Birth	After Birth
Umbilical vein	Brings arterial blood to liver and heart	Obliterated; becomes the round ligament of liver
Umbilical arteries	Brings arteriovenous blood to the placenta	Obliterated; become vesical ligaments on anterior abdominal wall
Ductus venosus	Shunts arterial blood into inferior vena cava	Obliterated; becomes ligamentum venosum
Ductus arteriosus	Shunts arterial and some venous blood from the pulmonary artery to the aorta	Obliterated; becomes ligamentum arteriosum
Foramen ovale	Connects right and left auricles (atria)	Obliterated usually; at times open
Lungs	Contain no air and very little blood	Filled with air and well supplied with blood
Pulmonary arteries	Bring little blood to lungs	Bring much blood to lungs
Aorta	Receives blood from both ventricles	Receives blood only from left ventricle
Inferior vena cava	Brings venous blood from body and arterial blood from placenta	Brings venous blood only to right auricle

Source: Williams, J. F.: *Anatomy and Physiology,* ed. 7. Philadelphia, W. B. Saunders.

way through the internal iliac, or hypogastric arteries, and so back through the cord to the placenta, where it is again oxygenated; but a small amount passes back into the ascending vena cava to mingle with fresh blood from the umbilical vein and again makes the circuit of the entire body.

Circulation Change at Birth

The fetal circulation is so arranged that the passage of blood to the placenta through the umbilical arteries and back through the umbilical vein is possible up to the time of birth, but it ceases entirely the moment the baby breathes and so begins to take its oxygen directly from its own lungs. During intrauterine life the circulation of blood through the lungs is for the nourishment of the lungs and not for the purpose of securing oxygen (Fig. 10-7).

In order to understand, even in a general way, the course of the blood current and how it differs from the circulation after birth, it must be remembered that in infants after birth, as in the adult, the venous blood passes from the two venae cavae into the right auricle of the heart, thence to the right ventricle and through the pulmonary arteries to the lungs, whence it gives up its waste products and takes up a fresh supply of oxygen. After oxygenation, the so-called arterial blood flows from the lungs, through the pulmonary veins to the left auricle, thence to the left ventricle and out through the aorta, to be distributed through the capillaries to all parts of the body and eventually collected, as venous blood, in the venae cavae and discharged again into the right auricle.

Circulation Path after Birth

As soon as the baby is born and breathes, the function of the lungs is established, and the placental circulation ceases. This change not only alters the character of the blood in many vessels, but also makes many of these vessels of no use as such: the umbilical arteries within the baby's body become filled with clotted blood and ultimately are converted into fibrous cords, and the umbilical vein within the body, after occlusion of the vessel, becomes the round ligament of the liver. After the umbilical cord is tied and separated, the large amount of blood returned to the heart and the lungs, which are now functioning, causes more or less equal pressure in both of the auricles—this pressure causes the foramen ovale to close. The foramen ovale remains closed and eventually disappears, and the ductus arteriosus and the ductus venosus finally shrivel up and are converted into fibrous cords or ligaments in the course of two or three months. The instantaneous closure of the foramen ovale changes the entire course of the blood current and converts the fetal circulation into the adult type.

The changes in the fetal circulation after birth are shown in Table 10-2.

PERIODS OF DEVELOPMENT

For the purposes of classification, human life has been divided into periods. The successive periods, with the duration of each, are indicated below.

THE PERIOD OF THE OVUM extends from fertilization to implantation, about the close of the first week of prenatal life. (The term ovum is used in a strict sense to denote the female germ cell and also to indicate the developing zygote, or fertilized ovum, prior to implantation.)

THE PERIOD OF THE EMBRYO extends from the second to the fifth weeks of gestation, during which time the various organs are developed and a definite form is assumed.

THE PERIOD OF THE FETUS extends from after the fifth week to the time of birth.

THE PERIOD OF THE NEWBORN (NEONATAL) extends from birth to the close of the first month of postnatal life.

THE PERIOD OF INFANCY extends from the close of the first month to the close of the second year of life.

THE PERIOD OF CHILDHOOD extends from the close of the second year to about the fourteenth year in females and to about the sixteenth year in males. Puberty ends the period of childhood.

THE PERIOD OF ADOLESCENCE extends from puberty to the last years of the second decade (late teens) in females and to the first years of the third decade (early 20s) in males.

THE PERIOD OF MATURITY extends from the end of the adolescent period to senility (old age).

Development goes on throughout life; during senility, retrogressive or degenerative changes occur.

SUGGESTED READING

Barnes, A. C.: *Intrauterine Development*. Philadelphia, Lea & Febiger, 1968.

Gruenwald P. *The Placenta*. Baltimore, University Park Press, 1975.

Moore, K. L.: *The Developing Human*. Philadelphia, W. B. Saunders, 1973.

Torpin, Richard: *The Human Placenta: Its Shape, Form, Origin and Development*. Springfield, Ill., Charles C Thomas, 1969.

Reproduction Control and Sexuality: Assessment and Management

Eleven

Common Concerns Related to Sexuality

*The Maternity Nurse as Sexual Counselor / Approaches
to Sexual Counseling / Common Sexual Problems
During Pregnancy and Postpartum / Educating Children
about Sex*

The area of human sexuality has become a specialty within the health care field. Professionals from various disciplines, including medicine, nursing, psychiatry, psychology, social work, and marriage counseling have undergone preparation with all degrees of formality to become equipped for handling sexual problems. A body of knowledge, a science, and an art have been developed for this specialty area of human sexuality, and they are growing rapidly. As more professionals participate in sex therapy, more research and empirical data are generated to expand the body of knowledge about sexuality. Across the country "institutes of human sexuality" are being formed by groups interested in this new branch of health care, offering services ranging from sex education to intensive therapy. Groups and individuals in private practice or associated with health care institutions are providing many other opportunities for diagnosis and treatment of sexual problems. Many resources are available with prepared specialists, although their therapeutic approaches often vary significantly.

Although the field of sexual therapy has become a sophisticated and complex specialty in certain ways, there are actually different levels of practice within the field related to the nature of the sexual problems. Because of changing public attitudes toward sex and a great increase in openness about sexuality in many channels of public communication and media, there is a greater expectation on the part of patients that health professionals will respond to sexual problems and concerns.

The nurse is an ideal member of the health care team to assume responsibility for counseling patients about sexuality, because of a background in the social, behavioral, and physical sciences as well as knowledge of counseling techniques. A comprehensive view of nursing care requires that nurses understand the relationship of sexuality to the particular patient's health needs or illness and the context of current living situations and sexual-affectional relationships in order to assess and utilize support systems. Patients need adequate sex information whether they are coping with an illness or striving to attain a higher level of health. The importance of a positive integration of one's sexuality has been repeatedly demonstrated:

Few authorities in human behavior would deny that sexual adjustment is prerequisite to an individual's maturation and successful adaptation to his environment. Indeed, history has demonstrated that the mental health of whole nations has been markedly influenced by the sexual attitudes and behavior of their citizenry—young and old, male and female alike. Scientific investigations

129

and clinical observations have confirmed the premise that sexual adjustment is positively correlated with well-timed, ongoing, accurate sex education presented in a wholesome, guilt-free manner.[1]

THE MATERNITY NURSE AS SEXUAL COUNSELOR

The care of the reproductive family is concerned with events intimately associated with sexual functioning and expression. This special area of nursing practice embraces a wide spectrum within the sexual-affectional system, although older concepts of "maternity care" viewed the processes in largely asexual terms. Pregnancy is a time of unusual sensuousness with increased feelings of masculine and feminine potency, voluptuous sexual expression in fantasy and behavior, and profound primitive satisfactions in bearing, nursing, and nurturing of children. Intuitively nurses have often sensed that the essence of the childbearing experience involves the mystery of life, as it springs forth in a sexual expression of creativity. Sexuality is undeniably an integral part of maternity nursing, and the nurse's vision must expand to recognize that sexuality is more than reproduction: it encompasses self-concept and roles and interpersonal relations as these relate to pregnancy, childbirth, parenting, contraception, abortion, and other specific facets of maternity care.

There are many opportunities for maternity nurses to provide sexual counseling as they work in prenatal, postnatal, and family planning clinics, physician's offices, hospital maternity units, and public health agencies. Nurses frequently conduct classes for expectant parents and classes in parenting or contraception. In any of these areas, concerns related to sexuality are likely to surface if the atmosphere is comfortable and accepting. The nurse who is prepared to deal with both information and feelings about sex will find no lack of opportunity to assist patients in a wide variety of settings.

The Nurse's Comfort with Sexuality

While it is always important for the nurse to be aware of his or her own feelings and attitudes toward a particular area of practice, human sexuality requires a level of self-understanding beyond that of most other areas. Nurses bring their personal experiences, values, and attitudes to the professional relationship; and these can either facilitate or obstruct the process of providing care to patients with sexual concerns and problems. A nurse who plans to provide sexual counseling must become comfortable with sexuality both generally and personally.

Becoming comfortable with sexuality can be undertaken as a deliberate process by the nurse. The first step involves gathering information through reading books and articles, viewing films, and attending workshops and symposia. It is a good idea to read popular as well as professional books, because this is where the public gets its information. Knowing the facts about sex enables the nurse to provide accurate information, teach with authority, and refute commonly held myths and misconceptions.

Examination and reexamination of personal attitudes is an ongoing part of becoming comfortable with sexuality. The nurse must identify prejudices and blind spots as well as positive and healthy feelings concerning various sexual practices. Personal definitions of normal and acceptable sexual expression must be carefully identified, and the extent to which these may affect the ability to assist patients in these areas assessed.[2]

The nurse-patient encounter is a constant feedback loop, and how the nurse is perceived by the patient when sexual matters come up is important in the nurse's effectiveness. Attitudes are communicated in numerous ways, both verbal and nonverbal, and people are always reading each other's subtle behavioral cues and responding accordingly. The nurse who is aware of her or his own attitudes and feelings, and is comfortable with sexuality, will be less likely to react with shock, ambivalence, or discomfort when patients reveal unusual or unexpected information related to sex. The ability to be accepting and understanding and to avoid passing judgment on others' sexual behaviors or concerns enables the nurse to provide care more effectively.

A Framework for Sexual Counseling

Sexual counseling is basically talking to people about their sex-related problems and concerns. This can occur at various levels of depth and complexity and involve problems of differing severity and character. The role of the maternity nurse in providing sexual counseling is determined by the individual nurse's background and expertise as well as the origin and severity of the sexual problem of the patient. Sexual problems range from those involving gender identity, such as hermaphroditism and transsexualism, to those resulting from misinformation, confusion about the normal sexual response cycle, and minor sexual dysfunctions. The different levels of sexual problems can be approached by dividing them into three (often overlapping) categories: problems of knowledge, relationship, and attitudes.

Problems of Knowledge

These are the most common and simple types of sexual problems, and usually arise out of misinformation or ignorance. A couple may fail to appreciate the erotic significance of the clitoris, be unaware of differing tempos of sexual arousal, have the idea that sex during pregnancy might injure or mark the baby, think that oral sex indicates latent homosexuality, expect the woman's sex drive to be decreased during pregnancy and be worried when it increases, and so forth. Lack of knowledge about changes in sexual drive and eroticism during pregnancy which often happen to both partners can be a cause of misunderstanding and conflict.

Fears created by minor unpleasant symptoms may lead to avoidance of sex when there is no understanding of the physiology or of what can be done. For the woman, the common symptom of painful intercourse during pregnancy can be related to a number of factors: vaginitis causing perineal or vulval irritation, insufficient vaginal lubrication due to inadequate foreplay, normal uterine contractions during orgasm setting off Braxton-Hicks contractions, or increased pelvic pressure due to the presenting part deep in the pelvis. These can be alleviated with proper medical treatment, explanation of physiological causes of the pain, and teaching of techniques to heighten arousal or increase comfort. In this way, a potential stressor to the relationship and the couple's adaptation to pregnancy can be removed.

Couples need specific information about practical matters regarding sex and pregnancy. For instance, there is no good reason in the absence of complications to avoid sex during late pregnancy or postpartum once lochia has ceased. The couple's own comfort and desires are their best guide when there is no physical pathology. However, understanding the vagaries of sexual drive during this time could prevent development of conflicts which might set up negative patterns as the couple tries to cope with the many demands of impending or new parenthood.

Nurses working with adolescents and young adults, as in family planning clinics, will find innumerable problems of knowledge related to sexuality. This is a setting in which provision of information can have an enormous impact on developing sexual practices and adjustments and can prevent many potential future problems involving unwanted pregnancy and sexual dysfunctions. Problems of knowledge related to sexuality are clearly within the scope of maternity nursing practice, and with the addition of specific factual content and a sense of comfort with sexuality to the nurse's repertory, this kind of sexual counseling can be readily carried out.

Problems of Relationship

A second level of sexual problems involves relationships between partners, and these may or may not fall within the scope of maternity nursing practice. This would depend largely on the nature of the given problem and the individual nurse's counseling skills. Communication problems between the partners are the most common types of relationship problems. The sending and receiving of messages between people is a highly complex symbolic process, with many variations of style and receptivity. Both sender and recipient must be attuned and ready for clear communication to take place; consequently there are often garbled messages and failures of communication.

In the area of sexual needs and preferences, good communication is even more difficult than in most interpersonal situations. People find it hard to talk about their own sexual feelings or to accept criticism or suggestions regarding sexual performance. Communication is often faulty concerning sexual practices which one partner may dislike but is embarrassed to discuss or may desire but is unable to ask for. Open and candid discussion of sexual preferences between partners can often dramatically improve satisfaction; but many fears about propriety, hurting the other's feelings, not knowing how to say it, or being embarrassed prevent this communication from occurring.

A first step, and one the maternity nurse could take in dealing with common sexual problems such as painful intercourse, lack of interest in sex, early ejaculation and nonorgasm, is to encourage the couple to talk with each other about what they like and do not like in sex. If they can settle on practices which are comfortable and enjoyable to both of them, often the problem will be resolved.

Many other factors complicate communication, however. The bedroom as a battlefield and sex with a hidden agenda are familiar syndromes to those involved in marital counseling. Perceptions of male and female roles may hamper communication: for example, the notion that the woman is there to serve the man sexually, that her enjoyment of sex is secondary and her sexual needs do not deserve much attention. Or a struggle for power and dominance may be raging between the pair, part of the game being frustrating the other sexually or doling out sex as a reward for compliance. Anger over real or imagined wrongs may interfere with giving oneself freely to the sexual experience or may be expressed in a desire to hurt the other partner, either mentally or physically.

Such situations create barriers to clear communication about sexual needs and preferences. They represent problems in the couple's relationship that must be worked out before the sexual problem itself can be resolved. If the maternity nurse is skilled in family or marital counseling, then she or he is equipped to deal with these relationship problems. Since sexual difficulties are part of the symptomatology, it is frequently necessary for the counselor to have an understanding of sexual physiology and be familiar with basic sex therapy techniques to be able to provide effective care.

Problems of Attitudes

Attitudes toward sexuality and the sexual self result from internalized beliefs and values, originating from earliest childhood and often rooted in the unconscious levels of the psyche. This represents the third and most complex level of sexual problems. Arising from the individual's psychological conflicts, the more common of these sexual problems include impotence, premature ejaculation, nonorgasm, vaginismus, and lack of arousal. The underlying mechanism in the great majority of these sexual dysfunctions is fear. Whether this fear has its origins in sociocultural values, religious inhibitions and guilt, negative early experiences, familial patterns of dominance and discipline, or temporary functional failures of performance, it is the catalyst which sets into motion the psychodynamics producing the sexual problem. This fear, the fear of inadequacy in sexual performance, is the most significant deterrent to effective sexual functioning because it completely distracts the individual from her or his natural responsiveness by blocking reception of sexual stimuli. Both partners eventually become self-conscious, worrying about his or her own and each other's sexual performance. Crippling tensions can develop in the relationship as frustrations and dissatisfactions mount. Obviously problems of attitudes and relationship often overlap. It is unlikely that the partner can remain uninvolved when a sexual problem occurs.

Numerous therapeutic approaches have been developed to help people with such sexual problems. These range from intensive residential sexual therapy to short-term behavior modification. Frequently a process of reeducation is used to modify negative attitudes and counteract inhibitive beliefs. Combined with teaching effective techniques for sexual stimulation, these approaches have a reasonably good success rate.

When deep anxieties, unresolved guilt or conflict, or other psychopathology is present, the person usually receives some kind of psychotherapy aimed at the specific problem. Many sex therapists prefer not to delve into old conflicts, however, but focus on changing the problematic behavior with a variety of sexual techniques. Whatever the cause, they reason, removal of the symptom will bring immediate relief and perhaps result in satisfactory long-term functioning without the need for extensive insight therapy.

Nurses have become involved in this type of sex therapy after undergoing additional education in human sexuality and training in specific techniques for treating sexual problems. This level of sexual counseling is specialty practice and is often provided by a team, using the cotherapist approach (one therapist of each sex) in an extensive program involving education, attitude change, setting a permissive environment for sexual experiencing, marital counseling or psychotherapy, and application of appropriate techniques of sex therapy. The scope of maternity nursing practice usually does not include this kind of sexual therapy, unless the nurse has been specially prepared and works in a setting that provides these services.

APPROACHES TO SEXUAL COUNSELING

Sexual counseling fits well into the nursing process, and the same principles and approaches apply to this area of nursing care as apply to others. The assessment phase concerns gathering information about the patient's past and current experiences with sex, how sexual knowledge was obtained, key attitudes toward sexuality, and difficulties as manifest in questions or symptomatologic behavior. The person's sexual self-concept, relationship with sexual partner(s), and health status of both partners are also explored in the history. From the assessment phase the nurse is able to form conclusions about the nature of sexual concerns or problems—in essence, to diagnose the problem. Identification of the problem provides the basis for planning care or intervention.

Nursing intervention is directed at assisting the patient or couple to find methods of alleviating their sexual difficulties. Many approaches may be utilized in this process, including the nurse providing facts about the sexual response cycle and the ranges of normal sexual experiences, teaching techniques to heighten sexual arousal or delay orgasm, facilitating better communication between partners, or assisting the couple to find sources of in-depth sexual therapy or marital counseling through referral. When illness or physical problems are involved, consultation with a physician is often necessary. A wide range of resources can be used to deal with problems ranging from economic relief to child care, as any of these may adversely affect sexual functioning.

Evaluation of the effectiveness of care is an essential component of the nursing process. This is accomplished through return visits in which progress is assessed. It is often necessary to alter approaches, try new approaches, or examine what factors are interfering with satisfactory resolution of the problem, which in itself is frequently therapeutic. Simple sexual problems may resolve surprisingly rapidly through the reassurance of accurate information, and altering the context in which sexual activity occurs. However, there may be many layers of difficulty, and dealing with an apparently simple problem may reveal more deep-seated conflicts, requiring specialty referral.

The Sexual History

A sexual history can be incorporated into the usual history taken in a given setting, such as the menstrual and contraceptive history, pregnancy history, and gynecologic history. It flows nicely when included in assessment of the reproductive system; in fact, it should probably be a standard part of data gathering regardless of setting or area of practice. In clinics or services dealing specifically with sexual problems, the sexual history will, of course, be more detailed and the center of focus. But, even in the absence of indications of sexual problems, the information gathered serves a number of purposes which enhance the nurse-patient relationship and provide a broader base for nursing care.

The most obvious outcome of taking a sexual history is provision of a base for identifying present or potential sexual problems, from which nursing intervention can be planned, either therapeutic or preventive. Additionally, gathering information about the couple's sexual experiences and attitudes demonstrates that the nurse is comfortable talking about sex. By taking the initiative in bringing up the subject, the nurse implicitly gives them permission to discuss sexual concerns. This legitimizes sexuality as an important component of health and an integral part of care for reproductive families and indicates that sexual counseling is an appropriate part of care they can expect to receive from health providers.[3]

Varying degrees of formality may be used in taking a sexual history, although it is generally best to have a flexible structure so the discussion can go in the direction the patient wants it to go. If forms are used, they should be relatively short and simple, to keep writing at a minimum and allow the nurse to focus attention on the interaction. Principles of conducting a sexual history include proceeding from more general to specific areas, from common to unusual, from simple to complex, and using conditional statements which assume a range of behavior.

Sexual History During Pregnancy

Sexual expression during pregnancy is influenced by the physical and emotional changes which happen at this time, as well as attitudes and beliefs about sex during pregnancy. Difficulties can arise as a result of myths, misconceptions, and a lack of understanding of the physiology and emotional dynamics of couples during pregnancy. Questions related to the sexual self-concept, relationship, physical status, and attitudes are included in the sexual history:

How does the pregnancy make you feel? (asked of both)

How do you feel about changes in appearance and emotions?

How do you feel about each other's experience of the pregnancy?

What are your feelings about sex during pregnancy?

Has the pregnancy made many changes in your life and sexual relationship?

How do you think having a baby will change your life? How do you plan to manage these changes?

What have you heard about that you should or should not do sexually during pregnancy?

How do you feel physically, what medications do you take, have you had any recent changes in your health?

Are there any concerns or worries about your sexual relationship during pregnancy or afterwards?

Even if there are no significant sexual problems associated with the pregnancy, most couples have many questions about sexual activities and their sexual responses during this time and appreciate the opportunity to discuss these. Openly discussing the many changes during pregnancy with implications for sexuality can prepare the couple for potential reactions and prevent the development of conflicts and tensions in their relationship stemming from misunderstandings of physiological changes and psychodynamics.

COMMON SEXUAL PROBLEMS DURING PREGNANCY AND POSTPARTUM

There are a wide range of sexual problems which couples may encounter during pregnancy. Sexual problems of a dysfunctional nature include dyspa-

reunia (painful intercourse), changing and conflicting sexual drives, and impotence.[4] These problems may be specifically related to the pregnancy and a function of the couple's psychobiological responses, or they may represent deeper-seated difficulties brought to the surface by the psychological effects of pregnancy. Other common problems include the avoidance of intercourse, breast feeding and erotic response, and lack of arousal or dyspareunia during the postpartal period.

Changes in Sex Drive

Alterations in the woman's level of sensuousness and sexual responsiveness are undoubtedly very widespread during pregnancy. These may be a problem for some couples and rather insignificant for others. In early pregnancy, some women experience a heightened sexuality, enjoy sex more, and seek it frequently. Their general level of sensuousness may increase, with heightened awareness and responsiveness to stimuli. Other women have decreased sex drive during the first two to three months of gestation, often because of nausea, bloating, breast soreness, fatigue, and the many other physical changes women experience at this time. As pregnancy reaches its midpoint, heightened sexuality becomes more common, with many women reporting an increase in erotic feelings, more interest in sex, active seeking of sexual encounters with partners, and, not uncommonly, occurrence of first orgasms. The physiologic changes of pregnancy, including increased pelvic vascularity and vasocongestion, contribute to this phenomenon.[5]

During the first trimester, the pregnant woman is very aware of her pelvis. The feeling of fullness, the sharpened sensations, and the round ligament twinges that may occur deep in the groin with sudden movement all give rise to some anxiety. Even though she may have had previous successful pregnancies and enjoyed sexual relations, she still tends to view these symptoms as possible threats to the pregnancy. If there is occasional (common) spotting, there is all the more reason for her to believe (however mistakenly) that the pregnancy is in danger. Very different sensations from those usually experienced occur with deep penile penetration with an enlarging soft uterus, although the uterus is still entirely in the pelvis. This does not imply that intercourse should not take place or that thrusting or movement need be curtailed. However, it does have implications for the woman's immersing herself in the pleasures of sexual stimulation, since she may be preoccupied with these other thoughts and sensations. Hence, she may not be orgasmic on all occasions or as often as is usual for her. This preoccupation may also give rise to unpredictableness in her general sexual desire. If there appear to be large changes from what is usual, concern may be generated in both partners. It is important for them to understand that the time of pregnancy can be one of the most anxiety-free, spontaneous sexual interludes of a couple's life. They can be counseled that intercourse poses no threat to pregnancy under normal circumstances. If they have been reasonably comfortable with their sexuality before the pregnancy, and there are no unusual problems, there is no reason to anticipate that their sexual *activity* need be curtailed.

If there are times when intercourse should wait a few days because of the psychic factor, there need not be a limitation of any of the other variations of sexual stimulation and orgasmic release for either the man or the woman. Sexual techniques may need modification due to the breasts' and genitals' increased sensitivity. As the secretions increase and change in character, there may be an accompanying odor which need not be unpleasant if standards of hygiene are maintained daily. Medication and/or douching may be required if there is the yeast overgrowth common to pregnancy. The physician will prescribe these as needed and the nurse can be helpful in eliciting the needed information about the existence of any of these problems in the patient.

In the second trimester, early in the fourth month, the uterus enlarges rather rapidly and becomes an abdominal organ rather than a pelvic organ. The expectant mother has usually adapted to the pelvic awareness and does not approach intercourse so gingerly. However, with the rapidly enlarging abdomen, new concerns are engendered regarding crushing the fetus. While these are not valid concerns, they are very real to both partners. The fetus is very well protected by the uterus and the abdominal wall, but the enlarging uterus can get in the way about the fifth month if the partners assume the top and bottom position for intercourse. Hence, modifications in positioning may be needed. Since the uterus is not pressing down in the vagina, there is not the feeling of hitting an immovable object with penetration.

Vaginal bleeding during the second trimester is very unusual. Even abortions and premature deliveries during this period are not generally preceded by bleeding, but by cramping and a gush of amniotic fluid. Stress incontinence of urine (losing urine with coughing, sneezing, or orgasm) may continue into this trimester, since the uterus is pressing on the bladder, although it is out of the pelvis. This incontinence is sometimes confused with a gush of amniotic fluid and can be frightening during intercourse.

Intercourse using the side position can be successful, and from a purely mechanical point of view, is necessarily gentle. As the uterus grows larger, the expectant mother is usually much more comfortable lying on her side, with her uterus supported by a pillow. If she is on her back for any length of time, with the enlarged uterus pressing on the great blood vessels in the abdomen, there may be problems with hypotension and lightheadedness. Using a pillow under the hips during intercourse can be helpful in avoiding hypotension.

It is well to remember that the maintenance of sexual activity does not have to include intercourse per se, and often the female genitalia are so sensitive that the woman is not interested in intercourse and many prefer alternate practices or caressing.

As the woman's abdomen increases in size, giving evidence of the pregnancy, the couple may respond with feelings of shame or of pride. To some women, the change in body image is an unwelcome development, making them feel unattractive; others take pleasure in this evidence of the growing fetus and feel a sense of heightened potency. These feelings affect sexual response. Men also react to the woman's changing shape: some feel their partner is more beautiful and sexy, others are turned off by the perceived distortion of the woman's body. Such feelings have a significant impact upon the man's sexual responsiveness, and naturally upon the woman's response to him. The woman's emotional lability and fluctuating sexual drives are often confusing for both the expectant father and mother. Fathers undergo psychological processes in pregnancy similar to the mothers' and may have symptoms and alternating periods of emotional stability and well-being and times of anxiety, unexplained fears, and compulsions.[6]

Communication between the expectant parents is very important if they are to understand their own and each other's responses to this time of emotional change and uncertainty. There is a tendency for women to withdraw as they become preoccupied with their physical and emotional changes and the psychological tasks related to incorporating and differentiating the baby, as well as preparations for motherhood. The father may at times feel excluded and seek other sources of understanding, support, and companionship.

Dyspareunia During Pregnancy

Painful intercourse during pregnancy can result from a number of causes. Pressure on the pregnant abdomen may cause a generalized discomfort. Deep penile thrusting may be painful when there is pelvic congestion, the presenting part is deep in the pelvis, or certain positions are assumed which exaggerate pressure. Although vaginal secretions are increased during pregnancy, in some instances there may be a relative lack of lubrication due to inadequate stimulation, leading to discomfort with intercourse. Irritation of the perineum or introitus secondary to vaginitis causes burning or pain on penetration and during intercourse. Cramps and backache may occur following coitus due to increased vasocongestion of sexual arousal combined with that of pregnancy. Orgasm may initiate Braxton-Hicks contractions, which may continue and cause considerable pain. Or aching postcoital pain may result from lack of orgasm to assist removal of the pelvic congestion associated with plateau levels of sexual arousal. If the woman experiences conflicts about having intercourse while pregnant, there may be a psychological overlay with the dyspareunia.

Avoidance of Sex

Misinformation and fears about the effects of intercourse during pregnancy on the mother and the fetus can prompt couples to avoid or abstain from intercourse. Common fears are that the baby will be injured or marked in some way or be aware of the parents having sex. If a previous baby was born with some kind of physical or mental impairment, this fear may be strong though rarely expressed. Some couples also fear injury to the mother, particularly if she experiences painful intercourse. The widespread practice of advising sexual abstinence

during the last part of pregnancy may reinforce these fears of injury. For couples accustomed to frequent, regular intercourse, prolonged abstinence can be a real hardship and may encourage extramarital relations. It is now generally accepted that intercourse poses no problems in late pregnancy if there are no complications. Once membranes have ruptured or labor has begun, or if there is vaginal bleeding, intercourse should be avoided. When premature labor threatens and intercourse is proscribed because orgasm can initiate uterine contractions, the couple must also be advised against oral or manual stimulation which can produce orgasm.

Impotence During Pregnancy

Occasionally men find themselves unable to attain or maintain an erection during their partner's pregnancy. This is a type of secondary impotence; it may be a situational phenomenon with no long-term repercussions, or it may indicate a more significant psychological problem with sexual dysfunction. Almost all men, at one time or another, will fail to have an erection during a sexual encounter for a vast complex of reasons. This does not signify impotence and is usually connected with being upset, tired, preoccupied, or having too much alcohol. As men experience emotional upheavals during pregnancy, they may at certain times be disinterested in sex because of other psychological processes. For some, a reawakening of maternal relationships and the projection of this relationship onto their pregnant wife create conflicts interfering with erotic response. If the woman's body is perceived as unattractive, sexual arousal may be blocked. This may also occur when the man fears injuring the mother or fetus, or if he is feeling a close identification with his partner in vicariously experiencing the pregnancy.

Inability to attain erection on occasion during pregnancy, as at other times, does not constitute a true sexual problem unless the couple perceives it as such. Expectations of male performance create enormous pressures on men and often exaggerate fears of inadequacy which further interfere with sexual arousal, perpetuating the difficulty in having or maintaining erections. Only when a man does not achieve penile erection in 25 percent of his sexual attempts, is he considered to be impotent.[7]

Breast Feeding and Erotic Response

The physiology of sexual responses includes changes in the breasts which have characteristic variations during lactation. The contractile tissues surrounding the milk ducts contract during orgasm and may result in milk spurting out during sexual arousal and orgasm. Sexual stimulation may produce a "let down" reflex, causing milk to leak or spurt. If this is a concern to the couple, the woman can wear a bra with absorbent pads, and pressure on the breasts can be avoided. Breast tenderness can also present a problem postpartally, but this is a temporary condition and the couple can avoid breast stimulation until the soreness subsides.

Another relatively common occurrence is sexual arousal in response to the baby's suckling. This may range from pleasant, mild excitation to orgasm. If women are aware that this is a normal response and does not indicate they are somehow perverted, they may become comfortable with this experience. Some women discontinue breast feeding, however, because they cannot accept these responses. Women who breast feed also tend to resume intercourse sooner postpartally than those who do not, presumably because of increased eroticism associated with breast feeding.

Postpartal Dyspareunia or Lack of Arousal

During the first six months following delivery, the vagina does not lubricate well because of relatively low levels of steroid hormones, which inhibit the vasocongestive response to sexual stimulation. There is also a time period of some three to six weeks needed for the healing process to occur after childbirth, involving episiotomy, cervical, vaginal or perineal lacerations, and the site of placental attachment. Couples are usually advised to resume intercourse by the third or fourth postpartal week, if the bleeding has stopped and the episiotomy is not painful. Their own comfort and sexual desires are used as the guide for resumption of intercourse in the absence of contraindications.

However, women are at times concerned with their lack of sexual response in the months following childbirth. Taking their mothering responsibilities into consideration, with the lack of sleep, fatigue,

and juggling of activities this usually requires, it is not surprising that their sexual interest might be low even without the additional factor contributed by their sexual physiology after delivery. Understanding this may alleviate fears and enable women to await full restoration of their hormonal and physical status. Residual tenderness of the perineum or vagina can also contribute to painful intercourse as well as lack of interest in sex. Vaginitis can result from low estrogen levels, further creating problems with dyspareunia. Fears that intercourse may be permanently affected by pregnancy, labor, and delivery grow out of the belief that these cause damage to the woman's genitalia. Painful intercourse and lack of arousal during the postpartal period can be taken as evidence that these fears have been realized unless the couple can be assisted to understand the physiological processes of childbirth and of the postpartal period and their true effects on sexual functioning.

EDUCATING CHILDREN ABOUT SEX

Parents are often concerned about sex education for their children, and a wide range of values are connected with where and who is responsible for this. Developing positive attitudes toward sexuality is very important, but so is conducting sexual activities responsibly. Guilt or conflicts arising from inadequate sex knowledge interfere with learning and schoolwork, happy relationships, and future adjustments with sexual partners. Anxiety due to lack of understanding and confusion about sexual feelings inhibits the freedom of the sexual response, which can lead to various types of sexual dysfunctions. The greater the amount of accurate sex information, the less the anxiety; therefore, sex education is an important method of preventing sexual problems.

Sex Education in the Schools. Public schools are assuming increasing responsibility for sex education, and about 71 percent of parents do favor this as part of school curricula.[8] Parents are often concerned about the quality of sex education in the schools, however. Some feel the information is presented in a dry, dehumanized way that does not assist children to understand the emotional com-

NURSING CARE: SEXUAL PROBLEMS IN PREGNANCY AND POSTPARTUM

Problem	Assessment	Intervention	Evaluation
Changes in Sex Drive	Stage of pregnancy and associated physical and emotional symptoms. Level of couple's understanding of psychophysiology of pregnancy. Attitudes toward sex in pregnancy. Communication patterns.	Reinforce accurate knowledge. Teach correct information, clear misconceptions. Reassure about normality of fluctuating sex drives. Support clear communication.	Concern decreased. Couple feels comfortable with changing sex drives.
Dyspareunia in Pregnancy	When this occurs, associated factors and symptoms. Techniques of intercourse. Adequacy of stimulation. Perineal irritation due to vaginitis.	Instruct on alternate techniques and positions. Discuss arousal patterns. Refer for treatment of vaginitis. Teach normal variations of pregnancy (Braxton-Hicks contractions with orgasm, backache).	Comfortable intercourse attained, or acceptable alternative found.
Avoidance of Sex	Reasons why sex is avoided (fears, misconceptions, told by physician, etc.). Difficulties this poses to the couple. Attitudes toward sex in pregnancy.	Correct misinformation and teach normal fetal-maternal development. Inform when sex should be avoided and reasons why. Discuss alternatives to intercourse.	Fears and misinformation cleared, no longer avoid sex when not medically necessary. Use acceptable alternatives if indicated.
Impotence	Extent of the problem, how often this occurs. Level of couple's concern. Level of understanding of the man's psychophysiology in pregnancy.	Teach about normal male reactions and psychological processes. Reassure normality of occasional inability to maintain or attain erection. Refer to specialist if problem is extensive.	Concern decreased. Able to have intercourse often enough to satisfy both partners.
Breast feeding and erotic response	Loss of milk with arousal or orgasm. Extent to which this poses problem to the couple. Arousal or orgasm with nursing, level of concern about this.	Advise regarding normality of milk loss. Suggest wearing bra with absorbent pads if a problem. Avoid pressure or stimulation of breasts. Advise of normality of arousal during nursing. Discuss discomfort and concern, meaning of this to woman.	Comfortable with methods to prevent milk loss from interfering with sex. Able to accept erotic feelings and continue nursing.
Postpartum Dyspareunia and Lack of Arousal	When symptoms occur, how often, associated with what factors. Weeks or months postpartum and stage of involution. Contraceptive use. Techniques of arousal and intercourse. Level of understanding of postpartal physiology. Perineal irritation due to vaginitis.	Teach normal postpartal physiology and hormonal effects. Reinforce that arousal levels are often lower at this time. Discuss techniques of arousal, advise lubricants if needed. Refer for treatment of vaginitis. Discuss approaches to managing home and family demands to provide the couple with private time.	Concern decreased. Comfortable with level of sexual arousal. Comfortable intercourse attained or acceptable alternative found.

ponents of sexuality. Others fear that too much will be presented too rapidly, and the children will not be well assisted to process this information or the ethical issues will not be addressed. Valid concerns over the qualifications of those teaching sex education are voiced, because few schools specifically train teachers for this sensitive subject. Teachers who are embarrassed, uncomfortable, and ill-in-formed, or who conduct their classes in a strained, mechanical manner will not enhance the development of healthy, positive attitudes toward sexuality.

Parental Responsibility. Parents need to assume a major responsibility in teaching their children about sex, recognizing that inevitably much information will come from such other sources as peers, older children, pornography, and mass media. One of the best ways of teaching is by the example of a caring, committed relationship between parents and the parents' comfort in answering sexual questions as they arise. Touching and physical expression of love among family members helps create a climate of acceptance of one's sexuality and body. Flexibility in habit training and weaning also prevents conflicts from developing over these primitive levels of sexuality and allows the young child's emotional and physical needs to unfold naturally.

Genital Exploration. Infants and small children touch their genitals as part of necessary exploration of the body, and parents need not discourage this activity. When the child is about three years old, parents can advise him or her that handling genitals in public is not polite. Children usually will not spend an inordinate amount of time with this self-stimulation if they are comfortable in their family environment. Any compulsive behavior which preoccupies a child can signify an emotional conflict, however, whether the behavior is masturbation, scratching, eating, talking, or something else. Giving the child the message that any part of his or her body or normal functions is bad or dirty can create guilt and conflicts later.

"Playing doctor" and other games involving genital exploration among children are very common. Parents occasionally find children at such games. Most feel the need to intervene in some way to assist children to learn the socially acceptable modes of sexual expression, but want to avoid causing a negative conditioning toward sexuality. Letting the children know this is not the time or place for such activities, without making them feel they are doing something terrible, can accomplish this goal.

Nudity in the home may be one way to dignify sexuality and body comfort. However, parents should be comfortable with nudity if they want to use this method, or else a negative or strained attitude might be communicated, which can confuse the child. Also, parents need to be ready to deal with the child's touching their breasts or genitals, which is a natural way children explore and learn. If parents act shocked or slap the child's hand, another double message is communicated; parents can limit touching with gentle expression of personal preferences and privacy needs.

Basic Explanations. When children encounter objects they do not recognize, their natural curiosity leads them to ask what these are for, as with sanitary napkins, tampons, or contraceptives. Simple explanations about normal body functions in a matter-of-fact tone are readily accepted by children. Usually short answers are enough, but if parents discuss more than they think the child can absorb, the child will not be dismayed as long as there is no sense of fear, embarrassment, or discomfort. Children will ask additional questions later to clarify what they have not fully understood.

Accurate explanations of the processes of menstruation, childbirth, erection and nocturnal ejaculations, development of secondary sexual characteristics, and sexual intercourse will enable children to attain comfortable sexual feelings. These explanations usually occur over many years, may be repeated several times at various levels of sophistication, and can occur spontaneously following the child's questions or be deliberately planned by parents. Actually, the process involves a combination of both, with reinforcements and clarifications as children process the information. Probably the basic sex education should be completed by about age nine, as girls may menstruate around ten to eleven and boys have wet dreams at this age also. More discussion of intercourse, sexual expression, and contraception is needed during the early adolescent years.

Sexual Terminology. Using correct anatomic and physiologic terms when discussing genitals or sexual matters aids understanding and prevents problems in communicating. It is no more difficult for a child to learn to say penis or vagina than such slang terms as pee-pee and ding-dong, and it gives more dignity and acceptability to the sexual parts of the body.

Children pick up sexual words from many sources and usually sense when such terms or expressions are provocative or inappropriate. They may test parents' responses by suddenly saying the word with a straight face. Again, a calm reply with a straightforward explanation of the meaning of the obscenity or sexual term is best. Then the child can be advised as to how the family feels about the use of the word or expression. By repeating the word, parents demonstrate that they are not upset or hurt by its usage or by other expressions, such as swear words or obscenities, and that it is useless to use them as a weapon or an attention-getting devise. Children also learn that parents are willing to respond to sensitive areas of sexuality in a comfortable manner.

Teenage Sex

Parents find teenage sex a thorny issue, and one they are often uncomfortable with. For many good reasons, they desire children to postpone intensive sexual involvements until they are emotionally mature enough to handle the powerful feelings associated with these kinds of relationships. Helping teenagers to recognize that there are many types of sexual expression not involving intercourse may be one approach, as is teaching sexual ethics about respecting the other person and relating with concern and caring. Teenagers can find a wide range of expression, through masturbation, close physical contact without intercourse, dating and doing activities together, kissing, daydreaming, and having caring friendships with each other. Postponing intercourse until they feel ready can do much to prevent conflicts and tensions or the establishment of dysfunctional sexual patterns that can later plague the individual's expression of sexuality. Parents need to communicate the idea of responsible sex to adolescents, in terms of avoidance of pregnancy, venereal disease, and emotional exploitation or injury to others.[9]

Objectives of Sex Education

Given that there are differences in religious traditions, philosophies, and personal-familial values related to sexual information and expression, the objectives for sex education set forth by the Sex Information and Education Council of the U.S. (SIECUS) provide an excellent framework for approaching this sensitive area. (See chart)

OBJECTIVES OF SEX EDUCATION*

To provide the individual with an adequate knowledge of his or her own physical, mental, and emotional maturational functions as they relate to sex.

To eliminate fears and anxieties regarding the individual's sexual development and adjustments.

To develop objective and understanding attitudes, in the individual toward the self and toward others, regarding sex in all of its various manifestations.

To give the individual insight concerning relationships to members of both sexes, and to help him or her understand obligations and responsibilities to others.

To provide an appreciation of the positive good that wholesome human relations can bring to both the individual and the family group.

To build an understanding of the fact that ethical and moral values form the only rational basis for making decisions regarding one's behavior.

To provide enough knowledge about sexual abuse and aberration so that the individual can protect him or herself against exploitation and damage to physical and mental health.

To provide an incentive to work for a society in which prostitution, illegitimacy, archaic sex laws, irrational sex-related fears, and sexual exploitation are nonexistent.

To provide the insight and the climate conducive to the individual's eventually utilizing his or her sexuality effectively and creatively in the roles of spouse, parent, community member, and citizen.

* Sex Information and Education Council of the U.S.

REFERENCES

1. James L. McCary:*Human Sexuality*. New York, D. Van Nostrand Company, 1973, p. 4.
2. Leonide M. Tanner: "The Maternity Nurse as Counselor in Human Sexuality," in *Current Concepts in Clinical Nursing*, Vol. IV. Edith H. Anderson (Ed.). St. Louis, C. V. Mosby Company, 1973, pp. 169–178.

3. Marianne K. Zalar: "Sexual Counseling for Pregnant Couples," *MCN—The American Journal of Maternal-Child Nursing*, 1:3, May-June 1976, pp. 176–181.
4. Zalar, op. cit.
5. Leonide L. Martin: *Health Care of Women*. Philadelphia, J. B. Lippincott, 1978, pp. 130–131.

6. Arthur D. Coleman and Libby L. Coleman: *Pregnancy: The Psychological Experience.* New York, Herder and Herder, 1971, pp. 31–40.

7. William H. Masters and Virginia E. Johnson: *Human Sexual Inadequacy.* New York, Little, Brown, 1970, p. 157.

8. McCary, op. cit., p. 17.

9. Sol Gordon: *Lets Make Sex a Household Word: A Guide for Parents and Children.* New York, John Day Company, 1975, pp. 83–132.

Twelve

Contraception

*Contraceptive Counseling / Oral Contraception /
Intrauterine Device (IUD) / The Diaphragm / The
Condom / The Safe Period or Rhythm Method / Jellies,
Creams, Suppositories, Foams / Withdrawal /Unreliable
Approaches / New and Experimental Methods /
Postpartal Contraception / Sterilization*

Changing attitudes and technological advances have given the majority of people in advanced societies the option of controlling reproduction. Contraceptive methods are widely utilized throughout most of the world, ranging from the ancient practice of coitus interruptus (withdrawal) to the use of chemical (hormonal) oral contraceptives by some 80 to 100 million women. Although governments may support a policy of limited population growth by encouraging use of contraceptives, decisions to control reproduction are based on individual choice and are made for highly personal reasons. The right of individual choice in fertility control has been emphasized by international bodies, as seen in the following statement made by the General Assembly of the United Nations in 1966: "The size of the family should be the free choice of each individual family."

The concept of the individual's right to choose freely has been expanded to include the right to have access to the means by which births may be safely and effectively limited or spaced. While, highly effective contraceptive methods are available, their effectiveness is often lowered by inappropriate use. In addition, their safety has not yet reached levels at which risk is truly minimal. The ideal contraceptive would be a method that is 100 percent safe and 100 percent effective, inexpensive, simple to use and understand, not directly connected to intercourse, totally reversible at any time, and readily available. No currently available contraceptive method meets all these criteria, nor does it seem probable that research will find such a method in the near future. Despite the risks involved, people desire the benefits of reproductive choice, and must therefore make decisions about methods based on personal values and a full understanding of the risks and benefits involved.

In the United States, there is a trend toward smaller families, with women in the childbearing years expressing increased support for the concept of the two-child family.[1] A number of factors are involved in the growing openness and acceptance of contraception, including social values, life styles, economics, and technology. Improved methods of mass communication have aided health professionals in making contraceptive information and methods available on a wider and more equitable basis. A better informed public, supported by changing social values that encourage individual choice and smaller family sizes, has demanded access to professional advice and contraceptive techniques as an integral part of health care services. Changes in family structures have placed greater emphasis on companionship and mutual growth and less on economic necessity, which in the past locked family members into separate role identities and stressed the importance of children as family workers. Traditional norms regarding children as an unquestioned duty to past or future generations have given way to the belief that children should be wanted and parenthood should be the result of deliberate choice. Modern urban life styles make large families an economic liability, and increasingly two-income families are needed to maintain high standards of living in an inflationary economy. The feminist movement and increasing numbers of women who work or pursue careers also significantly affect attitudes toward contraception.

The majority of American women, regardless of religious affiliation, approve of and utilize contraception, whether they are rich or poor, urban or rural, white or nonwhite. For the poor, having fewer children puts less strain on the family's resources and enhances the family's opportunities for economic and personal betterment. Black women have continued to use family planning clinics to meet their personal needs, despite accusations that this may constitute a form of genocide.[2] Although predominantly Catholic, Mexican-American women utilize family planning clinics and a range of contraceptive methods. Motives for contraceptive use are unique, and the choice of method and its meaning are highly individual. Therefore, differences must be respected by the nurse, without presumption based on external characteristics, and the full range of contraceptive possibilities discussed with each individual or couple so a fully informed and satisfactory choice can be made.

CONTRACEPTIVE COUNSELING

Both the maternity and the community health nurse play an important role in the care of the patient seeking contraceptive advice. While it is not necessary to advocate a particular method of contraception, the professional nurse has a responsibility to see that help, understanding, and guidance in family planning are available to all parents. The nurse who, in conscience, is unable to give general contraceptive advice should state this to the patient and provide referral to another source for the information which is sought.

Certainly, every nurse who will give contraceptive advice needs to be aware of all the available methods of birth control and should be conversant with the advantages and disadvantages of each method, both at the functional and the psychologic levels. The choice of a suitable contraceptive depends on many factors which vary even from year to year in any couple's contraceptive life span. These factors include expense, bathroom facilities, frequency of intercourse, number of children, the risk of pregnancy the couple wishes to accept, illness, and physical problems.

The nurse should also be acquainted with the increasing availability and acceptability of vasectomy and tubal ligation. Studies have shown that one-fourth to one-third of all couples look to this permanent method of contraception when their families are completed. Currently available methods of contraception are listed in Table 12-1.

General Approach to the Patient

A number of important principles should be observed when assisting couples to select a suitable means of contraception. Unlike other health measures, pregnancy prevention ideally involves the participation of both male and female partners. Good family planning programs should encourage participation of the male and provide an opportunity for him to share responsibility for fertility control. A discussion of some of the methods of male contraception, such as withdrawal, the use of condoms, vasectomy, or even rhythm when it is the method of choice should be included in the program.

Since family planning deals with the patient's sexuality, a private setting should be arranged whenever possible. The patient's feelings about contraception should be explored in a nonjudgmental way and the variety of choices summarized to allow selection of a method which fits the individual circumstance of the couple. There is no "best method" of contraception, but there is always a method which can work best in the circumstances at hand.

It should also be recognized that some patients appearing in a family planning clinic may be there because they may have an infertility problem or because they wish to have a Pap smear, a breast examination, or an evaluation for venereal disease. Family planning clinics often serve as a patient's

TABLE 12-1
METHODS OF CONTRACEPTION CURRENTLY AVAILABLE

Male and Female	Male	Female
ABSTINENCE	WITHDRAWAL	SPERMICIDES*
Total	CONDOMS	Foam, Cream, Gels
Periodic	VASECTOMY	Diaphragm with Gel or Cream
Rhythm		OVULATION PREVENTION†
Basal Body		Oral
Temperature (BBT)		Injectable
Nonvaginal Variations		Implanted
Masturbation		UNKNOWN ACTION
Solitary		Minipill
Mutual		Morning-After Pill
Oralgenital		Intrauterine Device
Anal Intercourse		Mechanical
		Chemical
		Hormonal
		Heavy Metals (Copper)
		TUBAL STERILIZATION‡

* Douching is not a contraceptive method.
† Breast-feeding is not a contraceptive method.
‡ Abortion is not a contraceptive method.
Source: Pierson, E. C.: *Sex Is Never an Emergency,* ed. 3. Philadelphia, J. B. Lippincott, 1973, p. 5.

initial introduction to the health care system and offer opportunities for general health maintenance

One of the optimal times for exploring methods of family planning is in the postpartal period following delivery. Choices can conveniently be reviewed with the patient at that time so that knowledgeable selection of a method can be made. It has been shown that availability of contraceptive advice has resulted in a marked increase in the number of patients returning for postpartal care.

Informed Consent and Contraceptive Risk

There is a certain amount of risk in every contraceptive method, whether related to the method itself or the risk of pregnancy due to contraceptive failure or misuse. It should be noted that the mortality associated with pregnancy is greater than that of any commonly used contraceptive method. Often the risk a given method poses for the individual

TABLE 12-2
EFFECTIVENESS AND RISKS OF CONTRACEPTIVES, PREGNANCIES PER 100 WOMEN PER YEAR

Method	Theoretical effectiveness	Use effectiveness	Continuing pregnancies	Deaths due to pregnancy	Deaths due to contraceptive	Major morbidity (%)	Minor morbidity (%)
No contraception	—	—	80	.016	0	—	—
Oral contraceptives	.1	3–4	.5	0	.003	1	40
IUD	2	5	3	.001	.001	1	40
Diaphragm	3	13–17	12	.002	0	—	—
Rhythm	14	35–40	25	.005	0	—	—
Early abortion*	0	0	0	0	.003	1	8
Laparoscopic tubal ligation	0	.04	.15	0	.03	.6	1
Vasectomy	0	.15	.15	0	0	1	5
Condom†	3	15	—	—	—	—	—
Spermicides†	3	13–17	—	—	—	—	—
Coitus interruptus†	3	15–25	—	—	—	—	—

* Abortion is not a method of contraception, but is included here for comparison.
† Data on continuing pregnancies, deaths due to pregnancy are not available, but use effectiveness figures indicate these would be in the range found for the diaphragm.
Adapted from R. A. Hatcher, et al., *Contraceptive Technology 1976–1977,* New York, Halstead Press, Division of John Wiley & Sons, 1976, pp. 25, 100 and S. L. Romney, et al., *Gynecology and Obstetrics: The Health Care of Women,* New York, McGraw-Hill, Blakiston, 1975, pp. 551, 552.

cannot be completely determined in advance, although in many instances contraindications can be identified for known health problems or personal characteristics. Still, an apparently healthy woman with no major contraindications to a given method can develop serious complications, some of which are life-threatening. Although the incidence of such complications is low, it is the patient's right to be well informed about the risks, benefits, and effectiveness of all contraceptive methods (Table 12-2).

Informed consent is both a safeguard for the patient and a way of increasing proper contraceptive use. When the women or couple fully understand the technique, have weighed the possible adverse effects against the convenience and acceptability of the method for them, and have made a choice based on which method best meets their needs, the likelihood of discontinuation and misuse is reduced. Guidelines for informed consent suggested by the U.S. Department of Health, Education and Welfare are indicated in the chart below.

GUIDELINES FOR CONTRACEPTIVE TEACHING

Informed consent is the voluntary, knowing assent from the individual on whom any procedure is to be performed after she or he has been given

1. a fair explanation of the procedures or method;
2. a description of attendant discomforts and risks, including all major (life-threatening) and all common minor risks;
3. a description of the benefits to be expected;
4. an explanation of alternative methods and effectiveness rates with indication that nothing is 100 percent, and that sterilization is permanent;
5. an offer to answer any questions about procedures or method;
6. an instruction that the individual is free to withdraw consent to the procedure or method at any time prior to the procedure, or to discontinue the method, without affecting future care or loss of benefits;
7. a written consent document detailing the basic elements of informed consent and the information provided. This should be signed by the patient, an auditor-witness of the patient's choice, and by the person obtaining the consent.[3]

ORAL CONTRACEPTION

Oral contraceptives ("the pill") are hormonal agents consisting most commonly of a combination of estrogen and a synthetic progestational agent. They act principally at the central nervous system level to inhibit ovulation through suppression of FSH and LH. There are secondary effects on endometrial development, tubal motility, and cervical mucus. Under the influence of the progestational agent, the cervical mucus becomes thick, viscous, and unreceptive to spermatozoa. However, the most important effect of standard dose combination pills is the inhibition of ovulation, which means that there is no ova to be fertilized.

Oral contraceptives are available in 21- and 28-day packages; in the 21-day packs a pill is taken each day for three weeks, followed by a week without any pills. In the 28-day pack, a pill is taken every day for four weeks, but only those taken during the first three weeks will have active hormonal ingredients; those pills taken during the last week consist of lactose or ferrous sulfate, but no hormones. The purpose of a week of nonhormonal pills is to keep the woman in the habit of taking a pill a day, and in some instances to provide an iron supplement for prevention of anemia. When the 21-day approach is used, the pill is taken daily beginning on the fifth day of the menstrual cycle through day 25. Two or three days after the last pill is taken there is usually a "withdrawal" menstrual flow.

There is a large number of oral contraceptives available, with differing combinations of estrogen and/or progestin doses (see Table 12-3). Basically there are two types: the combination pills which contain estrogen and progestin and are available at the standard or low (micro) dosage levels, and the progestin-only type (minipills). As the majority of serious side effects are due to estrogen, the trend has been toward reducing this hormonal agent from the original dosage of 80 to 100 mcg. to doses ranging from 50 to 20 mcg. However, use of 20 or 30 mcg. pills is associated with high rates of breakthrough bleeding and unpredictable menses, making them less acceptable to many women. Similar problems are encountered with progestin-only pills, and the increased amenorrhea, spotting, and irregularity of menses has discouraged their widespread use.

The theoretical effectiveness of the combined formulation pill approaches 100 percent. In fact, the method failure rate—failure when properly used—

TABLE 12-3
MOST CURRENTLY AVAILABLE COMBINATION MICRODOSE AND PROGESTIN ORAL CONTRACEPTIVES

Product/ Manufacturer	Type	Estrogen	Progestin
Enovid-E/Searle	Comb	100 mcg. mestranol	2.5 mg. norethynodrel
Ortho-Novum/Ortho	Comb	100 mcg. mestranol	2 mg. norethindrone
Norinyl/Syntex	Comb	100 mcg. mestranol	2 mg. norethindrone
Ovulen/Searle	Comb	100 mcg. mestranol	1 mg. ethynodiol diacetate
Ortho-Novum 1+80	Comb	80 mcg. mestranol	1 mg. norethindrone
Norinyl 1+80/Syntex	Comb	80 mcg. mestranol	1 mg. norethindrone
Norlestrin/Parke-Davis	Comb	50 mcg. ethinyl estradiol	2.5 mg. norethindrone acetate
Norinyl 1+50/Syntex	Comb	50 mcg. mestranol	1 mg. norethindrone
Ortho-Novum 1+50/Ortho	Comb	50 mcg. mestranol	1 mg. norethindrone
Norlestrin/Parke-Davis	Comb	50 mcg. ethinyl estradiol	1 mg. norethindrone acetate
Ovral/Wyeth	Comb	50 mcg. ethinyl estradiol	0.5 mg. norgestrel
Demulen/Searle	Comb	50 mcg. ethinyl estradiol	1 mg. ethynodiol diacetate
Ovcon-50/Mead Johnson	Comb	50 mcg. ethinyl estradiol	1 mg. norethindrone
Zorane 1+50/Lederle	Comb	50 mcg. ethinyl estradiol	1 mg. norethindrone acetate
Brevicon/Syntex	Comb	35 mcg. ethinyl estradiol	0.5 mg. norethindrone
Ovcon-35/Mead Johnson	Comb	35 mcg. ethinyl estradiol	0.4 mg. norethindrone
Modicon/Ortho	Comb	35 mcg. ethinyl estradiol	0.5 mg. norethindrone
Loestrin 1.5+30/Parke- Davis	Comb	30 mcg. ethinyl estradiol	1.5 mg. norethindrone acetate
Zorane 1.5+30/Lederle	Comb	30 mcg. ethinyl estradiol	1.5 mg. norethindrone acetate
Lo-Ovral/Wyeth	Comb	30 mcg. ethinyl estradiol	0.3 mg. norgestrel
Loestrin 1+20/Parke- Davis	Comb	20 mcg. ethinyl estradiol	1 mg. norethindrone acetate
Zorane 1+20/Lederle	Comb	20 mcg. ethinyl estradiol	1 mg. norethindrone acetate
Micronor/Ortho	Prog		0.35 mg. norethindrone
Nor-Q.D./Syntex	Prog		0.35 mg. norethindrone
Ovrette/Wyeth	Prog		0.075 mg. norgestrel

is negligible. When patient error is included—and this involves failure to take the pill for one or more days during the cycle—effectiveness falls to approximately 90 to 95 percent. The discontinuation rate has been reported to be from 20 percent to as high as 50 percent. The reasons for discontinuation include appearance of side effects and untoward symptoms, as well as variations in motivational factors in the populations studied.

Contraindications and Side-Effects

Generally accepted, absolute contraindications to oral contraception include a history of thrombophlebitis, thromboembolic disorders, or cerebral vascular accident or the presence of marked impairment of liver function, malignancy of the breast or of the reproductive tract, and, of course, pregnancy. Additional contraindications include migraine, hypertension, diabetes, gallbladder disease, sickle cell disease, undiagnosed vaginal bleeding, and less than four weeks postpartum.

Common side effects of the pill include accentuation of premenstrual symptoms, such as mastal-

gia, irritability, and edema. The most untoward side effect of any contraceptive modality—pregnancy—occurs very rarely and is generally related to failure to take the pill.

The side effects of oral contraceptives, according to the excess or deficiency of hormone responsible for the symptom or condition, are shown in Table 12-4.

Systemic Effects of Synthetic Hormones

Initially oral contraceptives were believed to affect only the reproductive system through suppression of ovulation and alteration of menstrual flow. However, there is increasing recognition that these powerful synthetic hormones affect many systems of the body, causing metabolic and endocrine changes with far-reaching impact. The possible long-term consequences and risks of taking the pill are creating a climate of real concern among women and health professionals and have led to a call for a more conservative and cautious approach involving careful selection and frequent monitoring. Some of the more significant systemic effects include the following:

Thrombotic Effects. Several factors seem to be involved in the increased risk of death or disability due to clotting disorders (stroke, pulmonary embolism, retinal vein thrombosis, myocardial infarction, thrombophlebitis) in women taking the pill. There is more rapid fibrin formation with increased clot firmness among pill users than among nonusers as well as an increase in certain blood factors associated with coagulation, an increase in platelet count with changes in electrophoretic mobility of platelets, and an increase in vascular lesions and venous stasis.[4,5] Women who use the pill have a seven to eight times greater risk of death from thromboembolic disease than nonusers. The incidence of complications is dosage-related, with a significant difference between women taking pills with less than 50 mcg. of estrogen as compared to those taking dosages above 50 mcg. of estrogen. The risk of death from clotting disorders secondary to oral contraceptive use is also age-related, increasing after age 35.

Effects of Cigarette Smoking. Evidence indicates that there is an increased death rate from cardiovascular complications among women over 35 who use oral contraceptives and smoke. Studies have shown that women over age 30 who both smoke and use oral contraceptives have a greater risk of fatal heart attack than younger women who use the pill and women over 30 who do not smoke. While other risk factors such as hypertension and high cholesterol are also associated with higher incidence of myocardial infarction, cigarette smoking was considered the most important factor. Apparently women without these risk factors can continue taking oral contraceptives with relative safety during the years of 30 to 44.[6] The Federal Drug Administration has required the following antismoking warning be added to package inserts accompanying oral contraceptives:

Cigarette smoking increases the risk of serious cardiovascular side effects from oral contraceptive use. The risk increases with age and with heavy smoking (15 or more cigarettes per day) and is quite marked in women over 35 years of age. Women who use oral contraceptives should be strongly advised not to smoke.[7]

TABLE 12-4
HORMONAL BASIS OF SIDE EFFECTS OF ORAL CONTRACEPTIVES

| Estrogen | | Progestin | | Androgen |
Excess	Deficiency	Excess	Deficiency	Excess
Nausea, vomiting	Amenorrhea	Acne, oily scalp	Hypermenorrhea	Acne
Fluid retention	Oligomenorrhea	Increased appetite	with clotting	Oily skin
(premenstrual	Early or midcycle	Weight gain	Late cycle spotting	Rashes
tension, irrita-	spotting	Fatigue	Delayed onset of	Increased hair
bility, breast	Loss of pelvic	Depression	menses	growth in male
tenderness, cor-	tone	Hair loss		pattern
neal swelling,	Hot flashes	Headaches when not		Increased interest
cramping, edema)	Nervousness,	taking pills		in sex
Increased vaginal	irritability	Increased breast size		Cholestatic jaundice
discharge	Decreased interest	Increased muscle		Increased appetite
Chloasma	in sex	mass		
Headaches		Increased monilial		
Increased breast		vaginitis (Candida)		
size		Breast tenderness		
Weight gain		not related to fluid		
Increased cer-		retention		
vical ectropion		Short menses		
Increased size		Relative endometrial		
of fibroids		atrophy		
Telangiectasia		Decreased interest		
Thromboembolic		in sex		
disorders		Cholestatic jaundice		
Reduction of				
lactation				
Possibly hyper-				
tension				

Liver and Gallbladder Effects. Changes in liver function due to oral contraceptives is related to estrogen dosage levels and is apparently reversible. There is an increased risk of liver adenomas developing after five years of pill use, predominately associated with mestranol (an estrogen).[8] There also appears to be a relationship between surgically proven cholelithiasis and oral contraceptives, with symptoms developing shortly after pill use is started.

Carbohydrate Metabolism. About 20 to 25 percent of women taking oral contraceptives have elevated fasting blood sugar, and an additional 20 percent show abnormal glucose tolerance test curves. Human growth hormone is significantly increased with a compensatory increase in insulin, which usually allows women to maintain a normal GTT even though blood sugar levels are increased. A history of diabetes or the presence of obesity places women at greater risk for abnormalities of carbohydrate metabolism with pill use. Although short-term studies show reversal of these changes after discontinuation of oral contraceptives, the long-term effects have not been established.

Lipids. Increases in plasma triglycerides and phospholipids among women taking the pill are related to dosage levels of estrogen. Possibly increased hepatic production of lipids is involved, and although the long-term effects are not yet known, it is speculated that these changes may be associated with cardiovascular disease and acute vascular accidents.[9]

Fetal Abnormalities. Although there appears to be no increase in fetal abnormalities among women who have used oral contraceptives prior to conception, studies have indicated an association between use of progestins in the first four months of pregnancy and congenital heart and limb reduction defects. There was a 4.7-fold increase in the risk of limb reduction defects in infants exposed to sex hormones in utero, including oral contraceptives, hormone withdrawal tests for pregnancy, or treatment for threatened abortion.[10] Cardiovascular malformations occurred at an increased rate of 8.6 per 1,000 among infants of women receiving progestins only during pregnancy.[11] These concerns are reflected in physician labeling and patient warnings that are now required by the FDA when progestational drugs are used during pregnancy.

Cancer. There is still much question about the relationship between oral contraceptives and cervical, endometrial, and breast cancer. Because women taking the pill tend to have more frequent visits to clinics or physicians' offices, frequency of incidence data is confounded by greater diagnostic opportunity. However, a relationship has been established between prolonged unopposed estrogen stimulation of the endometrium and endometrial hyperplasia and adenocarcinoma. Certain types of breast cancer are known to grow more rapidly under higher levels of estrogen stimulation, and breast cancer has been caused in animals with oral contraceptives. Because combination pills cause a hyperestrogenic state, there is concern about long-term effects on the breasts and endometrium.

Initiation of Therapy and Follow-Up

Patients on the pill should undergo regular check-ups, ideally at intervals of six months. The initial visit should include assessment of the patient for contraindications to the pill, a blood pressure determination, Pap smear, hematocrit or hemoglobin, urinalysis, and, when circumstances dictate, a culture for gonorrhea and a serologic test for syphilis. An alternate method of birth control should be reviewed thoroughly, against the possibility that the patient would discontinue the pill without prior consultation.

In many family planning centers, an early follow-up visit at six to twelve weeks is suggested. On that occasion, evidence of side effects and the patient's general attitude are reviewed with specific questions about headaches, blurred vision, chest pain, leg pain, as well as a blood pressure check and an evaluation to be sure the pills are being taken correctly.

When the pill is discontinued, ovulation and menstruation will usually return by the next monthly cycle. Some women, however, may experience a delay in ovulation and, therefore, of menstruation for several months. There is no evidence that future pregnancies are affected by the prior use of oral contraceptives.

INTRAUTERINE DEVICE (IUD)

This technique (actually an ancient practice but only recently validated scientifically) involves inserting a small, usually flexible appliance into the uterine

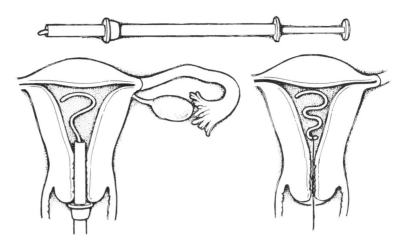

Figure 12-1. (Left) Method of insertion of a Lippes loop. Note location of head which protrudes beyond the cervix.

cavity (Fig. 12-1) and allowing it to remain in the uterus for as long as contraception is desired. Devices have been made in various shapes (spirals, loops, rings) and of various materials (plastic tubing, nylon thread, stainless steel). The most commonly used are the Lippes loop, Saf-T-Coil, Copper 7, Copper T, and Progesterone T. Although the mechanism by which these appliances prevent conception is not completely understood, there appears to be a local inflammatory effect on the endometrium making it unfavorable to implantation or causing cytolysis. An immunologic antifertility mechanism may also be operating, or a dislodging effect may occur mechanically.

IUDs are about 97 percent effective (three pregnancies in 100 users with the IUD in place). They rank second only to the oral contraceptives and probably equal the properly used diaphragm in the protection they afford. The advantages of intrauterine devices are that they are inexpensive and, once inserted, require no further attention, provided they remain in place. The main drawback of the appliances is that they are frequently expelled, and at times cause bleeding and cramps requiring that they be removed. Spontaneous expulsion or necessary removal occurs in from 15 to 20 percent of patients.

Many commonly used IUDs have a nylon string attached. This serves two purposes: 1) it aids in removal, and 2) it allows the patient to check for its presence by palpating the strings at the cervix. The nurse should emphasize to the patient that it is important to check for the presence of the IUD before each sexual exposure during the first several months of use. Beyond this time the chance of spontaneous expulsion without the patient's knowl-

edge is reduced, and it is at this time that the quoted 97 percent rate of effectiveness is valid.

The incorporation of metallic copper in intrauterine devices appears to be associated with a lower expulsion rate and an increased effectiveness. The copper is slowly delivered from the device into the uterine fluid. For this reason, it is recommended that the copper device be replaced every two to four years. Intrauterine devices which contain progesterone, slowly released from the device to provide a local effect on the endometrium, are also reported to increase effectiveness. However, these types have to be replaced at intervals because the progesterone is gradually dispersed.

Contraindications and Side Effects

The major *contraindications* to IUDs include active pelvic infection, recent or chronic pelvic infection, postpartum endometritis or septic abortion, pregnancy, endometrial hyperplasia or carcinoma, and abnormalities of the uterus such as myomata, polyps, or bicornate uterus making insertion problematic. In women with a small uterus (sounding to less than 6 cm.) or with marked anteflexion or retroflexion, insertion is more difficult but may be accomplished with the smaller devices.

Commonly reported side effects of the IUD include increased menstrual flow, dysmenorrhea, and intermenstrual spotting. Since flow is sometimes excessive, patients should be checked routinely for anemia. They should be instructed to report any fever, pelvic pain or tenderness, or unusual vaginal bleeding, since these may be signs of pelvic infection. If pregnancy occurs when the

IUD is in place, removal is recommended. An increased danger of intrapartum infection and deaths from sepsis have been reported among patients whose IUD was allowed to remain in place in pregnancy. The risk of spontaneous abortion is somewhat higher when the IUD remains in place (about 50 percent) than when it is removed at the time pregnancy is discovered (25 percent). Another major complication is uterine perforation which usually occurs at the time the IUD is inserted. When perforation through the uterine wall into the abdomen occurs, it is generally recommended that the IUD be removed. This can be done with the use of a laparoscope, avoiding an exploratory laparotomy.

Occasionally on insertion, the IUD may produce enough pain and stimulation to result in syncope. The nurse should be aware of this complication and should be ready to place the patient in a recumbent position if there are any signs of lightheadedness, sweating, or nausea.

Ectopic pregnancy may also be related to the presence of an IUD. The incidence of ectopic pregnancy is considerably higher with the Progseterone T (Progestasert) IUD than with unmedicated or copper containing IUDs. About 3 to 4 percent of women with unmedicated or copper IUDs who become pregnant have ectopic pregnancies, as compared with about 16 percent ectopic pregnancies with the progesterone IUD or no contraception. The FDA has alerted health professionals to carefully evaluate patients who become pregnant with progesterone IUDs in place to determine whether the pregnancies are ectopic.[12]

THE DIAPHRAGM

The diaphragm, a dome-shaped rubber cup ranging in diameter from 7 to 10 cm. is inserted into the vagina and over the anterior vaginal wall and cervix prior to intercourse (Fig. 12-2). The diaphragm, by itself, is not a contraceptive device; it must be used with a spermicidal jelly or cream which is placed in the diaphragm between it and the cervix. The use of the diaphragm insures the placement of spermicidal jelly over the cervix.

When the diaphragm is properly used—each time intercourse occurs, without exception—it is associated with a failure rate of three pregnancies per 100 women years, a very acceptable rate. In practice, however, the overall failure rate varies from 20 to 25 pregnancies per 100 women years of use, possibly because of inconsistent use. A diaphragm requires motivation and premeditation, but despite these drawbacks it has again gained favor as some of the disadvantages of the pill and IUD are weighed.

Advantages of the diaphragm include its safety and lack of side effects and its flexibility according to frequency of intercourse. Since it can be inserted up to 2 hours before sex, it is relatively separated from coitus. Once in place it is unobtrusive, as its presence cannot be felt by either partner if properly fitted, and less cream or jelly is left in the vagina than with a spermicide alone. Well-motivated women have used the diaphragm effectively to limit pregnancies since the end of the 19th century.

A common objection to the diaphragm is the vaginal manipulation necessary for insertion, a procedure which is repugnant to some women. This problem is easily solved if the patient is fitted with a flat or coil-spring diaphragm (in contrast to the arc flex diaphragm). These diaphragms may be used with an "inserter" which allows the patient to insert it like a tampon, without touching the genital area. The arc flex diaphragm cannot be used with an inserter. It was designed for ease of manual insertion and may, in some cases, give a better fit in the presence of a mild cystocele. Some women, after one or more pregnancies cannot be fitted with a diaphragm.

One of the stated disadvantages of prescribing a diaphragm is the office time consumed during fitting and instruction on its use. Increasingly the nurse is called upon to play an active role in both. Sample diaphragms or rings of known size are inserted until a size is found which will cover the cervix and fit snugly behind the symphysis pubis. The patient is then asked to remove the diaphragm by hooking a finger over it just beneath the symphysis and then to reinsert it. Before the patient leaves the office, she should be able to insert and remove the diaphragm with ease. She should be instructed always to use a spermicidal cream or jelly with the diaphragm, placing it around the rim and in the dome. If intercourse occurs a second or third time, additional spermicidal agent should be inserted for added protection. The diaphragm should be left in place for at least six hours following intercourse. A douche is recommended after removal to remove the remaining jelly or cream.

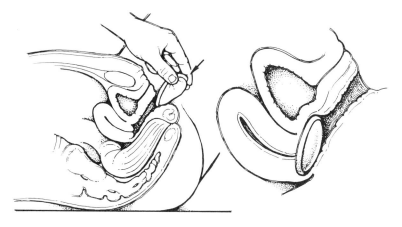

Figure 12-2. (*Left*) Method of manual insertion of diaphragm. Prior to insertion, contraceptive cream or jelly is placed over the dome around the edges of the diaphragm. Plastic inserters are also available for ease of insertion of the diaphragm. (*Right*) Diaphragm in place.

THE CONDOM

Condoms ("rubbers") are thin sheaths of rubber or processed collagenous tissue which are placed over the penis to act as a mechanical barrier to prevent sperm from entering the vagina. Also effective in preventing venereal infections, condoms are a male method of contraception which has been used since ancient times. The condom is applied over the shaft of the penis after erection. Before withdrawal of the penis from the vagina, the condom should be held in place on the penis so that it does not slip off into the vagina. Some condoms are packaged with a lubricant and some have a small pouch at the tip to collect the ejaculate, which reduces the danger of tearing. In some cases, lubricants cause an irritation at the introitus and an unpleasant "stinging" sensation. In general, a lubricant should not be necessary if there is suffcent foreplay to produce the natural lubrication associated with female sexual arousal.

If used properly, the condom is an effective contraceptive. However, it must be applied before any penile-vaginal contact. As for advantages, condoms are available without a medical prescription, are easy to use, do not present any serious side effects, are low in cost, and prevent transmission of sexual infections.

The major criticism of condoms is that they decrease sensation for both partners or, more commonly, for the man. In addition, their use requires that the sex act be interrupted to apply the condom, a disruption which can prove distracting for some couples. There is also frequent worry that the condom might break.

The nurse might point out that no method of contraception is perfect (all have some disadvantages

for one or both partners and have some anxiety-producing aspects). If used before any penetration, condoms are safe and rarely break. This information will help those couples who have anxiety over other forms of contraception.

THE SAFE PERIOD OR RHYTHM METHOD

The rationale of the safe period or the rhythm method is that when there are regular periods, ovulation occurs at approximately the same time in each cycle (i.e., 14 days prior to the beginning of the next cycle). The ovum is capable of being fertilized only for a period of 48 hours, at the most, after ovulation. Theoretically, therefore, abstinence from sexual intercourse on that day and for the two days before and after (a total of five days) should forestall conception.

In actual experience, however, even normal, regular cycles can be off by one to two days in either direction (e.g., 28 ± 2 days). This puts the day of ovulation in the same four day range ± two days, and the period of abstinence must then be, realistically, about eight days. For more accuracy the basal body temperature should be used.

The most important point about the rhythm method and its repeated failures really has more to do with the longevity of the sperm than with the day of ovulation. Sperm are found in the cervical mucus as soon as 20 seconds after ejaculation and as late as seven days after ejaculation. Any motile sperm must be regarded as capable of fertilizing an egg. There are many "day six and day seven" pregnancies that attest to this fact (i.e., that intercourse on day six or seven of a 28-day cycle resulted in pregnancy).

If rhythm is to work, there must be regular cycles and abstinence for at least 14 days out of each 28-day cycle. Intercourse during the first days of a cycle (menses) is not contraindicated, except on an aesthetic basis by some couples, nor is it contraindicated during the last five or six days of a cycle, if these can be determined accurately.

Rhythm methods are more effective if intercourse is avoided through the entire first half of the menstrual cycle, the preovulatory phase. Failure rates as low as 15 pregnancies per 100 woman years have been reported in constant, highly motivated users. In actual use, however, rates are nearer 40 pregnancies per 100 woman years. Many couples find the long times of abstinence and the need to have sex "on schedule" a deterrent to use of rhythm. An additional disadvantage is the implication that accidental pregnancies occurring when the ovum or sperm are deteriorating, as at their outer limits of functioning, are associated with increased fetal abnormalities. Because intercourse tends not to occur near ovulation when rhythm is practiced, fertilizations may occur when sperm or ova are past their optimum.

For the couple who has developed a degree of mutual understanding such that prolonged abstinence can be accepted and, especially, when an accidental pregnancy would not be a tragedy or constitute a health hazard, rhythm can be recommended, provided the drawbacks are recognized and accepted.

Ancillary Aids to Rhythm

Temperature Charts. Use of the basal body temperature provides variation of the rhythm method. Oral temperatures are recorded on a chart daily for three cycles and submitted to the physician or nurse for analysis (see Fig. 8-5 and Chapter 8). Special thermometers are sold at most drugstores for this purpose. An increase in basal body temperature which is sustained indicates that ovulation has occurred.

Temperature chart variation of rhythm is all the more useful if periods are irregular. In general, when a temperature rise of one degree or more is sustained for three days, it can be assumed that ovulation has occurred and that intercourse is safe.

Since the time of ovulation cannot accurately be forecast in a given cycle and since spermatozoa may survive several days, abstinence should begin shortly after the end of menses. When cycle length is prolonged, the method requires a long period of abstinence.

Changes in Cervical Mucus. Self-observed changes in the quality of the cervical mucus are also recommended to time ovulation. When daily observations of cervical mucus are combined with the basal body temperature chart, the approach is called the *symptothermal method*. Characteristically, in the ovulatory cycle there is a rapid increase in the quantity of cervical mucus just prior to ovulation. At that time, the mucus becomes clear and stringy. The patient may observe the presence of such mucus at the introitus or may wipe the cervix to obtain a sample for observation. Subsequent to ovulation, mucus becomes more viscous. When this change is associated with a rise in temperature, it is assumed that ovulation has occurred. Many workers in rhythm clinics have been successful in teaching patients to observe bodily signs associated with ovulation by encouraging increased awareness of such changes.

JELLIES, CREAMS, SUPPOSITORIES, FOAMS

These contraceptives are inexpensive and available without consulting a physician. They are relatively ineffective, however, because the woman cannot be sure of the placement or the retention of the spermicidal agent (Fig. 12-3). For proper use, the spermicidal agent should be inserted vaginally no more than one-half hour before intercourse, with a separate application made for each act of intercourse. In addition, the woman should not douche for at least eight hours after intercourse. The aerosol foams expand rapidly when inserted, covering the vaginal folds and seeming to disappear. They also leave less vaginal residual than jellies or creams, which take longer to spread over the vaginal surface.

The major disadvantage of spermicides is their low effectiveness when used alone. Many couples find them aesthetically unpleasant, and there is limited usefulness for repeated acts of intercourse. However, these preparations are particularly useful as short-term interim contraceptives, as in the following situations. In the postpartum period, spermicides are useful until the six-weeks checkup, when a more effective method can be instituted. They are frequently recommended for two weeks to one month after insertion of an IUD or initiation of an oral contraceptive regimen, as a precaution before these methods should be relied on alone. When the pill or IUD is discontinued, spermicides can be used for a few cycles until another method is begun or pregnancy attempted.

WITHDRAWAL

Withdrawal, or *coitus interruptus,* is an extensively used method of contraception and appears to be satisfactory for some couples. However, withdrawal as a method of contraception is a compromise at best. It requires concentration and willpower on the part of the male and trust on the part of the female. This trust is not always well founded and creates anxiety. Neither of these factors is conducive to relaxation and pleasure and may leave the couple with a distorted idea of what sexual pleasure is or can be. Also, preejaculatory secretion may contain motile spermatozoa, especially when there has been prolonged erection.

Withdrawal is one of the more ineffective contraceptive methods, with a failure rate of about 20 to 25 pregnancies per 100 woman years. However, it is always available and costs nothing. This method, often used by young people just beginning their sexual activities, can contribute to later sexual difficulties through a conditioning process. When intercourse occurs in circumstances associated with haste, fear, and guilt, and withdrawal is used in a way that interferes with communication and fulfillment, patterns of premature ejaculation in the male and orgasmic dysfunction in the female may be established.

UNRELIABLE APPROACHES

Douching after intercourse is actually not a contraceptive method. Sperm enter the cervix within 20 seconds of ejaculation, and it is highly unlikely that douching could occur before this time. The douche must be considered simply a method of cleansing

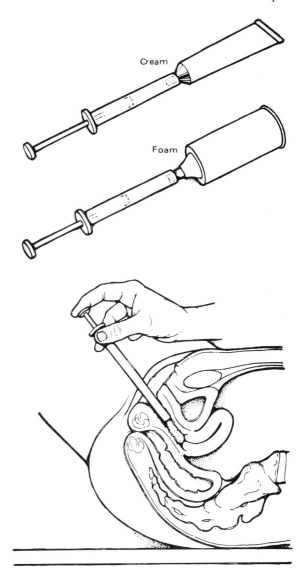

Figure 12-3. Insertion of foam or cream near the cervix.

the vagina, or a means of inserting a medicated solution to treat vaginal infections.

Lactation has been considered a method of postponing pregnancy by delaying ovulation. It is widely used in developing countries with some effectiveness for varying periods of months, probably related to the nutritional status of the mother. However, in the United States, women generally have good nutrition, and the lactation period is shorter since infants are given formula supplementation and solid foods at an earlier age. These factors contribute to an earlier and unpredictable return of fertility, making breast feeding an unreliable approach to contraception.

NEW AND EXPERIMENTAL METHODS

Hormonal methods of contraception involving injections of a long-acting progesterone (medroxyprogesterone acetate) every three months are available and seem to be as effective as oral contraceptions, although there are side effects such as irregular bleeding, amenorrhea, and possible delayed fertility after discontinuation. Several other new methods are under study. Subdermal Silastic capsules containing progestins are being tested as a method of reversible long-term contraception as are hormone impregnated Silastic endocervical devices and vaginal pessaries or rings. These devices are inserted each month after menstruation and left in place for 21 days, with dose-related effectiveness lower than that of combination pills. Major side effects are irregular bleeding and amenorrhea. Tests are also being conducted on a long-acting estrogen which is taken once a month, stored in body fat and gradually released (quinestrol). Effectiveness is comparable to that of minipills (progestin only) and nausea and amenorrhea are the major side effects. Another chemical approach to contraception is the use of prostaglandins which are currently used for abortion and are known to suppress corpus luteum activity necessary to maintain pregnancy.

As for male contraceptives, steroid hormones to suppress sperm production are being tested in a variety of forms—oral, injection, or subdermal implants. The main concern is reversibility, as return to adequate and active sperm production has not been established. Techniques for reversible male sterilization involving removable plastic devices or clips are also being explored.

POSTPARTAL CONTRACEPTION

In the absence of complications, intercourse is commonly resumed two to three weeks following delivery. The practice of advising couples to abstain from intercourse for six weeks has generally been discarded, since there is no reason to avoid sex once lochia has ceased and the episiotomy is adequately healed. Although the incidence of ovulation within the first six weeks postpartum is small, fertility does occasionally return and women are well advised to use a contraceptive method during this time. The condom is probably the most practical method to use during this period, since it does not involve introducing chemicals into the vagina. However, spermicidal foams and creams are frequently advised, either in combination with the condom or alone, if the condom is unacceptable. If foams and creams are not used too early in the postpartum period, there does not appear to be a problem with infection.

Insertion of an IUD within the first six weeks postpartum is generally not recommended, as the expulsion and infection rates are higher during this time. Oral contraceptives are contraindicated because of the increased incidence of thromboembolic complications associated with their use in the postpartum period. Nursing mothers are usually advised not to use oral contraceptives, since lactation may be suppressed and these synthetic hormones are excreted in breast milk.

STERILIZATION

Vasectomy in the male and tubal ligation in the female are being resorted to with increasing frequency as a means of limiting family size. Since both are permanent methods of contraception, the decision to undergo these procedures must be very carefully considered. In many settings, the role of the nurse in the decision-making process is pivotal. It is the responsibility of the counselor to be sure that both husband and wife are aware that these methods are considered irreversible. Total family circumstances which could influence the decision should be reviewed in depth and such factors as the number of children, stability of the marriage, age of marital partners, and ability to use nonpermanent methods should be considered.

Vasectomy

The *vas deferens* is a tube which leads from the testis to the urethra in the male and carries spermatozoa from the testis to the urethra. It is a firm structure somewhat less than .5 cm. in diameter which can be felt bilaterally in the scrotum, lateral to the base of the penis. *Vasectomy*, which involves surgical interruption and ligation of the vas, is a relatively minor operation. It can be carried out under local anesthesia and is associated with minimal risk and only slight morbidity. The procedure itself is simple, requires about 15 minutes, and can be done on an outpatient basis.

The major disadvantage is that it is permanent. Although surgical methods have been developed to reanastomose the ligated vas, the success rate is low. Even when a channel is recreated, the spermatozoa which subsequently appear in the ejaculate are not always normal, as they are affected by sperm antibodies which sometimes are produced after ligation.

Vasectomy failure is the result of recannulization of the ends of the ligated vas, and occurs in 0.15 per 100 cases. Additional pregnancies occur following vasectomy when unprotected intercourse takes place before the male reproductive tract is cleared of spermatozoa. Couples must be advised that the first few postvasectomy ejaculates contain active spermatozoa. Except for the absence of spermatozoa, vas ligation does not affect the ejaculate itself, nor does it affect the ejaculatory process.

The fear of a reduction of potency or masculinity prevents many men from accepting vasectomy. However, the vast majority of men who have had vasectomies are satisfied with their decision and report that sexual performance is unchanged. Less than 2 percent report decreased sexual pleasure or other dissatisfaction with vasectomy.

Tubal Ligation

Tubal ligation is, of course, designed to eliminate the passage along which spermatozoa and ova pass. A number of approaches have been used to interrupt the continuity of the fallopian tubes. The procedure may be carried out via an abdominal incision and is commonly done along with cesarean section or in the first few postpartal hours. Many workers in the family planning field now feel that patients should be encouraged not to accept a permanent form of contraception during emotionally charged intervals in their lives. An "on the spot" decision to have a tubal sterilization following an abortion or delivery should be explored with great care.

Coagulation and interruption of the fallopian tubes can be carried out using a *laparoscopic approach* (Fig. 12-4). In some centers this procedure is carried out under local anesthesia, but usually a general anesthetic is used. After the abdomen is distended with carbon dioxide, the laparoscopic trocar is

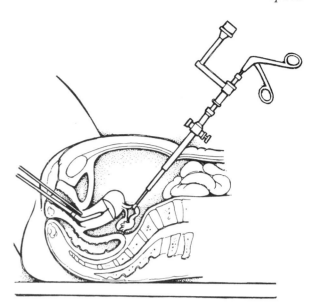

Figure 12-4. One-incision technique using the operating laparoscope.

introduced through a small incision in the umbilicus. The laparoscope is then passed into the peritoneal cavity. Visualization of the adnexae is usually complete. A coagulating instrument is used as the fallopian tubes are grasped, coagulated and severed.

Because the procedure is relatively simple, it can be carried out on an outpatient basis. Although it is associated with a relatively low morbidity, the morbidity is considerably higher than for vas ligation.

The *interval mini-laparotomy* is a sterilization technique in which a small suprapubic incision is usually made below the pubic hair line in order to enter the abdominal cavity. The fallopian tubes are isolated with grasping instruments and may be crushed, ligated, imbedded, clipped, or plugged as in other tubal ligation methods. About two days of hospitalization and a general anesthetic are required.

Most women who undergo tubal ligation are satisfied with their decision, but about 10 to 15 percent regret the termination of fertility or express other dissatisfactions, including diminished sexual enjoyment, dysmenorrhea, menorrhagia-metrorrhagia, and premenstrual tension. Although tubal interruption theoretically has no effects on hormone cycles, it is possible that interference with lymphatic and vascular drainage secondary to scar tissue formation could contribute to increased pelvic congestion.

Method	Assessment	Intervention	Evaluation
All types	Understanding of sexuality, characteristics of sexual activity (i.e., regular or occasional intercourse, one or several partners) Knowledge of contraceptives and understanding of their use Previous contraceptive practices, satisfaction/dissatisfaction Menstrual and pregnancy history General health history Expectations of benefits from contraceptive method Concerns about various methods related to religious affiliation, life style, and values such as naturalism	Reinforce accurate knowledge. Teach correct information, clear misconceptions. Provide information about methods not well understood. Provide feedback about effectiveness rates, reasons why method not effective. Provide feedback about risks and contraindications of various methods. Reinforce accurate expectations, clear misconceptions. Discuss various methods, mechanisms of action and implications.	Affirms understanding, no further questions Able to select method and feel comfortable with it Effective contraceptive use (i.e., no unwanted pregnancies)
Oral Contraceptives	Determine if contraindications are present from history and physical examination. Explore understanding of requirements for this method to be effective (i.e., regularity of pill taking).	Advise if contraindicated. Discuss regular use of medication, need for periodic checkup, blood pressure, and Pap smears. Explain how to begin and discontinue pills. Discuss side effects, serious complications, when to seek medical care, what to do if one or more pills are forgotten. Discuss advantages and disadvantages.	Finds method suitable and uses effectively
IUD	Determine if contraindications are present from history and physical examination. Explore understanding of requirements for this method to be effective (i.e., checking IUD strings).	Advise if contraindicated. Discuss techniques and experience of IUD insertion and removal, need for periodic checkup and Pap smears. Explain method, discuss side effects, serious complications, when to seek medical care. Note when IUD must be replaced if copper or hormone-containing. Discuss advantages and disadvantages.	Finds method suitable and uses effectively
Diaphragm	Determine if contraindications are present from history and physical examination. Explore understanding of requirements for this method to be effective (i.e., insertion/removal techniques, checking for tears, using with every act of intercourse).	Advise if contraindicated. Discuss insertion/removal techniques, instruct and have patient practice until correctly done. Explain method and necessity for constant use, applying more spermicide with additional acts of intercourse, leaving in 6–8 hours. Advise that diaphragm must be refitted after each delivery and if substantial amount of weight is lost or gained. Discuss advantages and disadvantages.	Finds method suitable and uses effectively
Rhythm	Explore understanding of requirements for this method to be effective (i.e., long periods of abstinence, regular menstrual periods, ancillary techniques to increase effectiveness).	Discuss methods to establish baseline menstrual patterns and identify ovulation. Instruct on calculating fertile period. Discuss advantages and disadvantages.	Finds method suitable and uses effectively
Spermicides and condom	Explore understanding of requirements for this method to be effective (i.e., timing of application, regular use, precautions to avoid leakage or decreasing spermicide effectiveness).	Instruct on proper insertion of spermicides and application of condom. Advise on repeated acts of intercourse and reapplications, care in condom removal, no douching for 6–8 hours with spermicides. Discuss advantages and disadvantages.	Finds method suitable and uses effectively
Sterilization	Determine understanding of procedure as ending fertility and nonreversible. Obtain childbearing history, ages and health of children, marital situation, values assigned to reproductive role.	Discuss permanence of sterilization, emphasize as end to fertility. Explore meanings to couple. Explain various procedures and required follow-up.	Affirms understanding of permanence, desire to end childbearing; accepts requirements of procedure; satisfied with outcome

Although tubal ligation must be considered a permanent method, surgical techniques have been developed to reunite the fallopian tubes. These are difficult procedures at best. The success rate is variable, depending upon the experience of the surgeon and the extent of the segment of tube which was damaged or removed. A decision to attempt reanastomosis is usually based on social circumstances—the death of a child, divorce and remarriage, or an agonizing reappraisal of an earlier decision which was made in haste.

REFERENCES

1. "Birth Expectation Among U.S. Wives," *Family Planning Perspectives,* 7, 1:5–6, January-February 1975.

2. W. A. Darity and C. B. Turner: "Attitudes Toward Family Planning: A Comparison between Northern and Southern Black Americans," *Advances in Planned Parenthood* 8:13, 1973.

3. Adapted from HEW guidelines for informed consent to voluntary sterilization, included in R. A. Hatcher et al.: *Contraceptive Technology 1976–1977,* 8th Ed. New York, Halsted Press, Division of John Wiley & Sons, 1976, pp. 131–132.

4. I. R. Fisch and S. H. Freedman: "Oral Contraceptives, ABO Blood Groups, and in Vitro Fibrin Formation," *Obstetrics and Gynecology* 46, 4:473–479, October 1975.

5. S. L. Romney et al.: *Gynecology and Obstetrics: The Health Care of Women.* New York, McGraw-Hill, Blakiston Division, 1975, p. 562.

6. "Digest: Cigarettes Plus Pill: Deadly for Women 30 and Over," *Family Planning Perspectives* 9, 1:36, January-February 1977.

7. "Drug Data Up-Date," *American Journal of Nursing* 79, 1:137, January 1979.

8. H. A. Edmondson, B. Henderson, and B. Benton: "Liver-Cell Adenomas Associated with Use of Oral Contraceptives," *New England Journal of Medicine* 294, 9:470–472, February 26, 1976.

9. M. Stern et al.: "Cardiovascular Risk and Use of Estrogens or Estrogen-Progestogen Combinations," *JAMA* 234, 8:811–815, February 23, 1976.

10. D. T. Janerich, J. M. Piper, and D. M. Glebatis: "Oral Contraceptives and Congenital Limb-Reduction Defects," *New England Journal of Medicine* 291:697, 1974.

11. O. P. Heinonen et al.: "Cardiovascular Birth Defects and Antenatal Exposure to Female Sex Hormones," *New England Journal of Medicine* 296:67, 1977.

12. "Progestasert IUD and Ectopic Pregnancy," *FDA Bulletin,* DHEW-PHS 8, 6:37, December 1978–January 1979.

Thirteen

Pregnancy Termination

Psychological Factors Affecting Abortion Decisions /
Abortion Counseling / Abortion Procedures

The elective termination of pregnancy is sought by women for a variety of reasons including health, economics, marital status, family stability, the circumstances of conception, personal goals, age, and many other social and psychological factors. Most societies control or regulate abortion procedures in varying degrees. Whether the society's approach is permissive or restrictive depends on several factors—cultural, economic, and ecological. For example, the existence of a predominant religion in a country can affect abortion laws and practices, as can the country's economic or sociopolitical system and its population trends, level of technology, and standard of living. In general, attitudes toward abortion and the availability of abortion procedures are strongly influenced by prevailing societal values.

Women have long sought abortion as a solution to unwanted pregnancy, regardless of whether their culture approved or disapproved of this practice. Although accurate abortion statistics are difficult to obtain, especially in countries where the procedure is illegal, it is estimated that from 30 to 55 million pregnancies are willfully terminated each year throughout the world. In the United States, the abortion ratio is reported at about 500 abortions per 1,000 live births, although this varies with the area of the country.[1] Scandinavia, Japan, and Eastern European countries preceded the United States in liberalizing abortion laws and making legal abortion widely available. Prior to 1973, the U.S. had restrictive abortion laws which generally allowed "therapeutic" abortion only when the mother's life or health were threatened by the pregnancy, or when the pregnancy had resulted from felonious intercourse (rape, incest). As each state had its own abortion laws, some also permitted the procedure when there was substantial risk that the child would be born with a serious physical or mental defect.

In 1973 a substantive change occurred in the legal status of pregnancy termination in the United States when the Supreme Court announced a decision to legalize abortion. This decision left the choice for abortion, before the end of the first trimester, to the judgment of the pregnant woman and her physician. During the second trimester, the state can regulate the circumstances of abortion to ensure safety, but cannot otherwise interfere with the decision. When pregnancy is advanced beyond the second trimester, state law determines what can and cannot be done. States can regulate and even proscribe abortion subsequent to viability, defined to be between 24 and 26 weeks gestation, except when necessary for the preservation of the life or health of the mother. As the result of the changed legal status, pregnancy terminations are now being sought and obtained in large numbers throughout the United States.

Availability of legal abortion has dramatically decreased the maternal mortality and morbidity previously associated with illegal, criminal abortion (see Chapter 31, Complications of Pregnancy).

Although abortion is now legal, it is still viewed with misgivings on the part of many, based mainly on religious and personal attitudes toward pregnancy termination. Most agree that abortion is not a happy substitute for pregnancy prevention and that the procedures necessary for bringing about termination, though generally safe, are associated with a higher morbidity than are most contraceptive methods.

The nurse must recognize that attitudes toward abortion are varied and personal and that there are strong religious and moral influences in these attitudes. One is entitled to one's own conclusions on this matter but the opinions of others should be respected. Personal convictions of health professionals in this area are generally respected, and those who do not feel that abortion is ethically acceptable should make their views known so that arrangements can be made well in advance for substitute medical personnel.

PSYCHOSOCIAL FACTORS AFFECTING ABORTION DECISIONS

Pregnancy is an event in a woman's life which is surrounded by many positive values, ranging from enhancement of the self-concept to social approval. The highest value placed on women in most societies is for their role as mothers, and powerful systems of reinforcement operate to make motherhood central to women's lives. A decision to terminate a pregnancy is rarely taken without some conflict, because of the complex meanings and values associated with reproduction and motherhood. Even if the outcome of pregnancy (a child) is consciously unwanted, the woman may on some level desire to be pregnant as a symbol of potency, vitality, or reconnection with primal inner forces. While pregnancy can be completely accidental, it is often used to affect relations with important people in the woman's life, such as parents, husband, or lover.

A teenage girl may become pregnant to demon-strate her maturity, prove her sexuality, or bolster her self-concept as a woman. She may become pregnant because her romantic ideals of motherhood and man-woman relations preclude the use of contraceptives which imply premeditated sexual activity. Or pregnancy may result from sexual experimentation when neither partner takes responsibility for avoiding unwanted consequences. A woman at any age may use pregnancy as a means of alleviating feelings of inadequacy or doubts about her femininity. A woman entering menopause may conceive to reinforce her sexual self-image or avoid facing the loss of reproductive capacity. Although pregnancy per se may be desired in these instances, the woman may find she cannot face the responsibilities of caring for and raising a child, and so elects abortion as the most reasonable solution.

Marital status can also affect the decision to continue or terminate a pregnancy. Many unmarried women feel incapable of raising a child outside of marriage, although there are increasing numbers of single parents and more social acceptance of this situation. The critical factor is the quality of the man-woman relation and meaning for the woman of commitment and dependability. Pregnancy has historically been used to force a man into marriage, but has proven to be a poor basis on which to build a lifetime relationship. In marriages which are in trouble and facing dissolution, pregnancy may be used as an attempt to prevent a break-up. A woman may also become pregnant, even though she does not truly desire a child, in order to meet her partner's expectation, for example, if the man's sense of masculinity or potency requires that "his woman" become pregnant. In many of these cases, however, the pregnancy does not produce the desired result, and the woman may seek abortion when she realizes that motives for pregnancy were not appropriate for her.

Poor physical or mental health can lead a woman to terminate her pregnancy if pregnancy poses a risk to her life or a drain on her already depleted energies. Or a life crisis and emotional upheaval may lead a woman to feel incapable of coping with pregnancy and motherhood until her life becomes less chaotic.

Abortion may also be the choice of action when a pregnancy is untimely. Education or professional goals may have higher priority at the time, or pregnancy may occur too early in a marriage or too soon after the birth of a child. Or the couple may feel emotionally or economically unable to manage parenthood. Couples frequently seek abortion for economic reasons. They prefer to strive for a higher standard of living and greater social opportunity for themselves and their children and are unwilling to be subjected to increased material hardship.

Abortion may be sought for eugenic reasons, even if pregnancy and the child are desired. Patients are becoming better informed about the hereditary genetic defects for which their offspring may be at risk and are taking advantage of screening programs to detect such conditions as Tay-Sachs disease, hemophilia, Down's syndrome, sickle cell disease, and other genetic abnormalities. Awareness of fetal anomalies caused by rubella, exposure to radiation, and teratogenic drugs may cause some women to elect abortion if exposure occurred during the first trimester.

Sociocultural factors play an important role in a decision to seek abortion. If abortion is illegal the woman risks criminal prosecution, and if social values condemn abortion she faces disapproval by peers, family, and community. When abortion is legal and there are generally accepting social values, deciding to have an abortion does not present such a traumatic experience and is usually well accepted emotionally. Studies have demonstrated that there are few negative psychological reactions to abortion when positive attitudes on the part of professional staff encourage acceptance.[2] It also has been shown that psychologic sequelae are usually of short duration and reflect the circumstances surrounding abortion and attitudes conveyed by peer group, family, and health providers.[3]

ABORTION COUNSELING

The nurse is often a key professional in providing counseling to patients considering abortion. The need to weigh alternatives and make responsible decisions about an unwanted pregnancy may become apparent in the prenatal or family planning clinic or other health care setting. As part of patient education and the supportive role, the nurse may offer initial discussion and assistance in problem-solving to women or couples facing the problem of an undesired conception.

The approach to pregnancy termination varies according to gestational age. Prior to the twelfth week, abortion is generally a relatively uncomplicated vaginal procedure. Beyond the eleventh to twelfth week, termination requires more complex procedures, often involving amniocentesis, for which one to three days of hospitalization are often necessary and the complication rate is considerably higher. Many physicians or hospitals will not perform abortions beyond the twentieth to twenty-fourth week of gestation.

First trimester abortion may be carried out as an outpatient procedure. Extra-hospital facilities have been established, and many hospitals have designed facilities for outpatient procedures. Personnel in such units should include counselors whose role it is to help the patient to evaluate the decision to terminate pregnancy, to review alternate possibilities—having the baby and placing it for adoption—and to provide contraception advice. Termination of a pregnancy is often an emotionally charged situation and must be handled with the greatest skill and delicacy.

Many women need assistance to help them think beyond their first reaction to the unwanted pregnancy. They need to be encouraged to consider other options available to them. Many women feel ambivalent and confused and are under pressure from family or their own social values. It is important that the nurse stress that the woman make the decision for herself, since there is less regret and emotional sequelae when the choice is not perceived as being forced by other people. Exploring alternatives realistically helps clarify the situation and place manageable boundaries within which the decision can be made. Thinking through what each choice means not only for present feelings and relations but also for future circumstances, goals, and needs, both from a practical and emotional-values standpoint, encourages a carefully weighed choice. While the counseling is in progress, tests are carried out to confirm the pregnancy and determine the length of gestation, and the type of abortion procedure indicated is discussed. These factors in and of themselves may influence the decision. Simply knowing that the pregnancy has progressed beyond the time when simple curettage can be used and that the abortion may actually involve labor and expulsion of the fetus may cause a woman to decline abortion. In any event, understanding the nature of the procedure required is essential to informed decision-making.

ABORTION PROCEDURES

The abortion procedure used will depend on the length of pregnancy. Pregnancies up to 12 weeks gestation are usually terminated by dilatation and evacuation (D&E, suction curettage) or by standard dilatation and curettage (D&C). In the early stages of pregnancy, prostaglandins may be used in the form of vaginal suppositories, intramuscular injections, or transcervical instillation to induce abortion. Or a suctioning method for menstrual extraction or regulation may be carried out by means of a very small cannula. This procedure is occasionally used during the first two weeks after a missed menstrual period, frequently before pregnancy is confirmed. When pregnancy has progressed to between 12 and 14 weeks, termination becomes more difficult. Suction curettage can be used, but the complication rate increases, and intraamniotic instillations of solutions to induce labor are not yet effective. Serial intramuscular injections of prostaglandins (the 15 methyl analogues) have been quite successful in inducing abortion during this time, but with the usual side effects involving temperature regulation and gastrointestinal symptoms. From 16 to 20 weeks gestation, intraamniotic instillation of hypertonic saline, urea, and prostaglandins are effective.

Techniques Prior to 12 Weeks Gestation

Suction Curettage

Increasingly the procedure of choice for the termination of early pregnancy is *suction curettage* (Fig. 13-1). A local anesthetic (paracervical block) or a light general anesthetic may be used. The cervix is dilated with graduated dilators and a suction curette is placed into the endometrial cavity to the fundus. Suction is applied, usually by electric pump, and the products of conception are evacuated into a container. These are usually sent to the pathology laboratory for confirmation of the pregnancy and to rule out unusual conditions such as hydatidiform mole (see p. 509). Generally, recovery takes from two to three hours, during which time the patient is observed for excessive bleeding.

In some circumstances, the cervix is prepared for the abortion by the use of *laminaria*. These are

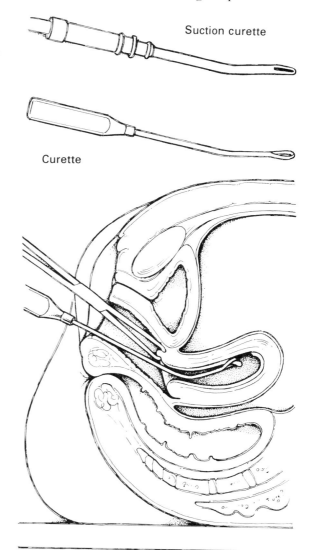

Figure 13-1. Curettage or vacuum aspiration for first trimester abortion.

lengths of sterile hydroscopic material, derived from seaweed, which absorb moisture at a rapid rate. When placed in the cervical canal, they expand in three to six hours and cause cervical dilatation. Insertion of laminaria several hours prior to a first trimester abortion can reduce the need for mechanical cervical dilatation. Some feel their use decreases the incidence of cervical lacerations.

Surgical (Sharp) Curettage

Standard dilatation and curettage, used for first trimester abortions, requires a general anesthetic and the usual preoperative precautions. The cervix must be dilated more than for suction curettage, and there is more danger of cervical laceration and blood loss. The advantage of this technique is that it is widely used and known to family physicians, general practitioners, and obstetrician-gynecologists.

Menstrual Extraction

Aspiration of the endometrium on an outpatient basis performed from five to seven weeks after the last menstrual period is called menstrual extraction, menstrual regulation, menstrual induction, minisuction, miniabortion, and interception. The procedure is simple and relatively atraumatic, as little or no cervical dilatation is required and no anesthetic usually given. A 4 to 6 mm. flexible plastic cannula and a syringe or other low pressure suction are used. The uterus need not be clinically enlarged, and often a pregnancy test is not required since one of the advantages of the procedure is that the woman need not know for certain if she is pregnant. Although this procedure has been taught and used among womens' groups as a self-administered technique, it is not safe to use it this way because of the dangers of hemorrhage, retained products, and infection.

Prostaglandins

Prostaglandins, a group of fatty acids found in the semen, are very effective abortifacients at any stage of pregnancy. The exact mechanisms by which they work are not clearly understood. Oral administration is impractical because of the high incidence of side effects, the most common being vomiting, diarrhea, fever, and shaking. Vaginal, intramuscular, and transcervical administration produce fewer side effects and serious complications are rare. Prostaglandins will no doubt be used with more frequency as preparations are refined and side effects minimized.[4]

Techniques after 12 Weeks Gestation

Hypertonic Saline

When pregnancy has progressed beyond the twelfth week, termination is often carried out by instillation of *hypertonic saline* into the amniotic cavity. This procedure is most easily carried out beyond the fourteenth week, when there is sufficient fluid in the amniotic cavity to be identified and aspirated. The bladder is emptied, and the patient is placed in the supine position. The skin is prepped and draped with sterile towels, and infiltrated with a local anesthetic over the injection site. An 18-gauge spinal needle is then inserted through the uterus into the amniotic cavity. When properly placed, clear amniotic fluid flows into the syringe attached to the needle. After a small amount of fluid is removed to verify proper placement of the needle, hypertonic saline is injected into the amniotic cavity. Initially a small amount is placed, and if there is no reaction, the remainder is delivered over approximately 15 minutes.

Following a latent period of several hours, labor usually ensues and the fetus with part or all of the placenta is delivered within 24 to 72 hours. If the placenta cannot be extracted completely after delivery, a curettage must be carried out to complete the abortion. During the course of labor, the contractions can cause considerable discomfort. As the cervix dilates, the patient should be medicated at intervals and generally a substantial amount of emotional support is needed during this process. The previable fetus is usually dead at the time of delivery, but at this late stage of gestation it has human form.

Oxytocin infusion is often used as an adjunct to saline abortion, to decrease the time needed for completion of the process. Oxytocin is used in a manner similar to that employed for induction of labor (see Chapter 31) except that a more concentrated solution is used. The oxytocin drip is begun six to twelve hours after amnio infusion of saline. Maximum time of oxytocin use should be limited to 24 hours. When used longer, there is an increased incidence of water retention which could lead to water intoxication.

In cases where the hypertonic saline fails to induce contractions, a repeat dose must be administered. In some circumstances, as in severe hypertension, infusion of hypertonic saline is contraindicated. Complications most often include hemorrhage, infection, and retained placenta. Occasionally more serious complications occur as a result of the intravenous injection of saline, including hypernatremia, amniotic fluid embolism, disseminated intravascular coagulation, and necrosis of the myometrium from saline entering the uterine musculature.

TABLE 13-1
MORBIDITY AND MORTALITY RATES FOR COMMON METHODS OF INDUCED ABORTION

Type of Complication	D and C	Suction	Saline	Hysterotomy
Hemorrhage	1.0	0.5	4.0	3.7
Infection	0.9	0.8	5.4	11.0
Perforation	1.9	1.3	0.2	5.1
Anesthesia	0.1	0.1	0.1	0.7
Shock	—	—	0.2	0.7
Retained products	0.5	0.5	14.7	1.5
Lacerated cervix	0.3	0.2	0.1	0.7
Other	0.3	0.3	1.0	4.4
Unspecified	0.1	—	0.2	—
Total morbidity*	5.1	3.7	28.3	27.8
Total mortality†	2.8	1.2	22.9	235.3

* Complications per 1,000 abortions
† Deaths per 100,000 abortions
Martin, Leonide L.: *Health Care of Women*. Philadelphia, J. B. Lippincott, 1978, p. 193.

Intraamniotic Prostaglandins

Instillation of prostaglandins into the amniotic cavity by a similar amniocentesis technique has become the preferred method of inducing midtrimester abortions, as its complication rate is lower than with saline and the onset of labor with subsequent expulsion is more rapid. Medication can be used to control the gastrointestinal side effects. Women with asthma or pulmonary disease are at increased risk, since the drug can cause marked bronchospasm. Other rare serious complications are arrhythmias, cardiovascular changes, and grand mal seizures. These complications are more frequent when the prostaglandins enter systemic circulation; therefore, careful placement in the uterine cavity reduces the incidence of such complications.

Over half of the women given intraamniotic prostaglandins abort within 24 hours, and 93 percent abort within 48 hours.[5] Although these drugs are more expensive than sodium chloride, this may be offset by shorter hospitalization and fewer complications.

Intramuscular Prostaglandins

Serial intramuscular injections of the 15 methyl analogues of prostaglandins are effective in terminating pregnancies of between 10 and 17 weeks gestation. Contractions begin rapidly and are intense within 40 minutes, with abortion completed within 12 hours in 76 percent of the patients and within 24 hours in 96 percent. One type of prostaglandin causes greater gastrointestinal symptoms, and the other type causes more temperature elevation, shak-

ing, and chills. This method is managed as an inpatient procedure, because repeated injections are necessary and labor must be carefully monitored.[6]

Hysterotomy

When there is failure of other methods of midtrimester abortion, or saline or prostaglandins are contraindicated for various reasons, a hysterotomy or mini-cesarean section may be performed. The operation is major surgery and may be done abdominally or vaginally, requiring the standard preoperative preparations and general or spinal anesthesia. The morbidity and mortality from this procedure are greater than for other techniques and delivery of a live fetus may occur. Advantages include the opportunity for concomitant sterilization by tubal ligation or hysterectomy, and treatment of pelvic disease. Table 13-1 summarizes morbidity and mortality rates for the commonly used methods of pregnancy termination.

Follow-up Care

After a first trimester abortion, the woman is instructed about signs and symptoms of complications and how to contact the clinic or physician should these occur. Fever and chills, foul-smelling discharge, heavy bleeding, severe abdominal pain, and nausea and vomiting can indicate complications. Abstinence from intercourse and avoidance of tampons and douching for two weeks are advised. Normal activity may be resumed in one or two days in most instances. Contraception is discussed

NURSING CARE: PREGNANCY TERMINATION

Assessment	Intervention	Evaluation
Menstrual history and last menstrual period, use of contraceptives. Assist in physical examination, collection of specimens, pregnancy tests to determine length of gestation. Circumstances surrounding unwanted conception. Understanding of physiology of conception, contraceptive methods. Level of ambivalence or certainty about abortion decision. Involvement of partner, family, parents and sources of support. Consideration of alternatives to abortion. Presence of crisis, need for further psychological counseling. Pregnancy and health history to identify special needs and risks.	Advise of length of gestation and what type of procedure this indicates. Discuss various types of abortion procedures, time in hospital or if outpatient, techniques and what the experience entails, risks and complications. Explore alternate choices (i.e., have abortion, continue pregnancy and either keep or give baby for adoption) and meanings these have for woman and partner/family. Assist during procedures, provide support, clarification, and keep patient informed of process. Advise of postabortion complications, when to seek medical care, preventive measures, when to resume activities and sex. Discuss contraception, follow-up visits, emotional reactions. Initiate referral to psychological counseling if indicated. For midtrimester abortion, monitor during labor, provide pain relief, supportive care, and facilitate presence of companion if desired.	Able to reach decision about pregnancy termination with which patient feels comfortable. Accepts requirements of various procedures as indicated by gestational age. Affirms understanding of process of conception and effective use of contraception. Returns for follow-up visit and institutes contraceptive method. Feels accepting of abortion if undertaken, no serious emotional problems. Seeks prenatal care if abortion decided against. Avoids future unwanted pregnancies. Initiates psychological counseling if emotionally distressed.

and occasionally an IUD inserted at the time of abortion, but perforation and expulsion rates are high. Oral contraceptives may be given with instructions that they be started one week after the abortion. It is standard to have a follow-up office visit in two weeks, at which time contraceptives are prescribed if not already begun. The patient's adjustment to termination of pregnancy, as well as her partner's or family's reactions, can be discussed and referral made if needed for psychological, social, or economic reasons.

Following midtrimester abortion, RhoGAM is administered to unsensitized Rh negative women. Instructions about signs and symptoms of infection and hemorrhage are given, and patients advised to avoid sex, tampons, and douches for two weeks. Since there is frequently some depression similar to postpartum blues, probably related to drastic hormonal changes, women need to be prepared for this. A return visit is scheduled for two weeks after the abortion, at which time uterine size should be normal and bleeding ceased. Contraception is usually initiated and reactions to the abortion discussed with referral as needed.

REFERENCES

1. C. Tietze: "Incidence of Legal Abortion," in A. R. Omran, ed.: *Liberalization of Abortion Laws: Implications.* Chapel Hill, University of North Carolina, Carolina Population Center, 1976, pp. 1–4.

2. J. D. Osofsky and J. H. Osofky: "The Psychological Reactions of Patients to Legalized Abortion." Paper presented at meeting of the American Orthopsychiatric Association, March 1971.

3. N. F. Woods: *Human Sexuality in Health and Illness.* St. Louis, C. V. Mosby, 1975, p. 83.

4. M. Bygdeman, et al.: "Outpatient Postconceptional Fertility Control with Vaginally Administered 15 (S)15-methyl-PGF$_2\alpha$-methyl ester," *American Journal of Obstetrics and Gynecology* 12, 5:495–498, March 1, 1976.

5. W. E. Brenner: "The Current Status of Prostaglandins as Abortifacients," *American Journal of Obstetrics and Gynecology* 123, 3: 306–328, October 1, 1975.

6. N. H. Lauersen, et al.: "Midtrimester Abortion Induced by Serial Intramuscular Injections of 12 (s)-12-methyl-prostaglandin E$_2$-methyl ester," *American Journal of Obstetrics and Gynecology* 123, 7:665–670, December 1, 1975.

SUGGESTED READING

Bendel, R. P., Williams, P. P., and Butler, J. C.: "Endometrial Aspiration in Fertility Control." *American Journal of Obstetrics and Gynecology* June 1, 1976, 328–32.

Brenner, W. E., et al.: "Suction Curettage for 'Menstrual Regulation.' " *Advances in Planned Parenthood.* Proceedings of the Annual Meeting, American Association of Planned Parenthood Physicians 9, 1974.

Burchell, R. C.: "Professional Perspectives on Abortion." *Journal of Obstetric, Gynecologic and Neonatal Nursing* 3:25–27, November-December 1974.

Gedan, S.: "Abortion Counseling with Adolescents." *American Journal of Nursing* 74: 1856–58, 1974.

Irani, K. R. et al.: "Menstrual Induction: Its Place in Clinical Practice." *American Journal of Obstetrics and Gynecology* 46, 5:596–598, November 1, 1975.

Sarvis, B. and Rodman, H.: "Social and Cultural Aspects of Abortion: Class and Race." In N. Ostheimer and J. M. Ostheimer, eds.: *Life or Death—Who Controls?* New York, Springer, 1976, pp. 104–118.

Tanis, J. L.: "Recognizing the Reasons for Contraceptive Non-Use and Abuse." *MCN—The American Journal of Maternal Child Nursing,* 2, 3:364–369, May-June 1977.

Fourteen

Infertility

Counseling Considerations | Standards for Infertility Studies | The Infertile Couple | The Seminal Factor | The Postcoital Test—Evaluation of Insemination | The Ovarian Factor | Tubal Factors | The Uterine Factor

Increased levels of technology have introduced an element of choice in reproduction. Yet, during the course of nursing practice, one will surely encounter patients who are pregnant when they do not wish to be or are infertile when pregnancy is consummately desired.

Regulation of fertility is most often expressed in demographic terms. Indeed, population pressures represent a major social force. For the practicing nurse or physician, however, the importance of understanding and controlling reproductive potential is perhaps more cogently expressed in individual terms. The right of choice of the individual has been emphasized by international bodies. The General Assembly of the United Nations has declared that, "The size of the family should be the free choice of each individual family." The concept was later expanded to include the right to the means to space and limit births.

At the other end of the spectrum, fertility is not always a matter of choice. The generally accepted estimate is that about 10 percent of couples are infertile. One can realistically project a rise in the incidence of infertility due to social causes. The increase in the prevalence of gonorrheal salpingitis, and recent changes in women's social orientation—with the concomitant trend toward postponement

of childbearing until the late reproductive years—will materially influence reproductive potential. A shortage of children for adoption has created additional pressures.

COUNSELING CONSIDERATIONS

Often the nurse is called upon to act as counselor in what inevitably is an emotionally charged situation—as a couple faces the prospect of a barren marriage. Ideally the nurse should be equipped to schedule and interpret the various tests used in an infertility investigation and to understand, in order to be able to explain to the patient, the physiologic basis for treatment.

In preceding chapters, basic reproductive mechanisms were discussed and events beginning with spermatogenesis and oogenesis and ending in the development of the term fetus were explored. This information will now serve as a basis for understanding the clinical approach to problems of human reproduction.

When one considers the complexity of reproductive processes, it is not surprising that unprotected coitus at about the time of ovulation does not always result in a pregnancy. In fact, under normal circumstances an average of six cycles of exposure is required. It is generally felt that infertility should be explored after a year's exposure without contraception. However, it is unwise to insist on an interval of one year before investigation is initiated in each case. A reassuring consultation is often helpful, if only to dispel doubts concerning the existence of major abnormalities. Since fertility declines with age, it would seem justifiable for couples in their thirties to seek advice somewhat earlier. Even among younger couples when the nurse or physician senses that there is anxiety over failure to conceive or when on cursory exploration there is an obvious reason for infertility, for example, amenorrhea, or a history of acute salpingitis or postabortal infection, early evaluation is in order.

STANDARDS FOR INFERTILITY STUDIES

Before selecting a method of treatment, efforts should be made in identifying the underlying cause of infertility. Appropriate therapy can be selected only after the cause for infertility is determined. Shotgun measures involving use of so-called fertility drugs are useless and are to be deplored. There is no quick substitute for a carefully planned investigative program. Minimal standards which are suggested for a complete infertility investigation include evaluation of seminal, cervical, ovarian, tubal, peritoneal, and uterine factors. In addition, the frequency and technique of intercourse should be explored. The ultimate goal of an infertility investigation is not solely that of a successful pregnancy. It is equally important to establish a prognosis and thus to enable couples who, after careful evaluation, are finally adjudged hopelessly sterile to plan their lives realistically.

THE INFERTILE COUPLE

Since infertility is usually caused by abnormalities in the anatomy and physiology of the male or female reproductive tract, management of the problem involves both marital partners. Male factors are responsible in at least 35 percent of infertility in couples, and evaluation of the husband early in the course of the investigation is mandatory.

In the initial interview, sexual habits should be reviewed with both husband and wife. Although the frequency of coitus varies greatly from one couple to the next, patterns of intercourse do influence fertility. Only about 16 percent of couples who are having intercourse less than once a week will conceive in less than six months. Over 80 percent conceive in the same interval when exposure occurs four or more times weekly. When intercourse occurs infrequently the sexual adjustment in the marriage should be explored. There is no evidence to suggest a relationship between female orgasm and conception. Nevertheless, the frequency of coitus is influenced by sexual satisfaction; intercourse may be infrequent because it is associated with discomfort (dyspareunia) or because it is simply not a pleasurable experience for the wife.

Patients who have made it a habit to arise from bed immediately after intercourse, spilling much of the ejaculate shortly after it is placed in the vagina, should be advised to remain in bed for at least 30 minutes following coitus. Occasionally, couples admit to using lubricants during intercourse which may interfere with sperm migration or to douching postcoitally. Petroleum jelly (Vaseline) and some of the water soluble lubricants have been shown to be spermicidal. These factors may not cause infertility when the husband's fertility potential is normal, but may play a role when sperm production is marginal. In the occasional patient, there is even anatomical evidence—an intact hymenal ring or a rigid perineal body—that normal intercourse is not occurring. Other sexual problems such as premature ejaculation may have resulted in failure of proper placement of sperm. Sympathetic and knowledgeable advice in these areas is often useful not only in the treatment of infertility but also in bringing about a better marital adjustment in this sexual sphere.

THE SEMINAL FACTOR

Because evaluation of the male is much less complicated than the series of tests required to explore female infertility, his reproductive potential should always be assessed initially. The postcoital test—examination of cervical mucus for the presence of spermatozoa—is useful in this regard. Unless adequate numbers of spermatozoa are seen in the cervical mucus following coitus, the semen should be evaluated. This involves assessment of the fresh ejaculate obtained by masturbation after at least three days of abstinence. The ejaculate is collected in a clean, dry container and brought to the laboratory as soon after collection as practical. The patient should be cautioned not to lose the first few drops of the ejaculate, since the majority of active spermatozoa are located in the first portion of the specimen. Normally, seminal fluid becomes coagulated immediately upon ejaculation. Liquefaction of the coagulum occurs within 20 minutes. Examination should be deferred until liquefaction is complete, because the coagulum interferes with the distribution of spermatozoa in the counting chamber.

The volume of the specimen, sperm density, percentage of motile forms, quality of the motility, and the percentage of abnormal spermatozoa are determined. The volume of the normal ejaculate ranges from 2 to 5 ml. A sperm count of more than 20 million/ml. is considered normal, provided the quality and percentage of motility in the specimen are also normal. The single most useful criterion is the actual quality of motility—the ability of spermatozoa to progress.

Because there is usually some variation in the quality of semen ejaculated at various times, assessment of the husband's fertility potential should never be based on a single analysis. Since maturation of spermatozoa within the testis occurs over a 60-day interval, the quality of semen could be influenced by an event, such as a viral infection, that took place many days before the spermatozoa appeared in the ejaculate.

If the postcoital test is abnormal, but the semen analysis is within normal limits, the possibility that semen is not being ejaculated deep in the vagina during intercourse should be considered. In such cases, further investigations of coital techniques and examination of the male genitalia is often helpful. Hypospadias, a condition in which the opening of the urethra is located along the shaft of the penis and not at the glans, may result in loss of the ejaculate high in the vagina. Discussion may uncover unsuspected sexual difficulties, such as premature ejaculation or even impotence. The diagnostic importance of a postcoital test in these situations is obvious.

When the semen analysis or postcoital test is abnormal, the male partner should be evaluated further for anatomical, genetic, or endocrine abnormalities. These evaluations are usually carried out by urologists with special interest in infertility. A recently emerging subspecialty, *andrology*—devoted to the study of male reproductive problems—places major emphasis on the diagnosis and treatment of the infertile male.

THE POSTCOITAL TEST—EVALUATION OF INSEMINATION

A couple is instructed to have intercourse during the 12 hours preceding the examination. The test is timed for within a day or two before expected ovulation, that is, day 12 or 13 in the 28-day menstrual cycle. At that time, the cervical mucus, under the influence of estrogen, is normally clear and abundant and is most receptive to spermatozoa. At other times in the cycle, the mucus is scanty, thick, and turbid and generally unreceptive.

A sample of cervical mucus is obtained as follows: The cervix is exposed with vaginal speculum, and after secretions and debris are gently wiped from the exocervix, mucus is removed from well within the endocervical canal. An instrument, such as a fenestrated intestinal forceps or a nasal polyp forceps may be used for this purpose, or the mucus may be aspirated from the cervix into a polyethylene tube. Its gross characteristics, quantity and clarity are evaluated, and its ability to form a thin continuous thread (a quality referred to as *spinnbarkeit*) is assessed. *Spinnbarkeit* is determined by stretching the mucus between the tips of the forceps until the thread breaks. Normal preovulatory mucus can be stretched for a distance of up to 10 cm. The sample is then placed on a clean, dry slide and a cover slip applied. The specimen is then examined microscopically for spermatozoa. The test is normal when there are more than 20 motile spermatozoa/HPF in areas of clear, abundant cervical mucus. In addition to allowing assessment of proper placement of spermatozoa during coitus, the postcoital test permits evaluation of the quality of cervical secretions and their ability to support the life of the spermatozoon—the cervical factor.

The Cervical Factor

In order to assess the quality of the cervical secretions and to diagnose abnormalities at that level, the timing of the recovery of the mucus in the cycle is critical. One should be mindful of the normal variations in mucus quality in the menstrual cycle. If the mucus never demonstrates the characteristics of normal ovulatory mucus after serial evaluation on alternate days during the presumed ovulatory period, the possibility that mucus production is deficient should be seriously considered. Inability of spermatozoa to penetrate and survive in such mucus may reasonably be inferred to be a cause of infertility.

Because little is known about the physiology of cervical mucus production, treatment of the cervical factor has not been uniformly successful. Local treatment of the cervix when there is a cervicitis and the use of small doses of estrogen prior to ovulation have been suggested to produce a mucus more favorable to sperm migration, but success with such treatment is limited.

Artificial Insemination

In selected cases, artificial placement of semen is an effective therapeutic modality. The technique involves insertion of a freshly ejaculated specimen at the cervical os with a cannula and syringe (Fig. 14-1) within a day or two of the estimated time of ovulation. Alternatively, the specimen can be injected into a plastic cervical cap placed around the cervix. The cap retains the specimen at the cervix and is removed several hours later. In order to be sure that ovulation has been covered, insemination is repeated on alternate days until it has been determined by the temperature chart that ovulation has occurred.

AIH. Artificial insemination with the husband's specimen (AIH) is especially useful in cases in which the postcoital test consistently reveals few or absent spermatozoa in cervical mucus of good quality. In selected cases, the use of a "split ejaculate" is recommended. Here, the specimen is collected into two containers. By and large, the first portion of the ejaculate contains a significantly higher portion of normal motile spermatozoa and it is this first portion which is used for the insemination.

AID. In cases of azoospermia (absence of spermatozoa in the ejaculate) or severe oligospermia (markedly decreased numbers) which has failed to respond to treatment, insemination of a specimen from a donor (AID) may be employed. AID is sometimes called "semi-adoption" and has gained increasing popularity and acceptability in recent years. Willingness of a couple to consider AID has been influenced to a large degree in recent years by the lack of availability of children for adoption. AID is also used in cases in which the husband suffers from a genetic defect or in cases of RH sensitization. In the latter instance, an RH negative donor is used.

The physician who wishes to use donor insemination should settle on an organized approach and must be willing to give this procedure the necessary time and attention it demands. Selection of the donor must be carried out with great care, with attention to general state of health, genetic background, RH type, and physical characteristics which at least to some degree resemble those of the husband. Those advising patients on this matter, should be aware of the social and ethical implications of the procedure and should allow adequate time to explore matters with the couple in depth before proceeding. On the positive side, when donor insemination is accepted by informed consenting partners, the end result is usually satisfactory. There is a remarkable marriage stability among properly

Figure 14-1. Technique for artificial insemination.

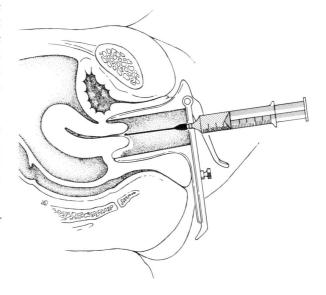

selected couples who have been treated with AID. Recently, freeze-stored semen has been used to increase the rate of availability of specimens for donor insemination.

THE OVARIAN FACTOR

Clearly, conception does not occur when there is failure of ovulation, and fertility is impaired when ovulation is infrequent. Thus, ovulation detection is an integral part of the infertility investigation. Clues as to the occurrence of ovulation are derived from menstrual history (see p. 89), evaluation of characteristic changes in cervical mucus, and by the basal body temperature chart (see p. 97). Additional parameters used to assess ovulation include histologic evaluation of a sample of endometrium obtained by biopsy and a plasma progesterone determination obtained late in the cycle.

Endometrial biopsy is a simple office procedure and offers the additional advantage of ruling out a chronic inflammatory condition in the endometrium. Any one of the available specially designed biopsy curettes may be used (Fig. 14-2).

After the position of the uterus is determined, a curette is gently introduced through the cervical canal to the level of the fundus and one or two samples of tissue removed. The endometrial sample is then sent to the pathologist's laboratory for evaluation.

Figure 14-2. Biopsy curettes for endometrial biopsy.

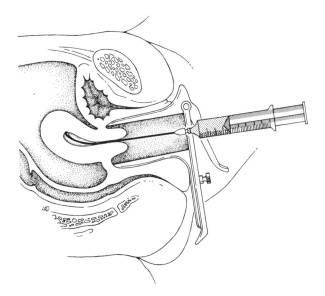

Following ovulation, the endometrium takes on "secretory" changes under the influence of progesterone. The changes in the endometrium after ovulation are progressive and predictable and timing of ovulation can be established retrospectively. Additional evidence of corpus luteum function and, therefore, indirect evidence of ovulation is obtained when plasma progesterone levels are greater than 4 ng. per ml.

Treatment of Ovulatory Failure

Treatment of anovulotory infertility depends on the underlying cause. When failure of ovulation is suspected, a thorough endocrine evaluation is in order. The defect may occur at the level of the hypothalamus, the pituitary, or the ovaries themselves. Ovulation is also influenced by the patient's general state of health and thyroid and adrenal abnormalities.

Ovulatory failure can be caused by a pituitary adenoma, a space-occupying tumor within the pituitary gland. Such tumors produce the breast-stimulating hormone, prolactin, and thus are often associated with secretions from the breasts (galactorrhea). Patients with ovulatory failure should be screened for this condition by careful examination of the breasts for secretions and if galactorrhea is present, a serum prolactin determination should be carried out. When prolactin levels are elevated, the pituitary must be evaluated further. Serial x-rays or tomograms of the sella turcica, the bony structure in which the pituitary gland is located, are useful in this regard. Any patient exhibiting galactorrhea with elevated prolactin levels should be evaluated with tomography before treatment with ovulation-inducing methods is considered.

Recent availability of effective agents for the induction of ovulation has made careful evaluation of patients suspected of anovulatory infertility all the more important. In properly selected cases, the use of an estrogen antagonist, *clomiphene citrate,* is associated with a success rate above 50 percent. In patients whose ovulatory failure is the result of a defect at the hypothalamic-pituitary level, the use of *human menopausal gonadotropin (HMG),* derived from the urine of postmenopausal women, is associated with some success. Multiple pregnancies, which have received considerable attention in the press, are usually the result of HMG treatment.

Even in expert hands, it is difficult to avoid over-stimulation of the ovary with HMG and induction of more than one ovulation in a given cycle.

TUBAL FACTORS

The clinical approach to tubal disease involves assessment of tubal and peritubal anatomy. Since the human tube is a conduit which provides a passage between the ovary and uterus, tubal obstruction, of course, results in infertility. In addition, since the fimbriated end of the tube is important in transferring the ovum from the rupturing follicle to the tubal lumen, when the relationship between it and the ovum is distorted by pelvic adhesions, fertility is diminished.

Anatomic defects in and about the fallopian tubes are generally a result of a past infection or pelvic irritation. Acute gonorrheal salpingitis, seen with increasing frequency, is a common offender. A ruptured appendix associated with pelvic peritonitis may also cause peritubal and periovarian adhesions.

Endometriosis, a condition in which the endometrium has been displaced into the peritoneal cavity around the tube and ovaries, may also result in pelvic adhesions and distortion of pelvic architecture. Treatment of anatomic tubal disease is surgical, involving lysis and excision of the adhesions and special techniques to reestablish the patency of the fallopian tubes.

The commonly used tests for evaluation of tubal function include uterotubal insufflation (the Rubin's test), hysterosalpingography, and finally endoscopy.

Uterotubal insufflation involves the introduction of carbon dioxide into the uterus via a cannula. If one or both of the tubes are patent, the carbon dioxide flows along the uterus and tubes into the peritoneal cavity. When the patient sits up, the carbon dioxide rises to the diaphragm, causing pain in the shoulder referred there via the phrenic nerve. This test is useful only as a screening measure and, increasingly, physicians have substituted other methods for it.

Hysterosalpingography involves introduction of radiopaque material into the uterus and fallopian tubes (Fig. 14-3). This is usually done under fluoroscopic visualization, and x-rays are taken at intervals to provide a permanent record. When the tubes are patent, the radiopaque material enters the peritoneal

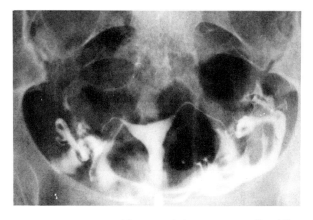

Figure 14-3A. A normal hysterosalpingogram revealing bilateral tubal patency with spill of radiopaque material into the peritoneal cavity. (Mastroianni, "Variations of Fertility.")

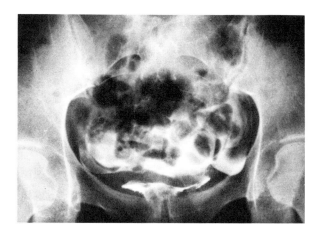

Figure 14-3B. Pelvic (peritubal and periovarian) adhesions associated with infertility. Ruptured appendix occurred at age eight. (Mastroianni, L., Jr.: "Variations of Fertility." In S. Romney, et al, (eds.): *Gynecology and Obstetrics: The Health Care of Women.* New York: McGraw-Hill, 1975.)

cavity and is evenly distributed there. When the tubes are closed, the peritoneal egress is prevented by the obstruction, and a diagnosis of tubal occlusion can be made without further delay.

Peritoneoscopy involves direct visualization of the tubes and ovaries with an endoscope. This may be carried out either through the cul-de-sac (*culdoscopy*) or through the umbilicus (*laparoscopy*). The former is carried out under local anesthesia with the patient in the knee-chest position. In expert hands, visualization is usually satisfactory. It is a more difficult procedure, however, than laparoscopy which has become the procedure of choice.

Diagnostic laparoscopy is generally carried out under general anesthesia (Fig. 14-4). This is the

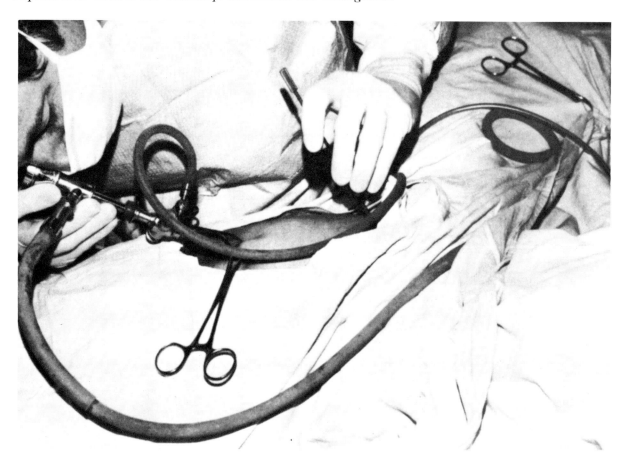

Figure 14-4. The double-puncture laparoscopic technique utilizing the probe to position the pelvic structures for optimum visualization. (Seitz, H. M., Jr., and Rosenfeld, R. L.: *Clin. Ob. and Gyn.* 17:86, 1974.)

same procedure as that used for tubal sterilization. In this case, however, tubal patency is evaluated by the introduction of a dilute solution of dye while the ends of the tubes are under visualization. Dye can be seen spilling from the ends of patent tubes. In addition, the area in and about the fallopian tubes can be evaluated directly for the presence of adhesions. When the latter are present, the condition is called the peritoneal factor in infertility. The treatment of adhesions is surgical.

THE UTERINE FACTOR

Pathologic conditions of the uterus associated with decreased fertility include uterine fibroids, congenital malformations, and intrauterine adhesions. Inflammatory lesions of the endometrium also occur.

Pelvic tuberculosis is usually first detected at the time of endometrial biopsy.

Congenital defects of the uterus as well as uterine fibroids are more often related to habitual abortion than to infertility. Fibroids may distort the endometrial cavity and if strategically located and large enough, presumably could interfere with implantation. If located adjacent to the tube, they may cause tubal obstruction. When a causal relationship is thought to exist, *myomectomies* (removal of the fibroids) with preservation of the uterus are usually technically possible. Treatment of congenital abnormalities, more commonly associated with habitual abortion than infertility, is also surgical.

Asherman's syndrome, or adhesions within the uterine cavity, are usually the result of a postpartal or postabortal infection or pelvic tuberculosis. There is often a history of a previous dilatation and curettage followed by a stormy postoperative course. Increasing use of abortion as a backup for contraceptive failure may be associated with an increased incidence of this uncommon but potential fertility-impairing lesion. Treatment of intrauterine adhesions is surgical, in association with the use of steroids and estrogens to decrease the incidence of repeat formation of adhesions.

Some patients, for reasons that are not understood, conceive during the course of the diagnostic evaluation for infertility. Occasionally conception occurs after not more than a preliminary examination and discussion of the diagnostic approach to follow. It is tempting to conjecture that, in some cases, the decision to seek aid for infertility is associated with a release of emotional tension followed, somehow, by improved reproductive performance. With the exception of ovulatory failure,

which may have a psychologic basis, and decreased frequency of intercourse which certainly has a psychologic basis, there is as yet no proved somatic basis for psychologically induced infertility. The general impression that adoption is often followed by conception has not been substantiated. Nevertheless, throughout the infertility investigation, the emotional support provided by those involved in patient management is especially important. Infertility is a threatening condition, and both husband and wife inevitably display anxiety. The role of the nurse in such situations is to understand the purpose of the various diagnostic procedures for infertility and to provide the couple with information so that both partners can cope with the problem knowledgeably.

SUGGESTED READING

Amelar, R. D., Dubin, L., Walsh, P.: *Male Infertility*. Philadelphia, W. B. Saunders, 1977.

Beck W.: Critical look at the legal, ethical and technical aspects of artificial insemination by donor." *Fertil Steril* 27:1, 1976.

Garcia, C. R., and David, S.: "Pelvic Endometriosis: Infertility and pelvic pain." *American Journal of Obstetrics and Gynecology* 129:740, 1977.

Mastroianni, L., Brackett, B. G.: "Internal environment of the tube," in *Progress in Infertility*. eds., S. J. Behrman, R. W. Kistner. Boston, Little, Brown, 1975.

Mastroianni, L.: "Potentials for fertility regulation at the tubal level." *Contraception* 13:447, 1976.

Speroff, L., Glass, R. H., and Kase, H. G.: *Clinical Gynecologic Endocrinology and Infertility*, 2nd ed. Baltimore, Williams & Wilkins, 1979.

Wallach, E., and Kempers, R. D., eds.: *Modern Trends in Infertility and Conception Control*, Vol. I. Baltimore, Williams & Wilkins, 1979.

Wheeler, J., Mastroianni, L.: "Pathology of the fallopian tube," in *Pathology of Female Genital Tract*. Ancel Blaustein, ed. New York, Springer, 1977, pp. 341–365.

Fifteen

Genetic Counseling and Diagnosis during Pregnancy

INTRODUCTION

Since 1956, when it was determined that human cells contain 46 chromosomes, the knowledge gained from research in human genetics has expanded rapidly. During that time, clinical genetics has developed as a medical discipline, which utilizes and integrates expertise from all other medical fields. More important, genetic information has been disseminated beyond the academic community and research laboratory to the practicing physician. Nurses, as an integral part of the health care team, should be cognizant of the need for, and content of, genetic services, especially in view of the fact that the amount of genetic information available to the lay public has increased markedly in the last few years. Magazine articles, newspaper stories, and television programs frequently discuss genetic diseases, often focusing on dramatic new advances in diagnostic methods. As a result, patients, as health care consumers, expect physicians, nurses, and other providers to respond to their increasing sophistication and needs in this area. Many more patients are requesting counseling and are willing to make decisions about their health care. These changes in information and attitudes facilitate the counseling process.

There are a variety of genetic services available. As a necessity, comprehensive programs employ a multidisciplinary approach to the care of patients and their families. A team composed of physicians (geneticists with specialty backgrounds such as obstetrics, pediatrics, internal medicine), nurses, genetics associates, laboratory personnel, and other support services is required.

As patients approach genetic counseling, they invariably feel anxious. Many have only a limited understanding of the inheritance of diseases and what the counseling process will involve. Often, these patients are in the process of dealing with grief over the birth of a malformed child or a serious illness in a family member. Guilt frequently compounds this anxiety. One or both parents may feel that there is something inherently wrong with themselves because a "defective" child has been born. On the other hand, they may blame the child's problems on the other partner or their "side of the family." The anxiety associated with counseling is easily exaggerated during pregnancy. It is, therefore, important that genetic counselors be particularly sensitive to the pregnant patient's concerns and family dynamics, so that disruption of the marriage or other family relationships may be avoided.

An Overview of the Nurse's Role

The nurse's role in genetic counseling often parallels that of the genetics associate with master's level preparation in human genetics and counseling. Both are involved in the initial patient contact, assessing clients for referral, and taking family histories. They perform preliminary counseling and coordinate appointments with physicians for evaluation and extended counseling. Throughout the counseling, the rapport which has been established permits them to serve as a patient advocate. Since they generally maintain contact after counseling, they are able to evaluate the patients' understanding of the information presented and their response to it. Through continued contact they may facilitate decision-making and identify resources for implementation of decisions.

A nurse-counselor or coordinator is especially suited to the prenatal genetic diagnostic team because of the procedures involved (e.g., ultrasonography and amniocentesis). In addition to having a basic knowledge of human genetics, the nurse has undergone educational preparation in reproduction and in obstetrical procedures, which makes her invaluable for both patient education and emotional support during prenatal diagnosis. The nurse's role is easily adapted to these services because nursing has traditionally espoused the philosophy of treating the whole patient and including family members in patient care, rather than focusing on the disease process or therapeutic regimen in itself. Additionally, in other areas of health care delivery, nurses often assume the role of coordinating total patient care.

GENETIC COUNSELING

Genetic counseling is a process in which individuals or families are given information that is needed to understand a hereditary disorder. This information may deal with a genetic disease in the individual, a family member, or future offspring. The aspects discussed during the counseling process include:

1. *medical considerations*—a description of the disease or defect including the clinical manifestations, therapy, prognosis, etc.;
2. *genetic mechanism*—the mechanism by which the disorder occurs and the risk of occurrence or recurrence;
3. *options*—during counseling any alternatives which may alter the risk for or the course of the genetic disease are discussed.

Counseling should enable patients to make decisions regarding a genetic disease in their present family or future generations. These decisions often involve selection of reproductive options (childless marriage, selective abortion of affected fetuses, artificial donor insemination, sterilization).

Identification of Risk

An important aspect of primary obstetrical care is identifying families at increased risk of having a child with a genetic disorder or birth defect. Ideally, these factors should be recognized prior to pregnancy; however, it cannot be assumed that couples are aware, or have been accurately informed, of a specific risk, no matter how obvious it may seem.

At the first obstetrical visit, the nurse's interview can identify patients who might benefit from genetic counseling. The aspects which should be reviewed are the following:

1. *Maternal age*—the risk of having a child with Down's syndrome increases significantly for the mother over 35.
2. *Ethnic background*—a number of rare genetic disorders occur with higher frequency in certain groups, Eastern European Jews have a ten times greater chance of carrying the Tay Sachs gene than the general United States population, descendants of Mediterranean forebears have a greater chance of carrying the gene for thalassemia, blacks have a much greater chance of carrying sickle-cell trait.
3. *Family history*—a specific disease (e.g., Huntington's chorea, hemophilia, etc.), birth defects (e.g., neural tube defects), or mental retardation may be hereditary.
4. *Reproductive history*—spontaneous abortions, stillborns, and previous liveborn children with birth defects, slow development or mental retardation may indicate an increased risk.
5. *Maternal disease*—several maternal disorders are

associated with higher frequency of birth defects (e.g., diabetes mellitus, seizure disorder) or with mental retardation (e.g., maternal phenylketonuria).

Referral Considerations

While any patient who requests genetic information should be referred for counseling, initiation of the referral by the health care provider is most appropriate for patients with more than one course of action available to them. Many patients who suspect that they might be at increased risk for a child with a birth defect use denial effectively until a pregnancy is established. The reality of the pregnancy and concerns for the fetus motivate them to seek information for the first time during early pregnancy. Occasionally, patients with the greatest anxiety are identified among those seeking pregnancy termination. Their concerns for having a malformed child may be based on misinformation. Genetic counseling in these circumstances should allow the patients to make an informed and appropriate decision for their family. Moreover, counseling may provide reassuring information.

Considerations in Prenatal Diagnosis

If prenatal diagnosis and selective abortion of affected fetuses are to be considered, several prerequisites should be met.

1. *Gestational age*—counseling should be offered as early as possible during pregnancy. Restrictions on pregnancy termination dictate the most advanced gestational age at which prenatal diagnosis can be initiated. Most often, procedures for genetic diagnosis are performed between 14 and 20 weeks gestation.
2. There must be a reasonably *reliable and safe method* for the diagnosis of the particular disorder. The testing, including its safety, limitations, and accuracy, should be explained in detail and accepted by the patient. In discussing risks, it may be helpful to contrast the patient's individual risk to the risk in the general population for the defect in question and birth defects in general.
3. The *value of the test results* must be established early in the course of counseling. While a

negative study will provide reassurance, the patients must consider in advance their options if a positive diagnosis is found.

DISORDERS AMENABLE TO PRENATAL DIAGNOSIS

Chromosome Disorders

The nucleus of a normal human cell contains 46 chromosomes (diploid number or 2N), which include 22 pairs of autosomes and one pair of sex chromosomes (XX in females and XY in males). Each chromosome is composed of DNA strands containing thousands of genes and a supporting protein structure. Due to the process of meiosis, the mature gamete contains only 23 chromosomes (haploid number or N); one member of each chromosome pair and one sex chromosome (an X in the ova and either an X or Y in sperm). At the time of fertilization, the diploid number is restored; one member of each chromosome pair is inherited from each parent.

The chromosomes of an individual may be examined by arresting the metaphase of dividing cells with colchicine or related agents. This can be performed on lymphocytes, cultured skin fibroblasts or amniotic fluid cells. After appropriate preparation, the chromosome content of the cell is analyzed microscopically, photographed, and karyotyped (see Fig. 15-1). Pretreatment of the chromosomes with a number of different chemical agents will cause distinctive staining patterns (banding) which allows the identification of each chromosome pair and definition of small subsegments of the chromosomes.

Numerical chromosome errors

An abnormal number of chromosomes (*aneuploidy*) in a conception results in major developmental defects. When there is an extra chromosome in each cell, the disorder is termed a *trisomy* and the individual is said to be trisomic for that chromosome. In the instance of a missing chromosome the disorder is termed a *monosomy*. These disorders may originate at conception, because the egg or sperm had an abnormal chromosome content, or after fertilization as a result of misdivision of the chromosomes to daughter cells during mitosis. *Nondisjunction,* in which there is unequal distribution of chromosomes to daughter cells during either meiotic or mitotic division, accounts for a large proportion of numerical chromosome abnormalities (Fig. 15-2B).

The cells of a conception may contain 69 (3N or triploid) or even 92 (4N or tetraploid) chromo-

Figure 15-1. G-banded chromosome spread shown. Karyotype of same spread above.

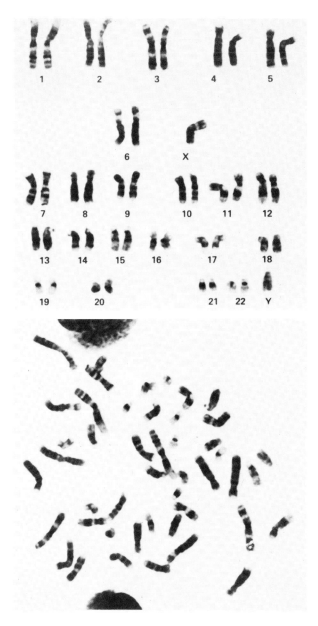

somes. These conditions, known as *polyploidy,* can be due to error in fertilization, for example, two sperm (dispermy) penetrating an egg, resulting in a triploid (3N) conception.

Frequency of Occurrence. The frequency of numerical chromosome errors in human conceptions is much higher than previously suspected, but the vast majority of these pregnancies are lost by spontaneous abortion. It is estimated that in at least 40 percent of early spontaneous abortions, there is an abnormal chromosome constitution. Autosomal trisomies, 45,XO (Turner's syndrome), and polyploidy are the most common abnormalities detected in early abortuses. The frequency of chromosome abnormality is also greater with late pregnancy loss, stillbirth, and perinatal death than in liveborn children. An abnormal chromosome constitution occurs in approximately 1 in every 200 live births. The most common numerical abnormalities encountered in newborn surveys are autosomal trisomies (trisomy 21, 18, 13) and sex chromosome aneuploidy (45,XO; 47,XXY; 47,XYY; 47,XXX).

Age Factor. The frequency of meiotic nondisjunction resulting in trisomic conceptions increases with maternal age. This is exemplified by the well-defined association between age of the mother and the birth of children with Down's syndrome (trisomy 21). This increase in frequency of Down's syndrome births is most dramatic in pregnancies of women over the age of 35 years (see Table 15-1). For this reason, it has become generally accepted that pregnant women in the late reproductive years should have the opportunity to consider amniocentesis.

Although the likelihood of bearing children having different autosomal trisomies (e.g., trisomy 13 or trisomy 18) increases with age, these are much less common abnormalities and the numerical risk is not as well defined as that for trisomy 21. Children with trisomy 18 and trisomy 13 most often do not survive the first year of life. Thus, the burden of these disorders differs from that of Down's syndrome, which is compatible with prolonged survival. Younger women who have had a child with trisomy 21 have a recurrence risk of 1 to 2 percent, irrespective of their age. These patients, as well as those who have had children with other trisomies, often request amniocentesis.

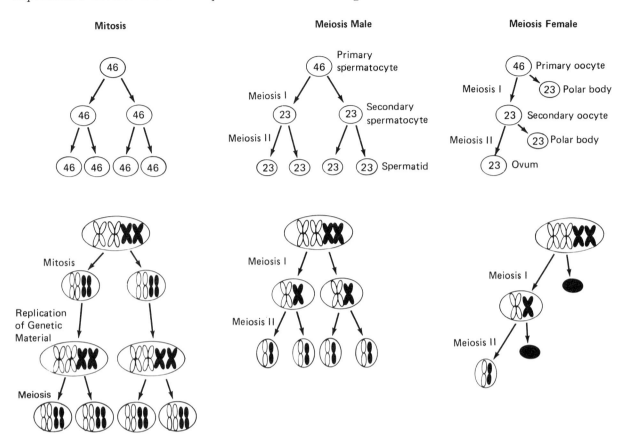

Figure 15-2A. Normal mitosis and meiosis: upper portion demonstrates the segregation of chromosomes numerically and lower portion depicts the segregation of two of the 23 chromosome pairs: 1. two normal mitotic divisions; 2. normal meiosis in the male; 3. normal meiosis in the female.

Structural Chromosome Abnormalities

Structural chromosome abnormalities occur as a result of breakage and reunion of chromosomes. Exchange of material between chromosomes of different pairs is known as a *translocation.* If all the

TABLE 15-1
INCIDENCE OF DOWN'S SYNDROME BIRTHS RELATED TO MATERNAL AGE

Age	Ratio	Age	Ratio
<20	1:2300	34	1:527
20–25	1:1600	35	1:413
25–30	1:1200	36	1:333
		37	1:266
30–35	1:880	38	1:183
35–40	1:290	39	1:135
		40	1:106
40–45	1:100	41	1:83
>45	1:46		

Retrospective data for maternal age related risk of Down's syndrome taken from: Collman, R. D., Stoller, A.: "A Survey of Mongoloid Births in Victoria, Australia 1942–1957." *American Journal of Public Health* 52:813, 1962; Hook, E. B.: "Estimates of Maternal Age—Specific Risks of a Down's-Syndrome Birth in Women Aged 34–41." *Lancet* 2:33, 1976.

genetic material is conserved, the individual is unaffected and is designated a balanced carrier of the rearrangement. The gametes produced by a balanced translocation carrier may contain a normal chromosome constitution, the balanced rearranged chromosomes, or a combination of the two chromosome pairs which would result in deleted or duplicated chromosome segments (see Fig. 15–3). In the latter case, spontaneous abortion may occur; however, liveborn infants with missing or extra chromosome segments are likely to have serious physical and mental defects.

Since the development of banding, which helps to identify chromosome regions, many more children are being diagnosed as having structural chromosome abnormalities. This may occur as a new event (*de novo*) or be secondary to a balanced translocation in one parent. Persons with translocations are usually detected because of a history of habitual abortion or the birth of a child with an abnormal chromosome constitution.

Translocations involving the number 21 chro-

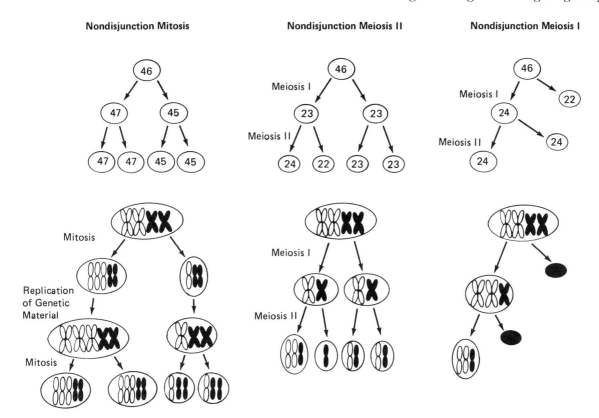

Figure 15-2B. Nondisjunction in mitosis and meiosis: upper portion demonstrates the segregation of chromosomes numerically, and lower portion depicts the segregation of two of the 23 chromosome pairs: 1. mitosis, two mitotic divisions with nondisjunction occurring in the first and the error passed through the subsequent division. 2. Meiosis in male, with nondisjunction occurring in the second division of meiosis resulting in normal and abnormal spermatids. 3. Meiosis in female, nondisjunction occurring in the first meotic division resulting in abnormal ovum.

mosome may result in an additional segment of that chromosome in children born with Down's syndrome. Because a balanced translocation may be passed from one generation to another, a family history of Down's syndrome should be investigated. Chromosome analysis of the affected child will indicate whether the abnormality is due to nondisjunction or secondary to a familial translocation. If an unbalanced translocation is found, chromosome studies to identify relatives who are translocation carriers are indicated. The reproductive risk when a parent carries a translocation varies with the sex of the carrier and chromosomal segments involved in the rearrangement. In these cases the parents may elect amniocentesis to determine if the fetus has an unbalanced chromosome constitution.

Mendelian Disorders

A large number of genetic disorders that follow the inheritance patterns described by Mendel (i.e., dominant, recessive) have been delineated. For some of

these diseases, the expression of the gene in cultured cells can be studied, permitting fetal diagnosis by amniotic cell culture.

Dominant disorders are those in which the presence of a single abnormal gene results in important phenotypic changes or disease, even though the other member of the gene pair is normal. Dominant disorders may occur in conception as a result of a new mutation of a gene or transmission of an abnormal gene from one of the parents. When a parent has a dominant disorder the chance that he or she will contribute the abnormal member of the gene pair to a fetus is 1:2 or 50 percent. Because the penetrance and expression of some dominant genes vary greatly, the diagnosis of the disorder in a parent may only be made after the birth of an affected child.

The biochemical expression of the gene for many dominant disorders is not known at the cellular level, which makes the disorders undetectable by amniocentesis. In some instances, major structural

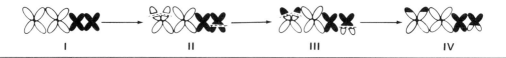

Figure 15-3A. Mechanism of reciprocal translocation. I. two normal chromosome pairs; II. breakage of one member of each pair; III. exchange of broken segments; IV. reunion to form balanced rearrangement (translocation).

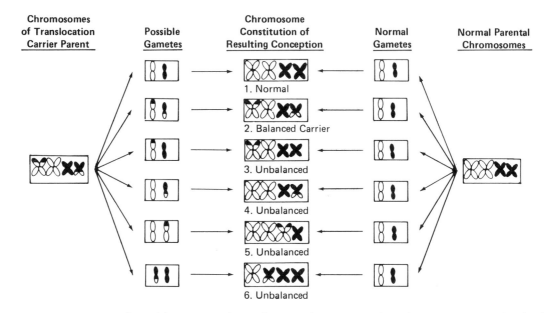

Figure 15-3B. Depicts gametes formed by parent with translocation shown in A and resulting conceptions after fertilization with normal gametes; 1. normal; 2. balanced translocation carrier; 3, 4, 5 and 6. conceptions with unbalanced chromosomal segments.

or anatomic defects associated with the disorder may be diagnosed by methods which define fetal anatomy (see p. 187). Prenatal diagnosis may be possible when the gene for a dominant disorder is linked (i.e., in close proximity) on the chromosome to other traits which can be studied. The use of linkage analysis to refine the estimation of the risk of a dominant disease is limited at present but may increase dramatically in the future.

Recessive disorders are those in which both members of the gene pair must be abnormal or deficient for expression of the disease state. When only one member of the pair is abnormal, the individual is unaffected but is heterozygous for, or a carrier of, the trait. The conception of children with recessive disorders can only occur when both parents are carriers of the same abnormal gene. In this instance there is a 50 percent chance (1:2) that the child will inherit the abnormal gene from either parent and be a carrier. The likelihood that the child will inherit the abnormal gene from both parents and, thus,

have the disease is 25 percent ($1/2 \times 1/2 = 1/4$) (see Fig. 15-4).

Everyone carries recessive genes for several rare disorders. Although these may be passed from generation to generation, the likelihood that we will reproduce with a carrier for the same rare gene is quite low. In some instances, a couple are carriers of the same abnormal gene because they are closely related (consanguinity). The genes for some disorders which are otherwise quite rare have a relatively higher frequency in certain geographic areas or ethnic groups. Common examples of this were previously cited (see p. 175). If laboratory testing can detect carriers for a recessive disorder, counseling and monitoring of pregnancies can be done prior to the birth of an affected child.

Screening programs for *Tay Sachs disease* (hexosaminidase A deficiency) are an example of this approach. The carrier frequency for this disorder in the U.S. population is about 1/300. Thus, the chance that both members of any couple are carriers of the gene is $1/300 \times 1/300 = 1/90,000$. Because the risk to a "carrier couple" for having a child is 1 in 4, the frequency of the disease is $1/90,000 \times 1/4 = 1/360,000$. The likelihood that a Jew of Eastern European origin carries this gene is 1 in 30. Thus, the frequency of "carrier couples" is $1/30 \times 1/30 = 1/900$ and the frequency of the disease is $1/900 \times 1/4 = 1/3,600$. Because reliable prenatal diagnosis is available for this lethal disease, many Jewish communities have supported *voluntary* screening programs for carrier detection. Most often, however, couples in which both members are carriers of the gene for a rare recessive disorder are not identified until birth of an affected child.

More than 50 recessive disorders may be diagnosed by amniocentesis (Table 15-2). For many of the disorders, the availability of diagnosis is limited to a few research laboratories.

X-linked recessive disorders The genes of X-linked recessive disorders are present on the X chromosome. In females, one X chromosome is inactivated in each cell. This inactivated X chromosome may be visualized as a chromatin mass in the periphery of the cell nucleus and is called a *Barr body* (Fig. 15-5). In women with Turner's syndrome (45, X0), the single X chromosome is active in each cell and Barr bodies are absent. Individuals with more than two X chromosomes (47, XXX) maintain one

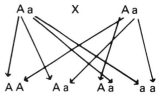

Genotype of parents Aa X Aa

Possible genotype of offspring   AA   Aa   Aa   aa

AA= Normal genotype   Aa= Carrier   aa= Disease

Figure 15-4. Recessive inheritance: A = normal gene; a = abnormal gene. Note frequency of aa children when both parents are Aa carriers is 1:4 or 25%.

active X in each cell and have double Barr bodies. Analysis of Barr bodies can be performed on nondividing cells (interphase) and provides a rapid screening test for identification of sex or disorders of sex chromosomes.

Inactivation of the X chromosome in normal women occurs randomly; that is, in some cells the maternally inherited X chromosome is active, and in the remainder the paternally inherited X chro-

Figure 15-5. Cell from buccal mucosa. Arrow points to Barr body.

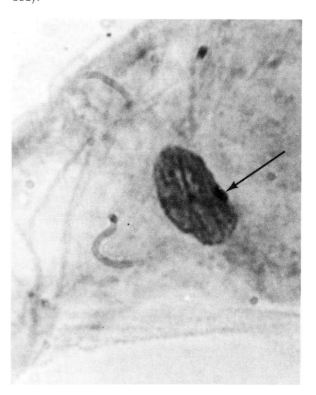

TABLE 15-2
EXAMPLES OF INBORN ERRORS OF METABOLISM
DIAGNOSABLE BEFORE BIRTH

Lipidoses	
Fabry's disease*	Niemann-Pick disease, Type A
Gaucher's disease	Wolman's disease
Krabbe's disease	Tay Sachs disease
(globoid cell leukodystrophy)	
Mucopolysaccharidoses	
MPS I—Hurler's syndrome	
MPS II—Hunter's syndrome*	
MPS IIIA—Sanfilippo A	
MPS IIIB—Sanfilippo B	
Amino Acid and Related Disorders	
Maple syrup urine disease	Proprionic acidemia
Argininosuccinicaciduria	Methylmalonic acidemia
Homocystinuria	
Disorders of Carbohydrate Metabolism	
Galactosemia	
Glycogen storage disease (types II, III, IV)	
Miscellaneous Hereditary Disorders	
Congenital nephrosis	I-cell disease
Hypophosphatasia	Lesch-Nyhan syndrome*

* Indicated X-linked recessive disorders, remaining examples are autosomal recessive.

mosome is active. When a woman has a gene for an X-linked recessive disorder on one of her two X chromosomes, it will be genetically active in only a portion of her cells. When this situation occurs, the woman is a carrier of the gene for the disorder. Unless the normal X happens to be inactivated in the vast majority of cells, the disease will not be manifested. In some instances, the X with the abnormal gene will be active in enough cells to allow laboratory identification of the carrier state.

The single X chromosome present in the male is active in each cell. When a gene for an X-linked recessive disorder is present on that chromosome, the male will manifest the disease. Commonly cited examples of X-linked recessive disorders are hemophilia (factor VIII deficiency) and Duchenne's muscular dystrophy. In some instances, a male child will have the disorder by new mutation. When the gene is inherited in the family, there may be a history of the disease in the mother's brothers and/ or her maternal uncles. Half of the daughters born to a carrier mother will also be carriers of the gene. Likewise, half of the sons born to a carrier mother will inherit her X chromosome with the mutant gene and will have the disease.

For a few X-linked recessive disorders amniotic fluid studies can detect the affected males. Examples of this are Lesch-Nyhan and Hunter's syndromes (Table 15-2). In the majority of cases when a woman is a carrier of an X-linked recessive disorder, the risk can only be refined by identifying the sex of the fetus. Sex identification is best performed by chromosome analysis.

Sex chromatin studies, i.e., examination for Barr bodies in female cells, although not as reliable, may provide rapid results as a screening test. In addition to Barr body analysis, the presence of a Y chromosome can be detected in the interphase nucleus of male cells by fluorescent dye staining. Hormone measurements in the amniotic fluid can also help confirm sex identification. The concentration of testosterone in amniotic fluid is higher when the fetus is a male, whereas FSH levels are higher when the fetus is female.

When the fetus of a mother who is a carrier for an X-linked recessive disorder is male, the risk that the child will have the disease is 50 percent. If the disorder cannot be specifically diagnosed by other methods, the patient and her husband face the dilemma of selective termination based on the sex of the fetus.

Multifactorial Disorders

Multifactorial defects occur when several genes predispose the fetus to an abnormality or lower the threshold for an abnormality in development. In addition to the genetic constitution, environmental factors are thought to play a part in the development of these defects. Many of the most common birth defects are multifactorial in origin. Most often, these are single defects such as cleft palate, pyloric stenosis, congenital heart diseases, or neural tube defect (anencephaly, myelomeningocele, etc.).

The occurrence risks in close relatives are based on empiric studies of families in which the defect has occurred. The risk to siblings is frequently in the range of 2 to 7 percent, and subsequently increases with each affected child. The risk to other close relatives (nieces and nephews, first cousins), although low, is often higher than that of the general population. More distantly related individuals (second cousins) are usually not at a substantially increased risk compared to the population. Advances in the methods used to detect structural abnormalities in the fetus, especially ultrasound and fetoscopy, may be useful for the diagnosis of some of these defects.

Neural Tube Defect

Only one group of the more common multifactorial disorders can be reliably diagnosed by amniocentesis at present. These are the neural tube defects (NTDs). These defects arise during early fetal development due to a failure of fusion of the neural tube, which will form the central nervous system. Although they may be associated with chromosome abnormalities or certain recessive disorders, the majority of NTDs are multifactorial in origin. The frequency of NTDs in the United States population is 1 to 2 per 1,000 live births. The risk of recurrence when there has been an affected child is 3 to 5 percent. Following two affected pregnancies, this risk increases to 10 to 12 percent.

Neural tube defects are described according to their location and anatomic structure. *Anencephaly,* failure of development of the brain and skull, is the most severe NTD and is incompatible with survival. *Myelomeningocele,* in which there is a defect in formation of the spinal cord, surrounding tissues and spinal column, is an example of a caudal neural tube defect.

Advances in neurosurgical techniques and aggressive medical management have improved the survival and quality of life for children with these defects. Nevertheless, the likelihood of serious handicaps remains quite high for a child with a neural tube defect.

The prenatal diagnosis of neural tube defects by amniotic fluid analysis is based primarily on measure of the *alphafetoprotein (AFP)* concentration in the amniotic fluid. Alphafetoprotein is produced in large quantities by the fetal yolk sac and liver during early fetal life. A small amount of AFP is normally present in amniotic fluid. When a highly vascularized, nonskin-covered defect such as a meningomyelocele is present, this protein may leak in excessive quantities from the fetal vessels into the amniotic fluid. Other abnormalities in which there are skin defects, such as omphalocele, may also be associated with elevated AFP levels in the amniotic fluid. To enhance the accuracy of this testing, methods to define the anatomic defect such as ultrasound or amniography are also employed.

Very low concentrations of AFP are measurable in maternal blood by sensitive radioimmunoassay techniques. Studies have shown that maternal serum testing is a reasonably reliable method of identifying a large percentage of fetuses with an open neural tube defect. The feasibility of large-scale maternal serum screening has been investigated in areas of the United Kingdom, where the frequency of these defects is several times higher than in the United States. It is likely that this type of screening may be offered in the United States in the near future on a voluntary basis, after the reliability and cost effectiveness are further evaluated in our lower risk population.

METHODS USED IN THE PRENATAL DETECTION OF BIRTH DEFECTS

Several techniques may be employed in the prenatal diagnosis of genetic disorders or birth defects. Ideally, these methods should define the genotype (genetic constitution) of the fetus; however, in some instances only techniques to delineate the phenotype (observable characteristics) of the fetus are available. The latter include fetal visualization by x-ray, ultrasound, and fetoscopy.

Roentgenograms (x-rays) performed as early as 20 weeks of pregnancy have been used to examine the fetus for skeletal manifestations of certain genetic disorders or birth defects. Because the fetal skeleton is rather poorly visualized at this gestational age, *amniography* is often employed. In this procedure, a water soluble contrast material is injected into the amniotic fluid to provide a more distinctive outline of the fetus and improve the identification of skeletal structures (Fig. 15-6). The usefulness of radiographic procedures is limited to the diagnosis of severe disorders with major skeletal manifestations early in development or, occasionally, large soft tissue defects (e.g., a bulging myelomeningocele). Unfortunately, many skeletal disorders can only be diagnosed so late in pregnancy that the option of termination is not feasible.

Ultrasound. Rapid advances in *ultrasound* have enabled the definition of fetal anatomy to a degree not imagined ten years ago. With this technique, fetal organs may be evaluated and single organ defects detected. Additionally, the examination of one or-

Figure 15-6. Amniogram outlining 16-week fetus with normal skull.

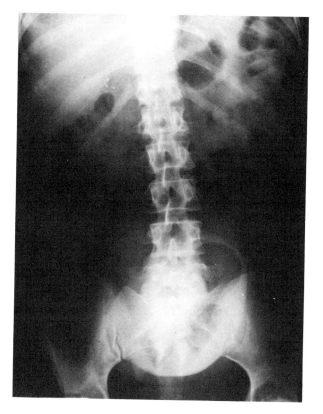

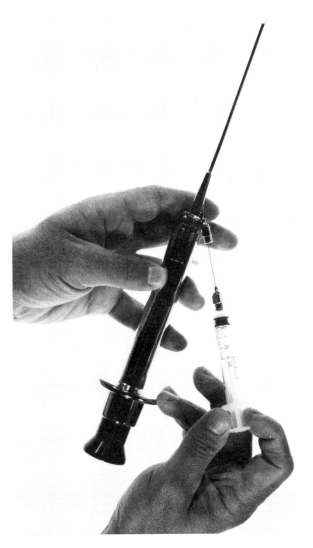

Figure 15-7. Amnioscope. Experimental endoscope for trans-abdominal amnioscopy with needle for aspiration.

gan may permit the diagnosis or refine the risk of certain multiple malformation syndromes. Examination of the cerebral ventricles for dilatation due to hydrocephalus, renal evaluation for the diagnosis of renal agenesis (Potter's syndrome) or polycystic kidneys, and evaluation for short-limbed dwarfism are only a few examples.

Fetoscopy. Delineation of other defects will require more direct examination of the fetus. *Fetoscopy* is currently an experimental procedure. Under local anesthesia, a fine caliber endoscope, about the thickness of a 14-gauge needle, is inserted percutaneously into the amniotic cavity to visualize the fetus (Fig.

15-7). Although it is easy to imagine the great potential of this instrument, its broad scale applicability for direct visualization awaits improvement in the optics of the system and further experience for evaluation of its safety. Recently, small amounts of fetal blood obtained from the placental vessels during fetoscopy have been used for fetal diagnosis.

Amniocentesis. Prenatal genetic diagnosis is most often performed when the fetus is at risk for a disorder which may be diagnosed by studying cells obtained by *amniocentesis.* This has become a relatively simple and safe outpatient procedure, which may be performed as early as 14 to 16 weeks of pregnancy (Fig. 15-8). Amniotic fluid contains desquamated fetal cells that are separated from the fluid by centrifugation. The supernatant fluid contains a number of hormones, proteins, and other elements which are useful for diagnosis. As mentioned earlier, AFP measurement for the prenatal diagnosis of neural tube defects is an example. Although the cells present in amniotic fluid come from a variety of sites—amnion, skin, gastrointestinal and genitourinary tract—all are of fetal origin. Since these cells are desquamated, a large proportion are dead or dying. Generally, enough viable cells are collected to permit cell culture. The cells are placed in plastic flasks or dishes containing a nutrient medium. The temperature, pH, and atmospheric conditions of the culture are adjusted and controlled in specially designed incubators. After a period of time, viable cells will attach to the plastic and begin to multiply by cellular division. Chromosome analysis, detection of enzyme defects, and, more recently, DNA isolation procedures can be done following adequate cell growth. With the latter methods, the absence or deletion of a gene may be detected by sophisticated molecular genetic techniques. (The details of the procedure for amniocentesis and the related counseling considerations are discussed on pp. 189–190.)

ROLE OF THE NURSE IN PRENATAL GENETIC COUNSELING AND DIAGNOSIS

While the majority of patients referred for genetic counseling and prenatal diagnosis are aware of the reason for referral, most are unsure of what to

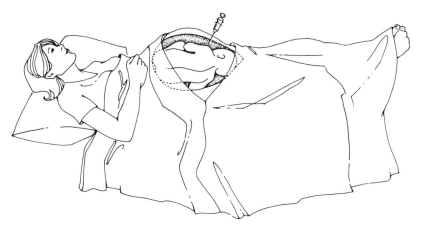

Figure 15-8. Technique for amniocentesis (From *Causes and Treatment for Genetic Disorders*. The American College of Obstetrician and Gynecologist, 1977.)

expect. Contact should be made as soon as possible after referral. Any delay can only serve to intensify the patient's anxiety, while the advancing gestational age may limit the options available to the patient.

The nurse-counselor must assume an attitude of calm reassurance from the beginning to ensure good rapport. At the outset, it is made clear that the decision to have a study performed will rest with the couple and a nondirective approach is maintained throughout the counseling.

History Taking

During the initial interview, it is useful to assess any factors which may alter the approach to counseling. It is determined how the referral was made and by whom (physician, nurse, advice of a friend or family member, or self-referred because of publicly available knowledge). The patient's response to the referral and her perception of prenatal diagnosis are discussed. The gestational age of the pregnancy is determined. The couple's feelings concerning the pregnancy are explored. The counselor should determine if the pregnancy was planned or if there is ambivalence about continuing the pregnancy. It is extremely important to allow the patient to express her ideas and anxieties prior to counseling. If the opportunity for this is not given, the focus during counseling may be diverted from the information presented and clouded by prior misinformation or denial.

To ensure comprehensive counseling, the nurse-coordinator obtains a detailed family history (pedigree) (Fig. 15-9). The outcome of all previous pregnancies and the health and development of liveborn children are reviewed. The health and

reproductive histories of the couple's parents and their siblings, as well as both sets of grandparents, are taken. In addition, the ethnic origin of the families and any possibility of consanguinity of families are noted.

If a family member is deceased, it is important to know the cause and approximate age at which death occurred. When there is a history of a birth defect or mental retardation, there may be a need to review medical records including autopsy reports, x-ray films, photographs, and pathology slides. This permits the most precise definition of identifiable genetic risks for the couple. If a hereditary disorder in the family is ascertained, this may have a great impact on the counseling. For example, if a woman is referred for prenatal cytogenetic diagnosis at age 35 with a 1 in 400 chance of having a child with Down's syndrome and it is learned from the pedigree that her father recently died from Huntington's chorea (a dominant disorder with late onset of neurologic deterioration) the entire focus of the counseling changes. In that instance, while the chance for a child with Down's syndrome is quite low, the chance that the child will develop Huntington's chorea is 25 percent (a 50 percent chance that the patient herself has the gene and will develop the disease and a 50 percent chance if she has the gene that the fetus will inherit it from her). Although prenatal diagnosis of Down's syndrome is available through amniocentesis, there is no predictive study for Huntington's chorea. Thus, this new information may become the most important factor for this couple in selecting options.

When review of family medical records becomes important because of the medical history, it is essential that they are requested in a nonthreatening manner. Many families with malformed or retarded

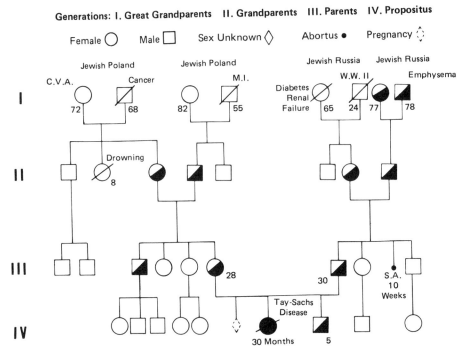

Figure 15-9. Sample pedigree—demonstrates recessive inheritance of Tay Sachs disease and the carrier state. Slanted line (/) through symbol represents deceased individual. Carriers depicted by partially blackened symbol. Affected individual depicted by totally blackened symbol.

children are very protective of these individuals. Often, their diagnosis is not discussed outside the immediate family and a long-standing silence about their problem has prevailed. Since medical records are confidential, permission is required to obtain them. The patient must understand the reason for and value of obtaining the records to elicit cooperation. The release forms are sent to the patient and forwarded by her to the relatives. While family members should not be contacted independently by the counselor, it is vital that the patient be assured that relatives should feel free to contact the counselor for any explanation or clarification. Through this approach, the counselor may create opportunities to offer services to the extended family, while maintaining the privacy of the individual.

A review of medical records may enable the nurse or the physician to determine that the health problems of other family members do not indicate an increased risk for the fetus. If there has been unspoken or denied anxieties about the medical problems of close relatives, the reassurance provided by the counselor is of great value to the couple and, frequently, to other family members.

Counseling

Once the background information has been gathered and the scope of the counseling established, the counseling process begins. In most cases, prenatal counseling can be done by the nurse-counselor. In the usual situation (advanced maternal age without significant family history), an explanation of chromosomes, genes, and their functions is given. The mechanism for, and the numerical risk of, having a child with Down's syndrome at the patient's age are explained and contrasted with the risk at other ages. The couple's knowledge of Down's syndrome is assessed and their information is clarified and supplemented. Studies in genetic clinics have shown that, in addition to numerical risk, the perception of burden is of paramount importance in the decision-making process. The presentation of burden must not be biased by the opinion or experience of the counselor, but must be well founded in fact.

The medical procedures involved in prenatal diagnosis, as well as their rationale, are explained. It is vitally important to conduct the discussion in terms that the patient can readily understand. The vocabulary must be individualized to each patient's level of comprehension. The risks and diagnostic limitations of the procedure are discussed in detail. For example, when ultrasonography is to be performed prior to amniocentesis, it is often necessary to distinguish this procedure from x-ray. The reasons for performing this test are explained. Ultrasonography allows localization of the placenta. Placental puncture or injury during amniocentesis may be avoided when the implantation site is defined (Fig. 15-10). Measurement of the biparietal diameter of the fetal skull by ultrasound confirms the gestational age. The detection of multiple gestation is also a benefit of the procedure. It is also explained that ultrasound is not painful and requires no special preparation by the patient (e.g., fasting); however, the bladder must be full during the study. The anatomic relationship of the bladder to the anterior lower segment provides a landmark for the evaluation of the uterus and its contents.

Counseling for Amniocentesis

Once the couple has been counseled regarding the particular disorder and the risk for having an affected child, the diagnostic procedure is explained. Following a description of the technical aspects of the test, the patient will want to consider the limitations, safety, and diagnostic accuracy of the procedure.

Limitations. It should be explained to the patient that amniocentesis is not invariably successful. If ultrasound or clinical examination indicates that the pregnancy is earlier than 14 to 16 weeks gestation, the procedure is postponed. When amniotic fluid is not obtained by the initial needle insertion, the physician may suggest another attempt or postpone the procedure for seven to ten days until a slightly more advanced gestational age. Once an adequate fluid sample is obtained, successful completion of the study depends upon the growth of cells in tissue culture. The patient is told that if culture failure occurs (less than 1 percent of cases) a repeat amniocentesis must be considered. Most important, the couple must understand that the study is not a general test for birth defects or mental retardation, but is designed to detect the specific disorder which has been discussed in the counseling. Chromosome analysis and AFP determination are usually offered to the patients, even when these are not the primary

studies being performed. The parents are told that if they wish to know the sex of the child when the chromosome studies are completed, the information will be available to them.

Risks. The risks of amniocentesis must be explained in detail. Concerns regarding spontaneous abortion related to the procedure prompted a collaborative controlled study by a number of centers in the United States. The frequency of pregnancy loss in approximately 1,000 patients undergoing midtrimester amniocentesis and in the controls was not significantly different; the incidence of pregnancy loss in both groups was approximately 3.5 percent. The results were confirmed by a similar study performed in Canada. These studies indicate that the risk of pregnancy loss related to midtrimester amniocentesis is probably considerably less than 1 percent. More important, if pregnancy loss occurs following amniocentesis, it is most likely unrelated to the procedure. Instances of septic abortion due to chorioamnionitis following midtrimester amniocentesis have been reported. Most often, parents express a fear of fetal injury by the needle. A few cases of neonatal scars, secondary to midtrimester amniocentesis injury, have also been reported. Because of the large number of studies being performed, it is reasonable to assume that the likelihood of serious fetal injury is exceedingly low.

Entry of fetal blood cells into the maternal circulation as a result of amniocentesis occurs in approximately 10 percent of cases. When the woman is Rh negative and the fetus is Rh positive, Rh sensitization may occur. Many centers administer Rh immunoglobulin prophylaxis to Rh negative women in conjunction with amniocentesis. When the potential for Rh sensitization is present, the rationale for this approach is explained.

Other complications following amniocentesis are spotting of blood or leakage of a small amount of fluid from the vagina. These occur in about 1 percent of cases and are generally limited to an isolated episode. Many patients will experience mild discomfort at the needle site for one to two days and a few may have ecchymosis or, more rarely, abdominal wall hematoma.

Accuracy. It is of paramount importance that prenatal genetic diagnosis be highly accurate. Nevertheless, every laboratory test has certain limitations. Every effort is taken to avoid human error, including

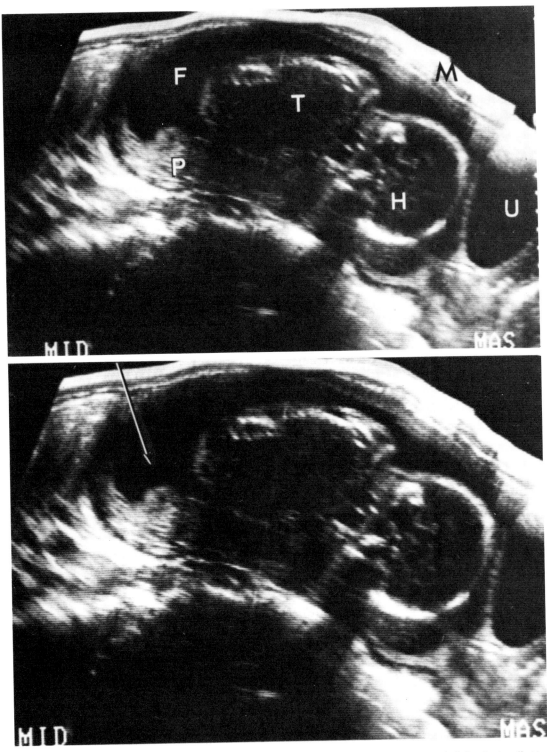

Figure 15-10. (*Top*) B-mode gray scale ultrasound of intrauterine pregnancy; M—maternal abdominal wall; H—fetal head; T—fetal trunk; P—posterior placenta; F—amniotic fluid; U—maternal urinary bladder. (*Bottom*) Same ultrasound; arrow shows site selected for amniocentesis.

independent duplicate analysis. When cultured amniotic fluid cells are used for testing, error due to maternal cell contamination may be unavoidable. In less than 1 percent of cases, maternal cells are "picked up" by the needle as it penetrates the abdominal wall, and these cells grow in the tissue culture. When this occurs, the study may reflect the genotype of the mother rather than of the fetus.

While amniocentesis is very safe and accurate for the prenatal diagnosis of a number of genetic disorders, it is important that the patients understand that the procedure has certain inherent risks and limitations. Most important, absolute guarantees of the validity of the results and especially of a "perfect" child cannot be given to the couple.

During counseling, it is not unusual for the patient to ask for the nurse-counselor's opinion or advice regarding the testing. The counselor must emphasize that the decision to have prenatal diagnosis is one that belongs only to the couple. The same information is interpreted differently by each couple based on personal factors. For example, a 40-year-old primigravida with a long-standing infertility problem may view any risk of spontaneous abortion associated with a procedure as unacceptable and her risk for having a child with Down's syndrome as low (99 percent chance that it will not occur). When patients ask for advice it should be explained that the opinion of the counselor may not be appropriate to their particular situation.

Post-counsel Follow-up

After counseling, the couple needs time to discuss all of the information presented with each other and to explore their feelings about the diagnostic procedure. Ideally, the counseling is given at a time when they have several weeks to make a decision regarding the testing. Even when the initial contact is made late in gestation (16 to 18 weeks), the couple should have at least several days to consider the procedure. It should be emphasized that both the husband and the wife must feel comfortable with their decision.

Several days after the counseling, the nurse contacts the patient. Any questions which have arisen are answered. If there is a great deal of ambivalence, difficulty, or disagreement about the decision, additional counseling is offered. It may be suggested that the couple speak with the physician either individually or together. Some couples wish to discuss the decision with other family members or advisors.

Procedure for Amniocentesis

Shortly prior to amniocentesis, the obstetrician reviews the counseling and answers any additional questions from the couple. The patient is asked to sign a consent form, which includes the risks and limitations of the procedure. Because of the rapport which has been established, the presence of the nurse-counselor during the procedure is invaluable in minimizing anxiety. The steps in the procedure and possible sensations which the patient will feel are anticipated by the nurse and explained to the patient.

After emptying her urinary bladder, the patient is instructed to rest on the examining table in a supine position with her legs extended. The site selected for needle insertion is determined by abdominal examination and the ultrasonic findings. The skin is prepared with antiseptic solution and a sterile field is established. Local anesthesia is injected into the skin and through the abdominal wall to the peritoneum. A stinging or burning sensation upon injection of the local anesthetic is usually the most uncomfortable aspect of amniocentesis. A number 18 or 20 gauge spinal needle is inserted through the anesthetized area and uterine wall into the amniotic cavity. The patient may have a sensation of deep pelvic pressure during the procedure.

Amniotic fluid will often spill spontaneously after the amniotic sac is entered with a needle. One to two cc's of fluid are discarded to help avoid contamination of the sample with cells from the maternal abdominal wall. If blood is obtained at first, the fluid may become clear again before the specimen is collected. The amount of fluid withdrawn varies with the studies to be performed, but generally ranges from 5 to 30 cc. The fluid specimen is collected in two or more separate, sterile syringes which are capped and labeled immediately. The samples are transported to the laboratory in these same syringes to avoid the possibility of bacterial contamination during transfer to another container. The volume of fluid withdrawn rapidly reaccumulates.

Following the procedure, the needle puncture site is dressed with a Band-Aid and the patient is asked to rest on the examining table for several minutes. There are usually no symptoms after the procedure. Although apprehension and anxiety levels are quite high prior to amniocentesis, most patients state that the whole experience involves less discomfort than a dental appointment.

At the conclusion of the procedure, the patient is often shown the labeled sample before it is transported to the laboratory. This helps to alleviate concerns regarding mislabeling of samples, especially if a positive diagnosis occurs. Signs or symptoms of complications, such as bleeding, leakage of amniotic fluid, and fever, are reviewed and instructions for contacting the nurse or physician are given. The length of time required for completion of the studies, usually two to four weeks, is discussed again and the mechanism for notifying the patient of the results is decided.

Counseling after Amniocentesis

Prior to amniocentesis, much of the patient's anxiety is focused on the procedure. Following amniocentesis, the patient's concerns shift to possible complications and the test results. Several days later, the nurse may contact the patient to determine if there are any unusual symptoms related to the procedure. Most often there are none. When necessary, an examination may be arranged. The patient is aware that the successful completion of the study depends on the adequate growth of fetal cells in culture, and that delays or, rarely, failure of culture can occur. Whether the cell culture was successful can usually be determined by the examination of the sample at seven to ten days, and the patient is notified immediately. If repeat amniocentesis is required, this should be discussed with the patient as soon as possible. The patient is reassured that failure or delays in establishing cell culture are not indicative of a problem with the pregnancy. If this occurs, or more commonly, if fluid is not obtained after the initial amniocentesis is attempted, the decision regarding a repeat amniocentesis must be made by the couple.

The anxiety during the interval between successful amniocentesis and final results is also accentuated by physiologic changes and social pressures. In some cases, the parents have not announced the pregnancy to relatives and friends and wish to wait until the diagnostic results are known. During the sixteenth to twentieth weeks of gestation, the uterus

grows and the pregnancy begins to "show" or be more apparent. The mother may feel fetal movement for the first time while awaiting the results of studies. This will intensify her fears of an abnormal result and her ambivalence about termination. It is interesting that many patients ignore or deny fetal movement until after the studies are completed. Perhaps the most important aspect of the nurse-counselor's role is giving emotional support to the parents during this waiting period. There should be ample telephone communication with the couple and they should feel free to call as frequently as necessary for reassurance.

Giving the parents the normal results following amniocentesis does not end the nurse-counselor's role; follow-up is also important. The accuracy of prenatal diagnosis is not confirmed until the baby is born. After delivery, the nurse may also wish to discuss the patient's reactions to amniocentesis once again.

When a positive diagnosis occurs, the nurse-counselor and physician notify the parents; preferably, this is done in person. Prior to informing patients of positive results, all studies should be completed and verified; most patients will ask about the certainty of the results. After counseling, these patients often desire termination of the pregnancy as rapidly as possible. The method of termination is selected with maternal safety as the greatest priority. Confirmation of the diagnosis for scientific purposes and parental information should be secondary. Because detailed information regarding pregnancy termination during the second trimester is not offered prior to the test results, this information must be presented to the patient at this time. The nurse-counselor maintains in-patient contact with the patient throughout the termination procedure and recovery.

Following selective abortion of an affected fetus, the parents experience grief. Observation of these patients has documented a high frequency of depression and marital discord. Because of the emotional stress following selective abortion of a wanted pregnancy, the couple is dissuaded from making permanent decisions about their future reproduction. Sterilization is not advisable at this time. Several weeks to months later, one or more visits are arranged for the couple to assess their resolution of grief, and if they wish, to discuss future reproduction. In the interval between these visits, the nurse-counselor maintains close contact with the patient. Often she may be the only person with whom the couple can freely discuss their feelings about the pregnancy and termination. Communication between the husband and wife is fostered, and psychiatric care or marriage counseling are offered when appropriate.

SUMMARY

The field of prenatal genetic diagnosis has developed rapidly over the past ten years. The number of genetic disorders and birth defects which can be diagnosed continues to increase dramatically. Public education has resulted in a large number of patients who consider having these studies performed. Nurses involved with the health care of women should also be aware of these services and be able to identify patients who might benefit from them. In an extended role of the maternal-child health nurse, the nurse-counselor is ideally suited to coordinate and deliver essential elements of this care.

SUGGESTED READING

Harris, H.: *Prenatal Diagnosis and Selective Abortion.* Cambridge, Mass., Harvard University Press, 1975.

Milunsky, A.: *Genetic Disease and the Fetus: Diagnosis, Prevention and Treatment.* New York, Plenum Press, 1979.

NICHD National Registry for Amniocentesis Study Group: "Midtrimester amniocentesis for prenatal diagnosis: Safety and accuracy." *JAMA* 236, 1976.

Simpson, N. E., et al.: "Prenatal diagnosis of genetic disease in Canada: Report of a collaborative study." *Canadian Medical Association Journal* 115, 1976.

Smith, D.: *Recognizable Patterns of Human Malformation,* 2nd ed., Vol. VII. Philadelphia, W. B. Saunders, 1976.

Thompson, J. S. and Thompson, M. W.: *Genetics in Medicine,* 2nd ed. Philadelphia, W. B. Saunders, 1973.

Antepartal Assessment and Management

Biophysical Aspects of Normal Pregnancy

Psychosocial Aspects of Normal Pregnancy

Parent Education

Nutrition in Pregnancy

Antepartal Care

Sixteen

Biophysical Aspects of Normal Pregnancy

Signs and Symptoms of Pregnancy | Presumptive Signs | Probable Signs | Positive Signs | Physiologic Changes of Pregnancy | Changes in the Various Systems | Endocrine Changes

This chapter is concerned with the anatomic and the physiologic adaptations of the human organism to pregnancy. Knowledge of human reproduction, presented in the previous unit, is essential to the understanding of this phase of the reproductive process. From a biologic point of view, pregnancy and labor represent the primary function of the female reproductive system and should be considered a normal process.

The length of human pregnancy varies greatly, but the average duration, if counted from the time of conception, is approximately 267 days or 38 weeks (see Chapter 10).

Many changes in maternal physiology occur during pregnancy. These adaptations to pregnancy, although most apparent in the reproductive organs, involve other body systems as well. Concomitant with these changes, the expectant mother usually has many emotional adjustments to make: sometimes fear, apprehension, worries (financial as well as physical), and family problems. The fact that delivery must be "faced," that there is no turning back or "changing one's mind," can in itself sometimes create an overwhelming crisis (see Chapter 17). However, these are all temporary alterations. Usually they are forgotten after the birth of the baby.

IMPORTANT DEFINITIONS

Gravida   A pregnant woman.

Primigravida   A woman pregnant for the first time.

Primipara   A woman who has given birth to her first child. Usage is not uniform.

Multipara   A woman who has had two or more children.

Para I   A primipara.

Para II   A woman who has had two children (and so on up numerically, para III, para IV, etc.).

The plural of these words is usually formed by adding "e," as "primigravidae."

The term *gravida* refers to a pregnant woman, regardless of the duration of pregnancy. In reference it includes the present pregnancy. The term *para* refers to past pregnancies that have produced an infant of viable age, whether or not the infant is dead or alive at birth. The terms *gravida* and *para* refer to pregnancies, not to fetuses.

195

SIGNS AND SYMPTOMS OF PREGNANCY

The first visit of the expectant mother to her physician is usually prompted by the query, "Am I really pregnant?" Oddly enough, this is the one question which the physician may answer equivocally after an initial pelvic examination, because even the most careful of examinations will rarely reveal clear-cut evidence of pregnancy until two menstrual periods have been missed. The availability of rapid, accurate, and easy-to-perform pregnancy tests has markedly improved our ability to substantiate the diagnosis.

Certain signs are absolutely indicative of pregnancy, but even these may be absent if the fetus has died in the uterus. Some so-called positive signs are not present until about the middle of gestation, and at that time the diagnosis of pregnancy can be made without them by the "circumstantial evidence" of a combination of earlier and less significant symptoms.

The signs of pregnancy are usually divided into three groups—presumptive, probable, and positive signs—as indicated by the chart below.

SIGNS AND SYMPTOMS IN PREGNANCY

A. Presumptive Signs
   1. Menstrual suppression
   2. Nausea, vomiting, "morning sickness"
   3. Frequency of micturition
   4. Tenderness and fullness of the breasts, breast pigmentation, discharge
   5. "Quickening"
   6. Dark blue discoloration of the vaginal mucous membrane (Chadwick's sign)
   7. Pigmentation of the skin and abdominal striae

B. Probable Signs
   1. Enlargement of the abdomen
   2. Changes in the uterus—size and shape and consistency (Hegar's sign)
   3. Fetal outline, distinguished by abdominal palpation and detection of a fetal part vaginally by ballottement
   4. Changes in the cervix
   5. Braxton Hick's contractions
   6. Positive pregnancy test

C. Positive Signs
   1. Fetal heart sounds
   2. Fetal movements felt by examiner
   3. Roetgenogram—outline of fetal skeleton
   4. Ultrasonographic demonstration of the presence of a conceptus

---

PRESUMPTIVE SIGNS

Menstrual Suppression

In a healthy woman who previously has menstruated regularly, cessation of menstruation strongly suggests that impregnation has occurred. However, not until the date of the expected period has been passed by ten days or more can any reliance be put on this symptom. When the second period is also missed, the probability naturally becomes stronger.

Although cessation of menstruation is the earliest and one of the most important symptoms of pregnancy, it should be noted that pregnancy may occur without prior menstruation and that occasionally menstrual periods may continue after conception. An example of the former circumstance is noted in certain cultures where girls marry at a very early age; here pregnancy may occur before the menstrual periods are established. Nursing mothers, who usually do not menstruate during the period of lactation, may conceive at this time from the first postpartal ovulation. More rarely, women who think they have passed the menopause are startled to find themselves pregnant.

Conversely, it is not uncommon for a woman to have one or two periods after conception; but almost without exception these are brief in duration and scant in amount. In such cases the first period ordinarily lasts two days instead of the usual five, and the next only a few hours.

Although there are instances in which women are said to have menstruated every month throughout pregnancy, these are of questionable authenticity and are probably ascribable to some abnormality of the reproductive organs. Indeed, vaginal bleeding at any time during pregnancy should be regarded as abnormal and reported at once.

Absence of menstruation may result from a number of conditions other than pregnancy. Any conditions which affects the function of the CNS–hypothalamic–pituitary–ovarian–endocrine axis may cause amenorrhea. Probably one of the most common causes of delay in the onset of the period is psychic influence. In addition, certain chronic systemic diseases, such as tuberculosis, advanced thyroid disease, chronic malnutrition, and the like may be associated with amenorrhea.

Nausea and Vomiting

About one-half of pregnant women suffer no nausea whatsoever during the early part of pregnancy. About 50 percent experience waves of nausea; of these perhaps one-third experience some vomiting. *Morning sickness* usually occurs in the early part of the day and subsides in a few hours, although it may persist longer or may occur at other times. When morning sickness occurs, it usually makes its appearance about two weeks after the first missed menstrual period and subsides spontaneously six or eight weeks later.

Since this symptom is present in many other conditions, such as ordinary indigestion, it is of no diagnostic value unless associated with other evidence of pregnancy. When the vomiting is excessive, lasts beyond the fourth month, begins in the later months, or affects the general health, it must be regarded as pathologic. Such conditions are termed *hyperemesis gravidarum,* or pernicious vomiting, and will be discussed with complications of pregnancy in Chapter 31.

Frequent Micturition

Irritability of the bladder with resultant frequency of urination may be one of the earliest symptoms of pregnancy. It is attributed to the fact that the growing uterus stretches the base of the bladder, so that a sensation results identical with that felt when the bladder wall is stretched with urine. As pregnancy progresses, the uterus rises out of the pelvis, and the frequent desire to urinate subsides. Later on, however, the symptom is likely to return, for during the last weeks the head of the fetus may press against the bladder and give rise to a similar condition.

Although frequency of urination may be somewhat bothersome, both at the beginning and at the end of pregnancy, it never should constitute a reason for reducing the quantity of fluid consumed.

Breast Changes

Slight temporary enlargement of the breasts, causing sensations of weight and fullness, is noted by most women prior to their menstrual periods. The earliest breast changes of pregnancy are merely exaggerations of these changes. After the second month, the breasts begin to become larger, firmer, and more tender. A sensation of stretching fullness, accompanied by tingling both in the breasts and in the nipples, often develops, and in many instances a feeling of throbbing also is experienced. As time goes on, the nipple and the elevated, pigmented area immediately around it—the *areola*—become darker in color. The areola tends to become puffy, and its diameter, which in the nulligravida rarely exceeds 3 cm. (1½ inches), gradually widens to reach 5 or 6 cm. (2 or 3 inches). Embedded in this areola lie tiny sebaceous glands which take on new growth with the advent of pregnancy and appear as little protuberances or follicles.

In a few cases, patches of brownish discoloration appear on the normal skin immediately surrounding the areola. This discoloration is known as the secondary areola and is a sign of pregnancy, provided the woman has never nursed an infant previously.

With the increasing growth and activity of the breasts, it is not surprising that a richer blood supply is needed; consequently, the blood vessels supplying the area enlarge. As a result, the veins beneath the skin of the breast, which previously may have been scarcely visible, now become more prominent and occasionally exhibit intertwining patterns over the whole chest wall.

The alterations in the breasts during pregnancy are directed ultimately to the preparation for breast-feeding the baby. After the first few months, a thin viscous yellowish fluid may be expressed by gentle massage, or may appear spontaneously, from the nipples. This is a watery precursor of breast milk, *colostrum.*

In primigravidae breast changes are helpful adjuncts in the diagnosis of pregnancy, but in women who have already borne children, particularly if they have nursed an infant within the past year, they naturally are of much less significance.

"Quickening"

Quickening is an old term derived from an idea prevalent many years ago that at some particular moment of pregnancy life is suddenly infused into the infant. At the time this notion was in vogue, the first tangible evidence of intrauterine life lay in the mother's feeling the baby move, and the conclusion was only natural that the infant "became alive" at the moment these movements were first felt. As is reflected in the Biblical reference to "the quick and the dead," the word quick used to mean alive, and the word quickening meant becoming alive. Hence, our forebears were accustomed to say that when fetal movements were first felt, the baby had quickened or come to life. We now know that the infant is a living organism from the moment of conception, but the old term quickening is still used in obstetric terminology, whereas the common synonym among the laity is "feeling life." As used today, quickening refers only, of course, to the active movements of the fetus as first perceived by the mother.

Quickening is usually felt toward the end of the fifth month as a tremulous fluttering low in the abdomen. The first impulses caused by the stirring of the fetus may be so faint as to raise some doubt as to their cause; later on, however, they grow stronger and often become disturbingly active.

Many fetuses, although alive and healthy, seem to move about very little in the uterus, and, not infrequently, a day or so may pass without a movement being felt. Inability to feel the baby move for brief periods of time does not mean that it is dead or in any way a weakling but, in all probability, that it has assumed a position in which its movements are not felt so readily by the mother. Should three or four days pass without movements, the nurse or physician should listen for the fetal heart sounds. If these are heard, it means that beyond doubt the fetus is alive and presumably in good condition.

It might seem that the sensations produced by the baby's movements would be so characteristic as to make this a positive sign of pregnancy, but, oddly enough, women occasionally misinterpret movements of gas in the intestines as motions of a baby and on this basis imagine themselves to be pregnant. Therefore, the woman's statement that she feels the baby move cannot be regarded as absolute proof of pregnancy.

Vaginal Changes

On inspection of the vagina, one is able to observe discoloration of the vaginal mucous membrane due to the influence of pregnancy. The mucosa about the vaginal opening and the lower portion of the anterior wall frequently becomes thickened and of a dark bluish or purplish congested appearance because vascularity is greatly increased. This increase in the blood supply of the genital canal gives a dark violet hue to the tissues (Chadwick's sign), in contrast with the ordinary pink color of the parts, and is often described as a valuable sign of pregnancy. As the result of the succulence of the parts, the vaginal secretions may be considerably increased toward the end of gestation. The increased vascularity extends to the various structures in the vicinity (i.e., tissues in the perineal region, skin, and muscle) and effects changes in preparation for labor.

Chadwick's sign is of no special value in women who have borne children; and, as it may be due to any condition leading to the congestion of the pelvic organs, it can be considered only a presumptive sign of pregnancy.

Skin Changes

Striae Gravidarum.   The abdomen naturally enlarges to accommodate the increase in size of the uterus. The mechanical effect of this distention of the abdominal wall causes (in the later months of pregnancy) certain pink or slightly reddish streaks, or *striations,* to form in the skin covering the sides of the abdomen and the anterior and the outer aspects of the thighs. These streaks, or *striae gravidarum,* are due to the stretching, rupture, and atrophy of the deep connective tissue of the skin. They grow lighter after labor has taken place and finally take on the silvery whiteness of scar or cicatricial tissue. In subsequent pregnancies new pink or reddish lines may be found mingled with old silvery-white striae. The number, size, and distribution of striae gravidarum vary exceedingly in different women, and patients occasionally are seen in whom there are no such markings whatever, even after repeated pregnancies.

Striae are not peculiar to pregnancy but may be found in other conditions which cause great abdominal distention, such as the accumulation of fat in the abdominal wall or the development of large tumors of rapid growth.

Striae gravidarum often develop in the breasts, the buttocks, and the thighs, presumably as the result of deposition of fat in those areas with consequent stretching of the skin.

Pigment Changes. Certain pigmentary changes also are common, particularly the development of a black line running from the umbilicus to the mons veneris, the so-called *linea nigra.*

The external genitalia and any pigmented nevi also darken. In certain cases irregular spots or blotches of a muddy brown color appear on the face. This condition is *chloasma,* or the "mask of pregnancy." Oral contraceptives may also cause chloasma in some women. These facial deposits of pigment often cause the woman considerable mental distress, but her mind may be relieved by the assurance that they will often disappear after delivery. However, the increased pigmentation of the breasts and the abdomen never disappears entirely, although it usually becomes much less pronounced.

All these pigmentary deposits vary exceedingly in size, shape, and distribution and usually are more marked in brunettes than in blondes.

Vascular Markings. Vascular spiders are minute, fiery-red blemishes on the skin with branching legs coming out from a central body. They develop more often in white women; however, they are of no clinical significance and will disappear.

Variations in Skin Changes. The changes in the skin which may accompany pregnancy (i.e., striae gravidarum, linea nigra, chloasma, pigmentation of the breasts, and so on) vary exceedingly in different persons, often being entirely absent. The pigmentation changes in particular are frequently absent in decided blondes and exceptionally well marked in pronounced brunettes. As already mentioned, this pigmentation may remain from former pregnancies and cannot be depended on as a diagnostic sign in women who have borne children previously.

Sweat Glands. In addition to the aforementioned skin changes, there is a great increase in the activity of the sebaceous and the sweat glands and of the hair follicles. The augmented activity of the sweat glands produces an increase in perspiration, an alteration which is helpful in the elimination of waste material.

PROBABLE SIGNS

Abdominal Changes

The size of the abdomen in pregnancy corresponds to the gradual increase in the size of the uterus, which at the end of the third month is at the level of the symphysis pubis. At the end of the fifth month it is at the level of the umbilicus, and toward the end of the ninth month, at the ensiform cartilage (Fig. 16-1). Mere abdominal enlargement may be due to a number of causes, such as accumulation of fat in the abdominal wall, edema, or uterine or ovarian tumors. However, if the uterus can be distinctly felt to have enlarged progressively in the proportions stated above, pregnancy may properly be suspected.

Changes in the Uterus

Changes in shape, size, and consistency of the uterus which take place during the first three months of pregnancy are very important indications. These are noted in the bimanual examination which shows the uterus to be more anteflexed than normal, enlarged, and of a soft, spongy consistency. About the sixth week, the so-called Hegar's sign, named for the man who first described it, is perceptible (Fig. 16-2). At this time, the lower uterine segment, or lower part of the body of the uterus, becomes much softer than the cervix. So soft does it become, that in its empty state (for it has not yet become encroached upon by the growing embryo) it can be compressed almost to the thinness of paper. This is one of the most valuable signs in early pregnancy.

The uterus increases in size to make room for the growing fetus. The growth of this organ in gestation is phenomenal. It increases in size from approximately 6.5 cm. long, 4 cm. wide, and 2.5 cm. deep to about 32 cm. long, 24 cm. wide, and 22 cm.

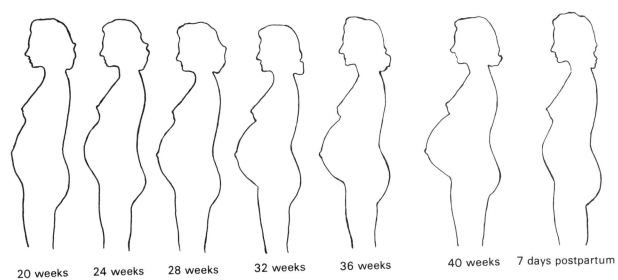

20 weeks   24 weeks   28 weeks   32 weeks   36 weeks   40 weeks   7 days postpartum

Figure 16-1. Changes in abdominal contour in pregnancy.

deep. The uterine wall thickens during the first few months of pregnancy from about 1 cm. to almost 2 cm., but thereafter it thins to about 0.5 cm. or less. By the end of pregnancy, the uterus becomes a soft-walled muscular sac which yields to the movements of the fetal extremities and permits the examiner to palpate the fetus easily. Its weight increases from 50 to 1000 gm. The small, almost solid organ which has a capacity of about 2 cc. increases to become a thin-walled muscular sac

Figure 16-2. Hegar's sign.

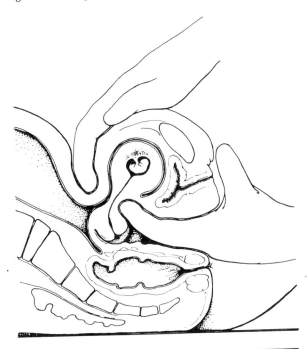

capable of containing the fetus, the placenta, and over 1000 ml. of amniotic fluid.

The tremendous growth is due partly to the formation of new muscle fibers during the early months of pregnancy, but principally to the enlargement of preexistent muscle fibers which are seven to eleven times longer and two to seven times wider than those observed in the nonpregnant uterus. Simultaneously, fibroelastic tissue develops between the muscle bands and forms a network around the various muscle bundles. This is of great importance in view of the function of the uterus in pregnancy and labor, because it strengthens the uterine walls. During early pregnancy, the hypertrophy of the uterus is probably due to the stimulating action of estrogen on muscle fibers.

The muscle fibers are arranged in three layers: the external hoodlike layer which arches over the fundus; the internal layer of circular fibers around the orifices of the fallopian tubes and the internal os; and the figure-8 fibers in the middle layer which make an interlacing network through which the blood vessels pass. This last group plays an important role in childbearing and will be referred to particularly in the care of the mother during labor and after delivery; for when these muscle fibers contract, they constrict the blood vessels.

Fetal Outline

After the sixth month, the outline of the fetus (head, back, knees, elbows, and so on) usually may be identified sufficiently well by abdominal palpation to justify a diagnosis of pregnancy. As pregnancy progresses, the outline of the fetus becomes more and more clearly defined. The ability to outline the fetus makes pregnancy extremely probable. In rare instances, however, tumors of the uterus may so mimic the fetal outline as to make this sign fallible.

Ballottement.   Another valuable sign suggesting the presence of a fetus is ballottement (from the French *balloter,* to toss up like a ball). During the fourth and the fifth months of pregnancy, the fetus is small in relation to the amount of amniotic fluid present; during vaginal examination, a sudden tap on the presenting part makes it rise in the amniotic fluid and then rebound to its original position and, in turn, tap the examining finger. When elicited by an experienced examiner, this response is the most certain of the probable signs.

Cervical Changes

Softening of the cervix usually occurs about the time of the second missed menstrual period. In comparison with the usual firmness of the non-pregnant cervix (which has a consistency approximate to that of the cartilaginous tip of the nose), the pregnant cervix becomes softened, and on digital examination the external os feels like the lips or like the lobe of the ear (Goodell's sign).

Softening of the cervix may be apparent as early as a month after conception. The softening of the cervix in pregnancy is due to increased vascularity, edema, and hyperplasia of the cervical glands.

As shown in Figure 16-3, the glands of the cervical mucosa undergo marked proliferation and distend with mucus. As a result they form a structure resembling honeycomb and make up about one-half of the entire structure of the cervix. This is the so-called mucous plug and is of practical importance for a number of reasons. First, it seals the uterus from contamination by bacteria in the vagina. Second, it is expelled at the onset of labor and along with it a small amount of blood; this gives rise to the discharge of a small amount of blood-stained mucus, or *show.* Frequently, the onset of labor is heralded by the appearance of show.

Braxton Hicks' Contractions

Uterine contractions begin during the early weeks of pregnancy and occur at intervals of from five to ten minutes throughout. These contractions are

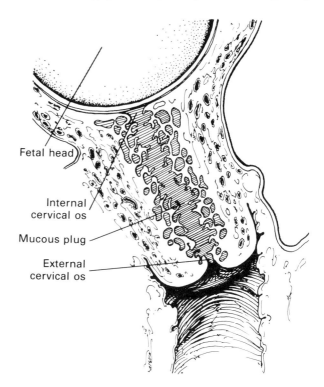

Fetal head
Internal cervical os
Mucous plug
External cervical os

Figure 16-3. Cervix with mucous plug.

painless, and the patient may or may not be conscious of them. They may be observed during the later months by placing the hand on the abdomen and during the bi-manual examination. By means of these contractions, the uterine muscles contract and relax, thereby enlarging in size to accommodate the growing fetus. These contractions are called the Braxton Hicks' sign, after a famous London obstetrician of the last century who first described them. They often account for false labor.

Pregnancy Tests

Since the dawn of civilization efforts have been made to devise a satisfactory test for pregnancy. The priest-physicians of ancient Egypt, in the earliest writings handed down to us, tell of a test then in vogue based on the seeming ability of pregnancy urine to stimulate the growth of wheat and barley seeds. The itinerant physicians of classical Greece employed similar tests, and during the Middle Ages the omniscient physician merely gazed at the urine and claimed in this way to be able to diagnose not only pregnancy, but also many other conditions.

Today, interestingly enough, as in the tests of old, urine is used in a large number of tests for pregnancy. The tests are based on the fact that the early chorionic villi of the implanted ovum secrete hCG, which appears in the maternal blood and is excreted in the urine. This hormone may be detected in maternal serum or urine by biologic or immunologic methods. Some of the biologic tests which were used extensively in the past include: 1) the Aschheim-Zondek test (immature female mouse), 2) the Friedman test (female rabbit), 3) the Hogben test (South African toad), and 4) the American male frog test.

Immunologic Pregnancy Tests. Numerous systems for immunologic pregnancy testing have been devised. Since hCG is an antigen capable of producing specific antibodies when injected into an animal, such as the rabbit, the serum of the animal so injected will contain an antibody or antihormone specific for hCG. This serum then can be used by reliable immunologic methods to establish the presence or absence of hCG in maternal serum or pregnancy urine.

Kits for immunologic pregnancy testing are available and have been simplified so that with a little practice the test can be carried out within minutes. Immunologic tests have two main advantages over the older biologic ones: 1) they provide an answer within a few minutes rather than many hours; 2) they eliminate the need for maintaining an animal colony. These tests are more accurate than the older biologic methods.

The great value of the endocrine test is that they become positive very early in pregnancy. The standard office pregnancy tests are usually positive about ten days after the first missed menstrual period, sometimes even a few days earlier than this. If any of the tests have been carried out properly, the results are accurate in more than 95 percent of cases. They are not, therefore, absolutely positive signs of pregnancy, but very nearly so.

Radioimmunoassay Test. Recently, very accurate tests to detect hCG in maternal serum by radioimmunoassay have been developed. These methods are capable of detecting from about the eighth postfertilization day on, and thus pregnancy can be diagnosed even before the skipped menstrual period. HCG is made up of an alpha and a beta subunit. The alpha subunit is common to the pituitary gonadotropic hormones. The beta subunit has molecular characteristics which are specific for hCG.

Antibodies specific for this subunit have been produced. These antibodies are used in a radioimmunoassay for hCG. This assay system has the advantage of being specific for hCG, and is capable of detecting minute amounts of hCG in blood. It is a much more elaborate assay than those used in the office to detect urinary hCG, and must be carried out in the laboratory with radioisotope techniques (radioimmunoassay).

Another radioimmunoassay for hCG, the radioreceptor assay, which is based on a slightly different principle, has been developed. In this system, antibodies against the combination of hCG and the intracellular receptor for hCG (the constituent in the cell to which hCG attaches when it exerts its effects) are used. This method is also highly sensitive, but is not quite as specific as the beta subunit assay. As there is some crossreaction with pituitary LH, LH levels are also detected by this method. These tests have found increasing use for the early diagnosis of pregnancy, and are especially useful clinically to diagnose abnormalities such as ectopic pregnancy, as well as to follow the course of early pregnancy when abnormalities of embryonal development are suspected.

POSITIVE SIGNS

Although certain of the signs mentioned above—notably, the hormone tests, ballottement, and palpating the fetal outline—are nearly positive evidences of pregnancy, they are not 100 percent certain; errors in technique occasionally invalidate the hormone tests, and on rare occasions the other signs may be simulated by nonpregnant pathologic states. If the term "positive" is used in the strict sense, there are only four positive means of detecting pregnancy, namely, the presence of fetal heart sounds, fetal movements felt by the examiner, the x-ray outline of the fetal skeleton, and delineation of a pregnancy by ultrasonography.

Fetal Heart Sounds

When heard distinctly by an experienced examiner, the fetal heart sounds can leave no doubt about the existence of pregnancy. Ordinarily, they become audible at about the middle of pregnancy, or approximately the twentieth week. If the abdominal

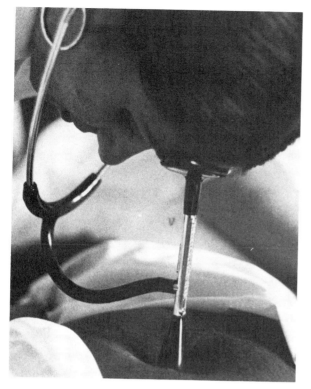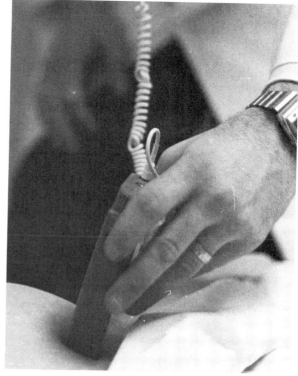

Figure 16-4. Auscultation of fetal heart beat by means of fetoscope (*Left*) and by ultrasound (*Right*).

wall is thin, and conditions are favorable, they may become audible as early as the eighteenth week, but obesity or an excessive quantity of amniotic fluid may render them inaudible until a much later date.

Although the usual rate of the fetal heart is approximately 140 beats per minute, it may vary under normal conditions between 120 and 160. The use of the ordinary bell stethoscope, steadied by rubber bands, is entirely satisfactory, but in doubtful cases the head stethoscope is superior, since the listener receives bone conduction of sound through the headpiece in addition to that transmitted to the eardrum (Fig. 16-4 left).

Office electronic fetal heart monitors which detect fetal heartbeat by ultrasound are now available. The heartbeat is transmitted to a monitor and amplified so that it can be heard by both the examiner and the patient (Fig. 16-4 right). The use of this instrument provides an exciting experience and can be appreciated by all, including the patient's mate who is present at the time.

Learning Technique.

It is advantageous to determine the fetal position by abdominal palpation before attempting to listen to the fetal heart tones, since ordinarily the heart sounds are best heard through the fetus's back (see Chapter 21). One method to use while learning the characteristics of the fetal heart sounds, is to place one hand on the maternal pulse and feel its rate at the same time that the fetal heart tones are heard through the stethoscope. Occasionally, the inexperienced attendant, particularly when listening high in the abdomen, may mistake the mother's heart sounds for those of the fetus. Since the two are not synchronous (fetal, 140; maternal, 80), the method suggested above will obviate this mistake; in other words, if the rate that comes to the ear through the stethoscope is the same as that of the maternal pulse, it is probably the mother's heartbeat; on the other hand, if the rates are different, it is undoubtedly the sound of the fetal heart.

Funic and Uterine Souffles.

Two additional sounds may be heard in listening over the pregnant uterus: the funic souffle and the uterine souffle. Since the word *souffle* means a blowing murmur, or whizzing sound, the nature of these two sounds is similar, but their timing and causation are quite different.

The word *funis* is Latin for umbilical cord, and, accordingly, the term *funic souffle* refers to a soft blowing murmur caused by blood rushing through the umbilical cord. Since this blood is propelled by the fetal heart, the rate of funic souffle is synchronous with that of the fetal heart. It is heard only occasionally, perhaps in one case out of every six.

The funic souffle is a positive sign of pregnancy, but it is not usually so listed, because it is almost always heard in close association with the fetal heart sounds.

The *uterine souffle* is produced by blood rushing through the large vessels of the uterus. Since this is maternal blood, propelled by the maternal heart, it is synchronous with the rate of her heartbeat. In other words, the rate of the funic souffle is ordinarily around 140 per minute (or the same as that of the fetal heart rate); the rate of the uterine souffle, near 80 (that of the maternal heart rate). The fetal heart

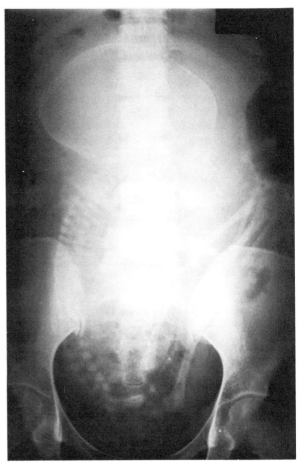

Figure 16-6. Normal breech position. (Bonner, K. P.: Radiography and Clinical Photography.)

may also be detected electronically or with ultrasound techniques described in detail in Chapter 37.

Fetal Movements Felt by Examiner

As already noted, fetal movements supposedly felt by the patient may be very misleading in the diagnosis of pregnancy. However, when an experienced examiner feels the characteristic thrust or kick of the fetus against the hand, this is positive evidence of pregnancy. Often this can be felt after the end of the fifth month.

Roentgenogram

A roentgenogram showing the outline of the fetal skeleton is, of course, undeniable proof of pregnancy. How early the fetal skeleton will show in

Figure 16-5. Normal vertex position. (Bonner, K. P.: Radiography and Clinical Photography, Eastman Kodak Company, Rochester, N.Y.)

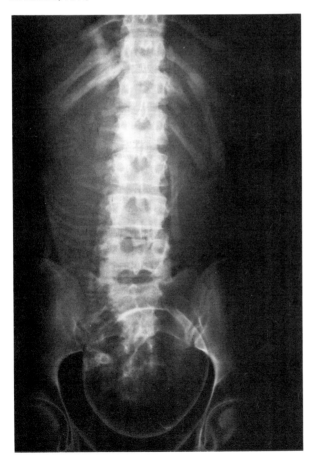

the roentgenogram depends on the thickness of the abdominal wall, the x-ray equipment and other factors. It has been demonstrated as early as the fourteenth week and is quite easily demonstrated as a rule after the twentieth week (Figs. 16-5 and 16-6).

Ultrasonography

The presence of an early embryo can be detected by the use of ultrasound techniques. This requires the use of an ultrasound machine and is most useful clinically when the diagnosis of intrauterine pregnancy is in question. A fetal sac within the uterus usually provides an unmistakable pattern on the ultrasonogram. Sonography is of great clinical use when tubal ectopic pregnancy is suspected. The test is increasingly accurate as pregnancy advances, and ultrasonographic outline of a fetus within the fetal sac constitutes a positive sign of pregnancy. This technique is described in greater detail in Chapter 36.

PHYSIOLOGIC CHANGES OF PREGNANCY

The physiologic changes of pregnancy are those alterations, both local and general, which affect the maternal organism as a result of pregnancy, but subside at or before the end of the puerperium. Such changes are to be regarded as normal, inevitable, and purely temporary. They are present in varying degrees in every instance, and in the case of a physically healthy woman there should be no significant traces of them after convalescence is complete. It must be remembered, however, that after pregnancy the uterus does not return to its normal nulliparous size, though it does return to a normal nonpregnant state. The adult parous uterus is slightly larger than that of a woman who has never borne children.

Bodily Changes Associated with Uterine Growth

Between the third and the fourth months of pregnancy, the growing uterus rises out of the pelvis and can be palpated above the symphysis pubis, rising progressively to reach the umbilicus at approximately the sixth month and almost impinging on the xiphoid process at the ninth month (Fig. 16-7).

In the majority of pregnancies the uterus is rotated to the right as it rises out of the pelvis. This dextrorotation is probably caused by the presence of the rectosigmoid on the left.

As the uterus becomes larger, it comes in contact with the anterior abdominal wall and displaces the intestines to the sides of the abdomen.

Coincident with the uterine and abdominal enlargement, the umbilicus is pushed outward until at about the seventh month its depression is completely obliterated and it forms merely a darkened area in the smooth and tense abdominal wall. Later, it is raised above the surrounding integument and may project, becoming about the size of a hickory nut.

When the abdominal wall is unable to withstand the tension created by the enlarging uterus, the recti muscles become separated in the median line—so-called *diastasis recti*.

About two weeks before term, in most primigravidae, the fetal head descends into the pelvic cavity. As a result, the uterus sinks to a lower level and at the same time falls forward. Since this relieves the upward pressure on the diaphragm and makes breathing easier, this phenomenon of the descent of the head has been called *lightening*. These changes usually do not occur in multiparas until the onset of labor. By palpating the height of the fundus, experienced examiners can determine the approximate length of gestation.

Effects on Posture. Since the full-term pregnant uterus and its contents weigh about 6000 gm. (12 pounds), a gravid woman may be likened to a person carrying a heavy basket pressed against the abdomen. Such a person will instinctively lean backward to maintain equilibrium. This backward tilt of the torso is characteristic of pregnancy. From a practical viewpoint it is important to note that this posture imposes increased strain on the muscles and the ligaments of the back and the thighs, and in this way is responsible for many of the skeletomuscular aches and cramps so often experienced in late pregnancy.

An additional contributing factor is a relaxation of the ligaments which support the joints of the spinal column and pelvis. This feature is increasingly

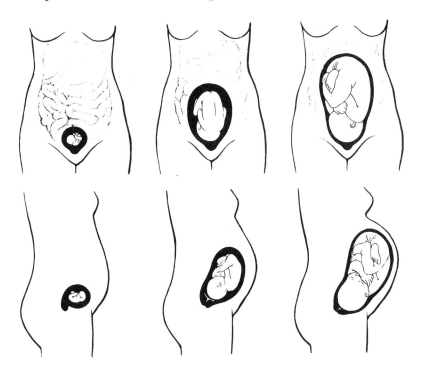

Figure 16-7. Relative size of the growing uterus, (*top*) front views, (*bottom*) lateral views, showing the fetus at four, six-and-a-half, and nine months of gestation. The fundus reaches a height between the symphysis pubis and the umbilicus by the fourth month, is about the level of the umbilicus at six-and-a-half months, and almost impinges on the xiphoid process at about the ninth month of gestation.

prominent as pregnancy progresses. Relaxation of the sacroiliac joints and the pubic symphysis creates a certain amount of pelvic instability, producing additional strain on the back muscles and thighs. These changes account for the waddling gait observed in late pregnancy and in the early postpartal period.

CHANGES IN THE VARIOUS SYSTEMS

Carbohydrate Metabolism

Pregnancy has a decided influence on carbohydrate metabolism. In general, the levels of fasting blood sugar are lower, and the secretion of insulin by the pancreas is increased. The stress of pregnancy may actually bring to light subclinical diabetes (see Chapter 32). In fact, diabetes is often detected for the first time during the course of prenatal care.

Blood

The total volume of blood in the body increases approximately 30 percent during pregnancy. The minimal hematologic values for nonpregnant women apply to pregnant women, namely, 12 gm. of hemoglobin, 3.75 million erythrocytes, 35 percent hematocrit. If there are adequate iron reserves in the body, or if sufficient iron is supplied from the diet, the hemoglobin, the erythrocyte count, and the hematocrit values remain within normal limits during pregnancy.

During pregnancy, there is an increased production of red blood cells by the bone marrow. At the same time, the maternal blood volume, the total amount of fluid circulating in the vessels, increases. Thus, under normal conditions, the actual concentration of red blood cells is relatively the same, and the normal values cited above apply.

Iron Needs. The marked increase in production of red blood cells places an inordinate demand on bodily iron stores. Iron stores in the female are often marginal anyway because of the normal loss at menstruation. Iron deficiency anemia is often present prior to pregnancy, especially when there has been inadequate dietary intake of iron, frequently the case among patients in poor socioeconomic circumstances. Iron deficiency is markedly aggravated by pregnancy because of the heavy demand for iron by the growing fetus, especially late in gestation. The increased demand for iron as a result of the changes associated with pregnancy should be kept in mind during the course of prenatal care, and the use of supplementary iron should be seriously considered.

Heart

An important aspect of this increase in blood volume relates to its effect on the heart. As a natural result of this change, the heart has more blood to pump through the aorta—about 50 percent more blood per minute than it did prior to pregnancy. This augmented cardiac output attains a peak at the end of the second trimester, then declines to the non-pregnant level during the last weeks of gestation. Immediately following delivery there is a sharp rise again. In women with normal hearts this is of no particular concern. However, in women with heart disease this increase in the work that the heart has to do may add to the seriousness of the complication (see Chapter 32).

Palpitation of the heart is not uncommon; in the early months of pregnancy this is due to sympathetic nervous disturbance, and toward the end of gesta-tion to the intraabdominal pressure of the enlarged uterus.

Respiration

In the later months of pregnancy the lungs are subjected to pressure from the underlying uterus, and the diaphragm may be displaced upward as much as 1 inch. As a consequence, shortness of breath at that period is common. It might seem that this upward displacement of the diaphragm would decrease the capacity of the lungs, but a concomitant widening of the thoracic cage occurs which more than compensates for the other change. Actually, the pregnant woman breathes in much more air than the nonpregnant woman. This is necessary, since the mother is called upon to oxygenate not only her own blood, but, by osmosis, that of her baby as well.

Digestion

The function of the digestive organs may be some-what altered during pregnancy. During the early months the appetite may be diminished, particularly if nausea exists. Since the nutritional requirements to meet the needs of the mother's body and the growing fetus demand quality of the diet rather than an appreciable increase in the quantity of food ingested, this temporary manifestation should not produce injurious effects. As pregnancy advances, and the digestive apparatus seems to become ac-customed to its new conditions, the appetite is increased and may be voracious. Heartburn and flatulence may occur at this time. Also, the pressure from the diaphragm and the diminished tone may delay the emptying time of the stomach.

Constipation is exceedingly common in preg-nancy; at least one-half of all gravid women suffer from this disorder. This suggests that the entire gastrointestinal tract is limited by diminished tone and pressure of the growing uterus during gestation.

Urinary System

The urine in pregnancy usually is increased in amount and has a lower specific gravity. Pregnant women show a tendency to excrete dextrose in the urine. Although a reduction in the renal threshold for sugar is often associated with pregnancy, the presence of any sugar in the urine should always be reported to the physician. Lactosuria may be ob-served at times, especially during the latter part of pregnancy and the puerperium. It is of no signifi-cance, being due to the presence of milk sugar which is absorbed from the mammary glands.

The *ureters* become markedly dilated in preg-nancy, particularly the right ureter. This change apparently is due in part to the pressure of the gravid uterus on the ureters as they cross the pelvic brim and in part to a certain softening which the ureteral walls undergo as the result of endocrine influences. These dilated ureters, the walls of which have now lost much of their muscular tone, are unable to propel the urine as satisfactorily as pre-viously; consequently, stasis of urine is common. Following delivery, the ureters return to normal within four to six weeks. The stretching and the dilatation do not continue long enough to impair the ureter permanently unless infection has devel-oped or pregnancies are repeated so rapidly that a subsequent pregnancy begins before the ureters can return to normal.

The *bladder* functions efficiently during preg-nancy. The urinary frequency experienced in the first few months of pregnancy is caused by pressure exerted on the bladder by the enlarging uterus. This is observed again when lightening occurs prior to the onset of labor.

ENDOCRINE CHANGES

Placenta

In Chapter 10 the placenta was considered as an organ designed to transmit nutritive substances from mother to fetus and waste products in the reverse direction. The role of the placenta as an important organ of internal secretion was also reviewed. As discussed previously, the early chorionic villi of the implanted ovum secrete a hormone, human chorionic gonadotropin (hCG), which prolongs the life of the corpus luteum. The result is the continued production of estrogen and progesterone, which are so necessary for the maintenance of the endometrium. During pregnancy this hormone appears in maternal blood and is excreted in the mother's urine. It makes possible the standard tests for pregnancy.

The chorionic cells of the placenta produce yet another unique protein hormone—*human chorionic somatomammotropin* or *human placental lactogen*. This hormone is detectable in placental cells as early as the third week after ovulation and is found in maternal serum by the sixth week. Its name suggests its actions. It influences somatic cell growth of the fetus and facilitates preparation of the breasts for lactation.

In addition to its function in the formation of hCG and human chorionic somatomammotropin, the placenta takes over the production of estrogen and progesterone from the ovaries, and after the first two months of gestation becomes the major source of these two hormones. The increase in these hormones in the maternal organism is thought to be responsible for many important changes that take place during pregnancy, such as the growth of the uterus and the development of the breasts. In the breasts, the development of the duct system is promoted by estrogen, and the development of the lobule-alveolar system by progesterone.

Pituitary Body

The pituitary gland enlarges somewhat during pregnancy, but, as such, is not essential for the maintenance of pregnancy.

Anterior Lobe. The *anterior lobe* of this small gland, located at the base of the brain, has already been referred to as the "master clock," which, under the influence of the hypothalamus, controls the menstrual cycle (see Chapter 8). In addition to gonadotropins, it secretes hormones which act on the thyroid and adrenal glands, and yet another hormone which influences the growth process. Production of these hormones continues during the course of pregnancy. Gonadotropins, on the other hand, are no longer released cyclically. The estrogen and progesterone produced by the placenta inhibit their release from the pituitary gland.

The Posterior Lobe. The *posterior lobe* of the pituitary secretes an oxytocic hormone, *oxytocin,* which has a very strong stimulating effect on the uterine muscle. That portion of extracts of the pituitary gland which contains oxytocin, is widely employed in obstetrics to cause the uterus to contract after delivery, thereby diminishing postpartal hemorrhage. It is sometimes used also to initiate labor and to stimulate contractions during labor when they are of poor quality. Oxytocin also has an influence on the breasts. It causes *milk let-down,* or ejection of milk from the nipples. This effect is of clinical use in the care of the nursing mother. Oxytocin is marketed under the names Pitocin and Syntocinon, the latter a synthetic product, and is administered either parenterally or, for milk let-down, by a nasal spray.

Other Endocrine Glands

It is quite clear that the placenta is the major endocrine gland in pregnancy. Other endocrine glands display alterations during normal pregnancy.

Thyroid. During the course of pregnancy, there is slight to moderate enlargement of the thyroid. It is now known that this hypertrophy of thyroid tissue is not associated with increased thyroid activity, although there is an elevation in the basal metabolic rate which increases throughout the course of pregnancy. This is merely a reflection of the increased oxygen consumption as a result of the metabolic activity of the products of conception.

Other parameters for the measurement of thyroid function also display changes. The serum protein-bound iodine (PBI), butyl extractable iodine (BEI) and thyroxine (T_4) levels increase, and the elevated levels are maintained until shortly after delivery.

The increase is due not to increased thyroid activity as such but, rather, to an elevation in the level of thyroid-binding protein normally present in the blood. Thus, although there is an increase in the amount of circulating thyroid hormones and, therefore, the total concentration of hormone is elevated, the actual amount of unbound or available hormone remains within normal limits.

The triiodothyronine (T3) uptake test displays decreased values in pregnancy. This, again, is the result of an increase in the binding of circulating triiodothyronine. A similar increase in the level of thyroid-binding proteins is seen in the nonpregnant patient following the administration of estrogen, and it is likely that in pregnancy the increase is a reflection of the high level of circulating estrogen.

Adrenals. The *adrenal cortex* hypertrophies during pregnancy, and it is believed that its activity increases. The actual secretion of cortisol by the adrenals is unchanged, although there are alterations in the metabolism of cortisol as a result of the influence of estrogen. There is clearly an increase in the production by the adrenal glands of aldosterone, the hormone responsible for the retention of sodium by the kidneys. This increase begins early in pregnancy and continues throughout. The net result of the increase is a decreased ability of the kidneys to handle salt during pregnancy. In the absence of proper dietary control of salt intake, there is often fluid retention, and either occult or overt edema.

Ovary. The *ovary,* except for the activity of the corpus luteum of pregnancy, remains relatively quiescent. Gonadotropin levels are low, inasmuch as their release is inhibited by the estrogen and progesterone produced by the placenta. Thus, follicular activity in the ovary remains in abeyance, and there is no further ovulation until after delivery.

SUGGESTED READING

Pritchard, J. A. and Macdonald P. C.: *Williams' Obstetrics*, ed. 15. New York, Appleton-Century-Crofts, 1976.

Quilligan, E. J.: "Prenatal care." In *Gynecology and Obstetrics; The Health Care of Women.* ed. Romney, S. L., et al. New York, McGraw-Hill, 1975.

Seventeen

Psychosocial Aspects of Normal Pregnancy

*Cultural Influences on Perceptions of Pregnancy /
Pregnancy in the American Culture / The Meaning and
Effect of Pregnancy on the Couple / Emotional Reactions
to Pregnancy / Implications for Health Providers*

CULTURAL INFLUENCES ON PERCEPTIONS OF PREGNANCY

As we have indicated previously, the family is society's most basic unit, surviving through the centuries as it has because it serves vital human needs. We have seen that there may be very different styles of family living and different ways of relating the family to the larger society. However, whatever the form, the family will no doubt continue to exist as long as humans continue to populate this planet.

In the family, as we have noted, each member assumes roles for which the culture dictates overt and covert behavioral expectations. Each member's perceptions of these roles also vary according to the manner of socialization and the kind of interaction he or she has had with others. As the society evolves and changes, so do the various role expectations. Each successive generation may hold different expectations as they adapt to changing times and needs, although there are always socially imposed limitations.

So it has been with childbearing. Pregnancy and birth are events that are treated as important in most cultures. However, attitudes toward these processes vary considerably among different cultures and even within one society. In some cultures, birth is a social

event, with open attendance by all friends and family; in other cultures it is conducted in secrecy.[1] Similarly, pregnancy may be seen as a normal uneventful preparatory phase to a desired change in status connoting achievement; conversely, it may be viewed as mysterious, crisis-ridden, and the harbinger of possible disaster. Again, it may be looked upon as atonement for simply being a lowly female.[2]

PREGNANCY IN THE AMERICAN CULTURE

There have been two competing views of pregnancy in our culture. One conceptualizes pregnancy and childbirth as a "crisis" situation, and the other regards these two processes as more of a role transition experience. Both of these attitudes have quite different assumptions and if carried to their logical conclusions have very different implications for the delivery of health care. Unfortunately, assumptions and terminology have not always been clearly articulated and when the rhetoric has been uncritically accepted and applied to the health care scene, some peculiar innovations and traditions have been incorporated into the delivery of care. In this chapter we will discuss these two orientations to pregnancy so that the implications of these attitudes for actual maternity care can be seen.

Pregnancy as Crisis

A couple's first pregnancy, in particular, constitutes a critical period in the evolution of a family. This fact has long been recognized. During the last three decades, there have been a variety of disciplines interested in this critical event. Psychologists and psychiatrists, notably Bibring, Hass, Larsen, Menninger, Caplan and Coleman and Coleman, have all written concerning the critical nature of this event and have at least alluded to the assumed crisis implications of such a stressful event.[3,4,5,6,7,8] Shainess, in fact, refers to this period as a "crucible tempering the self" and recognizes the possibility that the tempering process may go wrong, resulting in damage to the person and to the person's relationships with others.[9] Chertok speaks of pregnancy as a progressively developing crisis with the labor and delivery as the peak of the crisis since parturition results in separation of the mother and child and isolation from significant others.[10]

It is important to note that these writings are based largely on experiential and/or clinical impressions of individuals who have experienced difficulty. There have been no comparison studies with control groups.

Another tradition of research has led to the formulation of the "normal crisis of parenthood." While the focus here is on parenthood, the time of pregnancy was often included rather by default and so has become intermingled with the general research in this area.

Some of the early studies of parenthood focused entirely on this event as a crisis or extremely disruptive event.[11,12,13] From these early studies with their small skewed samples, inferences were drawn which were often unfounded. The inferences included pregnancy in the whole process, although this aspect was not studied per se. Moreover, there was some confusion as to the connotation of "crisis" and "normal crisis." In many of the conceptual formulations, both psychological and sociological, a crisis appears to be considered a critical event but not necessarily one that is totally psychologically or interpersonally disruptive. However, the true meaning of the authors' is often subverted since they do not precisely define their terms.

In the original stress research on the family as exemplified by Hill and Hansen[14] and Hill,[15] the term crisis connoted a sharp change. Specifically, crisis was defined as any sharp, decisive change for which old patterns (of behavior) are inadequate.[16] Thus, a crisis was considered an interruption in the routine of the family's social system and was sharp enough to render former patterns of interaction inadequate. There was also the implication that resolution and reintegration were not only possible, but quite normal and well within the family's capabilities. In sum, then, there has been some confusion, both semantic and conceptual over the way the term crisis has been applied to the events of pregnancy, childbirth and parenthood. This has led at times to the acceptance of pregnancy as always being disruptive and potentially damaging.

Pregnancy as a Role Transition

A decade ago, Rossi suggested that the term "normal crisis" was a misnomer as applied to parenthood because the concepts of "normal" and "crisis" are basically incongruous since one implies natural successful resolution and the other plainly indicates the possibility of nonresolution.[17] She suggested that parenthood be viewed as a role transition and be based on a stage-task conceptual framework such as is found in the work of Erickson, Benedek and Hill.[18,19,20] This type of orientation puts parenthood and other phases of the reproductive cycle, including pregnancy, into a developmental task formulation and allows these phenomena to be seen as essentially normal or usual, but also respects the fact that deviation, stress and/or disruption can occur depending on a variety of circumstances. In Chapter 27 we will discuss this concept as applied to the postpartum period when parenthood becomes very tangible. In this chapter we will limit the discussion to pregnancy.

If one views the total life span in terms of a developmental task-interaction, then we can view individuals' life spans as having cycles composed of stages or phases, each with its unique tasks. As the various cycles occur, social roles develop out of interaction with others in our social network. By analogy, social roles may be said to have cycles and each stage in the cycle has its set of tasks and adjustments. Rossi has outlined four broad stages in the role cycle that have implications for pregnancy as well as parenthood.[21]

1. *Anticipatory Stage.* Almost all social roles have some kind of formal or informal training, either through formal schooling, role modeling or watching others. This stage serves to socialize or train the potential actor for the role he or she is to assume. As its name implies, this stage precedes the assumption of the role and may take place years ahead of the actual role assumption.

2. *Honeymoon Stage.* This is the time period immediately following the full assumption of the role. Here intimacy and exploration occur as the person tries to adjust the "fit" of his or her personality to the role demands. Reality testing takes place rather than the fantasizing that often accompanies the anticipatory phase.

3. *Plateau Stage.* This is the protracted middle period of a role cycle during which the role is fully exercised. In this phase, the individuals validate themselves as adequate or inadequate depending on how well they and others see themselves performing in the role.

4. *Disengagement-Termination Stage.* This period immediately precedes and includes the actual termination of the role. For some roles, this stage is quite tangible. The marital role, for instance, ends abruptly with death or divorce. For other roles, such as parenthood or pregnancy, the distinction is much less clear since there is little cultural prescription about when the authority and obligations end.[22]

THE MEANING AND EFFECT OF PREGNANCY ON THE COUPLE

As we discuss the impact of pregnancy on the potential father and mother, we will relate some of the psychosocial aspects to the stages of the role cycle. We can see that pregnancy is a unique experience in which a sexual union between a male and female leads to the creation of a new life. This new life in turn will result in the creation of many new and unprecedented relationships.

For the Mother

Though the normal female may love her partner greatly and desire a child very much, there still are major developmental changes that she must make to become a mother. In the process of childbearing, she is creating from the union of herself and her mate, another individual *inside* herself which must ultimately grow to become a separate person *outside* herself. Hence the coming child represents the synthesis of three distinct entities: the mother's relationship to her partner, the relationship of the mother to the child as a representative of herself and the relationship to the unique individual which is the unborn child itself. As with puberty, when the individual can never again be a child, or with menopause when the individual can never again reproduce, with pregnancy the individual can never become a completely single unit again. As long as the child lives, it will never cease to exist as a representative of the woman, her mate and itself.[23]

The Psychological Tasks of Pregnancy

Several psychological tasks that the pregnant woman must accomplish have been delineated. First she must believe she is pregnant and incorporate the fetus into her body image.[24] Rubin has spoken of the two questions that the pregnant woman continues to ask during the course of her pregnancy—"Now?" and "Who me?" The woman questions if this is the right time to have the infant and acknowledges the ever-present surprise she feels being in the pregnant state.[25] As the mother feels the fetus move and her body change in both subtle and very apparent ways, she begins to realize that the fetus inside her is a real and separate being complete with its own boundaries and identity.[26] With this comes a lessening of the surprise and gradual integration. This is not to say there is no turmoil—mood swings, introspection, physical and psychic weariness; there is a great range of behavioral displays. Hence, we have many descriptions of the emotional lability of pregnancy. We must note, however, that there is ample evidence that the physiological and hormonal changes play an additional role in this lability.

The mother's second task is to prepare for the physical separation—the birth of the infant. As with all aspects of pregnancy, there are various responses.

Many women are eager to have the baby; they are "tired" of being pregnant. Some even state they are frightened to have this intrusive "invader" within them. However, others do not want to let the fetus go; they anticipate delivery as a loss of a loved object, and this anticipation may actually cause depression. Nevertheless, the task must ultimately be resolved, for every fetus lost is, in a moment, a baby gained.[27]

A third task is to resolve the identity confusions that accompany role transition and thus prepare for the smooth functioning of the family after birth. Coleman and Coleman suggest that, as the woman progresses in pregnancy, she becomes one with "mother"—the primitive memory of the omnipotent being who nurtured her. Moreover, she becomes increasingly prone to evaluate her partner with respect to his appropriateness as a father. She may criticize his current behavior patterns in order to bring them more into line with her idea of what constitutes an ideal father. Similarly, the pregnant father watches his partner become transformed into "mother" as her body changes, her behavior becomes more nesting and so on. He is simultaneously confronting his own feelings and aspirations as he metamorphoses into father. Pregnancy may be the first occasion in the relationship when the partners realize the extent to which they are interdependent psychologically, socially, and economically. On the one hand, this represents a physiological union which can be mystical; on the other hand, however, the merger may be experienced as a trap.[28] No wonder this resolution of identity confusions requires energy, commitment and work!

Emotional Reactions to Pregnancy

As indicated in the preceding pages, pregnancy is a time of change—both physical and psychological. Although the physiologic changes are overt manifestations of pregnancy, the psychological changes are more subtle but just as important.

At various times throughout pregnancy, a woman's emotional reactions have been described as ambivalence/uncertainty, introversion/narcissism, passiveness/dependency, and fear/anxiety. Certain of these feelings predominate at different periods of pregnancy; others fade in and out as pregnancy progresses.

First Trimester

Ambivalence. At the outset, many women experience ambivalent feelings about being pregnant. Even those who have planned their pregnancy are plagued by doubts as to whether this is the "right time" to have a child. A woman who is pregnant for the first time may wonder if she is really ready for a child. A frequently heard question, asked by both parents, is "What kind of parent will I be?" "How will I be able to cope with the total responsibility of a child—24 hours a day, seven days a week?" Assuming that these women will carry to term, there is no going back for them. Whatever their life style, a drastic change is in the making, which may account for some of the ambivalence they feel as a result of a reluctance to let go of old and familiar ways. For a woman who has other children and has already made the transition to parenthood, doubts may exist as to whether the spacing between that last child and the expected child is suitable. These basic uncertainties may be compounded by other concerns related to the timing of the pregnancy, the impact on the other children (if there are other children), the economic considerations of providing for another family member, the possibility of giving up a job and losing a second income—all of these doubts and concerns can contribute to the unsettling prospects of pregnancy. Added physical discomforts such as nausea and vomiting that frequently accompany early pregnancy only serve to underscore the sense of ambivalence felt by so many women.

This is not to say that a woman does not feel positive about her pregnancy. At the same time that she is struggling with her doubts she may also be experiencing joy and excitement as well as happiness and anticipation. The point is that in all likelihood her feelings will fluctuate between doubts and joys, and she may need to be reassured that what she is feeling is not unnatural and that she need not feel guilty about her ambivalence.

Fears and Fantasies. The first trimester is a time of speculation and anticipation on the part of the mother as she works her way toward accepting the fact that she is pregnant and deals with the physical changes and possible discomforts that she is experiencing. Much time is spent fantasizing about her pregnancy and the impact it will have on her life and the lives of other family members. Mixed with the sense of anticipation is a sense of concern over whether the baby will be normal and healthy, especially if the mother has been recently exposed to a questionable infection.[29]

Shereshefsky and Yarrow noted that mothers who visualized themselves with confidence and clarity during the first trimester tended to make satisfactory adaptations during the entire pregnancy.[30]

If the fantasies become moribund or are characterized by fear and despair, further intervention may be necessary. If concrete evidence for concern exists (the presence of genetic defects in the mother's or father's family, the exposure to infection, or the use of drugs or alcohol), the mother should be encouraged to discuss these conditions with the nurse and/or physician. In some cases, counseling may be necessary in order to consider alternatives with the parent. Perhaps the nurse will be able to allay the mother's fear by simply listening and clarifying misconceptions.

Sometimes, old wives' tales underlie the mother's concern. For example, some mothers believe that eating certain foods (strawberries or watermelon are common examples) will cause the baby to have birthmarks. Other mothers believe that, if they are frightened during the pregnancy, their babies will be adversely affected. Assessing the mother's fears, beliefs or notions provides the nurse with a framework from which to work. Adequate data collection allows the nurse to know what factors are likely to influence the mothers. This information allows the nurse to plan a more appropriate, individualized strategy for working with the expectant mother.

Second Trimester

The second trimester is often marked by a feeling of well-being as the body adjusts to the hormonal changes and some of the early discomforts of pregnancy (nausea and vomiting) subside. Usually, the woman has adjusted to the reality of the pregnancy and reconciled herself to whatever inconvenience it carries. Many of the fears regarding the health and well-being of the infant are forgotten temporarily. Feeling the baby move and hearing the heartbeat are immensely reinforcing and rewarding events for both the expectant mother and father. Allowing the father and the children to share in the experience of feeling fetal movement and hearing the fetal heart tone is a tangible way of incorporating the entire family into the pregnancy.

In the second trimester, mothers become particularly engrossed in fetal growth and development. Both parents become fascinated with pregnancy and the birth process and extremely conscious of the behavior of infants and children with whom they come in contact. At this time parents begin to plan for the actual birth of the baby. They may arrange to attend childbirth classes, read books on infant care and prepare in general to face the issues of parenthood.

It is during the second trimester that the mother can be described as becoming narcissistic, passive and introverted as she concentrates on her own needs and the needs of the fetus growing within her. As she prepares for her transition to parenthood she may reflect upon her own childhood and her relationship with her mother from whom she may draw her sense of maternal identity.

Because of her preoccupation with her own thoughts and feelings, the mother may seem to be self-centered and egocentric to those around her. Her moods may change drastically from happy to sad for no apparent reason. At times she may seem romantic and preoccupied with daydreams.

Because her preoccupations may be somewhat troublesome to both her and those around her, people close to the mother should be alerted to her passiveness and dependency needs. In this way they can provide the extra love and attention she needs. This, in turn, will enable her to give more of herself to others. Family members should also be reassured that the mother's behavior and emotional lability are not abnormal but are rather part of the reaction to pregnancy.

Third Trimester

The third trimester adds further psychosocial dimensions. As the woman's body changes, so does her self-image, reflected at times in a feeling of awkwardness and clumsiness. She may feel more unfeminine than at any point in pregnancy and worry about how her husband or mate perceives her.

The third trimester is a time of heightened introversion marked by periods of thinking back on her own childhood and projecting forward in thoughts of her yet-to-be-born child. New fears arise at this time concerning the health and well-being of the baby, as well as her own health and well-being as she contemplates the approach of labor. Mothers frequently distress family members by talking about the possibility of dying during labor. This may reinforce fears that the father is likely to have concerning the outcome of labor.

Furthermore, the mother is likely to wonder how she will "perform" during labor and will be interested in hearing about labor and what she can expect. She may wish to discuss the labor experience with other mothers or to read about it in books and pamphlets.

Regardless of the apprehension she may feel about labor, as the mother approaches the end of pregnancy, she wonders if "her time" will ever arrive. Many mothers cannot seem to wait for pregnancy to be over as they approach full-term. The obsession with delivery frequently finds expression in dreams about labor and the birth of the child. In conscious fantasies, the mother's thoughts center on the appearance of her infant. Toward the end of pregnancy, many expectant parents can clearly conceptualize what the baby will look like and imagine what characteristics he or she will have.[31]

As she contemplates her own labor, the mother may again wonder what kind of parent she will be. Since both father and mother may share the same feelings, some form of role playing may take place with the parents presenting each other with hypothetical situations in an effort to think out what their responses should be. Such "fantasies" seem to be useful to parents during the transition to parenthood. For the couple expecting their first child, the birth of the baby will signal the crossing of a one-way bridge—that of parenthood. No matter what happens, the new parents cannot go back developmentally to a time prior to the conception.

Pregnancy as a Social Role

While there have been positive attempts to describe the various stages of pregnancy together with the developmental tasks which need to be accomplished, we still do not have definite boundaries, expectations and prescriptions for the pregnant role. How are the incumbents supposed to act? What kind of behaviors are really expected? Does one act "ill" or is pregnancy essentially a well state? Is it "business as usual" or are there special restrictions or exemptions that may be claimed? There are several interesting explanations of the many and varied behaviors that we see in parents to be.

If we examine the stages we outlined in a role cycle transition, we find that being pregnant is, in fact, in itself an anticipatory stage in a role transition to parenthood. This can cause confusion at the outset. As she enters the anticipatory stage of the pregnant role, the woman attempts to learn the role by observing others, both family and friends, and she recalls how other significant people in her life acted as they became pregnant. She also takes cues from her physician, who may overtly or covertly influence her thinking, even to the extent of regarding pregnancy as a "sick" or "well" state.[32,33] It is interesting that, in our culture, we do not have any socialization or role modeling for the pregnant role—little girls play at being mothers, but not at being pregnant. Thus, although there are certain behaviors that directly relate to women and their fetuses during pregnancy, that are essential for the collective well being of the entire family (to say nothing of the happiness), the prescriptions for these activities are very amorphous and vary considerably in different social classes. These include such behaviors as positive, personal health habits, prompt and consistent attendance to prenatal care, and adequate nutrition practices.

The honeymoon and plateau stages of the role cycle come quickly upon the anticipatory stage. The round of showers, coffee klatches and increasing conversations with mother and pregnant friends or new mothers serves to help the woman adjust the "fit" of the pregnant state of her personality. Some women find that they adore being pregnant. They feel at one with the earth and sky and see themselves at the center of the universe. They find that they seem to bloom physically and emotionally. Others find the condition almost unbearable. They feel unwell, ugly and put upon and cannot wait to be "unpregnant." By far the more usual are those women who come to accept this condition and tolerate the discomforts and inconveniences. They see it as a necessary stepping stone to another larger role change.

With the infant's birth comes a relatively sudden disengagement stage. As we stated previously, there are few cultural norms concerning when the duties and privileges of pregnancy end and parenting begins. It is this role ambiguity that makes this condition difficult. The student is referred to the Suggested Reading for articles that examine this issue in depth.

For the Father

In our culture, being pregnant refers almost exclusively to the woman. In fact, if a man says "We're pregnant," he is still apt to raise eyebrows and be the target of some merriment. Men undergo far less social preparation than women do for parenthood and there is essentially nothing to prepare them for pregnancy per se. Experience with fathers who have actively involved themselves in pregnancy indicates that men, like women, go through various phases during the pregnancy.

The introduction comes with the confirmation of the diagnosis of pregnancy. This places fathers almost immediately into a honeymoon stage. As we know, the reactions are as many and varied as with the women. There may be very unclear feelings for the intellectual focus is on the impending fatherhood, rather than the immediate state of pregnancy.[34] Like his partner, he must assimilate the fact that the baby is his. He does not have the physiological changes to help him in this as the woman does, although some men do experience many of the same physical symptoms of early pregnancy.[35] How men accomplish this psychological task is still unclear and should be the topic of some fascinating research. We do know there may be guilt reactions about getting the partner pregnant or causing her to be sick and uncomfortable. On a more positive note, there may be feelings of pride at his virility or mutual pride that "We did it!"[36] There may also be feelings of distance between him and his partner as she continues through her introverted first trimester. Jealousy, worry about the change in sexual relationships, and concern about his own competence as a man and provider may occur.[37]

The first perceptible movement of the fetus generally creates a profound feeling that the fetus is real; most men, when questioned, recall the time and circumstances when "I first felt the baby move." In the second trimester, more thought is given to what it means to be a father and the plateau stage is entered. Men observe children and pregnant women more intently and become more acutely aware of their partner's growing uterus. A myriad of thoughts, concerns and downright worries may sweep over the father just as with the mother. Often these center on his ability to provide for the ex-

panding family. However, there is also concern and thought about how well he will be able to "father" the new progeny and meet the newly evolving expectations of the mother.[38]

As with pregnancy for the woman, there is a good deal of literature that describes this period as a crisis time for fathers. Yet there is evidence to indicate that psychologically healthy men cope without major problems.[39] What is clear, however, is that pregnancy requires as much adjustment for the father as it does for the woman.

As with the mother, labor and delivery mark the disengagement-termination stage of the role transition of pregnancy for the father. How these proceed can have a profound effect on the father. Most health providers who have had experience with pregnant couples believe that men who take an active part in the pregnancy by attending childbirth and parent education classes, participating in preparations for the infant, and so on, are more likely to particpate in the birthing with positive psychological outcomes and this, in turn, strengthens the building of the parental bond.[40]

IMPLICATIONS FOR HEALTH PROVIDERS

The nurse can function in collaboration with other members of the health team by providing emotional support together with counseling and teaching for the pregnant couple. As we have seen, regarding pregnancy as a role transition rather than crisis helps us emphasize the normality of the condition and avoid a search for illness and other negative aspects. We can then structure our care to support the resources of the couple rather than looking for problems which may not exist until we create them. The key to appropriate intervention in this instance is *family* assessment.

Family Assessment

There are certain extrafamilial stressors, both developmental and situational, that must be taken into account. Pregnancy and parenthood are examples of developmental stressors. Death, divorce, natural catastrophes, and loss of a job, are examples of situational stressors. These extrafamilial stressors work in conjunction with the intrafamilial stressors (inadequate communication, personal disorganization) to affect the role relationships within the family by producing varying amounts of difficulty in role transition. The amount of difficulty produced is related to how well the family is organized and how good their resources are.

The way the family is organized (their role structure) depends on each member's values, goals and ability to put a meaning on events (definition of the situation). On the basis of these goals and definitions, roles are given to the members and certain behaviors become associated with each role (role differentiation and allocation). Strength is gathered from the family resources which can be material (finances) or interpersonal (integration, cohesiveness, good communication, etc.). Appropriately structured roles and a reservoir of family resources serve to buffer the family from the impact of the various stressors and make role transition easier.

The following provides a guide for the development of a family care plan.

Assessment

A. Family Composition
   1. Who are the family members?
      a. What are their ages? What are their relationships to one another?
      b. Where do they live? Do they interact frequently?
      c. Are they "close" emotionally if not physically?
      d. What is the family's relationship to the larger community? Is the family involved in community affairs, church activities? What is its community support structure?
      e. Does the family have additional members in its social network? Are there other relatives or friends available for support?
B. Family Functioning
   1. How are the roles allocated and differentiated?
      a. Who does what in the house? Is this mutually satisfactory?
      b. Who makes decisions; how are they made?
      c. What are the changes that members would like?
      d. How do the parents see their roles being changed with the new infant?

   2. How do members usually define situations that happen?
      a. Does the family generally consolidate in time of trouble?
      b. Do they tend to be optimistic, pessimistic or do attitudes vary with situations?
      c. What are the communication patterns? Who talks to whom? Do problems usually get solved with discussion?
   3. What are the family's material and emotional resources?
      a. Who turns to whom for emotional support? Who is the mother's main support at this time? Who is the father's?
      b. Are finances adequate? Who contributes? Will the pregnancy make a difference?
   4. Are there interpersonal or intrapersonal difficulties?
      a. Are there long-term problems? What are the attempts to resolve them?
      b. Are there problems specific to this pregnancy?
      c. What alternatives for solution for the existing problems do the parents see?
   5. What are the specific plans for the baby and for themselves during pregnancy?
      a. What are their plans for themselves as parents?
      b. What are their plans for the infant?
      c. Are siblings anticipated (if this is the first child)?
      d. What are plans for siblings?

These questions illustrate the kinds of questions the nurse would include during an assessment.

Intervention and Evaluation

Intervention is aimed at helping the parents define possible stressors and resources within their family unit and developing strategies for coping with manifest or possible disruptive elements. By helping parents become aware of their resources and supporting them in their decision making, the nurse can minimize a great deal of stress associated with this role transition. Parents need to validate their impressions of what is happening to them, both physically and emotionally, with an outside person. Family, friends and health professionals all can be used in this way. The nurse will want to encourage the parents to use their network of family and friends if it is determined that this network can supply material and emotional support.

Intervention can be evaluated as effective if the family unit is perceived as drawing together (by the family as well as the nurse), there is open discussion of problems and experiences, concrete plans are made for the infant's arrival and the parents have a realistic perception that the infant will change their lives and that adjustment is possible for this momentous new role.

References

1. C. R. Phillips and S. J., Anzalone: *Fathering, Participating in Labor and Birth.* St. Louis, C. V. Mosby, 1978.

2. M. L. Brown: "A cross -cultural look at pregnancy, labor and delivery." *JOGN Nurs.* 35–38, Sept./Oct. 1976.

3. G. L. Bibring et al.: "A study of the psychological processes in pregnancy and of the earliest mother-child relationship." *Psychoanalytic Study of the Child,* New York, International Universities Press, vol. 16, pp. 9–72.

4. S. Haas: "Psychiatric implications in gynecology and obstetrics." In Ballak, ed.: *Psychology of Physical Illness.* New York, Grune and Stratton, 1952.

5. V. L. Larsen: "Stresses of the childbearing years." *Amer. J. Public Health* 56:32–36, 1966.

6. W. C. Menninger: "The emotional factors in pregnancy." *Bull. Menninger Clinic* 7:15–24, 1943.

7. G. Caplan: "Patterns of parental response to the crisis of premature birth: A preliminary approach to modifying the mental health outcome." *Psychiatry,* 23:365–374, 1960.

8. A. P. Coleman and L. Coleman: *Pregnancy: The Psychological Experience.* New York, Herder and Herder, 1971.

9. N. Shainess: "The structure of the mothering encounter." *J. Nervous and Ment. Dis.* 136:146–161, 1963.

10. L. Chertok: *Motherhood and Personality.* London, Tavistock, 1969.

11. E. E. Le Masters: "Parenthood as crisis." *Marriage and Family Living* 19:352–355, 1957.

12. E. D. Dyer: "Parenthood as crisis: A restudy." *Marriage and Fam. Living* 25:196–201, 1963.

13. D. J. Hobbs, Jr.: "Parenthood as crisis, a third study." *J. Mar. and the Family,* 27:367–372, 1963.

14. R. Hill and D. A. Hansen: "The identification of a conceptual framework utilized in family study." *Marriage and Fam. Living,* 22: 299–311, 1960.

15. R. Hill: "Generic features of families under stress." *Soc. Casework,* 39, 2–3:32–54, 1958.

16. Hill, op. cit., p. 33

17. A. S. Rossi: "Transition to parenthood." *J. Mar. and the Family,* 30:26–39, Feb. 1968.

18. E. Erikson: "Identity and the life cycle: Selected papers." *Psychological Issues,* 1:1–171, 1959.

19. T. Benedek: "Parenthood as a developmental phase." *J. Amer. Psychoanalytic Assoc.,* 7, 8:389–417, 1959.

20. Hill, op. cit.

21. Rossi, op. cit., pp. 29–30.

22. Ibid.

23. H. J. Osofsky: "Psychological and sociological aspects of normal pregnancy." *Medical Services J., Canada,* 23, 4: 512–521, 1967.

24. A. D. Coleman and L. Coleman: "Pregnancy as an altered state of consciousness." *Birth and the Family J.* 1, 1: 7–11, 1974.

25. R. Rubin: "Cognitive style in pregnancy." *Am. J. Nurs.* 3: 502–508, 1970.

26. Osofsky, op. cit.

27. Coleman and Coleman: "Pregnancy as an altered state of consciousness." op. cit.

28. Ibid.

29. Rubin, op. cit.

30. P. Shereshefsky and L. Yarrow, eds.: *Psychological Aspects of a First Pregnancy and Early Postnatal Adaptation.* New York: Raven Press, 1973.

31. M. E. Pharis and M. Manosevitz: "Parental models: A means for evaluating different prenatal contexts." In D. B. Sawin, R. C. Hawkins II, L. O. Walker, and J. H. Penticuff, eds.: *Exceptional Infant IV: Psychosocial Risks in Infant-Environment Transactions.* New York: Brunner/Mazel, in press.

32. W. Rosengren: "The sick role during pregnancy: A note on research in progress." *J. Health & Human Behav.,* 3, 3:213–218, Fall 1962.

33. W. Rosengren: "Social instability and attitudes toward pregnancy as a social role." *Soc. Prob.,* 9, 4:371–378, Spring 1962.

34. Phillips and Anzalone, op. cit.

35. Brown, op. cit.

36. K. Antle: "Psychologic involvement in pregnancy by expectant fathers." *JOGN Nurs.* 40–42, July/Aug. 1975.

37. Ibid.

38. Phillips and Anzalone, op. cit.

39. Ibid.

40. Ibid.

SUGGESTED READING

Antle, K.: "Psychologic involvement in pregnancy by expectant fathers." *JOGN NURS.* 40–42, July/Aug. 1975.

Brown, M. S.: "A cross-cultural look at pregnancy, labor and delivery." *JOGN Nurs.* 35–38, Sept./Oct. 1976.

Galloway, K. G.: "The uncertainty and stress of high risk pregnancy." *Amer. J. Mat. Child Nurs.* 294–299, Sept./Oct. 1976.

Hern, W. M.: "The illness parameters of pregnancy." *Soc. Science & Medicine* 9:365–372, 1975.

Rosengren, W. R.: "Social instability and attitudes toward pregnancy as a social role." *Soc. Prob.* 9, 4:371–378, Spring 1962.

Rossi, A. S.: "Transition to parenthood." *J. Mar. and the Family* 30:26–39, Feb. 1968.

Eighteen

Parent Education

*Teaching and Learning / Factors in Parent Education /
Types of Education for Childbearing / Guide for
Preparing Parents for Childbirth and the Puerperium /
Postpartum Teaching*

Education of the patient is a major component of the professional nurse's role. In this era of the consumer movement, greater emphasis must be placed on allowing the patient and family to fully understand the body processes and the rationale for medical and nursing management of health problems. Particularly in the area of maternity, patients and families are not only very interested in learning, but have come to view such knowledge as their right. They expect the nurse to be willing and able to assist them in acquiring knowledge and to take their individual wants and needs into consideration.

The increased involvement of childbearing couples in all phases of the reproductive cycle benefits not only the parents, as receivers of care, but also nurses, as givers of care. A concerned and knowledgeable woman will follow a more healthful regimen during pregnancy, including nutrition, exercise and rest, physical care, and psychological processes. A prepared woman and an involved partner can cope positively with the stresses of labor, enriching their relationship and promoting psychological maturation. Parents who are informed and who actively seek understanding of their child's numerous needs for comfort, security, and stimulation during the early formative years can attain a happier, more satisfying parent-child relationship and foster optimal growth and development of the child.

When the childbearing couple desires to learn, and the health professional is ready to teach, their shared experiences can be most satisfying to all involved. The roles of teacher and learner are not rigid, however, for often the nurse learns much of value from the parents, and gains deeper understanding of the reproductive experience through appreciating their perspectives.

The cornerstone of patient education is recognition and respect of the learning needs of patients. The nurse may design content, but if it does not meet the patient's learning needs, it is pointless and ineffective. A responsibility of the nurse is developing the skill to assess these learning needs accurately.

Parent education encompasses an enormous body of knowledge, only a portion of which is included in this chapter. Throughout the text additional information about teaching as a part of nursing intervention for specific parent/patient needs or problems will be found. Concepts related to the teaching-learning process, some approaches to group and individual teaching, and programs providing preparation for childbirth and parenting are discussed here.

TEACHING AND LEARNING

"Teaching is an interactive process between a teacher and one or more learners."[1] The teaching-learning process is a complex entity composed of various interrelated parts: 1) identifying the need or needs of the learner, 2) determining the motivation of the learner, 3) establishing the objectives of learning, and 4) evaluating the results in terms of desired learning. Learning may be defined as a (desired) change in behavior. Teaching is accomplished only when the learner learns, retains new knowledge, and is able to use it at the present or in the future.

Many factors affect the teaching-learning process, and the nurse must be aware of those which might either enhance or interfere with learning. The following concepts about learning illustrate some of these influences:

1. Learners (and teachers) bring with them to the classroom a cluster of understandings, skills, appreciations, attitudes, and feelings that have personal meaning to them and are in effect the sum of their reactions to previous stimuli.
2. Learners (and teachers) are individually different in many ways even when grouped according to ability.
3. Learners (and teachers) have developed concepts of self, which directly affect their behavior.
4. Learning may be defined as a change in behavior.
5. Learning requires activity on the part of the learner. The learner should not be passive.
6. Learners ultimately learn what *they* actively desire to learn; they do not learn what they do not accept or come to accept.
7. Learning is enhanced when learners accept responsibility for their own learning.
8. Learning is directly influenced by physical and social environment.
9. Learning occurs on successively deeper levels.
10. Learning is deepened when the learning situation provides opportunity for applying learnings in as realistic a situation as is feasible.
11. Learners are motivated when they understand and accept the purposes of the learning situation.
12. Learners are motivated by success experiences.
13. Learners are motivated by teacher acceptance.
14. Learners are motivated when they can associate new learnings with previous learnings.
15. Learners are motivated when they can see the usefulness of the learning in their own personal terms.[2]

The idea of educating women during pregnancy is probably very ancient. In Manchester, England, during the 18th century, Dr. Charles White wrote a book of instructions for the supervision of women during pregnancy and how to help them in labor and make them more comfortable. During the last few decades of this century, increased understanding of the psychodynamics of pregnancy and the puerperium has established a scientific basis for the content and structure of antepartal and postpartal education.

FACTORS IN PARENT EDUCATION

Psychologic Tasks of Pregnancy and Women's Interests

Nurses have long observed that pregnant women ask different kinds of questions and express different concerns in early pregnancy from those of later periods in gestation. The widely recognized receptiveness of women in the third trimester toward information about baby care and behavior led to the common practice of scheduling prenatal classes at this time. Women in the first or second trimester did not exhibit the same level of interest in "mothercraft" classes; thus they were largely omitted from prenatal education.

Professional interest in the many behavior changes characteristic of pregnant women led to identification of the specific and unique psychologic tasks which appear to be a universal phenomenon of pregnancy. Viewing pregnancy as a developmental process, involving profound endocrine and general somatic as well as psychologic changes, it can be understood as a period of disequilibrium and a significant turning point in the woman's (and probably her partner's) life.[3] Certain specific psychologic tasks are necessary to cope with the numerous changes, and these seem to occur at specific times during gestation.

1. The first, incorporation and integration of the fetus, occurs during the first trimester and is not evident during later stages of pregnancy.

2. The second, perception of the fetus as a separate object, seems to begin in the second trimester and to be quite well established by the third trimester.

3. The third task, readiness to assume the care-taking relationship with the baby, increases from the second to the third trimester and is not apparent in early pregnancy.

4. The fourth task concerns preparation for labor. The highest level of anxiety about labor is manifest during the second trimester, while women in the third trimester express more confidence about undergoing labor.[4]

This "time schedule" of involvement with different psychologic tasks suggests that pregnant women's interests and needs for information will vary according to stage of gestation. While research has not yet identified exactly what periods of time are involved in each psychologic task, nurses can utilize these data to plan appropriate antepartal education.

During early pregnancy, when the woman is working through the idea of being pregnant, informational needs center on validation of pregnancy, understanding physical changes, and recognition of normal emotions and feelings. In midpregnancy, a woman begins to identify the baby as a unique individual and is receptive to information about fetal growth and development and about maintaining her own and the baby's health. As pregnancy draws to an end, the woman becomes concerned about preparing for the baby's arrival, thus the interest in preparation for childbirth, infant behavior, and care-taking activities including feeding, handling, bathing, and so on. By tailoring the information presented to the different interests of each group and providing women with the opportunity to express their own learning needs, nurses can conduct meaningful antepartal educational programs.

Postpartum Processes and the Mother-Child Relationship

Although the experience of labor is undoubtedly significant for the woman's self-concept, maternal-infant bonding, and possibly the couple's relationship, few data are available to substantiate what impact nursing intervention during labor might have on these perceptions. Advocates of prepared childbirth believe women move more rapidly into the care-taking role when they are awake and actively participating in their labor. There is some empirical evidence that fathers who act as labor coaches develop stronger and more recognizable paternal feelings toward the babies of these labors than toward their other children. The work of some neonatologists in the area of high-risk infants strongly suggests that early and prolonged contact between mother and baby following labor and delivery enhances the bonding process. As with other mammals, humans seem to have a critical time for optimal mother-infant bonding, and this time probably is the first several hours after delivery. There also appear to be certain species-specific maternal behaviors which initiate and carry out the attachment process.[5]

On first contact with their babies, mothers seek an "en face" position in which their eyes are in the same vertical plane as the baby's. It has been suggested that this eye-to-eye contact may initiate or release maternal care-taking responses. Mothers then begin to explore the infant, first with fingertips touching the infant's extremities, then within a few minutes proceeding, with encompassing palm contact, to massage the infant's trunk. Some fathers have been observed going through these same steps. Kennell and Klaus[6] described this process as taking only a few minutes. Rubin, writing many years earlier, observed very similar behavior patterns in mothers as they moved from fingertip to palm touch, then encompassed their infants in their arms. However, this process took about three days according to Rubin's observations.[7]

Other physiologic and psychologic changes occur during the puerperium which are part of the process of regeneration undergone by the mother. There is a "taking-in" period which lasts for the first day or two, possibly three. During this restorative period the mother has a great need for sleep, may indeed have "sleep-hunger" for several days. Among other normal reactions associated with this taking-in phase is the mother's passive and dependent behavior. However, when the "taking-hold" phase follows, the mother is physically and psychologically ready to assume active care of her infant and seeks information and support to facilitate her mothering behaviors. Once her dependency needs have been met in the taking-in phase, she needs to move toward greater independence.[8] For further details of nursing care during the puerperium, refer to Chapter 28.

Effective patient teaching must take into account what is known about the processes occurring during labor and the puerperium, as well as individual variation and specific need. If the labor experience is as important as we suspect, health professionals have an obligation to assist parents to prepare for it and support them during this stressful time. When labor has started, a certain amount of teaching is possible, and sensitive care can be helpful, but this is not as effective as antenatal preparation. While parents have long recognized the significance of being together with their new baby in the hours right after birth, health professionals until recently have largely been oblivious to this in their concern for asepsis, technology, and immediate dangers to the newborn. Perhaps it is time to rethink delivery and recovery routines and educate both parents and professionals in the new data concerning mother-infant attachment.

During the few days the postpartal woman spends in the hospital, her needs may conflict with the nursing staff's needs to maintain the routine or provide the teaching they believe necessary. Mothers will progress at different speeds in their assumption of the care-taking role, and will have individualized concerns. Finding a way to respond to individual needs yet conduct an efficient postpartal educational program is a major challenge to postpartal nurses. Parent teaching activities must also extend into the community, to respond to the needs of families integrating a new member during the early years of childrearing.

Socioeconomic Factors

The learning process will vary according to culture and socioeconomic situation. Mothering practices in lower income groups are influenced by economic circumstances which limit equipment, supplies and mobility; by the organization of the family group and the authority structure; and by the accumulated folk knowledge which establishes specific practices for many common activities and problems of child-rearing. Standard educational programs about breastfeeding or formula preparation, clothing and supplies for the baby, integration of the baby into the family, and the mother's nutritional and rest needs are often meaningless to low income mothers

because of a lack of resources and a different value system. Family and friends are generally viewed as more reliable consultants for health concerns than professionals, whose assistance is sought only when community knowledge cannot solve the problem. Sometimes the use of language itself precludes useful exchange of information, as differences in terms used, accent, and speed of delivery vary substantially between middle-class nurses and low income mothers. In lower socioeconomic levels, the grandmother's word about baby care is often law, and she may be the major caretaker of the baby. Teaching given solely to the mother may thus be of little consequence to the actual care given to the baby. Different cultural groups also have their unique approaches to childrearing and patterns of assistance to new mothers. Values, language, style, and knowledge will exert influences within other cultural groups in a manner similar to that discussed above.

The nurse must come to understand different cultural and low income lifestyles if effective antepartal and postpartal teaching is to occur. The approach to teaching utilized with these groups will probably need to shift from the giving of information to assessing present practices, supplementing these practices when necessary with information presented in a form that can be understood and accepted.[9]

TYPES OF EDUCATION FOR CHILDBEARING

Preparation for motherhood actually begins with the woman's own birth or earlier, and is influenced by an accumulation of her experiences through infancy, childhood, adolescence, and maturity. The father's feelings and attitudes are influenced in a like manner by his previous experiences. There is an increasing tendency for schools to incorporate information about childbearing and parenthood into "health education" and "family life" courses. Classes about pregnancy, sexuality, and parenthood are becoming more common in college and university curricula, as well as more widely available in continuing education and private adult educational programs. Couples thus bring a wealth of previous learning to their experience of childbearing, some of it useful and positive and some frightening and inaccurate. With the advent of pregnancy, preparation for parenthood begins in earnest as the immediacy of the event escalates the need for information.

Individual Teaching and Counseling

One-to-one teaching is widely used in all nursing settings, and is frequently effective in assisting patients to understand and adapt to a variety of health problems. In most nurse-patient contacts, some individual teaching occurs. During pregnancy numerous opportunities are present for nurses to enhance the effectiveness of medical care through explanations of treatments and procedures, interpretations of what the physician tells parents, and specific instructions for carrying out the regimen of care. When the patient asks questions about symptoms or feelings or seeks general information, an on-the-spot response by the nurse meets that particular learning need.

Some clinics and offices have pamphlets or audiovisual material intended to provide individualized instruction to parents during the antepartal period. The amount of structure necessary to ensure that these materials are actually used varies widely. The effectiveness of written or media information without reinforcement through discussion is questionable.

Counseling, an interchange of opinions or giving of advice to help direct the judgment or conduct of others, is often hard to separate from teaching. While counseling is more personal and feeling-oriented, its use in combination with presentation of facts usually results in enhanced learning. Appropriate use of counseling takes into consideration the patient's viewpoint and works within an acceptable framework to bring about increased understanding, leading to a change in behavior in the desired direction through the patient's internalization of the new goals.

Individualized nursing care in which the woman is assisted to recognize her feelings and fears, reassured that such feelings are normal, and given certain facts to dispel myths or anticipate and prepare for coming events is a common example of how teaching and counseling are combined in antepartal care.

Although individual teaching and counseling will continue to be a major mode of nursing intervention,

concerns for more efficient utilization of the health professional's time have led to increased use of groups for antepartal education. Groups are also beneficial because the exchange of experiences among parents with common concerns provides support and encouragement, and expertise and knowledge of the group members combined often exceeds that of the professional alone.

Groups and Classes

Most institutions providing maternity care also offer some type of antepartal group instruction, but the goals and purposes of these groups vary widely. Many private organizations also offer programs in antepartal education, prenatal exercise and Yoga, and preparation for childbirth and parenthood. Classes may be affiliated with continuing education programs in colleges and universities, adult education programs in local communities and high schools, health professionals in private practice, or national health care organizations such as the Red Cross. The teachers in these groups or classes usually have some type of preparation or certification. They may represent one or, less commonly, several disciplines.

These educational programs can enhance, strengthen, and broaden the care and services provided by the physician and maternity nurse. Programs in parent education should be related segments in the total constellation of services provided to families. In order to make these sessions truly a preparation for parenthood and family-centered nursing, special attention has to be given to timing and availability of these courses. Sometimes hospitals and institutions arrange classes at times which are not feasible for the parents attending, especially for the father and often for the mother (e.g., in the middle of a busy day). Therefore, attendance is sparse and limited and many valuable aims of the programs may be thwarted.

Informational Groups

The informational group is the most widely used type of program in this country. These groups are planned to serve everyone in the community and place emphasis on a general type of "education for childbirth." Courses usually include the physiology of childbearing, general hygiene, including nutrition during pregnancy and lactation, preparations for the baby, and the care of the mother and baby after delivery. In this type of program a multidisciplinary approach may be used in the teaching, or the nurse may be responsible for teaching all of the content.

In general, the material is usually covered in a lecture format with time allowed for questions and discussion. At times a semistructured approach may be used, with certain topics being suggested by the participants and additional relevant information introduced by the nurse-discussion leader as it seems appropriate. Audiovisual materials such as films and slides are often used, with a film depicting actual childbirth a standard component. Tours of the hospital labor unit, postpartum floor and nursery are usually included.

Some of these classes are given for expectant mothers or fathers alone; in others the parents attend classes together. In the latter group the classes aid the parents in their mutual appreciation of the value of antepartal preparation and tend to promote the idea of sharing parenthood. The goals set for the parents in any of these classes are similar—namely, to gain increased knowledge about childbearing and increased understanding of ways to promote and to maintain optimum health through the practice of good health habits in daily living.

These classes are included as a part of the programs of private "public health" agencies such as the Visiting Nurse Association, official community health agencies such as the local and state departments of health, private organizations such as the Maternity Center Association in New York City, and many hospitals throughout the states.

Discussion or Counseling Groups

In this format no structured curriculum is set in advance. Group discussion is developed from the contributions of the group members. The leader is responsible for guiding the discussion and for opening essential areas not probed by the group members. The various areas described in informational programs (physiology of childbearing, general hygiene) are covered as the nurse-leader introduces these topics when they fit with the areas brought up by the participants.

The group situation demands that the nurse develop a new concept of self as a leader and acquire new skills. Knowledge and understanding of what material is relevant are essential so that it can be

drawn upon as the group needs it. Hence, the nurse must be totally prepared each time that the group meets since the discussion may range from nutrition in the first trimester of pregnancy to the physiology of labor. In addition, she must be skilled in communication techniques of listening, probing, and reflecting so that she can help the group to elaborate on germane comments and statements.

The nurse must recognize the importance and the implication of "iceberg questions," sometimes spoken of as "the question behind the question," knowing that such questions may indicate an underlying concern of the questioner. For example, an expectant mother in the last trimester of pregnancy asks, "How common is going crazy after having a baby?" In such instances the professional nurse should be able to explore and to sift alternatives until the real question can be asked and appropriate action may be taken. In this instance the patient really was not concerned with how often people became psychotic after childbirth but rather whether she is likely to experience this malady. Because of a history of mental illness in her family and her own extreme emotional lability during this pregnancy she was afraid that she might become psychotic after delivery.

Since training group leaders is a costly and time-consuming business (and it is essential that those who manage parents in this way be trained in the techniques), group education is not a commitment to be undertaken lightly by either the participating nurses or the sponsoring agencies. Unfortunately, many of these agencies rate the success of a program by the numbers attending; and in the group situation, by definition, only *small groups* can be served at any time.

Group discussion programs are usually well received by those who become involved on a continuing basis, with high levels of professional and patient satisfaction. Small groups are also quite effective in bringing about behavior change. Moreover, group education has the advantage of not limiting the discussion to certain topics usually discussed by particular class groups, and it can focus upon any of the aspects of pregnancy or childbearing which are of interest to the group.

Whatever the approach, the nurse who participates in parent classes is in a favorable position to help the patients and families to develop a better understanding of their immediate situations, together with a balanced view of the sociology of pregnancy and parturition, growth and development, and the psychologic and emotional aspects of family life.

Prepared Childbirth Groups

The interpretation of "labor" as "pain" has been held by women from time immemorial, with the result that many women approached childbirth in dread of a fearful ordeal. Orthodox Christian teaching considers pain the natural accompaniment of childbirth in partial reparation for Eve's enticing Adam into the original sin. As most body processes are free from discomfort, the question of labor pain as a social phenomenon is frequently raised. Whatever the basic causes and mechanisms of childbirth pain (see Chapter 24), concern developed gradually over finding a means to help relieve the suffering of women during labor.

The influence of the attitude of a woman toward her confinement upon the ease of labor was stressed for many years by the British obstetrician, the late Grantly Dick-Read. He emphasized certain psychological aspects of labor—that "fear is in some way the chief pain-producing agent in otherwise normal labor." The neuromuscular mechanism by which fear exerts a deleterious effect on labor is obscure, but the general validity of Dick-Read's contention is in keeping with common clinical knowledge. The woman builds up a state of tensions because she is frightened, and these tensions create an antagonistic effect on the muscular activity of normal labor, with resulting pain. The pain causes more fear, which further increases the tensions, and so on, creating a vicious circle.

Dick-Read's approach included an educational component to help the women comprehend the physiologic processes of labor, exercises to improve muscle tone, and techniques to assist in relaxation and prevent the fear–tension–pain mechanism. These three components are included in most childbirth preparation programs which developed after Dick-Read's work became well known.

The educational component during pregnancy is designed to eliminate fear. Facts which concern the anatomy and the physiology of childbearing and the appropriate care of the woman are taught. The woman not only learns how labor progresses but also is helped to gain an understanding of the sensations likely to accompany labor and methods of working cooperatively with them. The exercises which are included are designed for the muscles which will be used in labor, as well as those which will promote the general well-being of the body. In the performance of any skill the individual is more efficient if the muscles involved are in the best condition. The exercises are not strenuous and, for the most part, are ones that will contribute to improved posture, body balance, agility, and increased flexibility, strength, and endurance. The woman and her partner learn breathing techniques that will aid her ability to relax in the first stage of labor, and techniques that will help her to work effectively with muscles used in the delivery.

To enable the parents to better meet the needs of their baby after birth, information about growth and development also is included in these classes.

An important consideration throughout such programs is "to help the woman help herself," so that her pregnancy will be a healthy, happy experience and at the time of labor she will be better able to participate actively in having her baby. In former days when women often were given heavy sedation, they were unable to have this satisfying experience.

Currently most prepared childbirth programs include the father as an active participant, with a role in helping the woman cope with labor. In this way fathers are made to feel involved and useful, and through learning the physiologic and emotional processes of pregnancy, gain an appreciation of the woman's experience. They are also able to explore their feelings and role as parents and prepare psychologically for fatherhood.

Prepared childbirth is variously called *natural childbirth, participant childbirth,* or by the particular program's founder as with Lamaze and Bradley. Early in the movement in the United States, prepared childbirth earned a bad name through publicity about its more overzealous advocates. "Painless childbirth" was held up as a goal by some extremist groups, and the woman who did experience pain and resorted to pain medication during labor was made to feel a failure. This can be extremely destructive to the woman's self-concept at a time when she needs positive reinforcement in her abilities to achieve and perform competently. Fortunately, current thinking recognizes the variability in individual responses to stress and the differing character of individual labors and teaches that pain medication used judiciously may enhance the woman's ability to use relaxation techniques, thus helping her cope better with labor and achieve a satisfying outcome.

For some years many obstetricians and labor room nurses resisted prepared childbirth. Couples who had been trained in a particular method often had to buck staff pressures in their attempt to use the relaxation techniques they had learned. Medication was at times forced upon the laboring woman on the premise that the physician felt it would be best for her, even when she protested that it was not necessary. Such practices as laboring in a semi-upright position instead of lying flat, having ice chips or sips of water, eliminating the perineal shave, holding and putting the baby to breast immediately after delivery, and constant presence of the father throughout labor and delivery caused much staff consternation and were often vetoed.

Although prepared childbirth advocates had long been reporting the increased satisfaction the couple experienced, and the reduction of depressed babies when these methods were used, it took economic consumer pressure to bring about widespread acceptance of prepared childbirth. When childbearing couples began avoiding physicians and hospitals because they were not allowed to practice their method, the recalcitrants began to see the benefits of involvement and participation of the parents.

Lamaze or Psychoprophylactic Method (PPM)

The *psychoprophylactic,* or *Lamaze, method* is the most widely used prepared childbirth method in the United States today. It was first propounded by two Russian doctors, Nicolaiev and Velvovsky. The rationale of the program was based on Pavlov's concept of pain perception and his theory of conditioned reflexes (i.e., the substitution of favorable conditioned reflexes for unfavorable ones).

The theory intrigued a Paris obstetrician, Ferdinand Lamaze, who studied Russian-trained mothers-to-be in a Leningrad clinic. Lamaze returned to France and began to prepare his patients in *psychoprophylaxis* or *mental prevention* of pain in childbirth. He gradually introduced certain adaptations, the most important of which was the rapid shallow breathing which came to characterize the Lamaze method.

As the technique spread throughout Europe and Latin America the *Lamaze method* and psychopro-

phylaxis became synonymous. The late Marjorie Karmel was perhaps the most responsible for introducing this technique to America. There are now programs in psychoprophylaxis throughout this country. Many are under the auspices of the American Society for Prophylaxis in Obstetrics (ASPO) which was founded through joint efforts of Mrs. Karmel and a physical therapist, Elizabeth Bing, and others.

In general, the teaching in the program consists of combating the fears associated with pregnancy and childbirth by instructing the pregnant woman and her labor partner in the anatomy and the neuromuscular activity of the reproductive system and the mechanism of labor (Fig. 18-1). The underlying theory of these programs remains firmly based on the neurophysiology of cortical excitation and conditioned response. That is, the woman is taught to replace responses of restlessness and loss of control with more useful activity. Its usefulness lies in the fact that a high level of activity can excite the cerebral cortex sufficiently to inhibit other stimuli, in this case, the pain usually associated with labor.

In some programs nutrition and general hygiene are included. Exercises which strengthen the abdominal muscles and relax the perineum are taught, and breathing techniques to help the process of labor are practiced (Fig. 18-2). Thus, the mother is conditioned to respond with respiratory activity and dissociation (or relaxation) of the uninvolved muscles. She then controls her perception of the stimuli associated with labor and learns to work more effectively with the obstetric team.

Several changes have occurred in the Lamaze method as a result of experiences gained over many years of use. Class content, flexible breathing techniques, theories of learning and motivation, and emphasis on the childbirth team constitute the major changes. Class content originally dealt mostly with exercises, relaxation, breathing techniques, and the normal labor and delivery experience. Childbirth educators have added additional information such as prenatal nutrition, infant feeding, cesarean birth, and other variations from usual labor as well as discussions concerning sexuality, early parenting, and coping skills for the postpartum period.

The main modification in breathing technique has been to use a moderate shallow breathing rather than rapid panting. Shallow effortless breathing,

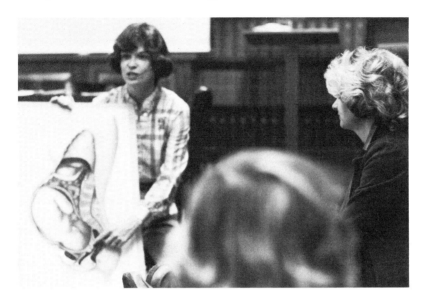

Figure 18-1. Prenatal class instruction.

moderate in pace and high in the chest, is now taught in combination with the slower chest breathing, to be used as labor intensifies when slow chest breathing is no longer effective by itself. Using this combined pattern, the woman begins her contrac-

tion with slow chest breathing, switches to shallow chest breathing for the peak of the contraction, and returns to slow chest breathing as the contraction declines. The shallow breathing itself has several variations, and an acceleration–deceleration pattern

Figure 18-2A. Couples practicing various methods of pushing, muscle relaxation and breathing in preparation for labor. (*B*) and (*C*), opposite page.

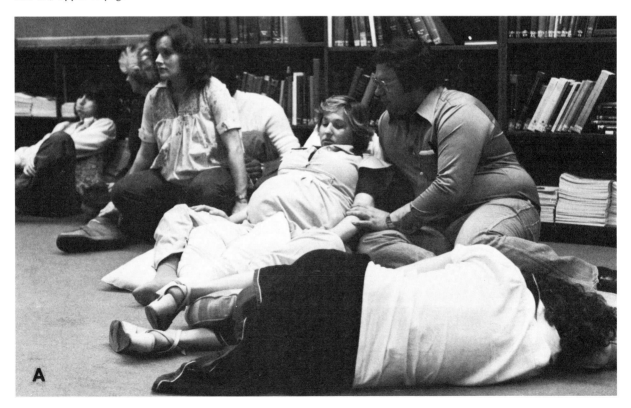

A

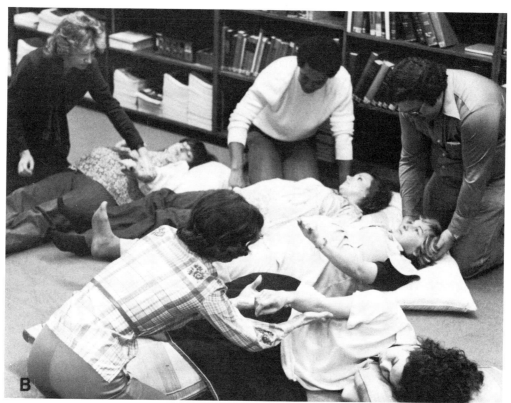

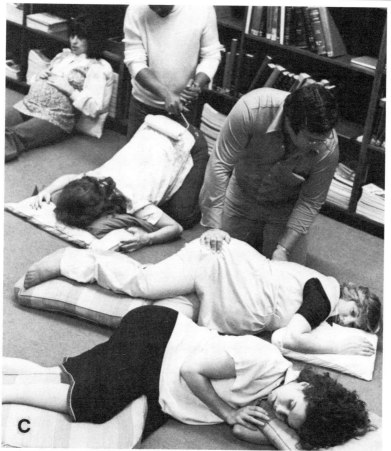

or a pant-blow pattern may be used as transition nears. In the second stage of labor, the woman may assume any comfortable physiologic position (a 35° semisitting position, squatting, or sidelying, as in Fig. 18-2A), take several deep breaths, and then hold her breath, bulge abdominal muscles, relax the perineum, and push out through the vagina. This pushing effort is repeated throughout the contraction, timed and coached by the partner. (For more specific techniques see Chapter 24, Table 24-2).

In the area of learning and motivation, Lamaze has progressed to a more individualized approach. The original psychoprophylactic training was rather rigid, with goals set by the teacher. Now, the couple set their own goals for labor and delivery, and the teacher assists them to learn ways in which these goals can be realized. This approach removes any set criterion for the success of the labor experience, avoiding the disappointment of externally imposed goals which may be unrealistic for the particular couple.

Greater emphasis is also given to the childbirth team, in which the couple, obstetrician, nurse, and Lamaze teacher are perceived as working together toward a satisfying labor experience. Rather than anticipating a thwarting of their goals, the couple is encouraged to discuss its goals with the physician so he or she can understand what they hope to do. They also gain appreciation of some of the physician's responsibilities and alternate plans, should labor not progress normally.

Labor room nurses tend to be better informed about methods of prepared childbirth and more committed to helping couples achieve their goals. Discussion of these goals with the nurses early in labor helps them understand and work more effectively with the couple. The theme of cooperation with the childbirth team has led to improved relations between prepared childbirth couples and health professionals.[10]

Other Childbirth Methods

Several other approaches to prepared childbirth are used throughout the country (see list in Chapter 24), some of which are popular in specific geographic regions or even specific areas of a particular city.

The *Bradley method,* also called husband-coached childbirth, emphasizes slow controlled breathing along with relaxation. The Academy of Husband-Coached Childbirth is the organization that trains teachers to conduct classes in the Bradley method.

The *Wright method* is based on psychoprophylaxis, but uses less active breathing than was taught in the Lamaze method. The breathing "levels" become more complex as labor progresses. Since Erna Wright promoted this method through her book and her travels, it has become known as the Wright method.

The *psychosexual method* of Shelia Kitzinger is not based on psychoprophylaxis but on a method using sensory memory as an aid to understanding and working with the body in preparation for birth. Included also is the Stanislavsky method of acting as a basis for teaching relaxation. Kitzinger advocates chest breathing but teaches release of the abdomen at the same time. Her method is called the psychosexual method because she saw sexuality as part of the larger whole encompassing family relationships, birth, cuddling, and feeding.[11]

Yoga, although not a method of prepared childbirth, has been used by numerous women in labor, sometimes in combination with other specific methods of childbirth preparation. Yoga teachings include relaxation, concentration, and a combination of abdominal and chest breathing called "complete breathing." It is not unusual to see childbirth educators teaching different techniques from several methods in an eclectic or "holistic" preparation for childbirth.

Although these programs may derive from different theories and may vary in specific techniques, they have many points in common including the basic beliefs that

1. Fear enhances the perception of pain but may diminish or disappear when the parturient knows about the physiology of labor;
2. psychic tension enhances the perception of pain but the parturient may relax more easily if childbirth takes place in a calm and agreeable atmosphere, and if good human contacts have been established between her and the personnel attending her;
3. muscular relaxation and a specific type of breathing diminish the pain of labor.

Hypnosis

This technique is to induce a state of extreme suggestibility in which the patient is insensible to outside impressions, except the suggestion of her attendant. There is no particular "program" associated with the use of this technique; rather, training in achieving a hypnotic state or autohypnosis is usually given by an obstetrician who is especially trained in this area. While there is no general regimen for learning this technique the conditioning required is usually presented in several individual sessions at the time of the antepartal visits, usually in the latter half of pregnancy.

The modus operandi of hypnotically induced relaxation has been explained by suggesting that whenever all the voluntary muscles are completely relaxed during labor, the uterus has a monopoly on available energy and hence can work more efficiently. In addition, it is likely that when fears are abolished or diminished, efficient uterine action is promoted. The utilization of comfort measures, such as low back massage, has also been suggested as enhancing the hypnotic state. The major drawback to this technique lies in the difficulty of securing adequately prepared physicians.

GUIDE FOR PREPARING PARENTS FOR CHILDBIRTH AND THE PUERPERIUM

Whether or not the maternity nurse is involved in offering classes for parents or group preparation, it is important that education for childbirth and the puerperium be part of the professional repertoire. This information can be used for individual teaching or to reinforce what has been learned from other sources. The guide for preparing parents presented here aims at helping the woman to manage her body well in activity and rest, to use her natural resources effectively during labor, and to achieve optimal postpartal restoration. Inclusion of the father in this instruction, when possible, will assist him to understand his partner's needs during the childbearing process and offer support.★

There are great similarities between the Maternity Centers' breathing techniques and those used in other prepared childbirth methods; therefore, we have presented this as a general guide. The nurse

★ The illustrative material and much of the information in the following section were provided through the courtesy of the Maternity Center Association, based upon their publication *Preparation for Childbearing*, ed. 4, New York, 1977.

must be aware, however, that this may vary somewhat in different parts of the country.

Comfort During Pregnancy

The majority of women can maintain their usual work and play activities during pregnancy. However, since changes do occur in weight and weight distribution, comfort in pregnancy can be significantly improved by good posture and body mechanics in everyday activities. It is often possible to reduce or overcome discomfort by correct positions, body movements and exercises (Table 18-1). Since the major postural changes begin in the second trimester of pregnancy, this is the logical time for learning. Correct posture for standing, sitting, and stair climbing, and good body mechanics for carrying packages or lifting objects must be reinforced.
(*Text contnues on p. 234.*)

TABLE 18-1
RELIEF OF COMMON DISCOMFORTS THAT MAY OCCUR DURING PREGNANCY

Discomfort	Exercise or Position
Swelling of feet, ankles	Leg elevating
Leaking urine when coughing, laughing	Pelvic floor contraction
Abdominal pain when coughing	Abdominal contraction
Heaviness in pelvis	Knee-chest; pelvic floor contraction
Hemorrhoids and swelling around vagina	Knee-chest; pelvic floor contraction
Low back pain	Knee-chest
Cramps in thighs, buttocks	Knee-chest
Cramps in legs	Leg elevating; calf stretching
Tired legs	Leg elevating; calf stretching
Varicose veins in legs	Leg elevating; calf stretching
Shortness of breath	Good posture; good body mechanics; rib cage lifting; shoulder circling
Low backache	Pelvic rocking; good posture; pushing posture; squatting
Middle backache	Pushing position
Upper backache	Shoulder circling; good posture
Numbness in arms and fingers	Shoulder circling; lying on side
Abdominal muscle spasm (stitch)	Squatting; pushing posture; lying on affected side

Complete Breath and Breath Control

A complete breath is one in which the chest wall expands and the diaphragm descends to its maximum extent. The breath is let out slowly under pressure so that a more complete exchange of oxygen and carbon dioxide can take place. It is used periodically during relaxation and should be followed by slow, quiet, easy respiration (Fig. 18-3).

1. Breathe in once as deeply as possible.
2. Hiss or blow the air out slowly, letting your whole body go limp.
3. Continue breathing quietly, easily, and rhythmically.
4. Let yourself go completely loose.
5. Soon your body will begin to feel very heavy and any exertion will be difficult.
   a. Gradually bend an elbow bringing your hand toward your chin. Notice the effort.
   b. Slowly lower your arm to its resting position. Again you will find yourself actually working to prevent its falling too quickly.

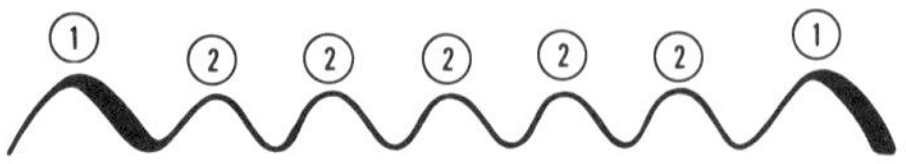

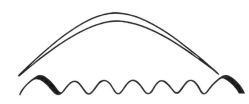

Figure 18-3. Complete breath and breath control.

The First Stage of Labor: Deep Breathing

1. Pretend that you are having a contraction lasting 30 to 45 seconds.
2. At the beginning of each contraction take a complete breath and hiss or blow it out.
3. Breathe deeply, slowly, and rhythmically throughout the remainder of the contraction.
4. When the contraction has ended, take another complete breath and hiss or blow it out slowly.
5. Breathe normally between contractions.
6. During labor, continue to use this pattern of breathing with contractions as long as it is helpful (Fig. 18-4).

Figure 18-4. Application of complete breathing to labor.

Modified Deep Breathing During Transition

As labor advances and contractions increase in strength, you often have a desire to keep the diaphragm as still as possible. Yet the uterus continues to need a good supply of oxygen. For this reason you should breathe deeply as the contraction begins and ends, and modify your breathing so that it is quiet and shallow at the peak of each contraction. To practice this:

1. Pretend that you are having stronger contractions, lasting almost a minute.
2. Breathe in deeply as the contraction starts. Then slowly hiss or blow out, letting yourself go completely limp.
3. Make each of the next 4 or 5 breaths a little shallower than the previous one. You will notice that you are breathing very lightly.
4. Light breathing is quiet and effortless, almost like a throat breath. Experiment to find your own comfortable rate and continue for 15 to 45 seconds. If you become dizzy or lightheaded, your breathing is too vigorous. If you have trouble getting enough air or difficulty maintaining the rhythm, try taking a quick, deep breath, and return to light breathing.
5. After the contraction has begun to subside, make each of the next four or five breaths a little deeper than the previous one.
6. End the breath pattern with one complete breath (Fig. 18-5).

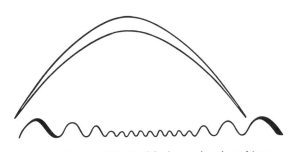

Figure 18-5. Modified complete breathing.

Further Adaptation for Transition

For the latter part of the first stage of labor (if you feel a tendency to hold your breath or to push during strong contractions) do the modified complete breath, but with one important change:

During light breathing, puff out gently as you exhale on every third or fourth breath (Fig. 18-6).

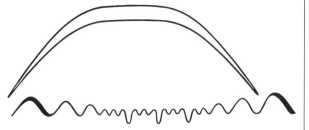

Figure 18-6. Modified complete breathing with adaptation for transition.

The Second Stage: Pushing

During the second stage of labor, you will find that pushing actively helps in the delivery of the baby. Contractions at this time last 60 to 65 seconds and generally are accompanied by a strong urge to push. (If regional anesthesia is used, however, the pushing sensation diminishes.) To practice for this (Fig. 18-7):

1. Lie on your back with head and shoulders elevated. Pillows may be used for practice at home. In the labor room the head of the bed may be elevated.
2. Bend your knees and separate your legs.
3. Take a deep breath and hiss or blow out.
4. Breathe in as quickly and deeply as you can; then hold your breath. (In labor, this "held" breath will help to fix your diaphragm so that your abdominal wall will make more effective downward pressure on the uterus and baby, aiding the baby's birth.)
5. Draw up your legs against your abdomen, in a squatting position, holding your thighs, ankles, or feet with your hands. If a delivery table is used, your feet and legs will be supported in stirrups so that you won't have to hold them, and there will be handles on which you pull. Raise head.
6. During practice, do *not* actually push. You will be able to do so in labor.

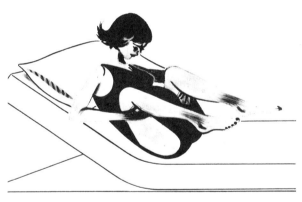

Figure 18-7. Pushing position.

7. Take *catch breaths* as needed. A catch breath is a short breath that may be taken whenever you can no longer hold your breath comfortably. Try to take no more than two or three catch breaths in each 60- to 65-second breath pattern (Fig. 18-8).
   a. Maintain the pushing position,
   b. Exhale, moving your head back.
   c. Take in a quick, deep breath.
   d. Tilt your head forward again and hold your breath.
8. When the contraction is over, relax completely, take a deep breath and sigh it out.

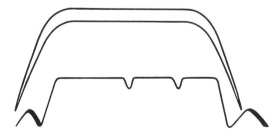

Figure 18-8. Catch breath.
Note: You may wish to practice breath holding and catch breaths without assuming the pushing position. You may do this while sitting in a chair by following the instructions relating to breathing described above.

BREATHING TECHNIQUES(Continued)

Panting

Your physician may tell you to pant or to stop pushing in the middle of a contraction. If so, begin panting immediately. This will make your diaphragm move up and down. Although this will not decrease the desire to push, it will physically prevent you from doing so. Forceful blowing will also accomplish the same purpose. To practice panting:

1. Start doing the exercise described in the section on The Second Stage: Pushing.
2. All at once, raise your head and shoulders, allowing your arms and hands to relax.
3. Breathe in and out very quickly, keeping your mouth open—like a panting dog.
4. Continue breathing this way until the contraction ends (Fig. 18-9).

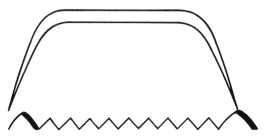

Figure 18-9. Diagrammatic breath pattern for panting.

The spinal muscles and joints should be protected from undue strain; thus the woman needs to know how her feet can be used efficiently for balance and for movement. (See chart: Principles for ADL During Pregnancy.)

For rest and comfort during pregnancy, the woman can learn the position for lying on her side, on her back, in the side relaxation position, and equally important, how to get up and out of bed without strain.

Backache is one of the most common complaints, and *pelvic rocking* performed daily will help to relieve abdominal pressure and low back pain during pregnancy and early labor. This exercise is useful also to firm the abdominal muscles following the birth of the baby.

Other exercises to promote comfort and give relief from some of the common discomforts of pregnancy include *rib cage lifting, shoulder circling, leg elevating, and calf stretching.*

Muscle Control

Two muscle groups undergo great changes during pregnancy, the abdominals and the muscles of the pelvic floor. The abdominal muscles stretch from the pressure of the enlarged uterus, and the pelvic floor muscles soften to prepare for the vaginal delivery. Loss of muscle tone can be minimized

PRINCIPLES FOR ADL DURING PREGNANCY

1. Activities need to be varied (walking, standing, sitting).
2. Time period should be of short duration.
3. Walking back and forth is preferable to standing still.
4. Standing posture—should be with one leg forward so that weight can be shifted easily and efficiently from foot to foot and the body turned comfortably.
5. Walking posture—head erect, back upright, and chin up and forward.
6. Sitting—a footstool is an invaluable aid.
7. Stair climbing—entire foot should be placed on stair and leg muscles used to lift self up each step without leaning forward.
8. Stooping and lifting should be avoided; if stooping is necessary, it is best to squat down and reach and lift, with feet wide apart and back straight.
   Alternate squatting position—one foot is placed forward; body is lowered slowly to the other knee. The front foot, which should be flat on the floor, will be used for lifting. The rear foot, flexed at the toes, will serve for pushing and will act as a balance.
9. Carrying bulky packages (groceries)—load should be divided and carried in two hands. A cart that rolls easily should be used for heavy loads.

during pregnancy and can be regained after delivery through proper exercise.

Abdominal contraction is an exercise which increases muscle tone and thus helps to strengthen the abdominal wall during pregnancy and the postpartal period. The exercise includes the following steps:

1. Assume any comfortable position (even standing and walking).
2. Tighten the abdominal muscles as much as possible.
3. Hold for a few seconds; then relax.

This should be repeated frequently throughout the day, and may be performed simultaneously with *pelvic floor contraction*. The latter exercise reduces congestion and general discomfort in the pelvic region and increases ability to control the muscles surrounding the orifice of the vagina, bowel, and bladder. It also improves muscle tone, thereby providing better support for the pelvic organs. Whenever exercises are taught to the patient with instructions to "repeat frequently throughout the day," the patient should understand about muscle fatigue and its consequences which may result from overdoing.

Conscious Relaxation

Relaxation is one of the most natural activities known to humans. However, human beings living in a civilized society, unlike their feline pets, seem to have forgotten how to relax naturally.

Relaxation enables a person to obtain maximum benefit from any rest period, it relieves bodily tensions that cramp muscles, producing fatigue, and promotes a feeling of physical and mental well-being.

Physical relaxation may reduce the pain of labor and, equally important, can put the woman in a calm frame of mind which permits her to cope more effectively with the demands of her situation.

The key to relaxation may be found in two principles—*correct posture* and *proper breathing*. Correct posture minimizes muscular stress and, coupled with this, controlled breathing makes it easier to relax. Techniques for breathing are described on pages 233 to 234.

Once the mother has developed the art of relaxing by using these techniques, she is advised to practice regularly and at other times when she is under pressure or excited. She may need to be reminded that her ultimate purpose in this preparation is to be able to relax during labor, when feelings of excitement and tension are apt to run high.

Avoiding Hyperventilation

Another reason for teaching correct breathing techniques is to avoid hyperventilation during labor. Nurses are often concerned about hyperventilation during labor when prepared childbirth breathing techniques are used. Undue fatigue, hyperventilation, and subsequent carpopedal spasm have been observed when breathing techniques are improperly used. Maternal respiratory alkalosis and a paradoxical acidosis in the fetus are also possibilities if hyperventilation is prolonged.

Hyperventilation and its complications can occur in any labor when the woman breathes improperly. Correct use of prepared childbirth breathing techniques can help prevent hyperventilation from occurring, which is another benefit of these programs.

Postpartum Exercises

During the puerperium, the six weeks following childbirth, the body undergoes major changes. The organs that had adjusted during pregnancy to make room for the growing baby gradually return to their original positions in the woman's body. The uterus, cervix, and vagina slowly return to the nonpregnant state. Important hormonal changes also occur. In effect, a bodily transformation that took nine months to complete is being reversed in the course of a few weeks.

Good nutrition and adequate rest are essential during this period. A new mother needs at least one rest period each day. Lying on the abdomen may help her uterus to return to good position (Fig. 18-10). A pillow under the hips when she is lying this way prevents back strain.

Postpartum exercises are important in restoring muscle tone and the woman's figure. In an uncomplicated delivery, these may be begun during the first few postpartal days, starting with the simpler exercises and progressing to the more strenuous ones. If the woman had an abnormal delivery or extensive perineal repair, exercises may need to be delayed. Practiced properly, the exercises should not be tiring, as they are done slowly and rhythmically, only a few times at first, and gradually increased (see Chart, pp. 238–239).

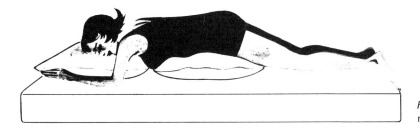

Figure 18-10. Prone position for rest and relaxation postpartally.

The pelvic floor contraction (Kegal exercise), used to strengthen and tone the muscles of the pelvic floor, can be started a few days postpartum and continued daily for the rest of the woman's life. The exercise can be done in almost any position, and no one need know it is being done. The steps of the exercise are as follows:

1. The muscles around the anus are tightened as if to control a bowel movement.
2. Next, the muscles around the vagina and urethra are tightened as if to stop urine in midstream.
3. These muscles are held tight for the count of 3 or 4.
4. The muscles are then relaxed.

This exercise should be repeated 50 to 100 times at least once a day. It is widely used for women with sexual dysfunction to increase their capacity for orgasm and is also helpful for minor degrees of cystocele. It is an excellent exercise to maintain life-long pelvic tone and enhance sexual enjoyment.

POSTPARTUM TEACHING

Parenthood often constitutes a stress in the developmental processes of both mothers and fathers. The postpartum period is particularly stressful because of the numerous physical changes the mother undergoes, the incomplete integration of her pregnancy and labor experiences, the changing roles which must occur within the family complex, and the uncertainty of the nature of the early mother-child relationship. Fatigue, confusion, feelings of helplessness and inadequacy, and depression often complicate this period. Isolation from the extended family, lack of community resources, economic strains, and pressures upon the woman to resume her full previous role within the family as rapidly as possible create additional stresses.

The nurse on the postpartum unit has a unique opportunity to intervene early in the developing mother-child relationship and assist the parents to anticipate and plan for the first few critical weeks at home. If the mother can attain a level of confidence in her ability to perform care-taking tasks, and begin to recognize her baby's behavioral messages, a good foundation can be laid and perhaps later difficulties minimized. Sources for continuing care and counseling need to be available to parents during the baby's first few months at home, and the postpartum nurse can direct them to such sources in the particular community.

Individual Teaching

Part of the postpartum nurse's daily responsibility is to provide individual instruction and support to those mothers to whom she provides care. This can range from information about infant sleep and activity patterns, growth and development, and how to dress the baby for different types of weather to sibling rivalry, contraception, and organizing the household to get the necessary tasks done. Mothers' concerns may be small and particular, such as getting the baby to stay awake and suck well, or they may be larger and more general, such as the changes in her own and the father's lifestyle after the advent of the baby. The nurse needs to be informed about a wide variety of topics including contraception, sexuality, and family dynamics as well as infant care and involutional physiology.

Individual teaching allows the nurse to respond to the personal questions and concerns of mothers, and relate information to that particular situation. Reinforcement of mothering skills is particularly effective on an individual basis, as is counseling regarding family problems or emotions. However, the nurse may not have the time to give each mother the amount of individual teaching and counseling needed. Certain types of teaching can be effectively done in groups, and the use of postpartum groups has increased on hospital postpartum units. Baby care classes seem well suited to group methods, because the more experienced mothers can add their wisdom and practices to the pooled knowledge available.

Postpartum Classes

The organization of classes for postpartum mothers, and sometimes for fathers as well, differs considerably from one institution to another. Each unit must work out the most convenient time for both staff and parents, and a method of communicating to ensure maximum attendance. At times a conference room on the unit is utilized, or a large patient room can be adapted and extra chairs brought in. The teachers may be postpartum nurses only, or may include nursery nurses, physicians, social workers, nutritionists, and public health nurses. A variety of media aids can be used, ranging from films to flip charts, books, or other printed material. Closed-channel television which can be viewed by each mother in her room has also been explored as a method of postpartum group instruction.

The content of postpartum teaching varies, but generally contains a section about the mother and one about the baby. Personal care of the mother includes information about perinatal care, breast care, involutional physiology, bathing and hair washing, medication and its effects, contraception, fatigue, and depression. In relation to the baby, mothers are instructed in the bath, breast- or bottle-feeding, holding and handling, dressing, care of the cord, the PKU test, care of the circumcision, sleep patterns, crying, individual behavior of babies, and sibling rivalry. During most classes, mothers have their babies with them, and can practice what they have just been taught with the nurse available for assistance and clarification.[12]

Special Classes

Some postpartum units organize special classes for mothers with particular needs. Breast-feeding classes, in which only breast-feeding mothers participate, are examples. The mothers are instructed in techniques of nursing and assisted to have successful nursing experiences, and possible problems and their prevention are discussed. Mothers whose babies are in the intensive care nursery, but who plan to nurse, may also be invited to these classes. More experienced mothers can be encouraged to

attend, as they are most helpful to new mothers who have never breast-fed before.

Common situations which breast-feeding mothers might encounter are brought up, and group solutions developed. Questions, such as what foods should be avoided, whether breast-feeding ruins the breasts, and what to do when the mother plans to be away for several hours, are elicited from the mothers. Answers to these questions can be provided by the nurse or other mothers in the group. Having the telephone number of the nurse for consultation if problems arise after discharge is very helpful to mothers and promotes continued success with breast-feeding.[13]

If the hospital is large enough to have a regular census of diabetic, adolescent, or low income mothers, postpartum classes to address their particular needs and concerns are helpful. Perhaps women who had a cesarean birth could make up another group, as their physiologic problems often affect accomplishment of mothering tasks. If, however, the maternity service is relatively small and cannot support many different postpartum groups, the common concerns of baby care can be taught to a group of varied composition, with needs for particular information handled on an individual basis.

Outpatient Groups

Nurses and other health professionals are increasingly aware of the need to extend services to parents after discharge from the hospital. This care may be provided through the public health department, hospital-affiliated clinics, private physician's offices, a community liaison nurse from the postpartum unit, or health professionals in private practice.

Parenting Groups

The importance of the first year of life in the child's development, both behaviorally and physically, has led to establishment of "parenting groups" in a variety of settings. Since most couples are caught unprepared for the realities of parenthood, there is a need to educate parents with respect to basic processes of parenting in order to foster more realistic expectations.

Such groups often meet prenatally and continue into the postpartum period. The goal is generally to promote healthy parent-child relationships by

POSTPARTUM EXERCISES

First day:
Lie on your back with your body and legs
  straight.
Inhale slowly, expanding your chest.
Pull your abdominal muscles in and press the
  lower part of your back to the floor.
Hold, then relax.
Repeat 5 to 10 times.

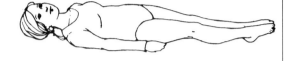

Second day:
Raise your head from the floor, bringing it as
  close to your chest as possible.
Try not to move any other part of your body.
Repeat 5 to 10 times.

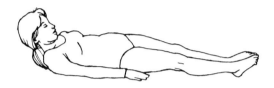

Third day:
Put your arms straight out at your sides, then
  raise them over your head until your hands
  meet.
Keeping your arms stiff, lower them again until
  they rest at your sides.
Repeat 10 to 15 times.

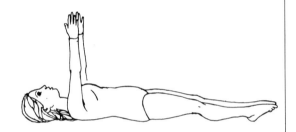

Seventh day:
Bring one leg up over your body until your
  foot touches your buttocks.
Straighten and lower it, then repeat the exer-
  cise with your other leg.
Repeat one more time each day.

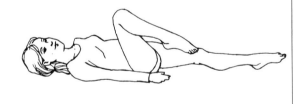

Seventh to tenth day:
Without using your hands, raise one leg at a
  right angle to your body. Keep your lower
  back on the floor.
Repeat, using the other leg.
Repeat 5 to 10 times.

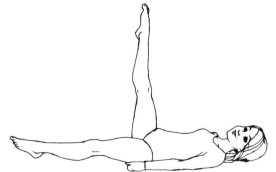

Fourteenth day:
Lying on your back, cross your arms on your
chest and raise your body upright, keeping
your legs close together on the floor.
Repeat one more time each day.

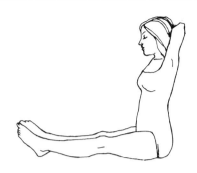

Next:
Bend your legs almost to a right angle and
raise your body, supporting it on your shoulders.
Press your knees together, but keep your feet
apart.
Contract the muscles of your buttocks at the
same time.
Repeat one more time each day.

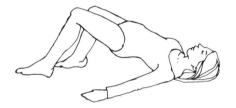

If ordered by your physician:
Turn on your stomach and raise your body so
that your knees and chest are close together.
Your chest should be against the floor, and
your legs about a foot apart.
Hold this position for two minutes.

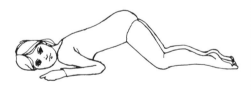

educating parents about the physical and psychological aspects of pregnancy, childbirth, infant care,
parenting, and child development. The group also
promotes independence and confidence in parents
by teaching problem-solving techniques and by
helping to establish and strengthen parents' support
systems.[14] Parents' sense of self-esteem and worth,
confidence in the parenting role, and realistic expectations regarding parenthood are key aspects in
determining parenting behavior.[15] Outcomes noted
for such groups are increased confidence of mothers
and fathers in their roles as parents, a more relaxed
feeling that makes them feel more in control of
parenting situations, and fewer behavioral problems
with the children.[16]

Mothers' Groups

Mothers' groups provided by local facilities can also
be helpful to new mothers. If mothers receive little
or no instruction in the hospital before discharge,
these groups can offer answers to many common
concerns about care of small babies and support in
mothering abilities. Cultural differences must be
respected and the structure informal and friendly if
such groups are to be effective.

The content of each class would vary, but information about infant nutritional needs and feeding
methods is important and should be covered in
detail, as inadequate nutrition and protein deprivation are common problems among this group,

with serious implications for the baby. General care of the infant, particularly bathing, diaper care, and causes of simple skin rashes, is another standard topic.

Sharing among the mothers can also enhance learning. If the atmosphere is comfortable, these mothers can be encouraged to examine practices that might be contributing to the baby's health problems, and possibly to modify these practices.

The nurse has the opportunity to observe the infants for signs of illness and refer them to the pediatrician if needed, as well as to identify serious emotional problems and make appropriate referrals.[17]

Cluster Visits

Cluster visits constitute a new approach to pediatric care that utilizes the group method. A small number of mothers and their babies, usually four pairs, are scheduled for a joint visit with the pediatric nurse practitioner or pediatrician. Each baby is examined with the mother standing by, findings explained, and instructions given for minor illness or problems. Subjects of general interest are postponed until discussion time, which follows the examinations. While one mother and baby are involved in the examination, the others are getting acquainted and comparing notes.

During the discussion period, the nurse and mothers talk about childbearing, feelings related to motherhood and baby care, changes in the family structure, or other topics relevant to the baby's age or the mother's needs. The groups are formed to include mothers with babies of about the same age. The mothers generally take the lead in the discussion and often provide specific information and teaching for one another. During the last ten minutes, the next cluster visit is planned and immunizations are given to the babies as needed.

These cluster visits are usually alternated with individual visits. They permit more care to be provided to mothers and babies using less professional time. The mothers involved tend to respond very positively, as they enjoy the camaraderie, sharing problems and anxieties, the chance to observe other babies, and the knowledge and support gained through the discussion. Increased confidence as parents and recognition that babies are individuals whose weights and development vary are also outcomes of the experience. There appears to be no increased cross-contamination. Cluster visits thus are one way to provide improved health care at a lower cost to parents.[18]

Parent Effectiveness Training

Other outpatient groups for parents are those that train parents in skills to prevent behavior problems in their children. Parent Effectiveness Training (P.E.T.) was started in the early 1960s by Dr. Thomas Gordon, a clinical psychologist from Pasadena, California. Parents attend class one night a week for eight weeks and learn active listening and other communication skills, behavior modification, and methods of resolving parent–child conflicts. Content also includes dealing with infants and toddlers. P.E.T. classes are available in many communities in all 50 states and are sometimes sponsored by schools, social agencies, or organizations serving parents as well as health professionals in private practice.[19]

REFERENCES

1. B. K. Redman: *The Process of Patient Teaching in Nursing.* St. Louis, C. V. Mosby, 1968, p. 11.

2. A. H. Gorman: *Teachers and Learners in the Interactive Process of Education.* Boston, Allyn and Bacon, 1969, p. 12.

3. G. F. Bibring, D. S. Huntington, and A. F. Valenstein: "A study of the psychological processes in pregnancy and of the earliest mother-child relationship." *Psychoanal. Stud. Child* 16: 9–71, 1961.

4. L. M. Tanner: "Developmental tasks of pregnancy." In Bergersen, B. S. (ed.): *Current Concepts in Clinical Nursing,* Vol. II. St. Louis, C. V. Mosby, 1969, pp. 292–297.

5. M. Klaus and J. Kennel: "Care of the mother." In Klaus and Fanaroff (eds.): *Care of the High-Risk Neonate.* Philadelphia, W. B. Saunders, 1973, pp. 98–118.

6. J Kennell and M. Klaus: "Care of the mother of the high-risk infant." *Clin. Ob. and Gyn.* 14: 926, 1971.

7. R. Rubin: "Maternal touch." *Nurs. Outlook* 11:829–831, Nov. 1963.

8. ———: "Puerperal change." *Nurs. Outlook* 9:753–755, Dec. 1961.

9. M. R. Spaulding: "Adapting postpartum teaching to mothers' low-income lifestyles." In

Bergersen, B. S. (ed.): *Current Concepts in Clinical Nursing,* Vol. II. St. Louis, C. V. Mosby, 1969, pp. 280–291.

10. J. L. Sasmor, C. R. Castor, and P. Hassid: "The childbirth team during labor." *Am. J. Nurs.* 73:444–447, March 1973.

11. C. A. Bean: *Methods of Childbirth.* New York, Doubleday, 1972, pp. 53, 54, 76.

12. E. G. Walker: "Concerns, conflicts, and confidence of postpartum mothers." In Anderson, E. H. (ed.): *Current Concepts in Clinical Nursing,* Vol. IV. St. Louis, C. V. Mosby, 1973, pp. 230–236.

13. I. S. Bird: "Breast-feeding classes on the postpartum unit." *Am. J. Nurs.* 75:456, March 1975.

14. D. Smith and H. Smith: "Toward improvements in parenting: A description of prenatal and postpartum classes with teaching guide." *J. Obstet., Gynecol. and Neonatal Nurs.* 7:22–27, Nov.-Dec. 1978.

15. M. Wuerger: "Stepping into parenthood." *Am. J. Nurs.* 76:1283–1285, Aug. 1976.

16. N. R. Shaw: "Teaching young mothers their role." *Nurs. Outlook* 22:695–698, Nov. 1974.

17. I. Cooper: "Group sessions for new mothers." *Nurs. Outlook* 22:251, April 1974.

18. M. Feldman: "Cluster visits." *Am. J. Nurs.* 74:1485–1488, Aug. 1974.

19. T. Gordon: *Parent Effectiveness Training.* New York, New American Library, 1975, pp. ix–2.

SUGGESTING READING

Bing, E.: *Six Practical Lessons for an Easier Childbirth.* New York, Bantam Books, 1977.

Dick-Read, G.: *Childbirth Without Fear.* New York, Harper & Row, 1972.

Goodwin, B.: "Psychoprophylaxis in childbirth." In Duffy, M. (ed.): *Current Concepts in Clinical Nursing,* Vol. III. St. Louis, C. V. Mosby, 1971, pp. 194–203.

Hassall, D.: "A home visit program for students." *Nurs. Outlook* 22:522–524, Aug. 1974.

Karmel, M.: *Thank You, Dr. Lamaze.* Philadelphia, J. B. Lippincott, 1959.

Salk, L.: *Preparing for Parenthood.* New York, Bantam Books, 1975.

Nineteen

Nutrition in Pregnancy

Importance of Nutrition During Pregnancy / Nutrition Counseling in Pregnancy / General Factors in Planning the Diet / Psychological Aspects of Nutrition / Daily Food Guide / Other Information on Nutrition / Digestive Problems and Diet

IMPORTANCE OF NUTRITION DURING PREGNANCY

In 1970, the National Academy of Sciences issued a report, *Maternal Nutrition and the Course of Pregnancy*.[1] This report reviewed reproductive experiences and concluded that adequate prenatal nutrition is one of the most important environmental factors affecting the health of pregnant women and their babies.

Studies conducted over the last several decades have shown that inadequate diet during pregnancy is associated with an increased incidence of difficult deliveries and complications. Stillborns, neonatal deaths, low birthweight infants, prematures, and infants with congenital defects occur more frequently.

One program to provide supplemental foods to pregnant women with deficient nutrition was carried out at the Montreal Diet Dispensary. The study showed a decrease in the incidence of toxemia and infant prematurity, morbidity, and mortality.[2]

All of these studies indicate that adequate prenatal nutrition is necessary for the maintenance of the woman's body tissues as well as for the growth and development of her baby.

NUTRITION COUNSELING IN PREGNANCY

Present-day antepartal clinics are utilizing the services of nutritionists for dietary counseling and planning whenever possible. When nutritionists are available, the nurse will find it helpful to work in conjunction with them to provide adequate guidance. The nurse's role in these cases may be to explore with the woman the extent of her need for nutritional counseling. However, when the services of a nutritionist are not available, the nurse may actually carry out the nutritional counseling.

The physician will regulate the patient's diet according to her needs and condition, and the nurse will follow through, planning with the woman how to best meet her nutritional requirements. If the patient's previous diet has been nourishing and well balanced, few changes will be necessary except to provide for the adjustment in protein, mineral, and vitamin intake.

Assessment in Nutritional Counseling

Each woman is an individual whose attitudes and beliefs toward emotional response to food, cultural

242

meaning of food, and knowledge of nutrition are unique. Creating a positive attitude toward nutrition during pregnancy requires patience, understanding, and respect for her particular nutritional patterns of behavior.

To deal with each patient's individuality, the physician and nurse must provide an opportunity and atmosphere for the woman to discuss her concerns about food and diet and to give information about her current dietary patterns. Nutritional evaluation requires information on not only what is eaten, but also the quantities and the method of preparation. Information will also be needed regarding purchasing practices as certain foods may not be purchased because of cost and more economical substitutions may be needed. Table 19-1 illustrates the type of nutritional assessment form that can be used to obtain adequate dietary information.

To provide appropriate guidance for the woman and to better assess her level of understanding and knowledge about her diet, a brief diet history can be taken to determine present eating patterns. The nurse may ask the woman to write down her usual daily and/or weekly meal pattern and any "extras" that she is likely to consume. These menus then are checked for an adequate intake of those foods that provide a substantial amount of the essential nutrients. As the nurse and the woman plan together, the patient's likes and dislikes are recognized, and those foods that provide the essential nutrients are encouraged. Suggestions may be given for the addition of certain foods or the modification of existing methods of selection and/or preparation.

Special Nutritional Considerations

There are certain circumstances which require special attention to nutritional needs during pregnancy. These situations may be listed as follows:

1. *Adolescence, high parity, and frequent conceptions* are factors related to the woman's physical readiness for her current pregnancy. Women under the age of 17, who become pregnant before finishing their own growth, have greater nutritional requirements than older women (see Fig. 19-1). Adolescent pregnancies have been associated with low birth weight, prematurity, and perinatal mortality. Similar problems may result from high parity and frequent conceptions because of depletion of maternal nutrient stores.

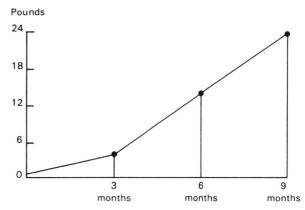

Figure 19-1. Recommended weight gain during pregnancy: 2 to 4 pounds (1–2 kg) during first trimester; 0.9 pound (0.5 kg) per week for second and third trimesters.

2. *Low prepregnancy weight, insufficient weight gain during pregnancy, and obesity* must also be considered high-risk problems. Women who have low prepregnancy weight for their height have a greater than average incidence of toxemia and a strikingly increased incidence of prematurity. In the instance of women who have insufficient weight gain during pregnancy, the result may be low birth weight infants.

   The major problem with the obese patient is the possibility of insufficient intake of specific nutrients because of unsound food habits. Food selections of some obese women are likely to emphasize "empty calorie foods, that are rich in carbohydrates and fats, and low in proteins, minerals, and vitamins."

3. *Previous obstetrical complications and existing medical complications* are a source of potential problems and affect the patient's health status and the outcome of her pregnancy. Nutrition-related factors in the obstetrical history include inadequate weight gain, preeclampsia and/or toxemia, anemia, diabetes, antepartum hemorrhage, multiple pregnancy, premature or small for gestational age infant, and fetal or neonatal death. Other preexisting medical conditions requiring special nutritional counseling are hypertension, cardiac disease, infections, gastrointestinal problems, liver and kidney diseases, and tuberculosis.

4. *Dietary faddism and pica* refer to the abnormal intake of specific substances. In the case of pica, the substance ingested is clay, dirt, cornstarch, or plaster. Nutritious food may be

(*Text continues on p. 246.*)

TABLE 19-1
DIET HISTORY AND EVALUATION FORM

Name _____ Date _____

_____ Due Date _____

Patient's childhood home _____ Height _____

   (State or country) _____ Present weight _____

Patient's occupation_____ Pregravid weight_____

Last year school completed_____

Husband's occupation _____ Birth date _____

Money available for food weekly_____ Number in household _____

Food currently bought by_____

Meals currently prepared by _____

Foods liked especially, including cravings _____

_____

_____

Foods never eaten and why (storage problems, equipment, and so on)_____

_____

_____

_____

Nutritional supplements currently used during pregnancy (kind and amount used) _____

_____

_____

_____

Diet modified previously or currently (type of diet and date) _____

_____

_____

Meals and snacks often eaten at these times:

Morning:_____

_____

_____

Midmorning: _____

Midday: _____

_____

_____

_____

Afternoon: _____

_____

Evening: _____

_____

_____

_____

Before bedtime: _____

_____

Prenatal diet prescribed and date _____

Instruction received on prenatal diet including materials given _____

_____

_____

Additional information_____   _____

_____

Follow-up remarks _____

_____

Prenatal dietary history recorded by: _____

_____

_____

_____

_____

It is desirable to obtain a dietary history as early as possible in pregnancy and before recommending a specific diet for an individual mother. This history should include: information concerning the expectant mother's usual food practices, meals often omitted, typical menu patterns, food likes and dislikes, cultural factors, methods of food preparation, financial situation, and so on. Nutritional gaps will be obvious from an evaluation of this information. During the process of taking a diet history, useful information is obtained concerning the patient's level of nutrition knowledge and clues to methods of counseling. Explaining any recommended changes will help the expectant mother understand her present needs. (If history is kept in patient's chart and information is recorded elsewhere, interviewer may prefer to omit some questions. Sample form may be changed to fit situation.)

Source: Cross, A. T., and Walsh, H. E.; Prenatal Diet Counseling, *J. Reproductive Med.* 7:269–270, Dec. 1971. From *Nutrition—During Pregnancy and Lactation,* Berkeley, Calif., California State Dept. of Public Health, 1971.

replaced by these craved items. In addition, iron and zinc intake may be reduced. The practice of pica is not restricted to any particular social or cultural group.

Women who, because of religious, philosophical, or other reasons, have limited their food intake to certain groups of foods as in macrobiotic diets, fruitarian diets, and the like are also at risk during pregnancy. In addition to being nutritionally inadequate, these food fads may induce harmful metabolic changes in the woman.

5. *Low income* has been related to an inadequate nutrient intake. Pregnant women with limited food budgets may be unable to purchase enough food to meet their nutritional requirements. As a result, low birth weight babies are more prevalent in low socioeconomic groups.

6. *Ethnic and/or language differences* may cause nutritional problems for the pregnant woman. The woman may be unable to obtain familiar foods, and, in an attempt to follow a specific cultural food pattern, she may replace these foods with less nutritious items found locally. If English is not a familiar language, the woman may not be able to read or understand information about foods eaten in this country. In many cases, ethnic and/or language differences have been associated with anemia and inadequate weight gain during pregnancy.

7. *Excessive smoking, alcoholism, and drug addiction* may diminish the amount of food eaten and are associated with adverse physiological changes.

8. *Psychological conditions* such as depression, anorexia, and other mental problems may result in reduced caloric and nutrient intake. This may lead to poor weight gain, low birth weight infants, and perinatal mortality.

GENERAL FACTORS IN PLANNING THE DIET

Calorie Intake and Weight Gain

Calories provide the energy requirements for the body and are needed to maintain bodily processes, thermal balance, and physical activity. Caloric allowances are established to provide for adequate energy requirements and to support growth and body weight levels for the fetus and mother which are commensurate with health and well-being.

In the past, it was generally recommended that weight gain be limited by caloric restriction with the purpose of preventing and controlling toxemia and eclampsia. This idea goes back to some observations that were made after World War I. It was noted that pregnant women in Germany and Austria-Hungary gained less because of protein and fat scarcity and seemed to have a lower incidence of toxemia. Subsequent studies were not done and from these unsystematic observations came the notion that caloric restriction to limit weight gain protected women from toxemia and other pregnancy complications. We now have evidence to indicate that the incidence of toxemia is significantly higher in women who are markedly underweight as compared to those who are extremely overweight. Moreover, it has been found that even an excessive weight gain of from 9 to 10 pounds at the end of pregnancy for very *underweight* women is still compatible with *minimum* risk for developing toxemia symptoms![3]

In pregnancy there is an increased need for calories to provide energy requirements necessary for building the fetal and placental tissue and for maintaining the woman's tissue requirements. An additional 300 calories above the woman's usual caloric intake are recommended during pregnancy. It is to be stressed, however, that these caloric requirements are to consist of quality foods, not "empty" or "junk food" calories.

We now have evidence that a strong positive association exists between the weight gain of the mother and the birth weight of the infant. A low birth weight is associated with increased incidence of neonatal death. Furthermore, prenatal malnutrition increases the incidence of neurological damage and mental retardation in the infant, since the fetal period is the initial phase of brain cell development. An analysis of approximately 1.5 million California births indicated that even among middle class whites, average fetal growth was less than optimum for gestational age.[4]

Among *healthy* women who have a *well-balanced* diet and eat "to appetite," the range in weight gains can be very wide. The Committee on Maternal Nutrition suggests that a range of from 24 to 27 pounds (11 to 12 kg.) is a reasonable target and is most consistent with favorable outcomes in pregnancy.

Generally, the distribution of added weight is as follows:

fetus	7½ pounds (3⅓ kg.)
placenta	1½ pounds (⅔ kg.)
uterus	2 pounds (1 kg.)
increased blood and fluids	8½ pounds (4 kg.)
body changes for breast feeding	4½ pounds (2 kg.)

However, as Cross and Walsh[5] point out, weight gain above the recommended range, if *proceeding at a regular rate,* should not be criticized *without consideration of cause.* Because of limited incomes, many women have to purchase a major portion of their protein and other nutrients in combination with large quantities of fats and carbohydrates. In these days of soaring and fluctuating prices, to restrict a woman's caloric intake would also restrict her intake of protein and other needed nutrients.

In addition, the Committee on Maternal Nutrition recommends that weight reduction programs should not be imposed during pregnancy as distortions in normal pregnancy weight gains are apt to occur. The focus should be on the birth weight of healthy infants and not on the maintenance of the woman's figure in accordance with the social norm.

The recommended weight gain of 2 to 4 pounds (1 to 2 kg.) during the first trimester and 0.9 pound (0.5 kg.) per week during the remainder of the pregnancy is commensurate with good health for both the woman and fetus *even if the woman is overweight at the beginning of pregnancy.* (See Fig. 19-1.)

"Every Calorie Should Count"

A more positive approach to the problem of caloric intake would be to advise the woman that "every calorie should count"; that is, calories eaten during pregnancy should provide an abundance of other nutrients as well. Table 19-2 lists the nutrient need of pregnancy for the various childbearing age groups recommended by the Food and Nutrition Board of the National Academy of Sciences, National Research Council, 1974.[6]

TABLE 19-2

RECOMMENDED DAILY DIETARY ALLOWANCES FOR PREGNANCY

	Age			
	11–14	*15–18*	*19–22*	*23–50*
Body size				
Weight kg	44	54	58	58
lb	97	119	128	128
Height cm	155	162	162	162
in	62	65	65	65
Nutrients				
Energy, kcal	2700	2400	2400	2300
Protein, gm	74	78	76	76
Vitamin A, RE[1]	1000	1000	1000	1000
IU[1]	5000	5000	5000	5000
Vitamin D, IU	400	400	400	400
Vitamin E, activity, IU	15	15	15	15
Ascorbic acid, mg	60	60	60	60
Folacin, μg	800	800	800	800
Niacin, mg[2]	18	16	16	15
Riboflavin, mg	1.6	1.7	1.7	1.5
Thiamin, mg	1.5	1.4	1.4	1.3
Vitamin B$_6$, mg	2.5	2.5	2.5	2.5
Vitamin B$_{12}$, μg	4.0	4.0	4.0	4.0
Calcium, mg	1200	1200	1200	1200
Phosphorus, mg	1200	1200	1200	1200
Iodine, μg	125	125	125	125
Iron, mg[3]	18+	18+	18+	18+
Magnesium, mg	450	450	450	450
Zinc, mg	20	20	20	20

1. RE = Retinal Equivalent; IU = International Unit. The recommended unit of measure is RE. 1 RE = 10 IU.
2. It is recognized that on the average 1 mg of niacin is derived from each 60 mg of dietary tryptophan.
3. This increased requirement for pregnancy cannot be met by ordinary diets; therefore, the use of supplemental iron is recommended.

Taken from: *Nutrition During Pregnancy and Lactation.* Maternal and Child Health Unit, California Department of Health, California, 1975, p. 28.

There are some specific suggestions that the nurse can make to help the woman attain the goal of making "every calorie count." In so doing, a high-quality diet can be maintained and an adequate weight gain can be achieved without excessive poundage due to "empty calories."

1. *The patient can be acquainted with the amazing fattening potentials of certain common nonessential foods—* most of which many people regard as mere snacks without perceptible effects on total caloric intake. Actually, taking these little extras between meals or at bedtime is one of the most common causes of excessive weight gain during pregnancy as well as at other times.

An 8 ounce glass of ginger ale or cola drink averages 100 calories. A chocolate bar approximates more than 300 calories. An 8 ounce cocktail or highball has 166 calories. A doughnut without icing plus a cup of cocoa yields 400 calories, and the average malted milk contains some 500 calories. Pie à la mode approximates 600 calories.

When it is recalled that 2,200 to 2,600 calories per day generally is recognized as a satisfactory allowance during pregnancy, it is plain that these "little snacks" loom tremendously large in relation to the total caloric allotment. Therefore, for between meal hunger, the mother may be advised to take the glass of milk scheduled for dinner, omitting it from her evening meal. Raw vegetables and fruit also are helpful in assuaging hunger pangs.

2. *The patient should be reminded that the way in which a food is prepared may affect its caloric value almost as much as the nature of the food itself.* Perhaps the simplest way to show how the preparation of a food affects its caloric value is to consider fried foods. Although a poached or boiled egg is about 80 calories and is so calculated in dietary lists, once that egg is fried, its caloric value jumps to around 120 calories because of the fat absorbed by the egg in cooking. A level tablespoon of fat, let it be emphasized, yields approximately 120 calories. With regard to soups and desserts, it is common knowledge that those made with milk are of much lower caloric content than those made with cream, and that those made with skim milk are still lower. When flour or cheese in addition to cream is used, as in escalloped or au gratin dishes, the calories soar to unbelievable heights; in general, for this group of foods, the smoother and the more delicious the taste, the higher the caloric value.

3. *The intrinsic caloric value of foods of the same type varies widely.* Fruits show considerable variation according to their degree of sweetness. For instance, canned fruit can be very high in calories because of the sugar in the syrup. Therefore, the woman can be reminded to use fresh fruits regularly, and, if for some important reason canned fruit must be served, the unsweetened varieties or those packed in light syrup are the only ones that should be taken. It might be added that these varieties are more economical than those packed in the rich heavy syrups.

Likewise, meats vary greatly in their caloric contents, lean meats being low and those with much fat in their substance being high. For example, one ounce of chicken or turkey (without skin) is 55 calories, while one ounce of any cheese, beef, pork, egg or cold cuts is equal to 100 calories, 45 of those calories coming from the additional fat. One frankfurter or two tablespoons of peanut butter is equivalent to 145 calories, 90 of those calories coming from the additional fat.

Balancing Food Needs and Appetite

In the later months of pregnancy, there may be an increase in the desire for all food or certain types of food. The woman may need help to discipline her appetite in accord with the amount of food needed. Thoughtful and cooperative meal planning with the patient, with specific and thorough direction as to quantity and quality of nutrients, does much to help the woman to maintain motivation and discipline during these times.

Also, it is well to counsel the woman early in her pregnancy to avoid sweets and high caloric desserts, as well as the habit of frequent nibbling, since these interfere with appetite for the more essential foods. Early pregnancy is a good time to institute health teaching of this sort, since many women are motivated to attain good health for themselves and their unborn child at this time. Appetite tends to be diminished, and therefore appropriate choosing of the quantity of food may be easier; later, when the "newness" of the pregnancy has worn off, and the appetite is unleashed, self-discipline is much harder, especially without previous reinforcement.

Occasional "cravings" for unusual types of food may occur. These sometimes indicate the lack of a certain element in the diet that the body demands. Any desires of this nature may be granted with safety, if they agree with the patient and are not exceptional in amount or content. If the diet supplies all the needs of the patient and the growing fetus, such cravings may not occur.

Salt Intake

There is one other consideration in planning the diet for the pregnant woman. That is the *deemphasis* in sodium restriction during pregnancy. Like the former calorie restriction, restriction of salt was thought to be an important factor in the prevention of toxemia. Clinical and laboratory data now indicate that sodium requirement is increased during pregnancy.[7] Restriction, therefore, can be harmful when imposed indiscriminately. Flowers[8] has noted that there is a mechanism present in pregnancy that increases sodium reabsorption and retention when there is a reduction in sodium intake during pregnancy. An adequate renal and placental blood flow demands an adequate circulating blood volume. When there is a stringent reduction in sodium intake, there is a reduction in circulating blood volume which is intolerable during pregnancy and causes damage to both the mother and fetus. Thus, the routine restriction of salt for the healthy woman is being questioned, as well as the indiscriminate use of diuretics for reduction of edema that was previously thought to be associated with sodium retention caused by excessive salt in the diet. Many physicians now advise their patients early in the pregnancy to simply "salt their food to taste" and not to cut down inordinately on their sodium intake. Patients should be advised to use iodized salt.

Food Preferences

During these planning sessions, it is important to remember that the woman is a member of a family, and although she plans the meals, many of her choices are dictated by the likes and dislikes of her family. The young teenage bride who has just learned to fry cheeseburgers and french fries for her spouse may not be persuaded easily to broil and bake instead; furthermore, she deserves recognition for accomplishing something as important as preparing a meal that is pleasing to her husband.

The religious, racial, and ethnic background of the patient and her family is another important consideration in nutritional counseling and other aspects of care. Many families are fond of their regional or national diet and prefer it to the American "meat and potatoes" regimen. Whenever possible, the preferred diet should be considered and planned through the use of "exchanges" for food groups (see Suggested Reading). Many nutrition books give a "basic national" diet for the various countries, which provide a springboard for planning. Table 19-3 gives sample menus that illustrate the common variations in diet found in this country.

A good deal of guidance is often needed to avoid food faddism and to meet nutritional needs. Those who choose alternate life styles for various philosophical, religious, or health reasons often follow vegetarian diets also, either pure or lacto-ovo. It is possible to meet the protein and mineral requirements of pregnancy on many of these various diets, but to do so requires considerable knowledge of the protein content of foods and continual attention to including these foods in the diet. However, some of the patients who subscribe to these diets do not have the requisite knowledge and resources to procure the appropriate amount of protein. Moreover, they may be swayed more by philosophical and religious considerations than by those which are nutritional.

Any health professional who tries to counsel those who belong to a strict vegetarian group must try to understand each group on its own terms and must appreciate the influences that govern food selection if he or she hopes to effect a stable and effective nutritional status (see Suggested Reading). Reinforcement of the positive aspects of the dietary practices helps to modify the more negative aspects of the vegetarian's belief system. In making attempts at education, there must be tolerance and a nonjudgmental attitude and respect for the client's rejections of dietary information if she chooses. These attitudes may be difficult to achieve as providers of care traditionally expect their advice to be followed. However, more may be gained in the long run by accepting the "client's right to choose" since she will be more likely to seek care from those whom she feels respect her views even if they differ considerably from the provider's views.

PSYCHOLOGICAL ASPECTS OF NUTRITION

Other aspects to be considered are the stage of growth and development of the patient and the psychologic factors involved in nutrition (e.g., the meaning that food has for the woman). We are aware, for instance, that foods enjoyed by adolescents are different from the foods enjoyed by older people; the "typical" hamburger-soda-french fry teenage diet has received wide publicity. It seems to meet some need in much the same way as peanut butter sandwiches do for the preschooler.

When people marry younger and become parents at an earlier age, they carry their eating patterns into marriage with them. In addition, adolescence is a time for developing independence, and this is healthy. However, many foods are rejected (milk, vegetables, cereal, and the like), because they are associated with "home" and a dependency period. The desire to be free and to select the "forbidden" foods is very strong.

TABLE 19-3
SAMPLE MENUS

	Regular	Mexican	Black	Oriental	American Indian	Lacto-Ovo
Breakfast						
2 Energy Foods	1 Cup Cream of Wheat	2 Corn Tortillas	1 Cup Grits	1 Cup Rice	1 Cup Corn Mush	1 Cup Brown Rice
	1 Tbsp. Sugar	2 Tbsp. Jelly	1 Tbsp. Sugar	1 Tsp. Sugar (in Tea)	1 Tbps. Sugar	1 Tbps. Honey
1 Calcium/ Protein Food	1 Cup Milk	½ Cup Evaporated Milk in Coffee	1 Cup Milk	1 Cup Milk	1 Cup Milk	1 Cup Milk
1 Vitamin C Food	1 Cup Orange Juice	1 Cup Orange Juice	1 Cup Orange Juice	1 Cup Orange Juice	1 Cup Orange Juice	1 Cup Orange Juice
Lunch						
1 Energy Food	1 Slice Bread	1 Tortilla	1 2″ Square Corn Bread	½ Cup Rice	1 Slice Indian Fried Bread	1 Slice Whole Wheat Bread
2 Protein Foods	2-1 oz. Slice Cheese	1 Cup Beans	1 Cup Pork and Beans	3½ oz. Tofu 1 Egg	1 Cup Pinto Beans	1 Cup Lentils
1 Calcium/ Protein Food	1 Cup Milk	½ Cup Evaporated Milk and Chocolate	1 Cup Milk	1 Cup Milk	1 Cup Milk	1 Cup Milk
1 Vitamin A Food	½ Cup Spinach	½ Cup Spinach 1 Green Pepper	½ Cup Collard Greens	⅗ Bok Choy	½ Cup Spinach	½ Cup Spinach
1 Vitamin/ Mineral Food	1 Banana	1 Banana	1 Banana	1 Banana	1 Apple	1 Banana
Dinner						
1 Energy Food	1 Small Baked Potato	½ Cup Spanish Rice	2 Halves Candied Yams	½ Cup Rice	½ Cup Fried Potatoes	1 Small Baked Potato
3 Protein Foods	3 oz. Beef Roast	1 Cup Beans 1 Cup Caldo	3½ oz. Fried Pork Chops	Okazu (Stewing Beef 3 oz. ½ Cup Broccoli) and 2 oz. Tofu)	3½ oz. Fish	3½ oz. Cheese (Cheddar)
1 Calcium/ Protein Food	1 Cup Milk	½ Cup Evaporated Milk and Coffee	1 Cup Milk	1 Cup Milk	1 Cup Milk 1 Stalk Brocolli	1 Cup Milk 1 Stalk Broccoli
2 Vitamin/ Mineral Foods	1 Stalk Broccoli 1 Cup Fruited Jello	1 Cup Fruited Jello	1 Cup Peas 1 Cup Fruited Jello	1 Cup Fruited Jello	1 Cup Fruited Jello	½ Cup Fruited Jello
Snacks						
1 Calcium/ Protein Food	1 Cup Custard	1 Cup Flan	1 Cup Custard	1 Cup Custard	1 Cup Custard	1 Cup Custard
1 Vitamin/ Mineral Food	1 Pear	1 Pear	1 Pear	1 Pear	1 Pear	1 Pear
1 Energy Food	2 Oatmeal-Raisin Cookies	2 Oatmeal-Raisin Cookies	2 Oatmeal-Raisin Cookies	2 Oatmeal-Raisin Cookies	2 Oatmeal-Raisin Cookies	2 Oatmeal-Raisin Cookies

The menus above show the cultural variations possible when planning a nutritionally adequate prenatal diet. All meet the Recommended Dietary Allowances for calories, provide a minimum of 90 gm. of protein, and exceed the Recommended Dietary Allowances for vitamins A and C and calcium. Only the black and Mexican dietary pattern meets the Recommended Dietary Allowances for iron, providing 21.9 mg. and 23.1 mg. The regular, American-Indian, and the Oriental pattern provide 15.3 mg., 15.8 mg., and 15.3 respectively. The lacto-ovo plan provides only 12.0 mg.
Source: Cross, A. T., and Walsh, H. E.: "Prenatal diet counseling." *J. Reproductive Med.* 7:274, Dec. 1971.

Permitting assertion of independence is important if the overall developmental task is to be accomplished and if there is to be a healthy adjustment in roles from that of the child to that of the adult. Yet limits often must be set if the health of the woman and the baby are to be safeguarded. Therefore, incorporating the woman into the planning and allowing her choices whenever possible, helping her to increase her knowledge of nutrients, encouraging and reinforcing correct choices or willing adaptations, and giving firm guidance when indicated all help the patient and the nurse to achieve their respective goals.

The psychologic aspects of nutrition lend themselves less well to clear-cut analysis. It has been said that people can survive a state of celibacy, however uncomfortably, but no one has been able to survive without food. Food is a basic need, according to the survival criteria, more basic even than the need for sex. We know that hunger is the most fundamental of all sensations. Related to hunger, but of a very different origin, is appetite. Appetite is Nature's primary defense for the prevention of hunger. Based on the anticipation of eating, the impulse is determined by the person's previous experience. Only by coincidence and training does appetite become associated with health-giving foods. Factors affecting food-seeking behavior are the main determinants of eating (i.e., hunger, appetite, and custom). The great deterrents to normal appetite are worry, fear, and preoccupation with troublesome or difficult problems—and these may be reflected in either an increase or a decrease of appetite. Some of the positive emotional stimulants include a situation of calm contentedness, a feeling of mild elation, or a condition of ego-stimulation.

Present-day cuisine is a potpourri of heritage, superstition, custom, knowledge, and opportunity. Subtle cravings are passed along from one generation to the next by the process of training and imitation. Unique methods of food preparation as well as food selection, combinations, and prejudices are embodied in this training. Congeniality and hospitality among normal people are enhanced by the serving of good food; and it has become the custom to serve food at practically all functions, business as well as social.

From infancy onward, food and closeness are associated with love and security. Food and eating, in and of themselves, are looked upon as symbolizing interpersonal acceptance, warmth, and sociability. Throughout all societies this symbolic undertone is unmistakable; from the "breaking of bread" in antiquity to the modern banquet the serving of food is a vehicle for expressing honor, joy or mutual bonds. It is easy to see why food has become associated with the symbolism of motherliness. Feeding is not only kindly and warm in its emotional meaning to those who receive food, but it is also essential to growth and well-being; hence it has become bound up with the idea of the mother, the one who originally nurtured, loved, and supported.

The pregnant woman makes a close identification with the concept of the mother, and selections and choices may be influenced profoundly by these symbolic meanings of food. She may respond to worry, frustration, or anxiety by overeating—either by nibbling or gorging. Conversely, another patient may develop anorexia. Or she may crave certain foods and reject others, and not because of physiologic factors. For instance, she may feel that certain foods will "mark" her baby or will give him strength. It is crucial that the meaning which food has for the patient be explored and that her feelings and attitudes be respected. Care must be taken not to make her feel deprecated or deprived while she is helped to understand the dynamics involved in hunger and appetite.

In summary, if counseling is to be effective and the results lasting, the nurse should strive to elicit wholehearted cooperation from the patient through involving her in the planning; considering her and her family's needs, background, preferences, and attitude; encouraging and reinforcing appropriate choices and preparation; and providing gentle but firm limit setting, when indicated, and careful, thorough explanation regarding the rationale behind the advice.

DAILY FOOD GUIDE

The following discussion and tables will provide guidelines in helping women plan their diet. Foods have been grouped according to six food types: protein foods, milk and milk products, breads and cereals, vitamin C rich fruits and vegetables, dark green vegetables, and other fruits and vegetables. This type of classification is a useful one to employ since most individuals have an understanding of the milk group, breads and cereals, and so on. Table 19-4 presents a Daily Food Guide for the nonpregnant, pregnant, and lactating woman. Table 19-5 lists examples of foods and the amounts to be used in planning meals.

Protein Foods

Four or more servings of beef, pork, lamb, veal, organ meats, fish, poultry, eggs, or cheese are recommended daily. Legumes (dried beans, peas) or nuts may be used as alternates. In addition, these foods contain vitamins and valuable minerals, but their main value is in their amino acids or "building stones," as they sometimes are called.

These are the elements that are needed not only by the mother, but also by the fetus for the development of all the delicate and intricate systems of his body. Meat, eggs, and fish contain complete proteins, with all the ten amino acids that are necessary to maintain life and support growth.

Often the family's budget restricts the quantity and the variety of these proteins, especially with respect to meat. The substitution of cheese, peanut butter, poultry, fish, or legumes then may be suggested. The mother may also need advice regarding the preparation and the utilization of the organ meats that are so rich in protein, vitamins, and minerals. Because some of these are relatively inexpensive, many women do not realize their nutritional worth and further avoid them because of the aesthetics that may be involved in the preparation—skinning, soaking, and so on. Taste also is sometimes a factor.

Nevertheless, with a little ingenuity and suggestions from a good nutrition or cookbook, the nurse can do much to help the family to utilize this valuable and inexpensive source of protein. Liver, for instance, can be lightly broiled, ground, and incorporated into a meatloaf or ground meat patties. The taste and looks are disguised, the nutritional value is retained, and the meat goes further.

Milk and Milk Products

The expectant mother needs a quart of milk or its equivalent daily. Milk is nature's most nearly perfect food and is invaluable as a nutrient. It contains all the different kinds of mineral elements that are

TABLE 19-4
DAILY FOOD GUIDE*

Food Group	Daily Servings		
	Non-pregnant	Pregnant	Breast Feeding
Protein Foods	4	4	4
Milk and Milk Products	2	4	5
Breads and Cereals	4	4	4
Vitamin C-rich Fruits and Vegetables	1	1	1
Dark Green Vegetables	1	1	1
Other Fruits and Vegetables	1	1	1

* Additions:
(a) 2 tablespoons (30 ml.) fats and oils each day; (vegetable oil, margarine, mayonnaise, salad dressing). Fats and oils provide essential nutrients such as fatty acids and vitamin E.
(b) Plenty of liquids: at least 6 8-ounce (240 ml.) glasses each day during pregnancy; plus 8 8-ounce glasses a day during breast feeding (water; milk, cocoa, fruit juice, soups, coffee, tea).
(From: *Eating Right for Your Baby*. Sacramento, Calif., California Department of Health Services, 1978, pp. 90–91.)

needed for fetal development. The high content of calcium and phosphorus in milk makes it almost indispensable for good growth of bone and teeth; it provides these minerals in the correct proportions and in a digestible form which permits optimum utilization by both mother and fetus. It is not only an excellent source of protein or tissue-building material, but also the most readily digested and easily absorbed of all food proteins. Milk is also rich in energy-providing values, so that one quart a day alone furnishes almost one-fourth of the total energy requirements. Finally, milk contains some of the most important vitamins, particularly vitamin A, which increases resistance to infection and safeguards the development of the fetus.

Unfortunately, many persons are not able to tolerate milk well or decidedly do not like it. If the woman is able to tolerate it, and if she can overcome her aversions, an effort should be made to have her drink two glasses a day. If ⅓ cup instant dry milk is added to each of two glasses of liquid milk, the daily calcium requirement can be met, or the remainder may be taken in some other form, such as soups, custards, and so on. Evaporated milk and instant dried milk are acceptable and may be substituted if fresh cow's milk is not available or desired.

Other dairy products, such as cottage cheese, ricotta cheese, farmer's cheese, hoop cheese, yogurt, and the hard cheeses are also adequate substitutes. Hard cheeses, such as cheddar, jack, swiss, and the like, are higher in calories than the soft cheeses—

TABLE 19-5
RECOMMENDED FOOD INTAKE

Protein Foods

Protein builds muscle and tissue for both you and your baby. Besides protein, PROTEIN FOODS provide B vitamins and iron. B vitamins help you obtain energy from food. Iron is need to form red blood cells.

Protein comes from both animal and vegetable sources. Each day eat a total of *4 servings*. Try to include 2 servings from animal protein foods and 2 servings from vegetable protein foods.

Animal Protein—A serving is 2 oz. (60 g) unless otherwise noted:

Beef (ground, cube, roast, or chop)	
Clams	4 large or 9 small
Eggs	2 medium
Fish (fillet or steak)	
Fish sticks	3 sticks
Frankfurters	2
Lamb (ground, cube, roast, or chop)	
Luncheon meat	3 slices
Organ meats: heart, kidney, liver, tongue	
Oysters	8–12 medium
Pork, ham (ground, roast, or chop)	
Poultry: chicken, duck, turkey	
Rabbit	
Sausage links	4 links
Shellfish: crab, lobster, scallops, shrimp	
Spareribs	6 medium ribs
Tuna fish	
Veal (ground, cube, roast, or chop)	

Vegetable Protein—Beans are the best choice from vegetable protein foods. A serving of beans contains more vitamins and minerals than a serving of nuts or seeds. A serving is any of the following:

Canned beans (garbanzo, kidney, lima, pork and beans)	1 cup (240 ml)
Dried beans and peas	1 cup (240 ml)
Nut butters (cashew butter, peanut butter, etc.)	¼ cup (60 ml)
Nuts	½ cup (120 ml)
Sunflower seeds	½ cup (120 ml)
Tofu (soybean curd)	1 cup (240 ml)

You can get the protein you need by eating only vegetable protein foods. However, these foods should be combined with eggs and milk. Ask your doctor or dietitian/nutritionist for further information.

Milk and Milk Products

Milk and Milk Products are the best food sources of calcium. Calcium builds strong bones and teeth in your baby. It also keeps your nerves and muscles healthy.

Milk and milk products also contain protein, several B vitamins, and vitamins A and D. Vitamin D helps your body use calcium. Vitamin A is needed for growth and vision. It also protects you from infection.

Choose *4 servings* of Milk and Milk Products each day if you are *pregnant*. Choose *5 servings* if you are *breast feeding*. A serving is 1 cup (8 oz. or 240 ml) unless otherwise noted:

Cheese (except camembert, cream)	1 slice (1 ½ oz. or 45 g)
Cheese spread	4 tablespoons (60 ml)
Cocoa made with milk	1¼ cups (10 oz. or 300 ml)
Cottage cheese	1⅓ cups (320 ml)
Custard (flan)	
Ice cream	1 ½ cups (360 ml)
Ice milk	
Milk	
buttermilk	
chocolate (not drink)	1¼ cups (10 oz. or 300 ml)
evaporated	½ cup (4 oz. or 120 ml)
goat	
low fat	
not fat	
non fat (made from dry milk powder)	
non fat dry milk powder	⅓ cup (80 ml)
whole	
Milkshake	
Pudding	
Soups made with milk	1 ½ cups (12 oz. or 360 ml)
Yogurt (plain)	

Not all milk and milk products contain vitamins A and D. Check the label!

Breads and Cereals

Breads and Cereals have several nutrients important for you and your baby including B vitamins and iron. These foods may be either whole grain or enriched. It's best to eat whole grains—they contain more vitamins and minerals. Whole grains also provide fiber which helps prevent constipation.

TABLE 19-5
RECOMMENDED FOOD INTAKE (*Continued*)

Choose *4 servings* of Breads and Cereals each day. A serving is any of the following:

Whole Grain Items

Bread: cracked, whole wheat, or rye	1 slice
Cereal, hot: oatmeal (rolled oats), rolled wheat, cracked wheat, wheat and malted barley	½ cup cooked (120 ml)
Cereal, ready-to-eat: puffed oats, shredded wheat, wheat flakes, granola	¾ cup (180 ml)
Rice (brown)	½ cup cooked (120 ml)
Wheat germ	1 tablespoon (15 ml)

In some communities you can also buy whole wheat macaroni, noodles, spaghetti.

Enriched Items

Bagel	1 small
Bread (all except those listed above)	1 slice
Cereal, hot: cream of wheat, cream of rice, farina, cornmeal, grits	½ cup cooked (120 ml)
Cereal, ready-to-eat (all except those listed above)	¾ cup (180 ml)
Crackers	4
Macaroni, noodles, spaghetti	½ cup cooked (120 ml)
Pancake, waffle	1 medium (5 inch or 13 cm diameter)
Rice (white)	½ cup cooked
Roll, biscuit, muffin, dumpling	1
Tortilla	1 (6 inch or 15 cm diameter)

Doughnuts, cakes, pies, and cookies are not included in the Breads and Cereals group. These foods contain mostly calories and very few nutrients.

Vitamin C Rich Fruits and Vegetables

Vitamin C Rich Fruits and Vegetables contain ascorbic acid (vitamin C). This vitamin is needed to hold body cells together and to strengthen blood vessel walls. Ascorbic acid also aids in healing wounds.

Choose *1 serving* of Vitamin C Rich Fruits and Vegetables each day. A serving is ¾ cup (180 ml) unless otherwise noted:

Vegetables

Bok choy	
Broccoli	1 stalk
Brussels sprouts	3–4
Cabbage	
Cauliflower	
Chili peppers (green or red)	¼ cup
Greens: collard, kale, mustard, turnip	
Peppers (green or red)	½ medium
Tomatoes	2 medium
Watercress	

Fruits

Cantaloupe	½ medium
Grapefruit	½ large
Guava	½ small
Mango	1 medium
Orange	1 medium
Papaya	½ small
Strawberries	
Tangerine	2 large

Juices

Fruit juices and drinks with vitamin C added

Grapefruit	½ cup (4 oz. or 120 ml)
Orange	½ cup (4 oz. or 120 ml)
Pineapple	1½ cups (12 oz. or 360 ml)
Tomato	1½ cups (12 oz. or 360 ml)

Dark Green Vegetables

Dark Green Vegetables are an excellent source of vitamin A and folacin. Your baby needs vitamin A for bone growth and tooth formation. Vitamin A is also important for vision and resisting infections.

Folacin, a B vitamin, is needed to form red blood cells and other body cells. Cooking temperatures destroy folacin, so eat dark green vegetables raw whenever possible.

Choose *1 serving* of Dark Green Vegetables each day. A serving is 1 cup (240 ml) raw or ¾ cup (180 ml) cooked:

Asparagus
Bok choy
Broccoli
Brussels sprouts
Cabbage
Chicory
Endive
Escarole
Greens: beet, collard, kale, mustard, turnip
Lettuce (dark leafy: red leaf, romaine)
Scallions
Spinach
Swiss chard
Watercress

TABLE 19-5
RECOMMENDED FOOD INTAKE (*Continued*)

Other Fruits and Vegetables

Other Fruits and Vegetables add vitamins and minerals to your diet. Those dark yellow in color contain vitamin A. Fruits and vegetables also provide fiber which is important for normal bowel movements.

Choose *1 serving* of Other Fruits and Vegetables each day. A serving is ½ cup (120 ml) unless otherwise noted:

Vegetables

Artichoke	1 medium
Bamboo shoots	
Beans (green, wax)	
Bean sprouts	
Beet	
Burdock root	
Carrot	
Cauliflower	
Celery	
Corn	
Cucumber	
Eggplant	
Hominy	
Lettuce (head, boston, bibb)	
Mushrooms	
Nori seaweed	
Onion	
Parsnip	
Peas	
Pea pods	
Potato	1 medium

Radishes	
Summer squash	
Sweet potato	1 medium
Winter Squash	
Yam	1 medium
Zucchini	

Fruits

Apple	1 medium
Apricot	2 medium
Banana	1 small
Berries	
Cherries	
Dates	5
Figs	2 large
Fruit cocktail	
Grapes	
Kumquats	3
Nectarine	2 medium
Peach	1 medium
Pear	1 medium
Persimmon	1 small
Pineapple	
Plums	2 medium
Prunes	4 medium
Pumpkin	¼ cup (60 ml)
Raisins	
Watermelon	

Dark yellow fruits and vegetables are an excellent source of vitamin A: carrots, sweet potatoes, yams, winter squash, apricots, persimmons.

From: *Eating Right for Your Baby.* Sacramento, Calif., California Department of Health Services, 1978, pp. 90–91.

cottage, ricotta, hoop; two exceptions are mozzarella and the Armenian string cheeses. Both of these are often made from skim milk.

One ounce of cheese contains approximately the same amount of minerals and vitamins as a large glass of whole milk. However, the total protein and fat content will vary and must be considered when making substitutions.

For some individuals, milk may cause distressing gastrointestinal symptoms, such as nausea and diarrhea. These symptoms indicate a milk allergy and intolerance and the product should not be encouraged. Substitutes can be found in other protein sources. For other patients, milk may be constipating, and, if amenable to treatment, an effort should be made to treat the constipation other than by omitting the milk. If the milk is merely distasteful without causing physical symptoms, it may be disguised in other foods as mentioned previously.

The instant nonfat and whole dry milks may be used in a quantity that provides an adequate intake.

Approximately five tablespoons of dried skim milk will equal one pint of fluid milk. The milk may be used dry and worked into meatloaf, mashed potatoes, cereals, sandwich spreads, baked articles, and so on. Reconstituted with less than the usual amount of water, it has a richer taste than the regular liquid skim milk. Certain condiments and flavorings (vanilla, nutmeg, instant coffee, cinnamon), when mixed with the milk, will enhance the flavor.

Some patients complain that milk is "fattening." In most instances the weight gain is due to the consumption of more food than is needed or an excess of such foods as bread, potatoes, and desserts. These should be the articles that are restricted, and not the milk. Occasionally, however, it will be necessary to substitute skim milk or churned buttermilk for whole milk. This is acceptable and will reduce calories. Most dairies nowadays reinforce skim milk with vitamins A and D, which otherwise would be deficient. Many companies now have another variety of skim milk, one that is fortified by the addition of nonfat milk solids, 400 USP units of vitamin D and 4,000 USP units of vitamin A per quart. It has a standardized 2 percent butterfat, so that the butterfat content in general is 1½ percent less than that of whole milk. To determine ingredients, the woman should be reminded to read the ingredients listed on the product label.

If the woman can be helped to realize the importance of this one article of food in relation to the development of her baby, the sacrifices or modifications that may be involved may be made more willingly.

Bread and Cereal

Four or more servings should be included from this group. Women should be counseled to eliminate white bread and cereals and to substitute the darker and whole wheat varieties. The darker varieties contain trace elements not found in white bread. When cereals are supplemented by milk, they become adequate for growth, as well as for maintaining life. Bread that is buttered increases the vitamin A intake. The coarse cereals and the dark breads add roughage to the diet. Vitamin B and roughage both help to counteract constipation.

Vegetables and Fruits

Three or more servings should be included from this group, especially the leaf, stem, green, and yellow varieties of vegetables, as well as the citrus fruits and tomatoes. It is desirable to serve at least one portion of each vegetable and fruit raw.

Vegetables, particularly, are rich sources of iron, calcium and several vitamins. At mealtimes there is no reasonable limit to the amount of lettuce, tomatoes, celery, string beans, carrots, beets, and asparagus which may be eaten. By increasing the quantity of such foods to several times the amount ordinarily taken, it is usually possible to satisfy the appetite without gaining abnormally in weight.

Fresh or frozen vegetables are a good alternate. Canned vegetables may be used if fresh are not available. Careful preparation and cooking of vegetables will help to retain the maximum vitamin and mineral content. Steaming or stir-frying is preferable to retain vitamins and minerals. Steamer baskets to fit standard size pans are widely available. Some vegetables contain several incomplete proteins which add to the total protein intake.

In addition to their value as nutrient agents, these vegetables deserve an important place in the diet as laxative agents, since their fibrous framework increases the bulk of the intestinal content and thereby stimulates the muscular, eliminative action of the intestines.

Fruits. Citrus fruits—oranges, lemons, and grapefruit—are the best sources of vitamin C. Most of these fruits also supply vitamins A and B. Tomatoes are also an excellent source of vitamin C, the amount, however, must be twice that of the citrus fruits to supply the same amount of vitamin. Other fruits, raw and cooked, such as prunes, raisins, apricots, contain important minerals (iron and copper) as well as vitamins. Fruits may stimulate a lagging appetite and counteract constipation. They may be used in many ways: as juices, combined in salads, additions to cereals, or plain yogurt, in-between meal refreshments and in desserts, such as gelatins and puddings. Fruits contain some incomplete proteins but only supplement the other proteins.

Fluids, Vitamins and Minerals

In addition to the basic food groups, special attention should be given to the following:

Fluids. Fluids should be taken freely, averaging six to eight glasses daily. Water aids in the circulation of the blood, body fluids, and the distribution of mineral salts, as well as in stimulating the digestion and the assimilation of foods. Fluids help to increase perspiration and to regulate elimination from intestines and kidneys. Tea and coffee may be included in the daily fluid quota in very moderate amounts if not found to be diarrhetic or sleep disturbing.

The intake of alcoholic beverages is to be discouraged during pregnancy. Not only is alcohol high in "empty calories," but recent studies have shown that alcohol can have a deleterious effect on the fetus. Since there is no definitive evidence as to the safe or unsafe limits of alcohol ingestion, it is best to advise the pregnant woman to abstain from alcohol during pregnancy.

Vitamins. Vitamins are the *live* elements in food and are essential to life. The best sources are the natural foods. To retain the vitamin value in foods, they must be fresh, carefully prepared, and not overcooked. During pregnancy and lactation the vitamin needs are increased, and so it is apparent that a well-balanced diet containing all the vitamins is of first importance. Some physicians add vitamin preparations to the diet to be sure that an adequate requirement has been met.

Vitamin A is essential in the diet for the maintenance of body resistance to infection. Foods which are good sources of this vitamin include whole milk, fortified skim milk, dairy products containing butterfat, eggs, green leafy and yellow vegetables, and liver.

The vitamin B complex is essential to good nutrition. During pregnancy, thiamine (B_1) is necessary in increased amounts, as the fetus readily depletes the mother's reserve. Milk, eggs, lean meat, and whole grain or enriched bread and cereal are good sources of thiamine. Riboflavin and nicotinic acid, absolute essentials in the diet, are found in such foods as meat, milk, eggs, and green vegetables.

Vitamin C is necessary for the proper development of the fetus. Since an adequate reserve of this water-soluble vitamin is not stored in the body, an abundant supply of this vitamin is needed daily throughout pregnancy and lactation. Fresh citrus fruits, berries, and green leafy vegetables (with the exception of lettuce) are foods which are a good source of vitamin C. These foods should be eaten raw as often as possible, since cooking destroys about half of their vitamin content.

Vitamin D is of great importance in safeguarding the mother and the fetus during pregnancy, since it bears some relationship to calcium and phosphorus metabolism. Liver, eggs, fortified sweet milk, and fish (particularly Atlantic herring and mackerel) are food sources of vitamin D. The National Research Council recommends a daily intake of 400 IU for the pregnant and lactating woman. This amount, the Council says, will protect all normal growing individuals from deficiency with an adequate margin of safety. In evaluating vitamin D intake, all fortified foods in the diet should be taken into account, since large doses of either vitamin A or D may be toxic.

Folacin. A daily supplement of 400 to 800 mg. folacin should be prescribed for all pregnant women. Dietary sources of folacin are inadequate to achieve the required amount for pregnancy. Folacin helps prevent the onset of megaloblastic anemia.

Minerals. Studies indicate that 13 or more mineral elements are essential for good nutrition. It is believed that if calcium, phosphorus, iron, and iodine are provided in adequate amounts, the others also will be present in sufficient quantities.

Calcium. Although two-thirds of the calcium in the fetus is deposited during the last month of pregnancy, the mother's daily requirement of calcium is increased during the entire course of pregnancy to prepare adequate storage for this demand. The principal foods from which calcium is obtained are cheese, eggs, oatmeal, vegetables, and milk. A quart of milk alone supplies 1.2 gm. of calcium.

Phosphorus. This element is an essential constituent of all the cells and the tissues of the body. Milk provides an abundant source of phosphorus. Actually, since phosphorus is an almost invariable constituent of protein, a diet which includes sufficient protein-rich foods, such as eggs, meat, cheese, oatmeal, and green vegetables, will provide also an adequate amount of phosphorus.

Iron. During the first two trimesters of pregnancy, iron is transferred to the fetus in moderate amounts, but during the last trimester, when the fetus builds up its reserve, the amount transferred is accelerated about ten times. Therefore, the diet should be balanced and nutritious as well as rich in iron-containing foods. But since dietary sources of iron and limited maternal stores of iron cannot supply the recommended amounts needed for pregnancy, supplementation is necessary. All pregnant women should receive 30 to 60 mg. of elemental iron daily. The elemental iron content of commonly used preparations varies and should be considered since constipation is a problem for some people and more than the 30 to 60 mg. elemental iron is not necessary. The elemental iron content is as follows: 30 percent for ferrous fumarate, 20 percent for ferrous sulfate (nonexsiccated), and 11 percent for ferrous gluconate. The patient should be advised to take her iron supplement with a citrus juice as this allows for maximum absorption.[9]

Iodine. Only very small amounts of iodine are needed for the health of the woman and the fetus.

PATIENT EDUCATION FOR DIGESTIVE PROBLEMS IN PREGNANCY

Nausea

Nausea or vomiting, sometimes called morning sickness, may occur during the early months of pregnancy. It usually disappears after the third month. If you have this problem, try the following:

- Before you get out of bed in the morning, eat a few crackers, a handful of dry cereal, or a piece of toast or dry bread. Put these within reach of your bed the night before.
- Get up slowly in the morning. Avoid sudden movements.
- Eat 5 or 6 small meals a day. Never go for long periods without food.
- Drink fluids, including soups, between rather than with meals.
- When you feel nauseated between meals, drink small amounts of apple juice, grape juice, or carbonated beverages.
- Avoid greasy and fried foods. These include butter, margarine, mayonnaise, bacon, gravies, pie crusts, pastries, fried meats, and french fries.
- Eat lightly seasoned foods. Avoid foods cooked with pepper, chili, and garlic.
- When you cook, open windows or use the exhaust fan to get rid of odors.
- Be sure to have plenty of fresh air in the room when you sleep.

Constipation

Certain changes which take place in your body during pregnancy may make you constipated. Little exercise or not enough fiber and liquids in your diet may also cause this problem.

The Daily Food Guide contains enough fluids and bulk to aid in elimination. If you are still constipated, the following may help:

- Eat more raw fruits and vegetables, including skins. Also dried fruits, stewed prunes and apricots, and prune juice.
- Use whole grain cereals and breads such as oatmeal, wheat bread, and brown rice. Try wheat germ on your cereal or have a bran muffin.
- Drink more liquids. Include water, milk, cocoa, fruit juice, and soups. A glass of warm water as soon as you get up may help.
- Eat meals at regular times.
- Exercise regularly.

If constipation continues, talk to your doctor. Do not take any over-the-counter drugs or home medications such as mineral oil.

Heartburn

Heartburn is sometimes a problem during the last months of pregnancy. As your baby grows, there is increased pressure on your stomach.

If you have heartburn, try the following:

- Eat 5 or 6 small meals a day.
- Limit fatty and fried foods.
- Avoid spicy foods.
- Wear clothes which are loose around your waist.

Over-the-counter drugs may be harmful to your baby. *Never* take a medication before talking to your doctor.

Source: *Nutrition During Pregnancy and Lactation.* Sacramento, Calif., Maternal and Child Health Unit, California Department of Health, 1975.

This mineral is obtained very readily from seafoods; cod liver oil is another good source. In certain localities around the Great Lakes and in parts of the Northwest the water supply and the vegetables grown are poor in iodine. Hence, daily use of iodized salt ensures an adequate intake and prevents deficiency.

OTHER INFORMATION ON NUTRITION

When consultation with a nutritionist is advisable and one is not available on the clinic or hospital staff, one may be found in the area through the local community health department or a home economist's office. Publications and visual aids, charts, and so on may be secured from city, county, and state health departments. The U.S. Government Printing Office is another invaluable source of publications. Certain professional organizations offer additional resources: Food and Nutrition Board, National Research Council, Council on Foods and Nutrition, American Medical Association, American Home Economics Association, American Public Health Association. The above associations are only a few of the resources that the nurse and the physician have to assist their patients in planning for adequate nutrition.

DIGESTIVE PROBLEMS AND DIET

Nausea, constipation and heartburn are problems which occur at different stages of pregnancy. All three can be greatly relieved by dietary measures as noted in the health teaching directives listed in the chart on page 258.

REFERENCES

1. Committee on Maternal Nutrition, Food and Nutrition Board, National Research Council: *Maternal Nutrition and the Course of Pregnancy.* Washington, National Academy of Sciences, 1970.
2. T. Primrose and A. Higgins: "A Study in Human Antepartum Nutrition." *J. Reprod. Med.* 7:257, 1972.
3. W. T. Tompkins et al.: "The Underweight Patient as an Increased Obstetric Hazard." *Am. J. Obstet. Gyn.* 69:898–919, 1955. M. Winich et al.: "Effects of Prenatal Nutrition Upon Pregnancy Risk." *Clin. Ob. and Gyn.* 16:184–198, March 1973.
4. R. L. Williams: "Intrauterine Growth Curves: Intra- and International Comparisons with Different Ethnic Groups in California." *Preventive Medicine* 4(2): June 1975.
5. A. T. Cross and H. E. Walsh: "Prenatal Diet Counseling." *J. Reprod. Med.* 7:265–274, Dec. 1971.
6. *Nutrition During Pregnancy and Lactation.* Sacramento, Calif., Maternal and Child Health Unit, California Department of Health, 1975.
7. Ibid., p. 21.
8. C. E. Flowers: "Editorial: Nutrition in Pregnancy." *J. Reprod. Med.* 7:264–274, Nov. 1971.
9. *Nutrition During Pregnancy and Lactation,* op. cit., p. 20.

SUGGESTED READING

California Department of Health Services: Nutrition for Pregnancy and Breastfeeding Series. *Eating Right for Your Baby, Using Vitamin/Mineral Pills and Salt, Your Weight and Weight Gain, Relief from Common Problems: nausea, constipation, heartburn.* Sacramento, California, 1978.*

Goodwin, M. T.: A New Technique for Nutrition Counseling: The Food Shield. *Birth and the Family Journal* 4:1, Spring 1977.

Lappe, F. M.: *Diet for a Small Planet.* New York, Friends of the Earth/Ballantine, 1971.

Nutrition During Pregnancy and Lactation, Sacramento, California, Maternal and Child Health Unit, California Department of Health, 1975.*

Streitfeld, P. P.: "Congenital Malformation: Teratogenic Foods and Additives." *Birth and the Family Journal* 5:1, Spring 1978.

Williams, E. R.: "Vegetarian Diets in Pregnancy." *Birth and the Family Journal* 3:2, Summer 1976.

Worthington, B. S. et al.: *Nutrition in Pregnancy and Lactation.* St. Louis, C. V. Mosby, 1977.

*Available without charge by writing to Department of Health, 714 P. Street, Sacramento, California 95814.

Twenty

Antepartal Care

Concepts of Prevention and Early Detection | Antepartal Management | General Health Maintenance in Pregnancy | Minor Discomforts | Preparations for the Baby | Use of Community Resources

Pregnancy is a normal physiologic process which only occasionally is complicated by pathologic conditions dangerous to the health or life of the mother, fetus or both. The vast majority of all births do not require active management by health professionals, as the natural reproductive process unfolds according to biologic patterns adaptive for the species. Normal pregnancy does, however, significantly alter the woman's physiologic systems and there is always the potential for reduction of general health status and the development of hazards for mother and fetus. The concept that pregnant women need special attention is ancient and interwoven into the social fabric of the culture. Modern prenatal care is a relatively recent development, in which the organized health care system assumes primary responsibility for the supervision of pregnancy and the conduct of labor and delivery. Nursing originated this practice around the turn of the century, when the Instructive Nursing Association in Boston began making house calls on mothers registered at the Boston Lying-In Hospital for delivery. Their goal was to contribute to the health of pregnant women, who then visited the physician only for confirmation of pregnancy and were not seen again until they appeared at the hospital in labor.

Antepartal care refers to the medical and nursing supervision and care given to the pregnant woman during the period between conception and the onset of labor. Opinions vary, but, generally in current practice adequate antepartal care is that care which considers the physical, emotional, and social needs of the woman and her unborn baby, her mate, and their other children. It attempts to provide the best of medical and nursing science to protect the life and health of the mother and fetus. In addition, it takes into consideration the social conditions under which the family lives (i.e., its economic status, educational level, housing, nutrition, and so on; see Chapter 5) so that the mother and fetus may pass through pregnancy, labor, and the puerperium with a maximum of mental and physical fitness. It is the former aspect, in particular, that is now being given more attention. Innovative styles in delivery of care, together with the utilization of personnel who have a better understanding of the lifestyles of the clients they serve, are gradually but surely improving utilization of health services. It becomes evident, then, that the goals of adequate antepartal care are accomplished through the combined efforts of the expectant parents, the physician, the nurse, and the various other members of the health team.

Adequate antepartal care also aims to increase the knowledge of the mother-to-be and her family, so that she and her infant may be kept healthy and happy after delivery.

Antepartal care may be considered the foundation for the normal development, adequate growth, and good health of the baby. During this formative period, the teeth, bones, and various systems of the body have their beginnings, as well as the foundations for the infant's future health. Adequate antepartal care also aids in stabilizing the daily health of the mother. As pregnancy advances, the demands of the fetus increase. Since individuals react differently to pregnancy, this supervision is of the utmost importance in detecting these reactions; for it not only helps to relieve discomforts and to prevent accidents and complications, but also aids in ensuring a more rapid convalescence and continued good health.

CONCEPTS OF PREVENTION AND EARLY DETECTION

Antepartal care is often thought of as preventive care, and the relationship between early and continued medical supervision during pregnancy and positive outcome for mother and fetus are well established. It is not clearly established which factors are really important within this complex interaction between the individual-family reproductive unit and the multiple-dimension prenatal component of the health care delivery system. To consider but a few aspects, there is patient self-selection for timing of entry into the system, degree of compatibility between personal values and goals and norms of professionals, physical and economic access considerations, the impact of patient education and monitoring on health-promoting behaviors, and the effects of early detection of potential problems on the incidence of complications. This last factor is probably responsible for most statistical correlates between antepartal care and infant and maternal morbidity and mortality. Early detection of such problems as anemia, urinary tract infections, and preeclampsia can have important effects upon preventing the serious consequences of these conditions which can occur if not treated in time.

The actual prevention of disease, and thus promotion of better health status, precedes the development of specific illnesses. Prevention involves macroecological issues that must be addressed on the societal level. Such factors as lifestyle and associated habits related to substance abuse, exercise and diet; poverty and its relations to education, housing, living conditions, nutritional status, and vital reserve; and environmental hazards such as air pollution, chemical toxins, noise and crowding have much more to do with health status of the population than the interventions of the medical care system. Real prevention means alleviation of the conditions leading to poor health and establishment of conditions which encourage health-promoting behaviors. The lack of a coordinated national health policy in the United States continues to fragment and render less effective our efforts to deal with these macroecological problems.

Quality and Equity Concerns

To a large degree, the structure in which antepartal care is delivered reflects values and assumptions of the middle class. For this group, it is quite effective in assuring healthy outcomes. However, there is a disparity in pregnancy outcomes of middle income and low income groups, which is usually taken to indicate that the prevalent model of antepartal care is not effective for certain segments of the population. Many factors are involved in this disparity, including quality of medical services, utilization and compatibility with cultural norms and values, ability to comply with remedies and treatments prescribed, and baseline health status often spanning several generations.

The lower socioeconomic groups, generally those in greatest need of good maternity care, with the highest death and sickness rates, often lack confidence in the community facilities for their care. They believe that adequate health care is a right of citizenship; however, when they seek it, they often find that two kinds of care exist: one for those who can pay and another for those who cannot. Since so many people now feel that proper health care is a right of citizenship, the provision of adequate health services for all requires a restructuring of present national priorities and an escalation of the public's social consciousness. Most health professionals agree that any worthwhile program should provide financial support and, in addition, should maintain the mother's dignity. The concept of comprehensive health planning by states and localities, including area health education centers, community clinics, and innovative programs in hospital clinics have been attempts to provide a better caliber of care for all segments of society.

Within the last ten years, the focus of service in many outpatient departments and clinics of hospitals has changed from dispensing first aid to giving ambulatory care. As a result, the ambulatory care department is now one of the most dynamic, change-oriented departments in many hospitals.

As part of this change, nursing service in these ambulatory care settings has discarded the managerial role and replaced it with a care-centered, more independent role in which nurses are expanding their functions of educating patients, providing supportive guidance, and making observations. In this role, the professional nurse becomes the health professional who is primarily responsible for maintaining continuity of health care for a specific patient population.

Increasingly, expanded nursing roles such as the nurse practitioner and clinical specialist are utilized to provide routine prenatal care in outpatient, ambulatory settings.

Distribution and Manpower Concerns

The maldistribution of health personnel characteristic of our urban specialty orientation in health care contributes to the disparity in outcomes noted among various population groups. Rural and geographically isolated communities have traditionally experienced difficulties obtaining adequate health and medical care, because professional socialization and economic considerations promote practice in highly populated metropolitan areas. Inner-city areas also suffer a lack of health care resources, largely due to economic factors and cultural differences between providers and patients.

It is now becoming more and more accepted that quality maternity care in the future will be provided by a closely integrated team of physicians, professional nurses, nurse-midwives or nurse practitioners, laboratory technicians, social workers, nutritionists, health educators, and homemakers. None of these are available in sufficient numbers at the present. However, the development of expanded roles for nurses, together with training programs for the education of paraprofessionals, are proving

to be viable efforts to ease this aspect of the present crisis. Research has indicated that when nurses utilize expanded roles and are integral members of the health care team, there are considerably fewer broken antepartal appointments, better postpartal clinic attendance, better utilization of family planning services and techniques, and reduction of infant mortality.[1,2]

Government programs have been developed to encourage health professionals to enter practice in medically underserved rural or inner city urban areas. Such efforts as the National Health Service Corps to support the start-up of team practices between physicians and nurse practitioners in rural communities, Medicare reimbursement of nurse practitioners and physician's assistants in rural clinics, scholarships and educational subsidies for primary care providers, and program grants for primary care to schools of nursing and medicine are steps toward ensuring greater availability and appropriate distribution of health personnel.

One of the most effective methods of providing care to underserved populations, whether geographically isolated or culturally unique, has been training of indigenous community members through decentralized educational programs. Utilization of indigenous populations often improves the quality of care. Their familiarity with the lifestyles of childbearing families, their knowledge of the socioeconomic factors to be considered and their willingness to provide whatever service is needed, be it transportation or referral for counseling, are salient factors in the improvement of reproductive outcomes. There is a very important message in the majority of the current research on the delivery of antepartal services to the various segments of society. Programs that are planned by outsiders and that do not consider the involvement of those whom they serve are doomed to failure and will in no way deliver the quality of care that they ostensibly were designed to give.

Lack of coordination and overlap in agencies presents another dimension of maldistribution of health services. For example, there may be several community health nursing services in one area, such as the health department, a voluntary nursing agency, and school nursing services. Many times they all serve one family, but seldom communicate with one another regarding the total needs of the family. Similarly, some hospitals may be overcrowded, while others have empty beds. Nothing is done to relieve the shortage because the first hospital may be governed by economic considerations to the exclusion of the comfort and safety of its patients.

The impact of Public Law 93-641, the National Health Planning and Resources Development Act of 1974, upon the distribution and quality of maternity services is the subject of considerable controversy. This act established Health Systems Agencies, which are regional organizations within states that have primary responsibility for health planning and development of health services, manpower, and facilities to meet the needs of their service areas. The HSAs are charged with:

1. improving the health of residents of a health service area,
2. increasing the accessibility (including overcoming geographic, architectural, and transportation barriers), acceptability, continuity, and quality of the health services provided them,
3. restraining increases in the cost of providing them health services,
4. preventing unnecessary duplication of health resources.[3]

Guidelines for implementation of this law have been issued by the Secretary of the Department of Health, Education and Welfare. The general thrust is to set a minimum number of deliveries per year for a hospital to maintain an obstetrical service, therefore promoting concentration of deliveries in larger regional centers to increase efficiency and cost-effectiveness. There are exception clauses for small, rural communities, isolated geographic areas, and transportation distances.

The development of innovations such as community clinics and alternative birth centers are attempts by the health system to respond to consumer needs. Community clinics are initiated and organized by the indigenous population and staffed largely by local people. Health professionals who share the ethnic and cultural background of the community are usually recruited. Supported largely by federal funds, community clinics can be very effective in responding to specific health care needs of the population served in a setting compatible with the values and style of the culture.

Alternative birth centers are special units associated with an acute hospital, which offer a more homelike atmosphere for labor and delivery. Low-risk mothers undergo labor in a comfortable room without the usual equipment and requirements of standard labor rooms and deliver in a natural position in the same bed. Companions may be present in varying mix, and there is a minimum of intervention by the health provider beyond basic safety monitoring (see Chapter 40, Alternatives in Childbirth).

Concerns Related to Economics of Health Care

Although the stated goals for health care on the national level include assuring quality, access and control of costs, methods of financing services continue to support disparities among population groups. The chief protection for the medical needs of most of America's young parents is voluntary and commercial prepayment insurance. Unfortunately, the maternity benefits traditionally have been distressingly low. Young people with low incomes are frequently saddled with a large medical and hospital bill at a time when they can least afford to pay. Many professionals feel that maternity care should be entirely covered, but the actuarials believe that the rates for this kind of coverage would be prohibitive. However, it might be noted that insurance companies have had this opinion about other forms of coverage and under public pressure have increased benefits. Many community health leaders feel that the resources of this country are so vast that full coverage is feasible if there is a public mandate to provide it.

Various bills for national health insurance have been introduced in the U.S. Congress, but conflicting goals and assumptions continue to make it very difficult for legislators to develop a comprehensive, widely acceptable plan. Many question the commitment of the majority to the concept that equitable health care is a right of all people. Certainly our values supporting individual rights and minimum government interference and our pluralistic governmental structure provide significant obstacles to a sense of national social purpose. The involvement of concerned health professionals in the governmental processes can help promote an equitable health care system, responsive to promotion of health and prevention of illness.

ANTEPARTAL MANAGEMENT

Maternity care is provided by a mixture of health professionals, including physicians, nurses, nurse practitioners or clinicians, nurse specialists, social workers, dieticians, and other specialized personnel. Although often thought of as a team, the actual interrelations vary from an integrated, collaborative arrangement to a loosely structured, referral-type situation.

In general, physicians are diagnosticians of normal and abnormal conditions associated with the childbearing cycle. They are also technical specialists in the sense that they carry through the technical medical procedures associated with the childbearing cycle, including, of course, delivery of the infant. The nurse-midwife also shares some of these activities. However, she works under the supervision of the physician and is not responsible for the complicated or abnormal patients. She can also be teacher, counselor, and coordinator for the patient. The role of the nurse as clinician or practitioner is somewhat newer in the health care spectrum. This nurse can be responsible for physical assessment of the patient as well as the teaching, counseling, and coordination aspects of care.

In some settings, family, OB-GYN, or maternity nurse practitioners assume primary responsibility for the management of uncomplicated pregnancies. Working in collaboration with a physician, who may be remote from the site, these nurse practitioners do the initial obstetrical workup, supervise the pregnancy and manage minor difficulties, coordinate other needed services, and may be involved in intrapartal care, although delivery is more commonly done by the physician or mid-wife. Well-infant care and postpartal follow-up are also assumed by the nurse practitioner.

The nurse is primarily the teacher, counselor, developer, and implementer of teaching programs and coordinator for assuring continuity of care in the total patient experience. It is apparent that all of these health professionals have some similar skills, but may differ somewhat in their orientations as to their primary responsibilities.

Several variables interact to determine who provides which services to the family. The number and availability of health professionals, for instance, is a crucial factor. In some rural areas, both physicians and allied health personnel are in short supply; hence, the nurse-midwives and nurses must truly fulfill every aspect of their roles. Usually a minimum of time is available and patients with the greatest need are seen in triage. This emphasizes the necessity for accurate and thorough patient assessments so that appropriate referrals can be made to other professional services. In some of the larger metropolitan clinics, there may be a surfeit of various personnel, but a large patient population, and the nurse will find that coordinating and providing continuity of care must be emphasized.

Another variable influencing who provides what services is the orientation of the nurse. A nurse who is technically oriented will concentrate on the technical aspects of the care. A nurse who is interested and skilled in the interpersonal and teaching aspect will spend time in supportive, interpretive, and counseling activities. The nurse's strong preparation in interpersonal communication and supportive techniques as well as formal and informal teaching techniques provides an ideal role for working with total families as they move through the reproductive cycle.

Initial Prenatal Visit

When the woman thinks she may be pregnant, she makes an appointment with the physician or clinic. The visit for confirmation of pregnancy may be combined with the prenatal workup, or two visits may be required depending upon office or clinic routines. The prenatal workup consists of a thorough history, a physical examination, and laboratory tests. Prenatal forms are used by most facilities to summarize data and serve as a flow sheet for continuing visits throughout pregnancy (Fig. 20-1). Frequently the nurse is responsible for obtaining the history, collecting specimens, participating in the physical examination, and providing initial patient education and orientation to the services which will be offered.

The initial contact with the patient is particularly important. By greeting the patient in a pleasant and professional manner the nurse can initiate a productive relationship that conveys interest and concern for the patient. In making a patient comfortable while she waits for her appointment with the

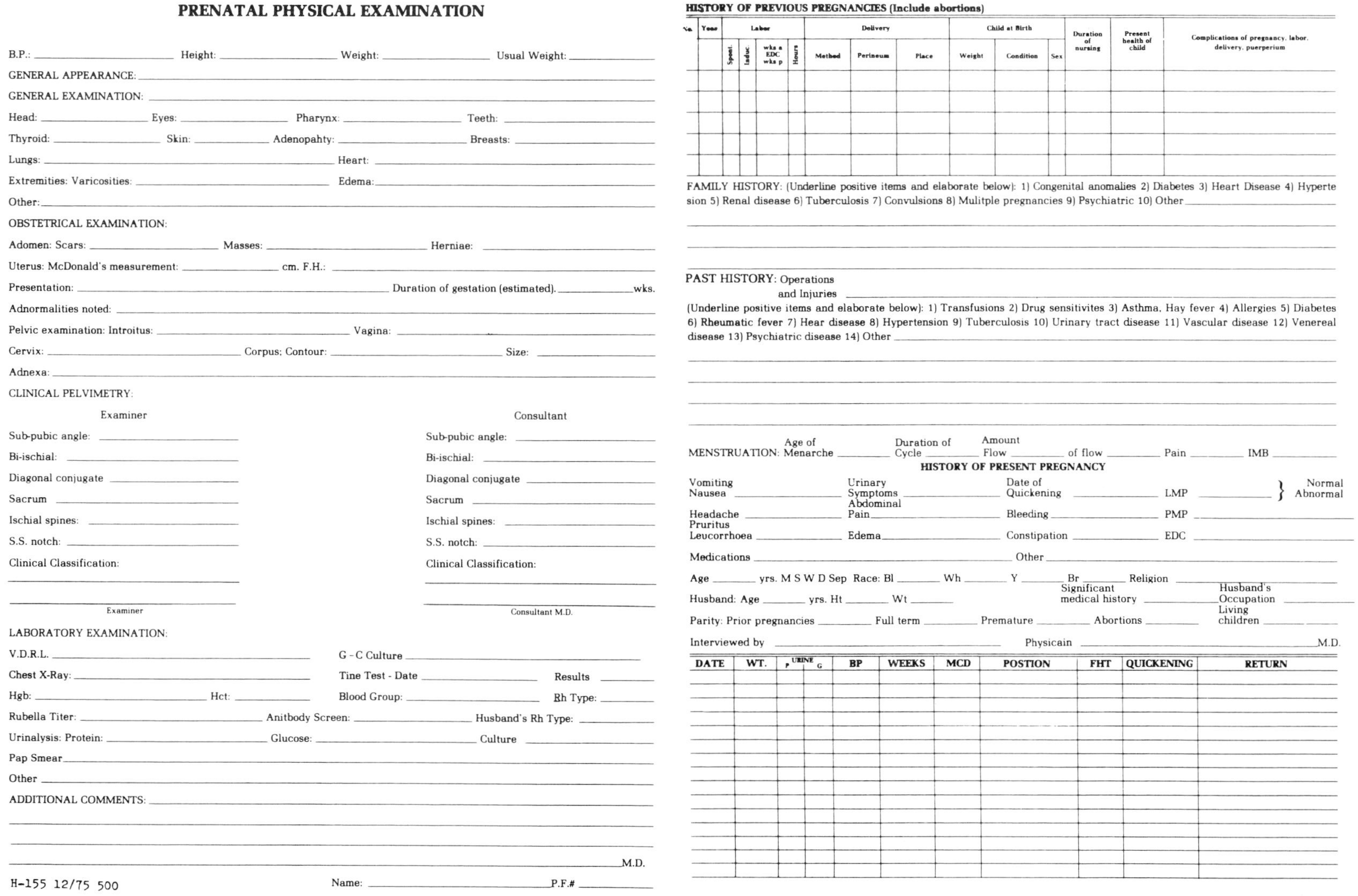

PRENATAL PHYSICAL EXAMINATION

B.P.: ______ Height: ______ Weight: ______ Usual Weight: ______

GENERAL APPEARANCE: ______

GENERAL EXAMINATION: ______

Head: ______ Eyes: ______ Pharynx: ______ Teeth: ______

Thyroid: ______ Skin: ______ Adenopahty: ______ Breasts: ______

Lungs: ______ Heart: ______

Extremities: Varicosities: ______ Edema: ______

Other: ______

OBSTETRICAL EXAMINATION:

Adomen: Scars: ______ Masses: ______ Herniae: ______

Uterus: McDonald's measurement: ______ cm. F.H.: ______

Presentation: ______ Duration of gestation (estimated). ______ wks.

Adnormalities noted: ______

Pelvic examination: Introitus: ______ Vagina: ______

Cervix: ______ Corpus; Contour: ______ Size: ______

Adnexa: ______

CLINICAL PELVIMETRY:

Examiner	Consultant
Sub-pubic angle: ______	Sub-pubic angle: ______
Bi-ischial: ______	Bi-ischial: ______
Diagonal conjugate ______	Diagonal conjugate ______
Sacrum ______	Sacrum ______
Ischial spines: ______	Ischial spines: ______
S.S. notch: ______	S.S. notch: ______
Clinical Classification: ______	Clinical Classification: ______
______ Examiner	______ Consultant M.D.

LABORATORY EXAMINATION:

V.D.R.L. ______ G - C Culture ______

Chest X-Ray: ______ Tine Test - Date ______ Results ______

Hgb: ______ Hct: ______ Blood Group: ______ Rh Type: ______

Rubella Titer: ______ Anitbody Screen: ______ Husband's Rh Type: ______

Urinalysis: Protein: ______ Glucose: ______ Culture ______

Pap Smear ______

Other ______

ADDITIONAL COMMENTS: ______

______ M.D.

H-155 12/75 500 Name: ______ P.F.# ______

HISTORY OF PREVIOUS PREGNANCIES (Include abortions)

No.	Year	Labor: Spont.	Labor: Induc.	Labor: wks a EDC wks p	Labor: Hours	Delivery: Method	Delivery: Perineum	Delivery: Place	Child at Birth: Weight	Child at Birth: Condition	Child at Birth: Sex	Duration of nursing	Present health of child	Complications of pregnancy, labor, delivery, puerperium

FAMILY HISTORY: (Underline positive items and elaborate below): 1) Congenital anomalies 2) Diabetes 3) Heart Disease 4) Hyperte sion 5) Renal disease 6) Tuberculosis 7) Convulsions 8) Mulitple pregnancies 9) Psychiatric 10) Other ______

PAST HISTORY: Operations and Injuries ______

(Underline positive items and elaborate below): 1) Transfusions 2) Drug sensitivites 3) Asthma, Hay fever 4) Allergies 5) Diabetes 6) Rheumatic fever 7) Hear disease 8) Hypertension 9) Tuberculosis 10) Urinary tract disease 11) Vascular disease 12) Venereal disease 13) Psychiatric disease 14) Other ______

MENSTRUATION: Age of Menarche ______ Duration of Cycle ______ Amount Flow ______ of flow ______ Pain ______ IMB ______

HISTORY OF PRESENT PREGNANCY

Vomiting Nausea ______ Urinary Symptoms ______ Date of Quickening ______ LMP ______ } Normal Abnormal

Headache Pruritus ______ Abdominal Pain ______ Bleeding ______ PMP ______

Leucorrhoea ______ Edema ______ Constipation ______ EDC ______

Medications ______ Other ______

Age ______ yrs. M S W D Sep Race: Bl ______ Wh ______ Y ______ Br ______ Religion ______

Husband: Age ______ yrs. Ht ______ Wt ______ Significant medical history ______ Husband's Occupation ______

Parity: Prior pregnancies ______ Full term ______ Premature ______ Abortions ______ Living children ______

Interviewed by ______ Physicain ______ M.D.

DATE	WT.	URINE P	URINE G	BP	WEEKS	MCD	POSTION	FHT	QUICKENING	RETURN

Figure 20-1. An example data sheet for the prenatal physical examination.

physician, the nurse can utilize the opportunity to find out any questions, symptoms, or problems that the mother may have and deal with them or report them to the proper person. This is an example of one way that the nurse can utilize limited contacts with the patient constructively.

The History

The name and address of the patient, her age and parity, and the date of the latest menstrual period are recorded, and the date of delivery is estimated. Inquiries are made into the family history, with special reference to any condition likely to affect childbearing, such as hereditary disease, tuberculosis, or multiple pregnancy.

The personal history of the patient then is reviewed not only with regard to previous diseases and operations, but particularly in relation to any difficulties experienced in previous pregnancies and labors, such as miscarriages, prolonged labor, death of infant, hemorrhage, and other complications.

Inquiry is made into the history of the present pregnancy, especially in relation to nausea, edema of the feet or the face, headache, visual disturbance, vaginal bleeding, constipation, breathlessness, sleeplessness, cramps, heartburn, lower abdominal pain, vaginal discharge, and varicose veins.

As time permits, the nurse can utilize the initial visit to expand upon historic information for assessment purposes, both nursing and medical. The following areas are generally included:

1. Social and personal characteristics of the patient: age, marital status, occupation, ethnicity, religion, height, weight, number of children in the home.
2. Information summary of spouse (father of baby): name, address, age, height, weight, ethnicity.
3. Characteristics influencing the course of pregnancy: EDC, LMP, blood type and Rh, pertinent medical conditions and/or hospitalizations, current medications and medication habits, usual bowel patterns, usual sleep patterns, resumé of dietary habits.
4. Attitudes toward the pregnancy:
   Was this child planned?
   What are the patient's goals and values regarding this pregnancy (and life in general)?

Does she view this pregnancy as a boon or interference in her life?
   What is her knowledge about health in general and pregnancy and childrearing in particular?
   Does she have any previous experience with pregnancy and/or childrearing?
   What are her expectations and concerns about this pregnancy, birth, and care of the infant?
   What is her apparent willingness or disinclination to prepare herself in the areas that need attention?
5. Resources:
   What appears to be her general level of intelligence and/or education?
   What is the level of economic stability?
   Is the family intact?
   Is there family available to her?
   Does she have sufficient friends from which she can get tangible help and emotional support if necessary?
6. Resumé of antenatal classes and instruction: antenatal classes and films attended, individual and group instruction and counseling.

Physical Examination

A thorough physical examination is usually performed to establish a baseline for the woman's general state of health and to evaluate the pregnancy. Vital signs including temperature, blood pressure, pulse, respiration, height and weight are done by the nurse or attendant. The physician or nurse practitioner then performs the physical examination, with attention to the teeth and throat, thyroid gland and lymph nodes, lungs, heart, breasts, skin, extremities and abdomen (Fig. 20-2). Characteristic changes of pregnancy are noted (see Chapter 16, Biophysical Aspects of Normal Pregnancy), and signs of infection or systemic disease identified if present.

Physical indicators of high risk pregnancy can often be determined in initial examination, such as obesity, hypertension, severe varicosities, preeclampsia, or uterine size inappropriate for dates.

Pelvic examination provides data relevant to confirming the pregnancy and determining the length of gestation, pelvic characteristics, and any abnormalities which might produce complications of

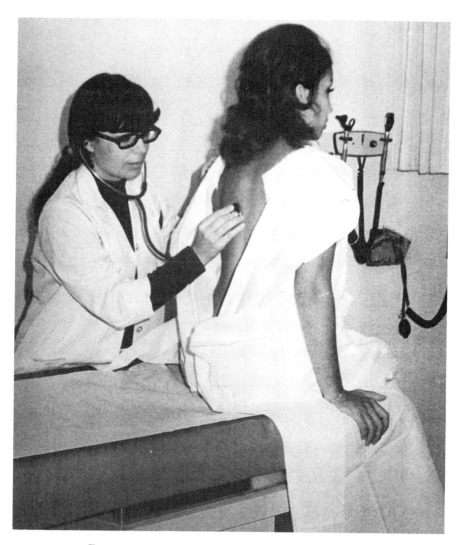

Figure 20-2. An important part of antepartal care is the initial physical examination.

pregnancy. At the same time specimens are obtained to screen for potential problems. The pelvic examination includes both speculum and bimanual examinations. On speculum exam, the characteristics of the vaginal and cervical mucosa are examined, and cervical discharge evaluated. Unusual lesions are identified and biopsies taken, as well as smears for vaginitis and cultures for gonorrhea. Papanicolaou smears to screen for cervical cancer are done routinely.

The bimanual examination provides information about the consistency of the cervix, the size, shape and consistency of the uterus, the condition of the fallopian tubes and ovaries, and the configuration of the bony pelvis. Uterine size is useful in deter-

mining length of gestation, and pelvic measurements enable a clinical appraisal of potential pelvic contractions which might lead to cephalopelvic disproportion in labor. Other abnormalities of the birth canal, such as soft tissue masses, can also be identified.

Abdominal examination is useful in providing information about the position of the fetus after the thirtieth week of gestation. Leopold's maneuvers help determine position and presentation of the fetus (p. 302), and auscultation of the fetal heart tones (FHT) can provide an indication of fetal conditions (p. 329). Fetal activity can be assessed, and the height of the fundus used to approximate the length of gestation by means of McDonald's technique. A

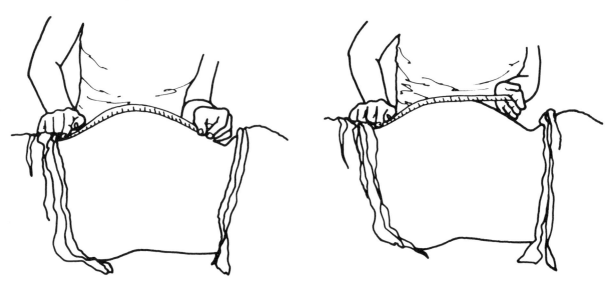

Figure 20-3. The McDonald technique for measuring the height of the fundus to approximate the length of gestation. The distance from the upper border of the symphysis pubis to the top of the fundus is measured with a tape measure. The tape measure may be curved over the abdomen as indicated on the left or held straight between the fingers with the hand at a right angle to the top of the fundus as shown on the right.

flexible tape measure is used to measure the distance from the upper border of the symphysis pubis to the top of the fundus. Frequently the tape measure is curved over the mother's abdomen (Fig. 20-3) although some providers hold it straight between the fingers with the hand at a right angle to the top of the fundus. The distance measured in centimeters, multiplied by two and divided by seven gives the duration of pregnancy in lunar months. Generally, up until about 32 weeks, this distance in centimeters corresponds to the length of gestation.

Role of the Nurse

While assisting the physician with the physical examination, the nurse has an opportunity to learn more about the patient's condition. Being alert to the cues and the events that transpire during this time will help the nurse interpret the physician's instructions or answer questions which the patient may ask afterward. Often a patient hesitates to discuss some matter with the physician, because she considers it too trivial, but she may feel comfortable in talking about it with the nurse. In turn, the nurse may consider this a problem of some importance, and on reporting it to the physician may find that it has a bearing on the course of treatment that is prescribed.

Another of the nurse's responsibilities is to prepare the patient for the physical examination. Since the initial examination is thorough, it is desirable that the patient disrobe completely and wear a gown that opens easily. In addition, the expectant mother should be covered with a small sheet to prevent unnecessary exposure and chilling. The nurse will want to instruct the patient to empty her bladder, since a full bladder is uncomfortable and may interfere with the manipulations carried out during the examination. A good footstool is imperative if the patient is to mount the table in safety and comfort. Many patients move somewhat awkwardly, especially as they near term, and the nurse can contribute a great deal to their safety and also help alleviate embarrassment by assisting the mother to move slowly but steadily when she changes position.

The vaginal or pelvic examination deserves special consideration, because often it is the most stressful part of the experience for the patient. This examination is carried out with the patient in the dorsal recumbent position. In this position the patient lies on her back with the lower extremities flexed and rotated outward. Her heels are supported in stirrups, which are level with the table, perhaps a foot in front of her buttocks. In this position the anxious patient, already under stress during the physical examination, is likely to tense her abdominal, pelvic and thigh muscles, attempting to adduct her thighs. Moreover, if the patient arches her back as her tension increases, her pelvis will be tilted downward, a position that makes the pelvic examination almost impossible to achieve.

The nurse can be most effective in assisting the patient to relax if she encourages her to keep breathing naturally, reminds her to breathe if she holds her breath, and helps her to let the small of her back press down on the table. Merely telling the anxious patient to relax is of no avail; thus the nurse needs to give the patient rather direct guidance, often step by step. For example, if the patient is clenching her fists, the nurse may say, "See, your wrists and hands are tense. Try to let them go limp—very limp—like a rag doll's. That's it—very limp." And a moment later, "Keep breathing naturally." Such short, explicit requests and instruction give the mother a simple task that she can do with guidance. This diverts her attention from the anticipated discomfort and promotes relaxation.

Steps in the Pelvic Examination

To see the cervix clearly, the examiner sits on a stool and focuses a good light into the vagina. Any equipment that is needed, such as vaginal speculum, swabs, cotton balls, slides, and lubricating jelly, should be within reach.

The pelvic examination will begin with an examination of the external genitalia, including the urethra and Skene's and Bartholin's glands. If any unusual discharge is present, a specimen may be obtained for culture or microscopic examination.

Usually, the next step is to insert a speculum into the vagina to distend the folds so as to provide a clearer view of the cervix. If a Papanicolaou smear is to be taken, no lubricating jelly will be used; instead, the speculum may be rinsed under *tepid* running water to facilitate the ease of insertion. Occasionally, the dilatation of the vagina by the speculum may cause an unpleasant sensation of stretching.

As the examination proceeds, the cervix is visualized, and the examiner will note its color and character. Normally, the cervix of the primigravida is pink or bluish and smooth, with a dimple for the os. The cervix of a multigravida may have an irregular os due to lacerations from previous deliveries. If erosions of the cervix are present, they may be treated with silver nitrate swabs. Any discharge that is purulent, greenish or frothy is considered to be abnormal, and a specimen may be secured for microscopic examination or culture.

After the cervix has been examined, the examiner will withdraw the speculum and proceed with the bimanual examination to evaluate the uterus and the adnexa. The size, consistency and contour of these organs, as well as the relationship of the uterus to the pelvis, are determined. At the same time pelvic measurements are taken. The examination is usually completed with an examination of the rectum to ascertain the presence of hemorrhoids, polyps, or other abnormalities.

At the completion of this examination, disposable tissues should be offered the patient to wipe the perineum adequately. Optimally, further activity and demands should be kept at a minimum, so that the mother may recoup the energy which has been dissipated through trying to absorb all the new experiences and information. Further specific health teaching and counseling is better postponed until a subsequent visit, when the patient is not so overloaded with new stimuli and fatigue.

Pap Smear. The Pap smear is obtained during speculum examination. The cervix is cleansed with a dry cotton ball to remove excess mucus, and a saline-moistened cotton-tipped applicator is introduced into the endocervical canal. It is rotated several times, withdrawn and rolled on a glass slide. The smear is fixed immediately with commercial fixatives or immersed in 95 percent ethyl alcohol to prevent drying of the specimen, which distorts the cells. Next, a wooden or plastic spatula is used to obtain the ectocervical sample. The shaped end is introduced slightly into the cervical os and turned firmly several times to scrape the tissue of the squamocolumnar junction (where the endocervical epithelium meets that of the ectocervix). This is the area where most malignancies arise and can be seen as a color change of cervical epithelium. This specimen is smeared on a glass slide and fixed as above. Some providers place both endo- and ectocervical specimens on one slide. A vaginal pool sample may also be taken by introducing the rounded end of the spatula into the posterior vaginal fornix. The smears should be accompanied by data about the woman's age, last menstrual period, pregnancy or postpartum, GYN surgery, and use of hormones.

Laboratory Tests

The laboratory tests carried out in antepartal care are the urine examination, the blood test for syphilis, complete blood count or hemoglobin, tests for the Rh factor and blood type, and often rubella titer (tests for the mother's status to rubella immunity), gonorrhea culture and antibody screening.

Urine Test.   At the first and subsequent examinations, the urine is tested for albumin and sugar. The patient is instructed to collect a part of the first urine voided in the morning before breakfast. The reason for this is that glucose may spill into the urine of a normal pregnant woman due to a decreased kidney threshold for glucose. Hence, it is more likely to appear in the urine after a meal. The test for sugar is the same as that used to test a diabetic's urine; several simple tests are available today and may be completed quickly and accurately in a matter of minutes.

Any positive reaction to sugar is reported so that the possibility of diabetes or a prediabetic condition can be ruled out.

The test for albumin also is simple. The principle involved here is the application of heat in chemical form, which solidifies any albumin present and causes a whitish precipitate. *The presence of albumin in the urine is another symptom of possible preeclampsia and should be reported immediately.* The sudden appearance of albuminuria is regarded as a symptom of preeclampsia.

Dipsticks with reagents for sugar, albumin, acetone and other urine constituents are widely used for their simplicity and convenience.

Blood Test.   Blood for the VDRL or other serologic tests for syphilis is usually obtained by venipuncture. A sufficient quantity of blood is drawn at this time so that a portion may be used for the Rh factor and CBC or hemoglobin estimation. Since many pregnant women develop anemia, the latter examination is highly important.

If the test for the *Rh factor* shows the patient to be Rh negative, it may be necessary to check the father and do serial antibody titers throughout pregnancy. It is also a wise precaution to obtain the father's blood type (see Chapter 36).

Return Visits

Regular return visits are scheduled throughout pregnancy to provide continuing monitoring of maternal and fetal status, to institute treatment and further diagnostic tests as necessary, and to offer ongoing opportunity for support and education.

The usual schedule of visits is:
once a month until the seventh month,
every two weeks during the seventh and eighth months,
weekly during the ninth month until delivery.
Visits are scheduled more frequently if problems arise. Routine return visits consist of follow-up history, physical examination, and patient education.

General inquiry is made about how the patient and family are feeling and the presence of any concerns or symptoms. New signs or physical findings, such as excessive weight gain or glycosuria, are explored through a series of questions. The woman is queried about any untoward signs and symptoms, including edema of the fingers or face, bleeding, constipation, and headaches. During these visits the woman is encouraged and given ample opportunity to ask any questions of concern to her.

Weight, blood pressure, fundal height, and fetal heart tones are taken during each return visit. Weight is plotted on a graph or flow sheet and deviations from expected progression noted and explored. The abdomen is examined for fetal position and measured according to McDonald's technique as described earlier. Legs and feet are examined for edema and development of varicosities. Other aspects of the physical examination are performed if indicated by signs or symptoms.

Vaginal examinations are usually not done on return visits until the patient nears term. Frequently vaginal exams are begun about two or three weeks from EDC (expected date of confinement) to assess the status of the cervix, fetal presentation, and the degree of engagement. The urine is tested on each return visit for sugar and protein (albumin), and hematocrit repeated at 32 to 34 weeks as a precaution against anemia.

Instructions to Patients

After the routine examination the patient may be instructed regarding diet, rest and sleep, daily intestinal elimination, proper exercise, fresh air and sunshine, bathing, clothing, recreation, and dental care.

It is usually possible and always desirable to assure the woman that the findings on examination were normal and that, barring complications, she may anticipate an uneventful pregnancy followed by an uncomplicated delivery. However, at the same time, she is tactfully instructed regarding certain danger signals which she must report immediately. These symptoms are as follows:

1. Vaginal bleeding, no matter how slight
2. Swelling of the face or the fingers
3. Severe continuous headache
4. Dimness or blurring of vision
5. Flashes of light or dots before the eyes
6. Pain in the abdomen
7. Persistent vomiting
8. Chills and fever
9. Sudden escape of fluid from the vagina

In addition to this detailed supervision the patient needs an explanation of the changes that are taking place within her body. This point cannot be stressed enough. Intelligent exploration with the patient regarding her concerns about these changes and appropriate instruction will give her greater reassurance and self-confidence. An understanding and empathic attitude will do much to buoy the patient's morale and to diminish unnecessary anxiety.

As the patient approaches full term, she can be instructed also about the signs and symptoms of oncoming labor, so that she may know when the process is beginning and when to notify the physician. At this time she will need to report the frequency of contractions and any other pertinent symptoms.

Most hospitals conduct routine tours of the maternity division for the expectant parents. It is advisable to encourage them to take advantage of this opportunity sometime during the pregnancy. Becoming familiar ahead of time with the surroundings where the mother-to-be will deliver the baby reduces the anxiety that may be experienced in going to a strange hospital for the first time after labor has begun. The details of the hospital admission routine are explained, so that the mother is familiar with this procedure before being admitted for delivery.

Weight

The routine estimation of weight at regular intervals during pregnancy is an important detail of antepartal care. And *marked gain* or *loss* in weight will be discussed by the obstetrician. At first the average gain in weight of the fetus is 1 gm. daily; nine-tenths of the weight is gained after the fifth month, and one-half of the weight of the fetus is acquired during the last eight weeks. Most specialists agree that a weight gain of about 25 to 30 pounds is desirable for a woman who is average or "normal" in her prepregnant weight. However, there is increasing evidence among investigators that the weight gain for pregnancy needs to be individualized for every patient, particularly those of under and over average prepregnant weights. In the former case, a gain of 30 pounds or more has had no deleterious effects on the mother and has resulted in a healthy normal weight infant. For all patients the emphasis is becoming less on gain per se than on a balanced nutritional status related to the patient's general physical condition.

Certainly no woman should try to lose weight during pregnancy, and even those who begin pregnancy significantly overweight must expect to gain additional weight. Explaining to the patient how pregnancy weight is distributed (see Chapter 19) helps her understand why it is necessary for normal progression of fetal development.[4]

Visual Aids; Teaching Groups. In hospitals and offices where the appointment system is used, the waiting time for the patient is minimized. In others the patient may have to wait longer periods. Waiting time in any setting may be utilized advantageously by providing reading material that will contribute to the patient's knowledge of her condition. Visual aids such as posters and charts may be both instructive and diverting. Flannelboard posters are excellent in this respect, since they can be changed frequently. These visual aids also provide an outlet for the creative ideas of the staff.

Some offices and more and more clinics are using a group approach for discussion, teaching, and guidance. These groups are usually under the leadership of the nurse and provide a maximum amount of instruction for a large number of patients in a short period of time. In addition, in the large, busy clinic, this group discussion technique provides patients with a feeling of continuity of care since the nurse leader remains a stable figure (Fig. 20-4).

Referrals. The problems that come to light are not always of a physical nature; emotional and social problems also may interfere with the patient's ability to derive full benefit from health services. It is the

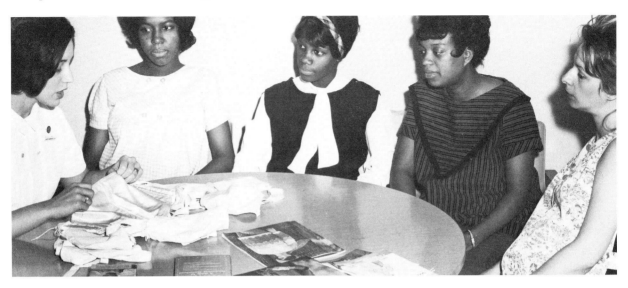

Figure 20-4. Group counseling by the nurse in the clinic.

responsibility of the nurse to find out in what ways the patient needs help and to make appropriate referrals when they are indicated (e.g., to the nurse in the community, to allied community services or to other members of the extended health team). This is one of her most important nursing activities, since through the use of referrals lines of communication can be kept open between the particular health agency, the community, and the members of the health team. Thus comprehensive care for the patient is assured.

Anticipatory Guidance. The nurse in the office or the clinic can devote much nursing care to health teaching and anticipatory guidance (i.e., informing mothers about what to expect regarding their pregnancy, delivery, postpartal and childbearing periods before they begin to worry or to make mistakes). Therefore, it is necessary to have broad knowledge and understanding about the physiology of pregnancy and childbearing, general hygiene, nutrition, the emotional, psychologic, and socioeconomic aspects of family living, and the part played by a family in the larger community. Teaching sessions are individualized for each patient, and should include 1) instruction in ways of maintaining good health habits in daily living, 2) interpretation of the reasons that these practices are important, and 3) suggestions of ways in which undesirable habits may be changed or modified.

The first step toward this goal is to identify the level of knowledge and understanding of the patient through exploration of what the patient knows and feels about the topic in question. Second, any misinformation or misconceptions must be clarified. The final step is to add to the base of knowledge and understanding through reinterpretation, clarification, reemphasis, and reinforcement.

GENERAL HEALTH MAINTENANCE IN PREGNANCY

Pregnancy ought to be a normal, happy, healthy experience for a woman. If a woman has a good general state of health, there is no reason why pregnancy should produce physical or emotional symptoms that would significantly interfere with her ability to function and participate in her usual activities. Women are encouraged to continue their usual habits with very little change, unless they have previously been living in ways not conducive to health and well-being. While pregnancy creates numerous physiological and psychoemotional changes, women with basically positive attitudes and good health are able to adapt without undue stress. Many find these changes intriguing and enjoyable—part of the mystery of the phenomenon of childbearing. During the months of antepartal care, the nurse has many opportunities to assist patients to attain healthier patterns of living and to reinforce health-promoting behaviors.

Rest, Relaxation and Sleep

Because rest and sleep are so essential to health, it is well to emphasize this detail in the parent-teaching aspect of the antepartal period. Pregnant women become tired more readily; therefore, the prevention of fatigue must be stressed emphatically. The body is made up of various types of cells, each of which has a specific function. Depletion of nerve-cell energy results in fatigue, and fatigue causes certain reactions in the body that are injurious. For all body processes, such as digestion, metabolism, working, playing, and studying, nerve-cell energy is utilized. Nature has made provision for some reduction in normal energy without injury to health. Beyond this limit the symptoms of fatigue are evidenced in irritability, apprehension, a tendency to worry, and restlessness. These symptoms are sometimes very subtle and misleading, but in contrast, human beings are very conscious of tired muscles. It is more important to avoid fatigue than to have to recover from overfatigue. The pregnant woman should rest to prevent this fatigue. Rest and sleep replenish the cell energy.

If patients cannot sleep, they can attempt to rest. Rest is the ability to relax. Patients often need to learn how to relax. There is no code so variable, so necessarily adapted to the individual, as that of rest and sleep. The final test is whether the day's work is done with zest and energy to spare.

The expectant mother ought to get as much sleep as she feels she needs. Some people need more than others. In addition to a good night's sleep, it is advisable that the mother take a nap or at least rest for a half hour every morning and afternoon. If this is not possible, shorter rest periods, preferably taken lying down (several times a day) are beneficial.

Not all mothers are able to follow the recommended rest periods to the letter. Both the woman who works throughout her pregnancy, and the mother of several preschool children need special attention in planning for adequate rest. Rigid recommendations are to be avoided, and the nurse can search with the mother for minutes in her busy day that can be utilized for rest; again, counseling the family may be necessary to maximize the mother's free moments. Although the nurse strives for flexibility, she also needs to emphasize the necessity of this aspect of general hygiene. It can be explained that rest means not only to lie down and perhaps to sleep, but also to lie down or to sit comfortably—to rest the body, mind, abdominal muscles, legs and back, and to stretch out whenever possible, and so make it easier for the heart to pump the blood to the extremities.

During the last months of pregnancy, a small pillow used for support of the abdomen while the patient lies on her side does much to relieve the discomfort common during this period and adds materially to the degree of rest that the patient gets in a given time.

It should be suggested that the patient sit whenever possible, even while doing her housework. Sitting to rest for other brief periods during the course of the day can be beneficial if the feet and legs are elevated.

Often certain minor discomforts of pregnancy can be overcome by rest. Rest and the right-angle position (see Fig. 20-7, p. 285) are advised for swelling, edema, and varicosities of the lower extremities. Rest and Sims's position (see Fig. 20-8, p. 286) are advised for varicosities of the vulva and the rectum. Even for the more serious abnormalities, the simple aids included in "diet and rest" may help measurably until more specific orders from the obstetrician can be obtained. In such instances, the nurse must be aware of the mother's interpretation of "rest," and, if indicated, she can provide the necessary guidance to help the mother to understand and to plan for it.

Exercise

Outdoor exercise during pregnancy is usually very beneficial, because it affords diversion in the sunshine and fresh air. However, the degree of exercise recommended depends on the individual woman, her general condition, and the stage of pregnancy.

There are differences in the amount of exercise for the early and late periods of pregnancy. When pregnancy is advanced, exercise may be limited in comparison with the amount advised previously. Exercise usually means diversion, and, of course, this phase is most important. Exercise also steadies the nerves, quiets the mind, promotes sleep, and stimulates the appetite, all of which are valuable aids to the pregnant mother.

Walking in the fresh air is quite generally preferred to every other form of exercise during pregnancy, because it stimulates the muscular activity of the entire body, strengthens some of the muscles used during labor, and is available to all women. Exercise of any kind should not be fatiguing; to secure the most beneficial results, it should be combined with fresh air and sunlight, as well as periods of rest.

The woman who does her own housework needs little or no planned exercise from the physical viewpoint. However, she does need fresh air, sunshine, and diversion. It is far better for the patient to be occupied than to sit idly, but standing for long periods of time should be avoided. Lifting heavy objects, moving furniture, reaching to hang curtains, any activity which might involve sudden jolts, sudden changes in balance which might result in a fall or the likelihood of physical trauma should be avoided. The more strenuous sports (i.e., horseback riding, skiing, hikes involving long climbs, rough water swimming) are subjects to be discussed. The pregnant woman who is accustomed to participating in certain sports and finds this participation an enjoyable form of recreation usually will be permitted to continue in moderation as long as it poses no risk to the pregnancy.

Employment

The same attitude of moderation can be maintained whether for work or play. Ideally, any activity, whether work or play, should not be continued to the extent of even moderate fatigue; however, it is not realistic to expect the mother to willingly discontinue her job because it is tiring, especially if it is essential to the family sustenance. If her employment is influencing her health adversely, the matter needs conscientious exploration by the health team to see what realistic adjustments can be made. A referral to a social worker may be indicated to better ascertain the economic situation of the family and/or the resources in the community that might be helpful. Different job opportunities can be discussed, and the patient's skills, satisfactions and preparation can be considered.

In general, jobs requiring moderate manual labor should be avoided if they must be continued over long hours, or if they require delicate balance, constant standing, or constant working on night shifts. Actually, the woman who has a "desk job" in an office often does less strenuous work than the average homemaker who does not go out to work. Nevertheless, positions which require the worker to sit constantly can be extremely tiring. Adequate rest periods should be provided for all pregnant women employed in such positions.

In some countries the time of discontinuing routine jobs has been regulated by law, and the limits, although arbitrary, are generally from six to eight weeks prior to the expected date of confinement.

Many women are employed in industry, and the problem of pregnancy for the working mother in this type of employment is a most important one. To safeguard the interests of expectant mothers so engaged, the Standards for Maternity Care and Employment of Mothers in Industry have been recommended by the U.S. Children's Bureau (see chart on p. 275).

Recreation

Recreation is as necessary during pregnancy as it is at any other time in life. The patient is preparing for one of the most important role changes that she will undergo during life, and concomitant with any such change is the production of anxiety. It is to be expected that a certain amount of concern about the impending labor will be present; the additional responsibility of having a helpless new baby in the household, plus caring for and integrating him into the family unit, is also anxiety-provoking. The parents will have occasion to wonder whether they are equal to the enormous responsibility of rearing children, and whether or not they will be "good" parents. Therefore, activities which are diverting, healthful, and relaxing help the patient and the family to keep things in their proper perspective. Hence, it is beneficial to discuss with the mother some types of recreation that are most relaxing and pleasing for her and her family. Family group activities still can be enjoyed, even though the mother's energy and dexterity may be somewhat curtailed.

Consideration and understanding on the part of the father, the family, the physician, and the nurse can do much to relieve any uncertainties or concerns that the mother may have. When the father, in particular, understands more about the processes involved in the pregnancy (see Suggested Reading), his helpfulness can be increased. If a "blue" day comes, the father can make it his particular responsibility to provide a means of counteracting it. On a home visit the nurse might discuss with the family ways in which they might help to diminish the

STANDARDS FOR MATERNITY CARE AND EMPLOYMENT

(U.S. Children's Bureau)

1. Facilities for adequate prenatal medical care should be readily available for all employed pregnant women; and arrangements should be made by those responsible for providing prenatal care, so that every woman would have access to such care. Local health departments should make available to industrial plants the services of prenatal clinics; and the personnel management or physicians and nurses within the plant should make available to employees information about the importance of such services and where they can be obtained.

2. Pregnant women should not be employed on a shift including the hours between 12 midnight and 6 A.M. Pregnant women should not be employed more than 8 hours a day nor more than 48 hours per week, and it is desirable that their hours of work be limited to not more than 40 hours per week.

3. Every woman, especially a pregnant woman, should have at least two 10-minute rest periods during her work shift, for which adequate facilities for resting and an opportunity for securing nourishing food should be provided.

4. It is not considered desirable for pregnant women to be employed in the following types of occupations, and they should, if possible, be transferred to lighter and more sedentary work:
   a. Occupations that involve heavy lifting or other heavy work.
   b. Occupations involving continuous standing and moving about.

5. Pregnant women should not be employed in the following types of work during any period of pregnancy, but should be transferred to less hazardous types of work.
   a. Occupations that require a good sense of bodily balance, such as work performed on scaffolds or stepladders and occupations in which the accident risk is characterized by accidents causing severe injury, such as operation of punch presses, power-driven woodworking machines, or other machines having a point-of-operation hazard.
   b. Occupations involving exposure to toxic substances considered to be extrahazardous during pregnancy, such as:
       Aniline
       Benzene and toluene
       Carbon disulfide
       Carbon monoxide
       Chlorinated hydrocarbons
       Lead and its compounds
       Mercury and its compounds
       Nitrobenzol and other nitro compounds of benzol and its homologs
       Phosphorus
       Radioactive substances and x-rays
       Turpentine
   Other toxic substances that exert an injurious effect upon the blood-forming organs, the liver, or the kidneys.

   Because these substances may exert a harmful influence upon the course of pregnancy, may lead to its premature termination, or may injure the fetus, the maintenance of air concentrations within the so-called "maximum permissible limits" of state codes, is not, in itself, sufficient assurance of a safe working condition for the pregnant woman. Pregnant women should be transferred from workrooms in which any of these substances are used or produced in any significant quantity.

6. A minimum of six weeks' leave *before* delivery should be granted, on presentation of a medical certificate of the expected date of confinement.

7. At any time during pregnancy a woman should be granted a reasonable amount of additional leave on presentation of a certificate from the attending physician to the effect that complications of pregnancy have made continuing employment prejudicial to her health or to the health of the child.

   To safeguard the mother's health she should be granted sufficient time off after delivery to return to normal and to regain her strength. The infant needs her care, especially during the first year of life. If it is essential that she return to work, the following recommendations are made:
   a. All women should be granted an extension of at least two months' leave of absence after delivery.
   b. Should complications of delivery or of the postpartum period develop, a woman should be granted a reasonable amount of additional leave beyond two months following delivery, on presentation of a certificate to this effect from the attending physician.

strain in this period. This may necessitate changes in attitudes, understanding and habits; certainly it will mean increased tolerance and forbearance on the part of those involved; yet this is one of the ways that others can make their contribution to a successful pregnancy. The father's gentleness and tenderness are especially appreciated and therapeutic at this time; the mother, for her part, can help him to maintain his supportive attitude and behavior by letting him know when his actions are helpful and gratifying. This type of "feedback" conveys her appreciation to the father and leads to reinforcement of his positive behavior. He is perhaps the key person in helping the mother to secure the kind of social relaxation that she enjoys most.

Books, radio, music, movies, sporting events, television, sewing clubs, church functions, visiting, drives, walks, and entertaining friends are some of the means of providing relaxation and diversion. However, the mother should avoid situations likely to cause discomfort. Amusements, exercise, rest, and recreation at proper intervals help to keep the pregnant mother well and happy in an environment conducive to her well-being and happy anticipation of the baby.

Traveling

This is perhaps a detail of antepartal care which most patients think very little about, unless they have a tendency to become nauseated or have had a previous miscarriage which precludes any extensive strain.

Even though there is little restriction on travel from a medical point of view, this topic is to be discussed with the mother, so that any of her concerns or misinformation may come to light. The general information usually given to a pregnant woman is to avoid any trip which will cause undue fatigue, since she is prone to tiring easily. For traveling long distances the railway or airplane is safest and provides greater comfort. If travel is by private automobile, rest periods of 10 to 15 minutes ought to be planned at least every two hours. This not only helps to avoid fatigue, but also benefits the general circulation by providing the chance to stretch and walk about.

If the woman has any questions about the safety of wearing seat belts while pregnant, she should be advised to use them. Seat belts have been found to decrease maternal mortality in severe car accidents. They should be worn low and comfortably under the abdomen and in conjunction with the shoulder strap if one is available. Both belts can be adjusted so that they are not too tight or pressing tightly against the neck and abdomen.

Thus, while traveling in general is not usually contraindicated during pregnancy, each expectant mother should seek individual consultation concerning the advisability of extensive travel at any time during the period of pregnancy.

Immunizations and Vaccinations

Another important topic that is interrelated with travel is that of immunization and vaccination protection for the pregnant woman. The diseases that she will be exposed to during her travels, as well as in the course of her daily life, must be considered. In *The Medical Letter on Drugs and Therapeutics,* the Advisory Committee on Immunization of Infectious Diseases of the American Academy of Pediatrics reviewed the following vaccinations and made these recommendations:[5]

1. Cholera. This is a killed bacterial vaccine and should be given only if there is danger of infection. As yet there is no definitive evidence of abortigenic effect.
2. Mumps and measles (rubeola). These are live viruses and should never be given to pregnant patients.
3. Poliomyelitis. Immunization during pregnancy is rarely indicated since this disease has been almost irradicated in *the United States.*
4. Rubella. Pregnancy is a contraindication for administration of the live rubella vaccine. This virus has been shown on occasion to infect both the placenta and the fetus and for this reason is to be avoided.
5. Smallpox. Vaccinia virus administered during pregnancy occasionally infects the fetus. This fetal vaccinia has almost always been associated with primary vaccination. Hence, primary vaccination should only be given in those cases where exposure in an endemic area has occurred.
6. Yellow fever. Since this is a live virus, it should be given to pregnant women only if there has been an exposure or if there is a great risk of exposure.

7. Other vaccines and immunizations. There were no recommendations made by the Committee regarding vaccination against influenza, epidemic typhus, and typhoid. Tetanus and diphtheria toxoids are considered safe and the tuberculin and histoplasmin tests are also permitted.

Since there is at least somewhat of a risk with many of these vaccinations, it is well to counsel patients regarding the spacing of conception well after receiving these injections. The patient can be counseled also to plan vacations and travels during pregnancy to minimize the opportunity for disease exposure and the consequent need for post hoc vaccination. In addition, all patients should be advised to report any illness, no matter how trivial, to their physician so that appropriate follow-up can be done.

Care of the Skin

The glands of skin may be more active during pregnancy, and there may be increased or decreased perspiration, resulting in irritation or dryness. Since the skin is one of the organs of elimination, bathing is obviously important, and baths should be taken daily because they are stimulating, refreshing, and relaxing. They not only act as a tonic and a general invigorator, but also favor elimination through the skin as well. Elimination through the skin is thought to lessen the strain of elimination by the kidneys.

During pregnancy, showers or sponge baths may be taken at any time. The old idea that tub baths should be avoided because the wash water enters the vagina and thereby carries infection to the uterus now is believed to have little validity. However, tub baths should not be taken after rupture of the membranes. There is only one objection to tub baths during the last trimester of pregnancy. At this period the heavy weight of the large abdomen may put pregnant women off balance and make climbing in and out of the tub awkward. Therefore, the likelihood of slipping or falling in the bathtub is increased.

Chilling the body should be avoided; thus, cold baths, sponges, or showers should be avoided if they produce this sensation.

Care of the Breasts

Special care of the breasts during pregnancy is one of the important preparations for breast-feeding.

During the antepartal period the breasts often have a feeling of fullness and weight and in fact do become larger, heavier, and more pendulous. A well-fitted supporting brassière which holds the breasts up and in may relieve these discomforts. It may also help to prevent the subsequent tissue sagging so often noticeable after delivery due to the increased weight of the breasts during pregnancy and lactation.

There may be sufficient secretion of colostrum from the nipples to necessitate wearing a pad to protect the clothing. The daily care of the nipples and the reason for it, as well as the actual procedure, should be explained to the patient.

Early in pregnancy the breasts begin to secrete. This secretion often oozes out on the surface of the nipple and in drying forms fine imperceptible crusts. If these crusts are allowed to remain, the skin underneath becomes tender; if left until the baby arrives and begins nursing, this tender skin area is likely to crack. With this condition there is always a possibility of infection. Nipples that are kept clean and dry do not have a tendency to become sore or cracked.

The breasts are to be bathed daily; this may be done at the beginning of the tub, shower, or the sponge bath. The patient ought to use a clean washcloth and warm water. Some studies have demonstrated that the use of soap, alcohol, and other such materials during the antepartal period and puerperium tends to be detrimental to the integrity of the nipple tissue, since they remove the protective skin oils and leave the nipple more prone to damage (see Suggested Reading). Therefore, the possible disadvantages of using these substances should be discussed with the woman in the early stages of antepartal care.

The woman should be taught to bathe her breasts as follows: She begins cleansing each breast by washing the nipple thoroughly with a circular motion, making sure that any dried material has been removed. She gradually continues working away from the nipple in this fashion until the entire breast is washed. The breast is then rinsed in this manner and dried with a clean towel. Rubbing the nipples with a rough towel during the last trimester of pregnancy may be helpful in attempting to toughen them.

Some specialists advise the use of nipple cream, a hydrous lanolin preparation, to prepare the nipples for nursing. This can be applied after the breasts are bathed. First, a small quantity of cream is placed on the thumb and the first finger; then the nipple is grasped gently between the thumb and this finger. With a rolling motion, the cream is worked into the tiny creases found on the surface of the nipple. The position of the thumb and finger should be gradually shifted around the circumference of the nipple until a complete circuit has been made. This procedure is limited to about 30 seconds on each breast.

A nipple which is flat or even slightly inverted in early pregnancy very probably will become protractile by delivery. If the nipples are inverted, special care can be started by the woman in the fifth or sixth month of pregnancy or earlier. In one such treatment, the thumbs are placed close to the inverted nipple, the breast tissue is pressed firmly while the thumbs are gradually pushed away from the areola. The strokes should follow an imaginary cross drawn on the breast and be done four or five times in succession on awakening each morning (Fig. 20-5). The nipple will assume an erect, projected position and then can be grasped as a unit and gently teased out a bit further. This is done daily, so that the nipples may be made more prominent for the baby to grasp.

Clothing

During pregnancy the clothes should be given the same or perhaps even a little more attention than at other times. The young mother who feels that she is dressed attractively and is well groomed will reflect this in her manner. Her clothing should be practical, attractive, and nonconstricting. Most women are able to dress in the manner to which they are accustomed in the nonpregnant state until the enlargement of the abdomen becomes apparent. Maternity specialty shops and department stores have made maternity fashions available, which has settled the problem of suitable clothing during pregnancy.

Today designers and stylists are giving consideration to the pregnant mother's clothing, so that she may dress attractively and feel self-confident about her appearance. The clothes are designed to be comfortable and "hang from the shoulders," thus avoiding any constriction; they are made in a variety of materials. The expectant mother can dress according to the climate and the temperature for her comfort.

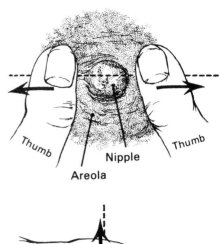

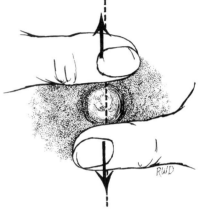

Figure 20-5. A suggested treatment for inverted nipples. The thumbs are placed close to the inverted nipple, pressed firmly into the breast tissue, then gradually pushed away from the areola. The strokes should be directed horizontally (*Top*) and vertically (*Bottom*) and be done four or five times in succession.

Abdominal Support. Women who have been unaccustomed to wearing a girdle will scarcely feel the need of abdominal support, especially during the early months of pregnancy. Later, however, a properly fitted maternity girdle often gives the needed support to avoid fatigue. The natural softening of the pelvic joints which accompanies pregnancy and the increasing weight of the abdomen may cause a change in posture and result in a severe backache.

If the mother's abdomen is large, or if previous pregnancies have caused her abdomen to become lax or pendulous, a properly made and well-fitting maternity girdle will give support and comfort. The purpose of the garment is support, not constriction of the abdomen.

Breast Support. It is advisable that every pregnant woman wear a well-fitted brassière to support the breasts in a normal uplift position. Proper support of the breasts is conducive to good posture and thus helps to prevent backache.

The selection of a brassière is determined by individual fitting and influenced by the size of the breasts and the need for support. It is important to see that the cup is large enough, and that the underarm is built high enough to cover all the breast tissue. Wide shoulder straps will afford more comfort for the woman who has large and pendulous breasts. The size of the brassière is, again, determined by the size of the individual being fitted, but in most instances the brassière is approximately two sizes larger than that usually worn. The mother who is planning to breast-feed will find it practical to purchase nursing brassières which can be worn during the latter months of pregnancy, as well as during the postpartal period for as long as she is nursing her baby.

Garters. Round garters or any tight bands (rolled stockings, elastic tops on knee-high stockings) that encircle the leg tend to aggravate varicose veins and edema of the lower extremities and should be discarded in favor of suspender garters or some form of stocking supporters attached to an abdominal support. If pantyhose do not aggravate any discharge that the mother may have, she may use these.

Shoes. A comfortable, well-fitting shoe is essential for the expectant mother. The postural changes which occur as the mother's abdomen enlarges may be aggravated by wearing high-heeled shoes, with resulting backache and fatigue. It is advisable that low-heeled shoes be worn during working hours and for busy daytime activities. For evening or more fashionable afternoon attire, a 2-inch heel is permissible if the patient does not develop backache from the increased lordosis induced by the heels, and if she can maintain adequate balance. Platform shoes contribute to precarious balance and are not advised.

The height of the heel is but one consideration; the support which the shoe gives the foot adds materially to the mother's comfort. Many flat-heeled shoes give little or no support to the feet and thus may cause fatigue and aching legs and backs. A simple method to check the support of a shoe is to place the shoe flat on the floor, and press the thumb down on the inner sole against the the shank (the part that would come under the arch of the foot). If the shoe gives under pressure, it will give weak support to the foot.

Care of the Teeth

Good dental care is necessary because the teeth are important for adequate mastication of food. This care need be little different during pregnancy from what is considered good general mouth hygiene for any person. The teeth should be brushed carefully on arising, after each meal, and before retiring at night. An alkaline mouthwash may be used, if desired. It is advisable for the expectant mother to visit her dentist at the very beginning of pregnancy and follow any recommendations made. Any extensive elective work is better postponed until after the pregnancy. The most favorable period for routine, minor procedures is from the fourth to the seventh month. The mother is usually less nauseated, not as yet very large and, in general, feeling well.

Diagnostic dental x-rays ought to be postponed until the latter half of pregnancy. A lead apron over the abdomen will give sufficient protection.

The old saying, "For every child a tooth," based on a belief that the fetus takes calcium from the mother's teeth, has no real scientific basis. It should be carefully explained to the mother that an adequate diet during pregnancy will supply the baby with lime salts and other necessities in sufficient amounts to build his bones and teeth. Therefore, this old adage need not be true if proper attention is given to the care of the teeth and nutrition during pregnancy.

Bowel Habits

The pregnant woman with regular habits of elimination usually experiences little or no change in the daily routine. Those who have a tendency toward constipation become noticeably more irregular during pregnancy due to 1) decreased physical exertion, 2) relaxation of the bowel in association with the relaxation of smooth-muscle systems all over the body, and 3) pressure of the enlarging uterus. Particularly during the latter part of pregnancy, the presenting part of the fetus exerts pressure on the lower bowel. Iron supplementation during pregnancy is an additional factor contributing to constipation.

Constipation may be prevented or alleviated by maintaining regular bowel elimination, drinking a large amount of fluids daily, and eating a diet that contains several daily servings of fresh fruit and raw vegetables, whole grain breads and cereals, and particularly products with whole bran. If these measures are not effective, a stool softener such as dioctyl sodium sulfosuccinate or a mild laxative such as milk of magnesia may be recommended. Harsh laxatives and purgatives are contraindicated. Mineral oil should not be used because it prevents absorption of fat-soluble vitamins from the gastrointestinal tract. Lack of vitamin K can lead to hemorrhagic disease of the newborn.

Hemorrhoids.   Pregnancy often precipitates the occurrence of hemorrhoids (anal varicosities) partially as a result of constipation. Maintaining regular bowel habits, keeping the stool soft, and avoiding straining at stool can help prevent or minimize hemorrhoids. Standing for long periods of time and wearing constricting clothing are aggravating factors. Passage of hard fecal material can injure the rectal mucosa and cause bleeding from fissures or hemorrhoids. Hemorrhoids may become thrombosed or protrude through the anus. The little bumps and nodules seen in a mass of hemorrhoids are the distended portions of the affected vessels. Like varicosities in other areas, they are caused by pressure interfering with return venous circulation and are aggravated by constipation. They often cause great discomfort to the pregnant patient and, due to pressure at the time of delivery, may cause great distress during the postpartal period.

The first step is the prevention and the treatment of constipation. The guidance that the nurse gives the mother in this respect cannot be stressed enough. In addition, when internal hemorrhoids protrude through the rectum, the mother can be instructed to replace them carefully by pushing them gently back into the rectum. Usually the patient can manage this quite well, after a thorough explanation and/or demonstration. She lubricates her finger with petrolatum or mineral oil to aid ease of insertion and to avoid trauma to the veins. If the patient wishes, a finger cot can be used to cover her finger. Also, taking either the knee-chest position or elevating her buttocks on a pillow facilitates replacement through gravity (see Fig. 20-8, p. 286).

The application of an icebag, or cold compresses wet with witch hazel or Epsom salts solution, gives great relief. The physician may order tannic acid in suppositories, or compresses of witch hazel and glycerin. If the hemorrhoids are aggravated the first few days after labor, the same medications usually give relief. Surgery is seldom resorted to during pregnancy.

Douches and Vaginal Hygiene

Vaginal douching, long considered a requisite of feminine hygiene by some women, should be kept at a reasonable minimum during pregnancy. If excessive vaginal secretion or infection exist, then the kind of douche and the frequency with which it is to be taken will be prescribed. In the absence of excessive secretions or infection, the nurse might reassure the patient that a washcloth and soap and water are quite adequate for general cleanliness, with emphasis on washing anteriorly first, and the rectal area last. The use of moist towelettes that are sold in foil packages is not contraindicated.

Deodorant "feminine hygiene" sprays are contraindicated as they have been found to cause severe perineal irritation in many women, as well as urethritis and cystitis in the more severe cases. During pregnancy, the sebaceous glands in the genital area are quite active and there may be a characteristic odor that some women find quite unpleasant. Plain soap and water are very effective agents to keep this odor under control. Any suggestions that the nurse might give for general cleanliness will usually be appreciated. Women may find that the genital area is a little more sensitive to heat and cold and pressure during pregnancy, but they should be reassured that regular cleansing procedures will not cause any harm.

Specific instructions about douching are to be given if the woman so desires. Having copies of the instructions for douching that agree with the philosophy of the office or clinic is an effective method of conveying this information. The instructions should be clear enough for the patient who has never douched and knows nothing about it.

The following points can be included in the instructions and stated in language and vocabulary that is understandable to the patient.

1. It is a four-minute procedure (after the initial few times).
2. It can be done while sitting on the toilet.
3. A gravity bag must be used (never a hand bulb syringe).
4. During pregnancy, the douche tip should not be inserted more than 3 inches.

5. The frequency and the solution are prescribed according to the needs of the patient.

6. The douche bag may be placed (hung or held) no higher than 2 feet above the level of the vagina.

7. The douche tip should be held at about the 3-inch length and inserted in the vagina, and the labial tissue in that area should be held around the douche tip with the same hand.

8. The solution is allowed to run in until there is a slight feeling of fullness, then it is expelled (the douche bag will hold enough solution to do this four or five times).

9. The bag and the tube should be rinsed and hung to dry with a towel underneath.

10. The solution, for comfort, should only be barely warm to the hand. Holding the labial tissue around the douche tip allows the water to flow in without flowing out immediately, and this, along with rapid expelling, enables the solution to get into the folds of the wall of the vagina. In the nonpregnant woman there is no contraindication to inserting the entire douche tip or as much of it as the vagina will accommodate.

Sexual Relations

From the standpoint of all parties involved —patient, nurse, and physician—the area of sexual relations, because of its intimate nature, often becomes one of the most difficult in which to give appropriate guidance. Many patients are reluctant to discuss sex in general, especially when the patient-physician-nurse relationship is new; yet they are disturbed because of the changes which may be taking place in their bodies and emotions, with consequent influences on their sexual relationship.

Because of this reluctance, nurses (and physicians) often avoid exploring with the patient the possibility of an existing problem. The counseling then consists mostly of prohibitions regarding the time and frequency of intercourse. However, when there is a need, most patients will discuss the subject with a little help, especially when the physician or the nurse conveys the idea that these are "expected" changes and that there is nothing "shameful" or unique about them. Thus the nurse should be prepared to fulfill this counseling activity and act as a resource person when called upon.

It is important to understand the anatomical, physiologic, and psychologic aspects involved, as well as the practitioner's attitudes regarding any particular advice relating to sex for this patient. The method of approach here is extremely important and requires adroit use of communication skills, especially those of listening, reflecting, and gentle probing. Finally, one's own feelings and attitudes about sexuality, pregnancy, and motherhood need to be examined in order to understand and better empathize with the patient's situation.

While sexuality has become a more open topic in today's society, there is a wide variety of views among people of different cultural backgrounds. Nonetheless, there is a growing expectation on the part of patients that health professionals will offer counseling related to sexuality as an integral part of health care. Particularly in maternity nursing, sexual concerns are close to the surface, providing a ready situation for intervention and satisfying sexual adjustments. Being willing to explore and respond to patient's sexual concerns and having knowledge of appropriate sources of referral for sexual counseling are part of the function of the maternity nurse. (See Chapter 11, Common Concerns Related to Sexuality, for a full discussion of this area.)

Smoking

The Surgeon General's report, as well as other recent studies, has indicated that cigarette smoking is a health hazard of sufficient importance in this country to warrant remedial action. Lung cancer, vascular thrombotic problems and heart disease have been linked significantly with cigarette smoking. With respect to pregnancy, several studies have found a relationship between smoking and lower birthrates, higher rates of prematurity, and higher neonatal mortality. The mechanism is somewhat obscure, but it is thought that the nicotine in the cigarettes causes peripheral vasoconstriction, with subsequent changes in the heart rate, blood pressure, and cardiac output that appear to have a detrimental effect on the development and the health of the fetus. Carbon monoxide also is found in higher concentrations in smokers, with a consequent decrease of oxygen; this also affects the fetus.

Data from a large perinatal mortality study revealed that birth weight distributions shifted downward as maternal smoking level increased. However, maternal weight gain distributions were the same for smokers and nonsmokers, indicating that smoking did not reduce maternal weight gain. Within each level of maternal weight gain, from below 5 pounds to over 40 pounds, the more the mothers smoked, the greater the percentage of neonates weighing less than 2,500 gm. Evidence supports a direct effect of maternal smoking on infant birth weight, possibly due to hypoxic effects of carbon monoxide, rather than an effect mediated through eating. Thus, efforts to prevent smoking should have greater benefits than efforts to increase maternal food intake.

Some disturbing observations from long-term studies indicate that low birth weight babies of smokers are small for dates at birth, and continue to grow at low percentiles for height and weight after birth. Also, at age 6 ½ years children of smokers have more neurological and electroencephalogram abnormalities, lower mean scores on 45 of 48 psychological tests, and slightly lower school placement than children of nonsmokers.[6]

The subject of smoking should be discussed thoroughly with the patient. Several "smoking clinics" have been developed around the country, and books and articles have been published on the topic of "how to stop smoking." A combination of motivation, education in the destructive effects of smoking for both mother and infant, and support seem to be the basic ingredients. The health team certainly can supply the last two; the patient is basically responsible for the first.

Alcohol

Until rather recently, moderate consumption of alcohol during pregnancy had been thought to cause no ill effects on the fetus, despite the known easy passage of alcohol across the placenta. However, there is presently a much more conservative attitude about the use of any drugs or toxic substances during pregnancy, as more evidence accumulates about the teratogenicity of many of these substances. It is known that infants of mothers who drink heavily are subject to alcohol withdrawal following birth and are at risk for the fetal alcohol syndrome (see Chapter 39). The effects of alcohol on the uterus have also been documented. Contractions are inhibited, even to the point of stopping premature labor when the mother is given alcohol (orally or parenterally) to the level of inebriation.

Current standards of medical practice indicate that pregnant women should be advised to avoid alcohol. Problems of alcohol addiction should be identified as early as possible, and treatment instituted to stop drinking or to minimize alcohol consumption.[7]

MINOR DISCOMFORTS

The minor discomforts of pregnancy are the common complaints experienced by most expectant mothers, to some degree, in the course of a normal pregnancy. However, all mothers do not experience all of these discomforts, and, indeed, some mothers pass through the entire antepartal period without any complaints of this type. While the discomforts are not serious in themselves, their presence detracts from the mother's feeling of comfort and wellbeing. In many instances they can be avoided by preventive measures, or entirely overcome by common sense in daily living, once they do occur.

Frequent Urination

One of the first signs the young woman may notice to make her suspect she might be pregnant is the frequent desire to empty her bladder. This is caused by the pressure of the growing uterus against the bladder and will subside about the second or the third month, when the uterus expands upward into the abdominal cavity. Later, during the last weeks of pregnancy the symptoms will recur.

Nausea

Nausea and vomiting of mild degree, the so-called morning sickness, constitute the most common disorder of the first trimester of pregnancy. Symptoms usually appear about the end of the fourth or sixth week and last until about the twelfth week. Nausea occurs in about 50 percent of all pregnancies; of these, about one-third experience some vomiting. Usually, it occurs in the morning only, but a small percentage of patients may have nausea and vomiting throughout the entire day.

Altered hormonal status, with high levels of HCG and progesterone, are involved in producing these symptoms through their effects upon gastrointestinal smooth musculature. Changes in carbohydrate metabolism and other metabolic processes may also contribute.

For many years it has been thought that this condition has an emotional basis. In all life's encounters, there are probably few experiences which are so anxiety provoking as the realization by a woman that she is pregnant. At first there is the anxious uncertainty before she can be sure of the diagnosis. Then, there are numerous adjustments that have to be made and responsibilities that may seem to be overwhelming. Emotionally, the implications of pregnancy extend far back into her childhood. It is understandable that women who cannot adjust to all these new circumstances could have problems. Moreover, whether causative or not, the stress of pregnancy and all its ramifications can contribute to the symptoms caused by the metabolic changes associated with pregnancy.

Manifestations. The typical picture of morning sickness starts with the woman experiencing a feeling of nausea on arising in the morning. She is unable to retain her breakfast, but by noon she has completely recovered and has no further episodes until the next morning. The nausea does not always occur in the morning, but may happen in the afternoon or in the evening. In a small percentage of women the nausea and vomiting may persist throughout the day and even be worse in the afternoon. With the majority of women this problem lasts from one to three months and then suddenly ceases. There may be a slight loss of body weight but no other signs or symptoms.

Management. Often this condition can be controlled, or at least relieved. Various before-breakfast remedies often are used. Taking a dry piece of toast or a cracker a half-hour before getting out of bed may produce relief. In some instances sips of hot water (plain or with lemon juice), hot tea, clear coffee, or hot milk have been tried, with success. However, the dry carbohydrate foods seem to be more effective. After remaining in bed for about a half hour after taking these remedies, the woman gets up and dresses slowly (meanwhile sitting as much of the time as possible). After this she is usually ready for her breakfast.

Greasy foods and those known to cause disagreeable aftereffects should be avoided in the diet. Other suggested remedies include eating an increased amount of carbohydrate foods during this period of disturbance or eating simple and light food five or six times a day instead of three regular full meals. Unsweetened popcorn during the morning is sometimes advised. Another helpful remedy is sweet lemonade, about half a lemon to a pint of water sweetened with milk sugar. Such a drink is usually welcome following a bout of vomiting. Small amounts of ginger ale or cola drink also may be helpful.

Nausea and vomiting, once established, are difficult to overcome; therefore, it is especially desirable to prevent the first attack, or at least to control this condition as soon as possible after it develops. Vomiting can deplete the system of necessary nutrients at a time when daily health should be maintained.

Pregnancies differ, and what may help one person may not benefit another. The trial-and-error method often is necessary to obtain results. If persistent vomiting develops, as it does with a small number of women, the condition is no longer considered to be a minor discomfort but a serious complication. (See Chapter 31, Complications of Pregnancy.)

Heartburn

This is a neuromuscular phenomenon which may occur any time throughout gestation. As a result of the diminished gastric motility which normally accompanies pregnancy, reverse peristaltic waves cause regurgitation of the stomach contents into the esophagus. It is this irritation of the esophageal mucosa which causes heartburn. It may be described as a burning discomfort diffusely localized behind the lower part of the sternum, often radiating upward along the course of the esophagus. Although referred to as heartburn, it really has nothing to do with the heart. Often it is associated with other gastrointestinal symptoms, of which acid regurgitation, belching, nausea, and epigastric pressure are most troublesome. Nervous tension and emotional disturbances may be a precipitating cause. Worry, fatigue, and improper diet may contribute to its intensity.

Very little fat should be included generally in the diet. Although fatty foods are especially aggravating in this disturbance, strangely enough, the taking of some form of fat, such as a pat of butter or a tablespoon of cream, a short time before meals acts as a preventive because fat inhibits the secretion of acid in the stomach. However, this will not help if the heartburn is already present.

Home remedies are not to be used to relieve this condition. Usually some alkaline preparation is prescribed because it gives the best results. However, *sodium bicarbonate is not to be used,* because the sodium ion tends to promote water retention. It is important to make sure that the patient understands this point. Equally effective medications are aluminum compounds, such as aluminum hydroxide gel, or this medication in tablet form with magnesium trisilicate.

Flatulence

This is a somewhat common and very disagreeable discomfort. Usually it is due to undesirable bacterial action in the intestines, which results in the formation of gas. Eating only small amounts of food which are well masticated may prevent this feeling of distress after eating. Regular daily elimination is of prime importance, as is the avoidance of foods that form gas; beans, parsnips, corn, sweet desserts, fried foods, cake, and candy. If these measures fail to relieve the condition, the physician should be consulted.

Backache

Most pregnant women experience some degree of backache. As pregnancy advances, the woman's posture changes to compensate for the weight of the growing uterus. The shoulders are thrown back as the enlarging abdomen protrudes, and, in order for body balance to be maintained, the inward curve of the spine is exaggerated. The relaxation of the sacroiliac joints, in addition to the postural change, causes varying degrees of backache following excessive strain, fatigue, bending, or lifting.

The woman can be advised early in pregnancy how to prevent such strain through measures such as good posture and body mechanics in everyday living and avoidance of fatigue. Appropriate shoes worn during periods of activity and a supporting girdle may be helpful (see Clothing, p. 278).

The key to good posture is to sit, stand, walk and lie in a way that minimizes the hollow or curvature of the lower back. To do this, the abdominal and gluteal muscles are contracted and those of the lower back relaxed, while the pelvis is tilted slightly upward and forward. Sitting posture can be improved by using armrests, foot supports, and a pillow for the back. The tailor position or lotus position used for yoga are useful for relief of back pain (Fig. 20-6). The mother should always bend from the knees rather than the back when lifting, keeping the spine straight. Avoiding forward leaning while doing chores helps prevent strain on the back and is facilitated by adjusting the height of the work surface or the mother's position to maintain proper posture when standing or sitting.[8]

A woman who has a pendulous abdomen, with a weak abdominal wall that allows the uterus to fall forward, will experience severe back pain, in addition to a "drawing sensation" in the abdomen and general discomfort in walking or standing. Relief measures for any persistent complaint can be prescribed as needed.

Dyspnea

Difficult breathing or shortness of breath occasionally results from pressure on the diaphragm by the enlarged uterus and may be sufficient in the last weeks of pregnancy to interfere considerably with the patient's sleep and general comfort. Usually it

Figure 20-6. Tailor sitting position to relieve backache.

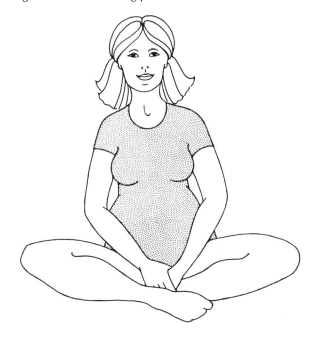

is not a serious condition, but unfortunately it cannot be wholly relieved until after "lightening" (the settling of the fetus into the pelvic cavity with relief of the upper abdominal pressure) or after the birth of the baby, when it will disappear spontaneously. It is most troublesome when the patient attempts to lie down, so that her comfort may be greatly enhanced by propping her up in bed with pillows. In this semisitting posture she at least will sleep better and longer than with her head low. It is well for the nurse to demonstrate how these pillows may be arranged comfortably so that the patient's back is adequately supported.

In patients with known heart disease, shortness of breath, especially of rather sudden onset, may be a sign of oncoming heart failure and should be reported at once to the physician.

Varicose Veins

Varicose veins or varices may occur in the lower extremities and, at times, extend up as high as the external genitalia or even into the pelvis itself. A varicosity is an enlargement in the diameter of a vein due to a thinning and stretching of its walls. Such distended areas may occur at short intervals along the course of the blood vessel; they give it a knotted appearance. Varicosities generally are associated with hereditary tendencies and are enhanced by advancing age, multiple pregnancy, and activities which require prolonged standing.

During pregnancy the pressure in the pelvis due to the enlarged uterus, which presses on the great abdominal veins, interferes with the return of the blood from the lower extremities. Added to this, any debilitating condition favors the formation of varicosities in the veins because of the general flabbiness and lack of tone in the tissues.

Naturally, the greater the pressure in the abdomen, the greater will be the tendency to varicose veins of the lower extremities and the vulva. Therefore, any occupation which keeps a patient constantly on her feet, particularly in the latter part of pregnancy, causes an increase in abdominal pressure and so acts as an exacerbating factor.

Symptoms. The first symptom of the development of varicose veins is a dull aching pain in the legs due to distention of the deep vessels. Inspection may show a fine purple network of superficial veins covering the skin in a lacelike pattern, although this does not always appear. Later, the true varicosities appear, usually first under the bend of the knee, in a tangled mass of bluish or purplish veins, often as large as a lead pencil. As the condition advances, the varicosities extend up and down the leg along the course of the vessels, and in severe cases they may affect the veins of the labia majora, the vagina, and the uterus.

Management. The treatment consists in promptly abandoning any constricting garters, stockings, or other clothing that will cause pressure, particularly on the legs or thighs. If varicosities persist in spite of this precaution, the patient can be taught to take the right-angle position, that is, to lie on the bed with her legs extended straight into the air at right angles to her body, with her buttocks and heels resting against the wall (Fig. 20-7). At first, this position is taken for two to five minutes several times a day, and that will soon demonstrate what can be accomplished. For some patients this position is very uncomfortable at first; but if it is explained, and the discomfort is therefore anticipated, the patient is less likely to discontinue the exercise. Late in pregnancy this position may be too difficult to assume because of pressure against the diaphragm.

Figure 20-7. Right-angle position for swelling, edema and varicosities of legs.

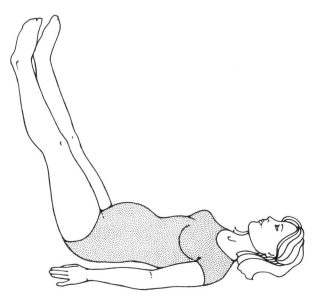

To give support to the weak-walled veins, either an elastic stocking or elastic bandage often is recommended. The initial cost of elastic stockings is somewhat more than that of bandages, but they are easier to put on, more effective, have a neater appearance and a longer usefulness than bandages. A regular nylon stocking put on over the elastic hose further improves the appearance. Many hosiery companies are manufacturing "support" hose which do not have the strength of the elastic stockings but are very effective in giving a moderate amount of support. This type of stocking is useful in cases in which the varicosities are very mild or may not even be apparent peripherally, but are suspected because of the ache they produce. Many women who must be on their feet a great deal and do not have the opportunity to rest frequently wear these stockings during working hours as a "prophylactic" measure. The nurse can be very helpful in apprising mothers of the varieties of hose now available which will meet the needs of individual patients.

The patient also must be told that the stocking or the bandage should be removed at night for greater comfort and reapplied in the morning after the legs have been elevated so that the vessels will be less dilated. The longer stockings or bandage is more satisfactory when the varicosities are above the knee. Both the elastic stocking and bandage are washable; indeed, washing helps to maintain their original elasticity. However, mild soap rather than detergent should be used.

Varicosities of the vulva may be relieved by placing a pillow under the buttocks and elevating the hips for frequent rest periods or by taking the elevated Sim's position for a few moments several times a day (Fig. 20-8). Patients suffering from this condition should not stand when they can sit, and they should not sit when they can lie down.

More important than the treatment of this condition is its prevention. Every pregnant woman should be advised to sit with her legs elevated whenever possible. And when the legs are elevated, care should be taken to see that there are no pressure points against the legs to interfere with the circulation, particularly in the popliteal space. Tight constricting garments, round garters, constipation, standing for long periods of time and an improper amount of rest all tend to aggravate this condition.

A varicose vein in the vagina may rupture during the antepartal or intrapartal period, but this is rare. The hemorrhage is venous and can be controlled

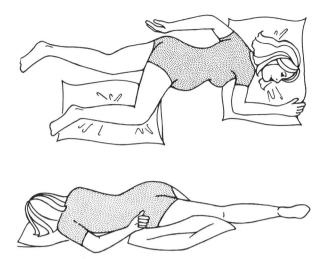

Figure 20-8. Sims's position for varicosities of vulva and rectum.

readily by pressure. The foot of the bed can be markedly elevated.

Cramps

Cramps are painful spasmodic muscular contractions in the legs. They may occur at any time during the pregnancy, but more generally during the later months due to pressure of the enlarged uterus on the nerves affecting the lower extremities. Other causes have been attributed to fatigue, chilling, tense body posture and insufficient or excessive calcium in the diet. They are commonly noted after the use of diuretics.

A quart of milk in the daily diet has been generally recommended to meet the calcium needs during pregnancy. However, studies show that large quantities of milk or dicalcium phosphate predispose to muscular tetany and leg cramps as a result of the excessive amount of phosphorus absorbed from these products. Some authorities suggest that small quantities of aluminum hydroxide gel be taken with the quart of milk because it removes some of the dietary phosphorus from the intestinal tract. Immediate relief may be obtained by forcing the toes upward and by making pressure on the knee to straighten the leg. Elevating the feet and keeping the extremities warm are preventives.

Cramps, while not a serious condition, are excruciatingly painful for the duration of the seizure.

If the husband has been taught the procedure for immediate relief, much pain will be prevented.

Edema

Swelling of the lower extremities is very common during pregnancy and is sometimes very uncomfortable. It is especially likely to occur in hot weather. Often it may be relieved by a proper abdominal support or by resting frequently during the day. Elevating the feet or taking the right-angle position often gives relief (see Fig. 20-7). If the swelling is persistent, the patient may have to stay in bed, but ordinarily this condition proves to be no more than a discomfort.

However, edema is one of the symptoms of toxemia, and it must never be overlooked.

When edema of the lower extremities is observed, careful investigation should be made to see if other parts are affected—the hands or the face, and so on. The condition should be reported to the physician at once.

Vaginal Discharge

In pregnancy there is increased vaginal secretion so that a moderately profuse discharge at this time usually has no particular significance. However, it is wise to instruct the patient to call any copious and/or yellow or greenish foul-smelling or irritating discharge to the attention of the physician. For instance, a profuse yellow discharge may be regarded as a possible evidence of gonorrhea or trichomonas (see Chapter 33), especially when it is accompanied by such symptoms as vaginal itching or burning, or by such urinary manifestations as burning on urination and frequency. A smear or culture may be taken, and the microscopic result will indicate whether or not definite treatment is necessary.

If any discharge becomes irritating, the patient may be advised to bathe the vulva with a solution of sodium bicarbonate or boric acid. The application of KY jelly after bathing often relieves the condition entirely. Instructing a patient to wear a perineal pad is sometimes all the advice that is needed. A douche never should be taken unless prescribed by the physician.

Trichomonas. A particularly stubborn form of leukorrhea in pregnancy is caused by the parasitic protozoan known as the *Trichomonas vaginalis.* It is characterized not only by a profuse frothy discharge (white or yellowish in color), but also by irritation and itching of the vulva and the vagina. The diagnosis is easily made by taking a small quantity of the fresh vaginal discharge and examining it under the microscope in a hanging-drop or wet prep. Here the spindle-shaped organisms, somewhat larger than leukocytes, with whiplike processes attached, can be seen in active motion.

Trichomonas vaginitis is treated with AVC cream, Vagisec suppositories or trichofuron cream. Although oral Flagyl (metronidazole) is highly effective, it is contraindicated during pregnancy because of its potential for fetal abnormalities.[9] Simultaneous treatment of the sexual partner is recommended, usually with oral Flagyl, as the infection is transmitted via sexual contact although males are generally asymptomatic.

Candidiasis. Candidiasis, a yeast infection caused by the *Candida albicans,* is another common cause of profuse vaginal discharge. The organism is frequently present in the vaginal canal without producing symptoms, but during pregnancy the physical changes in the vagina produce conditions that foster its development. It is characterized by white patches on the vaginal mucosa and a thick cottage-cheeselike discharge which is extremely irritating, so that burning or pruritus is present. Even the external genitalia often become inflamed, and occasionally extensive edema is observed. Bleeding may accompany the other symptoms if the patches on the mucosa are removed in any way.

It is not necessary to treat patients in whom *Candida* are found if signs and symptoms are not present. Specific fungicidal suppositories, such as mycostatin, are used to treat this condition. Although this treatment is effective, the infection is stubborn and likely to recur and require repeated treatment during the pregnancy. The *pruritus,* or itching of the skin, may be relieved to a marked degree if proper hygienic measures are employed to keep the area free of the irritating material being deposited on the skin surface.

The woman who has this infection may transmit it to her infant during the process of delivery. *Thrush* develops when the organisms attack the mucous membrane of the infant's mouth.

PREPARATIONS FOR THE BABY

Layette

The baby's layette and equipment are of real interest to all parents—in fact, they are interesting to almost everyone. The cost of the layette should be in keeping with the individual economic circumstances. The entire layette can be purchased ready-made or can be made at home quite inexpensively. Much or little may be spent in its preparation, but nurses who are teaching parents should know why certain types of clothes and equipment are preferable.

Baby clothing should have the following characteristics: it should be comfortable, lightweight and easy to put on and launder. Any clothing which comes in contact with the infant's skin should be made of soft cotton material. Wool should be avoided since it can irritate an infant's skin. Knitted materials are preferred because they are easy to launder and can stretch sufficiently to allow more freedom in dressing the baby. Caution should be taken that the materials are fire-resistant. Garments that open down the full length and fasten with ties or grippers are easier to put on. Ties or grippers are also safer than buttons.

The geographic location and climate will greatly influence the selection of the infant's clothing. Size 1 shirts and gowns are recommended, since the infant grows rapidly in the first six months and quickly outgrows garments. It is well to remember that clothing should not inhibit the baby's normal activities. The complete outfit of clothes that the baby wears need not weigh more than 12 to 16 ounces.

The mother can be advised to prepare a very simple layette. As she sees how fast her baby grows, and what is needed, the additional items can be secured. The complete layettes which can be purchased often contain unnecessary items and are often costly. Also, many articles may be received as baby gifts. Therefore, it is wise to choose only those things which are necessary for immediate use.

Layette necessities include:

five or six shirts

three to four dozen diapers (if diaper service is not used)

four to six receiving blankets (These are very versatile items and can be used in various ways. For instance, they can be rolled firmly and used

to support the back when the infant is on his side; in emergencies, they can be used as bathtowels, diaper pads, sheets.)

three to six nightgowns, kimonos, or sacques

six cotton covered waterproof diaper pads (11" x 16")

two waterproof protectors for under diaper pads

two afghans or blankets } (if climate is cold)
one bunting

two to four soft towels (40" x 40")

two to four soft washcloths

Nursery equipment should consist of:

basket, bassinet or crib

mattress (firm, flat and smooth)

mattress protector (waterproof)

sheets or pillowcases for mattress

chest or separate drawer

cotton crib blankets

bathtub

diaper pail

toilet tray—equipped

absorbent cotton—or cotton balls

baby soap (bland, white, unscented)

rustproof safety pins

soapdish

bath apron (for mother)

table, for bath or dressing

chair (for mother)

Additional suggestions for layette and equipment are:

sweaters	footstool
crib spreads	diaper bag (for traveling)
bibs	disposable diapers
clothes drier	nursery light
chest of drawers	carriage
nursery stand	

Some further suggestions in relation to the selection of specific items are as follows:

Shirts, Gowns, and the Like. The sleeves should have roomy armholes, such as the raglan-type sleeve. If a pullover-type garment is used, the neck opening should be so constructed that it is large enough to be put on easily over the feet or the head.

Diapers. Of the several varieties of diapers available, gauze diapers are most widely used. The selection of diapers should be considered from the standpoint of their comfort (soft and light in weight), absorbency and washing and drying qualities. The mother who plans to use a commercial diaper service may either use the company's diapers or her own. Disposable diapers are also available, but they are generally more expensive in the long run than cloth diapers or a diaper service.

Receiving Blankets. These should be made of cotton flannelette 1 yard square. This square is used to fold loosely about the baby. If properly secured, the baby may lie and kick and at the same time keep covered and warm. In the early weeks these squares take the brunt of the service and in this way save the finer covers from becoming soiled so quickly.

Afghans or Blankets. These can be of very lightweight cotton or polyester material. The temperature and the weather will determine the amount of covering needed.

Sheets. Crib sheets are usually 45″ x 72″ and are available in muslin, percale, and knitted cotton materials. The knit sheets are practical for bottom sheets and do not need to be ironed. Pillowcases are very usable for the carriage or the basket mattress. Receiving blankets may be used for top sheets.

Waterproof Sheeting. Various waterproof materials are suitable to protect the mattress and to be used under the pads. Even though the mattress may have a protective covering, it is necessary to have a waterproof cover large enough to cover the mattress completely—something that can be removed and washed.

Waterproof Pants. These offer protection for special occasions. If the plastic variety is used, they should not be tight at the leg or the waist. For general use, a square of protective material such as Sanisheeting or a cotton quilted pad can be used under the baby next to the diaper.

Bath Apron. This is a protection for both mother and baby and may be made of plastic material covered with terry cloth.

Nursery Equipment

In choosing the equipment, again the individual circumstances should be considered. Expense, space, and future plans all influence the selection. Most nurseries are planned for the satisfaction of the parents. Eventually the baby's room becomes the child's room; and if economy must be considered, furniture should be selected that will appeal to the child as he grows and develops.

Bed. A basket, bassinet, or crib may be used as the baby's bed. The trimming on the basket or the bassinet should be such that it can be removed easily and laundered. A bed may be improvised from a box or a bureau drawer, placed securely on a sturdy table or on chairs which are held together with rope. Many parents may have a carriage that may be used as a bed. However, after about the first two months, the baby will need a crib. The crib should be constructed so that the bars are close enough together to prevent the baby's head from being caught between them. If it is painted, a paint "safe for babies" should be used, that is, nonleaded.

Mattress. The mattress is to be firm (not hard) and flat. All mattresses, including the waterproof-covered, can be protected by a waterproof sheeting to prevent the mattress from becoming stained and from absorbing odors. The waterproof sheet is easily washed and dries quickly.

Bathtub. The plastic tub is safe and easy to keep clean. Some mothers adapt the kitchen or bathroom sink for the baby's bath.

Diaper Pail. This should be large enough for at least the day's supply of soiled diapers. It may be used also for boiling the diapers.

USE OF COMMUNITY RESOURCES

The nurse in the office or the clinic who is alert to such actual or potential health problems that affect both the woman and her family recognizes that a home visit by a community health nurse often is very helpful. If such a situation arises, she can tell the woman about available community health services and explain what this nurse might do while making a home visit and how such a visit can be beneficial. With the physician's knowledge and the woman's permission, she can institute a referral through the proper channels. Each institution or agency will have its particular method and procedure.

ANTEPARTAL NURSING CARE

Assessment	Intervention	Evaluation
Physiological status of pregnancy	Take general health history and obstetric history, physical examination and laboratory tests as part of antepartal workup; continuing surveillance at return visits.	Identification of EDC, minor health problems (i.e., anemia, UTI), complications of pregnancy, concurrent disease, high risk factors
Psychosocial status of pregnancy	Provide patient profile, identifying data, family composition, attitudes toward pregnancy, knowledge levels, expectations related to pregnancy, family and personal resources, coping mechanisms, economic situation.	Identification of actual and potential problems, sources of strength, resource networks, information gaps.
Health maintenance needs	Provide information about ways to promote health and well-being during pregnancy; i.e., rest, exercise, work, recreation, travel, medications and immunizations, skin care, breast care, clothes, teeth, bowel habits, douching, smoking, sexual relations, and alcohol use.	Identify areas needing improvement, inquire into changes in behaviors, determine if sense of well-being is improved following changes. Note areas that continue to be problems.
	Refer to appropriate health professional or agency when significant problems are identified.	Follow-through of referral and of recommendations and treatment plans.
Minor discomforts	Provide information and instruction about occurrence and alleviation of such discomforts as urinary frequency, nausea and vomiting, heartburn, constipation, flatulence, hemorrhoids, backache, dyspnea, varicosities, leg cramps, and vaginal discharge.	Identify present discomforts and determine whether remedies advised improved symptoms, or if understanding alleviated concern.
	Refer to physician or other health professional if difficulties persist or present significant interference with daily activities.	Follow-through of referral and of recommendations and treatment plans.
Prenatal educational needs	Provide specific information and instruction related to growth and development of the fetus,	Patient affirms understanding, has no further questions, has become involved in classes, has

ANTEPARTAL NURSING CARE (Continued)

Assessment	*Intervention*	*Evaluation*
	progression of pregnancy, physical and emotional changes, prenatal management routines, preparation for childbirth; or refer to sources providing these educational services (i.e., childbirth classes, nutritionist).	made preparations for labor and delivery and for infant care at home.
Indicators of complications of pregnancy (i.e., rising blood pressure, facial edema, bleeding, excessive weight gain, inappropriate fundal measurements for dates, etc.)	Notify physician, obtain additional physical data and laboratory tests as indicated, explain to patient the meaning of symptoms and signs and the plan of care.	Control or alleviation of signs and symptoms of complications. Patient affirms understanding and cooperates with treatment plans.
Indicators of stress and psychosocial problems (i.e., missed appointments, noncompliance, affect, direct expression of concerns, acting out behavior of children, complaints)	Determine sources of problems, whether economic, interpersonal, due to emotional illness, cultural discrepancies, conflicts with the system of health care, etc. Provide counseling according to level of skills, refer as needed for more intensive therapy. Utilize community resources for socioeconomic, cultural disparity problems. Work with agency and health team to improve patient relations if this is a problem.	Patient affirms improvement of the problem, follows through on referrals, implements suggestions and recommendations and reports these have been helpful. Some concrete indicators could be initiation of family therapy, application for social relief or medical care assistance, keeping appointments and complying with treatment.

Real value may be derived from a visit in which the nurse is able to see the woman in her usual surroundings. For instance, if the woman has the problem of excessive weight gain and is not responding to clinic therapy, the community health, nurse can visit the home and gain some insight into the basis of the problem. In her report to the clinic or the office staff, she would relate information that would contribute to both the medical and the nursing management of this pregnancy.

In situations in which the clinic program is limited in educational opportunities, such as parents' classes and/or individual guidance, the community health nurse's visit to the home may be necessary to supplement the health care teaching and anticipatory guidance done in the clinic.

Role of the Community Health Nurse

The nurse in the community is "home-based" in either an official or a voluntary agency. The official health agency may have an antepartal clinic offering complete antepartal services for those families who are having financial crises that may or may not be a result of the pregnancy.

If the woman and/or her family has a problem that the clinic nurse thinks needs follow-up in the home (between clinic visits), she will contact the community health nurse (CHN) and communicate the necessary information. In turn, the community health nurse will inform the clinic personnel of any pertinent findings. If complete comprehensive care is to be given to patients, open lines of communication and an expeditious interagency referral system are basic to the best service of all members of the health team, whatever their level of responsibility.

Home Visits.   The district community health nurse does not follow a stereotyped routine when she makes her home visits, since each visit involves an individual patient in her own home setting. She does not have the "captive audience" that the hospital nurse does; rather she is a guest in the woman's home, and this involves a somewhat different approach and orientation. In such a situation, it is especially important to orient the visit to what the woman wants and needs to know. Repeated visits based on the *nurse's* needs (to impart certain information, instruction, and so on) may very well result in a firmly closed door and a consequent severing of the nurse-patient relationship.

Astute assessment of the situation at each visit includes, first of all, finding out what the woman needs to know. Communication and observation skills (previously mentioned) are, of course, of paramount importance here. It is the wise nurse who takes her cues from the mother and handles each need as it arises without feeling compelled to "teach" a certain amount of material each visit. If the visits are managed in this way, topics may include basic information about pregnancy, hygiene, and nutrition, specific preparations for the baby, how to handle sibling rivalry, and so on. These subjects may come up naturally in the course of the visits, or the nurse can guide conversation around to them as she explores with the mother certain areas of need. By the end of the antepartal supervision period, all necessary counseling usually can be accomplished.

Opportunities for Family Health Supervision.
During the course of antepartal care, the nurse has many opportunities for family health supervision. In her observation of other children in the home, she may be the first person to notice a neglected orthopedic condition, to suspect a need for a chest roentgenogram, or to observe a possible vision or hearing difficulty. In addition, observation of the mother's interaction with her children may give valuable clues to the woman's mothering patterns. This will aid the nurse in planning more effective anticipatory guidance and health teaching.

The Medical Social Worker

Although nursing care is the primary consideration in this section, one member of the extended health team will be mentioned specifically since she works so closely with the nurse in the care of the pregnant woman. Most hospitals today have a substantial Social Service Department; it is hoped that more community health agencies will be able to take advantage of this service as more funds and personnel make this possible.

The function of Social Service workers is to help people to meet and to cope with problems that interfere with social functioning. These problems may include unmarried parenthood, divorce, desertion, placing older children during the mother's hospital stay, arranging for a working housekeeper, planning convalescent care for the mother, or arranging financial or material assistance.

In their professional role, social workers are called on to evaluate these problems. Then, with the patient's cooperation, they help her to mobilize her resources and assist her, when necessary, through referral and counseling to alleviate the condition. They may make home visits and interview the patient, and perhaps other family members, to aid them in diagnosing the extent of the problems.

Social problems may seem overwhelming if the patient's physical condition is affected, and these concerns, in turn, may interfere with the benefit that the patient may derive from medical services. The social worker may act as an understanding counselor between the family and the patient during her hospital stay. In many hospitals the need for a social service referral is apparent when the patient is registered early in pregnancy. In that event, the patient is interviewed after the initial medical examination, and from both the physical and the social findings plans are made with the patient to mobilize her resources.

By her observation, counseling, and liaison work, the social worker combines her efforts with the other members of the health team to see the patient not only as an individual maternity patient, but also as an important member of the family, and the family as an integral part of the community.

Summary

Comprehensive antepartal care, then, is a quality of patient care that is goal-directed toward the total health and the well-being of the pregnant woman and her family. With this as the central objective, the combined efforts of several disciplines, in addition to those of medicine and nursing, may be required in the cooperative plan to achieve the ultimate goals. The practitioner–patient relationship is reciprocal, involving one giving and the other receiving care, and, to be meaningful, it must be a positive interaction. This type of interaction can be achieved only if the patient and her problems are understood and viewed with respect. The patient, in turn, must be helped to understand the goals of the health practitioners.

A positive effort on the part of the health team becomes possible if each member has a clear understanding of his or her own role, appreciates and understands the contribution of the other professions represented on the team, knows something of the processes involved in the differing approaches, recognizes commonality of interest and skill, and has the intellectual and the emotional capacity to enter into a team relationship.

REFERENCES

1. L. M. Grimm: "Changed patterns of obstetric care: Maternity continuity clinic." *Am. J. Nurs.* 73:1723–1725, Oct. 1973.
2. H. E. Thompson, et al.: "Factors contributing to improved maternal care and fetal outcome in a medium-sized city-county hospital." *Am. Ob-Gyn.* 116:229–238, May 15, 1973.
3. Public Law 93-641, 88 Stat. 2236, 93rd Congress, S. 2994, January 4, 1975, pp. 6–7.
4. Elizabeth S. Holey: "Promoting adequate weight gain in pregnant women." *MCN, J. Maternal Child Nursing*, 2, 2:86–89, March/April 1977.
5. "Drugs and therapeutic information." In Safety of Immunizing Agents in Pregnancy. *Medical Letter of Drugs and Therapeutics* 18, 291:5, March 6, 1970.
6. Mary B. Meyer; "How does maternal smoking affect birth weight and maternal weight gain?" *Am. J. Obstet. Gynecol.* 131:888–893, Aug. 15, 1978.
7. Ralph C. Benson: *Current Obstetric and Gynecologic Diagnosis and Treatment*, ed. 2. Palo Alto, Calif. Lange Medical Publishers, 1978, p. 592.
8. Sandra B. Cooper: "Preventing back abuse in young mothers." *MCN, J. Maternal Child Nursing*, 2, 4:260–263, July/Aug. 1977.
9. "Is Flagyl dangerous?" *The Medical Letter* 17:53–54 1975.

SUGGESTED READING

Anderson, S. F.: "Childbirth as a pathological process: An American perspective." *MCN, J. Maternal Child Nursing*, 2, 4:240–244, July/Aug, 1977.

Bancroft, A. V.: "Pregnancy and the counterculture." *Nurs. Clin. North Am.* 8:67–76, March 1973.

Block, D.: "Some crucial terms in nursing: What do they really mean?" *Nurs. Outlook* 22, 11:689–694, Nov. 1974.

Erikson, M. P.: "Trends in assessing the newborn and his parents." *MCN, J. Maternal Child Nursing*, 3, 2:99–103, March/April 1978.

Jordan, A. D.: "Evaluation of a family-centered maternity care hospital program." *JOGN Nursing* 2, 1:13–35, Jan./Feb. 1973.

Kennell, J. H., et al.: "Attachments begin in fixed period after birth." *Ob. Gyn. News* 9, 20: 37, Oct. 15, 1974.

Kowalski, K. E.: "Changed patterns of obstetric care on call staffing." *Am. J. Nurs.* 73, 10: 1725–1727, Oct. 1973.

LaFage, W. L.: "A reversal of roles for the maternity nurse—New insights." *MCN, J. Maternal Child Nursing*, 2, 5:313–314, Sept./Oct. 1977.

244   Levine, M. M., et al.: Live-virus vaccines in
245 pregnancy: Risks and recommendations." *Lan-*
246 *cet* 2:7871, July 6, 1974.
247   Martin, L. M.: *Health Care of Women.* Philadelphia, J. B. Lippincott, 1978.

Otte, M. J.: "Correcting inverted nipples."
Am. J. Nurs. 75:454–456, March 1975.

Intrapartal Assessment and Management

Presentation and Positions
Phenomenon of Labor
Conduct of Normal Labor
The Nurse's Contribution to Pain Relief
Analgesia and Anesthesia for Labor and Delivery

Twenty-One

Presentations and Positions

Fetal Habitus / Fetal Head / Presentations / Positions /
Fetal Skull Measurements / Diagnosis of Fetal Position

FETAL HABITUS

Habitus, or attitude, of the fetus means the relation of the fetal parts to one another. The most striking characteristic of the fetal habitus is flexion. The spinal column is bowed forward, the head is flexed with the chin against the sternum, and the arms are flexed and folded against the chest. The lower extremities also are flexed, the thighs on the abdomen and the calves of the lower legs against the posterior aspect of the thighs. In this state of flexion the fetus assumes a roughly ovoid shape, occupies the smallest possible space, and conforms to the shape of the uterus. In this attitude it is about half as long as if it were completely stretched out. However, there are times when the fetus assumes many other positions.

FETAL HEAD

From an obstetric viewpoint the head of the fetus is the most important part. If it can pass through the pelvic canal safely, there is usually no difficulty in delivering the rest of the body, although occasionally the shoulders may cause trouble.

The cranium, or skull, is made up of eight bones. Four of the bones—the sphenoid, the ethmoid, and the two temporal bones—lie at the base of the cranium, are closely united, and are of little obstetric interest. On the other hand, the four bones forming the upper part of the cranium are of great importance; these are the frontal, the occipital, and the two parietal bones. These bones are not knit closely together at the time of birth but are separated by membranous interspaces called *sutures.* The intersections of these sutures are known as *fontanels* (Fig. 21-1).

By means of this formation of the fetal skull the bones can overlap each other somewhat during labor and so diminish materially the size of the head during its passage through the pelvis. This process of overlapping is called "molding," and after a long labor with a large baby and a snug pelvis, the head often is so definitely molded that several days may elapse before it returns to its normal shape.

The most important sutures are: the sagittal, between the two parietal bones; the frontal, between the two frontal bones; the coronal, between the frontal and the parietal bones; and the lambdoid, between the posterior margins of the parietal bones and the upper margin of the occipital bone. The temporal sutures, which separate the parietal and

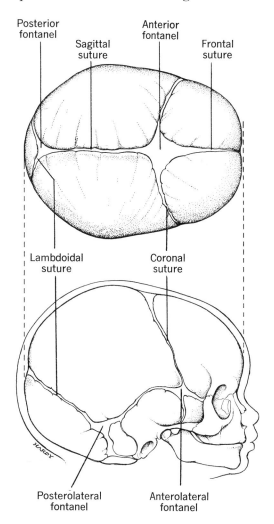

Posterior fontanel

Sagittal suture

Anterior fontanel

Frontal suture

Lambdoidal suture

Coronal suture

Posterolateral fontanel

Anterolateral fontanel

Figure 21-1. Fetal skull showing fontanels and sutures: *above,* superior aspect; *below,* lateral aspect. (From Chaffee, E. E., and Lytle, I. M.: *Basic Physiology and Anatomy,* ed. 4. Philadelphia, J. B. Lippincott, 1980.)

the temporal bones on either side, are unimportant in obstetrics because they are covered by fat parts and cannot be felt on the living baby.

The fontanels of importance are the anterior and the posterior. The anterior fontanel, large and diamond-shaped, is at the intersection of the sagittal and the coronal sutures, while the small triangular posterior fontanel lies at the junction of the sagittal and the lambdoid suture. The sutures and the posterior fontanel ossify shortly after birth, but the anterior fontanel remains open until the child is over a year old, constituting the familiar "soft spot" just above the forehead of an infant.

By feeling or identifying one or another of the sutures or fontanels, and considering its relative

position in the pelvis, one is able to determine accurately the position of the head in relation to the pelvis.

PRESENTATION

The term *presentation* or *presenting part* is used to designate that portion of the infant's body which lies nearest the internal os, or, in other words, that portion which is felt by the examining fingers when they are introduced into the cervix. When the presenting part is known, by abdominal palpation, it is possible to determine the relation between the long axis of the baby's body and that of the mother.

Head or *cephalic presentations* are the most common, being present in about 97 percent of all cases at term. Cephalic presentations are divided into groups, according to the relation which the infant's head bears to its body (Fig. 21-2). The most common is the *vertex presentation,* in which the head is sharply flexed so that the chin is in contact with the thorax; then the vertex is the presenting part. The *face presentation,* in which the neck is sharply extended so that the occiput and the back come in contact, is more rarely observed.

The breech presentation is the next most common, being present in about 3 percent of cases. In breech presentations the thighs may be flexed and the legs extended over the anterior surface of the body (*frank breech presentation*), or the thighs may be flexed on the abdomen and the legs on the thighs (*full breech presentation*), or one or both feet may be the lowest part (*foot or footling presentation*).

When the fetus lies crosswise in the uterus, it is in a "transverse lie," and the shoulder is the presenting part—*shoulder presentation.* The common causes of a "transverse lie" are: 1) abnormal relaxation of the abdominal walls due to great multiparity, 2) pelvic contraction, and 3) placenta previa. Shoulder presentations are relatively uncommon, and, with very rare exceptions, the spontaneous birth of a fully developed child is impossible in a "persistent transverse lie."

POSITIONS

In addition to knowing the presenting part of the baby, it is important to know the exact position of this presenting part in relation to the pelvis. This

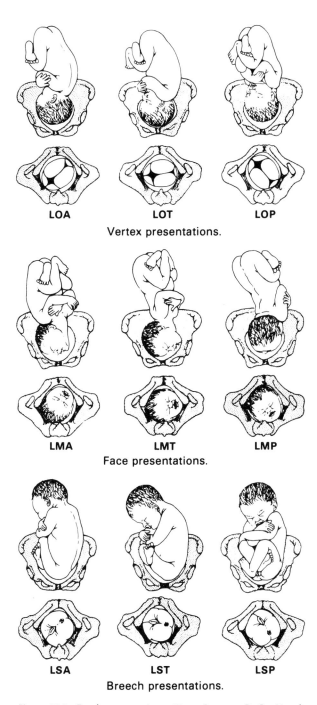

LOA LOT LOP
Vertex presentations.

LMA LMT LMP
Face presentations.

LSA LST LSP
Breech presentations.

Figure 21-2. Fetal presentations. (From Benson, R. C.: *Handbook of Obstetrics and Gynecology*. Los Altos, California, Lange Medical Publications.)

relationship is determined by finding the position of certain points on the presenting surface and relating these to the four imaginary divisions or regions of the pelvis. For this purpose the pelvis is considered to be divided into quadrants: left ante-

rior, left posterior, right anterior and right posterior. These divisions aid in indicating whether the presenting part is directed toward the right or the left side and toward the front or the back of the pelvis.

Certain points on the presenting surface of the baby have been arbitrarily chosen as points of direction in determining the exact relation of the presenting part to the quadrants of the pelvis. In vertex presentations the occiput is the guiding point; in face presentations, the chin (mentum); in breech presentations, the sacrum; and in shoulder presentations, the scapula (acromion process).

Position, then, has to do with the relation of some arbitrarily chosen portion of the fetus to the right or the left side of the mother's pelvis. Thus, in a vertex presentation, the back of the head (occiput) may point to the front or to the back of the pelvis. The occiput rarely points directly forward or backward in the median line until the second stage of labor, but usually is directed to one side or the other.

The various positions are usually expressed by abbreviations made up of the first letter of each word which describes the position (see list of abbreviations). Thus, left occipitoanterior is abbreviated L.O.A. This means that the head is presenting with the occiput directed toward the left side of the mother and toward the front part of the pelvis. If the occiput were directed straight to the left with no deviation toward front or back of the pelvis, it would be termed left occipitotransverse, or L.O.T. The occiput might also be directed toward the back or posterior quadrant of the pelvis, in which case the position would be left occipitoposterior, or L.O.P. There are also three corresponding positions on the right side: R.O.A., R.O.T. and R.O.P. (Fig. 21-2).

The occipital positions are considered the most favorable for both mother and baby, and of these, the L.O.A. position is preferred.

The same system of terminology is used for face, breech, and shoulder presentations, as indicated in the following list of abbreviations (S indicating breech; M, chin or face; and A, shoulder).

Although it is customary to speak of all "transverse lies" of the fetus simply as shoulder presentations, the examples of terminology sometimes used to express position in the shoulder presentation are listed. Left acromiodorso-anterior (L.A.D.A.) means that the acromion is to the mother's left and the back is anterior.

FETAL PRESENTATIONS:ABBREVIATIONS

Positions—Vertex Presentation

L.O.A.—Left occipitoanterior
L.O.T.—Left occipitotransverse
L.O.P.—Left occipitoposterior
R.O.A.—Right occipitoanterior
R.O.T.—Right occipitotransverse
R.O.P.—Right occipitoposterior

Positions—Breech Presentation

L.S.A.—Leftsacroanterior
L.S.T.—Left sacrotransverse
L.S.P.—Left sacroposterior
R.S.A.—Right sacroanterior
R.S.T.—Right sacrotransverse
R.S.P.—Right sacroposterior

Positions—Face Presentation

L.M.A.—Left mentoanterior
L.M.T.—Left mentotransverse
L.M.P.—Left mentoposterior
R.M.A.—Right mentoanterior
R.M.T.—Right mentotransverse
R.M.P.—Right mentoposterior

Positions—Shoulder Presentation

L.A.D.A.—Left acromiodorso-anterior
L.A.D.P.—Left acromiodorso-posterior
R.A.D.A.—Right acromiodorso-anterior
R.A.D.P.—Right acromiodorso-posterior

FETAL SKULL MEASUREMENT

Figure 21-3 shows the principal measurements of the fetal skull. The most important transverse diameter is the biparietal; it is the distance between the biparietal protuberances and represents the greatest width of the head. It measures, on an average, 9.25 cm.

There are three important anteroposterior diameters: the suboccipitobregmatic, which extends from the undersurface of the occiput to the center of the anterior fontanel and measures about 9.5 cm.; the occipitofrontal, which extends from the root of the nose to the occipital prominence and measures about 12.0 cm.; and the occipitomental, which extends from the chin to the posterior fontanel and averages about 13.5 cm.

In considering these three anteroposterior diam-

eters of the fetal skull, it is important to note that with the head in complete flexion and the chin resting on the thorax, the smallest of these, the suboccipitobregmatic, enters the pelvis, whereas if the head is extended or bent back (with no flexion whatsoever), the greatest anteroposterior diameter presents itself to the pelvic inlet. Herein lies the great importance of flexion; the more the head is flexed, the smaller is the anteroposterior diameter which enters the pelvis. Figure 21-4 shows this basic principle in diagrammatic form.

DIAGNOSIS OF FETAL POSITION

Diagnosis of fetal position is made in four ways: 1) abdominal palpation; 2) vaginal or rectal examination; 3) combined auscultation and examination; 4) in certain doubtful cases, the roentgenogram.

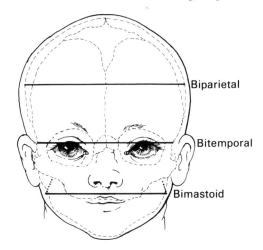

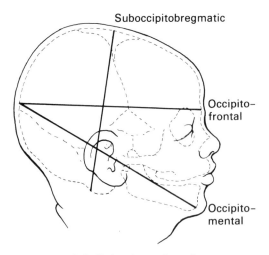

Figure 21-3. Fetal skull showing various diameters.

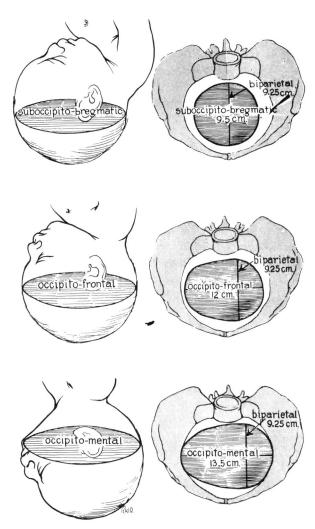

Figure 21-4. (*Top*) Complete flexion allows smallest diameter of head to enter pelvis. (*Center*) moderate extension causes larger diameter to enter pelvis. (*Bottom*) Marked extension forces largest diameter against pelvic brim, but head is too large to enter pelvis.

Palpation

It is extremely helpful to palpate the abdomen before listening to the fetal heart tones. The region of the abdomen in which the fetal heart is heard most plainly varies according to the presentation and the extent to which the presenting part has descended. The location of the fetal heart sounds by itself does not give very important information as to the presentation and the position of the child, but it sometimes reinforces the results obtained by palpation. To obtain satisfactory information by abdominal palpation for the determination of fetal

position, the examination should be made systematically by following the four maneuvers suggested by Leopold, often called the *Leopold maneuvers* (Fig. 21-5).

The patient should empty her bladder before the procedure is begun. This will not only contribute to the patient's comfort but also will aid in gaining more accurate results in the latter part of the examination. The first three maneuvers are conducted at the side of the bed, facing the patient; during the last one the examiner stands to the side, facing the patient's feet.

Although a diagnosis should not be made on the basis of inspection, actual observation of the patient's abdomen should precede palpation. For the examination the patient should lie flat on her back, with her knees flexed, to relax the abdominal muscles. The examiner should lay both hands gently and, at first, flat upon the abdomen. If done in any other manner than this, or if the hands are not warm, the stimulation of the fingers will cause the abdominal muscles to contract. One should accustom oneself to palpating the uterus in a definite, methodical way, and it will be found best to carry out the following four maneuvers.

First Maneuver

The examiner should ascertain what is lying at the fundus of the uterus by feeling the upper abdomen with both hands (Fig. 21-5A). Generally one will find there a mass, which is either the head or the buttocks (breech) of the fetus. Which pole of the fetus this is can be ascertained by observing three points:

1. Its relative consistency: the head is harder than the breech.
2. Its shape: if the head, it will be round and hard, and the transverse groove of the neck may be felt. The breech has no groove and usually feels more angular.
3. Mobility: the head will move independently of the trunk, but the breech moves only with the trunk. The ability of the head to be moved back and forth against the examining fingers is spoken of as ballottement.

Second Maneuver

Having determined whether the head or the breech is in the fundus, the next step is to locate the back of the fetus in relation to the right and the left sides

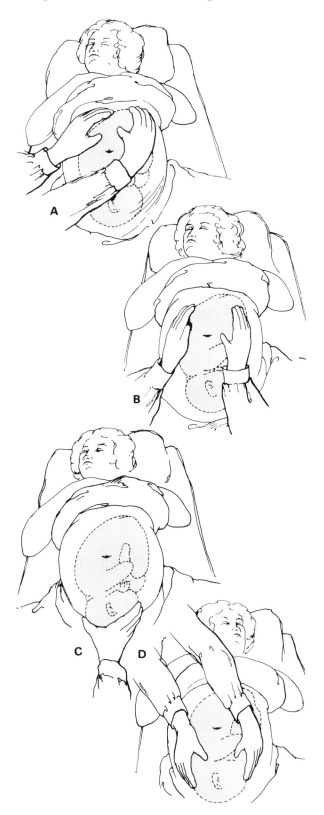

Figure 21-5. Leopold maneuvers: palpation of fetal position.

of the mother. Still facing the patient, the examiner places the palmar surfaces of both hands on either side of the abdomen and applies gentle but deep pressure (Fig. 21-5B). If the hand on one side of the abdomen remains still to steady the uterus, a slightly circular motion with the flat surface of the fingers on the other hand can gradually palpate the opposite side from the top to the lower segment of the uterus to feel the fetal outline. Then, to palpate the other side, the functions of the hands are reversed (i.e., the hand which was used to palpate now remains steady), and the other hand palpates the opposite side of the uterus.

On one side is felt a smooth, hard, resistant plane, the back, while on the other, numerous angular nodulations are palpated, the small parts; these latter represent the knees and the elbows of the fetus.

Third Maneuver

This maneuver consists of an effort to find the head at the pelvic inlet and to determine its mobility. It should be conducted by gently grasping the lower portion of the abdomen, just above the symphysis pubis, between the thumb and the fingers of one hand and then pressing together (Fig. 21-5C). If the presenting part is not engaged, a movable body will be felt which is usually the head.

Fourth Maneuver

This maneuver is conducted while facing the patient's feet. The tips of the first three fingers are placed on both sides of the midline about 2 inches above Poupart's ligament. Pressure is now made downward and in the direction of the birth canal, the movable skin of the abdomen being carried downward along with the fingers (Fig. 21-5D). It will be found that the fingers of one hand meet no obstruction and can be carried downward well under Poupart's ligament; these fingers glide over the nape of the baby's neck. The other hand, however, usually meets an obstruction an inch or so above Poupart's ligament; this is the brow of the baby and is usually spoken of as the "cephalic prominence." This maneuver gives information of several kinds:

1. If the findings are as described above, it means that the baby's head is well flexed.
2. Confirmatory information is obtained about the location of the back, as naturally the back

is on the opposite side from the brow of the baby, except in the uncommon cases of face presentation, in which the cephalic prominence and the back are on the same side.

3. If the cephalic prominence is very easily palpated, as if it were just under the skin, a posterior position of the occiput is suggested.

4. The location of the cephalic prominence tells how far the head has descended into the pelvis. This maneuver is of most value if the head has engaged and may yield no information with a floating, poorly flexed head.

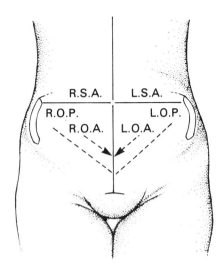

Figure 21-7. Fetal heart tone locations on the abdominal wall indicating possible corresponding fetal positions and the effects of the internal rotation of the fetus.

Vaginal Examination

During a vaginal examination, the fontanels and the suture lines of the fetal skull are identified. Prior to the onset of labor the vaginal examination gives limited information concerning the position of the fetus because the cervix is closed. However, during labor, after dilatation of the cervix, important information about the position of the fetus and the degree of flexion of its head can be obtained, by palpating and identifying the fontanels. When the head is well flexed, the posterior fontanel is easily identified by palpating the junction point of the sagittal suture and the two lambdoid sutures (Fig. 21-6). When the fetal head is well flexed, the anterior fontanel is located well within the birth canal. It is diamond-shaped, having four sutures which lead to it: the sagittal posteriorly, two coronal laterally, and the frontal. One can easily develop skill at identifying these landmarks on the fetal skull by palpating the skull of the newborn after delivery, first, with eyes closed, and then confirming their location visually.

Auscultation

The location of the fetal heart sounds, as heard through the stethoscope, yields helpful confirmatory information about fetal position but is not wholly dependable. Certainly, it never should be

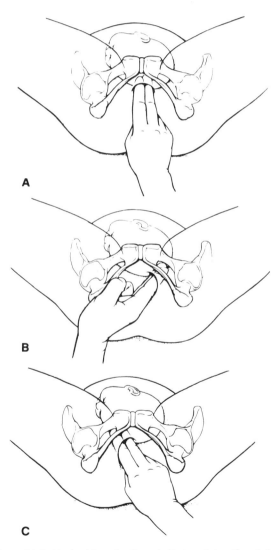

Figure 21-6. Vaginal Examination. *A.* Determining the station and palpating the sagittal suture. *B.* Identifying the posterior fontanelle. *C.* Identifying the anterior fontanelle. (From *The Lipppincott Manual of Nursing Practice,* ed. 2. Philadelphia, J. B. Lippincott Co.)

relied on as the sole means of diagnosing fetal position. Ordinarily, the heart sounds are transmitted through the convex portion of the fetus, which lies in intimate contact with the uterine wall, so that they are heard best through the infant's back in vertex and breech presentations, and through the thorax in face presentation.

In cephalic presentations the fetal heart sounds are heard loudest midway between the umbilicus and the anterosuperior spine of the ilium (Fig. 21-7). In general, in L.O.A. and L.O.P. positions the fetal heart sounds are heard loudest in the left lower quadrant. A similar situation applies to the R.O.A. and R.O.P. positions. In posterior positions of the occiput (L.O.P. and R.O.P.) often the sounds are heard loudest well down in the flank toward the anterosuperior spine. In breech presentation the fetal heart sounds usually are heard loudest at the level of the umbilicus or above.

Roentgenograms

Roentgenograms are of particular value in diagnosis of fetal position in doubtful cases, particularly in obese women or in those with abdominal walls so rigid that abdominal palpation is difficult. In such situations the roentgenogram enables the physician to recognize the existence of conditions which might otherwise have escaped detection until late in labor. They give accurate information concerning position, presentation, flexion and descent of the fetal head (see Fig. 16-6, p. 204).

SUGGESTED READING

Danforth, D. N.: *Textbook of Obstetrics and Gynecology,* ed. 2. New York, Hoeber Medical Division, Harper & Row, 1971.

Greenhill, J. P., and Friedman, E. A.: *Biological Principles and Modern Practice of Obstetrics.* Philadelphia, W. B. Saunders, 1974.

Pritchard, J. A., and MacDonald, P. C.: *Williams Obstetrics,* ed. 15. New York, Appleton-Century-Crofts, 1976.

Twenty-Two

Phenomena of Labor

Premonitory Signs of Labor / Cause of Onset of Labor / Uterine Contractions / Duration of Labor /The Three Stages of Labor

Labor refers to the series of processes by which the products of conception are expelled by the mother. Childbirth, parturition, accouchement, and confinement are also terms for thse processes. The actual birth of the baby is called delivery.

PREMONITORY SIGNS OF LABOR

During the last few weeks of pregnancy a number of changes indicate that the time of labor is approaching. Particularly in primigravidas, "lightening" occurs about 10 to 14 days before delivery. This alteration is brought about by a settling of the fetal head into the pelvis. This may occur at any time during the last four weeks, but occasionally does not occur until labor actually has begun. Lightening may take place suddenly, so that the expectant mother arises one morning entirely relieved of the abdominal tightness and diaphragmatic pressure that she had experienced previously.

But the relief in one direction often is followed by signs of greater pressure below, such as shooting pains down the legs from pressure on the sciatic nerves, an increase in the amount of vaginal discharge and greater frequency of urination due to pressure on the bladder. In mothers who have had previous children, lightening is more likely to occur after labor begins.

True Labor vs. False Labor For a varying period before the establishment of true labor, women often experience "false labor." The nurse can distinguish between this and effective uterine contractions, as true labor contractions will produce a demonstrable degree of dilatation of the cervix in the course of a few hours, while false labor contractions do not affect the cervix. The crux of the matter, then, between true and false labor is whether or not the uterine contractions affect cervical effacement and dilatation.

False contractions may begin as early as three or four weeks before the termination of pregnancy. They are merely an exaggeration of the intermittent uterine contractions which have occurred throughout the entire period of gestation but now may be accompanied by discomfort. They are confined chiefly to the lower part of the abdomen and the groin and do not increase in intensity, frequency, and duration. The discomfort is rarely intensified if the mother walks about and may even be relieved if she is on her feet. Examination will reveal no changes in the cervix.

The signs that accompany true labor contractions present a contrasting picture. True labor contractions usually are felt in the lower back and extend in girdlelike fashion from the back to the front of the abdomen. They have a definite rhythm and gradually increase in frequency, intensity, and duration. In the course of a few hours of true labor contractions, a progressive effacement and dilatation of the cervix is apparent.

Show. Another sign of impending labor is pink "show." After the discharge of the mucous plug that has filled the cervical canal during pregnancy, the pressure of the descending presenting part of the fetus causes the minute capillaries in the cervix to rupture. This blood is mixed with mucus and therefore has the pink tinge. It must be differentiated from substantial discharge of blood, which would indicate a medical complication.

Rupture of the Membranes. Occasionally, rupture of the membranes is the first indication of approaching labor. It used to be thought that this was a grave sign, heralding a long and difficult dry labor, but present-day statistics show that this is not true. Nevertheless, the physician must be notified at once; under these circumstances, the patient may be advised to enter the hospital immediately.

After the rupture of the membranes there is always the possibility of a prolapsed cord if the presenting part does not adequately fill the pelvic inlet. This is more likely if the infant presents as a footling breech, or by the shoulder, or in the vertex presentation when the fetal head has not descended far enough into the true pelvis prior to the rupture of the membranes.

CAUSE OF ONSET OF LABOR

In mammalian species, whether the fetus weighs 2 gm. at the end of a 21-day pregnancy, as in the mouse, or whether it weighs 200 pounds at the end of a 640-day pregnancy, as in the elephant, labor usually begins at the right time for that particular species, namely, when the fetus is mature enough to cope with extrauterine conditions but not yet large enough to cause mechanical difficulties in labor. The process responsible for this beautifully synchronized and salutary achievement has not yet been clearly identified.

The uterus during pregnancy consists of a large number of greatly hypertrophied smooth muscle cells. Each cell is activated by a series of chemical reactions to begin rhythmic contractions in a highly coordinated way, and with such force that the cervix is dilated and the baby expelled. The fundamental question is what stimulates these uterine cells, at a precise time in most pregnancies, to begin labor contractions. Various theories have been advanced to explain the onset of labor. It appears that several mechanisms are involved in initiating and maintaining labor, each having varying importance depending upon individual circumstances.

Progesterone Deprivation Theory

Progesterone, secreted first by the corpus luteum, and then by the placenta, is essential in maintaining pregnancy. Since the uterus is composed of smooth muscle, and most smooth muscle organs will contract when stretched, it is significant that the uterus remains quiescent throughout the greater part of pregnancy. This suggests that some substance is acting to inhibit uterine contractility. Progesterone is the most likely substance, and the role of a "progesterone block" in the maintenance and termination of pregnancy has been upheld by some investigators for many years. In several animal species, this theory is well supported by studies showing a drop in maternal progesterone with a rise in estrogen, which has opposite effects on uterine musculature, before labor begins. This could not be documented in humans until recently, when new methodology was able to identify a fall in circulating progesterone with a continuing increase of estrogen in a study population of women during the five weeks preceding labor. The onset of labor in humans is felt to result, then, from withdrawal of progesterone at a time of relative estrogen dominance.[1]

Oxytocin Theory

It has been clearly demonstrated that the human uterus is increasingly sensitive to oxytocin as pregnancy advances. Oxytocin is an effective stimulant of uterine contractions in late pregnancy and is commonly used to induce or augment labor. While oxytocin-like activity in the blood has been found in women during labor, with the highest concentration during the second stage, it is also present in both males and females having surgery. It is possible that any stress may release this hypophyseal hormone. Also, blood contains an enzyme which promptly inactivates oxytocin. Humans as well as several other mammals, still go into labor normally when the hypophysis has been removed or destroyed. While oxytocin alone seems unlikely as initiator of the labor process, it may well be significant in combination with other substances.

Fetal Endocrine Control Theory

At the appropriate time of fetal maturity, it appears that the fetal adrenals secrete cortical steroids which are felt to trigger the mechanisms leading to labor. Shortly before labor, the sensitivity of the fetal adrenal to ACTH, produced by the pituitary, increases. As a result, the production of cortisol increases. In laboratory studies with sheep, destruction of the fetal pituitary or hypothalamus (which would interfere with ACTH production) leads to prolonged pregnancy. In contrast, administration of ACTH or cortisol directly to the fetus leads to premature labor.[2]

Cortical steroids are released during periods of stress, which suggests one cause of premature labor in the instance when the fetus is compromised. Conditions which cause decreased blood flow to the uterus, such as toxemia or uterine overdistention due to multiple pregnancy or polyhydramnios, are known to be related to premature labor. These conditions also compromise the fetus, and thus could be implicated in fetal release of cortical steroids. The suggested mechanism of action is that fetal steroids stimulate the release of precursors to prostaglandins which in turn produce uterine labor contractions.

Prostaglandin Theory

Research has shown prostaglandins to be very effective in inducing uterine contractions at any stage of gestation.[3] Prostaglandins are formed by the uterine decidua, and their concentration in the amniotic fluid and blood of women increases during labor. Study of the mechanisms of prostaglandin synthesis has shown that arachidonic acid, the oblig-atory precursor to prostaglandin, increases markedly in comparison to the other fatty acids in the amniotic fluid of women in labor. Arachidonic acid injected into the amniotic sac during the second trimester is highly effective in producing abortion, while other fatty acids do not induce labor. It is hypothesized that initiation of human labor results from a sequence of events including the release of lipid precursors possibly triggered by steroid action, release of arachidonic acid from these precursors perhaps at the site of the fetal membranes, increased prostaglandin synthesis from the arachidonic acid, and increased uterine contractions as a consequence of prostaglandin action on the uterine muscle.[4]

UTERINE CONTRACTIONS

The degree of discomfort during labor varies considerably from patient to patient. The patient who anticipates a painful experience generally will have more pain than the patient who is properly prepared for what can be a good experience. To allay preexisting fear, one should refer to uterine contractions as *contractions,* not *pains.* The duration of these contractions ranges from 45 to 90 seconds, averaging about one minute.

Each contraction presents three phases: a period during which the intensity of the contraction increases (increment), a period during which the contraction is at its height (acme), and a period of diminishing intensity (decrement). The increment, or crescendo phase, is longer than the other two combined.

The contractions of the uterus during labor are intermittent, with periods of relaxation between, resembling, in this respect, the systole and the diastole of the heart. The interval between contractions diminishes gradually from about ten minutes early in labor to about two or three minutes in the second stage. These periods of relaxation not only provide rest for the uterine muscles and for the mother, but also are essential to the welfare of the fetus, since unremitting contractions may so interfere with placental functions that the resulting lack of oxygen produces fetal distress.

Another characteristic of labor contractions is that they are quite involuntary, their action being not only independent of the mother's will, but also of extrauterine nervous control.

During labor, the uterus is soon differentiated into two identifiable portions—the upper and lower uterine segments. The upper segment is the active, contractile portion of the uterus. Its function is to expel the uterine contents. It displays a decreasing gradient of intensity of contractions from the fundus downward. As labor progresses, a passive lower segment is developed. With each contraction, the muscle fibers of the upper segment retract, becoming shorter as the fetus descends. The upper segment, therefore, becomes thicker. Fibers of the lower segment stretch and, consequently, it becomes thinner. The distinct boundary between the upper and lower uterine segments is called a physiologic retraction ring.

DURATION OF LABOR

Although there is usually some degree of variation in all labors, an estimate of the average length of labor can be based on studies of records of some several thousand primigravidas and multiparas.

The average duration of first labors is about 14 hours, approximately 12½ hours in the first stage, 1 hour and 20 minutes in the second stage, and 10 minutes in the third stage.

The average duration of multiparous labors is approximately six hours shorter than for first labors: for example, seven hours and 20 minutes in the first stage, a half hour in the second stage, and ten minutes in the third stage.

During the first stage of labor full dilatation of the cervix (10 cm.) is accomplished, but for the greater part of this time the progress of cervical dilatation is slow. This has been clearly demonstrated in Friedman's study of 500 labors of primigravidas. From his study labor is divided into the latent phase and the active phase. The *latent phase,* from the onset of uterine contractions, takes many hours and accomplishes little cervical dilatation. But with the beginning of the *active phase,* cervical dilatation proceeds at an accelerated rate and then reaches a deceleration phase shortly before the second stage of labor.

The first 4 cm. of cervical dilatation occurs during the slow, latent phase. The remainder of cervical dilatation is accomplished much more rapidly in the active phase. Hence, 5 cm. of dilatation has taken the patient well past the halfway point in labor, even though 10 cm. represents full dilatation. In fact, at that point the average labor is more than two-thirds over.

THE THREE STAGES OF LABOR

The process of labor is divided, for convenience of description, into three distinct stages.

The first stage of labor, or the dilating stage, begins with the first true labor contraction and ends with the complete dilatation of the cervix. This stage may be further subdivided into the latent phase and the active phase.

The second stage of labor, or the stage of expulsion, begins with the complete dilatation of the cervix and ends with the delivery of the baby.

The third stage of labor, or the placental stage, begins with the delivery of the baby and terminates with the birth of the placenta.

The First Stage of Labor

At the beginning of the first stage the contractions are short, slight, 10 or 15 minutes or more apart and may not cause the woman any particular discomfort. She may be walking about and is generally quite comfortable between contractions. Early in the first stage the sensation is usually located in the small of the back, but, as time goes on, it sweeps around, girdlelike, to the anterior part of the abdomen. The contractions recur at shortening intervals, every three to five minutes, and become stronger and last longer.

When labor has progressed to the active phase, the woman usually prefers to remain in bed as ambulation is no longer comfortable. She becomes intensely involved in the sensations within her body and tends to withdraw from the surrounding environment.

As cervical dilatation progresses to 8 to 9 cm., the contractions reach peak intensity. This phase, between 8 to 10 cm. dilatation, is called *transition,* and is frequently the most difficult and painful time for the woman. At this time, there is usually a marked increase in the amount of show due to rupture of capillary vessels in the cervix and the lower uterine segment.

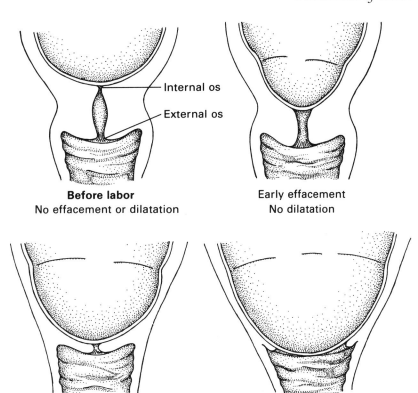

Before labor
No effacement or dilatation

Early effacement
No dilatation

Complete effacement
No dilatation

Complete dilatation

Figure 22-1. There are several stages in cervical effacement and dilatation.

As the result of the uterine contractions, two important changes occur in the cervix during the first stage of labor—*effacement* and *dilatation*.

Cervical effacement is the shortening of the cervical canal from a structure 1 or 2 cm. in length to one in which no canal at all exists, but merely a circular orifice with almost paper-thin edges. As may be seen in Figure 22-1, the edges of the internal os are drawn several centimeters upward, so that the former endocervical canal becomes part of the lower uterine segment. In primigravidas, effacement is usually complete before dilatation begins, but in multiparas it is rarely complete, dilatation proceeding, as a rule, with rather thick cervical edges.

The terms *obliteration* and *taking up* of the cervix are synonymous with effacement. Effacement is measured during pelvic examination by estimating the percentage by which the cervical canal has shortened. For example, in a cervix 2 cm. long before labor, 50 percent effacement has occurred when the cervix measures 1 cm. in length.

Dilatation of the Cervix. This means the enlargement of the cervical os from an orifice a few millimeters in size to an aperture large enough to permit the passage of the fetus—that is, to a diameter of about 10 cm. When the cervix can no longer be felt, dilatation is said to be complete.

Although the forces concerned in dilatation are not well understood, several factors appear to be involved. The muscle fibers about the cervix are so arranged that they pull upon its edges and tend to draw it open. The uterine contractions cause pressure on the amniotic sac and this, in turn, burrows into the cervix in pouchlike fashion, exerting a dilating action. In the absence of the membranes, the pressure of the presenting part against the cervix and the lower uterine segment has a similar effect.

Measurement of cervical dilatation is done during pelvic examination through digital estimation of the diameter of the cervical opening. It is expressed in centimeters, and often tactile charts are available in labor rooms to help the examiner translate into centimeters the mental picture obtained during this "blind" examination.

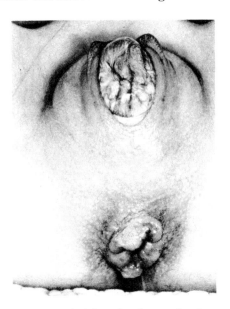

Figure 22-2. Extreme bulging of perineum showing patulous and everted anus.

Dilatation of the cervix in the first stage of labor is solely the result of uterine contractions which are involuntary. In other words, there is nothing that the mother can do, such as bearing down, which will help the slightest in expediting this period of labor. Indeed, bearing-down efforts at this stage serve only to exhaust the mother and cause the cervix to become edematous.

The Second Stage of Labor

The contractions are now strong and long, lasting 50 to 70 seconds and occuring at intervals of two or three minutes. Rupture of the membranes usually occurs during the early part of this stage of labor, with a gush of amniotic fluid from the vagina. Sometimes, however, membranes rupture during the first stage and occasionally before labor begins. In rare cases the baby is born in a "caul," which is a piece of the amnion that sometimes envelops the baby's head. According to superstitious beliefs this is considered to be a good omen.

During this stage, as if by reflex action, the muscles of the abdomen are brought into play; and when the contractions are in progress the woman will strain, or "bear down," with all her strength so that her face becomes flushed and the large vessels in her neck distended. As a result of this exertion she may perspire profusely. During this stage the mother directs all her energy toward expelling the contents of the uterus. There is a marked pressure in the area of the perineum and rectum, and the urge to bear down is usually beyond her control.

Toward the end of the secondstage, when the head is well down in the vagina, its pressure causes the anus to become patulous and everted (Fig. 22-2), and often small particles of fecal material may be expelled from the rectum with each contraction. This should receive careful attention to avoid contamination. As the head descends still further, the perineal region begins to bulge, and the skin over it becomes tense and glistening. At this time the scalp of the fetus may be detected through a slitlike vulvar opening. With each subsequent contraction the perineum bulges more and more, and the vulva becomes more dilated and distended by the head, so that the opening is gradually converted into an ovoid and at last into a circle. With the cessation of each contraction the opening becomes smaller, and the head recedes from it until it advances again with the next contraction.

The contractions now occur very rapidly, with scarcely any interval between. As the head becomes increasingly visible, the vulva is stretched further and finally encircles the largest diameter of the baby's head. This encirclement of the largest diameter of the baby's head by the vulvar ring is known as "crowning." An episiotomy is usually done at this time, while the tissues surrounding the perineum are supported and the head delivered. One or two more contractions are normally enough to effect the birth of the baby.

Whereas in the first stage of labor the forces are limited to uterine action, during the second stage two forces are essential, namely, uterine contractions and intraabdominal pressure, the latter being brought about by the bearing-down efforts of the mother. (The force exerted by the mother's bearing down can be likened to that used in forcing an evacuation of the bowels.) Both forces are essential to the successful spontaneous outcome of the second stage of labor, for uterine contractions without bearing-down efforts are of little avail in expelling the infant, while, conversely, bearing-down efforts in the absence of uterine contractions are futile. As explained in Chapter 23, Conduct of Normal Labor, these facts have most important practical implications.

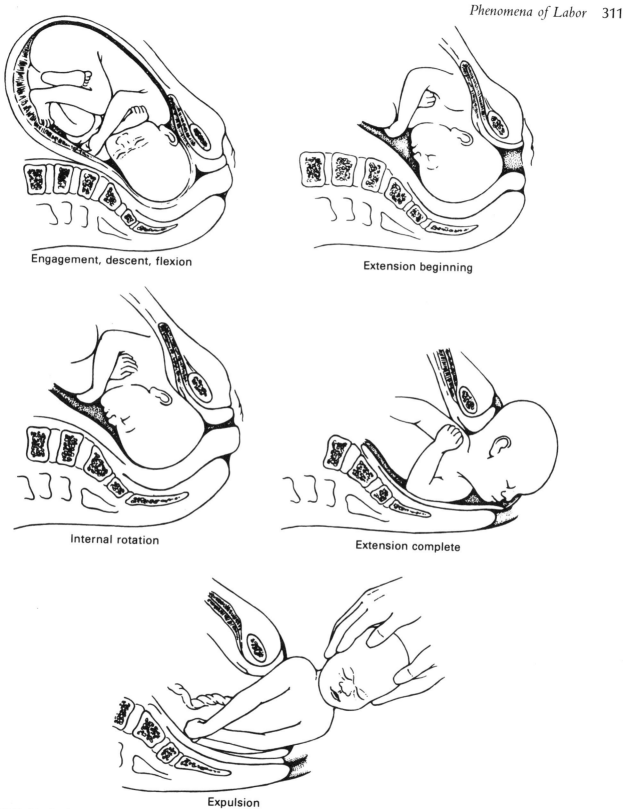

Engagement, descent, flexion

Extension beginning

Internal rotation

Extension complete

Expulsion

Figure 22-3. Mechanism of labor.

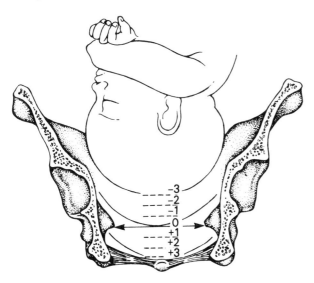

Figure 22-4. Stations of the fetal head.

The Mechanism of Labor

In its passage through the birth canal, the presenting part of the fetus undergoes certain positional changes which constitute the mechanism of labor. These movements are designed to present the smallest possible diameters of the presenting part to the irregular shape of the pelvic canal, so that it will encounter as little resistance as possible.

The mechanism of labor consists of a combination of movements, several of which may be going on at the same time. As they occur, the uterine contractions bring about important modifications in the attitude or habitus of the fetus, especially after the head has descended into the pelvis. This adaptation of the baby to the birth canal, as descent takes place, involves four processes, flexion, internal rotation, extension and external rotation (Fig. 22-3).

For purposes of instruction, the various movements will be described as if they occurred independently.

Descent. The first requisite for the birth of the infant is descent. When the fetal head has descended such that its greatest biparietal diameter is at, or has passed, the pelvic inlet, the head is said to be *engaged*. This provides a clear indication that the pelvic inlet is large enough to accommodate the widest portion of the fetal head and is, therefore, of adequate size. For the average fetal head, the linear distance between the occiput and the plane of the biparietal diameter is less than the distance between the pelvic

inlet and the ischial spines. Thus, when the occiput is at the level of the spines, its biparietal diameter has usually passed the pelvic inlet, and the vertex is therefore engaged. However, one cannot assume that engagement has occurred simply because the vertex is at the spines. When the fetal head has been molded markedly, with consequent increase in the distance between the occiput and the biparietal diameter, the vertex may be felt at the spines, but its greatest diameter may still be above the pelvic inlet.

SUMMARY OF STAGES OF LABOR

First Stage—Dilating Stage

Definition Period from first true labor contraction to complete dilatation of cervix.

What Is Accomplished Effacement and dilatation of cervix.

Forces Involved Uterine contractions.

Second Stage—Expulsive Stage

Definition Period from complete dilatation of cervix to birth of baby.

What Is Accomplished Expulsion of baby from birth canal—facilitated by certain positional changes of fetus: descent, flexion, internal rotation, extension, external rotation and expulsion.

Forces Involved Uterine contractions plus intraabdominal pressure.

Third Stage—Placental Stage

Definition Period from birth of baby through birth of placenta.

What Is Accomplished (A) Separation of placenta; (B) expulsion of placenta.

Forces Involved (A) Uterine contractions; (B) intraabdominal pressure.

The ischial spines are used as a landmark to describe the relative position of the fetal head in the pelvis (Fig. 22-4). When the vertex is at the level of the spines, it is at 0 station. If 1 cm. below, it is a +1 station; 2 cm. below, +2 station; 3 cm. below, +3 station. When the vertex is 1 cm. above the spines, it is a −1 station; 2 cm. above, −2 station; 3 cm. above, −3 station. This relationship is evaluated during the course of each pelvic examination and recorded, along with the assessment of cervical dilatation and effacement.

In primigravidas, engagement often precedes the onset of labor. This is the process of "lightening" described earlier. Because the vertex is frequently deep in the pelvis at the onset of labor, further descent does not necessarily begin until the second stage of labor. In multiparas, on the other hand, descent often begins with engagement. Once having been inaugurated, descent is inevitably associated with the various movements of the mechanism of labor.

Flexion. Very early in the process of descent the head becomes so flexed that the chin is in contact with the sternum, and, as a consequence, the very smallest anteroposterior diameter (the suboccipito-bregmatic plane) is presented to the pelvis.

Internal Rotation. The head enters the pelvis in the transverse or diagonal position. When it reaches the pelvic floor, the occiput is rotated and comes to lie beneath the symphysis pubis. In other words, the sagittal suture is now in the anteroposterior diameter of the outlet. Although the occiput usually rotates to the front, on occasion it may turn toward the hollow of the sacrum. If anterior rotation does not take place at all, the occiput usually rotates to the direct occiput posterior position, a condition known as persistent occiput posterior. Since this represents a deviation from the normal mechanism of labor, it will be considered in Chapter 33, under Abnormal Fetal Positions.

Extension. After the occiput emerges from the pelvis, the nape of the neck becomes arrested beneath the pubic arch and acts as a pivotal point for the rest of the head. Extension of the head now ensues, and with it the frontal portion of the head, the face, and the chin are born.

External Rotation. After the birth of the head, it remains in the anteroposterior position only a very short time and shortly will be seen to turn to one or another side of its own accord —*restitution.* When the occiput originally has been directed toward the left of the mother's pelvis, it then rotates toward the left and to the right when it originally has been toward the right. This is known as external rotation and is due to the fact that the shoulders having

entered the pelvis in the transverse position, undergo internal rotation to the anteroposterior position, as did the head; this brings about a corresponding rotation of the head, which is now on the outside.

The shoulders are born in a manner somewhat similar to that of the head. Almost immediately after the occurrence of external rotation, the anterior shoulder appears under the symphysis pubis and becomes arrested temporarily beneath the pubic arch, to act as a pivotal point for the other shoulder. As the anterior margin of the perineum becomes distended, the posterior shoulder is born, assisted by an upward lateral flexion of the infant's body. Once the shoulders are delivered, the infant's body is quickly extruded (expulsion).

The Third Stage of Labor

The third stage of labor is made up of two phases: *the phase of placental separation* and *the phase of placental expulsion.*

Immediately following the birth of the infant, the remainder of the amniotic fluid escapes, after which there is usually a slight flow of blood. The uterus can be felt as a firm globular mass just below the level of the umbilicus. Shortly thereafter, the uterus relaxes and assumes a discoid shape. With each subsequent contraction or relaxation the uterus changes from globular to discoid shape until the placenta has separated, after which time the globular shape persists.

Placental Separation. As the uterus contracts down at regular intervals on its diminishing content, the area of placental attachment is greatly reduced. The great disproportion between the reduced size of the placental site and that of the placenta brings about a folding or festooning of the maternal surface of the placenta; with this process separation takes place. Meanwhile, bleeding takes place within these placental folds, and this expedites separation of the organ. The placenta now sinks into the lower uterine segment or upper vagina as an unattached body.

The signs which suggest that the placenta has separated are:

1. the uterus becomes globular in shape and, as a rule, firmer;
2. it rises upward in the abdomen;
3. the umbilical cord descends 3 or more inches farther out of the vagina;

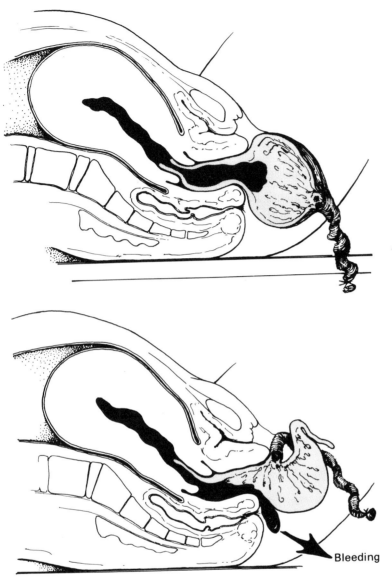

Figure 22-5. Expulsion of the placenta by (*Top*) Schultze's mechanism whereby the placenta is turned inside-out within the vagina and is delivered with the glistening fetal surfaces on the outside and (*Bottom*) by the Duncan mechanism whereby the placenta is rolled up in the vagina and is delivered with the maternal surface on the outside.

Bleeding

4. a sudden gush of blood often occurs.

These signs usually occur within five minutes after the delivery of the infant.

Placental Expulsion.   Actual expulsion of the placenta may be brought about by the mother bearing down if she is not anesthetized. If this cannot be accomplished, it is usually effected through gentle pressure on the uterine fundus. Excessive pressure should be avoided to obviate the rare possibility of "inversion" of the uterus (see Chapter 33).

The extrusion of the placenta may take place by one of two mechanisms. First, it may become turned inside-out within the vagina and be born like an inverted umbrella with the glistening fetal surfaces presenting. This is known as Schultze's mechanism and occurs in about 80 percent of cases. Second, it may become somewhat rolled up in the vagina, with the maternal surface outermost, and be born edgewise. The latter is known as the Duncan mechanism and is seen in about 20 percent of deliveries (Fig. 22-5). It is believed that Schultze's mechanism signifies that the placenta has become detached first at its center, and usually a collection of blood and clots is found in the sac of membranes. The Duncan mechanism, on the other hand, suggests that the placenta has separated first at its edges, and it is in this type that bleeding usually occurs at the time of separation.

The contraction of the uterus following delivery serves not only to produce placental separation but also to control uterine hemorrhage. As the result of this contraction of the uterine muscle fibers, the countless blood vessels within their interstices are clamped shut. Even then, a certain amount of blood loss in the third stage is unavoidable, commonly amounting to 500 cc. or more. It is one of the aims of the conduct of labor to reduce this bleeding to a minimum.

The Fourth Stage of Labor

The first hour postpartum is sometimes referred to as the fourth stage of labor. During this time *restoration of physiologic stability occurs,* following the tumultuous events of labor. It is a period of potential crisis, with increased incidence of hemorrhage, urinary retention, hypotension, and side effects of anesthesia; it requires careful monitoring of uterine contraction, vital signs, and other physiologic indices.

The first hour after the baby's birth is also considered critical for initial formation of the mother-child relationship and consolidation of the family unit.[5] The process of maternal-child attachment is still under study, but it is possible that early parental interactions with the new baby and each other set the tone for the quality of their relationships later. If so, this is a key time for nursing care which includes assessment of potential problems and support of satisfying interactions for the new family.

REFERENCES

1. A. C. Turnbull et al.: "Significant fall in progesterone and rise in oestradial levels in human peripheral plasma before onset of labour." *Lancet* 1:101–103, Jan. 26, 1974.
2. G. C. Liggens: "Adreno cortical related maturational events in the fetus." *Am. J. Obstet. Gynecol.* 126: 931, 1976.
3. S. M. M., Karim: *The Prostaglandins.* New York, Wiley-Interscience, 1972, pp. 73–164.
4. P. C. MacDonald et al.: "Initiation of human parturition. I. Mechanism of action of arachidonic acid." *Am. J. Obstet. Gynecol.* 44:629–636, Nov. 1974.
5. S. S. Rising: "The fourth stage of labor: Family integration." *Am. J. Nurs.* 74:870–874, May 1974.

SUGGESTED READING

Friedman, E. A.: "Patterns of Labor as indication of risk." *Clin. Obstet. & Gnyecol.* 16:172, 1973.
Pritchard, J. A., and MacDonald, R. C.: *Williams Obstetrics,* ed. 15. New York, Appleton-Century-Crofts, 1976.
Taylor, E. S.: *Obstetrics and Fetal Medicine.* Baltimore, Md., Williams & Wilkins, 1977.

Twenty-Three

The Conduct of Normal Labor

DIMENSIONS OF EFFECTIVE NURSING CARE

Perhaps at no other time during the maternity cycle is the nurse in such an advantageous position to give nursing care as during the time of parturition. It is a unique and humbling experience, this miracle of giving birth, not only for the mother and the father, the main participants, but also for the physician and the nurse who share this experience, and upon whom so much depends.

From the parents' point of view, labor looms as a critical period in the process of childbearing; often it is considered by them, and especially by the mother, as the end of a long-drawn-out process rather than the beginning of a new role. Hence they attribute enormous significance to events and people who are necessary and helpful to them at this time. They indicate repeatedly that they consider the nurse in particular to be one of those necessary, helpful people. Such indeed is the case if the nurse utilizes the opportunity.

Effective nursing care during labor provides for maximum well-being and comfort for both mother and infant and at the same time allows the father to participate in the process, insofar as he is able, and to derive a sense of satisfaction from that partici-pation. The nursing intervention is purposeful but flexible, based always on the needs of each individual patient, infant and father.

To execute such care, the nurse must have knowledge and understanding of the course of normal labor, ability to recognize deviations from the normal, and judgment and ability to cope with stressful and emergency conditions. Additional attributes include a mastery of certain skills, both technical and communicative, which can be applied appropriately to meet the exigencies of the situation. The importance of teamwork between physician and nurse should not be overlooked, and it is especially important to keep the physician informed through accurate reporting and recording of the progress of the mother in labor.

However, knowledge and technical ability are not sufficient in themselves, for the nurse must also be able to convey warmth and empathy if nursing care is to be really effective. The empathic nurse is able to enter into the feelings of the patient and at the same time to retain a sense of separateness. Thus, objectivity is maintained, which contributes to more effective care. Yet the worth and the individuality of each mother always are recognized.

In addition, the nurse ought to be accepting and nonjudgmental regarding the behavior of the mother or the father, realizing that this is a stressful period, and that their usual behavior may be drastically different. Sustaining the patient and reinforcing her confidence whenever necessary can help the mother to attain the greatest amount of comfort and satisfaction from the labor experience. By assisting the woman and her husband to mobilize their resources and strengths, the nurse is able to work with them in a positive way and to reinforce their concept of themselves as adequate people.

The mind of the nurse boggles a bit in the face of this considerable responsibility; certainly the young student has some trepidation when called upon to assume these duties. Yet with competent guidance and instruction, efficient means of fulfilling this role can be learned. To help the student and/or young graduate prepare for these responsibilities, the authors in this chapter have focused on both the woman and the nurse as they move through the successive stages of labor. Although it is the mother who truly delivers her infant, the other important people in this event—the husband, the physician, and ancillary personnel—are not to be forgotten, for they also play important roles.

PRELUDE TO LABOR

The prodromal signs heralding the onset of labor begin several weeks before true labor commences. As indicated in Chapter 22, lightening may occur any time during the last four weeks of pregnancy; in primigravidas it usually occurs about ten days to two weeks prior to labor. This phenomenon causes a sensation of decreased abdominal distention produced by the descent of the presenting part of the baby into the pelvis. In multigravidae this may not occur until the labor has begun. The usually painless Braxton Hicks contractions which have occurred intermittently throughout the latter part of pregnancy may increase so much that they become annoying. They may cause the mother many restless or sleepless nights that contribute to her gradually increasing tension and fatigue. Since the rise in the anxiety level contributes to heightened awareness, the mother becomes more sensitive to various stimuli: if the fetus is generally less active, she may worry; if the baby moves more than usual, she may worry. She wonders about the 2- to 3-pound weight loss that may occur three to four days before the onset of labor. Ordinarily this may be an occasion of great rejoicing, but now it may give her some concern. Even the increased vaginal mucous discharge may have an ominous significance for her. The spurt of energy that may occur one to two days before labor begins often leads her into activities that are overfatiguing, and she will need anticipatory guidance from the nurse and the physician to help her to set limits on activity.

This is the time to finish packing her suitcase and to simplify her housekeeping duties. She may want to complete meal preparations for the family's use when she is in the hospital; if this is done daily little by little, then it should not become bothersome. Last-minute details for the care of the other children or the functioning of the household can be taken care of at this time. Short walks in the fresh air are a good way to release extra tension without overfatigue. The mother should be encouraged to achieve a happy balance between activity and rest.

During the latter part of pregnancy the mother will have been instructed about what to do when she thinks labor has begun. As term approaches, it is wise for the nurse to explore with the mother her preparations for coming to the hospital. The mother and father should know approximately how long it will take them to reach the hospital and what alternate means of transportation are available if the father is not able to take her. What entrance to the hospital they should use and what admission procedures they must go through also are important. A tour of the ward for the parents can be arranged during the antepartal period so that they can become more familiar with the surroundings.

THE ONSET OF LABOR

Most physicians instruct their patients to notify them if the labor contractions become rhythmic and regular and/or the bag of water breaks. To adequately prepare the patient for what to expect, and to instruct her on an appropriate course of action, it is necessary that the nurse have an understanding of the physiology of labor as well as other factors.

The nurse, as the person who spends a great deal of time with the patient after admission, is expected to report on the general character of the labor contractions as well as the other manifestations of

TABLE 23-1
DIFFERENTIAL FACTORS IN TRUE AND FALSE LABOR

True Labor	*False Labor*
Contractions:	*Contractions:*
Occur at regular intervals	Occur at irregular intervals
Intervals gradually shorten	Intervals remain long
Intensity gradually increases	Intensity remains the same
Located chiefly in back	Located chiefly in abdomen
Intensified by walking	Walking has no effect; often gives relief
Show:	*Show:*
Usually present	None
Cervix:	*Cervix:*
Becomes effaced and dilated (this can be determined by digital examination)	Usually uneffaced and closed

labor. First, it must be determined whether the patient is actually in labor. Friedman has pointed out that there are no fixed or uniformly applicable rules that can be used at the bedside. We can assume that the patient is in true labor if her contractions continue uninterruptedly and result in dilatation of the cervix.[1] In practice, however, a variety of types of contractions may be apparent; thus the following differential points between true and false labor (Table 23-1) are to be used only as *guidelines* for assessing the state of the mother's labor.

Psychosocial Considerations

Since contact with the patient during the labor and delivery process is very short term, the nurse is faced with the problem of providing high quality care in a short space of time. The key to the problem appears to lie in the ability to utilize whatever time is available, whether it be five minutes or an hour, to provide an atmosphere of receptivity to the patients' needs. The ability to determine needs lies in the perceptions that underlie the collection and diagnosis portions of the nursing process. When effective care is implemented, the nurse's facility with therapeutic communication plus technical understanding and skill are key issues.

There has been a good deal of time and effort spent in nursing research to determine the needs of patients, especially the needs above and beyond those related directly to physiologic and pathologic conditions. These needs have generally been classified as "emotional" or "psychosocial." Whatever their label, they are especially important for consideration in the maternity patient.

Newman's study has indicated that patients when questioned expressed a preponderance of needs that were emotional in origin. These fell into the following general areas: the need to have one's *identity* recognized and maintained in the face of disability, the need to have some *control* over events relating to oneself, and needs deriving from *fear, anxiety* and *loneliness* which become translated into concern for *safety* and *comfort*.[2]

Aiken and Aiken point out that, if we as nurses look at patients' behavior as a probable consequence of our own behavior, and if we then view our own behavior as a force to facilitate patients' behavior, we will be in a better position to understand our patients' behavior. Moreover, we will then be better able to devise specific approaches to facilitate change.[3]

Encouragement. Accordingly, one of the first responsibilities of the nurse is to recognize that, in addition to the physical manifestations, there are these psychosocial factors which influence each mother's pregnancy and have a bearing on her individual needs for care (see Chapter 17). Therefore, every mother deserves encouragement that tends to inspire assurance during her labor. Her discomfort never should be minimized, and an effort can be made to help her to keep in control when her labor is painful. Attention can be directed to the fact that progress is being made and that her efforts to work cooperatively with her labor are helpful and necessary.

Establishment of the Nurse-Patient Relationship

For many a young woman in labor, admission to the maternity unit may mark her first acquaintance with hospitals as a patient. Her immediate reaction may be one of strangeness, loneliness and homesickness, particularly if the father is not permitted to stay with her in the labor room. Regardless of the amount of preparation for this event, whether she is happy or unhappy, whether she wants the baby or not, every mother enters labor with a certain amount of normal tension and anxiety. Moreover, some mothers are thoroughly afraid of the whole process. This may be attributed in part to the fact that the mother's preparation for childbearing has been limited, or she may have been reared in an environment fraught with mysteries and old wives' tales about childbirth. If she has had children previously, she may have had unfortunate and fear-producing experiences. All these factors make her fear understandable.

Rapport, Empathy and Identification

Rapport.   One of the most often talked about, yet not well understood, concepts deemed essential to an effective nurse-patient relationship is *rapport*. Rapport may be thought of as a relationship consisting of interrelated thoughts and feelings that include empathy, compassion, interest and respect for each individual as a unique human being.

Empathy.   One of the crucial components of this type of relationship is *empathy;* that is, the ability to enter into the life of another person, to accurately perceive her *current* feelings and their meanings.[4] The idea of currency is an important one here. Empathy must involve understanding the current feelings of a patient, not her feelings of sometime in the past. Previous perceptions based on earlier experiences with a patient or patients similar to her can be misleading if they block understanding of what the patient is currently experiencing.

Identification.   Perhaps the most important quality necessary for the nurse to begin to empathize with the patient is the ability to identify with the patient. Identification has been described as the mechanism which enables a person to take up any attitude toward another's mental life. Certain changes take place in the ego structure when this mechanism is employed resulting in an expansion of ego boundaries to include the attitude once observed in the other and now made a part of one's self. This type of identification is seen in children as they learn their various social roles, for instance.

However, in the therapeutic relationship, the altered ego structure is only a temporary experience and remains "ego segregated" but available for reality testing and further thought. Certainly to be able to identify and share with another and then revert to one's own identity requires flexibility of the ego boundaries, and this flexibility can become enhanced with repeated use of the mechanism.

After attempting to experience the patient's feelings, the nurse must be able to step back, that is, reestablish normal ego boundaries related to reality.

Intellectual processes can then be used to review what has occurred from three perspectives: 1) what is known about the patient, 2) what is known about herself, 3) what is known from theory. Thus, subjectivity is converted into objectivity and permits valid assessment of needs and problems.

In order for effective nursing therapy to be instituted, empathy must operate within a sound conceptual framework, backed by theoretical knowledge and clinical experience. It is a valuable aid in designing and implementing care, but is not to be considered a substitute for careful planning and rational evaluation. Unfortunately, we do not know if and how empathy can be taught or learned. We do know that the ability to utilize the identification mechanism has something very vital to do with the empathy process. It is to the identification-empathy-rapport linkage that more research needs to be directed.[5]

Positive Communication

In addition to the notion of empathy, the concept of rapport also involves positive communication that contributes to mutual understanding and acceptance. While no "method" or "rules" have yet been determined to establish this positive, therapeutic communication, the student may find the following general behavioral principles useful when attempting to institute an effective relationship.

1. The nurse's verbalization regarding an aspect of the patient's behavior or appearance confronts the patient with the nurse's perception of the immediate situation. This tends to elicit the patient's agreement or disagreement and any subsequent explanation, especially when nondirective probes are used. Here the nurse indicates attention and concern and the patient has the option of responding.

2. By being alert to the patient's cues regarding her various social roles (mother, wife, possible breadwinner, career woman) and by demonstrating a genuine interest in her roles, the nurse can collect more data upon which an evaluation of her immediate and future needs can be based. This allows the patient to keep her identity and gives her some feeling of control in the situation.

3. Communication can be facilitated when the nurse acknowledges an understanding of what

the mother is saying and asks for further clarification.

4. All members of the health team (and family also, if appropriate) ought to be informed of any needs of the patient that cannot be handled by the nurse alone; moreover, subsequent actions by personnel (and family) are to be communicated to the patient so that she may recognize that communication lines are open and her needs and problems are recognized and attended to as they arise. This retards feelings of helplessness and loss of control.

5. Therapeutic communication is more likely to be initiated and facilitated if the nurse assumes a relaxed and/or sitting position, *close* to the patient if possible. Standing at the foot of the bed or in the doorway is not conducive to satisfying conversation. In the hustle and bustle of the labor and delivery suite, the nurse often falls into the habit of "popping in and out" with the result that the mother may never have a chance for more than a routine answer to "How are you coming along?" This, of course, obstructs any attempts at positive communication and promotes the feelings that many mothers have of the delivery staff as being "too busy to care."

The nurse who establishes rapport with the patient will, then, demonstrate understanding and acceptance of the mother. The mother, in turn, is able to trust the nurse, and an effective nurse-patient relationship is facilitated.

Admission to the Hospital

As previously stated, the mother who has been given adequate antepartal care will have received instruction on what to anticipate when she comes to the hospital to have her baby. If this is the mother's first hospital experience, it will be much easier for her if she has been told about the necessary preliminary procedures, such as any vulvar and perineal preparation, the methods of examination employed to ascertain the progress of labor, and the usual routines exercised for her care in the course of labor.

If the mother has not had adequate antepartal care to prepare her, her labor may be rather advanced upon admission and she may not know what to expect. It will then fall to the nurse to reassure this mother and orient her as quickly as possible to the process of labor and the physical environment. In these instances, the ability to make decisive clinical judgments, especially with regard to establishing priorities of care, is extremely helpful and necessary.

The preparation for delivery will of necessity vary in different hospitals, since every hospital has its own admission procedure. Many of the details of management may be accomplished in a number of ways. Very few institutions employ precisely the same technique in preparing a mother for delivery. Actually, the differences are in details only, for the principles are the same everywhere—namely, asepsis and antisepsis, together with careful observation of the mother for any deviations from the normal.

First Impressions. The kind of greeting that the patient receives as she enters the delivery suite is extremely important and sets the tone for future interaction with the health team. Some institutions permit the father to accompany the mother to the area; others prefer to admit the mother first and then let the father remain with her. When the father is present, the nurse should be mindful that he is to be considered and welcomed in an appropriate way, as is the mother.

The mother can be made to feel welcome, expected and necessary (remember that it is she who delivers the baby). More hospitals are allowing not only the father to accompany the mother to the delivery suite, but also other significant persons whom the mother may want to have with her during her labor. Thus, the mother and her companion can be shown to the labor room that she will occupy. She can then be helped, if necessary, to change to the hospital gown and can be made comfortable in a chair or, if she wishes, she can get into bed.

In this chapter we will describe the environment and care that accompany a labor and delivery that is carried out in a conventional labor and delivery suite. A discussion of the environment and care found in alternate birth centers and facilities will be given in Chapter 40. The care given in a conventional setting tends to be accompanied by more technological intervention and more restriction on the patient's activity. However, even in these environments the nurse can still devise ways to maximize the mother's comfort and assist her in carrying out her prepared childbirth techniques.

Orientation

The mother and the father will need to know some of what will be expected of them, and what they in turn can expect as participants in this new situation. Hence, the nurse can begin an orientation to the process of labor as well as to the general environment. It is to be remembered that there is no set form or content for this orientation and no set time for the introduction and the continuation of this process; rather the nurse must first explore what the parents do know about the environment and the labor process, in order to judge what needs to be introduced, reinforced, and so on, and when the most appropriate time to do this would be. An easy conversational manner may be employed rather than a rapid-fire explanation of dos and don'ts.

The rationale for any procedures or restrictions is always given. The patient should not be overloaded with too many stimuli at one time and should be allowed to absorb any new information and explanation before additional material is presented. The nurse can structure the situation to allow the patient to "feed back" information, so as to reveal how much the mother really understands.

Generally, the mother and the father will need to know what procedures and activities will be performed and the reason for them. In addition, the couple should know the limits of the mother's activity and what restrictions of food and fluids there will be. What the patient and the father can expect regarding the progress of labor should be included also (i.e., what will be happening physically, how the mother will be feeling, and how she and her mate can participate in the labor experience). (See Table 23-2.) The father, if present, can be included in any explanations or information since he may be participating in the care of his mate.

As implied, this orientation will continue throughout the entire course of labor and possibly delivery. The nurse will determine when and how each phase will be instituted, according to the cues given by the mother and father.

Admission Information

After making the mother comfortable in the labor room, the nurse will need to find out some rather specific information regarding the mother's general condition (i.e., the frequency, the duration and the intensity of her contractions, the amount and the character of show, and whether the membranes have ruptured or are intact). At this point it is expedient to learn when the first signs of labor became apparent to the mother and the nature and timing of the uterine contractions from that time.

Since the mother's emotional status often has bearing on her physical labor, it is wise to be continuously alert to her behavior—whether she seems *unduly* apprehensive, or whether she is relatively relaxed or calm. Restlessness, excessive conversation, rapid, darting eye movements, arm and body rigidity, and plucking at the bedclothes are all signs of apprehension. The nurse reports all findings as soon as possible.

Although the nurse will want to avoid any outward display of rush or hurry, she should proceed with the admission as quickly as possible. It must be remembered that the mother's labor usually will become progressively stronger; hence the more procedures, orientation, and so on, that can be accomplished early in labor, while she can be more responsive with relative ease, will enhance the patient's comfort and well-being. Also, there generally will be several other people concerned with the care of the mother—the physician, intern, laboratory technician—and they often cannot carry out their activities until the patient is fully admitted. Finally, an expeditious completion of the admission procedures leaves more time for the mother and father to be together before the actual delivery.

Awareness of Physical and Behavioral Signs. The nurse will want to be constantly alert to the physical and behavioral signs associated with the progress of normal labor. She can be extremely helpful by giving the couple anticipatory guidance in this respect so that they will know what to expect during this experience. At the same time, she will watch vigilantly for any sign that may point to abnormal developments. For instance, an increase in pulse rate, a rise in temperature, excessive bleeding, changes in the character of uterine contractions, passage of meconium with a vertex presentation, or alterations in the fetal heart sounds are changes which may have profound implications for the mother's welfare.

Initial Assessment

Initially, the nurse takes the mother's temperature, pulse, respiration and blood pressure and listens to

TABLE 23-2
PARTICIPATION IN LABOR: GUIDELINES TO PARENTS

What is happening	Helping yourself	Breathing pattern in contraction	Other support
PRELUDE TO LABOR Lightening (2–4 weeks before first baby comes) Braxton Hicks contractions may increase Increased vaginal discharge Baby less active Excitement about labor may make sleeping difficult Spurt of energy (1–2 days before labor)	Simplify housekeeping Have hospital suitcase packed Conserve energy Try different relaxation positions		Husband can encourage continued practice of breathing and relaxation techniques
ONSET OF LABOR You may notice any one or a combination of: Regular contractions (felt as backache, pelvic pressure, gas, menstrual cramp, etc.) "Show"—vaginal discharge with pink or red tinge Leaking of fluid You may feel excited and relieved that labor has begun and yet somewhat apprehensive	Check signs; time contractions Call doctor. He will advise you when to go to the hospital Continue usual activity as long as comfortable		Husband can assist with timing of contractions Husband or other companion offers diversion and relieves possible tension-producing situations in the home
EARLY FIRST STAGE Cervix effacing, dilatation beginning Contractions become strong enough so that you feel need to do something Dilatation continuing; contractions becoming somewhat closer and stronger Contractions consume your attention Contractions may cause backache	When contraction starts, take complete breath and try to relax. Continue slow deep breathing through contraction Between contractions rest, read, watch TV, etc. Relax as much as possible in sitting or lying positions Lie on side, breathe deeply and slowly while rocking pelvis very gently throughout contraction		No distracting conversation during contractions Firm pressure against lower back or slow deep massage during contractions
LATE FIRST STAGE Dilatation continuing; contractions becoming closer, markedly stronger, and of longer duration May worry about ability to see labor through	Assume comfortable position Switch to modified breathing pattern, if desired Rest between contractions		Direction in control of relaxation and of breathing rhythm and depth Face sponged with cool cloth; lips moistened Use effleurage (Medication as indicated)
TRANSITION 10–20 strong, long contractions, close together but may be somewhat irregular. These contractions complete dilatation Rectal pressure may cause desire to bear down Possible tremors, nausea, heavy perspiration, hiccoughs, sense of panic	Concentrate on breathing control Use modified breathing Puff out occasionally if there is urge to push Don't hold breath! Don't push!		Reassurance about normality of sensations and probable limit of their duration Remind her this is transition; contractions not endless Understanding acceptance of possible expressions of irritability Do not leave her alone at this point!
SECOND STAGE Contractions change in character, remaining very strong but slightly further apart Continuing strong contractions pushing baby down against pelvic floor and causing stretching, perhaps burning sensation May be afraid to push despite desire Baby's head seen at vaginal opening As doctor slowly delivers head, there may be strong desire to push Shoulders are born one at a time. Relief is experienced as birth of baby is completed	Push toward vaginal opening as directed, relaxing pelvic floor and steadily reinforcing work of uterus Between contractions relax completely While being moved to delivery room, pant deeply through contractions When settled on delivery table, push as directed through contractions, remembering to relax pelvic floor and thighs Rest completely between contractions Pant to control pushing urge; relax thighs If requested to push, push very gently		Pillows arranged to support mother in comfortable position for pushing Direction of pushing effort and encouragement of relaxation between contractions; reassurance that progress is continuing Keep her informed of downward progress baby is making (Transfer to delivery room) (Anesthesia as indicated) (Episiotomy as indicated) Direction for controlled pushing and panting
THIRD STAGE Rhythmical contraction, less intense Abdomen sensitive Placenta delivered	Push as directed Lie back and enjoy baby!		

Maternity Center Association: *Preparation for Childbearing*, ed. 4. New York, 1977, pp. 38–39.

the fetal heart tones. A voided urine specimen will be obtained for the admission specimen and will be examined for protein and glucose content. If the patient is allowed to use the bathroom, a receptacle is placed under the toilet seat since whatever material may be passed per vagina should be examined along with the urine specimen. As soon as possible, a blood specimen is taken to check the hemoglobin or hematocrit concentration. Often the routine serologic testing is done and an additional tube of clotted blood is kept available for use by the blood bank to cross-match a donor if the occasion occurs. If the patient is in labor, the pubic hair may be clipped and the vulva cleansed as prescribed.

Enema

Until recently, an enema was a routine admission procedure. It was deemed a necessity to prevent the presence of stool in the rectum which might impede the descent of the presenting part and also to ensure that no stool would be expelled during delivery which might contaminate the sterile field. It was also thought to enhance the strength of the contractions. However, experience and research indicate that the enema is not so necessary as once believed. In some institutions, the decision to give an enema is left to the nurses on the basis of their clinical judgment. In other hospitals an enema is still required as prescribed. In any case, it is wise for the nurse to ascertain, during the history taking, the state of the mother's bowels. If she has had a normal evacuation that day, an enema is probably not necessary. If the mother is constipated, an enema can be helpful. However, if she is having diarrhea, the procedure is certainly not necessary and the possibility of an infection must be considered.

If an enema is ordered, the cleansing type is given. It may be a disposable type with a prelubricated tube which does not usually cause discomfort if care is taken on insertion and the contents are squeezed in gently. If a water enema is used via the more traditional enema can or bag with tubing, the nurse would use the same principles in administering it as for any other patient. However, it may be more difficult to insert the tube because of the pressure of the presenting part of the fetus or because of hemorrhoids that may accompany pregnancy. Hemorrhoids and/or the strength of the contractions may make the enema uncomfortable for the patient. It is essential that the mother be informed that the nurse is aware of the possible discomfort and that everything will be done to carry out the procedure carefully and comfortably. Giving a step-by-step explanation of the procedure will go far to alleviate the discomfort.

Vulvar and Perineal Preparation

The aim in shaving and washing the vulva is to cleanse and disinfect the immediate area about the vagina and to prevent anything contaminated from entering the birth canal. During labor, pathogenic bacteria ascend the birth canal more readily, and every effort should be made to protect the mother from intrapartal infection. In some hospitals a sterile gauze sponge or a folded towel is placed against the introitus to prevent contaminated matter, such as hair or soapy fluid, from entering the vagina during the preparation procedure.

Many physicians do not require that the mons pubis be shaved because of its distance from the episiotomy area and because of the discomfort that the regrowth of the hair causes; clipping the hair in this area often suffices. Some do not even wish the perineum shaved. However, the traditional perineal shave is frequently required.

The vulvar hair is lathered prior to shaving to facilitate the procedure and make it more comfortable for the mother. An ordinary safety razor is used. The shave is started at the top of the labia majora. The direction of the stroke goes from above downward as the area of the vulva and the perineal body is shaved. The skin can be stretched above each downward stroke and the razor permitted to move smoothly over the skin without undue pressure.

When the entire area anterior to an imaginary line drawn through the base of the perineal body has been shaved, the patient can be turned to her side to allow the anal area to be completely shaved. With the upper leg well flexed, the anal area is lathered and shaved, again with a front-to-back stroke. It must always be remembered that anything which has passed over the anal region must not be returned near the vulvar orifice.

The solutions as well as the techniques used in cleansing the genitals will vary in different hospitals, but warm water with soap is probably the most common one used.

In washing the genitals, the nurse cleanses thoroughly first the surrounding areas, using sterile sponges or disposable washcloths for each area, and gradually works in toward the vestibule. The strokes must be from above downward and away from the introitus. Special attention should be paid to separating the vulvar folds in order to remove the smegma which may have accumulated in the folds of the labia minora and/or at the base of the clitoris.

Finally, the region around the anus is cleansed. It should be emphasized here again that a sponge which has passed over the anal area must not be returned near the vulvar orifice but should be discarded immediately. The patient is instructed not to touch the genitals.

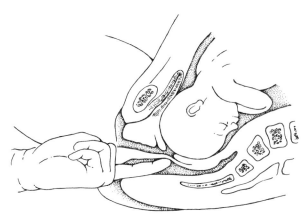

Figure 23-1. Rectal examination, showing how the examining finger palpates the cervix and the infant's head through the rectovaginal septum.

EXAMINATIONS IN LABOR

General. The pulse, respiration and temperature are taken, as previously stated, and are repeated every four hours. In cases in which there is fever, or in which labor has lasted more than 24 hours, it is desirable to repeat these observations every two hours. The blood pressure is recorded and is repeated every hour; in cases of toxemia of pregnancy, this may be done more frequently, according to the physician's instructions. As soon as possible after admission, a complete examination of the heart and the lungs is carried out by the physician to make certain that there are no conditions present which might contraindicate the type of analgesia or anesthesia to be used.

Abdominal. The abdominal examination is similar to that carried out in the antepartal period, comprising estimation of fetal size and position and listening to the fetal heart sounds.

Rectal and Vaginal Examinations

Both rectal and vaginal examinations may be performed during labor. They are generally done by the physician, although with special training in some institutions, nurses are given this responsibility. It was previously thought that rectal examinations were much safer than vaginal examinations, since they reduced the risk of carrying pathogenic bacteria from the introitus and the lower vagina to the region of the cervix and the lower uterine

segment. Studies and general experience show that this supposed advantage of rectal examinations over vaginal examinations has been exaggerated. Nevertheless, rectal examinations do have the advantage of not requiring preliminary disinfection on the part of the examiner or the patient.

For either rectal or vaginal examination the patient lies on her back with her knees flexed. The nurse should drape the patient so that she is well protected, but with the perineal region exposed. In making a rectal examination the index finger is used, the hand being covered by a clean but not necessarily sterile rubber glove. As shown in Fig. 23-1, the thumb should be fixed into the palm of the hand, otherwise it may enter the vagina and introduce infection. The finger is anointed liberally with a lubricating jelly and introduced slowly into the rectum. The cervical opening usually can be felt as a depression surrounded by a circular ridge. The degree of dilatation and the amount of effacement are noted. Very often the membranes can be felt bulging into the cervix, particularly during a contraction. The level of the fetal head is now ascertained and correlated with the level of the ischial spines as being a certain number of centimeters above or below the ischial spines. After the completion of the examination the patient's perineum is wiped, and the examiner's hands are washed. The rectal glove is discarded.

The frequency with which rectal or vaginal examinations are required during labor depends on the individual case; often one or two such examinations are sufficient, while in some instances more are required. The nurse who stays with the mother constantly will become increasingly skillful in the ability to follow the progress of labor to a great extent by careful evaluation of subjective and objective symptoms of the mother (e.g., the character of the uterine contractions and the show, the progressive descent of the area on the abdomen where fetal heart sounds are heard, the mother's overall response to her physical labor).

If the mother is to have a vaginal examination, she may be prepared by cleansing the vulvar and the perineal region in a manner similar to that used in preparation for delivery. The physician's hands are scrubbed and sterile gloves donned. Before the fingers are introduced into the vagina, the labia are opened widely in order to minimize possible contamination of the examining fingers if they should come in contact with the inner surfaces of the labia and the margins of the hymen. Then the index and the second fingers of the examining hand are gently introduced into the vagina (Fig. 23-2). Vaginal examination is more reliable than rectal, since the cervix, the fontanels, and other structures can be palpated directly with no intervening rectovaginal septum to interfere with the tactile sense. Some authorities feel that the danger of introducing infection into the birth canal is increased with repeated vaginal examinations and thus attempt to limit the number of times the examination is repeated, using it only as necessary.

CONDUCT OF THE FIRST STAGE

The first stage of labor (dilating stage) begins with the first symptoms of true labor and ends with the complete dilatation of the cervix. The physician examines the patient early in labor and sees her from time to time throughout the first stage but may not be in constant attendance at this time.

In normal labor, examination (fetal heart, vaginal, and so on) will show that the baby is in good condition and that steady progress is being made. Furthermore, the rate of progress often will give some indication as to when delivery is to be expected. During this stage, the nurse is in constant attendance, safeguarding the welfare of the mother and fetus and notifying the physician of the progress of labor.

Support During Labor

As already emphasized, it is important for the nurse to have an empathic supportive attitude toward the mother in order to interpret the progress of labor and perform certain technical procedures skillfully. It should be pointed out that "supportive care" includes not only emotional support but also aspects of physical care which in the total context of care contribute to the well-being and the comfort of the mother and hence to her emotional equilibrium. Thus, a sponge bath, oral hygiene, a backrub, an explanation before a procedure, and so on all enhance the mother's comfort and help her to feel that she is a special, worthwhile person.

The Effective Use of Touch

Many of the physical care activities that nurses perform consist, in part at least, of "laying on of hands," which is known to be necessary and helpful

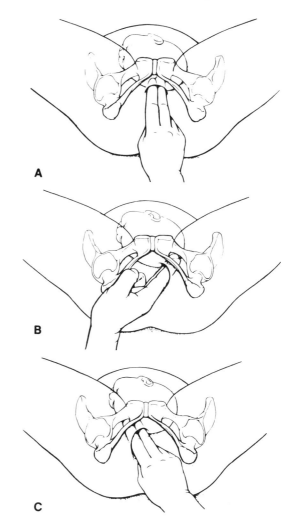

Figure 23-2. Vaginal Examination. *A.* Determining the station and palpating the sagittal suture. *B.* Identifying the posterior fontanel. *C.* Identifying the anterior fontanel.

to patients in maintaining or reachieving good health. These activities, then, can be valuable entrées in establishing and maintaining rapport and hence an effective relationship. Even the intrusive procedures which are so often painful or distasteful, if done with gentleness and skill, show the patient that her dignity and integrity are respected.

Related to this "laying on of hands" is the effectiveness of the use of touch. Although this has not been explored to any great degree scientifically, its importance was recognized as far back as the mid-19th century. More recently, research indicates that the patient's ability to work effectively with her labor contractions increased when extensive physical contact was introduced and then decreased when physical contact was withdrawn (see Suggested Reading). This contact can take the form of a backrub, allowing the patient to grasp the nurse's hand, stroking the patient's brow, and so on. Indeed, many of the relaxation techniques practiced in the prepared childbirth classes rely on the use of this sense.

However, touch need not be used indiscriminately, as excessive and/or inappropriate touching is offensive to many people. The need will vary from patient to patient, and the woman will indicate which type of touch is helpful and who will be the most appropriate person to give it. The nurse must use professional judgment regarding its use, and rapport with the patient will help to indicate a correct decision. This type of communication can be a way of demonstrating the nurse's concern and empathy, especially when verbal communication is difficult or impossible. It is also an effective means of incorporating the partner into the care and the support of his mate.

Providing Assurance

Once labor is well established, the mother should not be left alone. The morale of women in labor is sometimes hopelessly shattered, regardless of whether or not they have been prepared for labor during pregnancy, when they are left by themselves over long periods of time. During labor the mother is more sensitive to the behavior of those about her, particularly in relation to her perception of how much concern the personnel about her show for her safety and well-being. As labor progresses, there is a normal narrowing of the phenomenal field, an "inward turning," which results in easy distortion of stimuli and perception. For instance, careless remarks dropped in conversation often are misinterpreted as indicative of negligence or lack of feeling. It is well to remember that comments and laughter overheard in the corridor outside the patient's room may contribute to her uneasiness. Therefore, the nurse must be on guard against unfortunate happenings of this kind.

The nurse will want to be aware that her own anxieties in the situation may be communicated to the patient. The process of labor and the forthcoming delivery will produce normal anxieties which are no more than a healthy anticipation of the events to come (in both patient and nurse). Thus, most patients tolerate their labor much better if they are told the kind of progress that is being made and assured that they are doing a good job working with their contractions. This is part and parcel of the continuing orientation to the labor process that was mentioned earlier.

Another point that is apropos here is the usefulness and the effectiveness of suggestion for the mother in labor. The nurse can utilize this suggestibility to great advantage in her supportive care, since the mother responds very readily to suggestions, especially in early labor. The groundwork can be laid at this time for the more complicated instructions that may be necessary later in labor concerning relaxation, breathing techniques, and the management of pain.

The mother who has attended antepartal classes that have included exercise and relaxation techniques is usually better prepared for labor, but nevertheless she needs to be coached in utilizing the techniques which will enable her to cooperate with the natural forces of labor. During early labor the patient usually prefers to move about the room and frequently is more at ease sitting in a comfortable chair. She can be permitted and encouraged to do this and whatever else seems to be most relaxing and pleasant to her. If hospital policy permits the father to be in the labor room, his presence can be a valuable asset because of the support that it gives the mother. Research indicates that the presence of the father during labor is a major source of support for the mother (see Suggested Reading). This not only benefits the mother but also helps the father to feel that he has a more vital role in participating with her in the birth of their child.

Positioning

Since the introduction of the electronic fetal monitors (see Chapter 37), many hospitals now attach the monitors to mothers routinely even if there is no high-risk condition present. The mother must be in bed for this equipment to function appropriately. This, of course, limits the mother's mobility. The reason for the use of the monitor needs to be explained to the parents so that they can understand why their activity is restricted and will not become unduly alarmed.

It is well to remember that the usual comfort measures, including backrubs and position changes, need not be slighted if the mother has either an internal or external monitor attached. Very often patients are reluctant to move lest they disturb the monitor; the nurse can assure the patient that she may move and can see to it that the mother does, in fact, assume comfortable positions other than supine. Changes in position and transducer repositioning are to be noted on the graph paper.

If no monitors are employed, the patient can be encouraged to assume any position which is comfortable for her—side, squatting, all fours, sitting and so on. A mother needn't labor on her back. These other positions have been found to enhance the efficacy of the labor contractions and do not predispose to maternal hypotension as the supine position does.[6,7]

Progression of Active Phase of Labor

When the mother begins to be bothered by labor, she may need help to get into a comfortable position and to relax. During the contractions she can be coached as necessary in the application of the slow deep-breathing technique described in Chapter 24. Regardless of how diligently the mother has practiced the various breathing and relaxing techniques during pregnancy, or the level of her understanding about the physiology of labor, the situation is changed somewhat for her by active labor. Each mother may react in a slightly different way, for each is an individual. Some analgesic medication may be required for the mother's comfort after good labor is established. The nurse may observe in time that as the active phase progresses (i.e., the 7 to 10 cm. dilatation) slow deep breathing becomes difficult for the patient. The mother herself is aware that "her diaphragm won't cooperate." Rapid, shallow breathing (accelerated breathing) with the contractions is usually easier and more effective.

Uterine Contractions

Dealing with Discomfort

The term "pains" has been associated with uterine contractions of childbirth since time immemorial. One finds this term still in common usage, so that even today many young women approach childbirth with fear of pain. It is no easy task to dispel this age-old fear, but throughout the childbirth experience a conscious effort must be made to instill a wholesome point of view in the mother. The nurse will want to avoid the use of the word "pain" whenever possible because of the very connotation of the word. It is important to remember, however, that as labor progresses, the contractions often become painful. This is not just a figment of the patient's imagination. Therefore, it is the nurse's responsibility to help the mother to distinguish between the *fear and anticipation* of pain and the *actual* pain she may be experiencing, and to help her to cope effectively.

The contribution that the nurse can make in the management of pain during labor and delivery is discussed in Chapter 24. However, we would like to reiterate a few of the major points here in order to reinforce them. We know that studies of pain have demonstrated that the anticipation of pain raises the anxiety level significantly which lowers the pain reaction threshold. Thus, the patient reacts sooner to even minimal pain stimuli. The pain is subjectively intensified and even a slight amount of pain seems to be much greater. Furthermore, other sensations are misinterpreted as pain (e.g., pressure, stretching), which explains why the digital examinations and even the pressure of the nurse's fingers on the abdomen as she times contractions "hurt." Therefore, "everything" is painful, and the heightening of the anticipation of pain in turn increases the response to pain, and soon a vicious cycle is established.

The nurse can help to break this cycle or prevent it from becoming established by intervening at the anticipation-anxiety junction. This is done by reminding the patient when a contraction is over (and the pain is gone) and that another contraction is not expected for several minutes: thus, this is the time for the mother to rest and to relax. The anxiety related to the anticipation of pain is then lowered or eliminated (the mother knows now she will be free from pain for several minutes and can rest), and the subjective intensification is diminished. It is obvious that the nurse or some other reliable person must be in continuous attendance in order to do this.

Moreover, sociocultural factors play an important part in the meaning and interpretation of pain for patients. While pain is basically a physiologic phenomenon, the meaning pain has and the kinds of responses to pain that are deemed appropriate are matters of cultural prescription. Cultural orientations, social conditioning, and sociocultural sanctioning play a large part in molding patterns of

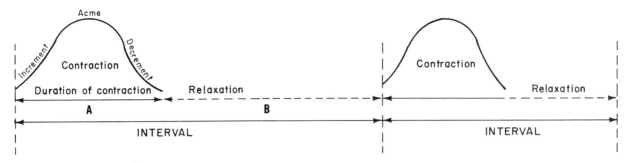

Figure 23-3. The interval and the duration of uterine contractions. The frequency of contractions is the interval timed from the beginning of one contraction to the beginning of the next contraction. The interval consists of two parts: (*A*) the duration of the contraction and (*B*) the period of relaxation. The broken line indicates an indeterminate period, since this time (*B*) is usually of longer duration than the actual contraction of (*A*).

response to painful experiences which are modal (i.e., occur most frequently) in a group, and these modal patterns are meaningful in terms of the values and beliefs of a particular group. Therefore, a culture or subculture from which a person comes conditions the formation of her particular reaction patterns to pain, and a knowledge of a group's attitudes toward pain is extremely important to the understanding of the reaction of a particular member of that group.

Characteristics of Contractions

The frequency, duration and intensity of the contractions should be watched closely and recorded.

The *frequency* of contractions is timed from the beginning of one contraction to the beginning of the next.

The *duration* of a contraction is timed from the moment the uterus first begins to tighten until it relaxes again (Fig. 23-3).

The *intensity* of a contraction may be mild, moderate or strong at its acme. Since this is a relative factor, intensity is difficult to interpret unless one is at the mother's bedside. For the sake of description, one might say that:

During a *mild* contraction, the uterine muscle becomes somewhat tense. During a *moderate* contraction the uterus becomes moderately firm. During a *strong* contraction, the uterus becomes so firm that it has the feel of woody hardness, and at the height of the contraction, the uterus cannot be indented when pressure is applied by the examiner's finger.

When the mother first becomes aware of the contractions, they may be 15 to 20 minutes apart and lasting perhaps 20 to 25 seconds. Since these are of mild intensity, she usually can continue with whatever she is doing, except that she is alert to time the subsequent contractions (to have specific information to report when she calls the physician). If this is her first pregnancy, she may be advised to wait until the contractions are five to ten minutes apart before coming to the hospital (depending on the other signs of labor). However, if she is a multipara, she will more than likely be told to come to the hospital as soon as a regular pattern of contractions is established (again, depending on other criteria).

Timing the Contractions

As labor progresses, the character of the contractions will change. They will become stronger in intensity, last longer (a duration of 45 to 60 seconds) and come closer together (at a frequency of every two to three minutes). One effective method the nurse can employ to time contractions is to keep her fingers lightly on the fundus. The fingers are recommended because they are more sensitive than the palm. However, for some people the whole hand is helpful. It should be emphasized that enough of the fingers should be used to ensure adequate contact with the abdomen; too slight a contact does not enable the nurse to ascertain the contractions accurately.

Assessing contractions in this manner will enable the nurse to detect the contraction, as it begins, by the gradual tensing and rising forward of the fundus, and to feel the contraction through its three phases until the uterus relaxes again. The inexperienced nurse can get some idea of how a contraction will feel under her fingertips by contracting her own biceps. First, the forearm should be extended and the fingertips of the hand on the opposite side placed on the biceps. Then the arm is gradually flexed until the muscle becomes very hard, held a few seconds, and gradually extended. This should take about 30 seconds to simulate a uterine contraction.

It is not reliable to rely on the mother to indicate when a contraction begins, because often she is unaware of it for perhaps five or ten seconds, sometimes even until the contraction reaches its acme. It is important to observe the rhythm of the contractions and to be assured that the uterine muscle relaxes completely after each contraction.

As the labor approaches the transition, the contractions will be very strong, last for about 60 seconds and occur at two- to three- minute intervals.

If any contraction lasts longer than 70 seconds and is not followed by a rest interval with complete relaxation of the uterine muscle, this should be reported to the physician immediately. The implications for both the mother and her infant can be severe (see Chapter 33).

Psychosocial Support during Contractions

Particularly during the late active phase the need for human contact—someone to hold on to—during the severe contractions will be seen. The mother responds less well to other physical contact, stroking, sponging, and so on; she may even say, "Leave me alone," meaning, of course, "Don't disturb me." However, if it is helpful for her to have someone's hand to hold, she should be allowed to do this if she indicates the need.

Since during the first stage of labor the uterine contractions are involuntary and uncontrolled by the patient, it is futile for her to "bear down" with her abdominal muscles, because this only leads to exhaustion. The mother who has been prepared for childbirth has been schooled in breathing techniques, such as diaphragmatic breathing or rapid shallow costal breathing, and with coaching from her partner or her nurse is usually able to accomplish conscious relaxation.

With the unprepared mother, a different situation exists. These mothers are often best helped to relax by encouraging and coaching them to keep breathing slowly and evenly during the early contractions and then to assume a pattern of more rapid and shallow breathing that is most comfortable to them during the late active phase. They will very often need to be reminded not to hold their breath during the contractions.

One cannot expect perfection in breathing techniques with these patients; however, this activity gives the inexperienced mother a point of concentration, and her feeling that she is actually participating and "controlling" her labor to some degree is helpful to her. Most mothers in labor, whether they are "prepared" or not, want to cooperate, and the calm, kind, firm guidance of an interested nurse can do much to help the mother utilize her contractions effectively.

Show

Show is a mucoid discharge from the cervix that is present after the mucous plug has been dislodged. As progressive effacement and dilatation of the cervix occur, the show becomes blood-tinged due to the rupture of superficial capillaries. The presence of an increased amount of bloody show (blood-stained mucus, not actual bleeding!) suggests that rather rapid progress may be taking place and should be reported immediately, particularly if associated with frequent severe contractions.

A perineal pad is not to be worn during labor because of the nature of the vaginal discharge. The tenacious mucoid discharge frequently comes in contact with the anus and could easily be smeared about the external genitalia and vaginal orifice when the patient moves about the bed or adjusts the pads. A quilted pad placed under the mother's buttocks serves very well to absorb material discharged from the vagina. This pad can be changed frequently and the perineum cleansed as necessary to keep the mother clean and dry.

Evaluation of the Fetal Heart Rate

The behavior of the fetal heartbeat in labor is of great importance. The heart rate can be monitored in a number of ways. The simplest, and still an effective method, is by frequent auscultation using a specialized head stethoscope. The widely used DeLee-Hillis stethoscope or the Leff fetal heart stethoscope are satisfactory for this purpose.

When checking the fetal heart sounds, the nurse listens and counts the rate for one full minute. Checking the rate before, during and after a con-

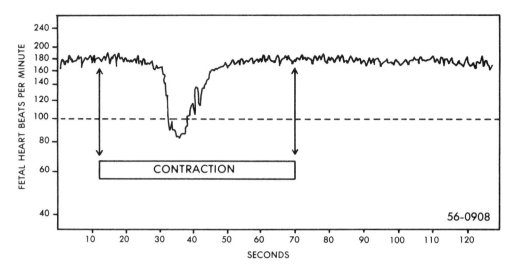

Figure 23-4. Electronic evaluation of fetal heart rates, showing normal slowing of the fetal heart rate during uterine contraction. (Hon, E. H.: Observations on "pathologic" fetal bradycardia, *Am. J. Ob. -Gyn.* 77:1084, 1959.)

traction is important so that any slowing and/or irregularities may be detected.

As previously explained, the fetal heart rate is normally between 120 to 160 beats per minute, except during and immediately after a uterine contraction, when it may fall to as low as 70 to 110. Hon found that in multigravidas the fetal heart rate might fall from 140 to 110–120 beats per minute at the acme of a contraction. In primigravidas the drop is greater, at times reaching 60 to 70 beats per minute (Fig. 23-4). This physiologic bradycardia begins after the onset of a contraction and ends 10 to 15 seconds prior to its end. It is believed to result from compression of the fetal skull by the partially dilated cervix rather than from fetal hypoxia. It appears to occur most commonly between 4 and 8 cm. of cervical dilatation.

It may be difficult to hear the sounds during a contraction, because the uterine wall is tense, and, in addition, it is more difficult for the mother to lie still during this period. But it is particularly important to listen at this time, since these observations inform the listener on how the fetus reacts to the contraction.

From a clinical standpoint any prolonged slowing should be reported to the obstetrician. *Should the slowing of the fetal heart rate be below 100 beats per minute, and should it last more than 30 seconds after the termination of a contraction, it is no longer considered to be physiologic and is taken as a sign of fetal distress.*

Occasionally, this prolonged slow rate is accompanied by the passage of meconium. It must be remembered that unless the membranes have ruptured, the meconium will not be apparent. Therefore, the passage of meconium is another sign of fetal distress if it occurs in a vertex presentation.

Any other unusual observations must be reported to the physician promptly so that measures can be instituted before permanent damage is done to the infant.

Repeated auscultation of the fetal heart sounds constitutes one of the most important responsibilities in the conduct of the first and the second stages of labor.

1. During the early period of the first stage of labor, the nurse records the fetal heart rate every hour and, once good labor is established, every half hour or even more often if indicated.
2. During the second stage, the fetal heart rate is checked every five minutes and recorded.
3. The fetal heart tones are checked immediately following the rupture of membranes, regardless of whether they rupture spontaneously or are artificially ruptured by the physician. With the gush of water that ensues, there is a possibility that the cord may be prolapsed, and any indication of fetal distress from pressure on the umbilical cord can thereby be detected.

In the last decade, the electronic fetal monitor has

been introduced and is often the method of choice for use in fetal auscultation and evaluation of contractions. A thorough discussion of this device can be found in Chapter 37.

Other Aspects of Care

Temperature, Pulse and Respiration. The pulse in normal labor is usually in the 70s or the 80s and rarely exceeds 100. Sometimes the pulse rate on admission is slightly increased because of the excitement of coming to the hospital, but this returns to normal shortly thereafter. A persistent pulse rate over 100 suggests exhaustion or dehydration.

The temperature and respiration should also be normal. If there is an elevation of temperature over 37.2° C. or 99° F. (orally), or the pulse and respiration become rapid, the physician is to be notified. The temperature is recorded every four hours, or more frequently if indicated. The pulse and respiration are taken every hour.

Blood Pressure. The blood pressure is recorded every hour during labor. During the first stage of labor there is little change in blood pressure between contractions, but during contractions an average increase of 5 to 10 mm. Hg may be expected. For this reason the blood pressure readings are taken between the contractions. Any unusual recordings of either systolic or diastolic pressure are reported immediately.

Fluid and Food Intake. The practice here varies greatly. Therefore, the wishes of the physician in charge need to be ascertained before proceeding. In general, it is customary to urge the mother to take water or clear fluids, such as tea with sugar, during the early phase of the first stage of labor, but she is not given solid or liquid foods because digestion is delayed during labor.

It may be necessary to administer a general anesthetic for the delivery; therefore, if the patient takes fluid or food shortly before delivery, vomiting and consequent aspiration may occur. On the other hand, in a prolonged labor, it is most important to maintain adequate fluid and caloric intake in order to forestall dehydration and exhaustion, in the event of which the physician may find it desirable to administer intravenous glucose solutions.

Bladder. The patient can be asked to void at least every three or four hours. The mother in labor often attributes all of her discomfort to the intensity of uterine contractions and therefore is unaware that it is the pressure of a full bladder which has increased her discomfort. In addition to causing unnecessary discomfort, a full bladder may be a serious impediment to labor or the cause of urinary retention in the puerperium. If the distended bladder can be palpated above the symphysis pubis, and the patient is unable to void, the physician is to be so informed. Not infrequently catheterization will be prescribed in such cases. Various techniques are used, all designed to maintain strict asepsis.

Analgesia. (See Chapter 25.) Before administering the medication prescribed to promote analgesia, the nurse informs the mother that she is about to receive medication which will make her more comfortable and help her in labor. The mother should be encouraged to rest and should be given reassurance that she will not be left alone. It may also be wise to remain quietly at the bedside and keep conversation to the very minimum to allow the medication to take maximum effect.

The mother may be asked to empty her bladder prior to receiving the drug, and the fetal heart tones and the mother's vital signs recorded before and after such medication is given. Once analgesic therapy has been instituted, the mother should not receive fluids or food by mouth and should remain in bed. The environment needs to be conducive to rest. Many institutions require that side rails be applied when the patient is medicated, even though there is someone in attendance. The necessity of this can be explained to both the patient and her partner to avoid any undue fears or misinterpretations. The father, especially, can be alerted to the importance of keeping the rails up if he is attending to any of his mate's needs.

If the mother has received scopolamine or other drugs in dosage sufficient to cause her to be heavily sedated, she *never* should be left unattended.

Signs of Second Stage

There are certain signs and symptoms, both behavioral and physical, which herald the onset of the second stage of labor. These signs and symptoms are to be watched for carefully. They are as follows.

1. The patient begins to bear down of her own accord; this is caused by a reflex when the head begins to press on the perineal floor.

2. Her mood of increasing apprehension which has been building since the contractions deepens; she becomes more serious and may appear bewildered by the force of the contractions.

3. There is usually a sudden increase in show that is more blood-tinged.

4. The patient may become increasingly irritable and unwilling to be touched; she may cry if disturbed.

5. The mother thinks that she needs to defecate. This symptom is due to pressure of the head on the perineal floor and consequently against the rectum.

6. Although she has been "working" successfully with her contractions during most of her labor, the uncertainty that she has been experiencing (since 6 to 8 cm. cervical dilatation) as to her ability to cope with the contractions may become overwhelming; she is frustrated and feels unable to manage if left alone.

7. The membranes may rupture, with discharge of amniotic fluid. This, of course, may take place any time but occurs most frequently at the beginning of the second stage.

8. The mother may be eager to be "put to sleep"; or if she is given appropriate help, she may narrow her concentration to trying to cope with the contractions and/or pushing according to instructions. It is important to remember that the mother's consciousness is somewhat altered because of the pain, her enforced concentration, and possibly medication; therefore, any coaching needs to be short and explicit and may need to be repeated with each contraction.

   The nurse also must be firm but gentle in setting limits with the mother, so that she can conserve her energy for the second stage. Thrashing about and continued crying only lead to exhaustion, and the mother needs the firm guidance of a skillful person to help her to maintain control.

9. The perineum begins to bulge and the anal orifice to dilate. This is a late sign, but if signs numbered 1, 3, 5, and 7 occur, it should be watched for with every contraction. Only rectal or vaginal examination (or the appearance of the head) can definitely confirm the suspicion. Emesis at this time is not unusual.

Reporting any or all of these signs promptly will allow enough time to transport the mother to the delivery room without a sense of rush and will provide an opportunity to cleanse and drape the mother properly. If these signs are overlooked, a precipitate delivery may occur without benefit of medical attention. In general, primigravidas are usually taken to the delivery room when the cervix is fully dilated, and multiparas when it is 7 or 8 cm. dilated.

CONDUCT OF THE SECOND STAGE

The second stage of labor (expulsion stage) begins with the complete dilatation of the cervix and ends with delivery of the baby. The complete dilatation of the cervix can be confirmed definitely only by rectal or vaginal examination. However, the nurse often is able to make a nursing diagnosis on the basis of her observations of the progress of labor, particularly if these findings are correlated with knowledge of the mother's parity, the speed of any previous labors, the pelvic measurements, and so on, noted in the antepartal record.

Although the general rule regarding the optimal time for taking a mother to the delivery room has been stated, it must be remembered that, in addition, the physician will be guided by such factors as the station of the presenting part and the speed with which labor is progressing. If on examination of a primigravida, the cervix is found to be fully dilated but the presenting part of the fetus only descended to the level of the ischial spines the mother most likely will remain in the labor room to permit the forces of labor to bring about further descent of the fetus before she is taken to the delivery room.

Method for Bearing Down

During this period the patient may be requested to exert her abdominal forces and "bear down." In most cases bearing-down efforts are reflex and spontaneous in the second stage of labor, but, occasionally, the mother does not employ her expulsive forces to good advantage, particularly if she has had epidural analgesia.

The nurse will be asked to coach and encourage the mother in this procedure.

1. The mother's head and shoulders can be raised to a 30° angle and supported firmly during the

contraction—the father is of great help in this regard and can provide the strength needed for this physical support.

2. The mother's thighs are then flexed on the abdomen, with hands grasped just below the knees when a contraction begins.

3. She should be instructed to take a deep breath as soon as the contraction begins and, with her breath held, to exert downward pressure exactly as if she were straining at stool.

4. Pulling on the knees at this time, as well as flexing the chin on the chest, is a helpful adjunct to maintain downward pressure of the diaphragm and to stabilize the chest and the abdominal musculature.

5. In addition, maintaining the legs flexed as for the "push" position deters the mother from pushing her feet against the table or bed. Avoiding such pressure on the feet is important, because it discourages tensing of the gluteal muscles and thus contributes to further relaxation of the pelvic floor. The bearing-down effort should be as long and sustained as possible, since short "grunty" endeavors are of little avail.

If at this time the mother is in the delivery room, but her legs as yet have not been put up in stirrups or leg holders, she can be coached in the same manner. In most hospitals the delivery tables have firmly attached hand grips which can be adjusted in position so that the mother can reach them comfortably to pull against, if she wishes.

However, in doing so her hands are not free to pull up on her knees with the contraction, so that the nurse or other person in attendance needs to assist her. This can be accomplished by assisting the mother to bring her legs up into position and exerting proper pressure against her knees as she bears down with the contraction. Care should be exercised to grasp the mother's knees from above, since doing so under the knees could exert undesirable pressure on the popliteal veins.

At the end of each contraction the mother is assisted to put her legs down and encouraged to rest until the next contraction begins. Usually, these bearing-down efforts are rewarded by increased bulging of the perineum, that is, by further descent of the head. The patient should be informed of such progress, for encouragement is all-important.

In certain instances it may not be desirable for the mother to bear down. In these cases, if the mother has an urge to bear down, she can be instructed to pant during each contraction; since it is impossible to push while panting.

Psychosocial Support

When the mother is ready to be transferred to the delivery room, it is more helpful if the same nurse who has been attending her in labor accompanies her to the delivery room. This transfer will mean a new environment for the patient to cope with under very stressful circumstances. Great physical and mental exertion may be called for with little preparation or practice. To the mother in labor who is unfamiliar with such surroundings, the "sterile" atmosphere of the delivery room can be strange, cold and uninviting, with its obstetric furnishings and supplies that become even more foreboding as they reflect the glittering lights of the room. Under such circumstances the sight of familiar faces and the sound of familiar voices, even though partially concealed and muffled by the surgical caps, masks and gowns, do give the patient some sense of continuity and security. Furthermore, by this time the nurse and the patient will have established a communication pattern, each able to pick up the other's more covert cues. Thus, the coaching, guidance and follow-through necessary in the second stage of labor will be expedited if the same person continues with the care.

The nurse will notice that the mother has become increasingly involved in the whole birth process. The seemingly panicky frustration of the late active phase subsides a bit (with appropriate coaching and reassurance), and the patient may experience a sense of relief that the expulsive stage has begun. The desire to push and to bear down is very strong now—uncontrollable, in fact—and the patient generally gets enormous satisfaction with each push. Some patients, however, experience acute pain and need all available help and encouragement to continue bearing down. The nurse will note that in most instances there is complete exhaustion after each expulsive effort, and the mother often drops off to sleep, only to be roused by the next contraction. Since consciousness is still altered, it may be difficult for the mother to follow directions readily even though she may want to. Again, repeated, short, explicit directions are required to encourage her to rest or to work, but especially to prepare the mother for the expulsive effort if she is sleeping between contractions and awakens abruptly.

Muscular cramps in the legs are common in the second stage because of pressure exerted by the baby's head on certain nerves in the pelvis. To relieve these cramps, the leg can be straightened and the ankle dorsiflexed by exerting pressure upward against the ball of the foot until the cramp subsides. Meanwhile, the knee is stabilized with the other hand. These cramps cause excruciating pain and must never be ignored.

Preparation for Delivery

Good obstetric care during the second stage of labor demands the closest teamwork among the patient, physician, nurse and anesthetist. By previous understanding, or more often by established hospital routine, each has his or her own responsibilities in the delivery room, and, if the best interests of the mother and her infant are to be fulfilled, the responsiblities of each must be carried out smoothly and efficiently.

Up to now, the primary focus for the nurse has been on direct patient care. Now she must enlarge her focus to include the obstetrician and other allied professionals; that is, there will be more activities which will require the actual assistance of these persons than was necessary during the first stage of labor. Thus, the nurse must be sensitive not only to the cues sent by the mother but also to those relayed by the other personnel.

Preparation of the Delivery Room. There are no two hospitals in which the delivery room setup or the procedure for delivery is precisely the same. Therefore observation and experience in a particular institution will serve as the basis for becoming acquainted with the physical layout and the method of care offered.

The following, however, gives a general idea of the equipment and materials used in the typical setting.

The delivery table is designed so that its surface is actually composed of two adjoining sections, each covered with its own mattress. This permits the patient to lie in the supine position (or be propped up at a 30° angle with pillows) until it is desired to put her legs up into stirrups, that is, put her in the lithotomy position. At this time the table is "broken" by a mechanical device. The retractable or

lower end of the table drops and is rolled under the main section of the table. Thus ready access is given to the perineal region. Or, if it is desired to deliver the patient in the dorsal recumbent position, the lower portion of the table can remain in place.

The instrument table opposite the foot of the delivery table contains the principal sterile supplies and instruments needed for normal delivery, including, among other articles, towels, sponges, catheter, solutions, basins and the "cord set." The cord set is a group of instruments used for clamping and cutting the umbilical cord; two hemostats, a pair of scissors, and a cord clamp. Other instruments often are included, because it may be necessary for the physician to perform an episiotomy or to repair lacerations (p. 354). Other instruments frequently included are two hemostats, two Allis clamps, one mouse-tooth tissue forceps, two sponge sticks, one vaginal retractor, two tenaculae, one needle holder, assorted needles and a pair of obstetric forceps.

A double-bowl solution stand or basin rack generally is used to hold the basins, one for wet sponges and the other to receive the placenta. Emergency instruments, a crib and a radiant warmer and resuscitator (Fig. 23-5) are part of standard delivery room equipment and should be in readiness at all times.

Asepsis and Antisepsis. Persons who have a communicable disease or persons who have been in contact with a communicable disease should be excluded from maternity service until examined by a physician. Only after the physician has certified that the employee is free from infections should he or she be allowed to return to duty. Personnel with evidence of upper respiratory infections or open skin lesions, diarrhea, or any other infectious disease also should be excluded. Furthermore, it is recommended that all persons working in the maternity area should have a preemployment physical examination and rubella titers, and such interim examinations may be required by the hospital.

Of prime importance in the conduct of the second stage of labor are strict asepsis and antisepsis throughout the entire delivery. To this end everyone in the delivery room wears a clean scrubdress, cap and mask, and those actually participating in the delivery are in sterile attire. Masking must include both nose and mouth. Caps are to be adjusted to keep *all* hair covered. If the nurse scrubs to assist the doctor, the strictest aseptic technique is ob-

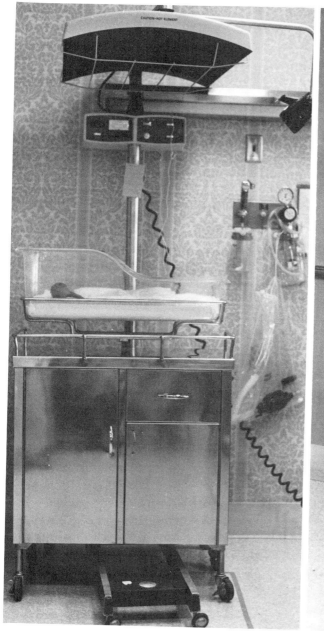 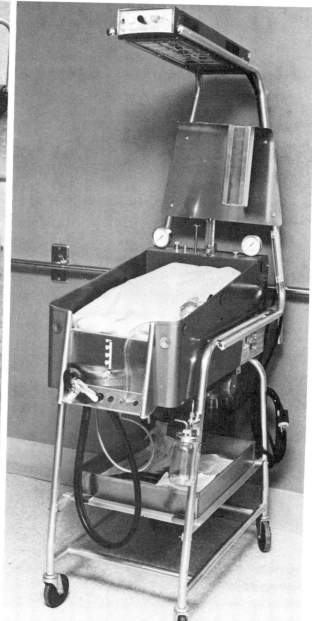

Figure 23-5. (Left) Radiant warmer; *(Right)* resuscitation unit.

served. The hands are disinfected as carefully as for a major surgical operation. Scrubbing the hands should be started sufficiently early to allot full time for the scrub, as well as to don gown and gloves.

Transfer of the Mother to the Delivery Room. When birth appears imminent, the mother will be transferred to the delivery room and prepared for delivery. If the father will not be accompanying the mother to the delivery room, then time is allowed for them to bid each other a temporary goodbye. This kind of planning not only is supportive but also enables both to cooperate more fully. Care should be taken to have only one person instruct or coach the mother at any one time. When delivery is imminent, her attention will necessarily be limited, as already illustrated, and the sound of several voices at one time is confusing.

Prior to the actual transfer to the delivery room, the nurse will find out what type of anesthesia will be used. Since the immediate positioning of the patient in the delivery room will depend on the type of anesthesia used, this preplanning will expedite activities during delivery and promote smoother functioning of the team.

Delivery

Positioning.   If regional anesthesia is to be administered, the patient is usually turned on her side. If she is given a saddle block, she may be placed on her side or assisted to a sitting position on the side of the delivery table, with her feet supported on a stool and her body leaning forward against the nurse. Her back should be toward the operator and bowed (the position requires flexion of the neck and the lumbar spine). This principle of cervical and lumbar flexion is used also in the side lying position (see Chapter 25). A caudal or epidural anesthesia may be started in the labor room.

Although the positioning and the administration of the anesthesia take only a few minutes, the mother may be extremely uncomfortable due to the severity of the contractions at this time; she can be assured that this discomfort is only temporary. The fetal heart tones and the maternal blood pressure are checked frequently—every five minutes or so. In addition, the mother's head should be elevated with two pillows to help prevent the anesthetic level from rising beyond the desired height. To allow the anesthetic level to stabilize, the nurse waits for instructions from the anesthetist before putting the mother's legs in stirrups or performing any other manipulations. If the mother is to receive general anesthesia, she lies supine on the table. Local or pudendal anesthesia is administered with the mother in the lithotomy position.

As has been previously stated, anesthesia should be administered only by a qualified physician or a nurse anesthetist. This entire subject is discussed in more detail in Chapter 25.

During the time that the anesthesia is being administered, the circulating nurse can uncover the sterile tables, check the resuscitator and attach a sterile suction catheter and oxygen mask, and perform other duties for which she is responsible. Once the anesthesia has been administered, the nurse resumes checking the FHR every five minutes.

Some hospitals and physicians do not require that the mother be placed in the lithotomy position for delivery. She simply grasps her legs at the knees as she did during the pushing phase of the second stage. This position allows visualization of the perineum and adequate prepping and draping of the area. Before the mother's legs are placed in stirrups or leg holders of some type, cotton flannel boots which cover the entire leg are put on. When the legs are placed in the stirrups or holders, care is taken not to separate the legs too widely or to have one leg higher than the other. Both legs are raised or lowered at the same time, with a nurse supporting each leg if the mother is unable to help in the positioning. Failure to observe these principles may strain the ligaments of the pelvis, with consequent discomfort in the puerperium. Care should be taken to avoid pressure on the popliteal space, and to angle the stirrups so that the feet are not dependent.

If stirrups are used during the delivery, the mother can be given handles to grip and pull on, which aid her in her bearing-down efforts. Wrist straps which are secured about the wrist allow some limited movement but prevent the mother from reaching up to touch the sterile drapes. The purpose of the handles and the cuffs should be explained to the mother, since many patients often complain about being "strapped down."

Preparing the Perineum.   With the patient in the lithotomy position, the nurse carries out the procedure for cleansing the vulva and the surrounding area. If the delivery is to be conducted with the mother in the recumbent position, this may be carried out with the knees drawn up slightly and the legs separated. Once the physician has scrubbed and donned sterile gown and gloves, the patient is draped with towels and sheets appropriate for the purpose.

After the patient has been prepared for delivery, catheterization, if done, is carried out by the physician. Sometimes it is difficult to catheterize a patient in the second stage of labor, since the fetus's head may compress the urethra. If the catheter does not pass easily, force never should be employed. Whenever it is possible and appropriate, all procedures, of course, should be explained to the mother as they occur.

The Delivery Process. As the infant descends the birth canal, pressure against the rectum may cause fecal material to be expelled. Sponges (as a rule with saline solution) may be used to remove any fecal material which may escape from the rectum.

Fundal pressure should not be used to accomplish spontaneous delivery or to bring the head deeper into the birth canal. Severe fundal pressure may cause uterine damage or rupture of the uterus.

As soon as the head distends the perineum to a diameter of 6 or 8 cm., a towel may be placed over the rectum while forward pressure is exerted on the baby's chin with one hand, at the same time that downward pressure is applied to the occiput by the other hand. This technique, called the Ritgen's maneuver (Fig. 23-6), provides control of the head as it is emerging and directs the extension phase of delivery so that the head is born with the smallest diameter presenting. The head usually is delivered between contractions and as slowly as possible. At this time the mother may complain about a "splitting" sensation caused by the extreme vaginal stretching as the head is born. All these measures (control of head by Ritgen's maneuver, extension and slow delivery between contractions) help to prevent lacerations. If a tear seems to be inevitable, an incision which is called an episiotomy may be made in the perineum. This will not only prevent lacerations but also will facilitate the delivery.

Immediately after the birth of the infant's head a finger is passed along the occiput to the infant's neck in order to feel whether a loop or more of umbilical cord encircles it. If such a coil is felt, it should be gently drawn down and, if loose enough, slipped over the enfant's head (see Fig. 23-7). This is done to prevent interference with the infant's oxygen supply, which could result from pressure of its shoulder on the umbilical cord. If the cord is too tightly coiled to permit this procedure, it must be clamped and cut before the shoulders are delivered; then the infant must be extracted immediately before asphyxiation results. The anterior shoulder usually is brought under the symphysis pubis first and then the posterior shoulder is delivered, after which the remainder of the body follows without particular mechanism. The exact time of the baby's birth should be noted. The infant usually cries immediately, and the lungs become expanded. About this time the pulsations in the umbilical cord begin to diminish.

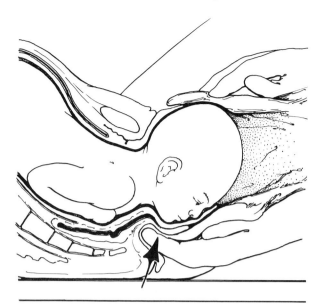

Figure 23-6. Ritgen's maneuver, as it appears in median section. Arrow shows direction of pressure.

Clamping the Cord. The cord usually is not clamped until this occurs, or for a minute or so if practicable, because of the marked benefit of the additional blood to the infant. The cord is then cut between the two Kelly clamps, which have been placed a few inches from the umbilicus; then the umbilical clamp or tie is applied (Figs. 23-8 and 23-9). The tie, a sterilized linen tape ligature, is usually applied about an inch from the abdomen, with care to secure it tightly enough to prevent bleeding without its cutting into the cord (Fig. 23-10). A second ligature may be applied for further protection if it is desired or if it is necessary because of any bleeding. There are several types of umbilical clamps, such as the Kane, the Hollister and the Hesseltine, which are used extensively in many institutions (Fig. 23-8). With these the possibility of hemorrhage is minimized.

Psychosocial Considerations

If the mother is awake, she will usually be eager to have a closer look at her baby and hold it, if this is possible. One should remember that, although she is quite tired, she is usually elated, proud of her accomplishment of giving birth and eager to share this with the baby's father. Whenever possible, all efforts should be made to allow the father, the

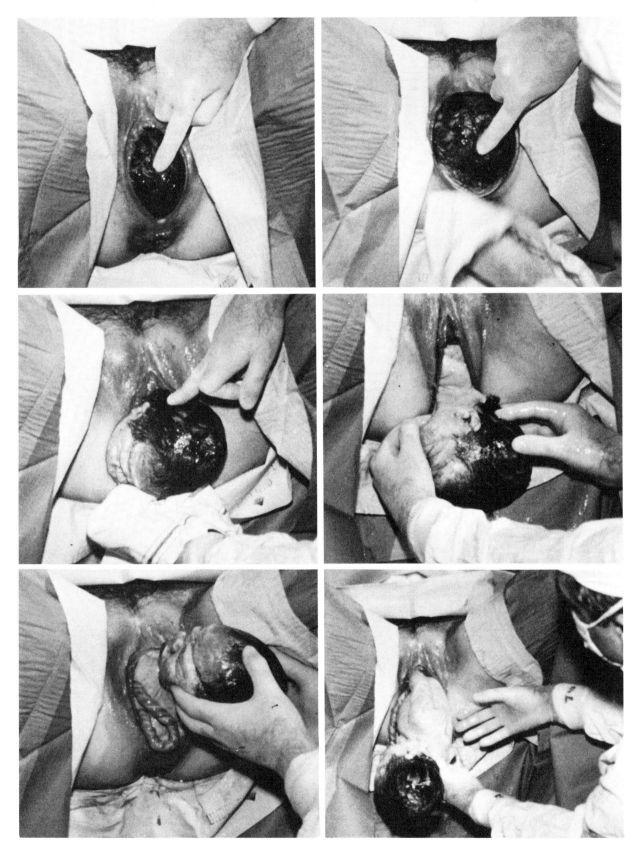

Figure 23-7. The normal birth process. (From the film *Human Birth,* published by J. B. Lippincott Co., Philadelphia.)

(*Continued opposite page*)

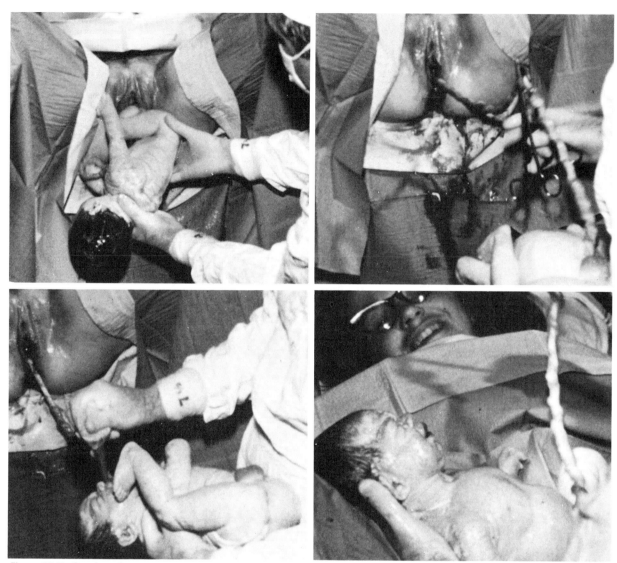

Figure 23-7. Continued.

mother and the infant to share this momentous time together if they so desire.

In some hospitals, the baby is placed in the mother's arms as soon as she is transferred to her bed and the father is permitted to remain at her bedside while she is in the recovery area. This type of arrangement provides an excellent opportunity to let both the mother and father have a close, thorough look at their baby and to let them begin the necessary process of incorporating it into their family unit.

The Leboyer Method of Delivery

In recent years a newer method of delivery has been advocated by a French obstetrician, Frederick Leboyer, who suggests that delivery room procedures be changed to make birth less of a traumatic event for the newborn. In his book and lectures he has described a method of handling infants during birth which includes a dimly lit and quiet delivery room, placing the infant on the mother's abdomen and stroking (massaging) it gently, delaying the clamping of the cord, and immersing the infant in a warm bath until it is relaxed and quiet.[8,9] Leboyer contends that the traditional method of delivery with all of its harsh, sudden sensory stimulation can be detrimental to the infant. The shock of birth produces jitteriness, interferes with eye contact between mother and infant, and may even prevent optimal bonding with the mother given the other restrictive practices followed in some hospitals.

There has been some controversy about this type of "gentle" birth mainly because of questions con-

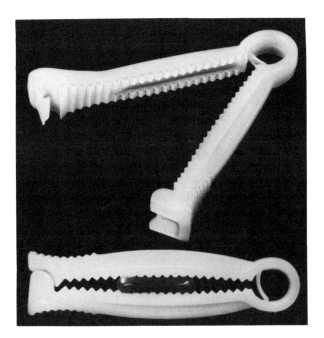

Figure 23-8. Umbilical cord clamp. A double-grip cord clamp in the opened and closed positions. (Hollister, Inc., Chicago, Ill.)

cerning possible threats to infant safety from undue chilling and possible infection. There has been no definitive research to either prove or disprove the efficacy of this method. Preliminary data do indicate that infants delivered by this technique do not tend to tremble or shudder as much and have more relaxed hand muscles. Morever, they spend more time with their eyes open in the period immediately subsequent to delivery. In addition, no greater risk for mother or infant of infection or chilling was found.[10] Many hospitals are offering at least a modified version of this technique and more parents are requesting it.

CONDUCT OF THE THIRD STAGE

Delivery of the Placenta

The third stage of labor (placental stage) begins after the delivery of the baby and terminates with the birth of the placenta. Immediately after delivery of the infant the height of the uterine fundus and its consistency are ascertained by palpating the uterus through a sterile towel placed on the lower abdomen. A hand is placed on the abdomen *under* the sterile drape and the uterus held very gently

with the fingers behind the fundus and the thumb in front. So long as the uterus remains hard, and there is no bleeding, the policy is ordinarily one of watchful waiting until the placenta is separated; no massage is practiced, the hand simply resting on the fundus to make certain that the organ does not balloon out with blood.

Since attempts to deliver the placenta prior to its separation from the uterine wall are not only futile but may be dangerous it is most important that the signs of placental separation be well understood. The signs which suggest that the placenta has separated are as follows:

1. The uterus rises upward in the abdomen; this is because the placenta, having been separated, passes downward into the lower uterine segment and the vagina, where its bulk pushes the uterus upward.
2. The umbilical cord protrudes 3 or more inches

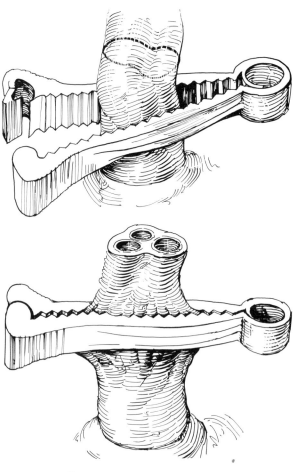

Figure 23-9. Clamp.

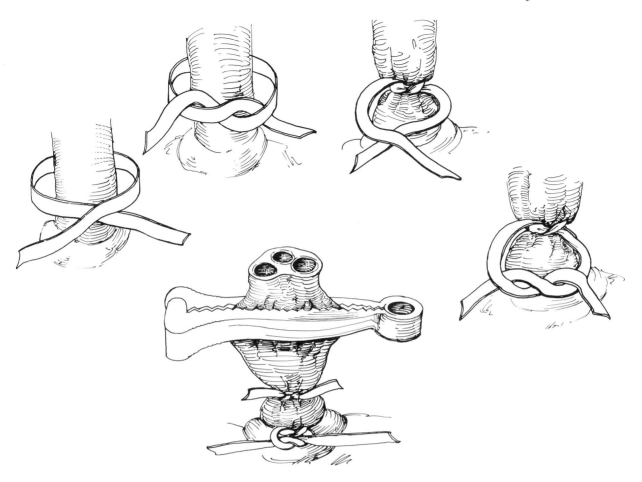

Figure 23-10. Tying off cord.

farther out of the vagina, indicating that the placenta also has descended.

3. The uterus changes from a discoid to a globular shape and becomes, as a rule, more firm.

4. A sudden trickle or spurt of blood often occurs.

These signs are apparent sometimes within a minute or so after delivery of the infant and usually within five minutes. When the placenta has separated and the uterus is firmly contracted, the patient is asked to bear down so that the intraabdominal pressure so produced may expel the placenta. If this fails, or if it is not practicable because of anesthesia, gentle pressure is exerted downward with the hand on the fundus and the placenta is gently guided out of the vagina. This procedure, known as placental *expression,* must be done gently and without squeezing (Figs. 23-11 and 23-12). It never should be attempted unless the uterus is hard; otherwise the organ may be turned inside out. This is one of the gravest complications of obstetrics and is known as

"inversion" of the uterus. Once the placenta is expelled, it is carefully inspected to make sure that it is intact (Fig. 23-13); if a piece is left in the uterus, it may cause subsequent hemorrhage.

Use of Oxytocics

Oxytocin and/or ergonovine, or their derivatives, may be administered at the physician's request to increase uterine contractions and thereby to minimize bleeding. These agents are employed widely in the conduct of the normal third stage of labor, but the timing of their administration differs greatly in various hospitals. These oxytocics are not necessary in most cases, but their use is considered ideal from the viewpoint of minimizing blood loss and the general safety of the mother.

Ergonovine is an alkaloid of ergot and is a powerful oxytocic; it stimulates uterine contractions and ex-

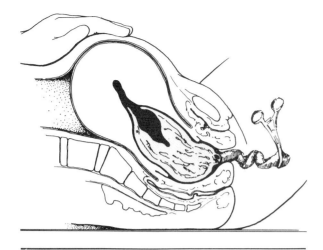

Figure 23-11. Expression of placenta is usually done by the physician, if necessary, but *on his instructions* may be done by an assistant. The *uterus must be hard* if this is attempted. Note that the uterus is not squeezed.

erts an effect which may persist for several hours. When it is administered intravenously, the uterine response is almost immediate, and within a few minutes of intramuscular or oral administration. This response is sustained in character with no tendency toward relaxation. *However, this drug will cause an elevation of blood pressure.*

More recently a semisynthetic derivative of ergonovine, *methylergonovine maleate,* has been employed because it possesses several advantages over the parent drug. Usually called by its trade name, Methergine, it has the ability to produce stronger and longer contractions and is less likely to cause elevation of the blood pressure. *However, it can cause a transient hypertension.*

Both drugs when given intravenously may cause transient headache and, to a lesser extent, temporary chest pain, palpitation and dyspnea. These side effects are less likely to occur with intramuscular administration of the drugs.

Oxytocin is another agent which, like ergonovine, causes a marked contraction of the uterus. However, the response of the uterus to oxytocin resembles the response to ergonovine for only the first five to ten minutes; then normal rhythmic contractions of amplified degree return, with intermittent periods of relaxation.

The oxytocic fraction separated from posterior pituitary extract is called oxytocin; it is widely used because it does not possess the strong vasopressor effects of Pituitrin, which was used more extensively in former years.

Oxytocin's most important side effect is its antidiuretic effect which can cause water intoxication if administered intravenously in a large volume of electrolyte-free aqueous dextrose solution. Fortunately the antidiuretic effect disappears within a few minutes after the infusion is discontinued.

A synthetic oxytocin injection has been developed and marketed under the brand name of Syntocinon.

Figure 23-12. Third stage of labor: the delivery of the placenta. (From the film *Human Birth,* published by J. B. Lippincott Co., Philadelphia.)

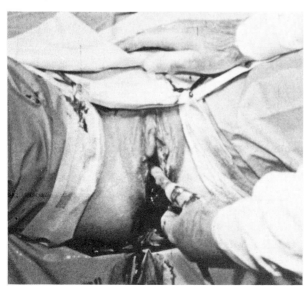
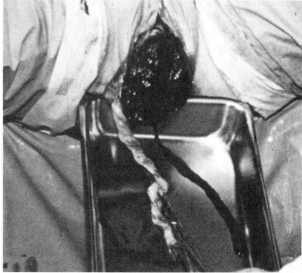

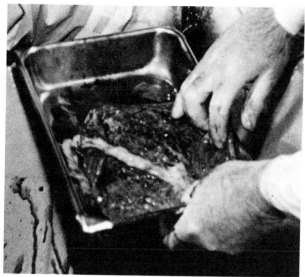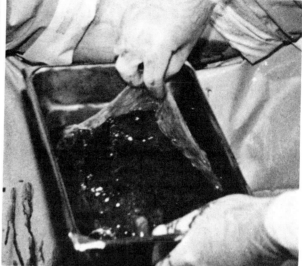

Figure 23-13. Inspecting the placenta. (From the film *Human Birth,* published by J. B. Lippincott Co., Philadelphia.)

Its action, dosage and indications are similar to those of oxytocin.

On the obstetrician's order the nurse administers the oxytocic intramuscularly, the intravenous medications being administered by a physician. The average doses of the drugs are as follows: oxytocin, 10 units (1 cc.) intramuscularly or intravenously; Syntocinon, 10 units (1 cc.) intramuscularly or intravenously; ergonovine, 0.2 mg ($\frac{1}{320}$ gr.) or 1 cc. IM or IV; and Methergine, 0.2 mg. ($\frac{1}{320}$ gr.) or 1 cc. IM or IV. Various institutions use the drugs separately or in conjunction as is necessary to produce the desired results. The choice of the oxytocic usually will depend on the anesthetic agent administered. Oxytocin is contraindicated for use with drugs that have a sympathomimetic action.

CONDUCT OF THE FOURTH STAGE

Physiological Considerations

These first hours after delivery have been described aptly as the "fourth stage of labor." The wearying work of labor per se is completed and the mother and father can look forward to a brief respite before assuming the forthcoming responsibilities of parenthood. This is truly a transition period and many important physical and psychosocial tasks will be begun at this time.

After the delivery has been completed and the episiotomy repaired, the drapes and the soiled linen under the mother's buttocks are removed, and the lower end of the delivery table is replaced. If stirrups have been used, the mother's legs are lowered *simultaneously* to prevent cramping or twisting of the extremities. A sterile perineal pad is applied and the mother given a clean, warm gown and covered with a blanket to avoid chilling. Usually she and the infant are then transferred to the postpartum recovery area. Some institutions still require that the infant be transferred immediately to the newborn nursery.

Management of Potential Complications

Hypothermic Reactions. Chilling accompanied by uncontrollable shaking often occurs in this early period after delivery. It is uncomfortable and sometimes embarrassing or frightening for the patient but is self-limiting (usually not over 15 minutes) and is not considered an ominous sign. The exact etiology has not been determined, although several explanations have been offered, which include sudden release of intraabdominal pressure after delivery, nervous and exhaustion responses related to the stress of childbirth, disequilibrium in the internal and external body temperature resulting from the waste products of muscular exertion, break in aseptic technique which predisposes to infection, minute circulatory amniotic fluid emboli and previous maternal sensitization to elements of fetal blood.

Clean, dry, warm gowns and blankets as well as a warm nondrafty environment help in the prevention and control of this phenomenon. Warm fluids by mouth can be given and are much appreciated for their hydrating and energy-giving effects.

Postpartum Hemorrhage. Constant massage of the uterus during this period immediately after delivery is unnecessary and undesirable. However, if the organ shows any tendency to relax, it is to be massaged immediately with firm but gentle circular strokes until it contracts effectively. *Relaxation of the uterus is a prime cause of postpartum hemorrhage, and surveillance of the uterus and the amount of bleeding is of extreme importance at this time.*

Since the prevention of postpartum hemorrhage is such a crucial factor in the health and well-being of the mother, those patients at risk (most likely) to develop this condition should be identified quickly. The following include the most predictive factors associated with postpartum bleeding:

1. Older age and high parity
2. Rapid labor
3. Prolonged first and second stages of labor
4. Operative delivery, i.e., forceps extraction
5. Overdistention of the uterus—polyhydramnios, multiple pregnancy, overly large infant
6. Previous uterine atony and/or associated previous postpartal hemorrhage
7. Other hemorrhagic complications such as abruptio placentae or placenta previa
8. Induced labor
9. Heavy medication during labor and/or general anesthesia
10. Preeclampsia and eclampsia

The nurse will want to have in readiness an intravenous infusion with an oxytocin for immediate administration in the event that the physician suspects hemorrhage is imminent.

Vital Signs. Thus, the first hour following the delivery is a most critical one for the mother, since it is at this time that postpartal hemorrhage is most likely to occur. *The fundus is to be checked every five minutes or so and massaged as necessary to ensure continued firmness and prevent its ballooning with blood* (Fig. 23-14).

It is also important to be alert not only to the condition of the mother's uterus but also to any abnormal symptoms relating to her general condition. Thus, checking the maternal vital signs are included in the nursing interventions.

Blood pressure and pulse are generally checked every 15 minutes until stable and then every half hour for one hour. Thereafter, they are continued every hour for several hours until the mother is definitely stabilized.

The flow is also checked about every half hour and the number of pads saturated is recorded.

Psychosocial Considerations

Emotional Reactions

Immediately after delivery, or perhaps later, the parents, particularly the mother, may relieve tension by giving way to some emotional displays such as laughing, crying, talking incessantly or expressing anger (if all has not gone well or as expected). These emotions often are quite unexpected and shock and embarrass those involved. A calm, accepting, nonjudgmental attitude on the part of the nurse is very effective in allaying any embarrassment and in helping the patient to gain control.

The nurse must remember that the patient is beginning a period that is enormously important; she is, in fact, now a "mother" with all its concomitant responsibilities; glimmerings of this already are reaching the consciousness. This is not the "end" but only the beginning of a whole new role! In addition, she is physically and emotionally exhausted from the great effort she has put forth; thus, there may be a temporary emotional upheaval.

Several comfort measures can be employed to restore calm and to help the mother to relax enough to get some much-needed rest and sleep. A soothing backrub, change of gown and linen, a quiet conversation with the nurse and/or the father in which the patient is allowed to ventilate her feelings, an environment conducive to rest—all are helpful. In addition, a warm beverage can be offered to help to allay undue excitement; since the mother is apt to be extremely hungry and thirsty, this is welcome nourishment as well as a therapeutic soporific.

Many mothers, of course, do not have an emotional outburst per se, although the majority do experience some degree of excitement and elation when the delivery is accomplished. Any of the above nursing activities are suitable also for them. Some patients experience a great need for sleep and drop off as soon as they ascertain that the baby is "all right." If the patient is sleeping continuously or intermittently, she should be allowed to do so, being disturbed only for those nursing observations which are necessary. When she indicates readiness, her baby can be presented, and she can be allowed to examine and to explore it to her heart's content.

The mothers who have not been conscious during the delivery may have rather different reactions from those patients who have participated in the birth process. Often they do not seem to believe that delivery has taken place or that the baby shown them "is really mine." They will question again and again: "Is it really all over?" "Tell me again, is it a boy or a girl?" "Did I have the baby?" The apparent alteration in awareness seems to be related to the anesthesia and the unconsciousness. These patients may need more firm reassurance and contact with their infants to help them realize that they have had a baby.

The Symbiotic Relationship and Mother–Infant Bonding

Even though the repeated questioning may become annoying, the nurse will recognize that this is necessary for the mother in order to begin the important process of disengagement from the symbiotic relationship that she had with her infant during pregnancy. She must now establish the baby as a real entity outside her body rather than inside. All mothers have this task to perform, but it may be harder for the mother who has been delivered under heavy anesthesia, for as far as she is concerned, she was not "there" when it all happened.

Maternal attachment feelings, as we know, do not spring unbound at the time of delivery. Rather, they are developed, often slowly, as in any other developmental process. It is now becoming recognized that the early encounters the mother has with her newborn (which often begin immediately after delivery) pave the way for later maternal responses in the postpartal period and, indeed, throughout life.[11]

Maternal attachment behavior has been defined as the extent to which a mother feels that her infant occupies an essential position in her life. Components of this phenomenon are feelings of warmth or love, a sense of possession, devotion, protectiveness and concern for the infant's well-being, positive anticipation of prolonged contact and a

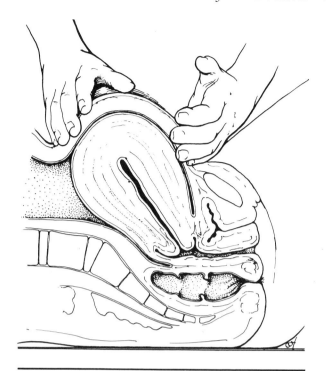

Figure 23-14. Proper method of palpating fundus of uterus during first hour after delivery to guard against relaxation and hemorrhage. The right hand is placed just above the symphysis pubis to act as a guard; meanwhile the other hand is cupped around the fundus of the uterus.

need for and pleasure in continuing transactions. As in other meaningful relationships, there is an acceptance of impositions and obligations intolerable with less important objects and a sense of loss experienced with the infant's actual or imagined absence.[12]

Assessment of Family Integration

Rising has pointed out that there is a certain openness about the fourth stage of labor that may not occur again during the postpartum period. This openness allows the nurse to make assessments regarding the couple's ability to proceed with integrating the infant smoothly into the family. She and other practitioners have suggested that it may be helpful to utilize a form to systematically record observations of the family unit during the fourth stage of labor (Table 23-3).[13] Such an assessment tool is invaluable in providing a focus for observations of behavior and can be further developed as a predictive tool to help determine those couples who may have difficulty in integration.

TABLE 23-3
OBSERVATIONS OF RESPONSES OF THE MOTHER DURING FOURTH STAGE OF LABOR

Patient's Name: _____

Please circle appropriate responses:

Verbal Responses

1. Calls baby by name
2. Calls baby affectionate terms
3. Comments on beauty of baby and on realistic defects
4. Voices unhappiness over sex of baby
5. Calls baby "it"
6. Uses unhappy or scolding inflections
7. Asks husband or nurse if baby is all right
8. Talks about baby
9. Answers in monosyllables
10. Complains of difficult labor and delivery
11. Doesn't talk about baby
12. Requests that baby be taken to nursery
13. Seeks considerable support for own discomfort

Nonverbal Responses

1. Looks, reaches out to baby
2. Hugs, touches baby
3. Smiles at baby
4. Kisses baby
5. Undresses baby
6. Doesn't touch baby
7. Doesn't look at baby
8. Pushes baby away
9. Tenses face, arms
10. Sleepy, not drug induced
11. Turns away from baby
12. Turns away from husband, nurse, visitor
13. Positive eye contact, emotional feeling with husband
14. Unresponsive to husband, nurse, visitor
15. Cries unhappily
16. Holds husband's hand
17. Breast feeds baby

First comments made in delivery room by mother about baby:
_____

Visitor with mother during fourth stage: _____
Involvement of husband or visitor: _____
Problems with baby: _____
Subjective opinion of response of mother: _____

Parity: _____
Age: _____
Marital status: _____
Feeding method: _____
Service: _____
Race: _____

Analgesia within last 4 hrs.: _____
Anesthesia: _____
Complications: _____
Significant social history: _____

Behavior of baby:
    Crying: None—periodic—almost continuous
    Affect: Difficult to arouse—dozes—eyes open—very alert

This form helped nurses at Yale focus their observations of mothers and infants the first one or two hours after delivery.
Source: Rising, S.: "The fourth stage of labor: Family integration." *Am. J. Nurs.* 74:873, May 1974.

If family units are so identified as potentially at risk for maladaptive integration, the nurse will want to set aside more time to be with the couple to reinforce any positive responses that they might demonstrate and to give as much encouragement as possible. Listening attentively as the couple relive their recent experiences (and perhaps their disappointments) and encouraging verbalization of these feelings, and at the same time pointing out to them whatever positive realities did occur in the recent event, can prove helpful. Most important, the nurse will want to pass on her observations and interventions to the postpartum personnel so that they may continue with positive interventions. These personnel, in turn, can work closely with community health nurses or arrange for other follow-up care to encourage subsequent adjustment. This is a time when the nurse needs to use all the observational skills, time and "laying on of the hands" to foster initial integration and to begin prescribing future care aimed at consolidating the family unit. The topic of parental–infant attachment will be discussed more thoroughly in Chapter 27, Psychosocial Aspects of the Postpartum Period.

IMMEDIATE CARE OF THE INFANT

Suctioning the Airway

As soon as the infant is born, measures are taken to promote a clear air passage before the onset of respiration. Often, as the head is delivered, it is necessary to wipe the mucus and fluid from the infant's nose and mouth before it has a chance to gasp and aspirate with this first breath. Babson and Benson recommend that the infant be kept in a face-down position immediately after delivery in order to facilitate the drainage of mucus, blood and amniotic fluid from the oropharynx.[14] A small rubber bulb syringe, or a soft rubber suction catheter attached to a mechanical suction or mouth aspirator, can be used promptly to suction the oropharynx and to remove fluids which may be obstructing the airway. If there seems to be much mucus present, the physician will hold the infant up by the ankles to encourage more mucus to drain from the throat. The mucosal surfaces of the palate and the posterior pharynx should not be wiped with gauze, since its rough texture can lead to abrasions and thus provide a portal of entry for pathogenic organisms. A

flexible rubber catheter may be passed by the physician to suction the larynx if the above measures do not clear the mucus well enough.

It is important *not to oversuction* at any time, because this merely deprives the infant of oxygen and irritates the mucous membrane. If further suctioning is necessary, the nurse may use the suction apparatus on the electric infant resuscitator, a bulb syringe, or a soft rubber catheter attached to a DeLee glass trap, which was designed especially for aspirating mucus in the treatment of newborn infants (Fig. 23-15). Care should be taken not to traumatize the tissues of the oropharynx with the tip of the catheter or with forceful suction. When the nasopharynx is obstructed by mucus which must be removed via the nostrils, a small French catheter may be passed into the nostril if force is avoided. The catheter must *not* be inserted far back. If the catheter is directed horizontally, as if passing over the roof of the mouth, instead of directing it upward as for the adult patient, it usually slips into the tiny infant nostril with more ease. If a bulb syringe is used, it should be collapsed before it is inserted in the baby's mouth; otherwise the material in the oropharynx will be forced into the bronchi and lungs when the bulb is collapsed.

Resuscitation

For the majority of normal newborns, there is little need for resuscitative measures beyond clearing the airway and applying warmth and gentle tactile stimulation. There are a small percentage of newborns who do require assistance, and for them it is life-saving assistance. Successful active resuscitation requires skilled personnel who have been trained in the procedure, a warm well-lighted work area, means to deliver oxygen by positive pressure, intubation if necessary and, finally, appropriate drug therapy.

Inadequate respirations that persist beyond a minute severely compromise the infant by leading to a falling heart rate, decreased muscle tone and greater possibility of acidosis. The airway must be cleared and oxygen delivered through a well-fitting mask at a pressure of about 20 cm. of water in 1- to 2-second spurts to deliver oxygen into the bronchi. The airway must be cleared well through suctioning, however, because the oxygen delivered under pressure will only force any foreign material deep into the infant's lungs. If this procedure (called "bagging") does not promptly stimulate breathing and correct the evidence of hypoxia, endotracheal intubation will be necessary under direct visualization with a laryngoscope. Further details of resuscitative measures can be found in Chapter 39.

Stimulating Crying

The baby may not "cry" at once, but it usually gasps or cries after the mucus has been removed, as oxygen by way of the lungs is now needed, since the accustomed supply was cut off when the placental circulation stopped.

If crying has to be stimulated, it is to be done with extreme care. As the infant is being held in the head-down position to promote the drainage of mucus from the respiratory passages, gentle rubbing of the infant's back is usually sufficient stimulus to initiate crying. And, in the act of crying, mucus is forced from the nose and the throat, thus enabling the infant to be better able to breathe.

Vigorous, external irritants are *unnecessary* and *dangerous* and should not be employed. These include harsh spanking on the soles of the feet and/or buttocks, forcible rubbing of the skin along the spine, alternate hot and cold tubbing of the infant, and dilatation of the anal sphincter. These obsolete procedures are shocking to the infant.

Preventing Hypothermia

A sterile receiving blanket is made available so that the infant may be wrapped securely to prevent heat loss. It must be remembered that any room, and particularly the delivery room, is much cooler than the mother's body, and if not properly cared for the infant can become dangerously chilled. Korones and others stress the importance of providing environmental warmth to minimize loss of the infant's body heat.[15] At birth, a major cause of heat loss is the evaporation of amniotic fluid from the infant's skin. Thus, the infant is to be dried rapidly by the nurse who takes the infant from the physician as soon as the infant's airway is cleared satisfactorily.

The baby can be placed in a slight Trendelenberg position (15°) or in a supine position for the immediate appraisal. There are various devices for preventing hypothermia in the infant. They include a warmed incubator, resuscitators that can be warmed, and overhead radiant lights. *The basic principle behind the use of this equipment is the same— to maintain the infant's body temperature which is related to the amount of oxygen needed by the infant, the control of apnea, and finally an acid-base balance.*

Assessment of the Newborn Infant

It cannot be stressed enough that the infant's condition be assessed accurately immediately after birth and that close observations be continued by the nurse. The information gathered concerning the baby's responses will provide valuable baseline data for subsequent care in the nursery.

The Apgar Scoring System

The Apgar score provides a valuable index for assessing the newborn infant's condition at birth. Every nurse who is responsible for the care of newborn infants, not merely those in the delivery room, should be familiar with the principles set forth by Apgar for infant assessment because they provide a simple, accurate and safe means of quickly appraising the infant's condition.

The Apgar scoring system is based on the following five signs (ranked in order of importance) each of which is evaluated at one minute of life and repeated again in five minutes. Each sign is evaluated according to the degree to which it is present and is given a score of 0, 1, or 2 (Table 23-4). The scores of each of the signs then are added to give a total score (10 is maximum).

Heart Rate. This sign is the most important and the last to be absent when the infant's condition is grave. It may be evaluated by palpating the pulsation

TABLE 23-4
THE APGAR SCORING CHART

Sign	0	1	2
Heart rate	Absent	Slow (less than 100)	Over 100
Respiratory effort	Absent	Slow, irregular	Good, crying
Muscle tone	Flaccid	Some flexion of extremities	Active motion
Reflex irritability	No response	Weak cry or grimace	Vigorous cry
Color	Blue, pale	Body pink, extremities blue	Completely pink

of the cord or by observing the pulsation where the cord joins the abdomen. Listening to the heartbeat with a stethoscope the most accurate method of ascertaining the beat. The beat may range from 150 to 180 beats per minute during the first few minutes of life; later, within the hour, it usually slows to between 130 and 140 beats per minute. Crying or increased activity will increase the number of beats. If the rate is 100 per minute or under, asphyxia is present, and resuscitation is indicated.

Respiratory Effort. A baby who is responding well cries vigorously and has no difficulty in breathing. "Regular" respiration usually is established in a minute or so. Depressed, irregular respiration or apnea indicates that respiratory difficulty is present, and these signs should be reported immediately so that prompt treatment may be instituted.

Muscle Tone. An infant who has excellent tonus will keep his extremities flexed and resist efforts to extend them. A baby who does not keep his extremities flexed consistently usually has only moderate tonus; one who is flaccid is in extremely poor condition.

Reflex Irritability. Although there are several ways to test this sign, the one most frequently used is a gentle slap on the sole of the infant's foot. This sign can be observed when a vigorous infant is suctioned for mucus by the way in which it resists the catheter. A baby who is in excellent condition will respond with a vigorous cry. An infant is judged to have a poor response if it cries weakly or merely makes a grimace. If there is a good deal of central nervous system depression, the infant will not respond at all.

Color. Cyanosis is seen in all infants at the moment of birth. As the infant's circulation makes the change from fetal to extrauterine existence and breathing begins, the body of a healthy infant usually will become pink within three minutes. Since acrocyanosis usually is present for a short while, even in infants who are in excellent condition, those who have scored 2 for each of the other signs may receive only a score of 1 for this part of the evaluation. This will, of course, influence the total score.

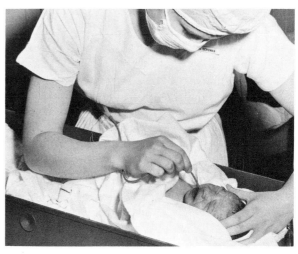

Figure 23-15. Suctioning the newborn in the delivery room.

Interpretation. An Apgar score of 7 to 10 indicates that the infant's condition is good. If the infant breathes and cries (or coughs) seconds after delivery, there are usually no special procedures necessary other than those of routine close observation, maintaining a clear airway, and supplying warmth as necessary.

A score of 4 to 6 means that the baby is in fair condition. There may be moderate central nervous system depression, some muscle flaccidity and cyanosis; respiration will not establish readily. *These infants must have their air passages cleared and be given oxygen promptly.* Administration of oxygen can best be done by mask, and the flow should not exceed 4 liters. Gentle patting and rubbing with the receiving blanket to dry the infant's body usually acts as an additional stimulus.

A score of 0 to 3 denotes an extremely poor condition. Resuscitation is needed immediately (see Chapter 39).

During the interval following the five-minute Apgar score, the nurse will continue evaluating the infant.

1. Auscultation of the chest will ascertain proper position of the heart and normal air exchange.
2. The head and body surfaces are scrutinized for trauma and for obvious congenital anomalies. These can include caput succedaneum, cephalhematoma, or forceps marks.
3. The anterior fontanel is checked for bulging or sunkenness and the head circumference for enlargement or smallness.
4. The skin is also checked for scaling or undue

wrinkling indicative of the maturity of the infant. Any jaundice is also noted.

5. The abdomen is palpated for masses and for enlargement of the liver, spleen or kidneys.

6. The genitalia are examined for normal sexuality and the anus for patency.

7. Each of the shoulders is moved while a finger is placed over the clavicle. A crunching sensation (crepitus) indicates a fracture.

8. Before the final clamp is applied to the cord, the physician or nurse will examine it closely to see if it contains the normal number of vessels (two arteries and one vein). The presence of only one artery suggests one or more major congenital malformations. The cut edges of the arteries are seen as two white papular structures, which usually stand out slightly from the surface. The vein is larger, often gaping so that the lumen and thin wall are easily seen.

The student is referred to Chapter 29 for details of the physical assessment and the nurse's responsibilities.

One further note of caution is appropriate at this time. Als and Brazelton have made the point that infants whose mothers have been heavily premedicated may respond at delivery with excellent function and optimal Apgar scores. However, these same infants arrive in the neonatal nursery as little as 30 minutes later in a dangerously depressed state of unresponsiveness. Their color, respirations, and muscle tone, as well as their ability to respond to life-threatening mucus in their airways, are so depressed that they need constant nursing care for this transient period of depressed function.[16] This fact has special relevance if the baby is to spend some time with the parents before being transferred to the nursery. The nurse will want to be especially watchful whenever the mother has had a good deal of medication throughout labor or just before delivery.

Other Aspects of Care

Care of the Cord

In most hospitals no dressing is applied after the cord has been clamped or ligated and cut. It is imperative that frequent inspection be done to note any signs of bleeding. The method of leaving the cord stump exposed has proved to be very satisfactory. If it is left free, it apparently dries and separates more quickly than when it is kept covered.

Care of the Eyes

As soon as the cord is cared for and the infant's respiration is well established, the eyes receive prophylactic treatment for protection against ophthalmia neonatorum (see Chapter 39). This treatment is so important that at the present time the use of some antibacterial agent is mandatory by statute in all states.

Penicillin and silver nitrate are the usual agents employed, although a nonirritating solution of 15 percent sulphacetamide is preferred by some physicians. When silver nitrate is used, it is supplied in wax ampuls containing a 1 percent solution especially prepared for eye instillation (Fig. 23-16).

Instilling drops in the infant's eyes is more easily accomplished if the infant's eyes are shaded from the light while the drops are put first in one eye, allowing time for the baby to recover from the shock and the discomfort before the drops are put in the other eye. One of the best methods is to draw down the lower lid gently and carefully instill two drops of the solution in the conjunctival sac, using great care not to drop it on the cornea. After two minutes, when it will have diffused itself over the entire conjunctiva, the lids should again be held apart and the conjunctival sac of each eye flushed gently with normal saline solution or sterile distilled water (Fig. 23-17). Prompt irrigation of the eyes following instillation of silver nitrate drops is said to reduce the incidence of chemical conjunctivitis without affecting prophylactic efficacy. Special precautions should be taken to avoid contaminating the eyes or dropping any silver solution upon the face. Silver nitrate prophylaxis may cause signs of irritation, such as redness, edema or discharge, but

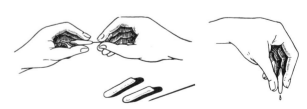

Figure 23-16. (Left) Silver nitrate 1 percent solution for the care of the eyes of newborn babies; needle puncture of wax ampule. *(Right)* Showing how to manipulate the ampule in administering the drug. (Eli Lilly and Company)

these manifestations are transient and in no way cause permanent damage if the silver nitrate solution used is in correct concentration.

Recently there has been some discussion concerning the timing of the silver nitrate instillation. Research has indicated that the instillation tends to blur the infant's vision temporarily and would thus interfere with the focusing and eye-to-eye contact deemed necessary for maternal–infant bonding in the first hours of life. Klaus and his coworkers have delayed the instillation for one to two hours after birth until the infant has had time to interact with the parents. They report that there has been no increase in infection as a result of this delay.[17]

If penicillin is to be used, it can be obtained in ophthalmic drops or ointment. The technique for instillation is similar to that for silver nitrate, except that there is no flushing with saline or water. Penicillin is also given intramuscularly for both prophylaxis and treatment of ophthalmia neonatorum. When gonorrheal ophthalmia does develop, it can be cured by penicillin within a few hours, whereas silver nitrate has long since been abandoned for treatment of this disorder. The incidence of chemical irritation with penicillin ointment or intramuscular injection is much less than with silver nitrate, and the irritation is generally milder. However, some sensitivity reactions have been reported; thus silver nitrate continues to be used.

Hypoprothrombinemia Prophylaxis

Many physicians prescribe that a single dose of phytonadione solution (AquaMEPHYTON) 1.0 mg. (0.5 cc.) be administered intramuscularly during the course of the immediate care of the newborn after delivery. This water-soluble form of vitamin K_1 acts as a preventative measure against neonatal hemorrhagic disease. Amounts of the medication in excess of 1.0 mg. may predispose to the development of hyperbilirubinemia and are to be avoided.

Identification Methods

Some method of identification of the newborn is applied before the cord is cut or before the baby is removed from the delivery room. Most hospitals use pliable plastic tapes which are applied to the infant's wrist and ankle. These contain the mother's name, physician's name, date, time of birth, and sex of the infant, and often the mother's hospital

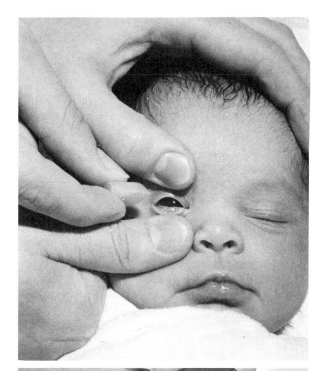
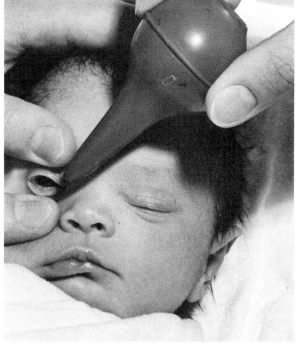

Figure 23-17. Silver nitrate prophylaxis. (*Top*) Instillation of two drops of silver nitrate 1 percent solution from a wax ampule into the conjunctival sac of each eye. (*Bottom*) After the medication has diffused over the entire conjunctiva (two minutes), the conjunctival sac of each eye is gently flushed with sterile distilled water or normal saline solution to remove the excess silver nitrate.

number. The baby's identification is checked against the mother's each time the baby is brought to her.

In addition, palmprints or footprints may be taken. This method of identification consists of a stainless procedure made on chemically treated, sensitized paper. It is designed to take the palmprints or footprints of the baby and the thumbprint of the mother at the time of delivery and may be repeated at the time of discharge from the hospital. It is a simple quick and permanent method.

Current practice emphasizes that the newborn should be discharged without removing the identification band. Several states now have laws making it mandatory not to remove the identification bands on hospital premises. The mother should be taught how to remove the band as part of the discharge instructions.

As already discussed in Chapter 2, the registration of the infant's birth is a legal responsibility. It is mandatory that a birth certificate, be filled out on every birth and submitted promptly to the local registrar.

After the Delivery

If the mother is awake after delivery, she may be anxious to have her baby brought near so that she may see it at close range. If she is drowsy, it may be better to wait until she is more alert. The nurse will be governed by each mother's response at this time.

If the infant is well wrapped and warm, it may be kept in a crib at the mother's side until the mother leaves the delivery room. The infant should be kept in a slight Trendelenburg position (at an angle of 15°) to promote drainage of mucus, and on his side to avoid aspiration of this mucus.

Care should be taken to avoid placing the infant in an exaggerated Trendelenburg position (almost directly downward), since the relatively large amount of abdominal contents will press against the diaphragm and the partially expanded lungs and may impede the infant's respiratory efforts.

The nurse observes the infant at frequent intervals to make sure that he is breathing properly, that the mouth and the nose are free from mucus, and that there is no bleeding from the cord. Because this period may be a critical one for the infant, many hospitals have facilities, such as a receiving nursery

on the labor and delivery division, where the infant is transferred at this time. This provides closer supervision for the infant and permits the nurse in the delivery room to devote her undivided attention to the mother. The chart on page 356 presents a care plan for the mother and infant during labor and delivery.

Baptism of Infant

If there is any probability that the infant is in imminent danger and may not live, the question of baptism should be considered in cases in which the religion of the family is Roman Catholic; this also applies to some of the other denominations of the Christian church. This is an essential duty and means a great deal to the families concerned, and thoughtfulness in this matter will never be forgotten by them. (It is to be understood that such baptism would be reported to the family.)

The following simple instructions, issued by a member of the clergy, may be followed:

The Catholic Church teaches that in case of emergency, anyone may and should baptize. What is necessary is to make the intention of doing what the Church wishes to do and then to pour the water on the child (the head by preference) saying at the same time, "I baptize thee in the name of the Father and of the Son and of the Holy Ghost." The water may be warmed if necessary but it must be pure water and care should be taken to make it flow. If there is any doubt whether the child is alive or dead, it should be baptized, but conditionally (i.e., "If thou art alive, I baptize thee . . .").

In the Book of Common Prayer of the protestant Episcopal church, it is stated: "In cases of extreme sickness, or any imminent peril, if a Minister cannot be procured, then any baptized person present may administer holy Baptism, using the foregoing form" (i.e., the form given above).

PRECIPITATE DELIVERY

In the course of labor one occasionally encounters the so-called *precipitate delivery*, a rapid spontaneous delivery in which the infant is born without benefit of asepsis. This may occur in certain multiparous women, particularly if the soft parts of the pelvis offer little resistance or if the contractions are unusually strong and forceful. It also can occur if the mother does not experience painful sensations during labor and thus has inadequate warning that the delivery is approaching.

The mother, of course, may suffer lacerations of the tissues as the result of tumultuous labor. The infant is endangered because, in its rapid progress through the birth canal, it may suffer cerebral trauma; or the umbilical cord may be torn in the process of the delivery. In addition, if the mother is unattended, the infant may be in jeopardy from lack of care during the first few minutes of life.

Whether the nurse is caring for a mother in the hospital labor room, making a home visit, or involved in some emergency situation, it is well to be prepared for a precipitate delivery. It seldom happens that the nurse is alone with the patient in the hospital when the delivery is imminent; but knowing what to do in such a situation is advantageous for all concerned.

It should be stressed that the nurse's composure and ability to convey calm is one of the cornerstones in a successful delivery. Whenever possible, the mother should be told what to anticipate and what she can do to cooperate effectively. Here teamwork with the mother is essential and can be accomplished if confidence is instilled by demonstrating competence in both the physical and the emotional aspects of care. If the father is present, he can be utilized in the care of the mother in whatever capacity seems most appropriate and in accord with his ability. He might help best by taking care of the other children or by calling the physician, or he might be involved directly in some aspect of the delivery. If it seems more desirable that he be away from the immediate vicinity, then the reasons for his leaving should be given. He is not to be dismissed summarily from the situation.

The nurse who is consistently conscientious about applying principles of asepsis and antisepsis will automatically apply them in this instance as much as is possible. Usually, there is inadequate time to cleanse the vulva properly or scrub and don sterile gloves, or drape the mother, all of which would be ideal. However, a clean delivery area should be maintained, and, if time and facilities permit, the nurse's hands should be cleansed.

Delivery of the Head. As the head distends the perineum at the acme of a contraction, gentle pressure is exerted against the head to control its progress and thereby to prevent undue stretching of the perineum. This kind of *control* applied during

each contraction will prevent the head from suddenly pushing through the vulva and causing subsequent complications. *The head must never be held back.* The mother should be encouraged to pant during the contraction to deter bearing-down efforts on her part, particularly as the head, which will be supported by the nurse, is being delivered. Whenever possible, the infant's head should be delivered between contractions. It is important to remember not to put the fingers into the vagina since this increases the chance of infection.

Rupture of the Membranes. If the membranes have not ruptured previously, they may remain intact until they appear as a smooth, glistening object at the vulva. If they protrude, they may rupture with the next contraction. But if the membranes have not ruptured before the head is delivered, they must be broken and removed immediately (by nipping them at the nape of the infant's neck) to prevent aspiration of fluid when the infant takes its first breath.

Precautions Concerning the Cord. As soon as the head is delivered, the nurse should feel for a loop or loops of cord around the neck and, if any is found, gently slip it over the baby's head, if this can be done easily. If the cord is coiled too tightly to permit this, it must be doubly clamped and cut (between the clamps) before the rest of the body is delivered. One or more loops of cord around the fetal neck occur in about a quarter of all deliveries.

Delivery of the Infant's Body. After external rotation of the head, which is usually spontaneous, there is no occasion for haste in the delivery of the body. Gentle downward pressure with the hands on either side of the head may be exerted to direct the anterior shoulder under the symphysis pubis, then reversed upward in order to deliver the posterior shoulder over the perineum. The infant's body now will follow easily and quickly and should be supported as it is born.

Immediate Care of the Infant. As soon as the face appears, mucus and fluids should be wiped from the nose and the mouth. Then, after the infant is born, if he does not cry spontaneously, or if there seems to be mucus in the respiratory passages, the infant should be held up by the ankles to encourage the mucus to drain from the nose and mouth. In doing this, care must be exercised to avoid any traction on the umbilical cord and, at the same time, to prevent the infant's head from pressing down against the bed. Drainage of mucus is stimulated when the infant cries but can be encouraged by "milking the trachea" (i.e., with the forefinger, stroking the neck from its base toward the chin). Further stimulation by gentle rubbing of the back may stimulate breathing.

Care of the Cord. There is *no* hurry to cut the cord, so this should be delayed until proper equipment is available. It is a good plan to clamp the cord after pulsations cease (but not imperative at the moment) and to wait for the physician to cut the cord later. One must always bear in mind that sterile conditions must exist for the cord-cutting procedure; otherwise the infant's safety is jeopardized. Also, the technique for applying the cord tie or umbilical clamp must be assiduously carried out to prevent bleeding from the umbilical stump.

Delivery of the Placenta. When signs of placental separation are apparent, the mother can be asked to bear down with the next contraction to deliver the placenta. Since the danger of hemorrhage is always to be guarded against, the fundus should be massaged after the delivery of the placenta if there is the slightest tendency toward relaxation of the uterine muscles.

When the infant is breathing satisfactorily, he can be placed on his side across his mother's abdomen (with his head kept low to promote postural drainage and his body covered to prevent chilling). This accomplishes several things: the mother is given her baby, she can touch him and is usually enthralled by the close physical contact with him; the warmth of the mother's body prevents the infant from being chilled; and the pressure exerted on the uterus by the weight of the infant helps it to contract.

One must remember to proceed slowly and carefully throughout the delivery. As stated earlier, the nurse's reaction to the situation undoubtedly will be transferred to the mother; if the nurse remains poised and unfaltering, the mother and other people involved are more likely to do so.

LACERATIONS OF THE BIRTH CANAL

During the process of a normal delivery lacerations of the perineum and the vagina may be caused by rapid and sudden expulsion of the head (particularly when it "pops" out), the excessive size of the infant and very friable maternal tissues. In other circumstances they may be caused by difficult forceps deliveries, breech extractions or contraction of the pelvic outlet in which the head is forced posteriorly. Some tears are unavoidable, even in the most skilled hands.

Perineal lacerations usually are classified in three degrees, according to the extent of the tear.

First-degree lacerations are those which involve the fourchet, the perineal skin and the vaginal mucous membrane without involving any of the muscles.

Second-degree lacerations are those which involve (in addition to skin and mucous membrane) the muscles of the perineal body but not the rectal sphincter. These tears usually extend upward on one or both sides of the vagina, making a triangular injury.

Third-degree lacerations are those which extend completely through the skin, the mucous membrane, the perineal body and the rectal sphincter. This type is often referred to as a complete tear. Not infrequently these third-degree lacerations ex-

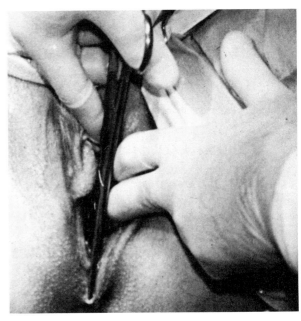

Figure 23-18. Median episiotomy. (From the film *Human Birth* published by J. B. Lippincott Co., Philadelphia.)

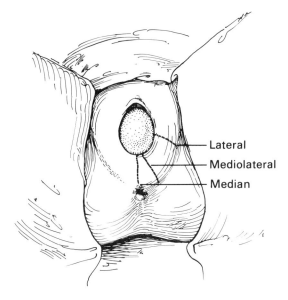

Figure 23-19. Types of episiotomies.

tend a certain distance up the anterior wall of the rectum.

First- and second-degree lacerations are extremely common in primigravidas; their high incidence is one of the reasons that episiotomy is widely employed. Fortunately, third-degree lacerations are far less common. All three types of lacerations are repaired by the physician immediately after the delivery to ensure that the perineal structures are returned approximately to their former condition. The technique employed for the repair of a laceration is virtually the same as that used for episiotomy incisions, although the former is more difficult to do because of the irregular lines of tissue which must be approximated.

EPISIOTOMY AND REPAIR

An episiotomy is an incision of the perineum made to facilitate delivery. The incision is made with blunt-pointed straight scissors about the time that the head distends the vulva and is visible to a diameter of several centimeters. The incision may be made in the midline of the perineum—a median episiotomy (Fig. 23-18). Or it may be begun in the midline and directed downward and laterally away from the rectum—a mediolateral episiotomy. In the latter instance the incision may be directed to either the right or to the left side of the mother's pelvis (Fig. 23-19).

As the infant's head distends the vulva, if a laceration seems to be inevitable, the physician undoubtedly will choose to incise the perineum rather than allow that structure to sustain a traumatic tear. This operation serves several purposes:

1. It substitutes a straight, clean-cut surgical incision for the ragged, contused laceration which otherwise may ensue; such an incision is easier to repair and heals better than a tear.
2. The direction of the episiotomy can be controlled, whereas a tear may extend in any direction, sometimes involving the anal sphincter and the rectum.
3. Inordinate stretching and tearing of the perineal musculature is avoided and the incidence of subsequent perineal relaxation with cystocele-rectocele may be reduced.
4. The operation shortens the duration of the second stage of labor.

In view of these advantages many physicians employ episiotomy routinely in the delivery of the primigravida.

There are many equally satisfactory methods utilized for episiotomy repair (Fig. 23-20). The suture material ordinarily used is a fine chromic catgut, either 00 or 000.

A round needle and continuous suture is used to

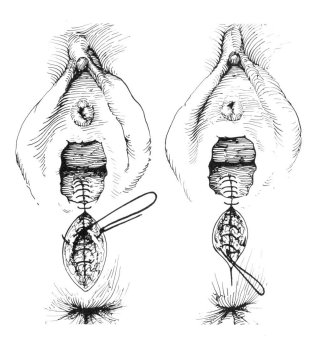

Figure 23-20. Episiotomy repair.

NURSING CARE DURING LABOR

Assessment	Intervention	Evaluation
	First Stage	
Greeting of parents	Convey that the parents are expected and welcome	Parents become familiar with the new environment and settle in.
a. Orientation to unit b. Orientation to labor	a. After finding out what they know, explain the expectations, restrictions (food, fluids, activity) of the environment and what will be happening during the labor process.	
Labor history	Interview and record and report information as appropriate	Mother and nurse begin to establish rapport.
a. When labor became apparent b. Frequency, duration and intensity of contractions c. Condition of the BOW d. Character and amount of show e. Vital signs: T.P.R. and BP f. Bowel and bladder patterns		
Admission procedures a. Enema b. Perineal clip c. Abdominal exam d. Vaginal exam e. General exam	Explain to parents the intended procedures a. Administer enema if necessary b. Complete perineal prep c. Palpate abdomen to ascertain presenting part d. Do or assist with remainder of examinations; record and report information	Parents have an understanding of the upcoming events. Mother assists examiners appropriately. Nurse-patient relationship continues to be built.
Continue to monitor labor: Contractions, FHR, vital signs, bladder distension, fluid intake, show. Determine need for electronic monitor.	Attach electronic monitor if necessary or time contractions, check FHR as indicated. Record and report information. Encourage voiding. Offer fluids if ordered early in labor.	Labor progresses. Mother works with her contractions. Bladder does not become distended, fluid intake appropriate.
Determine which comfort measures are necessary: back rub, oral hygiene, clean linen, etc.	Rub back, change mother's position and linen as necessary.	Mother relaxes between contractions. Father feels a part of the labor process; mother benefits by his presence and support.
Determine father's ability to coach/support the mother.	Allow parents time together; encourage father's participation in mother's care.	
Determine mother's need for explanations, emotional support as indicated as labor progresses.	Explain labor process as indicated—help mother change breathing patterns as indicated with onset of transition. Keep explanations, instructions short and simple.	Changes to shallow breathing with transition. Follows instructions with minimum of difficulty.
	Second Stage	
Continue to monitor labor: Determine appropriateness of bearing down.	Record and report as before. Monitor FHR every 5 minutes during delivery. Monitor maternal BP. Position mother correctly for "pushing"; coach as necessary.	Physician has a clear picture of mother's progress—infant's vital signs stable, mother's BP stable; mother works with contractions to enable delivery.
Transfer to delivery room	Instruct father in delivery room procedures if father will accompany mother.	Father coaches mother appropriately.
Assistance with anesthesia	Help with positioning for anesthesia if necessary. Assist with supplies, vital signs monitoring, intravenous infusions.	Anesthesia given on time and appropriately.

NURSING CARE DURING LABOR—Continued

Assessment	Intervention	Evaluation
Assistance with delivery	Continue coaching of mother in pushing and panting. Do perineal prep, draping as indicated. Check FHR, maternal BP as indicated.	A well infant delivered under aseptic conditions.
	Third Stage	
Postdelivery: The mother: Postdelivery observations: fundus, flow, bladder, vital signs, perineum	Administer oxytocin after delivery of placenta as needed. Gently massage fundus, if boggy; express clots as necessary. Record and report amount and character of flow, vital signs, hematoma/bleeding from episiotomy.	Uterus contracts after placental separation. Flow moderates. Vital signs stable. Bladder nondistended.
Determine need for comfort, rest.	Reposition mother as needed. Give warm and dry gown, blanket; provide adequate explanations, answers to questions; provide quiet environment for rest; provide light nourishment as indicated.	Mother warm and comfortable.
Post delivery: The infant: Determine general status	Apgar score at 1 min. and 5 min. Provide for warmth with radiant heat, blanket. Monitor airway and breathing. Eye prophylaxis. Weigh and measure height, head circumference. Examine body systems by thorough observation, inspection, palpation, and auscultation. Record, report as appropriate.	Infant adapts to extrauterine life with minimal trauma. Respirations stable, color and muscle tone good. No abnormalities or anomalies.
Family interaction	Enable father or companion to be with mother. Enable parents to explore infant if possible.	Mother interacts with partner and baby satisfactorily.
	Fourth Stage	
Postdelivery observations	Continue as before	Mother and infant's conditions stable.
Family interaction	See Chapter 27	Interaction mutually satisfactory.

close the vaginal mucosa and fourchet and then laid aside while several interrupted sutures are placed in the levator ani muscle and the fascia. Then the continuous suture is again picked up and used to unite the subcutaneous fascia. Finally, the round needle is replaced by a large, straight cutting needle, and the running suture is continued upward as a subcuticular stitch.

REFERENCES

1. E. A. Friedman: *Labor, Clinical Evaluation and Management*, ed. 2. New York, Appleton-Century-Crofts, 1978.
2. M. A. Newman: "Identifying and meeting patients' needs in short-span nurse-patient relationships." *Nurs. Form.* 5, 1:76–86, 1966.
3. L. Aiken and J. Aiken: "A systematic approach to the evaluation of interpersonal relationships." *Am. J. Nurs.* 73:863–867, May 1973.
4. B. J. Kalisch: "What is empathy?" *Am. J. Nurs.* 73:1548–1552, Sept. 1973.
5. Ibid.
6. Y. C. Liu: "Effects of the upright position during labor." *Am. J. Nurs.* 74:2202–2205, Dec. 1974.
7. J. E. Roberts: "Maternal positions for childbirth: A historical review of nursing care practices." *JOGN Nurs.* 8:24–32, Jan./Feb. 1979.

8. F. Leboyer: *Birth without Violence.* New York, Alfred A. Knopf, 1975.

9. M. Oliver and G. M. Oliver: "Gentle birth, its safety and effect on neonatal behavior." *JOGN Nurs.* 7:35–40, Sept./Oct. 1978.

10. Ibid.

11. C. R. Barnett et al.: "The maternal side of interactional deprivation." *Pediatrics,* 45:197, 1970.

12. D. S. Robson and H. A. Moss: "Patterns and determinants of maternal attachment." *Pediatrics,* 77:976–985, Dec. 1970.

13. S. Rising: "The fourth stage of labor: Family integration." *Am. J Nurs.* 74:870–874, May 1974.

14. S. G. Babson and R. C. Benson: *Management of High Risk Pregnancy and Intensive Care of the Newborn,* ed. 2. St. Louis, C. V. Mosby, 1971.

15. S. B. Korones: *High Risk Newborn Infants: The Basis for Intensive Care,* ed. 2. St. Louis, C. V. Mosby, 1976.

16. H. Als and T. B. Brazelton: "Comprehensive neonatal assessment." *Birth and the Family J.* 2:3–9, Winter 1974–75.

17. M. H. Klaus: "The biology of parent-to-infant attachment." Paper and discussion presented at the meeting: Technological Approaches to Obstetrics: Benefits, Risks, Alternatives. San Francisco, Feb. 3–4, 1979.

SUGGESTED READING

Auld, P. A.: "Resuscitation of the newborn infant." *Am. J. Nurs.* 74:68–70, Jan. 1974.

Chagnon, L. J., and Heldenbrand, C. L.: "Nurses undertake direct and indirect fetal monitoring at a community hospital." *JOGN Nurs.* 41–46, Sept./Oct. 1974.

Henson, D.: "Natural childbirth in the year, O." *Nurs. For.* 17, 3:228–244, 1978.

Korones, S. B.: High Risk Newborn Infants: The Basis for Intensive Nursing Care, ed. 2. St. Louis, C. V. Mosby, 1976.

Roberts, J. E.: "Maternal positions for childbirth: A historical review of nursing care practices." *JOGN Nurs.* 8:24–32, Jan./Feb. 1979.

Saltenes, I. J.: "Physical touch and nursing support in labor." Unpublished master's thesis. New Haven, Conn., Yale University, 1962.

Shields, D.: "Maternal reactions to fetal monitoring." *Am. J. Nurs.* 78:2110–2112, Dec. 1978.

Yunek, M. J. and Lojek, M.: "Intrapartal fetal monitoring." *Am. J. Nurs.* 78:2106–2190, Dec. 1978.

Cronenwett, L. R., and Newmark, L. L.: "Fathers' responses to childbirth." *Nurs. Res.* 23:210–217, May/June 1974.

Twenty-Four

The Nurse's Contribution to Pain Relief During Labor

Nature of the Pain Experience During Labor /
Definitions / Pain Mechanisms / Descriptions of Painful
Sensations of Normal Labor / Assessment of Labor Pain /
Nonpharmacological Pain Relief During Labor /
Assistance with Change in Expectations and Goals /
Aftermath Assimilation

NATURE OF THE PAIN EXPERIENCE DURING LABOR

Beliefs about Pain During Labor

Is childbirth painful or painless? Most laypeople expect pain to occur during childbirth. This expectation may evolve from a variety of sources, such as television, movies, books, comments from one's own parents, and reports from friends who have had babies. However, information about childbirth in general may be incomplete, if not inaccurate. Hence fear of pain may be anticipated by expectant parents as a result of their overall lack of knowledge about labor.

The fear of pain is second only to the fear of death. Understandably, then, some expectant parents are eager to examine and accept any information suggesting that childbirth need not be associated with pain. Such information may be forthcoming from several sources.

Reports of how childbirth is handled in some other cultures, especially the more primitive ones, often emphasize the lack of any expression of pain. In other words, there is an absence of the overt behavioral responses usually associated with pain, such as crying and moaning, inactivity or fatigue following pain, or requests for pain relief. Some women are noted to have their babies in the fields and resume work immediately following delivery. Other women are observed to remain quiet with relaxed facial expressions during childbirth.

From this information some people erroneously conclude that these women experience no pain and, therefore, that pain results *only* from anxiety or cultural expectations. However, *lack of expression of pain does not necessarily mean that pain is absent.* Indeed, a study of Samoan women revealed that while their expressions of pain were minimal during labor, they admitted afterward in interviews that they did experience pain or discomfort.[1]

Some methods of prepared childbirth may also suggest that labor is painless. One paperback book about a method of childbirth uses the phrase "painless childbirth" in the title.[2] Currently most methods of prepared childbirth do not purport to be painless, but they seem inadvertently to insinuate lack of pain in their films on childbirth and in the written narratives of couples who utilize the organization's particular method of childbirth. These films and reports focus on the techniques of a particular method and on the "peak experience" or ecstasy of giving birth while fully conscious. Expressions of pain are notably absent, often giving expectant parents the impression that childbirth is painless.

In answer to the question of whether childbirth is painful or painless, one must simply conclude that there are a number of very different responses to the event of childbirth. While some responses entail minimal expression of pain, this does not mean pain is absent. Certainly there are reports of painless labors, but these are infrequent. Untreated labors that are painless or minimally uncomfortable are certainly no higher than 14 percent.[3] In one study of both multiparae and primiparae, the women were asked how painful childbirth was in comparison to other pain they had experienced. Ninety-seven percent said it was the most painful experience they had ever had.[4] In another study of primiparae only, 35 percent rated their pain as intolerable; 37 percent, severe; and 28 percent, moderate. Various studies of both primiparae and multiparae reveal that between 35 and 58 percent of the women report pain that is intolerable or severe.[5]

Importance of Pain Control During Labor

The relief of pain and suffering is traditionally a humane and moral act. However, pain relief is often given a low priority by health team members, especially in regard to childbirth. It has been pointed out that during childbirth the two primary tasks of the mother and the staff are "to deliver a 'good' baby and to conclude that process with an unimpaired mother. . . . each takes precedence—as main tasks always do—over the relief of pain."[6] However, an analysis of the situation reveals that pain relief results in certain emotional and physiologic benefits that contribute to the health of the mother and baby. Further, information about nonpharmacological pain relief measures is now more readily available to parents and health professionals. Thus, pain relief can be a priority without harming the mother or child. In fact, pain relief may contribute to their physical and emotional well-being.

Emotional Advantages.   Control or relief of pain potentially allows the significant step toward becoming parents to be a positive experience for the mother and father. Ultimately one or both parents may be able to witness that moment which remains miraculous and awesome even to many obstetri-cians—the emergence of a new human being into the world. Even when the parents do not observe the delivery, there are other desirable outcomes. If the mother and father can handle the discomforts during childbirth, they can feel they are active participants in the actual birth of their own child. When people jointly plan for an event such as childbirth and are then able to carry through with these plans, the event will probably foster growth in the relationship between them. In the case of childbirth, a satisfying labor experience for both parents probably also fosters their relationship with their baby.

At least a childbirth experience in which pain is adequately controlled will not impede these relationships. Pain has the potential for eliciting anger and aggression, often referred to as the fight or flight response. Such feelings resulting from a miserably painful childbirth experience sometimes are projected onto the infant or the father. The mother temporarily may express hatred toward the infant or father, and she may withdraw from these relationships for a while. During and following very painful labors mothers have been quoted as saying they despise their partners. Fathers have been known to say they felt angry toward the baby because its birth caused the mother pain. One mother even commented that her labor was so painful it took her a year to forgive her child and establish a warm relationship with him.

It does not seem likely, however, that pain and suffering during labor could be the sole reason for permanent or prolonged impairment of mother-father-child relationships. Labor may be a convenient scapegoat. Other more significant factors operating over a long period of time have probably affected the relationships.

Physiologic Advantages.   The adequate relief of pain also results in physiologic benefits. The mother who experiences tolerable discomforts in labor is able to cooperate with examinations and to work with her contractions. Consequently she facilitates efforts of the health team members to obtain information and she avoids prolongation of labor. After childbirth she is less fatigued.

If she is able to utilize pain relief measures other than medication, she may eliminate the need for medication or reduce the amount necessary. This is of enormous physiologic benefit to the infant since many analgesics and anesthetics, including regional anesthesia, have untoward effects on the fetus, such as respiratory depression and bradycardia. There simply is no drug that has been proven entirely safe for the unborn child.

DEFINITIONS

Pain. Pain defies definition. It is always a personal and subjective experience, differing from one person to another and varying within the same person from one time to the next. Quite simply, pain is a localized sensation of hurt. But, for both the nurse and patient who work together to relieve pain, it seems more productive for the nurse to adopt the patient's definition of pain.

The nursing definition of pain may then be stated as whatever the experiencing person says it is, existing whenever he or she says it does.[7] A crucial aspect of this definition is that the nurse believes what the patient tells her. And, of course, the patient may communicate the pain experience in any number of ways besides verbalization. For example, in some patients a marked increase in rate and depth of respirations may alert the nurse to the intensification of discomfort.

Pain Experience. The phrase "pain experience" encompasses all the patient's sensations, feelings, and behavioral responses, including physiologic activities such as blood pressure changes. The pain experience may also refer to any or all of the three phases of pain—anticipation, presence, aftermath. And it may include not only the patient's actions, but also the impact that others have upon the patient during the pain experience.

Pain Expressions. People respond to pain in many ways. The manner in which an individual responds to pain is dependent upon numerous and varied factors such as the culture in which the person lives, the personal meaning of the pain, and the intensity of the pain. Hence pain expressions may be absent or minimal or not easily observed. For example, a slight and momentary frown may be the only sign that the patient is experiencing pain. Or the patient may be more expressive and engage in prolonged moaning.

Expressions of pain are usually observed in one or more of the following categories of behavioral response: physiologic, verbal, vocal, facial, body movement, physical contact with others, and general response to the environment.[8]

Pain Tolerance. It is very important to differentiate between the presence and intensity of a pain sensation, as indicated by expressions of pain, and the patient's tolerance for that pain. Pain tolerance may be defined as the amount of pain that the patient is willing to endure without pain relief.

Pain tolerance differs markedly from one person to another. Some patients will state that the pain sensation is severe, yet they are willing to tolerate the pain and do not request pain relief. Other patients will utilize or request pain relief measures when they rate the pain as mild. The latter group may be said to have a low tolerance for pain. While a high pain tolerance is valued by many people, the nurse should realize that a patient's tolerance for pain is not a matter of good or bad, or right or wrong. Indeed, none of the patient's responses to pain are to be judged in this way.

During childbirth, the mother is expected to endure or tolerate a certain amount of pain to ensure her own and her baby's good health.[9] However, some mothers have a low pain tolerance, and it is especially important for the nurse to help these mothers find a way to cope with their discomfort. Admonishing the mother to cope with the discomfort or leaving the room when she complains certainly is not helpful. Other techniques can be called upon in such instances. The nonpharmacological measures discussed in this chapter are especially appropriate for the mother with a low pain tolerance.

Suffering. Suffering is an affective state that may accompany pain. Copp, a nurse-researcher in the field of pain, pointedly uses the term suffering in reference to pain and defines it as "the state of anguish of one who bears pain, injury, or loss."[10] When pain cannot be eliminated, it is imperative that the patient receive whatever assistance is necessary to prevent or diminish feelings of suffering. While a painful experience is at best only unpleasant, in most cases it need not be unrelenting agony.

PAIN MECHANISMS

Two theoretical mechanisms that may produce pain will be considered here: 1) the gate control theory and 2) the endorphins.

Gate Control Theory

The mystery and complexity of pain are especially well demonstrated by the fact that no one really knows what neurophysiological mechanism underlies the sensation of pain. Through the ages a number of theories have been advanced, and the most recent of these is the gate control theory. It was first proposed in 1965 by Melzack and Wall, and has since been debated and expanded.[11,12,13,14] Like all theories, it is not absolute truth. Rather, it uses available information to explain the phenomenon of pain, suggesting reasons for known facts and offering possibilities where facts are absent.

There are numerous facets to the theory and many ways to categorize them. The following discussion will focus only on those aspects which seem most pertinent to a basic understanding of the mechanisms of pain and its relief in childbirth.

As its name implies, the gate control theory proposes that there is a gating mechanism involved in the transmission of pain impulses. A closed gate results in no pain; an open gate, pain; a partially open gate, less pain. This gating mechanism is probably located in various places throughout the central nervous system. When the gate is closed, the transmission of pain impulses is stopped and pain does not reach the level of awareness.

The transmission of pain impulses to the level of cortical awareness can be affected in at least three general ways:

1. *The activity in large and small sensory nerve fibers.* The gate is opened by excitation of small-diameter fibers that carry pain impulses. However, these pain signals can be blocked (i.e., the gate can be closed to prevent or decrease their transmission to the cortex) by stimulation of large-diameter fibers. Since many cutaneous fibers are large-diameter fibers, stimulation of the skin by rubbing or other means may result in pain relief.
2. *Projections from the brain stem reticular formation.* The reticular activating system regulates or adjusts incoming and outgoing signals, including the amount of sensory input. Somatic inputs from all parts of the body, as well as visual and auditory inputs, are monitored by the reticular system. Although it is not well understood, it appears that a sufficient amount of sensory input may cause the reticular system to project inhibitory signals to the gate; that is, the reticular formation may cause the gate to be closed to the transmission of pain impulses. Hence, pain signals would not reach the level of cortical awareness (no pain), or fewer pain signals would reach the brain (less intense pain). Thus, distraction, for example, may inhibit pain impulses whereas monotony (unvarying sensory input) would increase pain.
3. *Projections from the cerebral cortex and thalamus.* Signals from the cortex or thalamus can open or close the gate to transmission of pain impulses, either indirectly by projecting through the reticular formation or directly by projecting to the gate. Cognitive and affective processes are subserved at least in part by neural activity in the cortex and thalamus. Therefore, the individual's own unique thoughts and feelings can influence the transmission of pain impulses from the gate to the level of cortical awareness. Such thoughts and feelings may include the meaning of the pain, the person's beliefs, anxieties, memories of past painful experiences, and any number of other factors. Thus, input to the gating mechanism is evaluated by the individual *before* it is felt as a sensation as well as afterward.

Perhaps the most important contribution of the gate control theory is the possible explanation it offers for the individuality of the pain experience. One thing has been clear for many years—comparable stimuli (or lesions) in different people do not produce comparable sensations of pain. In other words, when comparable stimuli are applied to several people, one person may perceive intense pain, another moderate pain, and still another no pain at all. The gate control theory suggests mechanisms by which a myriad of factors may determine the existence of pain and influence the nature of a painful experience. In summary, these factors may include not only stimulation of pain fibers but also cutaneous stimulation, other sensory input, thoughts, and feelings.

The gate control theory also provides a basis for understanding and devising pain relief measures, as will be discussed.

Endorphins

Recently it has been discovered that opiatelike substances occur naturally within the body. These substances have been called *endorphins,* a combination of the words endogenous and morphine.[15,16] To date more than five endorphins have been discovered. Their role in the cause and alleviation of pain has yet to be clarified. Possibly a person's level of naturally occurring endorphin will influence the severity of pain or his tolerance for pain. Some pain relief measures probably relieve pain partially or wholly because they increase the production or release of endorphins.

DESCRIPTIONS OF PAINFUL SENSATIONS OF NORMAL LABOR

Uterine Contractions

During the first stage of normal labor, pain or discomfort may result from the involuntary contraction of the uterine muscle. The contraction tends to be felt in the lower back at the beginning of labor. As labor progresses the sensation encircles the lower torso, covering both back and abdomen.

Contractions are frequently described as wavelike: they come and go rhythmically, each one increasing to a certain height or intensity and then decreasing, finally disappearing. Contractions last from about 45 to 90 seconds. In early labor the contractions are not necessarily uncomfortable. As labor progresses the intensity of each contraction increases, resulting in a greater possibility or intensity of discomfort.

The quality of the discomfort is difficult to describe and certainly is varied. Basically there appear to be three possible qualities to any painful sensation—burning, pricking, and aching. Also, pain can be either deep or superficial. Consequently one may say that a labor contraction is felt as deep aching.

The intervals between contractions shorten as labor proceeds. Early labor contractions are about 20 minutes apart. Then for several hours they occur three to five minutes apart. During about the last hour prior to delivery the intervals between contractions may be only a few seconds long. This period, when the cervix is dilating from about 7 cm. to 10 cm., is referred to as transition.

Uterine contractions are at their highest intensity and greatest frequency during transition. This is usually when the mother will experience the most discomfort and will have the most difficulty handling her discomfort.

Back Labor

In addition to uterine contractions, approximately 25 percent of women in labor will also have to cope with the discomfort of *back labor*. This occurs when the fetus is in an occipitoposterior position (see Chapter 33). With each contraction the occiput presses on the mother's sacrum, causing extreme discomfort as the intensity of contractions increases. Back labor is considerably more painful for the mother than labor in which there is an anterior occipital position.

Delivery

A common but false assumption about labor is that the most painful part is the expulsive stage. However, mothers report a decrease in pain during this stage. Apparently the mother's more noisy behavior during expulsion efforts has been interpreted by observers as indicative of more pain.[17]

Of course, the mother certainly may experience discomfort during delivery but it is generally much less intense than what she felt during transition.

The predominant sensations during delivery occur in the vaginal and perineal area and can be described as pressure, stretching or splitting, and sometimes burning. Most of the time the mother has an overwhelming desire to push. Pushing may relieve whatever discomfort is felt. Also, the pressure of the baby's head causes a degree of numbness in the perineum. If desired, the physician can take advantage of this numbness during a contraction and perform a painless episiotomy.

The foregoing is a description of the painful or uncomfortable sensations often felt during normal labor. Considerably more pain may be experienced with certain complications of labor, such as hypertonic uterine dysfunction, delivery of an oversized baby, or a contracted pelvis.

Uniqueness of Pain During Childbirth

Most of the pain experienced by the general patient population is characterized by one or more of the following anxiety-producing factors. The patient may not know what causes the pain, may not have expected pain to occur, and may not know how to predict the course of the pain, e.g., how long it will last, how severe it will become. Pain may cause the patient to fear some dreaded illness or a long-term change in his lifestyle.

The discomfort and pain of childbirth are unique in that in most cases these common sources of anxiety need not be present. In fact, there are elements inherent in childbirth that are just the opposite of these sources of anxiety. Hence the childbirth experience has a high potential for the achievement of satisfactory pain relief. Following is a brief discussion of those elements which render childbirth a more manageable pain experience.

Anxiety-Reducing Knowledge. Studies suggest that anxiety is reduced if the person knows when a painful event will occur and how long the discomfort will last.[18] Ordinarily the mother knows the approximate date of confinement and she has some idea of the approximate length of labor. In other words, she knows labor will occur, she knows the expected date within a few weeks, and she knows labor usually lasts a matter of hours, not days.

Even more helpful is the information the mother has once labor has actually begun. With the assistance of a watch she can determine the usual length of her contractions and predict when the next one will occur. In addition she knows that contractions generally become more intense and more frequent as labor progresses. And although her discomfort may increase in intensity, she is not usually in constant discomfort. Between contractions there are periods of relative comfort even during the final phase of labor contractions.

The mother also knows in general the cause of her discomfort. At least she knows it is a normal process that has something to do with the expulsion of her baby and that parts of her body are contracting

and stretching to accomplish this event. This is quite different from the knowledge possessed by the person who suddenly experiences his first myocardial infarction. Most mothers recognize the onset of labor and do not fear that something harmful or life-threatening is happening.

An End-Product. The discomfort of labor is also unique in that there is a tangible end-product—the baby. This outcome, the birth of the baby, is something in which there has been deep personal involvement, both emotional and physiologic. The involvement may have been positive and desirable or unpleasant and unwanted. Nevertheless, when the baby is born, the discomfort of labor subsides markedly and the event is characterized by physical and psychological closure. Few episodes of pain end so dramatically.

ASSESSMENT OF LABOR PAIN

Prejudices that Hamper Assessment of Pain

Signs of Acute Pain. Precautions must be taken to avoid certain prejudices that may hamper the nurse's assessment of the pain experience. There is a tendency to recognize the existence of pain only in those patients who show signs of acute pain, such as perspiration, muscle tension, or moaning. The absence of these expressions of pain, as noted previously, does not necessarily mean the patient is not in pain. In fact, the patient may suffer greatly but exhibit only minimal pain expression.[19]

In childbirth there appear to be two major reasons for minimal pain expressions: 1) the mother may have learned that minimal pain expressions are the expectations of the culture, or 2) activities learned from a method of prepared childbirth may preclude expressions of pain. For example, practicing relaxation techniques may preclude muscle tension as a sign of acute pain; use of a breathing pattern or mouthing the words of a song may preclude the behavior of moaning.

It is often quite difficult, if not impossible, to rely upon signs of acute pain in assessing the laboring mother who is using one of the methods of prepared childbirth. Usually she simply is too busy to show signs of acute pain.

Physical Cause of Pain. We also tend to be prejudiced in favor of believing patients only when we know the physical cause of pain.[20] This hampers our understanding of the subjective pain experience. Hence, when the mother states, for instance, that she feels severe pain, her statement must be believed even if there seems to be no physical cause for such a painful labor. The temptation to judge the mother's discomfort by the results of electronic monitoring of intrauterine pressure must also be avoided.

Values of Mother or Father. The mother or father may also harbor prejudices or values that make it difficult for the nurse to assess the pain experience. Either or both of the parents may feel that responses to pain should be minimized. The only appropriate response may be a verbal description of the pain. Some mothers may not even volunteer this much, so they have to be questioned directly and at regular intervals. Still other mothers may want to avoid using the word pain or will resist any tendency to say they feel pain. They may prefer to use other terms, which may be deceptive if taken at face value. For example, the mother may verbalize feeling "enormous pressure" but refuse to call it painful. Yet the mother may need assistance in coping with this sensation, so that measures designed to relieve severe pain may be very appropriate.

Still another type of problem may arise with a father who forcefully tries to impose his own goals upon the mother who does not share his values. In the situation where the father does not want the mother to admit pain or to seek assistance with pain relief measures, the nurse may find that she obtains more accurate information when the father is absent from the room. She may also discover that the mother asks the father to get the nurse, but the father merely stands in the hall and then reports to the mother that the nurse is not available. Of course, the opposite type of situation may exist. The mother may feel perfectly capable of handling the pain and discomforts of labor, but the father may become insistent that she be "put out of this misery."

Agreement Between Health Team Members. There is a tendency for health team members to rate the mother's pain as less intense than the mother rates her pain. This is particularly true of the first stage of labor. Health team members also tend to agree with each other about the degree of the mother's pain.[21,22] In other words, the staff observing the patient may agree with one another that the patient's pain is not as severe as the patient actually experiences it. We must guard against letting agreement among ourselves about the patient's pain cause or reinforce any doubts about the intensity of the mother's pain.

Nursing Assessment of Pain and Pain Relief Measures

When the laboring mother is admitted to the hospital, the nurse identifies several factors important to the management of pain (Table 24-1). Since a thorough assessment is inextricably related to intervention, some pain relief measures will be mentioned in the discussion of assessment. Actually, the manner in which the nurse assesses the patient often contributes to pain relief. When the nurse conveys to the mother that she believes her and that she desires to understand the mother's experience as completely as possible, this can reduce anxiety and thereby relieve pain.

Contractions

When labor is discussed with the mother, the sensations should be referred to as contractions, not pains. Although many laypeople continue to use the term pains, the nurse should attempt to help the parents substitute the word contractions, because the word pain tends to suggest not just discomfort but an unbearable sensation. The initial contractions are not necessarily uncomfortable, and pain is usually a misnomer. Later in labor the contractions may be uncomfortable but not unbearable. Most mothers probably are not so suggestible that they would actually feel unbearable pain during contractions simply because the nurse used the term pains rather than contractions. But the use of the term pains may generate needless anxiety about the sensations of labor.

When assessing the characteristics of uterine contractions (onset, frequency, duration, intensity, description of sensation, and attitude toward contractions) it is important to note the time when labor begins (*onset*) since prolonged labor intensifies the painful experience. Not only is a longer time spent in discomfort, but a lengthy labor often fatigues and

TABLE 24-1
TOOLS FOR ASSESSING THE PAIN EXPERIENCE DURING LABOR

I. Contractions
　　Onset
　　Frequency
　　Duration
　　Intensity
　　Description of sensation
　　Attitude toward contractions

II. Pain Relief Methods Employed by Parent(s) for Labor
　　Person(s) to assist or be present during labor
　　Positioning
　　Relaxation techniques
　　Distraction (or concentration) methods
　　Breathing patterns
　　Physical activities
　　Medication

III. Current Discomforts of Mother Other than Labor
　　Pregnancy
　　Chronic illness
　　Recent illness or injury
　　Methods of handling above; effectiveness of methods

IV. Parents' Current Concerns Other than Labor
　　Activities or plans interrupted by labor
　　Care of children at home
　　Financial arrangements
　　Condition of mother or unborn child
　　Plans for care of infant
　　Unexpected change in childbirth plans
　　Plans and needs for assistance regarding above

V. Parents' Goals and Expectations Regarding Labor
　　Presence and intensity of pain
　　Provisions for pain relief (if any)
　　Father's (coach's) presence
　　Episiotomy
　　Differences between mother and father regarding above
　　Which of above not possible or not discussed with physician

discourages the parents, making it more difficult to cope with labor (see Part I of Table 24-1).

Regularity and increasing *frequency* of contractions along with increasing intensity of contractions indicate a normal labor. Such information can be used to assure the parents that progress is being made.

To obtain more detailed and useful information about *intensity of contractions,* the nurse may ask the mother to rate the contraction on a scale such as: mild, moderate, intense (strong), very intense (very strong).

It is also helpful to encourage the mother to *describe* other characteristics of the contraction, such as where the sensation begins and where it is felt most intensely. This information often suggests the need for specific pain relief measures. For example,

if the contraction begins in the lower back and is felt most intensely there, rubbing that area and applying pressure may provide considerable comfort.

At the same time that the mother is discussing her contractions she may reveal her *attitude* toward labor in general. Of special importance is the degree of fear or anxiety experienced, because these feelings have a profound effect upon pain. They decrease pain tolerance and increase the perceived intensity of pain. Anxiety or fear also increases muscle tension, and may increase painful stimuli during labor by interfering with contractions.

Anxiety or fear during labor may be related to worry about how pain will be managed and how labor is progressing. To alleviate such anxiety, the nurse may inform the mother of the various pain relief measures that may be employed. Concern over the progression of labor, or the effectiveness of the contractions, may be partially diminished if the nurse keeps the mother informed of signs of progress such as increasing cervical dilatation or regularity of contractions. It is sometimes helpful to assure the mother that it is possible to stop or correct ineffective or dysfunctional uterine contractions.

Pain Relief Methods Employed by Parent(s) for Labor

Whether or not the parents have any special or well-defined method of handling childbirth (e.g., Lamaze method), the nurse questions them about how they have handled the discomforts of labor thus far and what their plans are for the remainder of labor. In the United States there are many methods of preparation for childbirth, based on different techniques and philosophies. Some of the techniques and pain relief methods employed in prepared childbirth may seem odd. Sometimes mothers feel foolish doing them and nurses may be surprised to observe such techniques. However, a woman should be encouraged to use whatever method works for her. Some mothers intuitively devise their own special way of handling childbirth.

The following alphabetized list offers some idea of the existing methods of preparation for childbirth.
Gamper method (Margaret Gamper)
Husband-coached childbirth (Robert A. Bradley)
Maternity Center Association

Psychoprophylactic method (PPM, Lamaze method)
Psychosexual method (Sheila Kitzinger)
Read method (Grantly Dick-Read)
Wright method (Erna Wright)

It is difficult to list all the variations in *methods of childbirth* and to keep abreast of the constant changes taking place within each method, but the nurse can be reassured by the fact that in any single hospital labor suite one or two basic methods will be used. This is partially because physicians using one particular method of childbirth tend to congregate at the same hospital where they can share ideas and know that the nursing staff is reasonably familiar with the method. Also, certain methods tend to be popular only in certain geographical areas. Thus the nurse is likely to be able to identify quickly which methods are most common and can then study them in greater depth.

Part II of Table 24-1 lists some common pain relief methods employed during childbirth, such as comfortable positioning, relaxation techniques, and awareness of the persons who will be in attendance during labor.

Persons Present During Labor

With regard to the *person or persons to assist or be present during labor,* the father is almost always included if the couple has attended classes on one of the methods of prepared childbirth. Sometimes the couple's children are allowed an occasional and brief visit to the labor room. When the father is absent or does not want to attend labor or when the mother is unwed, the person in attendance may be a childbirth educator or the mother's friend or relative.

After identifying this person the nurse finds out if that person has been with the mother prior to hospital admission and if the mother wants that person to remain with her in the labor and delivery rooms. She also assesses the attending person's attitudes and desires. It is possible, for instance, that the mother might want the father to remain with her, but the father may be quite reluctant and fearful. (For convenience the person the mother brings to the hospital to be with her during labor henceforth will be referred to as the father.)

In addition, the nurse determines what the father has done for the mother prior to admission, what is planned for the remainder of labor, what (if any)

preparation the mother and father have had, and whether they have practiced what they plan to do. Sometimes the father simply stays near the mother, touching her gently and offering verbal encouragement. In other cases the father is expected to take a very active role in the following pain relief measures, such as massaging the back or abdomen or applying counterpressure.

Positioning

A variety of *positions* may be assumed during the course of normal labor. At the beginning of labor the mother may walk around between contractions, and during a contraction she may remain standing but bend forward, leaning on her husband's arms or back for support. As labor progresses she may be more comfortable sitting or lying in bed. Ordinarily the mother is encouraged to assume any position that is comfortable, with the possible exception of lying flat on her back. Some mothers may be more comfortable "on all fours" with gentle pelvic rocking during a contraction.

When the mother is admitted the nurse asks her which positions have been comfortable and which have not and which positions she may wish to consider later in labor. Some positions require additional pillows which the nurse can then obtain in advance. For pushing during delivery, most childbirth educators teach the father to stand behind the mother and to prop her up with pillows at a 35° to 45° angle.

Relaxation

Numerous techniques are utilized to achieve and maintain total skeletal muscle *relaxation.* To support the limbs, a pillow may be placed between the mother's legs when she is on her side. For general relaxation, the mother may smile, yawn, or take deep breaths at regular intervals. Or relaxation may be achieved by simulating sleep or imagining the contractions as soothing ocean waves. The father may aid by giving tactile or verbal cues to induce relaxation.

Again, the nurse finds out what techniques are used for relaxation so as to accurately interpret the mother's behavior. Knowing that the mother intends to keep her eyes closed, for example, will prevent the nurse from mistakenly concluding that this laboring mother is sleeping most of the time.

Distraction

Distraction and concentration are frequently used for coping with pain. Distraction techniques are also the most individualized and therefore the most varied of all the techniques a mother may employ during childbirth. Some women will bring with them a personal "concentration point"—an object to be stared at during a contraction. This can take any form, such as a mobile hanging from the ceiling, a seashell on the bed, a drawing pinned to the drapes, or a brilliant circle taped to the wall. Concentrating on this point or object helps the mother distract her thoughts from discomfort.

There are several other ways to employ concentration. For example, toward the end of labor, the mother may distract herself from discomfort by emphatically mouthing the words to a song and tapping her finger to the rhythm or slapping her thigh in rhythm. Some mothers may close their eyes and distract themselves with mental relaxation, such as visualizing previously selected pleasant childhood experiences. The father may participate in this technique by whispering predetermined messages in the mother's ear during a contraction to help call up the visual image.

Breathing Patterns

Controversy and change are characteristic of many of the *breathing patterns* employed in the various methods of prepared childbirth. The two basic types of breathing are 1) chest and 2) abdominal or diaphragmatic.

Some childbirth educators feel that abdominal breathing places more pressure on the uterus by forcing the diaphragm down and the abdomen out. However, other educators feel that abdominal breathing prevents pressure on the uterus by relaxing and lifting the abdominal wall off the uterus. They also feel that it enhances relaxation because it is the type of breathing used during sleep. Some mothers tend to find it difficult to breath abdominally as labor progresses, while others find it comfortable throughout labor.

Chest breathing with panting and rapid breathing is also a subject of controversy. Some instructors are modifying the panting or rapid superficial breathing because it is difficult to learn or because it may become fatiguing during labor and has caused hyperventilation in a few mothers during labor.[23,24]

Hence, some childbirth educators have abandoned panting and substituted another breathing rhythm, while others have simply solved the problem by teaching a more moderate rate of shallow breathing.

Mothers may be taught to use either abdominal breathing only, chest breathing only, a combination of both, or simply a pattern of breaths with no special attention directed at either abdominal or chest breathing. In general, the rate of breathing increases as labor progresses. Also, during a contraction the rate of breathing may accelerate as the contraction intensifies and decelerate as the contraction subsides.

The mother may breathe only through the mouth or she may inhale through the nose and exhale through the mouth. Any number of combinations of this technique may be used by any one mother. In addition, breathing may be accompanied by sounds or body movement. One mother may whistle upon exhalation; another may actively and rapidly turn her head to the right as she whispers "he" and back to the front as she says "who."

The nurse may be able to obtain information about the breathing patterns from some mothers simply by asking. Others may not be aware of the breathing pattern they are using. In such cases the mother should be observed closely to ascertain the breathing patterns being used. A thorough assessment of breathing patterns helps the nurse anticipate the needs of the mother. If a breathing pattern is not helpful, the nurse can suggest another. If the mother will be breathing through her mouth, the nurse can obtain ice chips or a damp cloth to alleviate dry lips and mouth. Some mothers are taught to use a lollipop for this purpose. If the mother uses rapid breathing, the nurse can remind her to report any tingling in the hands and other initial signs of hyperventilation (carbon dioxide insufficiency). In anticipation of these signs, the nurse can have a paper bag available. The patient can breathe in and out of the paper bag to inhale enough carbon dioxide to reverse the hyperventilation.

Physical Activities

Physical activities other than those which fall into the above categories may be used during labor. During a contraction the mother or father may rhythmically massage the abdomen, using some preparation such as talcum powder to keep the skin smooth. The father may rub her lower back between and during contractions. Or, he may employ a maneuver with his hands (learned from a childbirth educator) to raise the abdominal wall during a contraction. The mother may rock her pelvis while standing or lying on her side. The latter appears to be particularly helpful during back labor. Counterpressure is also useful. To achieve this the father may place tennis balls, a rolling pin, his knee or his fist against the lower back.

Medications

When the mother is admitted, the nurse also asks whether or not she has taken medication or any other substance for pain relief, such as aspirin, codeine, an alcoholic beverage, or even paregoric, prescribed for false labor. If medication was taken, the nurse notes the time, type, and amount.

It is always possible that the mother has taken some illegal drug such as marijuana, heroin, or a black market drug of unknown composition. The mother who uses illegal drugs may fear legal action against her or disdain from the health team. Therefore, to increase the likelihood of obtaining an honest answer from a mother who has used an illegal drug, the nurse should always stress that the questions about medication are asked for important reasons, such as determining what other medication can be used safely.

It is also important to inquire about what analgesics and anesthetics are being considered for use during labor. The mother may have no knowledge at all about medication, or she and the father may have discussed several possibilities with the obstetrician.

Current Discomforts Other Than Labor

The process of labor may not be the only source of discomfort for the mother. Indeed, there are other diseases or symptoms that may be much more irritating and painful than the concurrent labor. Such discomforts may be associated with the pregnancy itself or may represent a chronic illness or a recent illness or injury (see Table 24-1, III). For example, pregnancy may cause or increase heartburn, hemorrhoids, or varicose veins in the legs or vagina, all of which can be extremely uncomfortable.

As for chronic illness, any one of a number of disorders (arthritis, allergy) may result in pain and discomfort. The same is true of a recent illness or injury, such as influenza or an accident resulting in a broken bone, lacerations, or sprained ankle.

The nurse assesses sources of discomfort extraneous to labor so that appropriate actions can be taken to provide relief. For example, if a mother is experiencing heartburn, the simple administration of an antacid may enable her to devote her attention and energy to the process of childbirth. At the same time, any treatment instituted prior to the onset of labor should be identified. If the mother has found effective means of handling discomforts, it obviously is expedient for her to use the same methods during labor whenever possible.

Current Concerns Other than Labor

Since the precise time for the onset of labor is rarely predictable, significant activities or plans may be interrupted by labor (see Part IV of Table 24-1). If the mother was preparing dinner and left the house without turning off the stove, she and her husband may be so worried about a possible fire that they are more concerned with locating a neighbor to turn off the burner than concentrating on the directions being given. Or the onset of labor may interfere with the requirements of the father's occupation and cause him to worry over the possibility of losing his job if he does not report to work.

If the parents have other children, they may be anxious about what will happen to them during their absence. The parents may have had to leave for the hospital without knowing the exact whereabouts of an older child or without being able to calm the sobbing of a younger child.

The parents may also be concerned about financial arrangements related to hospitalization and the physician's fee, particularly if complications arise such as prematurity or if there is an unexpected multiple birth. More simply, perhaps the parents failed to make recommended financial payments to the hospital during the weeks prior to admission and are now afraid the hospital will not allow them to stay.

For some reason, realistic or not, the parents may be fearful about the condition of the mother and/or the unborn infant. Because a relative is mentally retarded the parents may be afraid the baby will be born with brain damage. They may fear infant anomalies on the basis of the mother's having had viral infections during pregnancy or having taken certain drugs before she realized she was pregnant. Or, the mother may have a cardiac condition, and both she and her husband may be concerned that she cannot live through labor.

The mother and/or father may be considering giving up the baby for adoption. Onset of labor may precipitate many feelings about this.

Unexpectedly there may have been a change in some aspect of the parents' plans for childbirth. Their obstetrician may be out of town, or labor may have progressed so rapidly they were unable to reach the hospital of their choice.

It is important for the nurse to realize that such concerns can stir anxiety and will interfere with the parents' ability to concentrate on handling discomforts, responding to directions, cooperating with examinations, and dealing with all the other aspects of labor. The nurse is frequently in a position to assist the parents in solving the problem or directing them to obtain appropriate assistance.

Goals and Expectations Regarding Labor

Parents generally have certain expectations regarding labor (Table 24-1, Part V). The nurse may encounter extremes in parents' expectations related to pain and pain relief. One mother may expect severe pain and desire that the physician render her practically unconscious throughout labor. Another mother may expect no pain at all and, therefore, no pain relief measures. When discomfort and pain are expected, the parents may believe that the techniques they have been taught to use during labor, such as breathing patterns, will be sufficient assistance for the mother. Their goal may be a completely unmedicated labor. Or the parents may expect to use the methods they were taught in combination with some type of medication if they desire it.

Mention has already been made of some of the possible persons expected to assist during labor. In some cases the father will be expected to remain with the mother from the beginning of labor, during delivery, and through the recovery period following delivery. In other instances the mother will not want the father present. Parents' expectations of the nurse and physician also need to be determined.

Some parents, particularly mothers, want very much to observe the effects of their pushing and the delivery of the baby. Many delivery rooms have mirrors for this purpose. The parents may have brought a camera to take pictures in the labor room and in the delivery room. They may also want someone to take a picture of them with their baby immediately after delivery. Some parents want to tape record the delivery.

An episiotomy is done in most deliveries, but some parents hope for or expect no episiotomy. To achieve this the mother may have done certain exercises daily for weeks prior to labor.

A fully conscious mother almost always wants to touch the newborn as soon as possible. The mother may plan on holding the baby before the cord is cut. She may also expect to be allowed to breast-feed the baby on the delivery table.

In helping the parents express their goals and expectations the nurse is alert to differences between the desires of the mother and father. For example, the father may not want to witness the delivery although the mother wants him in the delivery room. Or, the father may think the mother is unrealistic in her plans for little or no medication. When the nurse observes such differences she helps the parents become aware of them and hopefully formulate compatible goals.

In her assessment of the parents' goals the nurse also notes whether or not these goals have been discussed with the physician. Some goals may be contraindicated for medical reasons. Other goals may require the awareness and cooperation of the physician. In addition hospital policy sometimes places limitations on the parents. For instance, some delivery rooms are so small the hospital must have a policy of excluding the father.

As labor progresses the nurse continues to monitor the patient for any changes in the items listed in Table 24-1. Some aspects of the labor situation may change dramatically, such as the nature of the contractions. There may be a sudden need for modification of pain relief methods. Also, the discomforts and concerns extraneous to labor may be resolved or suddenly may appear when none had existed before.

NONPHARMACOLOGICAL PAIN RELIEF DURING LABOR

This discussion of pain relief measures is focused on those other than medication. These pain relief methods may be used either instead of or in addition to analgesics and anesthetics. The focus is purposefully limited to what the nurse may do for the mother or what she may assist the mother or father to do. Nursing activities related to the use of pharmacologic agents are discussed elsewhere.

Methods of Prepared Childbirth

A partial list of methods of prepared childbirth appears on page 366-367; and in the discussion of assessment of the patient in labor some of the examples are taken from these various methods. Methods of prepared childbirth do not necessarily have as their primary objective the management of pain during labor. They encompass preparation for and assistance with much more than labor.

Nevertheless, pain management is inherent in the preparation of the mother and/or father if other objectives are to be met. These objectives may be reduced need for analgesia and anesthesia, an awareness of the birth, or simply a personally satisfying experience for the parents. In any event, each method takes into account that some control of pain is essential. Hence it behooves the nurse to be acquainted with the nature of preparation. Many methods of prepared childbirth require a considerable investment of time and energy on the part of the parents.

The particular method of prepared childbirth used by a mother during labor may have been recommended by her physician, or she may have chosen it herself. Typically the mother and father attend a series of six or more two-hour classes during the last trimester of pregnancy. The classes are usually small, about ten couples, and they are taught by an instructor specially trained in that method. In addition to attending classes and performing other related tasks, the mother and father daily practice certain activities to be used during labor. Some of these activities assist the mother to tolerate pain, or reduce the intensity of pain. Information about the processes of labor is also given in the classes. This tends to reduce anxiety in the mother and father and thereby assist them to cope with pain.

The number of parents seeking childbirth education is increasing. In a 1973–74 survey of 54 university hospitals in the United States, almost three-fourths reported that some form of psychoprophylaxis or natural childbirth was practiced during labor for the purpose of relieving pain. Most of the time these methods were used in combination with other techniques such as regional anesthesia.[25]

The method of prepared childbirth growing most rapidly throughout the United States is the psychoprophylactic method (PPM) or Lamaze. In 1966 there were 77 Lamaze childbirth educators nationwide.[26] That number increased to 2,500 in 1976.[27] In 1975 more than 190,000 couples were trained in the Lamaze method of childbirth. This represented 7 percent of the pregnant population in the United States.[28]

Because of the growing popularity of the Lamaze method among laypeople, Table 24-2 summarizes those activities the nurse generally might expect to be used by Lamaze-trained couples during labor for the purpose of handling discomfort or pain. The nurse will encounter variations in these activities since instructors are always making efforts to improve the method and since the individual mother may adapt the method to her own particular needs.

Sometimes the nursing staff tends to spend very little time with Lamaze-trained or otherwise prepared couples. While it is true that some couples may manage quite well on their own, most couples will need some type of assistance. Knowledge of how a mother and father may attempt to cope with pain and discomfort enables the nurse to provide appropriate help. For example, when a breathing pattern has ceased to be effective, the Lamaze-trained mother may need assurance that labor has progressed sufficiently to warrant changing to the next breathing pattern. Or when the father must leave the labor room the nurse will know how to assume some of his responsibilities such as counting or breathing with the mother.

Goals and Principles of Pain Relief

Good pain relief does not necessarily mean the total elimination of painful sensations. In fact, complete abolition of pain is rarely a realistic goal. It is significantly helpful to the patient and often more reasonable to aim at a decrease in the intensity of pain and/or a decrease in the degree to which pain bothers the patient. The latter is closely related to another possible goal of increasing the patient's tolerance for pain.

Two important principles that underlie the accomplishment of these goals are 1) decreasing the pain impulses that reach the cortex of the brain, and 2) managing anxiety. The transmission of pain signals may be interrupted in a number of ways

(continued on page 374)

TABLE 24-2 SUMMARY OF PAIN RELIEF MEASURES

Aproximate Progress of Labor	Position	Relaxation	Mother's Activities During Massage
Onset to 3 cm., or contractions 5 to 20 min. apart.	Supported comfortably sitting or lying on side. Between contractions, may walk; during contractions, may stand and lean on object.	Inhales deeply at beginning of contraction and relaxes totally upon exhalation. Also takes a deep breath at end of each contraction.	Hands move slowly from pubic area up to umbilicus and out around abdomen down to pubic area. Or other body areas such as thighs may be massaged.
Dilates from 4 to 7 cm., or contractions 2 to 4 min. apart.	Same as above.	Same as above.	Same as above.
Dilates from 8 to 10 cm., or contractions 1 min. apart.	Same as above.	Same as above.	Omitted.
Delivery. (fully dilated)	Same as above except when pushing. For pushing in labor room: may conserve energy during pushing by elevating and supporting legs on pillows, or by lying on side with back curved and top knee pulled up. For pushing in delivery room: semipropped position with back curved, head and shoulders supported by pillows, head forward. If legs not in stirrups, she holds legs under knees with elbows out and brings knees as close to shoulders as possible.	Same as above except omitted when pushing.	Omitted.

USED BY LAMAZE-TRAINED PARENTS DURING LABOR

Eye Focus	Each Contraction in Relation to Breathing Pattern	Thoughts	Father's Activities Either During or Between Contractions
Eyes open and focused on one particular object ("concentration point," "focal point").	Slow chest breathing, 6 to 9/min., inhale through nose, exhale through mouth.	On inhalation, "In, 1, 2." On exhalation, "Out, 1, 2."	Times frequency of each contraction. Helps her get in comfortable positions. Checks for state of relaxation by moving parts of her body. As need arises may give signals to help increase relaxation, do abdominal massage for her, or rub her lower back.
Same as above.	Shallow chest breathing through mouth. Begins slowly, accelerates as contraction intensifies, decelerates as contraction subsides. Breathing is 4/4 rhythm.	Counts each breath in 4/4 rhythm emphasizing count of one, e.g., "1, 2, 3, 4, 1, 2, 3, 4," etc., or silently sings Yankee Doodle, a 4/4 song.	Same as above plus the following.\n\nDuring contractions: At 15-sec. intervals he calls off time that elapses, i.e., "15 sec., 30 sec., 45 sec., 60 sec." until contraction is over. As need arises, may breathe in rhythm with her, count aloud in rhythm to her breathing or sing song in rhythm, remind her of eye focus, remind her to breathe deeply at end of contraction. If "back labor," may try deep counterpressure to lower back.
Same as above. Or focuses eyes on father.	Shallow chest breathing through mouth. Rhythm of 4, 6, or 8 breaths and then one blow. Begins slowly, accelerates and decelerates with intensity of contraction. If not allowed to push but feels urge to push, blows repeatedly. If uncomfortable between contractions, uses slow chest breathing.	Counts each breath according to rhythm selected, e.g., "1, 2, 3, 4, 5, 6, blow."	Between contractions: Offers encouragement; wipes face with cool wet cloth; moistens lips and mouth with water, ice chips or lollipop. Reminds her to void q2h.
Same as above except when pushing. Then may focus on mirror or perineum, if visible, to see results of pushing.	Same as above except when pushing. For pushing: 2 or 3 deep breaths, inhale, hold breath, lean forward, slowly count to 10, release breath. Repeat inhalation and holding to count of 10 until contraction is over or until instructed to stop pushing.	Same as above except when pushing. For pushing: slowly counts to 10 during each breath holding.	Same as above except when pushing. For pushing: stands at mother's back to support her in pushing position. Counts aloud to 10 during each breath holding, tells her to take a deep breath and hold it, then counts to 10 again. Reminds her to relax pelvic floor and "push through vagina."

such as decreasing the source of noxious stimuli or closing the gate (see gate control theory, pp. 362-363). Likewise there are numerous ways of managing anxiety.

An appreciation of the variety of potentially effective pain relief methods available is enhanced by understanding the relationships between anxiety and pain sensations. It has long been recognized that most types of pain cause some degree of anxiety or fear and that anxiety increases the intensity of pain, or at least renders pain less tolerable and more bothersome. The gate control theory suggests that anxiety opens the gate to pain impulses, thereby actually increasing the intensity of pain. Anxiety may also increase the intensity of pain directly by causing muscle tension. In labor it is obvious that tension in the muscles of the abdomen, perineum, and lower back will increase discomfort.

The interaction between anxiety and pain may become a spiraling process. Pain may cause anxiety, and this anxiety may increase the intensity of pain by causing muscle tension or by opening the gate to pain impulses. In this way mild pain and anxiety can eventually become severe pain and panic.

Pain Relief Measures During Labor

Pain relief measures are aimed at reducing either anxiety or pain impulses. Following is a discussion of specific nursing activities to accomplish this. Some guidelines to the effective utilization of these pain relief measures are:

1. Use a variety of pain relief measures.
2. Use pain relief measures *before* pain becomes severe. (It is easier to prevent severe pain and panic than to alleviate them once they occur.)
3. Include those pain relief measures which the patient believes will be effective.
4. Take into account the patient's ability to be active or passive in the application of the pain relief measure.
5. Regarding the potency of the pain relief measure needed, rely on the patient's experience of the severity of pain rather than the known physical stimuli.
6. If a pain relief measure is ineffective the first time it is used during a contraction, encourage the mother to try it at least one or two more times before abandoning it.

Some of the pain relief methods discussed below will not be possible or acceptable in conventional labor rooms or when external monitoring is used. However, there is growing public demand for more natural childbirth and nonpharmacological methods of pain relief during childbirth. Alternative Birth Centers (ABCs) are one response to that demand. Thus, in the future the following low risk, nonpharmacological pain relief measures may be increasingly acceptable to both health professionals and expectant parents.

Support During Labor

From the beginning of labor the mother needs to have someone with her at increasingly frequent intervals and to know that someone is available at all times. Toward the end of labor she needs to have someone with her constantly. The presence, actions, and words of this person can be very supportive to the mother. This person may be the nurse, the father, or someone else. At times the nurse's greatest contribution is to support the father so that he can in turn support the mother. Specific ways the mother may be supported during labor are discussed on pages 366 to 369.

Support during labor lowers anxiety and increases the mother's ability to handle discomforts. It also enhances the effectiveness of other pain relief methods. Hence, it is important that other pain relief measures be implemented within the context of this type of relationship with the mother.

Giving Information

As mentioned previously, part of the uniqueness of labor pain is that the mother may possess anxiety-reducing knowledge. If the mother does not obtain this information for herself, the nurse can supply it. For example, the nurse may tell the mother approximately how long it will be before the next contraction and how long that contraction will last. During intense contractions the nurse may "count down" at 15-second intervals until the end of the contraction, telling the mother how long it will be until the contraction is over. Or the nurse may time the contraction so she can reassure the mother by telling her when the contraction has reached its peak and will begin to subside. Information about the progress of labor, such as cervical dilatation and descent of the baby, is also important. It serves as a reminder that there is a purpose to labor, that labor does end, and that the end is getting closer and closer.

Such information not only reduces anxiety but may also motivate the mother to tolerate pain. Especially toward the end of labor when discomfort increases, the knowledge that the ordeal is almost over may enable the mother to tolerate an intensity of pain that she would otherwise find unbearable.

Knowing that she and her baby are not in danger is also, of course, anxiety-reducing. Sometimes the mother finds the forces of labor so unexpectedly powerful that she is fearful of harm. The nurse should periodically reassure the mother that she and her baby are doing well (provided, of course, that this is true). She may say, for example, that the baby's heartbeat is strong and regular. Remembering that discomfort is associated with a normal process and not a life-threatening illness may be helpful to the mother. Briefly and in simple terms the nurse can remind the mother of what is happening, for example, that each contraction enlarges the opening for the baby.

Understanding what is happening during labor seems to increase the mother's sense of control over the event. Feelings of powerlessness can be anxiety-provoking, so it is important to further feelings of control. This may be done through instructions and explanations that help the mother cooperate with examinations and with the process of labor such as effective pushing. In particular the mother's feelings of control can be strengthened by teaching her about pain relief measures as early as possible. When this has not been done prior to labor the nurse can begin in early labor to explain certain of the following pain relief measures. The mother then knows that pain relief is available, that there are several possibilities, and that to some extent she may choose from among them.

Decreasing Sources of Noxious Stimuli

One source of noxious, or painful, stimuli is abdominal pressure on the contracting uterus. Total skeletal muscle relaxation, discussed in more detail later, relaxes the abdominal muscles and contributes to relieving pressure on the uterus.

Breathing Methods. Pressure may also be prevented by either abdominal breathing or chest breathing. While there is controversy as to which breathing method best relaxes abdominal muscles, the fact seems to be that it depends largely upon the individual mother. Hence, regardless of the breathing method the mother may be using, if she feels it is exerting uncomfortable pressure on her uterus, it seems wise for the nurse to help her learn the other method.

Between contractions the nurse can assist the mother to differentiate between abdominal and chest breathing and learn to use one or the other of the methods. While the mother is lying on her back, she places one hand on her chest, the other on her abdomen. The nurse points out that during an abdominal breath, the abdomen will rise as air is inhaled. During a chest breath, the chest will rise as air is inhaled. The nurse can have the mother practice each breathing method several times. Then the mother can choose the method that seems the most comfortable and/or the easiest. However, there may be no need for the nurse to assist the mother to differentiate between chest and abdominal breathing as long as the abdominal muscles are not contracted and the mother finds breathing easy and comfortable.

Abdominal Lifting. Another obvious method of reducing abdominal pressure is simply to lift the abdominal wall. The nurse may do this for the mother, or the father may be taught to perform this maneuver. A hand must be kept on the uterus to identify the beginning of the contraction. The instant the uterus begins to contract, the nurse places both hands at waist level with the fingers pointing toward the spine. She quickly slides her hands down and under the mother's back until the fingertips meet at the spine. The nurse then firmly and gently *lifts* until her hands rest between the pelvic bone and rib cage. As the hands are drawn from underneath the back, the hands are turned gradually (without releasing the upward lift) until the fingertips point toward the rib cage. The upward lift must be completed before the contraction reaches its peak. There should be lifting only and *no inward pressure*. When the contraction is over, the upward lift is released slowly.[29]

A more simple method of abdominal lifting is possible, but it is equally strenuous for the nurse or father. At the beginning of the contraction the fingers are hooked under the ribs and the distended abdomen lifted as the mother inhales. In both methods of abdominal lifting it is important that the mother not arch her back, since this would cause discomfort. Depending upon the amount of pressure exerted by the hand, the latter method may also result in lifting the baby, thus removing the pressure of the uterus on the back.[30]

Position.   Decreasing the weight of the uterus and baby on the muscles and bones of the mother's back can lessen considerably the amount of noxious stimuli. This is an especially important and effective pain relief measure when the mother experiences "back labor," that is, when the occiput of the fetus presses on the mother's sacrum. Regardless of the position of the fetus, a mother in normal labor probably will be more comfortable if she avoids the supine position.

One study compared the 30° upright position with the recumbent position during labor. The upright position was recommended for several reasons. Although the intensity of contractions was higher in this position, the contractions did not last any longer, the uterus relaxed more completely between contractions, and the first two stages of labor were shorter.[31] Thus, the duration of discomfort may be shortened by the upright position. This has the added advantage of reducing the danger to mother and infant that usually attends prolonged labor.

Unless there are complications such as a prolapsed cord, the mother should be allowed to choose the position she finds most comfortable. However, if she wants to lie on her back, the head of the bed should be somewhat elevated and her thighs slightly flexed.

Besides the 30° upright or semisitting position, other positions which may provide comfort during labor are the lateral Sim's and the tailor-sitting position. An unusual but increasingly popular position for mothers with back labor is the up-on-all-fours position. This position may even succeed in rotating the baby's head to an anterior position. If the baby's head is not in the posterior position, this crawl position may still produce pain relief, especially during transition, when labor is so often felt in the back.

Pushing.   As delivery approaches, most mothers feel the urge to push. However, unnecessary noxious stimuli can be eliminated if the mother understands that it is futile to push early in labor. Painful stimuli may also be avoided during delivery if the mother obeys instructions as to when she should and should not push. The urge to push can be almost irresistible. Thus the mother may need some techniques such as blowing or rapid breathing to help her refrain from pushing.

Relieving External Pressure.   When external electronic monitoring is used, the transducer may be a source of discomfort if it is secured in the same position over a period of time. The sensations of discomfort or heaviness may be decreased by moving the transducer at little as ¾ inch.

Distraction

Research studies as well as personal experiences confirm that distraction is an effective method of pain relief. As indicated earlier, the gate control theory provides some possible explanation. When the cerebral cortex is involved in activity (cortical excitation), the gate may be closed to pain. The cortex may signal a decreased attention to pain impulses. Or the reticular system in the brain stem may register that there is sufficient incoming stimuli and therefore signal the gate to be closed to further stimuli—painful stimuli in this case.

Regardless of the theoretical mechanism, common sense suggests that pain will be more tolerable if the patient becomes less aware of it—in short, distracted from it. Distraction places pain on the periphery of awareness. A person may be distracted from pain in an almost limitless variety of ways.

Instructors of methods of prepared childbirth have devised and taught many means of distraction for use during contractions. It is interesting to note that a large number of these are rhythmic in nature, such as "riding the wave," tapping out the rhythm of a song, rhythmic head movements, and rhythmic breathing.

The method of distraction tends to change as labor progresses, seemingly taking into account the increasing intensity of pain and the increasing effort the mother must exert to engage in any activity not related to labor. Thus, as demonstrated by the Lamaze method (see Table 24-2), during transition abdominal massage is eliminated and a relatively more easy breathing pattern is adopted. As a rule, the more intense the pain the more involved the patient must become in the distraction to achieve pain relief. However, the involvement must be compatible with the patient's ability.

Table 24-2 provides examples from the Lamaze method of activities that may serve as distracters. Many of these activities have other purposes as well. The breathing rhythms and purposeful thoughts undoubtedly serve as distracters, but maintenance of rhythmic breathing is also thought to relieve pain by providing adequate oxygenation of the uterus.

While relaxation, too, serves other purposes such as anxiety reduction and prevention of abdominal pressure, the mother may find that her concentrated efforts to relax provide a significant distraction. Changing positions and massaging the abdomen require both motor and cognitive effort, and therefore may be distracting. Keeping the eyes open and focused on a particular point is perhaps the purest and simplest distracter. Altogether, the Lamaze-trained mother consciously performs several varied activities with the end result of distraction from pain.

Other breathing patterns for use during contractions are suggested by Maternity Center Association and are described in Chapter 18, pages 232 to 234.

A brief comparison of the Lamaze method and the Maternity Center Association method reveals some of the ideas common to most methods of prepared childbirth—concentration on relaxation and a rhythmic breathing pattern during contractions.

The nurse needs to be familiar with a variety of distracters that she may suggest to the mother. What is sufficiently distracting for one mother may not be for another. And a mother may need assistance with distracters even if she has attended classes in a method of prepared childbirth.

Emphasis here will be placed on distracters that are of some proven effectiveness and also relatively easy to teach the mother. Most of the techniques taught in the Maternity Center Association (MCA)

method and the Lamaze method meet these criteria. (A review of the information in the page numbers mentioned above and Table 24-2 will assist the reader in the following discussion of these distracters.) Some distracters used in the various methods of prepared childbirth are extremely distracting but difficult to teach quickly once labor is in progress.

Early in labor the mother may be able to distract herself by "walking and talking" through a contraction. As labor progresses, some form of rhythmic breathing pattern is usually helpful. Slow rhythmic breathing is both relaxing and distracting, examples being either the "complete breathing" of the MCA or the "slow chest breathing" of Lamaze. If this is not effective, the nurse may suggest adding some of the distracters of the Lamaze method, such as a concentration point, counting during inhalation and exhalation, and abdominal massage.

When discomfort intensifies and a more powerful form of distraction is needed, the nurse may teach the mother the "modified complete breathing" of MCA or the accelerating and decelerating "shallow chest breathing" of the Lamaze method. Either of these may result in hyperventilation, so the nurse should caution the mother to inform her of any dizziness or tingling. Hyperventilation may be treated by having the mother breathe into a paper bag and suggesting that henceforth she breathe more slowly. Again, more distraction may be added to these breathing patterns by incorporating one or more of the distracters of the Lamaze method—the concentration point, abdominal massage, silent counting, or singing in rhythm with breathing. Another effective and relatively easy distracter to employ is finger tapping the rhythm to a 4/4 song, coordinating the rhythm with breathing.

Of all the breathing patterns suggested here, the one most likely to be difficult for the mother to learn during labor is the accelerated and decelerated aspect of the Lamaze "shallow chest breathing." If the mother finds this or any other distracter too difficult or fatiguing, it should be abandoned.

During transition the mother's focus tends to become extremely narrow because of the great increase in the intensity of contractions. Whereas earlier in labor the distracters could be suggested and taught between contractions, there is little time now and it is difficult for the mother to focus on anything but labor. Therefore distracters to be used during transition should be more simple and must be taught prior to the onset of transition. The Lamaze method suggests rhythmic, shallow chest breathing with blowing. Although this breathing pattern includes acceleration and deceleration with the intensity of the contraction, it is an easy breathing pattern to learn and use. The MCA suggests "modifed complete breathing" with the further modification of puffing out gently upon exhalation of every third or fourth breath. Simple additions to these breathing rhythms include coordinated and silent counting and use of a concentration point.

When the nurse wishes to assist the laboring mother with pain relief measures in the form of distracters, it is only reasonable to approach the mother between, not during, contractions. The nurse can describe briefly one or two possibilities. This needs to be accompanied by some explanation, such as, "It may seem silly at first, but many mothers find that it makes the contractions less bothersome because it forces them to think of something else." The mother should be asked to decide which one she would like to try first. It usually is most helpful if the nurse first demonstrates the pattern and then has the mother do it. If a song or counting is to be used, it is often much easier for the mother if the nurse counts or sings for her during the first contractions in which the pattern is used.

Certainly not everyone deals with pain in the same way. That is why it is so necessary to involve the mother in a decision about which distracters she would like to use. If the mother does not like any of the distracters discussed in this section, the nurse may creatively invent some others or simply ask the mother for suggestions. Some mothers prefer a form of distraction that involves an inward focus rather than the outward focus of the distracters described here. For example, the mother may stare into space or close her eyes and focus on the forces of her body, concentrating on the contraction being a wavelike force that she envisions herself on top of.

We have not yet begun to uncover and understand fully the various strategies people use to cope with pain. These strategies include much more than distraction, but within the area of distraction there are numerous approaches.

Whatever type of distracters the mother may choose to use during a contraction, the nurse and others must take care not to prevent her from using them. Early in labor it may be a helpful distraction to the mother to have someone to talk with during a contraction, but later she may find this irritating because it interferes with other strategies for coping with pain. In any event, the nurse needs to find out from the mother what, if anything, she wants the nurse to do for her during a contraction.

Cutaneous Stimulation

Rubbing a painful body part is a universal means of relieving pain. The gate control theory provides a possible reason for the effectiveness of this and other forms of cutaneous stimulation. As discussed previously, the theory suggests that stimulation of large-diameter nerve fibers may partially or completely close the gate to the transmission of pain impulses to the cortex. Because many cutaneous (skin) fibers are large-diameter fibers, stimulation of the skin may result in pain relief.

Several types of cutaneous stimulation may be used during labor and may prove to be effective pain relief measures. Rubbing the lower back is common. The Lamaze method describes a type of abdominal massage. The application of heat or cold (with the physician's permission) may be especially comforting to the patient with "back labor."

Creams or gels containing menthol may also be rubbed on the lower back for pain relief.

The above are examples of relatively moderate stimulation of cutaneous fibers. Mild to moderate stimulation is ordinarily more effective than intense stimulation. However, one notable exception is the use of intense pressure over the sacrum during a contraction. The pressure may be applied with the knee or fist, or the mother may lean back (in a semisitting position) on a tennis ball or rolling pin. It has been estimated that pressure so applied during a contraction is equivalent to the pain relief potential of 50 to 100 mg. of meperidine.[32]

Rubbing of any part of the body, even between contractions, possibly may contribute to pain relief. This not only encourages relaxation, but experimentation with cutaneous stimulation shows that it may help close the gate to painful impulses long after its usage and that the painful area need not always be the area of stimulation.[33] For example, if an external monitor prevents abdominal massage, the thighs may be massaged instead. Some mothers find that foot massage by the father or nurse brings considerable comfort.

Transcutaneous electric nerve stimulation (TENS) is a newer form of cutaneous stimulation that has been used successfully for pain relief during the first stage of labor. A mild electric current is applied to the skin via electrodes connected to a battery-operated device with controls to regulate the sensation. The patient usually feels a buzzing, tingling, or vibrating sensation. In one study of labor pain, two pairs of electrodes were placed on either side of the spinal column over the sacral and thoracic regions. Low intensity stimulation was provided continuously, and the mother increased the stimulation during a contraction. Of the 147 women treated, 44 percent considered TENS pain relief to be good to very good. No complications occurred except that in a few cases sacral stimulation interfered with monitoring the fetal heart rate. These researchers recommended TENS as a primary method of pain relief during labor, noting that it is low risk, nonpharmacological, and can be interrupted at any moment.[34]

Nursing responsibilities when TENS is used might include placing and securing the electrodes, explaining the use of the controls to the mother, and evaluating the effectiveness of TENS in relieving pain.

Relaxation

Virtually every method of prepared childbirth heavily emphasizes total skeletal muscle relaxation during labor. Relaxation contributes to pain relief in a variety of ways. Some of these have already been mentioned, such as relaxing the abdominal muscles to decrease the noxious stimuli of pressure on the uterus.

But even when noxious stimuli are not affected directly, skeletal muscle relaxation itself may be a pain relief measure. It relieves pain by interrupting the spiraling process of pain and anxiety. Muscle tension is a response to pain and anxiety. Since relaxation is the opposite of muscle tension, it prevents or diminishes tension. The behavioral response of relaxation, therefore, is incompatible with pain-anxiety responses. Some research suggests that a person's evaluation of the intensity of pain is in part a function of her evaluation of her own overt behavioral response to pain.[35] Possibly when the patient observes herself relaxed instead of tense, she evaluates her pain as less intense. Or

relaxation may cause the cortex to send signals to close the gate to the transmission of pain impulses.

Undoubtedly relaxation provides pain relief for other reasons, depending upon the individual patient. For some patients efforts to relax can serve as a distraction from pain. In other patients a state of relaxation may increase suggestibility, causing the patient to accept explicit and implicit suggestions of comfort.[36]

How can the patient achieve total skeletal muscle relaxation? Possibly the most frequently used but most unproductive method is for the nurse to say, "Relax." The verbal cue "relax" may be used effectively with patients who have been trained in relaxation, but to the untrained patient such a command often sounds impossible, if not absurd. The patient's inability to follow such an instruction may engender feelings of powerlessness, failure, and more tension.

People may be trained in relaxation techniques in many different ways and for many reasons besides childbirth, such as handling the tensions of daily living.

When the nurse encounters a mother who has been trained in relaxation techniques, she simply finds out how best to assist her. It is particularly helpful to identify cues that will encourage relaxation if the mother becomes tense. These cues may be verbal, such as "relax," or tactile-kinesthetic, such as touching or moving the tense body part.

If the mother has not been trained in relaxation, the nurse may use some simple techniques that can make a significant difference in the mother's level of relaxation. The nurse first explains to the mother that relaxing during a contraction is very important because it can decrease abdominal pressure on the uterus and also help her feel more calm and generally comfortable. The quickest and easiest ways to promote relaxation are to instruct the mother to take a deep breath or to yawn and to "go limp" or relax as she exhales. The nurse suggests that the mother try one or both of these at the beginning and end of contractions and anytime during contractions that she feels the need to relax. (The patient who chooses to yawn may find it becomes spontaneous and more frequent.)

These techniques are effective because they take advantage of conditioned responses. Both a big sigh (deep breath) and a yawn are associated with relaxation.

Relaxation may be furthered by providing support to comfortably positioned and slightly flexed extremities. Also, the nurse may gently move extremities and the head to test for the degree of relaxation. This slight movement enables the mother to feel tense muscles and helps her to relax them.

ASSISTANCE WITH CHANGE IN EXPECTATIONS AND GOALS

During the relatively brief and rapidly moving events of labor, any unexpected change in the parent's goals or expectations must be handled quickly. Otherwise anxiety may persist or increase, resulting in an increased intensity of pain. Some items listed in Part V of Table 24-1 are examples of areas in which a disturbing change may occur.

Sometimes the mother's personal obstetrician is not available, and a physician unknown to the parents must manage labor and delivery. Or the mother and father may have expected to be together throughout labor, but perhaps the father cannot be located or is unable to get to the hospital. In some instances the labor suite is too crowded to accommodate the father. Parents may have planned to use the alternative birth center (ABC) but the facilities may be occupied.

If external or internal electronic monitoring of the fetus is used, this may be disconcerting to parents for several reasons. The parents may be very fearful if they associate its usage with possible complications. Some hospitals monitor only high-risk situations, but others routinely monitor all patients. Regardless of the reason for electronic monitoring, the parents may strongly object to the use of such equipment because it renders childbirth a less natural experience. In addition, external monitoring in particular will make it difficult for the parents to use certain pain relief measures such as abdominal lifting, abdominal massage, and some positioning. Often external monitoring requires that the mother lie quietly on her back. If this is disturbing to the parents, the nurse should, if possible, remove the external monitoring equipment for a few contractions so that the parents can employ some of their pain relief activities.

When a situation occurs that disturbs the parents, the nurse encourages them to express their feelings and indicates an appreciation of their disappoint-

ment. She then explains the reasons for any rules, policies, or circumstances that prevent them from achieving their goals or expectations.

One of the more difficult problems is assisting the parents who are not able to achieve their "ideal" of labor and delivery. This ideal may vary considerably from one couple to another and may consist of any one or combination of goals referred to previously. Inability to achieve this ideal labor may cause profound feelings of failure in the mother or father. Also, they may refuse or be very reluctant to accept measures incompatible with their ideal.

Patients who have specific expectations or goals associated with an ideal labor may have arrived at these in a number of ways. But these parents seem most often to be a product of classes that prepare them in a specific method of childbirth. One of the most common criticisms of methods of prepared childbirth is that the mother and father are taught to strive for a particular kind of labor and delivery experience, such as medication-free delivery or ecstasy over the delivery. Not all childbirth educators state such goals. Yet parents, especially mothers, tend to adopt these goals and feel a sense of failure if they are not achieved. The reason for this is not necessarily related to what the childbirth educator says. Rather the goals are implicit in personal narratives and films to which the mother is exposed.

Written personal labor experiences are found in books and may be available from the childbirth educator's collections from former students. Some methods of childbirth use their own particular film to introduce their method to the parents. Examples are "The Story of Eric," showing the use of the Lamaze method, and "Childbirth for the Joy of It," showing the use of Husband-Coached Childbirth. Viewing these films, it is easy to understand why the mother or father would desire the same "ideal" experience. The films focus not on pain but on the techniques of the particular method of childbirth and on the parents' extreme happiness immediately following delivery. These films are emotionally appealing and very persuasive.

At the end of the film, with tears of joy in her eyes, the pregnant woman is not likely to want to settle for less than what she has just seen. She may reason, "If those women can give birth that way, I should be able to do it, too." Hence, the feeling of failure or not being "good at childbirth" may result if the mother finds that she is unable to go through her own labor as she saw it portrayed in film or in written narratives.

How does the nurse help the mother and father minimize feelings of failure and accept a change in their goals? Throughout childbirth, and particularly when goals must change, the nurse praises the mother and father for their efforts and abilities to handle labor. This promotes feelings of success. For example, the mother may have the goal of an unmedicated labor, but she may find the discomfort intolerable and request medication. If medication is given, the nurse can say that she knows medication was not planned. She can allow the mother to express her feelings and then praise the mother for the success of her efforts up to now and for the length of time medication was not necessary. She may add that the mother's continuing efforts may reduce the amount of medication required. She may also stress to the father that his approval and support are extremely valuable.

The mother may, however, choose to handle the above situation in a different manner. She may decide it is in the best interests of herself and her baby for her not to request medication, in spite of how intolerable she finds the pain. Such pain may cause her to become extremely tense and unable to cooperate with examinations or the forces of labor. This may prolong labor and increase the possibility of complications. If medication seems highly desirable, the nurse may find it necessary to use a direct approach with the mother to modify her perceptions of the situation. This may be accomplished by stating how the health team views the situation and pointing out differences in this view and the mother's perceptions. One thing the nurse may point out is that the mother wants to avoid both medication and complications, but the two goals are now incompatible.

This direct approach tends to cause unpleasant psychological tension, called cognitive dissonance. In other words, the mother's goals are at odds with one another and with the knowledge received from the nurse. Cognitive dissonance may motivate a person to change. One way the mother may reduce dissonance in this case is to adjust her thinking so that she will accept other pain relief measures.[37]

Another approach to this type of situation is to employ analogy. This may disrupt the mother's denial of what is actually happening, assist her with a clearer understanding of the situation, and/or foster feelings of normality about her childbirth experi-

ence. Explaining the situation by comparing it with something else allows the mother to distance herself from the actual situation. She is able to understand the problem but avoid the anxiety associated with looking directly at the problem.[38] For example, the nurse may compare labor to a menstrual cycle. She may say that no two labors are exactly alike, just as no two women have exactly the same menstrual cycle. She may add that some women normally experience more pain than others. Or she may cite some other symptom or sign that explains the need for a change in the mother's goal.

AFTERMATH ASSIMILATION

After anticipation of pain and the presence of pain, a third and final phase of the pain experience occurs—the aftermath. The pain experience does not end with the cessation of the painful sensations. The patient does not necessarily immediately forget about the pain, especially if it was severe, frightening, or in any way disconcerting.

On the maternity unit it is a common observation that mothers talk a great deal about their childbirth experiences. It is a frequent topic of conversation regardless of whether the mother experienced "ecstasy," "failure," or simply relief mixed with satisfaction. Not only may the mother want to talk about the pain, but a variety of feelings resulting from the pain may be present, such as nausea, vomiting, chills, anger, or embarrassment. The mother may even have nightmares about the pain.

Clearly, at least some mothers will need assistance during the aftermath phase of the pain experience. The most appropriate nursing action may be to assist the mother with the intellectual and emotional assimilation of her childbirth experience. In a sense the nurse helps the mother relive her labor. The nurse can ask the mother questions that help her discuss her discomforts, emotions, thoughts, overt responses, and the reactions of others during her labor. The nurse needs to be particularly alert and responsive to the mother's needs for support, such as praise, confirmation that her perceptions of discomfort are believed by others, or reassurance that her behavior was acceptable. Some patients will need information to help them fill in memory gaps or to correct understandings that are inaccurate and anxiety-provoking.[39]

It is particularly important to encourage assimilation in mothers who may harbor feelings of failure about childbirth. But assimilation may help maintain or restore a positive self-concept for any mother and aid in her ability to deal with mothering and other impending tasks.

REFERENCES

1. A. L. Clark et al.: "MCH in American Samoa." *Am. J. Nurs.* 74:700–702, April 1974.
2. F. Lamaze: *Painless Childbirth: The Lamaze Method.* Chicago, Henry Regnery, 1970.
3. H. Potter and R. D. Macdonald: "Obstetric consequences of epidural analgesia in nulliparous patients." *Lancet* 1:1031–1034, 1971.
4. B. Davenport-Slack and C. H. Boylan: "Psychological correlates of childbirth pain." *Psychosom. Med.* 36:215–223, May-June 1974.
5. P. Nettelbladt, C-F. Fagerstrom, and N. Uddenberg: "The significance of reported childbirth pain." *J. Psychosom. Res.* 20:215–221, 1976.
6. S. Y. Fagerhaugh and A. Strauss: *Politics of Pain: Staff-Patient Interaction.* Menlo Park, Calif., Addison-Wesley, 1977, pp. 223–224.
7. M. McCaffery: *Nursing Management of the Patient with Pain,* ed. 2. Philadelphia, J. B. Lippincott, 1979, p. 11.
8. Ibid., p. 284.
9. Fagerhaugh and Strauss, op. cit., pp. 222–237.
10. L. A. Copp: "The spectrum of suffering." *Am. J. Nurs.* 74:491, March 1974.
11. R. Melzack and P. D. Wall: "Pain mechanisms: A new theory." *Science* 150:971–979, 1965.
12. ———: *The Puzzle of Pain.* New York, Basic Books, 1973.
13. P. W. Nathan: "The gate-control theory of pain: A critical review." *Brain,* 99:213–258, 1976.
14. P. D. Wall: "Modulation of pain by non-painful events." In Bonica, J. J. and Albe-Fessard, D. (eds.): *Advances in Pain Research and Therapy,* Vol. 1, pp. 1–16. New York, Raven Press, 1976.
15. "Brain hormones help explain mind-body interface." *Brain Mind Bull.* 4:1, 3, Dec. 1978.
16. S. H. Snyder: "Opiate receptors and internal opiates." *Scientific Am.* 236:44–56, March 1977.
17. R. Cogan: "Comfort during prepared childbirth as a function of parity, reported by four classes of participant observers." *J. Psychosom. Res.* 19:33–37, 1975.
18. A. Jones, P. M. Bentler, and G. Petry: "The reduction of uncertainty concerned future pain." *J. Abnorm. Psych.* 71:87–94, April 1966.
19. McCaffery, op. cit., pp. 13–14.
20. Ibid., pp. 14–17.
21. Nettelbladt, Fagerstrom, and Uddenberg, op. cit.
22. B. Winsberg and M. Greenlick: "Pain response in Negro and white obstetrical patients." *J. Health Soc. Behav.* 8:222–227, Sept. 1967.
23. J. L. Sasmor, C. R. Castor, and P. Hassid: "The childbirth team during labor." *Am. J. Nurs.* 73:444–447, March 1973.
24. P. R. Ulin: "Changing techniques in psychoprophylactic preparation for childbirth." *Am. J. Nurs.* 68:2586–2591, Dec. 1968.
25. K. Osanai and M. Nishijima: "Comparison of analgesia and anesthesia for labor between the university hospitals of the U.S.A. and Japan, including our own." *Acta. Obst. et Gynaec. Jap.* 21:76–85, 1974.
26. M. Gandy: "Ten years ago in ASPO." *Conceptions,* Fall 1976.
27. N. Stotland: "What has ASPO done for me?" *Conceptions,* Winter 1976–77.
28. E. Declerck: *National Teachers Survey.* Washington, D.C., The American Society of Psychoprophylaxis in Obstetrics, 1977.
29. M. Gamper: *Preparation for the Heir Minded.* Illinois, Margaret Gamper, 1971, p. 48.
30. C. A. Bean: *Methods of Childbirth.* New York, Dolphin Books, 1974, pp. 103–104.
31. Y. C. Liu: "Effects of an upright position during labor." *Am. J. Nurs.* 74:2202–2205, Dec. 1974.
32. J. B. Pace: "Psychophysiology of pain: Diagnostic and therapeutic implications." *J. Fam. Practice* 1:4, May 1974.
33. McCaffery, op. cit., pp. 133–135.
34. L-E. Augustinsson, et al.: "Pain relief during delivery by transcutaneous electrical nerve stimulation." *Pain* 4:59–65, 1977.
35. R. J. Bandler, Jr., G. R. Madaras, and D. J. Bem: "Self-observation as a source of pain perception." *J. Pers. Soc. Psych.* 9:205–209, July 1968.
36. L. Chertok: *Motherhood and Personality: Psychosomatic Aspects of Childbirth.* Philadelphia, Tavistock Publications and J. B. Lippincott, 1969, pp. 13–16.
37. J. Miller: "Cognitive dissonance in modi-

fying families' perceptions." *Am. J. Nurs.* 74: 1468–1470, Aug. 1974.

38. M. S. Wacker: "Analogy: Weapon against denial." *Am. J. Nurs.* 74:71–73, Jan. 1974.

39. McCaffery, op. cit.

SUGGESTED READING

Abouleish, E. and Depp, R.: "Acupuncture in obstetrics." *Curr. Res.* 54:83–88, 1975.

Aleksandrowicz, M. K. and Aleksandrowicz, D. R.: "Obstetrical pain-relieving drugs as predictors of infant behavior variability." *Child Dev.* 47:294–296, 1974.

————: "Obstetrical pain-relieving drugs as predictors of infant behavior variability: A reply to Federman and Yang's critique." *Child. Dev.* 47:297–298, 1976.

Angelini, D. J.: "Nonverbal communication in labor." *Am. J. Nurs.* 78:1220–1222, July 1978.

Augustinsson, L-E. et al.: "Pain relief during delivery by transcutaneous electrical nerve stimulation." *Pain* 4:59–65, 1977.

Baer, E., Davitz, L. J., and Lieb, R.: "Inferences of physical pain and psychological distress. I. In relation to verbal and nonverbal patient communication." *Nurs. Res.* 19:388–392, Sept./Oct. 1970.

Bean, C. A.: *Methods of Childbirth.* New York, Dolphin Books, 1974.

Benson, H., Beary, J. F., and Carol, M. P.: "The relaxation response." *Psychiatry* 37:37–46, Feb. 1974.

Bing, E.: *Six Practical Lessons for Easier Childbirth.* New York, Grosset and Dunlap, 1967.

Bonica, J. J.: "The nature of pain in parturition." *Clin. Obstet. Gynec.* 2:499–516, 1975.

Bonica, J. J.: *Principles and Practice of Obstetric Analgesia and Anesthesia,* Vols. I, II. Philadelphia, F. A. Davis, 1967, 1969.

Bowes, W. A. et al.: "The effects of obstetrical medication on fetus and infant." *Mono. Soc. Res. Child Dev.* 35:1–55, 1970.

Bradley, R. A.: *Husband-Coached Childbirth.* New York, Harper & Row, 1974.

Chertok, L.: *Motherhood and Personality: Psychosomatic Aspects of Childbirth.* Philadelphia, J. B. Lippincott, 1969.

Clark, A. L. et al.: "MCH in American Samoa." *Am. J. Nurs.* 74:700–702, April 1974.

Cogan, R.: "Comfort during prepared childbirth as a function of parity, reported by four classes of participant observers." *J. Psychosom. Res.* 19:33–37, 1975.

Corah, N. L., and Boffa, J.: "Perceived control, self-observation, and response to aversive stimulation." *J. Pers. Soc. Psych.* 16:1–4, Sept. 1970.

Cronenwett, L. R. and Newmark, L. L.: "Fathers' responses to childbirth." *Nurs. Res.* 23: 210–217, May-June 1974.

Davenport-Slack, B., and Boylan, C. H.: "Psychological correlates of childbirth pain." *Psychosom. Med.* 36:215–223, May-June 1974.

DeLyser, F.: *A Professional's Guide to Prepared Childbirth.* Washington, D.C., American Society for Psycho-Prophylaxis in Obstetrics, Nov. 1973.

Dick-Read, G.: *Childbirth Without Fear.* New York, Harper & Row, 1972.

Diers, D. et al.: "The effect of nursing interaction on patients in pain." *Nurs. Res.* 21: 419–428, Sept./Oct. 1972.

Eppink, H.: "Catheterizing the maternity patient." *Am. J. Nurs.* 76:829, May 1975.

Fagerhaugh, S. Y. and Strauss, A.: *Politics of Pain Management: Staff-Patient Interaction.* Menlo Park, Calif., Addison-Wesley, 1977.

Federman, E. J. and Yang, R. K.: "A critique of 'obstetrical pain-relieving drugs as predictors of infant behavior variability.' " *Child Dev.* 47: 294–296, 1976.

Field, P-A.: "Relief of pain in labor." In Jacox, A. K. (ed.): *Pain: A Source Book for Nurses and Other Health Professionals,* pp. 427–434. Boston, Little, Brown, 1977.

Fisher, D. E. and Paton, J. B.: "The effect of maternal anesthetic and analgesic drugs on the fetus and newborn." *Clin. Obstet. Gynecol.* 17: 275–287, 1974.

Gamper, M.: *Preparation for the Heir Minded.* Illinois, Margaret Gamper, 1971.

Grad, R. K. and Woodside, J.: "Obstetrical analgesics and anesthesia: Methods of relief for the patient in labor." *Am. J. Nurs.* 77:242–245, Feb. 1977.

Hackett, T. P.: "Pain and prejudice: Why do we doubt that the patient is in pain?" *Res. Staff Physician* 18:100–109, May 1972.

Haire, D.: *The Cultural Warping of Childbirth.* Seattle, Wash., International Childbirth Education Association Supplies Center, 1974.

Hassid, P.: "Focus . . . on the behavioral responses." *Am. J. Nurs.* 76:1244, Aug. 1976.

————: *Textbook for Childbirth Educators.* New York, Harper & Row, 1978.

Henneborn, W. J. and Cogan, R.: "The effect of husband participation on reported pain and probability of medication during labor and birth." *J. Psychosom. Res.* 19:215–222, 1975.

Hill, S. Y., Schwin, R., Goodwin, D. W., and Powell, B. J.: "Marihuana and pain." *J. Pharm. Exper. Ther.* 188:415–418, 1974.

Hunter, M., Philips, C., and Rachman, S.: "Memory for pain." *Pain* 6:35–46, 1979.

Johnson, J. E., and Rice, V. H.: "Sensory and distress components of pain: Implications for the study of clinical pain." *Nurs. Res.* 23:203–209, May/June 1974.

Joseph, S. S.: "Whatever happened to prepared childbirth?" *JOGN* Jan./Feb. 1975, pp. 48–49.

Karmel, M.: *Thank You, Doctor Lamaze.* Philadelphia, J. B. Lippincott, 1959.

Kitzinger, S.: *Experience of Childbirth.* London, Victor Gollancz Ltd., 1972.

Kroger, W. S.: *Childbirth with Hypnosis.* Hollywood, Wilshire Book Company, 1965.

Lennane, K. J., and Lennane, R. J.: "Alleged psychogenic disorders in women—A possible manifestation of sexual prejudice." *N. Eng. J. Med.* 288:288–292, Feb. 1973.

Leppert, P. and Williams, B.: "Birth films may miscarry." *Am. J. Nurs.* 68:2181–2183, Oct. 1968.

Liu, Y. C.: "Effects of an upright position during labor." *Am. J. Nurs.* 74:2202–2205, Dec. 1974.

Lubic, R. W. and Ernst, E. K. M.: "Psychological analgesia: Natural childbirth and psychoprophylaxis." *Clin. Obstet. Gynecol.* 2:2–16, Dec. 1975.

Maternity Center Association: *Preparation for Childbearing.* New York, The Association, 1972.

McCaffery, M.: *Nursing Management of the Patient with Pain,* ed. 2. J. B. Lippincott, 1979.

Melzack, R.: *The Puzzle of Pain.* New York, Basic Books, 1973.

Nettelbladt, P., Fagerstrom, C-F., and Uddenberg, N.: "The significance of reported childbirth pain." *J. Psychosom. Res.* 20:215–221, 1976.

Neufeld, R. W. J. and Davidson, P. O.: "The effects of vicarious and cognitive rehearsal on pain tolerance." *J. Psychosom. Res.* 15:329–335, Sept. 1971.

The Pregnant Patient's Bill of Rights. Distributed by Committee on Patient's Rights, Box 1900, New York, NY 10001, ND.

Redland, A.: "Perineal splinting." *Am. J. Nurs.* 76:1258, Aug. 1976.

Rowbotham, C. J. F.: "Obstetric pain." *Physiotherapy* 60:103–106, April 1974.

Sasmor, J. L., Castor, C. R., and Hassid, P.: "The child-birth team during labor." *Am. J. Nurs.* 73:444–447, March 1973.

Scott, J. S.: "Patient-controlled intravenous narcotic administration during labour." *Lancet* 1:251, Jan. 31, 1976.

Shealy, C. N. and Maurer, D.: "Transcutaneous nerve stimulation for control of pain—A preliminary technical note." *Surg. Neurol.* 2:45–47, 1974.

Siegele, D. S.: "The gate control theory." *Am. J. Nurs.* 74:498–502, March 1974.

Smith, B. A., Priore, R. M., and Stern, M. K.: "The transition phase of labor." *Am. J. Nurs.* 73:448–450, March 1973.

Stevens, R. J.: "Psychological strategies for management of pain in prepared childbirth: A study of psychoanalgesia in prepared childbirth." *Birth and the Family J.* 4:4–9, Spring 1977.

Swartz, R.: "A father's view." *Children Today* 6:14–17, March/April 1977.

Tanzer, D.: "Natural childbirth: Pain or peak experience." *Psych. Today* 2:17–21, 69, Oct. 1968.

Ulin, P. R.: "Changing techniques in psychoprophylactic preparation for childbirth." *Am. J. Nurs.* 68:2586–2591, Dec. 1968.

White, J. R.: "Effects of a counterirritant on perceived pain and hand movement in patients with arthritis." *Phys. Ther.* 53:956–960, Sept. 1973.

Williamson, J.: "Hypnosis in obstetrics." *Nurs. Times* 71:1895–1897, Nov. 27, 1975.

Winsberg, B. and Greenlick, M.: "Pain response in Negro and white obstetrical patients." *J. Health Soc. Behav.* 8:222–227, Sept. 1967.

Wright, E.: *The New Childbirth.* New York, Hart Publishing Co., 1966.

Twenty-Five

Analgesia and Anesthesia for Childbirth

General Principles / Cause of Discomfort During Labor and Delivery / Selection of Anesthesia and Analgesia / Nonpharmacologic Methods / Pharmacologic Analgesia and Anesthesia / Anesthesia for Cesarean Section / The Role of the Obstetric Nurse in the Safe Practice of Obstetric Anesthesia

The discomfort and suffering endured by women during childbirth has been recounted in historical records since the time of early civilizations. In Europe and in colonial America, women were imprisoned and even put to death for either seeking or providing pain relief during parturition. It was not until November 8, 1847, that James Young Simpson, a courageous 36-year-old obstetrician, reported to the Edinburgh Medical and Chirurgical Society on the efficacy of chloroform to alleviate the pain associated with childbirth. For his work, Simpson was harshly criticized on theological grounds based on the the Bible passage, Genesis 3: 16:

Unto the woman He said, I will greatly multiply thy sorrow and thy conception; in sorrow thou shalt bring forth children. . . .

It was not until six years later that obstetric anesthesia was accepted and respectable. In 1853, the first fulltime physician anesthetist, John Snow, introduced "chloroform à la reine" when he attended the birth of Queen Victoria's eighth child, Prince Leopold, and administered chloroform analgesia for 53 minutes during labor. Snow again used chloroform for the anesthetic needs of his queen at the birth of Princess Beatrice in 1857. The monarch herself ended the need for women to suffer

in childbirth by saying, "Dr. Snow gave that blessed chloroform and the effect was soothing, quieting and delightful beyond measure."

Despite the acceptance of obstetric anesthesia, pain relief during childbirth was administered by persons untrained in the art and science of anesthesia. Anesthetic practices varied tremendously from area to area. Little thought was given to tailoring the anesthesia or analgesia to the specific needs of the laboring mother and the welfare of the fetus. New drugs producing analgesia, sedation and anesthesia were often used for the first time in the parturient after few, if any, controlled studies. The concept of "twilight sleep," in which the mother was drugged to the state of oblivion (oftentimes lasting hours if not days into the postpartum period), came into vogue. To this, general anesthesia was frequently added at the time of delivery, primarily for the convenience of the obstetrician. Its administration usually fell to the labor floor nurse or the nearest medical student, who was completely untrained and unaware of the dangers associated with general anesthesia. In some more "enlightened" centers, conduction or regional anesthesia was utilized by farsighted obstetricians who lacked training and support from their colleagues in anesthesia. Indeed, as late as 1962, it was estimated that in the United States 100 women died each year from pulmonary aspiration of stomach contents during the administration of general anesthesia for childbirth.

In the early 1950s, Dr. Virginia Apgar, then the Director of Anesthesia at Columbia Presbyterian Hospital in New York City, effectively addressed this problem. Although Virginia Apgar is better known for her evaluation of the newborn with the Apgar score, her realization that trained anesthesia personnel had as important a role to play on the labor floor as in the operating room is a greater contribution. Apagar's labors resulted in the first effective multidisciplinary teaching and research program devoted to obstetric anesthesia. Her program encouraged the interest of many young anesthesiologists in the neglected area of obstetric anesthesia. The program also provided the impetus for other well-known teaching institutes to establish similar fulltime anesthesia coverage for the labor floor and adequate training in obstetric anesthesia for both nurses and physicians specializing in anesthesia.

In the past two decades there have been great improvements and advances in the field of obstetric anesthesia. The Joint Commission on Accreditation of Hospitals has come to require that adequate and competent anesthesia coverage be available at all times on the labor floor. The American Board of Anesthesiology requires all residents to have adequate exposure to obstetric anesthesia in order for a residency program to gain approval. Obstetricians and patients alike are recognizing the desirability of fulltime anesthesia coverage for parturition. Yet we still have a long way to go before anesthesia on the labor floor is on a par with that in the operating room.

GENERAL PRINCIPLES

. . . The application of anaesthesia to midwifery involves many more delicate problems than its mere applications to surgery. New rules must be established for its use, its effects upon the action of the uterus, upon the state of the child and on the puerperal state of the mother. These and other questions all require to be accurately studied and to be duly answered.

These words were spoken over a century ago by Sir James Y. Simpson. Many of the guidelines covering anesthesia for the surgical patient have little place on the labor floor. The psychologic status of the obstetric patient is usually different from her surgical counterpart. Furthermore, unlike the surgical patient, the parturient is an active participant and her cooperation is needed in a vaginal delivery.

The administration of anesthetic and analgesic drugs affects not only the mother, but also the fetus and newborn.

Despite the fact that pregnancy, labor and delivery are considered normal physiological processes, the changes wrought by these physiological processes have profound implications for anesthetic techniques.

1. Pregnancy is associated with an increased sensitivity to most anesthetics, analgesics and tranquilizers, which make overdose more likely.
2. Because of the edema of the upper airway normally present in late pregnancy, the possibility of airway obstruction is increased.
3. Changes in pulmonary function and an increased oxygen requirement predispose the parturient to the rapid development of hypoxia, particularly in the second stage of labor or during induction of anesthesia. A 40 percent increase in pulmonary minute ventilation at term, which may increase further to 300 percent in the second stage of labor, makes induction of anesthesia with inhalation drugs rapid.
4. The effects of the use of medications during labor, and the fact that the maternity patient may have recently eaten, subject her to an increased risk of pulmonary aspiration of gastric contents with its devastating morbidity and mortality.
5. Changes in the cardiovascular system, particularly those associated with aorta caval compression by the gravid uterus, predispose the obstetric patient to sudden hypotension and cardiovascular collapse and her fetus to hypoxia and acidosis at the time of general or major conduction anesthesia.

Pregnancy alters, and often exacerbates, the pathophysiology of many disease states, particularly those involving the cardiovascular and endocrine systems. Obstetric emergencies, especially fetal distress and maternal hemorrhage, demand the rapid induction of anesthesia. Thus, although the parturient is usually considered a healthy young female undergoing a physiologic process, she becomes a high anesthetic risk requiring markedly different considerations from those applied to the surgical patient. Failure to take these factors into account can result in a disaster for the mother and her fetus.

CAUSE OF DISCOMFORT DURING LABOR AND DELIVERY

The discomfort experienced during labor and delivery comes from two distinct sources. The pain associated with the first stage of labor is visceral and results from uterine contractions. As the uterus contracts, it causes dilatation (stretching) and effacement (thinning) of the cervix by the presenting part. In addition, uterine contractions constrict the arterial blood supply to the myometrium, causing uterine ischemia. It is the stretching of the cervix and uterine ischemia that causes discomfort. The pain is experienced over the lower abdomen and the lumbar area of the back and it may radiate into the thighs. Between contractions, the mother is pain-free. Only a relatively small part of labor is uncomfortable, during the peak of the contractions.

In the second, or expulsive, stage of labor, uterine or *visceral* pain decreases as the cervix is completely dilated and effaced and is overshadowed by perineal or *somatic* pain. As the presenting part navigates the birth canal, it causes stretching of the vagina and perineum. When the uterus contracts in the second stage forcing the presenting part down the birth canal, the mother has a reflex urge to bear down, bringing into play the secondary or ancillary forces of labor necessary to propel the fetus down the birth canal for a vaginal delivery.

Oversedation, general anesthesia or regional anesthesia of the perineum may delay or even prohibit vaginal delivery by abolishing the bearing-down reflex.

SELECTION OF ANESTHESIA AND ANALGESIA

Three factors should play a major role in deciding the anesthetic management of labor and delivery:
1. The desires of the mother.
2. The amount of discomfort experienced during labor and delivery.
3. The anesthesia personnel and facilities at hand.

Ideally, the most appropriate form of pain relief should be available for each individual parturient.

Anesthesia is best tailored to the conditions surrounding the labor of each individual parturient. However, it is unwise for the obstetrician or the delivery room nurse to promise any particular type of analgesia. Furthermore, the mother should approach her labor with an open mind toward anesthesia. The patient should be aware that intervention with pharmacologic analgesia at times may be necessary in the best interest of both her and her fetus. She can be reassured that there is *no* evidence that modern techniques of analgesia and anesthesia, properly administered, have any prolonged or deleterious effects on the newborn. To the contrary, there is much evidence that properly conducted analgesia throughout labor may help to maintain a better respiratory, cardiovascular and metabolic status for the mother. Routine use of any particular type of pain relief is also to be discouraged. When the woman arrives on the labor floor in early labor, she should be visited by those who will administer anesthesia and given further counseling and reassurance that her anesthetic needs will be met, as much in accordance with her own desires as possible. Only when this approach is used by all involved will optimal anesthesia be employed and contribute to a successful and fulfilling outcome.

Ideal analgesia or anesthesia for labor and delivery satisfies the following conditions:
1. It provides satisfactory alleviation of pain for the individual parturient.
2. It does not interfere significantly with the normal mechanics or progress of labor and delivery.
3. It is not associated with undue risk to the mother.
4. It is associated with minimal fetal and newborn depression.
5. It allows early interaction between the mother and her newborn, preferably in the delivery room.
6. It provides safe and satisfactory conditions for the delivery.

No single technique of pain relief fulfills all of the above objectives for every mother.

NONPHARMACOLOGIC METHODS

Natural childbirth

This term applies to a rather broad and general philosophy of labor management. Such methods are based upon the principle that, with careful prenatal education, along with support from the father and those attending the delivery, and the application of controlled breathing and voluntary muscle relaxation, the need for anesthesia and analgesia can be minimized if not eliminated. The effectiveness of these methods is not based primarily on the physical techniques employed, but rather on the total involvement and acquired knowledge of the patient and the father, and the interest of the people supporting her.

The methods outlined by the British obstetrician Grantly Dick-Read have more recently been replaced in popularity by the Lamaze method, or psychoprophylaxis, an approach involving controlled breathing and active participation by the husband. Instructions in the use of such an approach are available in most areas through private tutors or an organization known as the Childbirth Education Association. If such instruction is not available, there are a number of books which may be used. Such an approach is not applicable to all patients, and the key to a successful application of the technique is motivation. Those interested only because of intellectual curiosity, or those talked into the idea, generally do poorly.

In recent years, prepared or natural childbirth has become increasingly popular in the United States. Much of this growth is due to the desire of mothers to experience birth and to be able to relate to their newborn shortly after birth. In addition, both the medical profession and the lay public have come to realize that heavy sedation and narcosis used during labor may have prolonged and pronounced deleterious effects on the neonate.

Childbirth classes vary tremendously in emphasis and the material taught, but despite their diversity they have certain basic principles in common. The father or a trusted companion attends the classes with the mother. During labor and delivery this companion will be with the mother to encourage and coach her. The mother is taught certain exercises, usually related to breathing and to bearing down, which she will use during contractions and delivery. The specific exercises and conditioning vary and, in general, serve to distract her from the painful aspects of childbirth. In the classes, which are usually attended during the latter half of pregnancy, the mother and her companion are taught the principles of labor and delivery. Attempts are made to correct misconceptions, to allay fears and to make childbirth a fulfilling experience for both the mother and father. Finally, the prepared or natural childbirth classes seek to minimize the need for the use of medications which can decrease the mother's awareness and cause newborn depression. Patients who select this approach should understand that, even though they may fail to get through their entire labor without anesthesia, they have still accomplished something and should not feel guilty. When used successfully, this approach can be a very rewarding experience for all concerned. (See also Chapter 18.)

Hypnosis

Hypnosis has been used sporadically for pain relief in both obstetric and surgical patients. Hypnosis per se is not associated with maternal and neonatal depression. Enthusiasts claim its use results in better maternal cooperation, reduces or eliminates the need for depressant drugs, decreases blood loss, provides postpartum analgesia and aids in milk letdown in nursing mothers. The use of formal hypnosis requires that the subject enter a state of trance which is essentially a state of altered and focused attention and hypersuggestibility. The trance state is not associated with sleep but rather increased attention. Narcotics, sedatives and tranquilizers decrease the ability to reach a state of trance by decreasing the ability to concentrate. The depth of the hypnotic or trance state varies tremendously from individual to individual. A rare individual may be placed sufficiently deep to allow surgery with no other anesthesia. In others, the depth of trance state is minimal or nonexistent. The use of formal hypnosis requires preparation by a medical hypnotist well before the onset of labor and may require his or her presence throughout parturition. Some patients may be taught autohypnosis or self-induction of trance.

While formal hypnosis may not be available, informal hypnosis or hypnoidal techniques involving suggestion, encouragement and reassurance are most valuable and can be safely used by both the nurses and physicians responsible for the care of the parturient. Examples of such techniques include using the term uterine "contractions" rather than uterine "pains," reassuring the mother that she can relax and rest between contractions, and having concerned and experienced medical personnel present throughout labor and delivery. The injection of one's understanding presence and encouragement may do far more than the injection of pharmacologic substances to alleviate anxiety and pain.

PHARMACOLOGIC ANALGESIA AND ANESTHESIA

The pharmacologic techniques which are used to relieve pain during labor and delivery fall into four general categories: (1) systemic medication with narcotics, sedatives, tranquilizers and amnestics, (2) inhalation analgesia with subanesthetic concentrations of inhalation drugs, (3) general anesthesia, and (4) regional or conduction anesthesia (i.e., nerve block with local anesthetics).

Systemic medication

Systemic medications, given intravenously or intramuscularly, are frequently used to decrease the pain and anxiety of the first stage of labor. In the past, this form of pain relief was selected because it is simple to administer. Small doses of systemic medications can be used with relative safety for the mother, although certain aspects of newborn neurobehavior may be modified for several days following their use in labor.

The keystone of systemic medications is the narcotics or analgesics. In general, equal analgesic doses of various narcotics produce equal amounts of depression in both mother and newborn. The major difference among the various narcotics is the duration of their action. Knowledge of the duration of action allows the rational selection of the appropriate narcotic. If prolonged duration is desired as, for example, in early labor, narcotics such as meperidine (Demerol) or morphine are indicated. If the narcotics are administered late in labor, when only a short duration of action is desired, short-acting narcotics such as fentanyl (Sublimaze) or alphaprodine (Nisentil) are appropriate.

Both the analgesic and the depressant properties of all the narcotics can be rapidly antagonized in mother and newborn by the use of naloxone (Narcan), a specific narcotic antagonist. Unlike the previous narcotic antagonists, nalorphine (Nalline) and levallorphan (Lorfan), naloxone has no narcotic or depressive activity of its own. It is useless in antagonizing depression from causes other than narcotics. The effective duration of naloxone is only about one hour. After its use, both the newborn and the mother must be carefully observed for signs of renarcotization, which can be treated with additional doses of the drug.

Naloxone should not be used in the mother to treat narcotic depression in the fetus shortly before birth unless another form of analgesia is first instituted because it will rapidly antagonize the analgesic activity of the narcotic. Furthermore, the effects of its use in a patient who has received a narcotic are unpleasant; its use is often associated with dyspnea as well as nausea and vomiting. It must be used with great caution in mothers who take narcotics chronically or habitually and in their newborns, as it can cause sudden and severe narcotic withdrawal. The usual dose of naloxone in the adult is 0.4 mg intramuscularly or intravenously and, in the newborn, 0.01 mg/K similarly given.

Frequently a tranquilizer or sedative is administered with a narcotic. These drugs may produce sedation and alleviate anxiety. However, they add little, if any, analgesia and, if given in the presence of pain without adequate alternative analgesia, produce confusion, disorientation, delirium and uncontrollable behavior during contractions. Tranquilizers and sedatives also add to the depressant effects of narcotics in both mother and newborn. Finally, many of the commonly used tranquilizers, particularly the phenothiazines such as promethazine (Phenergan), have a long duration of action (six to eight hours) and should not be repeated each time a narcotic is used. Scopolamine, a belladonna alkaloid and an anticholinergic, may be used in labor to produce sedation and amnesia. In the past, the desire for amnesia was common, but is much less popular with maternity patients today. If administered in the presence of pain without adequate analgesia, scopolamine frequently produces delirium, excitement and even hallucinations. When used, precautions must be taken to prevent patient injury. Scopolamine, while not associated with newborn depression, may cause fetal tachycardia, decreased fetal heart rate, beat-to-beat variability and may modify certain fetal heart rate decelerations. The anticholinesterase, physostigmine, antagonizes the maternal sedation and delirium associated with the use of scopolamine. It has also been claimed to antagonize these effects associated with the use of other tranquilizers such as the phenothiazines (e.g., promethazine) and diazepam. Physostigmine is usually administered to the mother intravenously in 1-mg doses until the desired effect is obtained or the maternal heart rate falls below 70 beats per minute. Its efficacy and safety in the newborn have as yet to be determined.

In recent years the use of ketamine, a dissociative intravenous anesthetic, has found its way into obstetric anesthesia. Given in intravenous doses of 0.25 mg/K (10 to 15 mg), it produces profound analgesia lasting for 2 to 5 minutes. Used in these quantities, the dosage may be repeated as needed, but not exceeding 1.0 mg/K total before the birth of the baby. It is associated with minimal newborn depression, no appreciable effects on uterine activity, and few bad dreams or hallucinations. When ketamine is given alone or in combination with inhalation analgesia in doses of 0.25 mg/K, the mother remains awake with upper airway reflexes intact. Larger doses are associated with newborn depression and loss of maternal consciousness, which predisposes the mother to the catastrophe of pulmonary aspiration of gastric contents unless her airway is protected with a cuffed endotracheal tube. Ketamine in analgesic doses is most often indicated at the time of delivery. Its use in combination with a pudendal block will frequently allow the obstetrician to employ low forceps without the use of general anesthesia.

Inhalation Analgesia

Inhalation analgesia requires that the mother breathe subanesthetic concentrations of inhalation anesthetics. Properly administered the mother remains conscious, yet has profound analgesia. Numerous inhalation anesthetic drugs have been used, including chloroform, ether, nitrous oxide, ethylene, cyclopropane, trichloroethylene (Trilene), methoxyflurane (Penthrane), and, more recently in this country, enflurane (Ethrane). Today in the United States, the two most commonly used inhalation drugs to produce analgesia in obstetrics are nitrous oxide and methoxyflurane.

Methoxyflurane.   Inhalation analgesia may be administered in the first stage of labor. Because of its potency, methoxyflurane is usually administered in air in concentrations between 0.2 to 0.6 percent. The drug may be self-administered through a calibrated vaporizer such as the Duke Inhalor or the Cyprane Inhalor, held in the mother's hand and set at the desired concentration. A disposable inhalor, the Penthrane Analgizer, is also available for use with methoxyflurane. When the contraction begins, the mother breathes through the vaporizer until the contraction ends. After two or three contractions an adequate blood level is maintained to provide profound analgesia in a conscious patient who remains responsive and cooperative. This analgesia may be continued through delivery of the newborn, delivery of the placenta and the immediate postpartum examination. The total amount of methoxyflurane administered throughout labor and delivery should not exceed 15 ml of liquid to avoid renal toxicity secondary to its breakdown in both mother and newborn to inorganic fluoride.

Nitrous Oxide.   Since nitrous oxide is a gas at atmospheric conditions, it is stored under pressure in steel gas cylinders and must be administered through a calibrated anesthesia machine with oxygen by a trained physician or nurse. As 30 to 50 percent nitrous oxide is required to produce analgesia, it is given in a mixture of 50 to 70 percent oxygen. In the United Kingdom (during labor and delivery) midwives often will give a 50 percent nitrous oxide, 50 percent oxygen mixture called Entonox that has been premixed in cylinders. In the United States, nitrous oxide analgesia is usually administered in the delivery room by a nurse or physician during the latter part of the first stage of labor and for delivery of the baby, the placenta and the immediate postpartum examination. While intermittent administration of nitrous oxide analgesia during contractions is still used, it is more effective when administered continuously in 30 to 50 percent concentration with oxygen.

Advantages and Disadvantages.   Inhalation analgesia provides profound but not complete analgesia for labor and delivery. Used alone, it often produces adequate pain relief for labor and uncomplicated vaginal delivery without episiotomy. If an episiotomy is to be performed and repaired or use of forceps is anticipated, the obstetrician should supplement inhalation analgesia with local infiltration of the perineum, or better still a bilateral pudendal block. In addition to analgesia, inhalation analgesia often provides amnesia, particularly for painful events.

Properly administered, inhalation analgesia has many advantages and is extremely safe for mother and newborn. Maternal and newborn depression is not produced in measurable degree by subanesthetic concentrations of inhalation drugs, regardless of the duration of their administration. The mother remains awake with upper airway reflexes intact and is protected from catastrophe of pulmonary aspiration of gastric contents without the need for intubation. The mother's reflex urge and ability to bear down in the second stage of labor are little affected. The onset of inhalation analgesia is rapid and the degree of analgesia can be altered quickly by changing the inspired concentration of the inhalation drug. It can be given safely to nearly every parturient and may be used to supplement other forms of analgesia, particularly regional or conduction anesthesia.

Despite its advantages, however, inhalation analgesia does have drawbacks. The amount of inhalation drug required for adequate analgesia varies from mother to mother and indeed for the same mother throughout the various phases of labor. She may pass from the stage of analgesia and amnesia (first stage anesthesia) into the stage of delirium and excitement (second stage of anesthesia) or even into the stage of surgical anesthesia (third stage of anesthesia), with loss of protective airway reflexes, subjecting her to the danger of pulmonary aspiration and her fetus to newborn anesthetic depression. *It is imperative that a fully trained nurse or physician always be present when inhalation analgesia is used.*

Inhalation analgesia does not produce complete analgesia. Except for the uncomplicated vaginal delivery, it must be supplemented. Even then, adequate analgesia and patient cooperation may not be satisfactory. Increasing the concentration of the inhalation drug often results in excitement and activity or general anesthesia with its attendant problems. When a patient receiving inhalation analgesia is delirious and uncooperative, this is often an indication that too much inhalation drug is being administered; this can be corrected rapidly by decreasing the concentration of the inhalation drug.

General Anesthesia

General anesthesia is rarely, if ever, indicated for uncomplicated vaginal delivery. Indeed most vaginal deliveries are more safely performed with other forms of analgesia or anesthesia. Obstetricians today are coming to realize that vaginal delivery with general anesthesia is fraught with many serious complications. Fortunately, women of the childbearing age are now less inclined to request that they be "put under" for delivery. Rather, they want to take part in the delivery and frequently wish the baby's father to be present in the delivery room to share the joy of birth. These changing attitudes deserve to be encouraged and supported by all those involved in the care of the mother-to-be.

Disadvantages. The disadvantages of general anesthesia in obstetrics are many. General anesthesia prevents the mother from participating in the birth of her baby and relating with her newborn at birth. When used for vaginal delivery, it cannot be administered until the baby is deliverable since it will immediately stop the bearing down reflex of the second stage of labor. In addition, the newborn, like the mother, is depressed by the anesthetic. Despite occasional statements to the contrary, controlled studies indicate that neonatal depression following general anesthesia for delivery is directly proportional to the depth of anesthesia and the length of the interval from induction of anesthesia to the delivery of the baby. While this depression from general anesthesia is usually rapidly overcome by ventilatory support of the newborn, it may compound depression from other sources. If the interval from induction of anesthesia to the delivery of the newborn is kept to less than 10 minutes with "light anesthesia," newborn depression from well administered general anesthesia will be minimal.

General anesthesia predisposes the parturient to the dreadful complication of pulmonary aspiration of gastric contents. Every parturient is at risk to this catastrophe because: (1) her stomach is rarely empty, (2) the gastroesophageal junction may not function as a result of changes in gastric position caused by the gravid uterus, and (3) the gravid uterus and lithotomy position increase intragastric pressure.

General anesthesia for any woman in the third trimester of pregnancy necessitates intubation with a cuffed endotracheal tube. The endotracheal tube

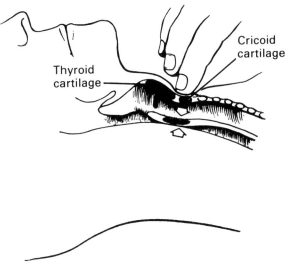

Figure 25-1. Technique of cricoid pressure (Sellick's maneuver) to prevent pulmonary aspiration of gastric contents during anesthesia induction. The esophagus is compressed and occluded between the cricoid ring of the trachea and the bodies of the cervical vertebrae. Pressure is maintained from loss of consciousness until successful tracheal intubation with a cuffed endotracheal tube. (From Hamelberg, W. and Bosomworth, P. B.: *Aspiration Pneumonitis.* ed. 1. Springfield, Ill., Charles C Thomas, 1968, p. 26. Courtesy of Charles C Thomas, Publisher, Springfield, Illinois)

should be inserted either before induction or immediately after a rapid induction during which cricoid pressure (Sellick's maneuver) is applied from the time of the loss of consciousness until intubation (Fig. 25-1). General anesthesia for the parturient without endotracheal intubation is unacceptable anesthetic practice today.

Indication for General Anesthesia

Despite the numerous disadvantages and problems associated with the use of general anesthesia for delivery, its proper use with rapid induction by a skilled anesthetist may result in the delivery of a healthy baby and the prevention of maternal morbidity and mortality. In certain circumstances, general anesthesia is the only form of anesthesia that can provide adequate conditions for the obstetrician to deliver the newborn rapidly and safely. The immediate availability of a skilled anesthetist provided with proper equipment and assistance in the obstetric suite is a primary requirement for good obstetric care.

The indications for general anesthesia for vaginal delivery include:

1. Fetal distress which demands immediate delivery and which can be safely accomplished by the vaginal route. Often the use of inhalation analgesia supplemented by local infiltration of the perineum or pudendal block provides satisfactory conditions for such a delivery.
2. When a parturient becomes uncontrollable during delivery.
3. When a parturient refuses regional or other forms of analgesia or anesthesia, or when these forms of pain relief are contraindicated.
4. The need for rapid depression of uterine activity.

Depression of uterine actvity may be indicated to abolish a tetanic uterine contraction, usually the result of too large a dose of oxytocin given during induction or augmentation of labor. It may also be required to allow intrauterine manipulation for the extraction of a distressed second twin or removal of a retained placenta. Although ether and all of the halogenated inhalation anesthetic drugs can depress uterine activity, halothane, given initially in 2 percent concentration, or enflurane, given initially in a 3 percent concentration, is usually favored because the onset of its effect is rapid and its action is predictable.

Techniques for General Anesthesia

While the scope of this chapter does not allow a discussion of techniques of general anesthesia, certain points concerning its use should be emphasized.

1. Patients in the third trimester of pregnancy requiring general anesthesia need to be intubated during anesthesia to protect against the risk of pulmonary aspiration of gastric contents. The time interval from the last ingestion of food or the onset of labor to the time of induction of general anesthesia is of no value in determining the risk of aspiration. The use of oral antacids during labor does not lessen the need for intubation when general anesthesia is used.
2. The extent of newborn depression is directly proportional to the induction-to-delivery interval. General anesthesia is induced only when the obstetrician is ready and delivery should be accomplished as rapidly thereafter as is in keeping with good obstetric principles. Nothing is gained by delaying delivery after induc-

tion to allow the drug to be removed from the fetus. Such delay will only expose the fetus to more depressant anesthetic drug.

3. The plane of anesthesia sought before delivery is that which will provide maternal analgesia and amnesia. Favorable surgical conditions and prevention of movement are provided by the use of minimal amounts of skeletal muscle relaxants such as succinylcholine and curare. If used in large doses, nondepolarizing relaxants such as curare may cross the placenta in amounts sufficient to depress newborn skeletal muscle activity.

4. Oxygen should make up greater than 50 percent of the inspired maternal anesthetic mixture before birth, to assure more vigorous and better oxygenated newborns. To ensure maternal analgesia and amnesia, the addition of low concentrations of potent inhalation drugs such as 0.5 percent halothane, 0.75 to 1 percent enflurane or 0.2 to 0.5 percent methoxyflurane added to 30 to 40 percent nitrous oxide is required.

5. While adequate maternal ventilation is to be assured, marked maternal hyperventilation as regulated by the anesthetist must be avoided until birth of the newborn, since hyperventilation is associated with decreased uterine blood flow and fetal acidosis.

6. Left uterine displacement must be maintained at all times until the birth of the newborn to avoid aorta-caval compression with its associated decreased maternal cardiac output and hence depressed uterine blood flow.

7. Following delivery, the depth of maternal anesthesia may be increased by increasing the concentration of nitrous oxide and giving narcotics. The concentration of the potent inhalation drugs should not be increased, since this may cause depressed uterine contraction and may be associated with increased maternal blood loss.

8. The same quality of anesthetic care must be available to the parturient as is to the surgical patient. This includes adequate monitoring during anesthesia and adequate postoperative observation.

9. When general anesthesia is required in an emergency, it is usually in the mother's interest to wait until qualified anesthesia personnel are available or to proceed with an alternative form of anesthesia. Nurses and physicians not

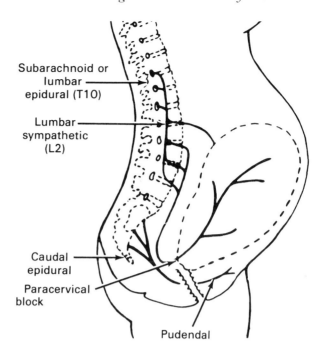

Figure 25-2. Pain pathways of labor with appropriate techniques of nerve block (Modified from Bonica, J. J.: *Principle and Practice of Obstetric Analgesia and Anesthesia.* Philadelphia, F. A. Davis, 1967, p. 492.)

fully trained and competent in anesthesia should not attempt the administration of general anesthesia.

Regional Anesthesia

Regional or conduction anesthesia is ideally suited to vaginal delivery. If the complications of hypotension and local anesthetic toxicity are avoided, it is associated with minimal newborn depression and a mother who is awake and free from pain and capable of relating to her newborn baby immediately following birth. Awake, she is unlikely to aspirate gastric contents and can cooperate with the obstetrician. Except when uterine relaxation is required, regional analgesia can provide complete pain relief and suitable conditions for both vaginal and abdominal delivery.

The primary neuropathways of pain and methods of effectively blocking them with local anesthetics are illustrated in Fig. 25-2. Uterine pain, resulting from dilatation and effacement of the cervix and from uterine contractions, is conveyed by small nerve fibers which pass from the cervix diffusely through the pelvis, join the sympathetic chain at L_2

to L$_5$ and enter the spinal cord at T$_{10}$ to T$_{12}$. These pain fibers can be blocked effectively by a paracervical block at the cervix, by a bilateral lumbar sympathetic block at L$_2$ or a segmental lumbar epidural block from T$_{10}$ to T$_{12}$. Vaginal and perineal pain, associated with the second and third stages of labor, is mediated primarily through the pudendal nerve originating from S$_2$ to S$_4$. There is additional perineal innervation from the genitofemoral, ilioinguinal and lateral femoral cutaneous nerves. Pudendal nerve block, true "saddle block" (subarachnoid or "spinal" block) (S$_1$ to S$_5$) and low caudal epidural block (S$_1$ to S$_5$) will alleviate most of the vaginal and perineal pain. A combination of blocks or a subarachnoid, lumbar epidural, or caudal epidural block from T$_{10}$ to S$_5$ will provide relief of all pain during labor and delivery.

Disadvantages. Despite its many advantages, regional anesthesia has disadvantages and requires constant observation of the mother if it is to be both safe and effective. Recent work has suggested that both the local anesthetics lidocaine (Xylocaine) and mepivacaine (Carbocaine) may be associated with minimally depressed neonatal tone at birth which resolves rapidly. This has not been observed with the use of the local anesthetics bupivacaine (Marcaine) and 2-chloroprocaine (Nesacaine).

The newer amide local anesthetics lidocaine, mepivacaine and bupivacaine have a prolonged half-life in maternal and neonatal blood due to their slow metabolism by the liver. This causes no difficulty in routine use, as levels usually remain well below toxic levels. However, repeated injection of these drugs, as in the case of continuous lumbar and caudal epidural anesthesia, can result in increasing blood levels in both mother and fetus. This is not a problem with the older ester type local anesthetics, such as procaine and 2-chloroprocaine, which are rapidly metabolized to nontoxic products by the enzyme pseudocholinesterase, normally found in both maternal and fetal blood.

Local anesthetics administered during labor may decrease fetal heart rate beat-to-beat variability, making fetal heart rate evaluation more difficult. This action of local anesthetics has not been associated with deleterious effects on the newborn and is shared by other drugs including the narcotics, tranquilizers and anticholinergics.

Nursing Implications. The use of regional anesthesia in the obstetric patient requires constant monitoring during labor, delivery and in the postpartum period by a trained obstetric nurse in constant attendance. An accurate record of maternal vital signs must be kept (Fig. 25-3). A reliable intravenous infusion must be maintained at all times. The personnel and means to assure a clear airway and apply positive pressure ventilation with oxygen and the ability to treat local anesthetic reactions, high levels of block and maternal hypotension must be immediately available if serious problems to both mother and fetus are to be avoided. Continuous recorded electronic monitoring of fetal heart rate and uterine contractions should be considered when regional anesthesia is used in the first stage of labor. Such monitoring is indicated in the high-risk pregnancy or when regional anesthesia is used for the mother receiving oxytocin stimulation.

Paracervical Block

Paracervical block is produced by injection of small quantities of dilute local anesthetic solution into the parametrium at sites in the cervix of 3 and 9 o'clock or 4 and 8 o'clock (Fig. 25-4). It provides rapid complete relief of uterine pain with minimal maternal side effects. Paracervical block does not affect vaginal and perineal sensation and hence does not interfere with the bearing-down reflex of the second stage of labor. Unfortunately, paracervical block has been associated with fetal bradycardia, fetal acidosis and even fetal death. These untoward fetal effects are thought to be caused by the local anesthetic passing rapidly through the placenta to the fetus secondary to absorption through the uterine artery. There is also evidence that proximity of the local anesthetic to the uterine artery may result in vasoconstriction of the uterine artery with decreased uteroplacental perfusion. The danger to the fetus can be minimized by using minimal doses of the less toxic local anesthetics such as 2-chloroprocaine

Figure 25-3. Obstetric anesthesia record during the course of continuous epidural anesthesia for labor and delivery. Note frequency of recordings of maternal vital signs.

SEEN 7 ³⁰/AM - D.D.

HOSPITAL OF THE UNIVERSITY OF PENNSYLVANIA - OBSTETRIC ANESTHESIA RECORD

Patient's Name	M B					
		B.P. 110/80 -12480	Pulse 88	Temp 99 40 F	Drug Reactions NONE	

History No. 335726 - 2111

Race BLACK	Height 5' 8"	Weight 193 lbs	Consent SELF

Age 24   Date NOV 22, 1974

Hct. or Hgb. 34%	Rh. Factor O+	Grav. III	Para. I

Procedure OUTLET FORCEPS DELIV. EPIS REPAIR

Time and Nature of Last Oral Intake SOLIDS 7⁰⁰AM NOV 22   E.D.C. NOV 20, 1974

Anesthetists D.D / BBC

Location DR #2   Onset of Labor 5⁰⁰AM NOV22   Signif. Meds. AEP. ASTHMA

Physical Status I   **Emergency** NO

Pre-Anesthetic Condition HISTORY OF SEASONAL ASTHMA, RX c̄ A.E.P. LAST ATTACK SEPT 74'. MODERATE OBESITY -30LB WT. GAIN c̄ PREGNANCY

Times: X 9⁴⁵/AM ⊙ 3⁴/AM ⊗ 12⁰⁵/PM

Obstetricians R.R /R.P

Obstetric Diagnosis TERM INTRAUTERINE PREG.

Medications During Labor

Time	45	10⁰⁰/AM	30	11⁰⁰/AM	30	12⁰⁰/N	30	Drug and Dose	Route	Time
Cervical Dilatation	5	6		10				DEMEROL 50 IV		8³⁰/A
O₂	10 LIT. NRB MASK			1——1				PHENERGAN 25 IV		8³⁰/A
Anesthetics ml	¼ To MAR 2+8									
ml	½ To MAR			2+10						
Fluids	D5 ½ NS 500——		—1000—			—1300				
Level of Block		T₁₀		T₉-55		T₉				
Maternal Position	♀ ⊙ I (L.U.D.)			♀ ⊙ F		♀⊔				
Monitoring	EXT U.C. INT. F.H.R. ————									

Infant Data

	Infant #1	Infant #2
Weight (GM)	3090	
Sex	MALE	
Time of Delivery	11 ³⁴/AM	
Time To Sust. Resp.	< 30 SEC	

	Apgar	1 Min.	5 Min.	1 Min.	5 Min.
	Heart Rate	2	2		
	Respiration	2	2		
	Reflex	2	2		
	Muscle Tone	1	2		
	Color	1	1		
	Total (0-10)	8	9		

Blood Pressure graph: values 180, 160, 140, 120, 100, 80, 60, 40, 20, 0

Mat. Pulse Rate •   Fetal Heart Rate ▲

Start Stop Anes. X   Start Surgery ⊙   End ⊗

Markings: X 1   2 ⊙   ⊗3 RR

Time Placenta Expressed

Abnormalities NONE   Manual ___ Spont. 11 ³⁸/A

N.B. Resuscitation, Methods, Drugs, Congenital Abnormalities
SUCTION, O₂ BY FACE MASK, STIMULATION

Condition on Leaving O.R. GOOD (REC NUR)

Agents	¼ To MARCAINE 10 CC TOTAL	½ To MARCAINE 12 ml TOTAL	EPHEDRINE 10 MG IV
Tech.	VIA EPIDURAL CATH		HYPOTENSION

OXYTOCICS	Dose	Rte.	Time
PITOCIN	5 U	IV PUSH	11 ³⁴
PITOCIN	15 U	IV BOT	11 ³⁴

Remarks: X BEGIN CONTINUOUS EPIDURAL I₂ c̄ ALCOHOL PREP. LOC ENFILT 5 MG MARCAINE. ENTER EPIDURAL SPACE c̄ EASE AT L3-4 18 9 HUSTEAD NEEDLE, INSERT CATH. REMOVE NEEDLE. NO HEME OR CSF ASPIRATED

1) EPHEDRINE 10 MG IV FOR MAT HYPOTENSION

2.) COMPLETE DILATATION - SITTING DOSE - TAKE TO DEL RM.

Airway	Nat. (circled)	OP.	NP.
Intub.		OT	NT
Blade		CR	ST

3) REMOVE EPIDURAL CATH. INTACT

Complications of Labor & Delivery NONE

Obstetric Complications NONE

Est. Bl. Loss 350 MI.

Length of Labor Stages 1st (Hr) 6 2nd (Min) 2 3rd (Min) 3

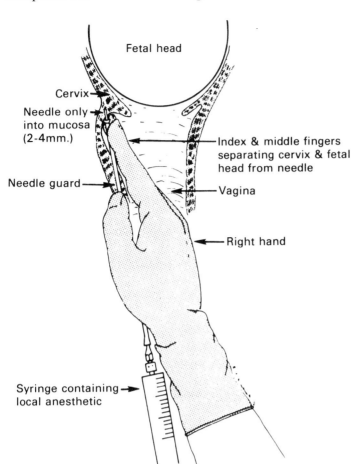

Fetal head

Cervix

Needle only
into mucosa
(2-4mm.)

Needle guard

Index & middle fingers
separating cervix & fetal
head from needle

Vagina

Right hand

Syringe containing
local anesthetic

Figure 25-4. Technique of paracervical block. Five ml. of dilute local anesthetic solution is injected superficially in the vaginal fornix at 3 and 9 o'clock *or* at 4 and 8 o'clock. (From Abouleish, E.: *Pain Control in Obstetrics.* Philadelphia, J. B. Lippincott, 1977, p 344.)

and by injecting them superficially and laterally in the parametrium.

The use of paracervical block is a good indication for continuous electronic fetal heart monitoring. Paracervical block is best avoided in the premature fetus and in the fetus at high risk.

Lumbar Sympathetic Block

Like paracervical block, a bilateral lumbar sympathetic block at L_2 abolishes uterine pain only. While this mode of anesthesia is associated with maternal hypotension, such a reaction is usually minimal and can be avoided by providing adequate hydration and left uterine displacement. Lumbar sympathetic block is associated with minimal, if any, fetal and newborn depression, which makes its use acceptable in the high-risk pregnancy. Bilateral sympathetic block may result in improved uterine contraction because it interrupts the sympathetic innervation of

the uterus that inhibits uterine activity. Since the block is rather complicated and somewhat painful to administer, it has been not used widely.

Pudendal Block

Of all the regional anesthetic blocks for vaginal delivery, bilateral pudendal nerve block is perhaps the safest and one of the most useful available. Although pudendal block provides no relief of uterine pain and no analgesia for cervical or uterine manipulations, it does alleviate most of the vaginal and perineal pain associated with delivery. It produces adequate analgesia for episiotomy and repair and allows most uncomplicated outlet forceps deliveries. When supplemented with inhalation analgesia, it usually produces adequate analgesia for other types of forceps deliveries. Since pudendal block does not completely anesthetize the perineum, it does not completely abolish the bearing-down reflex of the second stage of labor. It is relatively painless to administer and when local anesthetic toxicity is avoided, it has essentially no ill effects on the mother or her newborn. Pudendal block is not associated with maternal hypotension and is the only technique of conduction anesthesia which does not affect autonomic innervation of the uterus.

The pudendal nerve runs just lateral to the tips of the ischial spines, the obstetric landmarks which determine the station of the presenting part. It may be blocked from either the transvaginal approach (Fig. 25-5), most commonly used in obstetrics, or from the trancutaneous route. A bilateral block requires only 10 to 20 ml of a dilute local anesthetic solution, such as 1 percent lidocaine or 1 percent 2-chloroprocaine, and is usually administered by the obstetrician or midwife delivering the baby.

Spinal Anesthesia

Subarachnoid or "spinal" block is one of the most useful blocks for obstetrics and is technically easy to administer (Fig. 25-6). The amount of drug needed is less than that required for any other block used in obstetrics—about one-fifth that required to produce the same level of anesthesia by the epidural route. Thus, local anesthetic toxicity in both mother and fetus is not a problem. Onset of anesthesia is very rapid, usually complete within 5 minutes. Essentially every obstetric procedure not requiring depression of uterine activity can be accomplished with subarachnoid block. Late in labor a true saddle block of the perineum (S_1 to S_5) allows forceps delivery and repair of episiotomy. If a modified saddle block (T_{10} to S_5) is produced, both uterine as well as perineal discomfort are completely abolished. Long-acting local anesthetics such as tetracaine (Pontocaine) with epinephrine produce 3 hours of pain relief when injected into the subarachnoid space, permitting elimination of all pain in the latter part of labor and for delivery. Increasing the level of block to T_4 or higher produces satisfactory anesthesia for cesarean section.

Disadvantages. The major disadvantages of subarachnoid block are its potential for causing (1) maternal hypotension, (2) total spinal block, (3) postspinal headache, (4) the abolishment of the reflex urge to bear down in the second stage of labor, and (5) early relaxation of the perineal mus-

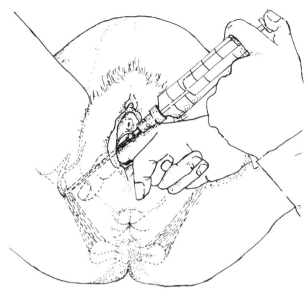

Figure 25-5. Pudendal block technique by the transvaginal approach. Note the examiner's fingers guiding the needle to the ischial spine. The pudendal nerve lies laterally to the spine at its tip.

culature, which can result in persistent occiput posterior presentation.

Severe and sudden maternal hypotension leading to fetal distress and maternal cardiovascular collapse due to vasodilatation secondary to sympathetic block is still a significant cause of maternal mortality. Prophylaxis includes left uterine displacement and hydration with a liter or more of balanced salt solution administered intravenously 15 to 30 minutes before the block is instituted. Treatment of hypotension includes these two steps as well as the use of a central acting vasopressor, such as ephedrine 10 to 25 mg given intravenously, and the administration of high concentrations of oxygen. Potent peripheral vasoconstrictors such as norepinephrine (Levophed), phenylephrine (Neo-Synephrine), and methoxamine (Vasoxyl) rapidly correct maternal hypotension but are to be avoided because they cause further decline in uterine perfusion, resulting in additional fetal distress.

Total or dangerously high levels of subarachnoid block usually result when the subarachnoid injection is made just before or during a uterine contraction or when too large a dose of local anesthetic is used. The same level of block can be obtained in the obstetric patient with only two-thirds of the amount of drug required to produce a given level in her

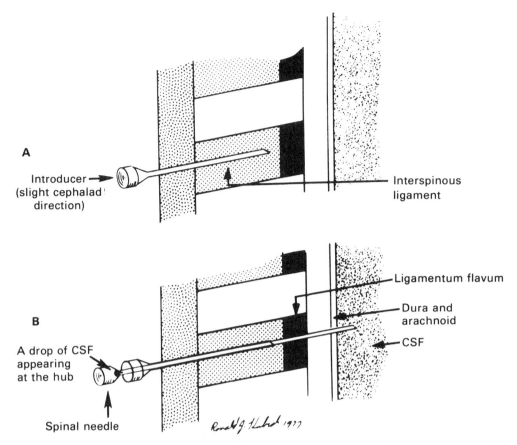

A

Introducer →
(slight cephalad
direction)

Interspinous
ligament

B

Ligamentum flavum

Dura and
arachnoid

CSF

A drop of CSF
appearing
at the hub

Spinal needle

Figure 25-6. Technique of subarachnoid (spinal) block. Note that the small 25 or 26 gauge spinal needle transverses the epidural space and pierces the dura and arachnoid to enter the subarachnoid space which contained the cerebral spinal fluid. Local anesthetic injected subarachnoid acts on the spinal nerve roots contained within the subarachnoid space. (From Abouleish, E.: *Pain Control in Obstetrics.* Philadelphia, J. B. Lippincott, 1977, p. 322.)

nonpregnant counterpart. Treatment of a high block consists of (1) immediate correction of hypotension, (2) support of maternal ventilation with positive pressure oxygen and, if necessary, (3) protection of the upper airway with a cuffed endotracheal tube. With proper therapy a high or total spinal need not delay delivery and should not be associated with increased maternal or fetal morbidity or mortality.

The incidence of postspinal headache is highest in the postpartum patient. An incidence of over 40 percent can be expected when the subarachnoid space is entered with a 20-gauge or larger bore needle. The headache usually occurs within 24 to 72 hours of the subarachnoid block, may last a few days to several weeks, and can be mild to incapacitating. The headache inevitably resolves. It is positional and is characteristically exacerbated in the upright position and relieved by assuming the supine po-

sition or by increasing abdominal pressure. It is caused by loss of cerebral spinal fluid through the hole made in the dura mater and pia-arachnoid by the spinal needle. Steps to prevent the spinal headaches include using small-gauge needles (25 gauge or less), adequate hydration during the postpartum and using a tight abdominal binder when the patient is in the upright position. Treatment consists of appropriate analgesics, bedrest, preferably in the prone position with the head down, hydration, a tight abdominal binder and reassurance. When the headache is incapacitating, "epidural blood patch," which consists of sealing the hole in the dura by injecting the patient's own nonanticoagulated blood into the epidural space, can result in a dramatic cure.

Abolishment of the reflex urge to bear down in the second stage of labor results from the complete perineal analgesia produced by subarachnoid block. It does not prevent the parturient from bearing down voluntarily when asked to do so with each contraction. In cases of occiput posterior presentation, the tone in the muscles of the perineum causes the occiput to rotate to the anterior presentation. As subarachnoid block does produce profound relaxation of the perineum, an increased incidence of persistent occiput posterior presentations can be expected with its use. Since perineal relaxation occurs, the occiput can usually be easily rotated manually or delivery accomplished in the occiput posterior position.

Technique.   Because of its rapid onset, subarachnoid block is usually given just prior to delivery in the delivery room. A modified saddle block to provide a T_{10} sensory level provides ideal conditions for forceps delivery and often allows uterine exploration or curettage. When indicated, lidocaine (40 to 50 mg) in dextrose gives the necessary T_{10} level, with anesthesia lasting about an hour. Tetracaine (5 to 6 mg) in dextrose with epinephrine added provides more than 3 hours of effective analgesia. The subarachnoid injection is usually made at the L_{3-4} or L_{4-5} lumbar interspace.

Epidural Anesthesia

Lumbar epidural anesthesia has achieved great popularity in both the United States and Great Britain. Using a continuous catheter technique, a segmental block with an upper level of T_{10} can be established with the onset of painful contractions and then maintained throughout the first stage of labor. In the second stage of labor, the block can be extended to give perineal analgesia. If a cesarean section becomes necessary, the level of the block can be elevated to T_4. Thus, as with subarachnoid block, lumbar epidural block can provide adequate anesthesia for all obstetric procedures not requiring depression of uterine activity. Its use allows a pain-free labor in an alert and cooperative mother who will require no additional medications for pain. Since it follows the logical sequence of labor, lumbar epidural anesthesia has largely replaced caudal epidural anesthesia. The latter provides perineal analgesia initially, requires about twice as much drug, and cannot be reliably extended to provide adequate analgesia for c-section. Caudal epidural is technically more difficult and more painful to perform and produces less reliable results than lumbar epidural.

The epidural space (Fig. 25-7) is a potential space filled with loose fatty tissue and a marked plexus of veins. It is the space in the vertebral canal surrounded by the ligamentous and bony structure of the vertebral canal on the outside and the dura containing the cerebrospinal fluid and the spinal cord on the inside. The uppermost limit of the epidural space is the foramen magnum at the base of the skull; interiorly it ends at the sacral hiatus at the base of the sacrum. It may be entered at any of the intervertebral spaces from the cervical area C_{1-2} to the L_5 to S_1 interspace or through the sacral hiatus. Injection of local anesthetic through the sacral hiatus is referred to as *caudal epidural block*.

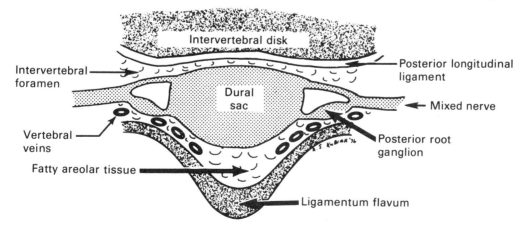

Figure 25-7. Diagrammatic cross section of the vertebral canal showing the contents of the epidural space. Note the prominent epidural veins. Local anesthetic injected in the epidural space acts primarily to block conduction of the nerve roots as they transverse the epidural space. (From Abouleish, E.: *Pain Control in Obstetrics.* Philadelphia, J. B. Lippincott, 1977, p. 261.)

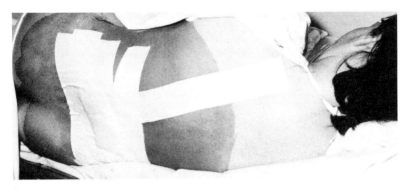

Figure 25-8. Caudal epidural block.

In obstetrics, the epidural space is usually entered at L_{2-3}, L_{3-4}, or L_{4-5} where it is largest and most easily identified. Once the needle is properly placed, a catheter can be threaded through it. The needle is then withdrawn, leaving the catheter in place (Fig. 25-8). Local anesthetic solution is introduced through the catheter as needed to initiate, maintain, or extend the level of anesthesia. As the nerve roots leave the spinal cord, they pass through the epidural space and hence are exposed to a local anesthetic injected in the epidural space.

Advantages and Disadvantages. There are two primary advantages of lumbar epidural anesthesia over subarachnoid anesthesia. Since the dura is normally not entered, the problem of postspinal headache is avoided. Second, the epidural technique allows the placement of a catheter for reinjection of local anesthetic drug as required.

The major drawback of epidural block as compared with subarachnoid block is that close to five times the amount of drug is required with the epidural technique. As an example, 150 to 200 mg of lidocaine are required by epidural injection to provide complete anesthesia for vaginal delivery, whereas by the subarachnoid route only 40 to 50 mg of lidocaine are needed. Epidural anesthesia necessitates careful control of the amount of local anesthetic drug used, particularly when the slowly metabolized amide-type drugs are employed, to avoid local anesthetic toxicity. When it is necessary to use large amounts of local anesthetic drug with epidural technique, one can employ the rapidly metabolized ester-type local anesthetics, such as procaine and 2-chloroprocaine.

Like subarachnoid block, epidural block does block sympathetic outflow and can result in vasodilatation and maternal hypotension. Although the onset of hypotension is slower with the epidural technique, it can be as serious as with subarachnoid block if unrecognized and untreated. Prevention and treatment of hypotension resulting from epidural block is the same as with subarachnoid block and includes left uterine displacement, intravenous hydration with balanced salt solutions, the use of small intravenous doses of ephedrine and oxygen administration. As the onset of hypotension is slower with epidural block, so also is the onset of analgesia. The onset of analgesia following subarachnoid injection occurs within a minute and is usually complete in 5 minutes, whereas the onset of analgesia with epidural block requires about 5 minutes and is not complete for 15 to 20 minutes. This slow onset of block can be partially overcome by initiating the block with a short-acting rapid onset local anesthetic such as 2-chloroprocaine, then using longer acting local anesthetics such as bupivacaine through the epidural catheter for later injections. Like subarachnoid block, epidural block, by providing complete perineal analgesia, eliminates the urge to bear down in the second stage of labor.

Since the amount of local anesthetic required for epidural block is five times greater than that required for subarachnoid block, accidental subarachnoid injection of the epidural drug will produce a sudden, extremely high or total spinal. This is avoided by always preceding each epidural injection with a small test dose and waiting a minute or two to ascertain that a subarachnoid block does not ensue before completing the injection. In pregnancy the epidural veins are markedly dilated and can easily be entered by the epidural needle or catheter. Due to the nature of these veins, blood frequently cannot be aspirated. Injection of local anesthetic into the veins in a dose needed for epidural analgesia could produce sudden local anesthetic toxicity in the mother with the onset of grand mal convulsions. This complication is avoided by injecting the first

4 or 5 ml of local anesthetic slowly, and then waiting a minute while observing for signs and symptoms of toxicity. These include ringing or buzzing in the ears, a metallic taste, perioral numbness, tremor and a feeling of lightheadedness or discomfort by the patient. If any of these signs or symptoms occur, no further injection is made, the needle or catheter is withdrawn and the procedure is repeated. With a small dose, the signs and symptoms of toxicity rapidly abate and no further problems will arise. The anesthesiologist administering epidural analgesia in the labor room must have immediately available the equipment and drugs necessary to treat the patient should these complications of high block or local anesthetic toxicity occur. Failure to be so prepared can rapidly result in the unnecessary death of the mother and her fetus.

Since epidural block is frequently started during the first stage of labor, its effect on the progress of labor must be assessed. While there is great debate on this issue, it is generally felt that once active labor is achieved, epidural anesthesia will not slow its progress. In the primigravida active labor is usually present when the cervix is 5 to 6 cm dilated. In the multipara active labor is usually present when the cervix is 4 to 5 cm dilated.

Lumbar epidural anesthesia has revolutionized the field of obstetric anesthesia. In hospitals with adequate personnel, its use has become widespread because of its ability to alleviate all maternal pain associated with labor and delivery in an alert, cooperative mother with minimal danger of neonatal depression. If complications are to be avoided, the same expertise in both administration and peripartum care as would be afforded the surgical patient is required. If this care is not available, epidural anesthesia should not be used.

ANESTHESIA FOR CESAREAN SECTION

Cesarean section can be performed under local infiltration, major conduction anesthesia (subarachnoid or epidural block) or general anesthesia.

Local infiltration was used widely in the past because of the apparent lack of depression in the newborn. Unfortunately, local infiltration seldom produces complete and satisfactory maternal anesthesia, and frequently the mother required supplemental general anesthesia following delivery. Other problems with local infiltration include the time required to produce analgesia and the large amount of local anesthetic drug required. With the refinements in major conduction anesthesia and general anesthesia, there is seldom justification for using local infiltration unless no skilled anesthetist is available.

Major conduction anesthesia is now widely used for cesarean section, particularly when trained anesthesiologists are available. The advantage of this type of anesthesia is the absence of associated newborn depression. In addition, there is evidence that the induction-to-delivery interval is not as important with conduction anesthesia in causing newborn depression, provided normal maternal physiology is maintained. The pressure for a quick delivery is eliminated. Major conduction anesthesia allows the mother to be wide awake, to be comfortable, and to see and relate early with her baby. Provided hypotension and local anesthetic toxicity are avoided, the risk of pulmonary aspiration is minimal.

The disadvantages of conduction anesthesia for cesarean section include: 1) it provides inadequate analgesia, 2) it involves the risk of maternal hypotension, 3) the time required for its onset may delay urgent surgical intervention, and 4) it is contraindicated in certain maternal conditions. Inadequate analgesia is usually the result of low level of block, compounded by traction on the perineum. A minimum of solid T_4 sensory block is required to avoid maternal discomfort unless the obstetrician is extremely gentle and quick. Sensory levels of less than T_4 frequently allow delivery, but then general anesthesia or heavy sedation is required for closure. Without proper prophylaxis, producing such high levels of block, particularly in the parturient, will uniformly result in significant maternal hypotension that will be associated with fetal and newborn acidosis secondary to a depressed uterine perfusion. The prevention and treatment of this hypotension has been dealt with in the section concerned with regional anesthesia.

Despite the fact that subarachnoid block produces complete analgesia in less than 5 minutes, performing the block requires several minutes even in the most skilled hands. General anesthesia can be induced in less than 1 minute. The minimal time required to induce general anesthesia is extremely important when an emergency cesarean section is indicated. As the anesthetist is preparing the patient for general anesthesia, the obstetrician can be preparing and draping the abdomen. In patients who have a functioning epidural catheter in place with a T_{10} sensory, injection of a rapid-acting local anesthetic such as 2-chloroprocaine will usually produce an adequate level of sensory block in about 3 to 5 minutes. Thus, if the mother's condition is stable, an epidural can often be used for emergency c-section. However, in a true emergency situation, one should not delay the cesarean section while waiting for the onset of adequate epidural analgesia.

There are several conditions which contraindicate major conduction anesthesia. An unstable maternal personality or cases in which the newborn is to be given up for adoption constitute relative contraindications. Maternal fear of or refusal to have major conduction anesthesia is an absolute contraindication. Maternal hypovolemia or shock from any cause is a contraindication because these conditions are exacerbated by the sympathetic block associated with subarachnoid or epidural anesthesia. Sepsis or localized infection at or near the site of injection is an absolute contraindication because of the danger of causing an epidural abscess or arachnoiditis. Abnormal coagulation of maternal blood contraindicates the use of conduction anesthesia because of the risk of forming an epidural hematoma. Certain neurologic conditions, such as multiple sclerosis, meningomyelocele and spina bifida, contraindicate the use of major conduction anesthesia.

In general, major conduction anesthesia is ideal for elective cesarean section or cesarean section that is urgent but not emergent. It provides ideal conditions for the father to be present with the mother in the delivery room. If an adequate level of block is obtained, ensuring freedom of pain, nearly all mothers will opt for major conduction anesthesia for repeat cesarean sections.

General anesthesia, properly administered, can be used safely for almost every cesarean section. Unlike major conduction anesthesia, there are few absolute contraindications for its use. It is possible to induce anesthesia and to allow the obstetrician to commence surgery in less than 1 minute if the mother has a functioning intravenous line and the anesthetist has drugs and equipment ready. It is the method of choice in cases of hypovolemia, shock, abnormal blood coagulation, septicemia and a fearful mother or mother who refuses major conduction anesthesia. For anesthetists not trained or allowed to use major conduction anesthesia, it is the method of choice for cesarean section anesthesia.

General anesthesia for cesarean section has three major disadvantages. It denies the mother immediate contact with her baby at birth. Second, it is associated with a higher incidence of newborn depression. With modern techniques of light balanced general anesthesia, however, the obstetrician usually has at least 10 minutes from induction to delivery of the baby before depression from anesthesia is significant. And even when the baby is depressed from general anesthesia alone, there is no associated acidosis, provided the mother has been maintained in good physiologic balance during the anesthetic. Resuscitation of anesthetic-depressed babies is usually easy and consists largely of support of the respirations and maintenance of the airway until the anesthetic gases and vapors can be eliminated through the newborn's lungs.

The third disadvantage is that general anesthesia exposes the mother to the potentially lethal complication of pulmonary aspiration of gastric contents. However, proper protection of the airway with cricoid pressure (Sellick's maneuver, see Fig. 25-1) from the time consciousness is lost until the trachea can be intubated with a cuffed endotracheal tube will essentially eliminate this catastrophe.

THE ROLE OF THE OBSTETRIC NURSE IN THE SAFE PRACTICE OF OBSTETRIC ANESTHESIA

For safe and effective analgesia or anesthesia to be available to all parturients, the obstetric nurse is required to play an active role. Unfortunately, it is impracticable today to have qualified anesthesiologists or nurse anesthetists remain in the labor room with the parturient throughout labor. However, the parturient deserves to have constant, competent observation and support throughout labor, delivery, and in the immediate postdelivery period. The administration of any form of anesthesia or analgesia during parturition demands constant observation if anesthetic morbidity and mortality are to be minimized.

It is usually the responsibility of the obstetric nurse to adequately monitor and record important observations of the patient receiving analgesia in labor. While generally she is not responsible to administer most forms of analgesia or anesthesia, the obstetric nurse must appreciate the complications of various techniques of pain relief, be able to recognize the signs and symptoms of the complications early, and know what action to take until an anesthesiologist or anesthetist is available. Without this kind of support, the use of conduction anesthesia cannot be safely used during labor.

The obstetric nurse may have to assist the anesthesiologist in the performance of regional anesthetic techniques. The nurse may be asked to administer various drugs under supervision, to apply cricoid pressure for the intubation of a mother who requires general anesthesia and to evaluate the newborn and take initial appropriate steps in its resuscitation in the delivery room. Postpartum, the obstetric nurse may have to observe and support the patient until the effects of anesthesia have dissipated.

To help women through childbirth is to share a mystery and a miracle. . . . It is also to touch life at a key point. . . . There the opportunity is taken to grow in understanding and in love. There is more to having a baby than simply pushing an occiput-anterior out into the world. Birth is also implicitly an assent to life. Those who help women in childbirth have the privilege of sharing that act of assent.

(Kitzinger, S.: *Education and Counselling for Childbirth.* London, Balliere Tindall, 1977, p. xii.)

SUGGESTED READING

Abouleish, E.: *Pain Control in Obstetrics.* Philadelphia, J. B. Lippincott, 1977. (An excellent and recent text on obstetric anesthesia with emphasis on the indications, advantages, disadvantages and complications of obstetric anesthesia.)

Albright, G. A.: *Anesthesia in Obstetrics, Maternal, Fetal and Neonatal Aspects.* Menlo Park, Calif., Addison-Wesley, 1978. (Another recent text devoted to the problems in obstetric anesthesia and their solutions. Has a good chapter on psychoanalgesia.)

Bonica, J. J.: *Principles and Practice of Obstetric Analgesia and Anesthesia.* Philadelphia, F. A. Davis, 1969. (The most complete text written on obstetric anesthesia. Techniques beautifully described and illustrated. Unfortunately, the text is rather dated now.)

Hartland, J.: *Medical and Dental Hypnosis and Its Clinical Applications,* ed. 2. Baltimore, Williams & Wilkins, pp. 3058325, 1971. (A good description of hypnosis for obstetrics.)

Heardman, H. and Ebner, M.: *Relaxation and Exercise for Natural Childbirth,* ed. 4, New York, Churchill Livingston, 1975.

Shnider, S. M. and Moya, F.: *The Anesthesiologist, Mother, and Newborn.* Baltimore, Williams & Wilkins, 1974. (A well-written short book dealing with many aspects of obstetric anesthesia, fetal and newborn evaluation and newborn care.)

Wylie, G.: "Psychological analgesia." In *Obstetrical Anesthesia, Current Concepts and Practice.* Ed. Shnider, S. M. Baltimore, Williams & Wilkins, 1970, pp. 57–59.

Postpartal Assessment and Management of the New Family

Biophysical Aspects of the Postpartum Period
Psychosocial Aspects of the Postpartum Period
Postpartal Care
Care of the Newborn Infant
Infant Nutrition

Twenty-Six

Biophysical Aspects of the Postpartum Period

---

*Anatomical Changes / Clinical Considerations /
Postpartal Examinations*

This chapter deals with the study of the anatomical and the physiologic changes that normally occur during the puerperium. Knowledge of the reproductive process in pregnancy and labor will serve as a basis for understanding how the generative organs and the various systems of the human body adapt following the delivery.

The term puerperium (from *puer,* a child; and *parere,* to bring forth) refers to the six-week period elapsing between the termination of labor and the return of the reproductive organs to their normal condition. This includes both the *progressive changes* in the breasts for lactation and *involution* of the internal reproductive organs. Although the changes brought about by involution are considered normal physiologic processes, they closely border on a disease condition, for under no other circumstances does such marked and rapid involution of tissues occur without a departure from a state of health. For this reason, the quality of the mother's care at this time is important to ensure her immediate as well as her future health.

ANATOMICAL CHANGES

Involution of the Uterus

Immediately following the delivery of the placenta the uterus becomes an almost solid mass of tissue. Its thick anterior and posterior walls lie in close opposition, leaving the center cavity flattened. The uterus remains about the same size for the first two days after delivery but then rapidly decreases in size by a process called involution. This is effected partly by the contraction of the uterus and partly by autolytic processes in which some of the protein material of the uterine wall is broken down into simpler components which then are absorbed.

The Process of Involution. The separation of the placenta and the membranes from the uterine wall takes place in the outer portion of the spongy layer of the decidua, and, therefore, a remnant of this layer remains in the uterus to be partly cast off in a vaginal discharge called the lochia. Within two or three days after labor, this remaining portion of decidua becomes differentiated into two layers, leaving the deeper or unaltered layer attached to the muscular wall from which the new endometrial lining is generated. The layer adjoining the uterine cavity becomes necrotic and is cast off in the lochia. The process is very like the healing of any surface; blood oozes from the small vessels on this surface. The bleeding from the larger vessels is controlled by compression of the retracted uterine muscle fibers.

The process of regeneration is rapid, except at the site of former placental attachment, which requires six or seven weeks to heal completely. Elsewhere, the free surface of the endometrium is restored in half that time.

The Progress of Involution. The normal process of involution requires five or six weeks, and at the end of that time the uterus regains its normal size, although it never returns exactly to its nulliparous state.

One can realize more fully the rapidity of this process by comparing the changes that occur in the weight of this organ. Immediately following the delivery the uterus weighs approximately 1 kilogram (2 lbs); at the end of the first week, about 500 gm (1 lb); at the end of the second week, about 350 gm (12 oz); and by the time involution is complete, it should weigh only about 60 gm (2 oz).

By observing the height of the fundus, which may be felt through the abdominal wall, the nurse is able to appreciate more fully these remarkable changes. Immediately after the delivery of the placenta the uterus sinks into the pelvis, and the fundus is felt midway between the umbilicus and the symphysis, but it soon rises to the level of the umbilicus (13 to 14 cm—5 or 5½ in—above the pubes); and 12 hours later it probably will be found a little higher. Day-by-day careful measurements will show that it is diminishing in size, so that at the end of 10 days or so it cannot be detected by abdominal palpation.

The approximate rate of decrease in the height of the fundus is a little over a centimeter (½ in) or one fingerbreadth a day. Observation of this rate of involution is very important; the physician will want to be informed about any marked delay, especially if accompanied by suppression of the lochia or retention of clots. In measuring the height of the uterus, care should be taken that the observations are made after the bladder is emptied, as a full bladder will raise the height of the fundus.

Apparent indications that involution is not occurring satisfactorily are: the uterus fails to decrease progressively in size, it remains "flabby" and causes the mother much discomfort (see Subinvolution in Chapter 35).

Changes in the Cervix

After delivery the cervix is a soft, flabby structure but, because it is retracting, by the end of the first week it becomes so narrow that it would be difficult to introduce anything the size of a finger. Simultaneously, any lacerations are healing. Once a mother has delivered a child vaginally, the cervix does not assume its pregravid appearance, but the external os remains open in varying degrees, although the internal os is closed. This is one of the characteristics of the uterus of a multiparous woman.

The Lochia

A knowledge of the healing process by which the lining of the uterus becomes regenerated is valuable in understanding and interpreting the lochial discharge. At first the discharge consists almost entirely of blood with a small amount of mucus, particles of decidua and cellular debris which escape from the placental site. It should not contain large clots or membrane or be excessive in amount. The discharge lasts about three days and is called *lochia rubra.*

As the oozing of blood from the healing surface diminishes, the discharge becomes more serous or watery and gradually changes to a pinkish color, the so-called *lochia serosa.* Toward the tenth day the lochia is thinner, greatly decreased in amount and almost colorless, the so-called *lochia alba.* By the end of the third week the discharge usually disappears, though a brownish mucoid discharge may persist a little longer. Lochia possesses a peculiar animal scent which is quite characteristic and should never, at any time, have an offensive odor.

Assessment. The quantity of lochia varies with individuals, but generally it is more profuse in multiparas. It is to be expected that when a mother is out of bed for the first time there may be a definite increase in the amount of discharge. *Nevertheless, the recurrence of fresh bleeding after the discharge has become dark and diminished in amount, or the persistence of bright blood in the lochia or the suppression of the discharge should be reported to the obstetrician.* The daily observation of the amount and the character of the lochia is of the greatest importance as an index of the progress of healing of the endometrial surface.

The Pelvis

The vaginal walls, the vulva and all other tissues which have become hypertrophied during pregnancy also undergo a process of involution in their return to normal. The *vagina* requires some time to recover from the distention brought about by delivery. This capacious passage gradually diminishes in size, although it rarely returns to its nulliparous condition. The *labia majora* and the *labia minora* become flabbier than before childbearing. Any abrasions and lacerations of the genital canal caused by the passage of the fetus should heal completely during the puerperium. The *ligaments* that support the uterus, the ovaries and the tubes, which have also undergone great tension and stretching, are now relaxed and will take considerable time to return almost to their normal size and position.

Abdominal Wall

The abdominal wall recovers partially from the overstretching but remains soft and flabby for some time. The striae, due to the rupture of the elastic fibers of the cutis, usually remain but become less conspicuous because of their silvery appearance. The process of involution in the abdominal structures requires at least six weeks. Provided that the abdominal walls have retained their muscle tone, they gradually return to their original condition. However, if these muscles are relaxed because they have lost their tone, there may be a marked separation or *diastasis of the recti muscles,* so that the abdominal organs are not properly supported. Rest, diet, prescribed exercises, good body mechanics and good posture may do much to restore the tone of these muscles.

The Breasts

During pregnancy, progressive changes occur in the breasts in preparation for lactation. The breast lobules have developed under the stimulation of the estrogen and progesterone produced by the placenta while the lactiferous ducts have undergone further branching and elongation. Prolactin, released from the anterior pituitary, cortisol from the maternal adrenal, and insulin, all of which appear in increasing amounts during gestation, also contribute to breast changes. Although all of the essential factors are more and more available as gestation progresses, milk production per se is held in abeyance. Its appearance is delayed until three or four days after delivery, when estrogen and progesterone levels have decreased.

Colostrum. On delivery, the breast produces increased amounts of a thin yellow fluid, colostrum. Women who carry out special breast care preparation during the last weeks of pregnancy often are able to express manually small amounts of it before birth. Colostrum contains more protein and inorganic salts, but less fat and carbohydrate than does breast milk. It also contains demonstrable levels of antibodies, and its immunoglobulin content (IgA) may offer the newborn protection against enteric infections. The nutritive value of colostrum is lower than that of breast milk.

Lactation. On the third or fourth day postpartum the breast milk usually "comes in." There is an obvious change in the color of the secretion from the nipples; it becomes bluish-white, the usual color of normal breast milk. At this time the breasts suddenly become larger, firmer and more tender as lacteal secretion is established, causing the mother to experience throbbing pains in the breasts extending into the axillae. This congestion, which usually subsides in one or two days, is caused in part by pressure from the increased amounts of milk in the lobules and the ducts, but even more by the increased circulation of blood and lymph in the mammary gland, producing tension on the very sensitive surrounding tissues. This is sometimes referred to as *primary engorgement.*

The efficiency and maintenance of milk production is, in large measure, controlled by the stimulus of repetitive nursing. The dermis on and about the nipple is richly endowed with sensory end organs. Their stimulation triggers a neuroendocrine reflex and results in sudden release of oxytocin from the posterior pituitary gland. Oxytocin stimulates contraction of the alveolar ducts of the breast, resulting in the ejection of milk. This suckling reflex also brings about a burst of prolactin, released from the anterior pituitary, which may play a role in maintaining milk production. The oxytocin released by suckling also stimulates uterine contractions, which explains the mild abdominal cramps often associated with the initiation of breast feeding.

Supply of Breast Milk. Breast milk varies markedly in its quality and quantity, not only in different individuals, but also in the same individual at various times. In general, the amount of breast milk increases as the infant's need for it increases. Nature seems to have coordinated carefully the mother's need for rest and the infant's need for food during the first two days, when only colostrum is secreted. But during this time lactation is definitely stimulated by the infant's sucking, and although the secretion of breast milk would occur naturally, without this stimulation and the complete emptying of the breasts the secretion of breast milk would not continue for more than a few days.

If the infant is put to breast consistently, by the end of the first week a healthy mother usually has about 200 to 300 ml (6 to 10 oz) of breast milk a day. By the end of four weeks this amount almost doubles, so that she produces about 600 ml (20 oz) a day. Breast milk is produced on the basis of "supply and demand" (i.e., the amount secreted gradually adjusts in relation to what the baby takes at an average feeding). In time, as the baby grows, the mother may have about 900 ml (30 oz) of breast milk a day.

The supply of breast milk is dependent on several factors, such as the mother's diet, the amount of exercise and rest she gets, and her level of contentment. An adequate diet for lactation requires increased amounts of protein, calcium, iron and vitamins as well as an ample fluid intake. The mother who is breast-feeding needs a good night's sleep, a rest period in the middle of the day and normal exercise. Worry, emotional tension and too much activity (overexertion and fatigue) have an adverse effect on lactation (see Chapters 20 and 30).

In relation to lactation, the actual size of the breast is not as important as the amount of glandular tissue, since the secreting tissues of the mammary gland produce the breast milk and not the fat. It has been verified that certain drugs, if administered to the lactating mother, are excreted in the breast milk, for example, large doses of salicylates, certain cathartics, iodides, bromides, quinine, atropine, and opium.

CLINICAL CONSIDERATIONS

Early Ambulation

The normal patient should be encouraged to get out of bed as soon as practical, and certainly within the first 24 hours postpartum. In general, patients feel stronger and psychologically better as a result of early limited activity, and constipation and bladder complications are less frequent. Most important, the incidence of thrombophlebitis and pulmonary embolus has been decreased materially in recent years as a result of early ambulation.

Temperature

Slight rises in temperature may occur without apparent cause following the delivery, but, in general, the mother's temperature should remain within normal limits during the puerperium, that is, below 38° C. (100.4° F.) when taken orally. Any mother whose temperature exceeds this limit in any two consecutive 24-hour periods of the puerperium (excluding the first 24 hours postpartum) is considered to be febrile.

It was formerly believed that an elevation of temperature naturally occurred with the establishment of lactation on the third or the fourth day after delivery; the so-called *milk-fever* was considered a normal accompaniment of this process. At the present time this is considered to be a fallacy. On rare occasions a sharp peak of fever for several hours may be caused by extreme vascular and lymphatic engorgement of the breasts, but this does not last longer than 12 hours at the most.

In judging the significance of a rise in temperature, the pulse rate provides a helpful guide, for in a puerperal patient with a slow pulse, a slightly elevated temperature is not likely to signify a complication. Nevertheless, any rise of temperature in the puerperium should excite the suspicion of endometritis (see Chapter 35).

Pulse

In the early puerperium a pulse rate which is somewhat slower than normal is a favorable symptom. The rate usually averages between 60 and 70 but may even become a little slower than this in one or two days after the delivery. This is merely a transient phenomenon, so that by the end of the first week or 10 days the pulse returns to its normal rate. On the other hand, a rapid pulse after labor, unless the mother has cardiac disease, may be an indication of shock or hemorrhage.

Blood

Most of the blood and metabolic alterations characteristic of normal pregnancy disappear within the first two weeks of the puerperium.

After-Pains

Normally, after the delivery of the first child, the uterine muscle tends to remain in a state of tonic contraction and retraction. But if the uterus has been subjected to any marked distention, or if tissue or blood clots have been retained in the cavity, then active contractions occur in an effort to expel them, and these contractions may be painful. In multiparas a certain amount of the initial tonicity of the uterine muscle has been lost, and these contractions and retractions cannot be sustained. Consequently, the muscle contracts and relaxes at intervals, and these contractions give rise to the sensation of pain, the so-called "after-pains."

These after-pains are more noticeable after a pregnancy in which the uterus has been greatly distended, as with multiple births or hydramnios. They are particularly noticeable in the breast-feeding mother, when the infant is put to breast (because sucking causes release of oxytocin from the posterior pituitary which stimulates the uterus to contract), and they may last for days, although ordinarily they become quite bearable in about 48 hours after delivery. They also occur with increased intensity, following the administration of oxytocic agents such as ergotrate. Often after-pains become so sharp that the administration of a sedative is necessary. Any time that they are severe enough to disturb the mother's rest and peace of mind, the physician should be notified.

Digestion

Although the mother's appetite may be diminished the first few days after labor, the digestive tract functions normally in the puerperium. Thirst is considerably increased at this time due to the marked diaphoresis associated with puerperium. Moreover, the fact that the mother may have gone without fluids for some hours in labor undoubtedly increases her thirst.

Loss of Weight

In addition to the 5- or 6-kg (10 or 11 lb) loss of weight at delivery, there is generally a still further loss of about 2 kg (5 lb) of body weight early in the puerperium due to marked diuresis, with its associated loss of body fluid.

Kidneys

The amount of urine excreted by the kidneys in the puerperium is of particular significance. During pregnancy there is an increased tendency of the body to retain water, so that now the tremendous output of urine represents the body's effort to return its water metabolism to normal. Diuresis regularly occurs between the second and the fifth days after delivery, sometimes reaching a daily output of 3,000 ml. After the delivery, in particular, the bladder may distend without any awareness on the part of the mother, especially if she has received any form of analgesia. *Therefore, it becomes a major responsibility of the nurse to be alert to signs of a full bladder and thus to prevent distention from occurring.*

During the first few days after labor there may be an increase in the amount of nitrogen in the urine. This excretion is due to the breakdown of protein material of the uterine wall during involution. Concerning acetone in the urine—as long as the regimen of "starvation" is not included in the management of labor, the presence of acetone in the urine, related to the incomplete metabolism of body fat, would not occur. Occasionally, during the first weeks of the puerperium the urine contains substantial amounts of sugar, which has no relationship to diabetes but is due to the presence of lactose, milk sugar, absorbed from the mammary glands.

Intestinal Elimination

The mother is nearly always constipated during the first few days of the puerperium. This is due to the relaxed condition of the intestinal and the abdominal muscles, in particular, and to the inability of the abdominal wall to aid in the evacuation of the intestinal contents. In addition, if hemorrhoids are present, the mother often is afraid to have a stool because of the discomfort these varicosities cause during elimination.

Skin

It is to be expected that elimination of waste products via the skin is accelerated in the early puerperium, often to such a degree that the mother is drenched with perspiration. These episodes of profuse sweating, which frequently occur in the night, gradually subside and do not require any specific treatment aside from protecting the mother from chilling when they occur.

Menstruation

If the mother does not breast-feed her infant, the menstrual flow probably will return within eight weeks after delivery. Ordinarily, menstruation does not occur so long as the mother is breast-feeding, but this is not a certainty. During lactation the first menstrual period may occur as early as the second month but usually occurs about the fourth month following the delivery. It has been known not to reappear until as late as the eighteenth month.

Studies have shown that failure to menstruate during lactation is due to suppression of ovulation. Since some mothers have been known to become pregnant in the course of breast-feeding an infant, we know that suppression of ovulation does not occur uniformly.

POSTPARTAL EXAMINATIONS

The condition of the mother is confirmed before she is discharged from the hospital to make sure that her progress has been satisfactory during the early puerperium. In addition to verifying her vital signs and present weight, observations are made to determine the condition of her breasts, the progress of involution and the healing of the perineal wound. A pelvic examination is deferred, since findings made by palpation of the uterus and inspection of the lochia will give satisfactory evidence as to the progress of involution at this time.

Follow-Up Examinations

As has been mentioned previously, the reproductive tract should return to its normal condition by the end of the puerperium. In order to investigate the general physical condition of the mother and determine with what normality she has completed her maternity experience, she should return for examination about six weeks postpartum.

During the visit the weight and the blood pressure are taken, the urine is examined for albumin, and a blood count may be done. The condition of the abdominal walls is observed, and the breasts are inspected. If the mother is breast-feeding, the condition of the nipples and the degree of lacteal secretion are a significant part of the observation. If the mother is not breast-feeding, the breasts should be observed to see that physiologic readjustments have occurred.

A thorough pelvic examination is carried out to investigate the position of the uterus, the healing of perineal wounds, the support of the pelvic floor, and whether involution is complete.

In addition, this return examination provides an opportunity to discuss any other problems relating to this maternity experience and to discuss methods of family planning (see Chapter 28). If abnormalities are found, they may be treated at this time and arrangements made for further examinations and treatments as necessary.

The postpartal visit is an ideal time to emphasize the importance of periodic examinations at six-month to yearly intervals for continued health care and advice on family planning.

SUGGESTED READING

Barden, T. P.: "Perinatal care," in *Gynecology and Obstetrics, The Health Care of Women.* Ed. Romney et al. New York, McGraw-Hill, 1975, pp. 657-712.

Willson, J. R., and Carrington, E. R.: *Obstetrics and Gynecology*, ed. 6. St. Louis, C. V. Mosby, 1979.

Twenty-Seven

Psychosocial Aspects of the Postpartum Period

Transition to Parenthood / Assumption of the Parental Role / Influences on Parental Behavior / Responding to Family Developmental Changes

In discussing psychosocial aspects of pregnancy in Chapter 17, we made the point that pregnancy and parenthood can be thought of as a role transition. We noted the tremendous change that comes with childbirth and the assumption of the new role, and the concomitant instability that can occur until new roles are allocated and the new member is integrated. In this chapter we will continue our exploration of the psychosocial needs of the new, expanded family as they assume their responsibilities as parents.

The discussion is based on the underlying assumption that the degree of ease and satisfaction with which individuals make the transition to parenthood is directly affected by how successfully they have defined and accepted their relationship with each other. If they have developed an ability to see each other as they are (not as they ought to be), if they can allow for divergence of values and behaviors, work collaboratively toward a flexible power base for each and develop norms that allow for mutual growth, then they will be more likely to move smoothly into the new role.

This assumption is identified specifically here because much of the literature on parenting singles out either the content of the parent-child relationship per se or the parents' own childhood relationships as the primary determinants of the family's progression through this phase. This neglects two other

vital areas: 1) the needs of each person within the system as an individual and 2) the needs of the parents as a couple. Use of this assumption does not negate the importance of the parent-child relationship or the parents' own background, but it does provide some focus on the marital couple as an entity. In reality it is the balancing of the three areas of needs within the family that is the ultimate task of the new family. Moreover, it is these areas that the nurse must be aware of and respect when working with families undergoing the transition to parenthood.[1]

TRANSITION TO PARENTHOOD

The student will recall that we have used Rossi's formulation of phases in the process of role transition. Specifically, these were the anticipatory phase, the honeymoon phase, the plateau and disengagement phases (see Chapter 17). In the puerperium, it is the honeymoon phase of the transition that will have the most bearing on the nursing care that the maternity nurse will render. However, we shall also review briefly the anticipatory phase since we previously focused primarily on its relevance to pregnancy rather than to parenthood.

The Anticipatory Phase

We noted previously that pregnancy is itself an anticipatory stage to becoming a parent and we outlined tasks that the parents must accomplish during this time. We spoke of decision making and expectations which have bearing on later parenting. Another aspect is the division of labor in the family. This becomes extremely crucial when the baby arrives. The mundane activities of family maintenance are often indicative of how comfortable the parents are in accepting their changing roles. This also gives a clue as to what later role assignments the child may have in the family. It is important that the nurse note in making an assessment whether there is any negotiation for task assignment or some indication of a flexible allocation and sharing of tasks. If one partner unilaterally appoints the other to a responsibility or if there is a rigid "his work, her work" attitude, there may be subtle sabotage or task overload as responsibilities mount with the addition of the infant.[2,3] Thus, how the family uses the time of pregnancy to work out or rework their division of labor in the family will have a large impact on their transition.

Overall, couples in the anticipatory phase experience many intense feelings, challenges and responsibilities. If used correctly, this can be an opportune time to test skills in preparing to accept and integrate the new family member into the system. The nurse can be very helpful in aiding the couple to examine and understand what they are experiencing by providing accurate information and feedback of perceptions and offering validation of the dynamics that are emerging.[4]

Honeymoon Phase

This phase refers to the postchildbirth period during which, through prolonged contact and intimacy, an attachment between the parents and child is achieved.[5] It should be noted that this is a "psychic honeymoon" and not necessarily a time of romanticized peace and joy. Rather, it is a period of intensity when both the mother and the father are exploring the new family member and where they stand in relation to him or her. The couple's personal relationship is no less important at this time, but with the limited energy, emphasis is often placed on development of the new relationship.

Bonding and Attachment

Much has appeared in the literature regarding the fourth stage of labor—the time immediately after delivery when there appears to be an optimum time for close contact between parents and child to initiate the process of bonding the trio together. The terms "bonding" and "attachment" are often used interchangeably to describe this process of parent-child affiliation. Brazelton has pointed out, however, that there is a difference in the connotation of these terms. Bonding refers to the initial attraction and desire to "make it" with another person. Attachment, on the other hand, is the long, hard work of staying in love.[6] Thus, bonding can be thought of as the initial step in a process, the mutual attractiveness and response *between parents and child* that paves the way for the later development of love and affiliation. In everyday usage, however, the two terms are interchangeable.

Until quite recently health providers and the public in general have viewed the newborn as essentially passive. Many medical schools still teach that the newborn infant has limited perceptual abilities as if only the mid-brain is functioning. This misconception has directly and indirectly affected the delivery of maternity care at all levels. If, instead of using the "lump of clay" model of the infant, we think of the child as organizing around various positive stimuli and experiences, we can readily see that the present tendency toward overstimulating and noncontingent care (care-taking timed *asynchronously* with the infant's responses) is not conducive to the organization of the infant's central nervous system and hence to expeditious positive parent-infant interaction. Care for the newborn needs to be timed to his activity and responses, not to schedules preordained by professionals.[7]

As we explore more carefully the amazing newborn, our research indicates that neonates are very adaptive, not only to survive in an often unwelcoming or uncomfortable environment but also to capture the important adults around them. They will, for instance, demonstrate a marked ability to habituate to different stimuli. If a light is flashed repeatedly into the eyes, the baby will startle the first two or three times, then gradually settle down and no longer respond. The same response occurs with the stimuli of a rattle, bell and pinprick. Moreover, there are definite auditory and visual orienting responses. If one talks and begins to play with the baby, he will become alert and will search for a face (Fig. 27-1). When he finds it, he softens, and as long as the face moves, the baby will follow it. If it becomes still, however, the infant will frown and avert his face. The immobile face has no attraction for the newborn!

Responses to auditory stimuli also demonstrate the ability of the neonate to make choices. If a man and woman stand on opposite sides of the baby and begin to talk, the infant will stop moving, his face will knit, and he will turn toward the female's voice again and again. There is also a differential response to human and nonhuman, machine sounds even if their qualities are exactly alike. When you present a baby who is sucking with a nonhuman sound, he will stop sucking and then quickly resume. If, however, he is offered a human sound, he will stop, and then resume with a pattern of suck, suck, pause, suck, suck, pause, indicating by this different, complex pattern a preference for the human sound.[8]

These manifestations of the infant's ability to control and console himself are powerful reinforcers for parents who are ready to move beyond the initial bonding and continue their attachment. The nurse, during both the immediate and later postpartum period, can be very helpful to parents and facilitate bonding by pointing out and *reinforcing parents' perceptions* of their infant's ability to interact

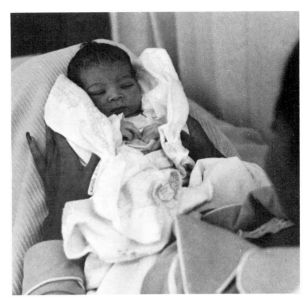

Figure 27-1B. The infant establishes eye contact with the mother. (*Continued on p. 416*)

with them. One reinforcer to attachment that can be shown to the mother and father is the manner of consoling the baby. When a baby is crying, even at the top of his voice, he can be quieted by insistently saying "baby, baby, baby . . ." Simply by using the voice, one can get the infant to turn his head, put his fist in his mouth and start looking for you. When this and other behaviors we have mentioned are shown to parents, they usually react by saying such things as "Now I know what I must do to mother," or "You have shown me how to father!" Parents will also turn to the nurse for validation of their impressions. "Do you think she really sees (or hears) me?" When you confirm this impression, their faces light up and another link is forged in the bond.[9]

Principles of Bonding

The work of Robson, Rubin, Moss, Brazelton, Klaus, Kennell, Bowlby and many others has begun to shed light on the fascinating subject of how infants and parents first develop their acquaintance. While we still do not have many of the answers and some of the information that we do have must still be considered tentative, there appear to be several vital principles of the bonding process. Again, these are not to be regarded as definitive; rather they reflect the state of the art in thinking and research

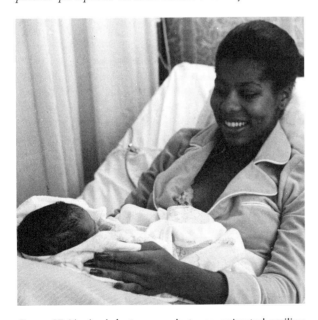

Figure 27-1A. An infant responds to an animated smiling face. Note the infant's different expressions as the mother smiles and talks and the manner in which he moves his mouth in response to the mother's voice and smile.

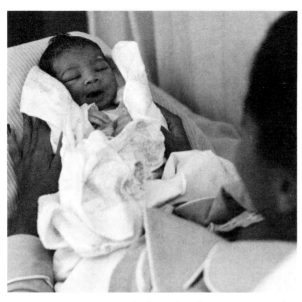

Figure 27-1C. (Continued) The infant begins to move his mouth as the mother smiles and talks.

in the area. Based on their work, Klaus and Kennell specify the following crucial principles:

1. There appears to be a sensitive period in the first minutes and hours after birth when it is necessary for the mother and father to have close contact with their infant for later development to be optimal.
2. There appear to be species-specific responses to the infant in the human mother and father when the infant is first given to them.
3. The attachment process seems to be structured so that the parents will become attached to only one infant at a time. In 1958, Bowlby stated this principle as *monotropy*.
4. For attachment to occur appropriately, it is necessary for the infant to respond to the mother and father by some signal such as body or eye movements. This principle has been called the "You can't love a dishrag" phenomenon.
5. Individuals who witness the birth process become strongly attached to the infant.
6. It is difficult (but not impossible) to simultaneously go through the processes of attachment and detachment. Thus, it is difficult (but not impossible) for parents to attach to an infant while mourning the loss or threatened loss of another person.
7. Some early events may have a long-lasting effect. For instance, anxiety over an infant

with a temporary disorder in his or her early days may result in long-term concerns and/or behavior that will have implications for future development.[10]

ASSUMPTION OF THE PARENTAL ROLE

As the parents continue in their transition, certain behaviors become apparent. It is important to note that there is much more information on maternal behavior than on paternal behavior.

Paternal Behavior

While most researchers agree that more studies need to be done regarding paternal behavior, we are still in the very early stages of this type of research. Parke, a pioneer in this area, has concluded in his studies that there are not significant behavioral differences between fathers alone with their infants and mothers alone with their infants. If, however, the trio are together, the father tends to hold the infant twice as much as the mother, he vocalizes more, touches the infant slightly more, but smiles significantly less. Thus, the father plays a far more active role than the passive cultural stereotype suggests.[11,12] The term *engrossment* has been used by Greenberg and Morris to describe the behavior pattern noted in fathers when they are involved and interacting with their newborn (Fig. 27-2). They conclude that there are identifiable aspects of paternal bonding similar to maternal bonding that are enhanced by newborn behavior and normal reflex activity.[13]

Lamb and Howells, on the other hand, contend that mothering and fathering are separate entities and may be dissimilar. Lamb proposes the following thesis: 1) the mother-child relationship is originally based on the infant's dependence and helplessness and gradually diminishes in importance as the child becomes older and more independent and 2) the father-child relationship revolves around not only caretaking activities but also many outside enjoyable activities. Hence, the father introduces and socializes the child to the world outside the home. Female parents could function in the paternal role but would have to dissociate from the mothering, nurturing tasks. Thus, the reason for the dissimilarity of the two roles.[14] Why the father can caretake and socialize outside the home at the same time and the mother cannot is not clear in Lamb's formulation.

Howells also believes that both fathering and mothering are equally important but may have dissimilar components. According to his formulation, the relationship of both parents to a child is unique and is dependent on the sum total of the variables that make up the psychosocial dynamics of each family.[15]

In view of the similarities found in the better research studies and society's recent trend toward a more flexible masculine-feminine role definition, the utility of breaking apart maternal and paternal behavior may well be called into question.

Maternal Behavior

A pioneer in first delineating parental behavior was Reva Rubin, who focused on the mother and identified various phases of maternal behavior, particularly relating to maternal touch and the infant. She contends that, mothering is composed of a set of interpersonal and production skills designed to foster the emotional, intellectual and physical development of the child. Thus, Rubin described the tasks of mothering as 1) identifiying the new child, 2) determining one's relationship to the child, and 3) guiding and reconstructing the family constellation to include a new member. In general, this formulation is still accepted.[16]

Certain behaviors have been found to accompany these various tasks and the assumption of the maternal role. These behaviors have also been found to be specific to three phases which Rubin also classified. The time spans for these phases may vary, particularly if the parents are permitted immediate contact with the newborn. The following discussion derives from Rubin's classification.[17]

The Taking-In Phase

In this phase the mother is oriented primarily to her own needs. She may be quite passive and dependent. This phase may last a day or two and it is important that the nurse try to help meet the mother's dependency needs so that she can move into more complex mothering tasks. The mother does not usually initiate contact with the infant. This is not out of disinterest, but rather because of her own

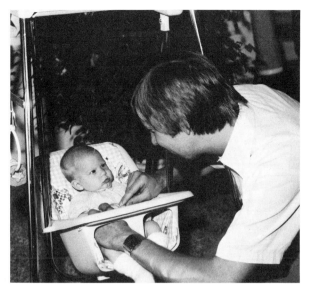

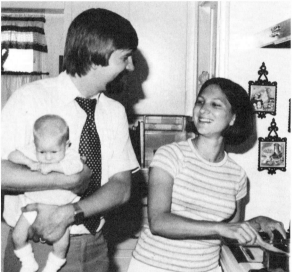

Figure 27-2. Fathering. Paternal involvement may be described as engrossment and can be satisfying to everyone.

immediate dependency. Although she is not indicating much interest in assuming responsibility for the baby's care, she is taking in information which helps her identify the infant. In this phase *finger-tip touch* with the infant can be observed (Fig. 27-3). The mother may lay the infant on her lap or bed and gently explore him or her with her fingers. This is one of the first steps in the identification process and an indication of awakening interest in the newborn. One may also note that she holds the baby facing her, so that they mutually explore each other's faces. This has been called the *en face* position.

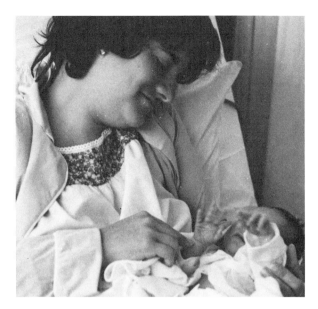

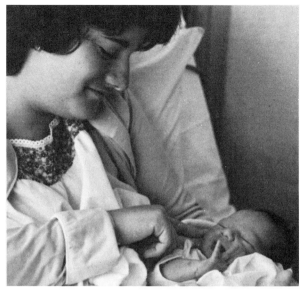

Figure 27-3. Identification process through maternal touch. A. Exploring the infant with fingertip touch.

B. The mother continues her exploration progressing to the infant's face.

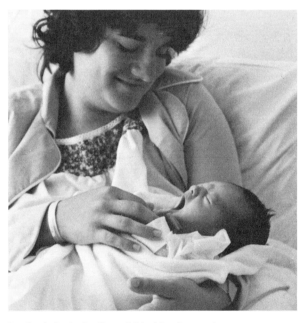

C. The baby is finally enfolded by the mother.

Sleep and Food play an important part during this phase. The mother is far more able to begin the activities required of her if she is allowed to have a well-earned refreshing sleep. If this necessary rest is disrupted, the mother may experience a "sleep–hunger" which may last for several days; this results in irritability, fatigue and general interference with

the normal restorative process. Thus, the necessity of appropriate intervention by the nurse to allow the mother to get adequate sleep cannot be stressed enough.

The nurse will note, also, that the mother usually has a good appetite and, in fact, may talk a good deal about either the adequacy or the inadequacy of her meals. Between-meal nourishment is appreciated and needed (especially by nursing mothers). The concern about food seems to be a part of the mother's general need to be restored. Food, as we know, has tremendous psychological significance for care-asking and care-giving. The nurse should be especially cognizant of the mother's need for hearty meals and should expedite extra nourishment whenever possible. Moreover, she will want to be aware that a poor appetite often is one of the first symptoms that all is not proceeding normally in the puerperal period.

Integrating the Experience. During the "taking-in" phase the mother begins to relive the delivery experience in order to integrate it fully into reality. She is apt to be very talkative at this time, and she may want to know certain specifics and details so that she can form a total picture of what "really happened" during delivery. As she obtains this information, she is able to realize more fully that the pregnancy and the delivery are truly over and that her baby now is born and is an individual outside of and separate from herself. This is a considerable task and involves rather profound changes in attitudes and feelings. The symbiotic relationship between mother and infant during pregnancy is at an end, and the mother now must identify her child as a separate individual.

Taking-Hold Phase

The second phase in the puerperal period has been described as a "taking-hold" phase; that is, the mother strives for independence and autonomy and finally begins to be the initiator. One of her main concerns at this point seems to be with her ability to control her bodily functions; her bowels and bladder must perform well, and she takes an active part in seeing that they do. If she is nursing her infant, she is concerned about producing an acceptable quantity and quality of milk. She often will ask the nurses and the doctors anxiously (referring to the milk), "Has it come in yet?" And later she wants to know: "Do you think I have enough?" She cannot have enough explanation and reassurance that she is "performing" well at this time. She wants to walk, to sit, to move as she did before delivery and is very anxious and impatient if she cannot make her body behave as it once did. It is as though she is thinking, "How can I possibly assume all my responsibilities for others if I cannot control my own body?"

Her first mothering tasks are especially important to her, and "failures" (inability to elicit a bubble from her infant, poor sucking response on the part of the baby, her awkwardness in handling her child), no matter how small and expected (by the staff,), can send her to the depths of despair. Even the skillful intervention of the nurse seems only to point up her "inadequacy" as a mother. She often will voice her feelings with an "Oh, I'll never be able to bathe her as easily as you do." Or another mother may say, "He always seems to take his milk better when *you* feed him." Conversely, when she succeeds at a task, her delight and relief are wonderful to behold. It is difficult to imagine (for anyone other than a new mother) how thrilling a hearty bubble from a small infant can be.

Since there is a good deal of anxiety as well as activity in this phase, fatigue and exhaustion may occur if the mother is not helped to set realistic expectations and limits for herself. Since this "taking-hold" phase lasts about ten days, much of it will take place at home.

The nurse can be invaluable in giving the mother, as she appears able and ready to accept it, anticipatory guidance about what to expect and how to manage. During the hospital stay the mother profits greatly from reassurance and explanation regarding the various processes and hour-by-hour events. She finds guidance and reinforcement of appropriate behavior particularly helpful when she attempts to perform her mothering tasks.

When assisting the mother, the nurse must be careful not to impose herself between the mother and her baby (no matter how awkward or maladroit the mother seems). Rather, the nurse should allow the mother to perform the actual task (after necessary demonstration or instruction) and then encourage or reinforce whatever behavior was appropriate. This is one way of demonstrating confidence in the mother's ability to cope with new tasks. In order to gain skill and confidence in her mothering ability, the mother needs the opportunity to make decisions about the baby's needs as well as guidance regarding his physical care. When she is allowed to find answers to her questions (again with guidance as necessary) and is reassured that her judgment is correct, she is able to feel confident in her ability to perceive needs accurately and to make decisions. Thus, she is better able to meet problems in the future.

As the mother becomes more comfortable with her infant, she moves to the second stage of maternal touch, *total hand contact,* and finally the third stage, *enfolding* (Fig. 27-3B,C). In general, the more competent she feels and the more satisfying her relationship with the infant, the greater the enfolding. These touching behaviors can be observed in fathers also if they are given the opportunity to handle and care for the infant. They, too, can be observed placing the infant in the *en face* position.

The mother who remains distant and aloof may not be attaching to her infant as optimally as she should. The nurse will want to be alert for such signs.

The Letting-Go Phase

As her mothering functions become more established, the mother enters the letting-go phase. This generally occurs when the mother returns home. In this phase there are two separations that the mother must accomplish. One is to realize and accept the physical separation from the baby and the other is to relinquish her former role of childless person. As

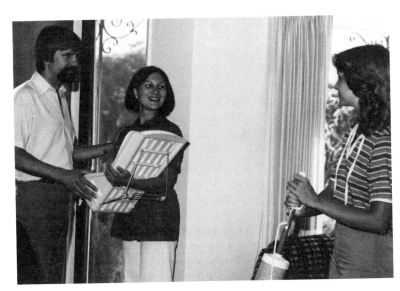

Figure 27-4. Utilizing responsible teenagers as "mother's helpers" allows parents to enjoy outing with their infant.

we pointed out in Chapter 17, she will never again be childless until the death of those whom she has borne. The implications are enormous. She must now adjust her life to the relative dependency and helplessness of her child. If she stops working, she must adapt at least temporarily to less freedom, autonomy and social stimulation. If she does continue working, she and the father will have to handle the complex details of finding mother substitutes and other household caretakers (Fig. 27-4). Her work load is such that there is almost always some role strain and overload even when the father is helpful and/or outside help is found. This can be managed by appropriate anticipatory guidance from the nurse, but nearly all mothers find the adjustment at least somewhat difficult.

Thus, during the puerperium (for no apparent reason, the mother thinks) she may experience a let-down feeling accompanied by irritability and tears. Occasionally her appetite and sleep patterns are disturbed. These are the usual manifestations of the postpartal or "baby" blues. This depression is usually temporary and may occur in the hospital. It is thought to be related in part to hormonal changes and in part to the ego adjustment that accompanies role transition. Discomfort, fatigue and exhaustion certainly contribute to this condition if not cause it. Crying often relieves the tension, but if the parents are not knowledgeable about the condition, the mother, especially, may feel rather guilty for being depressed. Understanding, anticipatory guidance will help the parents be aware that

these feelings are a normal accompaniment to this role transition. (This aspect of postpartal care is explored more extensively in Chapter 28.)

INFLUENCES ON PARENTAL BEHAVIOR

Figure 27-5 presents a schematic diagram of the major influences on parental behavior and their outcomes, including some disorders that have been hypothesized to arise from them. The diagram has been adapted from Klaus and Kennell.[18] We note that, at the time of the infant's birth, some of the influences or determinants are fixed and unchangeable (solid line), such as the genetic endowment of the parents, the type of mothering they received, previous pregnancies and the like. Other determinants can be altered, however (dotted line), such as practices of hospital personnel, separation of infant and mother and future parental relations. Klaus and Kennell feel that many of the disturbances and disorders can be directly attributed to separation of the infant from the mother after birth and the consequent interference with the bonding process. They point out that the separation of mother and infant is the one variable that is most easily manipulated and urge that hospitals reexamine their policies to bring them in line with more current findings regarding bonding and attachment.[19] As more research is done on this fascinating topic, we should

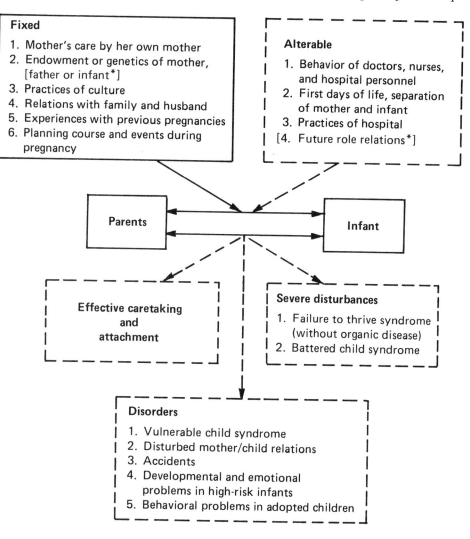

Fixed
1. Mother's care by her own mother
2. Endowment or genetics of mother, [father or infant*]
3. Practices of culture
4. Relations with family and husband
5. Experiences with previous pregnancies
6. Planning course and events during pregnancy

Alterable
1. Behavior of doctors, nurses, and hospital personnel
2. First days of life, separation of mother and infant
3. Practices of hospital
[4. Future role relations*]

Parents   **Infant**

Effective caretaking and attachment

Severe disturbances
1. Failure to thrive syndrome (without organic disease)
2. Battered child syndrome

Disorders
1. Vulnerable child syndrome
2. Disturbed mother/child relations
3. Accidents
4. Developmental and emotional problems in high-risk infants
5. Behavioral problems in adopted children

*Not in original Klaus/Kennell diagram.

Figure 27-5. Hypothesized diagram of the major influences on maternal behavior and the resulting disturbances. Solid lines represent unchangeable determinants; dotted lines represent alterable determinants. (Adapted from Klaus, M. H., and Kennell, J. H.: Material Infant Bonding. St. Louis, The Mosby Co., 1976.)

gain more insight into how we can better help the family to make the parental role transition more smoothly.

RESPONDING TO FAMILY DEVELOPMENTAL CHANGES: NURSING IMPLICATIONS

One key element of nursing intervention with the expanding family is the teaching of parenting skills that will promote the child's maturity, autonomy and competence. If the parents have a realistic conception of the infant's needs and their resources, they need not expend all their energy on their parenting responsibilities at the expense of their own personal needs and growth.

We have seen that skill in task performance is a cornerstone in both the mothering and fathering. Thus, promoting the development of infant-care skills is a vital aspect of the nurse's teaching role. Heretofore, we have focused on coaching parents about childbirth and we have found that planned learning has value. Similarly nursing's involvement in the recent trend toward health maintenance and promotion has set the stage for an expansion of these types of classes to include information and skill development needed after the infant is born. Teaching styles and format for parenting classes resemble those utilized in prenatal instruction.[20]

Learning needs of the parents can be determined by assessing the following areas: 1) expectations of childrens' performance ability; 2) lags in development task fulfillment; 3) social isolation; 4) immobilization due to role overload; 5) ability to set limits and carry them out. When these learning needs are diagnosed, the nurse can develop a teaching plan aimed at preventing and alleviating problems in this area. Active participation by the parents enhances the learning process and a variety of activities such as role-playing, group discussions, and readings will enhance the movement of the class. Strengths of the couple always should be delineated and worked with. When deficits are found, verbal and behavioral skills can be developed to cope with the problem. If the deficit is related to outside institutions, the nurse will want to be aware of community institutions and agencies where she can refer the parents.[21]

The nurse will recognize that it is impossible to teach all of the skills necessary to parenting. However, if she can help parents sort out problems, examine options and resources and negotiate outcomes, she will have accomplished a great deal for her patients and will be instrumental in this momentous role transition!

REFERENCES

1. D. M. Hrobsky: "Transition to parenthood." *Nursing Clinics of N. Am.* 12:457–468, Sept. 1977.
2. R. H. Turner: *Family Interaction.* New York, John Wiley & Sons, 1970.
3. Hrobsky, op. cit.
4. Ibid.
5. A. Rossi: "Transition to parenthood." *J. Marriage and Family* 30:26–39, Feb. 1968.
6. T. B. Brazelton: "The remarkable talents of the newborn." *Birth and the Family J.* 5:187–191, Winter 1978.
7. Ibid.
8. Ibid.
9. Ibid.
10. M. H. Klaus, and J. H. Kennell: *Maternal-Infant Bonding.* St. Louis, C. V. Mosby, 1976, p. 14.
11. R. Parke: "Father-infant interaction." In M. Klaus et al., eds. *Maternal Attachment and Mothering Disorders, A Roundtable.* Sausalito, Calif., Johnson & Johnson Co., 1974.
12. R. Parke: "The father's role in infancy: A re-evaluation." *Birth and the Family J.* 5:211–213, Winter 1978.
13. M. Greenberg, and N. Morris: "Engrossment: The newborn's impact upon the father." *Am. J. Orthopsychiatry* 44:520–531, July 1974.
14. M. E. Lamb: "Fathers: Forgotten contributors to child development." *Human Development* 18:245–266, 1975.
15. J. G. Howells: "Fathering." In *Modern Perspective in International Child Psychiatry.* J. G. Howells, ed. Edinburgh, Oliver and Boyd, 1969, pp. 125–156.
16. R. Rubin: "Basic maternal behavior." *Nurs. Outlook,* 683–686, Nov. 1961.
17. R. Rubin: "Puerperal change." *Nurs. Outlook,* 753–755, Dec. 1961.
18. Klaus and Kennell, op. cit., p. 13.
19. Ibid.
20. B. J. Perdue, et al.: "Mothering." *Nursing Clinics of N. Am.* 12:491–503, Sept. 1977.
21. Ibid.

SUGGESTED READING

Lazoff, B. et al.: "The mother-newborn relationship: Limits of adaptability." *J. Pediatrics* 91:1–13, July 1977.

Hrobsky, D.: "Transition to parenthood, a balancing of needs." *Nursing Clinics of N. Am.* 12:457–468, Sept. 1977.

Kiernan, B. and M. A. Scoloveno: "Fathering." *Nursing Clinics of N. Am.* 12:481–489, Sept. 1977.

"Parent to infant attachment," Special Issue. *Birth and the Family J.* 5:4, Winter 1978.

Twenty-Eight

Postpartal Care

Immediate Postpartum Care / Ongoing Care in the Hospital / Parental Guidance and Instruction / The First Weeks at Home / The Six-Weeks Checkup

The postpartal period is a time of major physical and psychological transition for the new mother. During the six weeks following delivery, her body undergoes restoration as involution of the reproductive organs returns them to their nonpregnant condition. If the mother is breast feeding, progressive changes occur with the beginning of lactation. The new mother also experiences psychological processes related to the ending of pregnancy, separation from the fetus, and development of a caretaking relationship with the infant, as discussed in Chapter 27. The father experiences similar psychological processes in initiating and developing his relationship with the infant. Both parents must adapt to a new family structure, integrate the infant into their family, and develop different interactional patterns within the family unit. The postpartum period is usually stressful, and sensitive professional care can be very helpful to new parents.

Providing optimal maternal care requires a thoughtful approach to the many facets and factors responsible for high-level wellness of the maternity patient. Her needs for physical care have been greatly modified by the advent of early ambulation following delivery and the subsequent evolution of more simplified maternity nursing procedures. Newly delivered mothers need certain kinds of physical care related to evaluating the progressive changes which occur in the breasts prior to lactation, as well as the involutional changes of the internal reproductive organs (Fig. 28-1). New mothers need nourishment, rest and sleep, and activity tempered with purposeful use of early ambulation.

Increased insight into the psychosocial needs of the newly delivered mother has resulted in greater attention to the emotional aspects of her care. This does not in any sense negate the need for physical care. As has been emphasized previously, the mother, the infant, the father and other children are considered as a family unit.

A very important consideration is the need that the mother and her newly born infant have for each other; and in today's highly organized hospitals, such times do not always coincide with hospital policy or routine. Increased awareness of the importance of the first few days after birth for development of appropriate bonding and attachment between mother and baby has led many hospitals to alter routines. Modified rooming-in procedures and other family-centered approaches generally provide mother and infant with longer time periods spent together, during which the identification and claiming phases of maternal-infant attachment may occur. Progressive policies for visits by fathers and

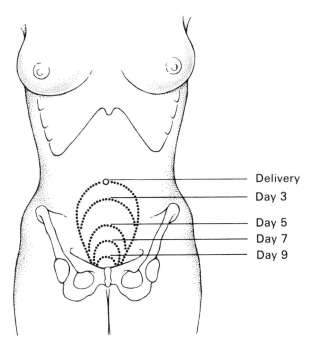

Figure 28-1. Involution of the uterus.

other family members in many hospitals encourage integration of the new infant into the family.

Nursing care takes the physical and psychological needs of mothers and families into consideration during the postpartum period. The mother's physiologic functioning must be observed accurately, her dependency needs must be met, anticipatory guidance and health teachings must be given according to the mother's readiness to learn, and the developing relationship between the mother and infant should be appropriately observed, guided and nurtured.

IMMEDIATE POSTPARTUM CARE

Immediately after labor, the mother usually experiences a sense of complete fatigue comparable to that which would normally follow any strenuous muscular activity. At the same time, she may be so exhilarated by the experience and the feeling of relief which accompanies it that she is not aware of being exhausted. She is interested in seeing and holding her baby and visiting with the father. Although this first visit of the family together may be rather brief, it is an experience which is particularly gratifying to the parents. Following this,

every effort should be made to help the mother to rest. With little encouragement she usually falls into a sound natural sleep. The discomforts and activities which may interfere with sleep, such as soreness of the vulva, hemorrhoids, "afterpains," and frequent postpartal observations, should be expedited or mitigated as much as possible.

Many mothers complain of feeling chilled immediately after labor; some actually shake with the chill. Such chills may be due in part to neurologic excitation and exhaustion. There is some disturbance of equilibrium between internal and external temperature caused by excessive perspiration during the muscular exertion of labor. Some authorities believe that the "chill" may be due partly to the sudden release of intraabdominal pressure which results as the uterus is emptied at delivery. This reaction may be alleviated if the mother is made comfortable in a warm bed and given a warm beverage when possible. If her body does begin to quiver, an extra cotton blanket should be placed over her or tucked close around her body for comfort. Many mothers (and their partners) are frightened or disturbed by the chill; thus, reassurance by the nurse that this is not an unusual occurrence following delivery is extremely helpful.

Postdelivery Observations

During the first few hours after birth, nursing care focuses on evaluating the mother's physical condition, since the risk of complications is greatest at this time. Hemorrhage is the major danger to the mother, and the condition of the uterus must be carefully monitored and bleeding assessed. Observations of vital signs and the condition of the bladder are also part of postdelivery care.

Considerable information can be gained by palpating the fundus through the abdominal wall to be assured that the uterus remains firm, round and well contracted. At the same time it is also important to inspect the perineal pad for obvious signs of bleeding, as well as to take the pulse and the blood pressure. During the first hour these observations should be made at least every 15 minutes, or more often if indicated.

As long as the bleeding is minimal and the uterus remains firm, well contracted and does not increase in size, it is neither necessary nor desirable to stimulate it. However, if the uterus becomes soft

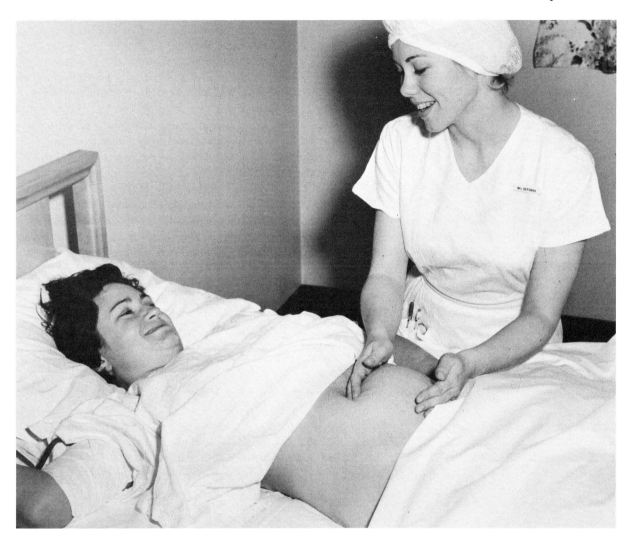

Figure 28-2. Palpating the fundus.

and boggy because of relaxation, the fundus should be massaged immediately until it becomes contracted again. This can be best accomplished by placing one hand just above the symphysis pubis to act as a guard, as the other hand is cupped around the fundus and rotated gently. It should be remembered that the uterus is a sensitive organ which, under normal circumstances, responds quickly to tactile stimulation.

Care must be taken to avoid overmassage, because, in addition to causing the mother considerable pain, this may stimulate premature uterine contractions and thereby cause undue muscle fatigue. Such a condition would further encourage uterine relaxation and hemorrhage.

If the uterus is atonic, blood which collects in the cavity should be expressed with firm but gentle force in the direction of the outlet, but only after the fundus has been first massaged (Fig. 28-2). Failure to see that the uterus is contracted before pushing downward against it could result in inversion of the uterus, an extremely serious complication.

Although excessive postpartum bleeding can happen to any mother, the nurse can identify those at increased risk as evidenced by factors related to their pregnancy or labor. A multipara who has had several deliveries has an increased tendency for heavy postpartum bleeding, as does the woman whose uterus was excessively distended by hydramnios, multiple pregnancy, or a large infant. Operative deliveries with lacerations of the cervix, vagina or perineum also predispose toward hemorrhage. Patients with a history indicating increased risk require more frequent observation for bleeding.

If the mother's bladder becomes distended, this can interfere with uterine contraction and produce atony, leading to heavy bleeding. With each 15-minute check of the condition of the uterus, the bladder should also be assessed. It is not unusual for the mother to need to void within one to four hours after delivery. If she is unable to void spontaneously and there is bladder distention, catheterization is necessary to prevent both bladder and uterine atony.

At the end of the first hour after delivery, if the uterus remains well contracted, bleeding is normal and vital signs stable, observations can be made less frequently, usually every four hours. Temperature is taken at this time also. The mother is allowed to rest as much as possible and kept comfortable. Liquids are usually provided if the mother's condition is stable.

Family Interactions

The immediate postpartum period, also called the fourth stage of labor (see Chapter 23), is important for the development of parent-infant relations as well as for the mother's physiologic status. When there is no contraindication due to the infant's condition, the infant is usually placed in the mother's arms and the two allowed to visit with the father in a private area for a short time. The infant's state of alertness immediately after birth facilitates eye contact with parents and is felt to be important in establishing the parental bond.[1]

After the excitement and strain of labor and delivery, the parents also appreciate this quiet time together. Needs for information or support will vary during this time, and care must be individualized. People of various cultural backgrounds will also respond differently during the immediate postdelivery period. In some cultures, the mother's female relatives assume the major supportive role during childbirth and thus will want to be with her after delivery. The extent of the father's involvement can vary considerably even among families where fathers have a significant part in the childbearing process. Flexible policies in hospitals permit the nurse to respond individually to these different cultural practices and family structures.

ONGOING CARE IN THE HOSPITAL

The daily routine procedures for the postpartal patient vary in different hospitals, but the principles of care are essentially the same. Certain observations should be made and recorded daily. These would include such findings as temperature, pulse and respiration; urinary and intestinal elimination; the physical changes which occur normally in the puerperium. One should note the changes in the breasts, the height and consistency of the fundus, the character, the amount and the color of the lochial discharge and the condition of the perineum and episiotomy. Furthermore, it is equally important for the nurse to be alert to the mother's general comfort and well-being—how she rests and sleeps, her activity, her appetite, her emotional status and, particularly, because of its vast influence, how she is adjusting to her role as a new mother.

Temperature, Pulse and Respiration

The temperature is carefully watched during the first few days of the puerperium, since fever is usually the first symptom of an infectious process. The pulse rate provides a helpful guide in determining the significance of a rise in temperature. These observations are usually made and recorded every four to eight hours for the first few days after delivery, omitting the 2 A.M. observations, which would disturb the mother's sleep. If the temperature rises above 37.8° C. (100° F.) or the pulse rate above 100, the physician should be notified immediately. Usually, the blood pressure is checked daily unless there has been some abnormality. Then observations and recordings are made every two to four hours or more frequently, as indicated.

Nutrition

Very shortly following the delivery, after having gone without food or fluids for some hours, the mother may express a desire for something to eat. Unless she has received a general anesthetic or is nauseated, there is usually no contraindication to giving her some nourishment. She usually enjoys a normal diet.

The two factors to bear in mind when considering the mother's diet are: 1) providing for her general nutrition and 2) providing enough nourishing foods to supply the additional calories and nutrients required during lactation. If these nutritional requirements are provided for, the mother's convalescence will be more rapid, her strength will be recovered more quickly, and the quality and quantity of her milk will be better. She will also be more able to resist infections.

Mothers in general, and particularly mothers who are breast-feeding, usually have good appetites and become hungry between meals. For this reason it is advisable to see that they receive intermediate nourishment consisting of a nourishing beverage or a snack three times a day. If the nourishment is in the form of a glass of milk or some milk product, this helps to incorporate the additional milk requirement for the nursing mother.

Rest and Sleep

During the puerperium the mother needs an abundance of rest and can be encouraged to relax and sleep whenever possible. This can best be accomplished if she is comfortable and free from worry and other anxiety-producing situations. The need for rest has even more significance for the mother who is breast-feeding, because worry and fatigue inhibit her milk supply. With the exception of the father, visitors can be limited during the first few days because they can be tiring. A mother who is not getting sufficient rest is usually anxious, and worries over minor things that otherwise might cause her little concern. Furthermore, many emotional problems are often precipitated by sleeplessness and fatigue.

It becomes the nurse's responsibility to adjust the hospital routine whenever possible to provide the mother with uninterrupted periods of rest. Routine procedures can be delayed or rearranged to meet the mother's needs. A bottle-fed infant may be fed occasionally by the nurse if the mother is sleeping and does not want to be awakened. If the mother is unable to nap during the day (and she may not, due to excitement and fatigue), she can be encouraged to rest as quietly as possible for certain periods. The need for rest and sleep may have to be explained and reiterated, especially during the "taking-hold" phase (p. 419), as she is eager to be up and about and may tend to overdo.

Early Ambulation

Early ambulation has intrinsic health-promoting value for the newly delivered mother. With this increase in exercise, circulation is stimulated, and there are fewer complications of thrombophlebitis. Moreover, bladder and bowel functions are improved, with the result that bladder complications leading to catheterization are greatly reduced. Abdominal distention and constipation occur less frequently. The majority of healthy mothers are allowed out of bed in four to eight hours.

If the patient has had a conduction anesthesia which involves entering the dura, she may be kept in a recumbent position for about the first eight hours. It is felt by many physicians that keeping the patient flat in bed for this time helps to prevent the occurrence of a postspinal headache, since headache is precipitated and aggravated when the head is elevated. Postspinal headache is thought to be caused by a leakage of the spinal fluid through the puncture hole of the dura, with subsequent decrease in cerebrospinal fluid volume and pressure. Therefore, having the patient in a recumbent position while the puncture hole is sealing, and encouraging the patient to force fluids (to hasten fluid replacement) may help this condition.

The first time that any mother is out of bed she can "dangle" for a short time before actually getting up. Then usually she can walk a few steps from the bed and sit in a chair for a brief period. On succeeding times up, she can increase her activity gradually. The newly delivered mother needs someone to assist her in and out of bed and to go with her when she walks to the bathroom. The nurse will want to remain close at hand while the mother is in the bathroom so that she can give immediate assistance if the mother becomes weak or faint.

It is important that the nurse explain the purposes of early ambulation to the mother and help her to learn how she can achieve an effective combination of sitting, walking and lying in bed. All too many mothers feel that once they are out of bed they are "on their own," and expected to take care of themselves entirely. Most of them are afraid of being a nuisance and hesitate to ask for help, whereas others do not realize that help is available. The nurse's attitude is important. Acting interested in the mother, demonstrating a desire to help her and making her feel comfortable will encourage the mother to ask for help. New mothers, in particular, are sensitive to the attitudes of those responsible for their care. Many of them are experiencing an enforced dependency for the first time in their adult lives and find this difficult. Others become resentful because they feel that they are being forced toward independence too quickly. By recognizing each patient as an individual the nurse is able to gain insight in providing for the mother's total nursing needs.

Although it is customary for mothers to be discharged home on the second or third day, it should be remembered that early ambulation and the duration of the hospital stay are two entirely different matters. Regardless of the day of discharge, mothers need to be cautioned to proceed slowly at home during the puerperium, resting a large part of the time. If teaching about "getting back to routine gradually" was begun early in the antepartal period, the mother will be better prepared.

Bathing

The mother is prone to have marked diaphoresis in the early puerperium, so that she will find a daily shower refreshing and a source of comfort. When the mother showers for the first time, the nurse usually will give the self-care instructions for breast care, perineal care and other aspects of physical care. The nurse will be guided by the mother's readiness to learn as well as by the realization that the mother can absorb only so much information at one time. Subsequently, when the mother is able to absorb the information, the nurse can explain about breast care, perineal hygiene, elimination, general activity and hospital routines.

Showers usually are permitted as soon as the patient becomes ambulatory. The first time or two that the mother takes a shower, the nurse or the attendant should remain nearby for safety. It is particularly important that a patient who has had a cesarean section be instructed regarding her bathing. Usually, these patients are not allowed to shower even though they are ambulatory, since the incision should be kept dry until it has closed, and the sutures have been removed. Tub baths usually are allowed in two weeks.

Urinary Elimination

The newly delivered mother may not express a desire to void, in part because the bladder capacity is increased as a result of reduced interabdominal pressure. In addition, if the mother has received analgesia or anesthesia during labor, the sensation of a full bladder may be further diminished. The mother should be encouraged to void within the first six to eight hours following the delivery. It is not prudent, however, to adhere to a designated time for the mother to empty her bladder, but rather on evidence indicating the degree of bladder distention. It is well to keep in mind that there is an increased urinary output during the early puerperium. Moreover, mothers who have received intravenous fluids are very likely to develop a full bladder. As the bladder fills with urine, it gradually protrudes above the symphysis pubis and can be observed bulging in front of the uterus. If the bladder is markedly distended, the uterus may be pushed upward and to the side and may become relaxed. When a hand is cupped over the fundus to massage it and to bring the uterus back to its midline position, the bladder will protrude still further. When the hand is removed, the uterus will return to its displaced position.

Further evidence of bladder distention can be gained by palpation and percussion of the lower abdomen, which will reveal a difference in consistency between the uterus and the bladder. The latter will be ballotable and filled with liquid in contrast with the uterus, which will have a firm tone. Such observations are of extreme importance and demand immediate attention.

A full bladder is considered to be one of the causes of postpartal hemorrhage, and if the bladder is permitted to become distended, urinary retention will inevitably follow.

Some mothers have difficulty in voiding at first. As a result of the labor itself, the tone of the bladder wall may be temporarily impaired, or the tissues at the base of the bladder and around the urethra may be edematous. When the mother is allowed early bathroom privileges, urinary elimination may present no problem. On the other hand, some efforts may be needed to excite normal urination. Running water so that the mother can hear it, letting the mother dabble her fingers in water or offering a beverage (preferably warm) may help to initiate voiding.

If the mother must be on bedrest, the nurse can assist the mother in voiding by helping her assume a comfortable position on the bedpan, providing privacy and giving her assurance that she will soon be able to urinate. The nurse will want to offer the mother a bedpan at intervals of two to three hours at first and measure the urine at each voiding during the first day (or days) until it has been established that the mother is emptying her bladder completely. A voiding must measure 100 ml. to be considered satisfactory.

At the first voiding, it may be apparent that the bladder has not been entirely emptied. If the bladder is not distended, the mother may be allowed to wait for an hour or so, as the second voiding usually empties the bladder. If, however, the mother continues to void small amounts frequently, one may suspect that she has residual urine, and these voidings are the result of the overflow of a distended bladder. If all attempts fail and the mother cannot void a sufficient quantity, catheterization will be necessary. Because of the risk of hospital-induced infection, it is very important to avoid this procedure unless the mother is absolutely unable to void, despite astute and persistent nursing intervention.

Catheterization. Although the procedure for catheterization varies to some degree in different hospitals, the principles involved are essentially the same. Aseptic technique must be maintained throughout to avoid introducing bacteria into the bladder or contaminating the birth canal. If the mother is given routine perineal care prior to the catheterization procedure, the potential danger of infection is further reduced.

Because there is a certain amount of soreness of the external genitalia, it is important to proceed with extreme gentleness and convey an awareness of the additional tenderness. As the labia are separated to expose the vestibule, care should be exercised so as not to pull on the perineal sutures. The meatus may be difficult to locate due to the edema and consequent distortion of the tissues; therefore a good light is imperative.

The urinary meatus and surrounding area are cleansed prior to the insertion of the catheter. The cleansing procedure is carried out in a gentle manner with just enough friction to allow proper cleansing of the area. None of the cleansing solution is permitted to run into the vaginal orifice because of the danger of contaminating the birth canal. Immediately following the cleansing, a dry cotton ball can be placed at the introitus to prevent excretion from the vagina (i.e., blood or lochia) from spreading upward to the urinary meatus, from which it can be carried into the bladder when the catheter is inserted.

Intestinal Elimination

Constipation. Because the bowel tends to remain relaxed in the early puerperium (as in pregnancy), intestinal elimination may be somewhat of a problem. In view of the sluggishness of the bowels during this time, constipation can be anticipated unless certain measures are instituted to prevent it. It is common to give a stool softener each night after delivery and/or a laxative or mild cathartic on the evening of the first or second day following delivery. If a bowel evacuation has not occured by the morning of the second or third day, a cleansing enema or a suppository may be prescribed. The latter is very effective and less traumatic for most patients.

If there has been no elimination and especially if the mother has had more extensive perineal repair done, an oil retention enema, followed some hours later by a cleansing enema, sometimes is prescribed.

The mother who is breast-feeding will be advised to follow her physician's prescription if laxatives are required to encourage proper elimination after she is discharged from the hospital. Certain laxatives are excreted in breast milk and therefore affect the infant. In addition, the usual measures employed to encourage good bowel habits (i.e., adequate fluid intake, roughage foods in the diet, establishing a habit time, and so on) are to be included in the health teaching.

Hemorrhoids. Hemorrhoids are a common problem for women during the postpartal period, as a result of pressure exerted on the pelvic floor by the presenting part and the straining of the expulsive phase of labor. They are most painful during the first two to three days after delivery, then gradually reduce in size and regress. Painful hemorrhoids are treated with sitz baths, anesthetic sprays, and cool astringent compresses (such as witch hazel or Tucks). Comfort is promoted by wearing perineal pads loosely and lying on the side in Sim's position while in bed. Prevention of constipation is the main measure to relieve ongoing difficulties with hemorrhoids.

Care of the Perineum

Observations of the condition of the vagina, perineum and perianal area are made regularly. The kind of lochia is noted, whether rubra, serosa, or alba, as well as its odor and whether clots are present. Lochia has a characteristic odor but should not smell foul. Presence of clots indicate heavy flow. Observing the lochia provides evidence of the progression of involution and enables the nurse to identify infection, hemorrhage and other complications. The mother is informed about the changes which should occur in lochia and the signs which would indicate problems. The difference between lochia and a menstrual period is explained.

The perineum is observed for healing and signs of complications, such as hematoma, bruising, swelling and tenderness. If an episiotomy has been done, the status of the stitches is assessed, particularly for infection and hematoma. The anal area is inspected for hemorrhoids and fissures. Usually some method of perineal cleansing is used after voiding and defecation, with the patient instructed in the method and the proper removal and application of perineal pads. Cotton balls, soap and water, or medicated wipes may be used, or a method employed such as use of the surgitator which directs a spray of solution onto the perineum while the patient sits on the toilet (Fig. 28-3).

The woman is instructed to cleanse and wipe from front to back in one motion, to prevent contamination of the vagina and urinary meatus with fecal material. She should wash her hands before applying a perineal pad and should not touch the inner surface of the pad before applying it from front to back. Pads should also be removed with this motion.

Perineal Discomfort. Following a spontaneous vaginal delivery without laceration, mothers usually do not experience perineal discomfort. It is most likely to be present if an episiotomy has been performed, or if lacerations have been repaired, particularly if the perineum is edematous and there is tension on the perineal sutures. Almost all primigravidas experience some degree of discomfort from an episiotomy, depending largely on the extent of the wound and the amount of suturing done. For the most part, during the first few days, local treatment in the form of dry heat, analgesic sprays or ointments is all that is necessary to alleviate the discomfort. But if the pain is more severe in the first day or so, such treatment may not be sufficient, and analgesic medications may have to be administered by mouth or hypodermic injection. Later

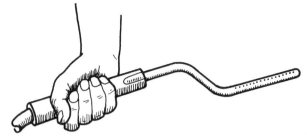

Figure 28-3. Surgitator for perineal care. With patient seated on toilet, nozzle is held several inches from perineum, solution flow is started, and flow directed against perineum. Nozzle does not touch perineum; each patient uses a new nozzle. Perineum is dried with gentle front-to-back blotting motion.

on, sitz baths may be ordered if the discomfort persists.

A perineal heat lamp may be used for 20 minutes three times per day. When the mother has assumed the dorsal recumbent position, the lamp can be easily slipped between her legs and placed about 10 to 12 inches from the perineum. After the perineum is exposed, the bulb is adjusted so that the light shines directly on it. The mother can be completely covered during the treatment, because the arch of the lamp frame acts as a cradle to support the top bedclothes.

Mothers who have discomfort from perineal sutures usually will find it uncomfortable to sit for the first few days. Many of them will be observed sitting in a rigid position, bearing their weight on one side of the buttocks or the other, with obvious discomfort to the back as well as the perineum. Therefore, it is important to teach the mother how to sit comfortably with her body erect.

In the sitting position, the perineum is suspended at the lowermost level of the ischial tuberosities, which bear the weight of the body. Thus, in order to achieve a greater measure of comfort, the mother must bring her buttocks together to relieve pressure and tension on the perineum, in the same manner as that described in the exercise for contraction and relaxation of pelvic floor muscles. After assuming a sitting position the mother is instructed to raise her hips very slightly from the chair, only enough to permit her to squeeze her buttocks together and contract the muscles of the pelvic floor, and hold them this way momentarily until after she has let her full weight down again. This exercise will also be helpful to the mother when she is reclining in bed.

Lower Extremities

The lower extremities are observed for varicosities, symmetry, edema, shape, size, temperature and color, and range of motion. Signs of thrombophlebitis include unilateral swelling, erythema, tenderness and pain in the calf when the foot is flexed with the leg extended (Homans' sign). Pulses in the lower extremities may be absent in thrombophlebitis. The mother is advised to avoid constricting garters or clothing which interferes with circulation.

Afterpains

Uterine contractions following delivery continue as part of involution and in some instances are felt as cramps similar to that of a menstrual period. Intermittent uterine contractions with subsequent afterpains occur more frequently in multiparas than in primiparas, because in primiparas the uterus remains tonically contracted. Afterpains are also more common and severe when there has been excessive distention of the uterus due to a large baby, hydramnios or multiple pregnancy. Breast-feeding mothers notice afterpains occurring when the infant nurses, because suckling stimulates release of oxytocin which increases uterine contractions. These cramps gradually diminish and are usually quite mild within 48 hours of delivery. Often simply explaining the cause of afterpains and their functional purpose enables the mother to tolerate them. If afterpains are severe, an analgesic is usually ordered to provide relief.

Breast Care

Routine breast care is directed at maintaining cleanliness and adequate breast support necessary for the normal function of the breasts and the comfort of the mother. The breasts should be handled gently and precautions given to avoid rough rubbing, massage or pressure on these organs.

The mother who is bottle-feeding her infant can bathe her breasts daily with mild soap and water; this is done most conveniently at the time of the daily shower or bath. No other special care need be given.

If the mother is breast-feeding, her nipples may be cleansed with clear water if cleansing is thought necessary. It is also recommended that soap not be used on the nipples; even the use of water is unnecessary under most circumstances since the nipple skin itself is cleansed by the natural antiseptic, lysozyme. It is important to instruct the mother not to use any drying agent (such as alcohol, etc.) on her nipples since it tends to remove the secretions of sebum, a physiologic emollient. Under normal circumstances, the best nipple care is provided by the body itself, without outside interference.[2] Additional cleansing before each nursing need not be done, but the mother is to be instructed to wash her hands with soap and water, as they will come in contact with the nipples and breast during nursing. In this way precautions can be taken against infection.

The mother can be encouraged to wear a well-fitting supportive nursing brassiere as soon as her milk begins to come (in about the second to fourth day but sometimes earlier). It is wise that she become accustomed to lowering the flaps of the bra occasionally during the day for 15 to 30 minutes to permit air to come in contact with the nipples. The brassiere should not have plastic liners in the cup to occlude air from the nipples. If there is leaking of milk the mother may use disposable breast pads and change them every time they become damp. This will promote the integrity of the nipples and inhibit infection since milk is a perfect medium for many bacteria.

Mothers who are not breast-feeding will also need breast support with a well-fitting brassiere. Usually these mothers will be given some type of lactation-suppressing hormone to help the breasts dry up, and engorgement is not a problem. Occasionally, however, they do suffer this phenomenon and may experience throbbing pains in the breasts which extend back into the axillae. During this time, analgesic medication may be required for pain relief until the condition subsides in one or two days. Ice bags to the breasts and axillae also are often helpful.

Engorgement

Breast discomfort several days after delivery has been attributed to venous and lymphatic engorgement, which mothers experience in relation to initiation of lactation. It has been proposed that postpartal breast discomfort can be attributed to two factors: 1) venous and lymphatic engorgement and 2) filling of the acini with milk. Most studies indicate that breast discomfort occuring during the first three or four postpartal days (the "initial breast engorgement") is due to venous engorgement. The breast discomfort appearing after the third or fourth postpartal day is due to the acini becoming filled with milk, called "late engorgement."

The peak incidence of discomfort seems to occur on the fourth or the fifth day postpartum. It is believed that the engorgement is caused by the pressure from the increased amount of milk in the lobes and ducts.

Symptoms.   When the milk "comes in," the breasts suddenly become larger, firmer and more tender; consequently, many mothers experience varying degrees of discomfort. Some do not seem to be bothered by this transitory condition (and produce a large quantity of milk), but the majority usually have at least a moderate amount of tenderness and pain. A few experience a great deal of discomfort, with throbbing pains in the breast, extending to the axilla.

The engorgement may distend the breasts so much that the skin appears to be shiny. The tissue surrounding the nipple may also become taut to the extent that it actually retracts the nipple, making it extremely difficult for the baby to grasp the nipple and the areola adequately. It used to be thought that fever was a normal consequence of this condition; however, engorgement is *not* an inflammatory process, and if fever occurs, some other cause should be suspected. Still the breasts may be reddened and feel warm to the touch. They can be very painful, and they become more so when touched or moved.

Although this condition is transitory and usually disappears in 24 to 48 hours, prompt treatment is to be instituted, not only for the mother's comfort but also to prevent the condition from progressing. If engorgement is allowed to become marked, then emptying of the breasts (which is the basis of treatment) becomes very difficult because the ducts become occluded by the surrounding congested tissues and the thick and tenacious character of the retained secretions. Secondary lymphatic and venous stasis may occur because the milk cannot be emptied.

Prevention of engorgement is preferable to treatment and is generally possible with good management. Early and regular nursing is considered by many to be the best preventive measure. When the mother and infant are together around the clock as in rooming-in, engorgement tends to occur less since the baby can nurse in response to the mother's needs as well as his own. If rooming-in is not available, the infant can be taken to the mother as soon as her breasts begin to fill and as often thereafter as is necessary to maintain her comfort. It is important that the mother's requests for her infant be met promptly and with friendliness; she can be reassured that even if the infant may not be hungry immediately, he soon will be.

Management.   Engorgement may be relieved by removing the milk, supporting the breast, applying hot packs and/or ice bags and administering analgesics for the relief of pain. Removal of the milk may be facilitated by the use of oxytocin before the baby nurses to encourage the let-down reflex. Interestingly enough, this drug sometimes is used to relieve discomfort from engorgement in mothers who are not nursing. The way in which the drug relieves pain in breasts that are not being emptied is unclear. In addition, manual expression of the milk and pumping, as well as the use of a nipple shield (to help the baby to grasp the nipple), may be recommended. Some mothers find the use of hot packs 15 to 20 minutes before nursing improves the flow of milk. Often ice packs between nursing periods are very useful in alleviating discomfort. The importance of a good uplift support for the breasts cannot be stressed enough, particularly during the period of engorgement. Analgesics such as aspirin, propoxyphene (Darvon) or codeine frequently are used for pain relief. These should be given in adequate dosage and with appropriate timing so that the mother can be relatively comfortable during nursing. Since engorgement is transitory, the drugs are needed for a very short time; hence any danger to the infant is minimal.

Care of the Nipples

Too much emphasis cannot be placed on the care of the nipples to facilitate breast-feeding. Cleanliness is a cardinal principle. Thus, keeping the nipples clean and dry is basic to keeping them in good condition.

Sore nipples are a frequent complaint during the mother's early breast-feeding experience; she can be instructed to report any discomfort so that corrective measures may be instituted at once.

Sore nipples can be treated after each nursing period with the application of a bland cream or ointment, such as lanolin or a commercially prepared compound (e.g., Massé Nipple Cream or Vitamin A and D Ointment). Many hospitals advocate the use of a thermalite (therapeutic) lamp for tender or cracked nipples; the affected breast is exposed for 20 to 30 minutes twice a day. The mother can be advised that even the exposure of the breast to fresh air for similar periods is beneficial.

When a sore nipple is examined, it may be found to be fissured (cracked) or to have a small erosion or blister. Interestingly, more frequent feedings day and night have been recommended in these cases to prevent overstrenuous sucking and to keep the breasts from becoming too full and thus making the nipple difficult to grasp easily.[3] Letting the nipples dry after nursing by exposing them to air and the judicious use of a nipple cream have also been recommended for helping control this condition. Manual expression of the milk to relieve engorgement can also be instituted if the sore nipples are a result of this problem. Cracked and raw nipples afford an easy portal of entry for pathogenic bacteria to gain access to the breast and to cause infection. If mastitis or abscess occurs, the physician usually suggests that breast-feeding be terminated. This is not always the case, however, since with the aid of antibiotics some women are permitted to continue.

Postpartum Exercises

Exercises may be initiated postpartally to hasten recovery, prevent complications, and strengthen the muscles of the back, pelvic floor and abdomen. By toning the muscles, these exercises assist the mother to restore her figure and can be psychologically beneficial. Exercises can be started on the first postpartum day and increased gradually. The mother must take care not to overexercise and to allow slow progression in adding to the routine. A new exercise can be added daily, with each done five to ten times per day for at least six weeks after

delivery (see Chap. 18, chart on postpartum exercises).

Kegal's exercises can be taught to increase vaginal tone which may be flaccid and distended following delivery. This exercise consists of contracting the muscles of the perineum with enough force to stop a stream of urine. The contraction is held for a few seconds and then released. The exercise is repeated 50 to 100 times and can be done several times per day.

PARENTAL GUIDANCE AND INSTRUCTION

Each mother's understanding and ability in providing infant care will vary, depending largely on her background and previous experiences. Undoubtedly, the primipara who has not been accustomed to infants will have much to learn about the care and handling of her new baby. On the other hand, the multipara may feel uncertain about the response of an older child to the new baby and thus require guidance in understanding and dealing with sibling rivalry. Many mothers need to know more about their own care; others need to know how to facilitate certain adjustments within the home or the family group. If the mother knows what she can expect and what to do, she usually can handle simple problems that might otherwise cause fear or apprehension.

Proper care for the mother during the puerperium emphasizes the need for rest, nourishing food and protection from worry. Parents, as a rule, seem to be under the impression that once the delivery is over, things return to "normal," allowing them to resume their usual activities immediately. However, it is agreed that it may be weeks before the generative organs have returned to normal size and position and the emotional and endocrine adjustments made.

One of the most important points to be emphasized is that the mother should proceed *as slowly as possible* in the postpartal period at home. The general feeling of well-being and the excitement of having the baby, together with the emotions aroused in the "taking-hold" phase, all too often provide so great a stimulus that the mother has a tendency to overdo. If there are other children in the household, especially toddlers, the demands on the mother may be considerable.

If it is at all possible, the major responsibilities of housekeeping should be taken over by a "helper," so that the mother can be more relaxed and devote herself primarily to caring for her new infant and spending more time with the immediate family. At this time family relationships can be strengthened if the mother is not overwhelmed with apprehension and fatigue. The subject of household assistance needs to be explored thoroughly with the mother (and if necessary, the father).

The parents may need help in realizing what possibilities and alternatives they have in this matter. Some parents, for instance, manage very nicely when the father takes some vacation time and assumes management of the household. However, it must be remembered that not all fathers are able (or willing) to shoulder this considerable task. Other couples can rely on parents, in-laws or relatives for a time. Still others must hire outside help; in these cases the expense and consequent budgeting may have to be discussed.

If outside help is employed, then the mother may have some question as to whether a housekeeper or a "nurse" (to take care of the baby) would be more desirable. This, of course, will depend on many factors. Most mothers find that when they are relieved of the heavy housekeeping chores, the "care" of the baby is relatively easy and provides an opportunity to get thoroughly acquainted with the new addition to the household.

By the time the mother leaves the hospital, she should have at least a basic understanding of her own condition and status, and she ought to know what physical and emotional changes to expect. In addition, she should be familiar with the daily care of her baby and know what to expect of him, as well as any other important details related to infant care. Parents also need to know how and where to contact the physician if any medical problem pertaining to either the mother or the infant should arise before the next scheduled visit.

Since the present-day maternity stay is rather short, some type of follow-up service often is desirable and necessary. Therefore, parents need to be offered information about the services of the public health nursing agency in the community and how they may use these services. In cases of obvious need a referral to an agency should be instituted before the patient leaves the hospital.

Individual Teaching

Regardless of the fact that a mother may attend all the group classes offered in the maternity hospital, each mother should be given individual help to learn how to handle and care for her infant while she is in the hospital, particularly if this is her first baby. Many new mothers are timid at first because they do not know what to expect of their infants, or they are afraid of what they will do to them because of their own feelings of inadequacy. A mother who has had no previous experience with infants will need some guided practice in changing diapers, dressing her baby and handling the infant in general (Fig. 28-4). Rooming-in units provide an environment in which the mother can have such an experience over an extended period of time. However, even in situations in which the infants are kept in a central nursery, the nurse will want to plan to spend some time with the mother, in addition to the regular feeding periods, to help her learn to care for her baby. If hospital staffing permits the time, it may be desirable for some mothers to bathe their own infants at the bedside, under the nurse's guidance, before leaving the hospital. There is no reason that such practices should violate the "clean nursery technique" if they have been properly planned.

A rooming-in experience is undoubtedly beneficial for mother, father and baby. But when this is not possible because of hospital facilities or policies, a daily extended visiting period can be extremely helpful. In this way the parents and the baby can become better acquainted in the security of the maternity division, where experienced personnel are near at hand to answer the parents' questions and to offer advice.

Sexuality and Contraception

Postpartum sexuality is affected by the degree to which the mother's steroid hormones have been depleted following delivery. This is discussed more fully in Chapter 11. Postpartum instructions are given regarding resumption of intercourse, with the couple advised that sex is appropriate after lochia has ceased and the perineum has healed to the point that intercourse is not painful, and as long as there are no contraindicating factors such as hematoma or infection.

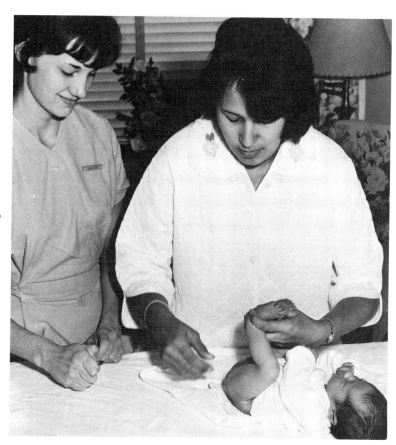

Figure 28-4. Helping mother to learn how to handle her infant.

Sexual adjustment following birth of a baby is a major concern of new parents, and often a source of conflict and confusion. The mother's interest in intercourse is usually less than her partner's in the first month or so after delivery, and her physiologic responses diminish[4] because of low hormonal levels, the adjustment to the maternal role, and fatigue due to lack of sleep and rest. Lochia has generally ceased or progressed to the alba stage by two to four weeks postpartum, and the perineal area and episiotomy are well healed and not painful. If intercourse causes discomfort, the couple is advised to wait somewhat longer or use noncoital sexual practices if they find this acceptable. Positions for intercourse which avoid the penile shaft pressing posteriorly on the perineum can also alleviate discomfort. In addition to the emotional benefits to the parents' relationship, intercourse after childbirth can promote perineal healing by softening the episiotomy scar.[5]

For most couples, intercourse is resumed before the six-weeks checkup, so it is important to provide contraceptive information before the mother leaves the hospital. Although it is unlikely that she will ovulate and become fertile before 6 weeks, it is possible. Many hospitals provide a supply of contraceptive vaginal cream and condoms and instruct the parents on their use before discharge.

THE FIRST WEEKS AT HOME

The process of integration of a new baby into the family is a stressful period and one in which there is little professional help available. Many parents have no contact with health providers during the time between discharge from the hospital and the six-weeks checkup, although they are contending with major changes and adjustments in what is often a new experience in their lives. In contrast to the cultural ideals of joyful parenthood and fantasies of blissful motherhood, many women find the first few weeks of their child's life to be extremely disillusioning.[6] The household is often disorganized and untidy, with greatly increased work related to diapers, feeding and care of the new baby, while the mother copes with fatigue and frustration in trying to learn the baby's patterns and ways of communicating. Within the first six weeks, many mothers find that they have yelled at and spanked their infants, that they cannot cope with or understand the baby's crying, that they feel trapped spending the greatest part of their lives caring for the baby, and that they wish they had not had the baby because they feel unsuited for such responsibility.[7]

The concerns of new mothers in the first weeks after delivery cover a wide range, and there seem to be few resources to assist them in coping with problems and providing information and support. The most common concerns expressed by new mothers are in the following areas: changes in their figures, fatigue and lack of sleep, infant care, changing roles and life styles, and nursing care.

Changes in Body Image

One of the most frequently expressed concerns of the postpartum involves return of the figure to normal. This concern appears to be more than just a minor anxiety. Although new mothers are initially delighted when their abdomens decrease in size after delivery, this positive feeling turns to dismay in the days and weeks following when the abdominal wall remains soft and flabby and part of the weight gained during pregnancy is retained, making it impossible to wear clothes that fit before pregnancy. Frequently, the mother feels as though she is still several months pregnant.

Although mothers may want to lose weight and tighten up muscles, they often find that the baby's demands and their own fatigue interfere with these attempts. A flabby postpartum figure, and the feeling that one lacks the control or ability to improve it, can be a source of depression.[8] Partners, too, are often disappointed because of the time it takes for the figure to become slim again, and both partners may fear that the figure changes are permanent. Another source of concern is the lack of tone in the vaginal introitus which carries many implications for the couple's sexual relationship.

The first few weeks at home can also be a time of continued physical discomfort, much to the woman's dismay, especially if she has anticipated a quick return to normal. Persistent discomforts—from episiotomy pain which lasts about two to three weeks, breast engorgement, which is a source of discomfort for both breast-feeding and nonbreast-feeding mothers, nipple soreness and the annoyance of leaking milk—all are troubling in themselves and a drain on energy at a time when added strength is needed to respond to the infant's constant demands. The continued discharge of lochia may also be disconcerting, particularly if it is compared to a menstrual period.

Fatigue and Lack of Sleep

Fatigue appears to be a consistent problem for new mothers. Labor and delivery are hard, exhausting work, followed immediately by the demands of caring for a totally dependent infant. The short stay in the hospital is insufficient to restore energy levels, as excitement, the strange environment, and physical discomforts often interfere with rest and sleep. Most women have also not slept well during the last weeks of pregnancy. This leaves them with a tremendous deficit of energy and sleep, which increases sharply during the first weeks at home with the baby.

Sleep deprivation is to some degree a part of living for all new mothers, and it can be severe. The mother's sleep needs are curtailed by the baby's needs for food and attention. It may be difficult for new mothers to obtain more than 30 to 45 minutes of uninterrupted sleep per night, particularly if there are other small children who frequently need attention at night. Increased bodily tension as a result can lead to insomnia when there is the opportunity to sleep. Mothers may find themselves resenting their partner's ability to sleep uninterrupted. Sleep deprivation can also produce changes in mood and mental functioning, with the mother experiencing increased anxiety, apathy, depression, withdrawal, irritability, illogical thought patterns, mental confusion and aggression and decreased sociability.[9]

Infant Care

Concerns about caretaking activities for the infant vary. Many primiparae have had little previous contact with infants and possess small knowledge of procedures and the common behaviors expected. Often care is learned by trial and error because there are few sources of expert advice. Infants are quite different in their patterns, so even multiparae may find that their prior experience does not apply to this infant. Babies range from quiet to active and respond in different ways to attempts to console and comfort them. A new mother must learn her baby's particular patterns and why he cries and fusses at various times. The greatest part of this learning occurs during the first few weeks after birth, and the difficulty is compounded by such concerns and problems as fatigue, discomforts and worries about restoration of the figure.

Mothers are concerned about how normal their infant's behaviors are, particularly in the areas of weight gain and loss, crying, bowel movements, feedings, and sleeping patterns.[10] There is little written information which can help identify ranges of normal, and health professionals often do not discuss specific changes that may occur during the first months of life. Parents are often surprised at the range of behaviors among infants. Conflicting advice regarding how frequently the baby should be fed, when to add solid food, when to pick up a crying baby, what clothes to put on the baby, who should be allowed to visit and when, and so forth leads to further confusion.

The processes for successful mothering have apparently been set in motion by the end of the first month following birth. The way a mother perceives her one-month-old infant is an indication of the child's subsequent growth and development and reflects the degree to which the mother is satisfied with her interaction with the infant. If she feels rewarded, she has a more positive perception of the infant and reinforcement of her own identity as a mother. This, in turn, fosters a nurturing relationship.[11] Clearly, nursing intervention before maternal perception is set should be aimed at increasing the mother's sense of mastery and satisfaction in infant care, thereby promoting healthier infant development.

Changing Roles and Life Styles

Few parents are prepared for the amount of change required in their roles, relationships and life styles as the infant is integrated into the family. Many parents may actually "grieve" over the passing of former life patterns. The mother particularly may have to make major changes in career and other activities, although the gratifications of motherhood

may be enough to compensate for these relinquishments. Changes occur in the family constellation, with problems related to jealousy among the other children and marital problems between spouses arising from relative neglect of their relationship. With less time for each other, and possible strain in their sexual relations, many couples report stress in their relationship following the birth of a new baby. Social isolation, lack of recreational activities, and financial concerns can compound family stresses.

Nursing Care

The structure of the health care provided during childbearing makes it difficult to respond appropriately to concerns and problems which can occur during the first few weeks at home. This period represents a gap in health care services, with limited resources available to patients and families. However, the nurse can provide some anticipatory care during that phase of the prenatal period when the mother will be most responsive to this type of information. Prenatally, the woman primarily focuses attention on the pregnancy and preparation for labor and delivery. During the third trimester, however, there is increased interest in caretaking activities, so that teaching related to infant behavior and infant care can be productive at this time. As the mother expresses some anticipated concern, the nurse can discuss these problem areas with the prenatal patient, including such topics as preparing other children for the new baby, exploring ways to meet the increased demands of a new baby for attention and continuous care, considering sources of potential stress to the marital and family relations and ways of coping with these problems.

Reinforcing the importance of some kind of help with household tasks during the first few postpartal weeks at home may encourage the mother to arrange for such help to alleviate fatigue and sleep deprivation. If the mother can appreciate that she will need time to regain her energy levels to compensate for the numerous drains that will occur in late pregnancy and postpartally, she may be more realistic in her expectations. Also knowing that her figure will take time to return to its prepregnant form and that physical discomforts will exist for a time after delivery will prepare the parents and reduce the dissonance which occurs when expectations are not borne out by reality.

Assessment	Intervention	Evaluation
Postdelivery observations Fundal checks Bleeding Status of bladder Vital signs Condition of perineum	Give gentle massage of fundus if boggy Express clots from fundus Report and record amount and character of bleeding Report and record increase in pulse rate or decrease in blood pressure, elevation of temperature Encourage voiding if bladder becomes filled; catheterize if distended and unable to void Report development of hematoma or bleeding from episiotomy	Fundus maintained well contracted Bleeding, normal amount without clots Vital signs stable Bladder emptied as needed Episiotomy remains intact
Family interactions Comfort and rest Mother-infant contact Contact with partner or companion	Comfort measures (position, keep clean and dry, provide fluids as appropriate, encourage rest by doing observations efficiently) Enable mother to hold and explore infant, if condition permits Enable partner or companion to visit mother and infant Respond to questions about labor and delivery, status of infant, postpartum status	Mother rests well between observations Mother holds and explores infant Partner or companion visits, able to interact satisfactorily Questions answered adequately
Hospital postpartum observations Vital signs Fundal checks Lochia Condition of perineum Elimination Ambulation and rest Nutrition Comfort Breast care	Record progress of involution, report signs of hemorrhage, infection, hematoma, thrombophlebitis Instruct in perineal and breast care Administer stool softeners, laxatives as needed Provide supportive measures to enjoy nutritious diet, snacks Measure first voiding, check for bladder residual, catheterize as needed Assist patient to ambulate and shower first time Plan procedures to provide rest times without interruptions	Involution progresses normally without complications Bowel and bladder elimination maintained Patient able to do perineal and breast care Patient's appetite good Ambulates without tiring Able to rest and sleep well
Development of mothering relation	Provide opportunity for extended mother-infant contact Answer questions about infant behavior and care, feeding Provide specific instruction in areas of infant care as needed	Able to feed and care for infant satisfactorily No further questions
Integration of infant into family	Discuss family adaptation to new baby, changes in routines, response of father and other children Provide information, referrals as appropriate to individual needs Assist in planning for care of infant at home, management of tasks and sources of assistance	Mother's questions are answered and concerns responded to Expresses comfort with family's ability to adapt to new baby Identifies specific sources of help Follows through on referrals
Sexuality and contraception	Discuss postpartum sexual responses and alterations Instruct on when to resume intercourse, signs of problems Advise on contraceptive method until six-weeks checkup	Validates understanding of changes in sexual response, when to resume intercourse, use of contraception Uses contraceptive measure successfully
Six-weeks checkup Progress of involution Family adaptation to new baby Contraception	Examine reproductive organs, provide specific treatment for problems Discuss routines of infant care, responses of family, concerns and problems, resumption of activities Discuss contraceptive methods, benefits and risks	Involution complete, reproductive organs returned to prepregnant condition Family adaptation and routines are stable and functional Contraceptive method instituted and used successfully

Postpartally, there is limited time for teaching and providing supportive care in the aforementioned areas of concern. Priorities must be set, and focus set on information concerning bodily changes and methods for relieving physical discomforts. Exercises and diet assume an important place and specific instruction is helpful. During hospitalization, the mother may not be very receptive to learning about infant care, as her needs are directed more toward identification and claiming, or getting to know, her baby than toward details of caretaking. The best time to instruct and reinforce specific techniques in infant care will be when the mother is engaged in feeding her infant and attending to his needs. Providing the mother with written brochures and instructions in infant care procedures is another effective way of offering information at a time when she is more receptive and will feel the need directly.

Most women can benefit from professional contact within the first one to two weeks after leaving the hospital. By this time, they have experienced most of the demands and difficulties in integrating the new baby into the family and have specific questions and concerns. Mothers can be assisted to recognize and respond appropriately to their baby's unique patterns and ways of communicating and to identify various states of consciousness of the infant and its particular needs for stimulation, sleep and feeding. When able to respond more smoothly to her infant, the mother's satisfactions are increased and the development of a healthy relationship encouraged.[12]

Community health nurses may be available to visit new mothers and provide this teaching and support during the first few weeks at home. For many others, however, there is no clearly identifiable resource and they are often reluctant to call the hospital or physician's office with these kinds of concerns. Even provision of such contact by telephone as part of postdischarge care would be helpful.[13]

THE SIX-WEEKS CHECKUP

A follow-up visit in the physician's office or clinic is scheduled for six weeks after delivery, to evaluate the process of involution and the woman's and family's adaptation to the new baby. At this visit, weight, blood pressure, breast, pelvic and perineal examinations are done. The amount and character of lochia is assessed, along with the size and position of the uterus and cervix and the condition of the breasts and nipples, especially if the mother is breast feeding. Problems with healing or infection are treated if present. The family's response to the new baby is discussed, and questions related to behavior, patterns of feeding, sleep and elimination, crying, weight gain and so forth are explored. The need for further care or referrals is identified.

Contraception is discussed at this visit, and a suitable method decided upon if the parents wish to prevent another pregnancy. The method is instituted at this time and the couple instructed in its uses and risks. The mother's concerns about rest and exercise, weight, diet, her energy level, household tasks, relations with relatives and friends, sexual relations, and physical needs or discomforts are discussed. If weight continues to be a problem, a suitable weight reduction diet and other measures can be started. If desired, the woman can resume full employment or activities at this time, if there are no complications and she feels psychologically ready.

REFERENCES

1. M. H. Klaus and J. H. Kennell: *Maternal-Infant Bonding*. St. Louis, C. V. Mosby, 1976, pp. 12–14, 50–66.

2. B. Countryman: "Breast care in the early puerperium." *JOGN* 2:36–40, Sept./Oct. 1973.

3. Ibid.

4. K. Kyndely: "The sexuality of women in pregnancy and postpartum: A review." *JOGN* 28–31, Jan./Feb. 1978.

5. A. L. Clark and R. W. Hale: "Sex during and after pregnancy." *AJN* 74:1430, 1974.

6. F. Roberts: *Perinatal Nursing*. New York, McGraw-Hill, 1977, pp. 165–167.

7. A. L. Clark: "Recognizing discord between mother and child and changing it to harmony." *MCN—Am. J. Maternal Child Nursing* 100–106, March/April 1976.

8. M. Gruis: "Beyond maternity: Postpartum concerns of mothers." *MCN—Am. J. Maternal Child Nursing* 182–188, May/June 1977.

9. Roberts, op. cit.

10. M. S. Brown and J. T. Hurlock: "Mothering

the mother." *Am. J. Nurs.* 77:439–441, March 1977.

11. Clark, op. cit.
12. A. L. Clark and D. D. Affonseo: "Infant behavior and maternal attachment: Two sides to the coin." *MCN—Am. J. Maternal Child Nursing* 95–99, March/April 1976.

13. Brown and Hurlock, op. cit.

SUGGESTED READING

Ludington-Hoe, S. M.: "Postpartum: Development of maternicity." *Am. J. Nurs.* 77: 1171–1179, July 1977.

Smith, D. and Smith, H. L.: "Toward improvements in parenting." *JOGN* 22–27, November/December 1978.

Rubin, R.: "Binding-in in the postpartum period." *Maternal-Child Nursing J.* 6, 2:67–75, Summer 1977.

Barnard, M. A.: "Supportive nursing care for the mother and newborn who are separated from each other." *MCN—Am. J. Maternal Child Nursing* 107–110, March/April 1976.

Weir, R., and Feldman, W.: "A study of infant feeding practices." *Birth and the Family J.* 2: 64–65, Spring 1975.

Twenty-Nine

Care of the Newborn Infant

Physiology of the Newborn / Assessment of the Newborn / The Environment of the Newborn / Nursing Care of the Newborn

The care of the newborn infant presents an interesting challenge to those in maternity nursing. In a very short period of time, usually a matter of seconds, the fetus, who has been completely dependent on the mother to supply all his physiological needs, suddenly becomes an "independent" being. The physiological changes that occur at this time and during the next few hours and days are more profound than at any other period of life.

Although independent of the mother for vital functions, the new baby is, of course, still very dependent in other ways. He could not survive long without a caretaker. In the immediate postnatal period this caretaker is often the nurse.

Since these first days and weeks are so critical, the care given by the nurse is very important. The nurse must use the utmost care in handling the baby, keeping him warm and protecting him from exposure and injury, at the same time making accurate observations and recording and reporting them. Communication and teaching skills are utilized in contributing to the infant's future well-being by helping the parents to develop an understanding of their baby's needs and acquire skill in his care. In this way their concept of themselves as adequate parents is reinforced. The nurse also must be aware that some parents need assistance in developing healthy attitudes regarding childrearing

practices, so that the infant can make a satisfactory emotional and social adjustment. A close parent-infant relationship must be fostered (and provision made for this in the hospital environment), and communication must be maintained between the nurse and the parents.

PHYSIOLOGY OF THE NEWBORN

Before adapting to extrauterine life, the infant passes through several phases. This transitional period must be negotiated successfully if the infant is to survive and develop normally. The transition begins with labor when the fetus is stimulated by uterine contractions and pressure changes due to the rupture of the membranes. At birth a variety of foreign stimuli are encountered, such as light, sound, heat, cold and gravitation. Breathing then must start and profound changes and reorganization in the functioning of the organ systems and metabolic processes begin. Respiration must be initiated, circulation must shift from fetal to neonatal, hepatic and renal function must be altered and meconium passed. The final phase of the transition involves further reorganization of the metabolic processes to achieve a viable, steady state. This includes changes in blood oxygen saturation, reduction of enzymes, diminution in postnatal acidosis, and recovery of the neurologic tissues from the trauma of labor and delivery. Since these changes take time, it is no wonder that the infant's natal day is so crucial to his life and future well-being.

Respiratory Changes

Prior to birth, the oxygen needs of the fetus are met by the placenta. While the fetal lungs do not function as organs of respiration, it has been confirmed in recent years, that respiratory-like movements do occur. The function of this "fetal breathing" is not known, but some of the hypotheses are that it is "prenatal practice" for later breathing; may aid in the development of alveolar and bronchial structures; or might have some relationship to the synthesis, release, and distribution of surfactant.[1]

For the newborn to survive extrauterine life, adequate maturation of the lungs is essential. The lungs are in a continuous state of development structurally throughout fetal life and early childhood. About the twentieth week of gestation, canals begin to develop in the bronchial tree and primitive air sacs begin to form. By the twenty-eighth week, these are in close enough proximity to the developing blood vessel structures for gas exchange to be possible and surface-active lipoproteins (surfactant) to be detected for the first time, so there is a potential for independent survival. If born this early, though, the infant will have many possible respiratory problems as a result of the limited amount of surfactant and the incomplete development of the alveoli.[2] (See Chap. 38 for discussion of respiratory problems of the preterm infant.)

At the time of birth, the normal, full-term fetus is ready for the initiation of effective breathing. For example, fetal respiratory movements have prepared the lungs for this activity and the complex interrelationships of swallowing and breathing have been developed. With everything in readiness, the question is often asked, "What keeps the fetus from taking real breaths before it is born?" Some important inhibitory mechanisms have been identified. One of these is facial immersion. Another is the inhibition of respiration by the presence of fluid in the laryngeal area. This emphasizes the importance of clearing fluid from this area after birth. Also the fetal lungs are constantly filled with fluid thought to be secreted by the alveolar cells, and this fluid in the deep respiratory tracts stimulates inhibitory stretch receptors.[3]

Initiation of Respiration. A multiplicity of factors is probably involved in stimulating the infant's initial respirations. This would seem to provide a margin of safety for the infant. Physical, sensory, and chemical factors are involved, but precisely how each of these influences the other and to what degree is not known exactly. There is some evidence to indicate that the change in pressure from intrauterine to extrauterine life may produce enough physical stimulation to prompt respiration.

Of the sensory stimuli that have been thought to play a role, such as cold, pain, touch, light, sound and gravity, cold seems to be the most important. In animal studies, cold stimulation has induced breathing in fetal sheep.[4] This should not be taken to mean that the infant needs to be in a cold environment. Just being in normal room air of about 22° C (72° F) is a drop of more than 15° C (25° F) below the mother's normal body temperature which the neonate has been used to. (See p. 445 for discussion of thermal regulation of newborn.)

The chemical changes that occur in the blood as a result of the transitory asphyxia during delivery seem to be of paramount importance. These include a lowered oxygen level, an increased carbon dioxide level, and a lowered pH. If the asphyxia is prolonged, depression of the respiratory center ensues rather than stimulation, and resuscitation is usually necessary (see Chap. 38). A vigorous infant often breathes seconds after birth and certainly within one minute of delivery.

A great effort is required to expand the lungs and to fill the collapsed alveoli. Surface tension in the respiratory tract, as well as resistance in the lung tissue itself, the thorax, the diaphragm, and the respiratory muscles must be overcome. Moreover, any obstruction (i.e., mucus, and so on) in the air passages has to be cleared. The first active inspiration comes from a powerful contraction of the diaphragm, which creates a high negative intrathoracic pressure, causing a marked retraction of the ribs because of the pliability of the baby's thorax.

This first inspiration distends the alveolar spaces and on expiration a residual volume of nearly 20 ml. of air remains as molecules of pulmonary surfactant diminish surface tension. Therefore, the second breath will take less effort than the first, and the third breath even less, since by this time most of the small airways will be open. Fluid is rapidly removed from the lungs by drainage, swallowing, evaporation and pulmonary capillary and lymphatic circulation. After several minutes of breathing, lung expansion is usually complete.[5]

Respiration in First and Second Periods of Reactivity. A healthy infant begins life with intense activity. This phase has been designated by some authorities as the first period of reactivity. In this phase the infant exhibits outbursts of diffuse, purposeless movements which alternate with periods of relative immobility. At this time respiration is rapid (reaching as high as 80 breaths per minute), and there may be *transient* flaring of the alae nasi; retraction of the chest and grunting are not uncommon. Tachycardia also is present, at times reaching 180 beats per minute in the first minutes of life and thereafter falling to an average of 120 to 140 beats per minute.

After this initial response, the baby becomes relatively quiet and does not respond intensely to either internal or external stimuli. He relaxes and may fall asleep. His first sleep occurs on an average of two hours after birth and may last anywhere from a few minutes to two to four hours.

When he awakens, he is again hyperresponsive to stimuli, and he begins his second period of reactivity. His color may change rapidly (from pink to moderately cyanotic), and his heart rate responds to stimulation, becoming rapid. Oral mucus may be a major problem in respiration during this period. Choking, gagging, and regurgitation alert the nurse to the presence of mucus, and appropriate intervention must be taken (see Chap. 38). Since the length of the second period of reactivity is variable, the nurse must be particularly alert for the first 12 to 18 hours of the infant's life.

Character of Normal Respiration. As the infant adapts successfully to extrauterine life, his respiration usually ranges from 35 to 50 breaths per minute. They are easily altered by internal and external stimuli. Normally, his respiration is quiet and shallow. This can be observed most accurately by watching the movement of the abdomen, since his respiratory activity is carried out largely by the diaphragm and the abdominal muscles.

Periods of dyspnea and cyanosis may occur sud-denly in an infant who is breathing normally, even after the transition period is over. This *may* indicate some anomaly or other pathologic condition and should be reported promptly. Therefore, the nurse should notify the physician if the respiration drops below 35 or increases beyond 50 when the infant is at rest, or if dyspnea or cyanosis occurs.

Circulatory Changes

The anatomical changes that occur with birth have been discussed previously in Chapter 10. It will be recalled that a rapid change takes place with closure of several fetal structures and with the redistribution of oxygenated blood to a circulation similar to that of an adult. Since all changes are not immediately complete, this time of conversion may be called a period of *transitional circulation.*

Total Blood Volume. It is difficult to give accurate values for the total blood volume of the newborn because of the variables involved, such as time of clamping the umbilical cord, weight and gestational age of the infant, type of delivery (vaginal or cesarean section), and the time after delivery the determination is made.

For example, an additional 50 to 100 ml. of blood may be added to the circulation if the infant is placed below the level of the placenta and the clamping of the cord is delayed several minutes until the cord stops pulsating. Many studies have been done to help decide the issue of early or late clamping, but it is still unclear whether this placental transfusion that occurs with late clamping is advantageous for the infant. The rapid increase in blood volume might stress the heart and pulmonary vasculature, but according to some reports, incidence of neonatal respiratory distress is decreased with delayed clamping. The infants who receive this extra blood will gain an increased storage supply of iron, resulting from the breakdown of the additional hemoglobin. This may contribute to hyperbilirubinemia during the first week of life, but the iron stores may be utilized to good advantage later when iron is needed for rapid growth or when the dietary intake of iron is inadequate.[6]

The Peripheral Circulation. Peripheral circulation in the newborn is somewhat sluggish. It is felt that this accounts for the residual cyanosis of the infant's hands, feet, and circumoral area. These areas often remain mildly cyanotic for one or two hours after delivery. The general circulatory lability probably accounts for the mottled appearance of the baby's skin when it is exposed to air and for the "chilliness" of the infant's hands and feet.

The Pulse Rate. Like the rate of respiration, the pulse rate also is labile and generally follows a pattern similar to that of the respiration. When the respiration is rapid, the pulse tends to be rapid; similarly, when the respiration slows down, so does the pulse. Since the pulse is affected by both internal and external stimuli, taking the *apical* pulse rate while the baby is quiet will provide a more accurate evaluation of the infant's pulse rate. The normal rate is usually 120 to 150 beats per minute, but it may rise to 180 for short periods with crying and other intense activity, or drop to 100 during deep sleep.

The Blood Pressure. The blood pressure is not routinely checked on term newborns in most nurseries. It is difficult to get accurate blood pressure readings on newborn infants for several reasons. When the palpation method is used or auscultation with a stethoscope, only the systolic pressure is obtained. With the color change (flush) method, the result is the midpoint between the systolic and the diastolic pressure. Direct recording through an arterial catheter is more accurate, but usually is only used when there is reason to have an arterial catheter in place. A newer method using a Doppler-shift ultrasonic device for auscultation has shown good correlation with the direct method and has confirmed that the newborn's blood pressure is characteristically low, with a mean value of 71/49 at birth, rising slowly for the first week.[7]

Erythrocyte Count and Hemoglobin Concentration. The newborn infant has a much higher erythrocyte, hemoglobin and hematocrit level than an adult. The erythrocyte level ranges between 5,000,000 and 7,000,000 per microliter, the hemoglobin level is usually 15 to 20 gm. per 100 ml. of blood, and the hematocrit values average about 55 percent.[8]

A number of factors influence these values:

1. *Duration of gestation:* During the final weeks of intrauterine life, hemoglobin concentration rapidly increases. The infant born before term will not have the benefit of this increase and will have a low concentration compared to the full-term infant.
2. *Time of cord clamping:* In infants who receive the additional blood that is added to the circulation with delayed cord clamping, increased hemoglobin and hematocrit levels can be demonstrated for at least three to four days.
3. *Site of blood sample:* In the first week, capillary blood samples usually show higher hemoglobin values than venous samples drawn at the same time. The venous samples are considered to be more accurate.[9]

The higher blood values are needed by the fetus in utero for adequate oxygenation. After birth, the need no longer exists, since the lungs are functioning, and a gradual decrease takes place. Immediately after birth there is an increase in erythrocyte count from cord blood levels because of a decrease in plasma volume. This reaches a maximum at two to six hours of age, then decreases to cord level at about one week. Red blood cell production (erythropoiesis) is suppressed for several months after birth and this, added to the increased blood volume caused by the infant's rapid growth, results in a progressive decline in the hemoglobin concentration. A low point of 10 to 11 gm./100 ml. may be reached after two to three months, producing a physiologic anemia which does not represent any abnormality or nutritional deficiency in the infant and is not affected by giving iron or other hematinics. Active erythropoiesis resumes about this time and, if iron supplies are adequate, the hemoglobin concentration gradually increases to an average of 12.5 gm./100 ml., where it stays during early childhood.

Physiologic Jaundice. The newborn's high erythrocyte count and the shorter life span of these fetal red blood cells lead to an increased breakdown of red blood cells, which contribute to the increased bilirubin load presented to the liver in the first days of life. There is also a marked deficiency of glucuronyl transferase, an enzyme, which is necessary to change the unconjugated, fat-soluble form of bilirubin to the conjugated, water soluble form which can be excreted. These factors partly account for a rise in the serum concentration of unconjugated bilirubin from approximately 2.0 mg./100 ml. in cord blood to a mean peak of 6.0 mg./100 ml. between 60 and 72 hours of age. Then there is usually a rapid decline to 2.0 mg/100 ml. by the fifth day of life and a slower decline until normal adult levels of less than 1.0 mg./100 ml. are reached by about the tenth day. Jaundice is the visible evidence of this rise in serum concentration of unconjugated bilirubin to levels of 5 to 7 mg./100 ml. or above.[10] Approximately 40 to 60 percent of full-term newborns (and a higher number of preterm infants) develop jaundice between the second and fourth days of life, and, in the absence of disease or specific causes, this has been called "physiologic" jaundice. Appearance during the first 24 hours of levels greater than 12 mg./100 ml. are two indications for considering jaundice "pathologic." (See Chap. 39 for discussion of pathologic jaundice and treatment.)

There seem to be some genetic and ethnic influences on the incidence of physiologic jaundice. Oriental infants and some other isolated groups have mean maximal serum unconjugated bilirubin levels between 10 and 14 mg./100 ml., which is approximately double that of nonoriental populations. Kernicterus is also significantly increased in oriental neonates. The reasons for these increases are not known, but there may be a genetic predisposition to slower maturation of hepatic bilirubin metabolism or a possible relationship to ethnic food or herbal medicines.[11]

Careful assessment of the newborn for jaundice is an important part of nursing care. The red color of the blood or the pigment in the skin of dark-complected babies sometimes hides the yellow color.

1. Blanching the skin over a bony area such as the chest or forehead by pressing with a finger and observing the area before the color comes back will often allow the yellow to be seen.
2. The sclera or the buccal mucosa are also good places to look.

The nurse should not be lulled into a false sense of security by the term "physiologic." Any baby who develops observable jaundice should be closely watched for symptoms of other possible problems.

Blood Coagulation. Immediately after birth the intestinal tract of the infant does not harbor the bacteria necessary to help to synthesize the very important substance vitamin K. Other substances important in blood coagulation are manufactured in the liver and are under the influence of vitamin K; these substances are temporarily diminished. Thus the infant suffers from a transitory deficiency

in blood coagulation. This condition occurs between the second and the fifth postnatal days and returns to normal spontaneously in several more days.

This deficiency can often be minimized or prevented by administration of water-soluble vitamin K to the infant on the day of birth. This is now done routinely in many nurseries.

White Blood Cells. The normal newborn has a wide range in the total number of white blood cells. A leukocytosis (15,000 to 45,000 cells per microliter) is present at birth, with polymorphonuclear cells accounting for a large percentage of the total count. During the first few days after delivery there is a considerable decrease in the total count, as well as a shift in the type of predominating cell. The polymorphonuclear neutrophils decrease, and the lymphocytes increase, so that by the end of the first week the lymphocytes predominate.

Temperature Regulation and Metabolic Changes

The infant is born into an environment which is considerably cooler than the one encountered in the uterus. Because of this rapid change in environmental conditions, the newborn's temperature may drop several degrees after birth. In recent years attention has been focused on the effects of hypothermia on the newborn and increasing efforts have been made to prevent this temperature drop in the delivery room and in the nursery. Neonates are predisposed to heat transfer between themselves and the environment because they have a limited supply of subcutaneous fat and a large surface area in relation to body weight.

Heat Loss. Evaporation, conduction, convection, and radiation are four ways in which the newborn can lose body heat to the environment. Excessive loss by *evaporation* occurs most often in the delivery room when the infant is wet (see Chap. 23), but it can also occur when the infant is being bathed. Heat evaporation may also occur from the lungs if the infant is tachypneic or if the humidity is low. Heat loss by *conduction* involves the transfer of heat from a warm object to a cooler one by direct contact and can occur when the infant is placed on a cold surface, or when cool blankets or clothing are used. Through *convection,* the transference of heat is from a body to the surrounding air, the infant's temperature is affected by the air currents in the environment, such as those caused by air conditioners. The fourth mechanism, *radiation,* occurs when heat is transferred from a warm object to a cooler one when the objects are not in direct contact. This type of heat loss can occur in infants if the walls of an incubator are cool or if the crib is placed close to a cool outside wall or window. Each of these mechanisms with the exception of evaporation can be responsible for an increase in the infant's temperature as well as the losses described.

Heat Production.   To maintain a normal temperature when exposed to a cool environment the newborn increases his rate of heat production in an attempt to replace what is lost. Shivering is the most common mechanism of heat production in an adult, but the neonate rarely shivers although there may be an increase in voluntary muscular activity. The primary mechanism of heat production in the newborn is nonshivering thermogenesis whereby a chemical reaction occurs in brown fat, breaking down triglycerides into glycerol and fatty acids and thereby producing heat. Brown fat cells contain many small fat vacuoles in contrast to the single large vacuole of white fat. There is also a richer blood supply which helps to account for its darker color and aids in the distribution of the heat produced. Brown fat is usually not found in adults, but in the newborn it accounts for 2 to 6 percent of the total weight and can be found between the scapulae, at the nape of the neck, in the axillae, in the mediastinum, and around the kidneys and adrenals.[12]

Heat Conservation.   Conservation of body heat in the infant occurs through peripheral vasoconstriction and through assumption of a flexed or fetal position which decreases the surface area from which heat may be lost.

Effects of Cold Stress on the Newborn.   The increased metabolic rate associated with nonshivering thermogenesis necessitates an increase in both oxygen and calorie consumption. To replace the heat lost during a temperature drop of 3.5°C. (6.3°F.), it has been found that the infant requires a 100-percent increase in oxygen consumption for more than one and one-half hours.[13] Even vigorous full-term infants may develop matabolic acidosis if

allowed to become hypothermic. It is obvious that cold stress can be detrimental or even fatal to an infant who is having difficulty with metabolism or oxygenation.

Efforts should be made to keep an infant in a neutral thermal environment, which means an environment where the infant's metabolic rate, and therefore oxygen consumption, is minimal but the body temperature remains within the normal range.

Neurologic Changes

The nervous system of the newborn is immature; that is, it is neither anatomically nor physiologically fully developed. Although all neurons are present, many remain immature for several months and some for years. Thus, the infant is uncoordinated in his movements, is labile in his temperature regulation, and has poor control over his musculature: he "startles" easily, is subject to tremors of the extremities, and so on. However, during the neonatal period, development is rapid, and as the various nerve pathways controlling the muscles are used, the nerve fibers connect with one another. Gradually, more complex patterns of behavior emerge, and the higher cerebral levels begin to function.

Reflexes.   The reflexes are important indices of the baby's normal development, for their presence or absence at certain times reflects the extent of normality in the functioning of the central nervous system. (Individual reflexes will be discussed in the section on Physical Assessment.)

Gastrointestinal Changes

The gastrointestinal tract functions in a very limited capacity during fetal life. The fetus is known to swallow amniotic fluid and a fecal material called meconium is formed, but the GI tract is not responsible for the digestion or absorption of nutrients. By 36 to 38 weeks, though, it is mature enough to adapt readily to extrauterine life. The various enzymes necessary for digestion are active and the muscular and reflex development provide the capability of transporting the food.

In order for the infant to swallow, food must be placed well back on the tongue, since the infant does not have the ability to transfer food from the lips to the pharynx. This means that the nipple should be placed well inside the infant's mouth. Sucking is facilitated by strong sucking muscles and ridges or corrugations in the anterior portion of the mouth. In addition, the *sucking pads* (deposits of fatty tissue in each cheek) prevent the collapse of the cheeks during nursing and further make sucking effective. This fatty tissue remains (even when fat is lost from the rest of the body) until sucking is no longer essential to the baby's getting food. The salivary glands are immature at birth and manufacture little saliva until the infant is about three months old.

The newborn's intestinal tract is proportionately longer than that of an adult. Although it contains a large number of secretory glands and a large surface for absorption, its elastic tissue and supporting musculature are poor and not fully developed. This increases the likelihood of distention. Furthermore, nervous control is variable and inadequate. Nevertheless, the infant digests and absorbs a tremendous amount of food in proportion to body weight.

Most of the digestive enzymes seem to be present and adequate, with the exception of pancreatic amylase and lipase. These last are somewhat deficient for several months but eventually reach a normal amount. The infant can digest simple foods easily, but has a difficult time with the more complex starches. Protein and carbohydrates are easily absorbed but fat absorption is poor.

Changes in Kidney Function and Urinary Excretion

The kidneys become functional during fetal life, as evidenced by the presence of urine in the bladder as early as the fourth month of gestation. However, kidney function is fairly low until immediately after birth when the kidneys must replace the placenta as the organ responsible for excretory and regulatory functions. Due to the relatively low rate of glomerular filtration at birth, excess water and solute cannot be disposed of rapidly and efficiently. The limitations in tubular reabsorption that are also present, may cause inappropriate substances from the glomerular filtrate, such as certain amino acids and bicarbonate, to appear in the urine.[14] In the healthy neonate these limitations do not have a

detrimental effect, but they do restrict the ability of the newborn to respond to stress. As the kidneys grow and mature, function increases.

Ninety-two percent of healthy infants void within 24 hours, but the first voiding may occur shortly after delivery and not be noticed. Voidings during the first days after birth may be scanty and somewhat infrequent unless the infant was edematous at birth, but as the fluid intake increases so does the output. Frequency usually increases from 2 to 6 times on the first and second day to 5 to 20 times per 24 hours after that until the infant begins to develop bladder control and the number of voidings per day decreases.

The urine of the newborn may appear cloudy due to high mucus and urate content, but with increased fluid intake the urine becomes clear, straw-colored and nearly odorless. Uric acid crystals in the urine may cause a reddish "brick-dust" stain on the diaper that is sometimes confused with blood in the urine.

Changes in Hepatic Function

During fetal life, the liver performs an important role in blood formation, and it is thought that it continues this function to some degree after birth. Later in the neonatal period the liver produces substances that are essential in the coagulation of the blood (see p. 445). If the mother's iron intake has been adequate during pregnancy, enough iron will be stored in the infant's liver to carry him over the first months of life when his diet (primarily milk) is iron-deficient. About the fifth month, however, the baby's iron reserve is depleted, and unless foods containing iron are given, a deficiency will ensue.

ASSESSMENT OF THE NEWBORN

During the first few days of life, the newborn will undergo numerous assessments to help determine how well he is coping with all the changes that are occurring. Which evaluations are done, and by whom, will depend on the setting and the infant's condition. The physical examination has traditionally been done by the physician. In recent years many nurses have learned physical assessment skills and in some hospitals a pediatric nurse practitioner *(Text continues on page 450.)*

NEWBORN PHYSICAL ASSESSMENT

Initial Evaluation

1. General Appearance: Color _____ Muscle Tone _____
2. Respiratory Effort: Retractions _____ Gasping _____
   Grunting _____ Quality of Cry _____
3. Temperature: _____
Comments: _____
_____

Assessment of Head and Neck

1. Observe and palpate the infant's *head* for symmetry; note absence or presence of:
   Molding _____ Caput Succedaneum _____ Cephalhematoma _____
2. Palpate the *fontanels* and *sutures* for: Fullness _____ Depression _____
   Overriding _____ Shape _____
3. Measure circumference of *head*: _____
4. Evaluate *ears*: Position _____ Shape _____ Location _____
5. Evaluate symmetry of *face*: _____
6. Observe *eyes* for: Shape _____ Position _____ Size _____
   Appearance of Pupils _____ Presence of Hemorrhage _____ Red Reflex _____
7. Evaluate *mouth* for: Clefts _____ Teeth _____ Frenulum Linguae _____
8. Observe *neck* for: Length _____ Relationship to Body _____
   Mobility _____ Presence of Webbing and/or Fat Pad _____
9. Observe skin of *scalp, face* and *neck* for: Abrasions and/or Contusions _____
   Other Breaks or Marks _____
10. Observe *nose* for: Symmetry _____ Septum _____ Flaring _____
Comments: _____
_____
_____

Assessment of Body

General Appearance
1. Measurements: Weight _____ Length _____ Circumference of Chest _____
2. Observe throughout evaluation for: General Activity _____
   Posture _____ Responsiveness _____
3. Observe *skin* for: Lanugo _____ Vernix _____ Meconium Staining _____
   Texture _____ Hydration _____ Color _____ Rashes _____
Comments: _____
_____

Thorax

1. Palpate *clavicles* for masses and intactness: _____
2. Inspect *thorax* for: Size _____ Symmetry _____ Shape _____
3. Auscultate for: Breath Sounds _____ Heart Sounds _____ Rhythm _____
4. Count: Respiratory Rate _____ Apical Pulse _____
Comments: _____
_____

Abdomen

1. Inspect shape of *abdomen*: _____
2. Palpate: Liver _____ Spleen _____ Kidneys _____
3. Observe *Cord* for Number of Vessels: _____
4. Palpate: Femoral Pulses _____
Comments: _____
_____

Genitals

1. Observe visible *genitals* for: Appropriateness with Stated Sex _____
2. Observe female infant for: Maturation of Labia _____ Vaginal Discharge _____
3. Observe male infant for: Position of Urethral Opening _____
   Maturation of Scrotum _____ Presence of Testes _____
4. Note Elimination: (should occur within 24 hours)
   Urine _____ Color _____ Amount in 24 Hours _____
   Stool _____ Color _____ Type _____ Number/24 Hours _____
Comments: _____

Posterior of Body

1. Palpate and inspect spinal column for: Masses _____
   Symmetry of Vertebrae _____ Intactness _____
2. Determine patency of anus: _____
3. Observe pilonidal dimple for intactness: _____
Comments: _____

Extremities

1. Note for all extremities: Symmetry _____ Abnormalities _____
   Ability to Move _____
2. Count digits on: Hands _____ Feet _____
   Observe for Polydactyly _____ Syndactyly _____
3. Evaluate rotation of hips: Abduct Thighs to Bed _____
   Rotate Hips Through Full Range of Motion _____
   Observe leg length, front and back (Are they equal?) _____
   Observe Symmetry of Leg Creases _____
4. Note position of feet _____
   Can they passively be returned to normal? _____
Comments: _____

Assessment of Neurological Function—Reflexes—Elicit and Evaluate:

1. Rooting and Sucking: _____

2. Grasp: Palmar _____ Plantar _____

3. Traction: (Pull to sitting position, noting head and arm position) _____

4. Moro: _____

5. Stepping: _____

Comments: _____

Items that require manipulation, such as palpation of the abdomen and abduction of the hips, require care in performance to avoid injury to the infant and should not be attempted for the first time without supervision by a trained examiner.

(Based on NAACOG Technical Bulletin Number 2, "Physical Assessment of the Neonate.")

will carry out the physical examination of some of the newborns. The NAACOG Technical Bulletin #2, "Physical Assessment of the Neonate," suggests that since "the registered nurse is usually the first health care professional to assess the neonate's adjustment during this transition to extrauterine life, the nurse must possess both the knowledge and skills to carry out a comprehensive evaluation of the newborn's physical status."[15]

Assessments will continue throughout the infant's hospital stay. Vital signs, general activity, color changes, feeding status, elimination, and condition of skin, eyes and cord will probably be checked at each shift, and the infant will usually be weighed daily. Although the infant's physical condition is most important, assessment of other areas such as the infant's behavior and the interaction between the parents and the infant are gaining increasing attention.

Physical Assessment

The Newborn Physical Assessment Form (pp. 448–449) and the discussion of newborn characteristics that follow are based on the NAACOG suggestions. The format could be used for an admitting assessment or for a later one. This is not intended to be a complete physical examination, but should give the nurse a good idea of the status of the infant. Practice and experience will improve the ability to recognize the range of normal. Discussion of abnormalities will be found in Chapter 38.

Methods used in physical examination are inspection, auscultation, palpation, and percussion, usually in that order. Percussion is not specifically used in this form. The examination is written for use in evaluating the infant in a cephalocaudal direction, but the items can be used in the order that works best for the examiner as long as a definite plan is followed so that nothing is missed.

When any assessment of the newborn is carried out, the parents should be included as much as possible. If they cannot be present for the examination it should at least be discussed with them. Being there, though, is a good way to help them get better acquainted with their infant.

Physical assessment will begin with the Apgar scoring in the delivery room (see Chap. 23). When the infant is brought to the nursery, the delivery room nurse will report pertinent information on the mother's antepartum history, labor and delivery course and the care given the infant while in the delivery room.

The nursery nurse will then make an initial evaluation of the infant's general condition.

1. The first thing to observe is the infant's appearance. Is the color ruddy, pale, cyanotic, or jaundiced? Is the color evenly distributed? The infant usually is in a flexed position with good muscle tone. A "floppy" baby will need careful observation.
2. The infant's cry can also be an indicator of general condition. A lusty cry is usually a good sign, but a weak or shrill cry can be indicative of central nervous system problems and grunting sounds mean that the infant is having to work harder to get oxygen.
3. Other signs of increased respiratory effort such as retractions, gasping or flaring of the nostrils should also be noted.
4. The vital signs should be taken.

From the foregoing observations the nurse can make a decision about whether the infant needs some immediate treatment, needs time for the temperature to stabilize, or if the assessment can continue.

It is important to remember that certain symptoms which might be cause for concern in an older child (e.g., rapid rate and rhythm of respiration), when observed in a newborn infant, may merely represent normal neonatal physiology. Also, it is well for the nurse to look at the baby from the parent's viewpoint. The healthy newborn infant has many characteristics which momentarily may look unusual to them. The nurse should be ready to talk with the parents about their baby and to answer their questions.

Assessment of Head and Neck

The infant's head is large, comprising about one-quarter of his size, and with cephalic presentations may initially appear to be asymmetrical because of the molding of the skull bones during labor (Fig. 29-1). If there has been extended pressure on the head, caput succedaneum (a swelling of the soft tissues) or cephalhematoma (an accumulation of blood between the bone and the periosteum) might be present (see Chap. 39).

The suture lines between the skull bones and the anterior and the posterior fontanels can usually be

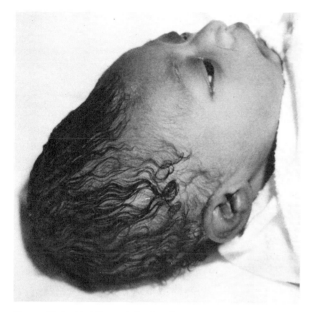
Figure 29-1. Molding of the head.

palpated easily (see Fig. 21-1, p. 298). When the hand is passed over the fontanels, the areas should feel soft but neither bulged nor depressed. The anterior fontanel, the diamond-shaped and larger of the two (normally 2 to 3 cm. wide and 3 to 4 cm. long), may feel smaller for the first several days when there is marked overriding of the skull bones. It usually closes by 12 to 18 months. The posterior fontanel is triangular and is located between the occipital and the parietal bones. It is smaller than the anterior fontanel and may be almost closed at birth, and completely closed by the end of of the second month.

The circumference of the head is measured by placing a nonstretchable tape measure just above the eyebrows and over the most prominent part of the occiput (Fig. 29-2). Normally the head circumference is 2 cm. larger than the chest circumference, but an accurate measurement may not be obtained at first if molding is present. The normal range is 33 to 37 cm. (13 to 14½ in.), depending on the general size of the infant.

The face is small and round, and the lower jaw appears to recede. Facial asymmetry is sometimes seen, especially of the chin and mandible. This can be the result of posture in utero when the flexed head is tilted to one side and presses against the shoulder. The nose may also be asymmetrical or have a deviated septum from intrauterine pressure. It is important that the nose not be obstructed, since

infants are nose breathers, and have difficulty breathing through their mouths.

The scalp, face and neck should be observed carefully for any abrasions, contusions or breaks in the skin. These can result from application of internal fetal monitor electrodes, forceps or other instruments used in delivery. Any opening in the skin is a potential site for bacterial invasion and should be watched for signs of infection.

Eyes. The eyes are closed much of the time but may open spontaneously if the infant's head is lifted or rocked gently (a valuable point to remember when one wants to inspect the eyes). From birth the infant can see and discriminate patterns as the basis for form perception. This capacity is rather limited by imperfect oculomotor coordination and inability to accommodate for varying distances. Moreover, the eye, the visual pathways, and the visual part of the brain are poorly developed at birth. Nevertheless, although the baby's vision is much less acute than an adult's, a good deal of visual experience is possible for him.

Most mothers do not realize that their infants can see as well as they do, and they appreciate being informed of this fact. In addition, some mothers become exceedingly anxious when they observe strabismus or nystagmus in their infants, but they should be reassured that this lack of coordination is normal during the first few months of life.

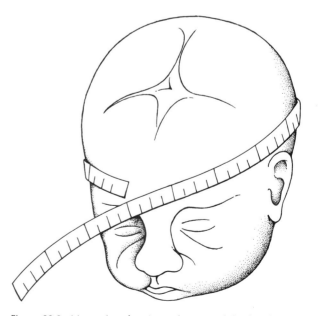
Figure 29-2. Measuring the circumference of the head.

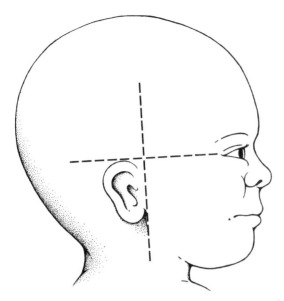

Figure 29-3. Assessment of ear position in the newborn. The top of the ear should lie on or above an imaginary line drawn between the outer corner of the eye and the most prominent point of the posterior occiput.

All babies' eyes are blue or a slatey gray color at birth. By the time the infant is three months old, most have achieved their permanent color, although complete pigmentation of the iris does not occur until the infant is about one year old. Since the lacrimal glands may not be functioning at birth, the baby does not usually shed tears when he cries. Tears may not appear for several weeks and sometimes for several months. There may be some edema of the lids and/or purulent discharge caused by the silver nitrate (see p. 467). The changes in the vascular tension of the eyes during delivery sometimes cause small areas of subconjunctival hemorrhage. These areas disappear spontaneously in one or two weeks and are not significant.

If an ophthalmoscope is used in examining the eyes, the pupil should appear as a small red-orange circular spot when the light is directed at it. This is the red reflex, caused by the light shining on the retina, and any opacities of the lens or other obstructions would be visible if present.

Ears and Hearing. The ears should be inspected for size, shape, position and anomaly. The top of the ear should fall on or above an imaginary line drawn between the outer corner of the eye and the most prominent point of the posterior occiput (Fig. 29-3). Abnormal positioning of the ears is frequently associated with kidney or extensive chromosomal abnormalities.

The ear and the nerve tracts for hearing are anatomically mature at birth, and the newborn can hear after his first cry. Hearing apparently becomes acute within several days as the eustachian tubes become aerated, and the mucus in the middle ear disappears.

Hearing can be tested by sounding a bell or rattle near the baby's head, but out of eyesight. Hearing the sound will cause blinking of the eyes, momentary cessation of activity or a startle response. This is not an accurate test, but may be helpful in alerting the examiner to a possible problem.

Neck. The newborn infant generally appears to have a short neck, which sometimes makes it difficult to tell if webbing or other problems are present. The head should be gently rotated to determine the range of motion of the neck and the muscles should be palpated for any masses.

Lips, Mouth, Cheeks. The rounded, thickened areas often present on the lips (particularly on the center of the upper lip) are known as labial tubercles or "sucking blisters" although they are not true blisters since there is no fluid in them. Sucking (fat) pads are usually present in the cheeks. The lips, gums, and palate should be examined to see that they are intact. Epstein's pearls, small white cysts which may be seen on the hard palate or gums, are not abnormal. Occasionally a tooth is present, which may be pulled to avoid the possibility of its being aspirated.

At this early age, the tongue does not extend far beyond the margin of the gums because the frenum is normally short. A mother's concern that her baby is tongue-tied is usually unwarranted.

General Appearance

The average term infant weighs 3,500 gm. (7½ lb.), and 95 percent weigh between 2,500 gm. (5½ lb.) and 4,250 gm. (9½ lb.). There is usually some weight loss in the first three to five days, possibly as much as 10 percent of the infant's birth weight. This is usually regained by the eighth to twelfth day.

Length should also be measured soon after birth to serve as a baseline from which to judge future growth. The average length of a full-term infant at

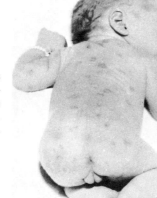
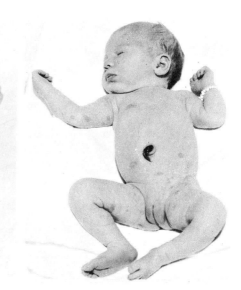

Figure 29-4. Erythema toxicum. This "newborn rash" develops more frequently on the back, the shoulders and the buttocks. (MacDonald House, The University Hospitals of Cleveland, Cleveland, Ohio)

birth is 51 cm. (20 in.), with 95 percent between 46 and 56 cm. (18 and 22 in.). Since the newborn infant usually assumes a somewhat flexed position, it can be difficult to get an accurate measurement from the top of the head to the heels.

Skin. The infant's skin appears to be thin and delicate and is often dry and peeling. The baby's color may be pink, reddish, or pale, becoming very ruddy when he cries. Initially, the hands and the feet are quite blue, due to the sluggish peripheral vascular circulation, but this cyanosis of the extremities soon disappears, often within a few hours.

Vernix caseosa, a white cheesy material which was a protection to the skin while the fetus floated in amniotic fluid in the uterus, may be apparent, particularly in the creases of the body. Also, on the body there may be large areas of fine downy hair called lanugo. Milia may be present on the nose and the forehead (see below) and small flat hemangiomas may be apparent on the nape of the neck, the eyelids or over the bridge of the nose. These so-called stork bites, clusters of small capillaries, usually disappear spontaneously during infancy.

Gray-blue pigmented areas are seen most often in dark-skinned infants, especially in the lumbosacral area, although other sites are not uncommon. These "mongolian spots" have no relationship to mongolism and will disappear spontaneously during late infancy or early childhood.

ERYTHEMA TOXICUM. Sometimes referred to as the newborn rash, or "flea-bite" dermatitis (although

no fleas are involved), erythema toxicum is a blotchy erythematous rash which may appear in the first few days of life (Fig. 29-4). The erythematous areas, which develop more frequently on the back, the shoulders and the buttocks, have a small blanched wheal in the center. The cause of this skin disturbance is obscure, and no treatment is necessary. The rash is transient and likely to change appreciably within a few hours, and it may disappear entirely within a day or so.

MILIA. Milia are pinpoint-sized, pearly white spots which occur commonly on the nose and the forehead of the newborn infant. When touched gently with the tip of the finger, these spots feel like tiny, firm seeds. They are due to retention of sebaceous material within the sebaceous glands, and if they are left alone, will usually disappear spontaneously during the neonatal period. Mothers often mistake milia for "whiteheads" and may attempt to squeeze them if the nurse or the physician has not warned them against such practice.

Thorax. The infant's chest is round and the circumference, measured just above the nipple line, is slightly smaller than the head. Engorgement of the breasts is common during the neonatal period in both male and female infants (Fig. 29-5). It is due to the same causes that bring about mammary engorgement in the mother—that is, endocrine influence. In the case of the infant, the breasts have been acted on throughout pregnancy by the estrogenic hormone which passes to them through the

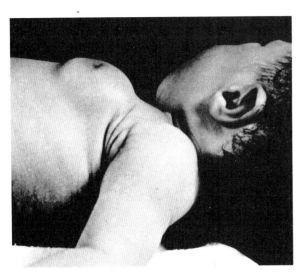

Figure 29-5. Hypertrophy of breast in infant developing in the neonatal period.

placenta from the mother. This is the same hormone which prepares the mother's breasts for lactation. When it is withdrawn after birth, changes in the infant's breasts similar to those in the mother take place.

Mammary engorgement in the newborn subsides without treatment, but sometimes it persists for two or three weeks.

Sometimes a small amount of fluid that has been called "witches' milk" will be secreted. Mothers should be cautioned against massaging the breasts or trying to express the fluid, because handling predisposes to infection such as breast abscess or mastitis.

Early experiences in listening to the newborn's chest can be confusing because both the heart rate and respirations are so much faster than an adult's and the infant often wiggles and fusses. With practice the student will learn how to quiet the infant and to be able to distinguish between the different sounds.

Abdomen. The abdomen is round and slightly protuberant, due to the relative size of the abdominal organs and weak muscular structures. The liver edge is usually palpable just below the right rib margin. The tip of the spleen may sometimes be palpated in the left upper quadrant. The kidneys may be palpated, but are more difficult to feel after four to six hours.

The umbilical cord stump is checked for bleeding or oozing (Fig. 29-6). The number of vessels is noted if not already recorded (see Chap. 23).

Genitals. Female genitalia should be inspected for presence and size of the labia majora, labia minora, clitoris, and vaginal opening. Enlarged labia or vaginal discharge may be present due to in utero stimulation by maternal hormones. The discharge is sometimes blood-tinged but need cause no special concern. The swelling and discharge will disappear spontaneously.

In boy babies the scrotum usually appears relatively large. At term in most infants the testes can be palpated in the scrotum or can be easily brought down. The prepuce (foreskin) covers the glans penis and is usually adherent at birth. During the first few months it becomes less adherent and can be manually retracted. When the opening in the foreskin is so small that it cannot be pulled back at all, the condition is called *phimosis*. There is some difference of opinion as to whether this is an indication for circumcision. Many doctors feel that it is, but others feel that as long as urination is not interfered with it is a normal condition of the newborn and the foreskin will gradually become retractable as the child grows (see p. 470 for discussion of circumcision). The penis should be inspected to determine the location of the urinary meatus. If the opening is covered by the foreskin, observing the infant while he is voiding will help in locating it.

Posterior. With the infant in the prone position, the entire posterior surface of the body should be inspected and palpated. Any masses or abnormal curvatures of the spine should be noted. Tufts of hair or small indentations, especially in the sacral area, may be an indication of spina bifida occulta.

The perineal area should be inspected to determine the patency and location of the anus. A pilonidal "dimple" resulting from an irregular fold of skin is sometimes seen in the midline over the sacrococcygeal area. It should be examined for intactness to make sure no sinus is present.

Extremities. Throughout the exam, the infant's ability to move all four extremities is evaluated and the limbs compared as to size, shape and movement. Webbing (syndactyly) or extra digits (polydactyly) should be noted also.

To check for congenital problems of the hip, the

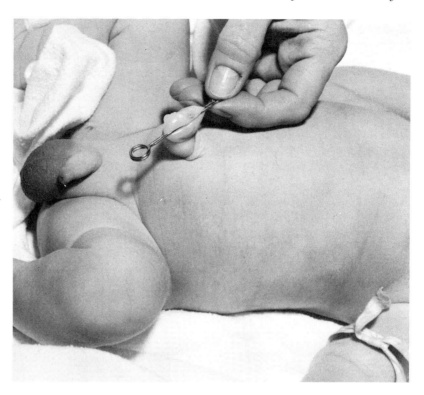

Figure 29-6. Inspection of cord stump.

infant is placed in the supine position, the legs are flexed on the abdomen and then abducted laterally toward the bed. With congenital dislocation, there may be uneven or limited abduction, uneven leg length, or a "hip click" might be felt. Unsymmetrical skin folds on the posterior aspect of the thigh are not diagnostic, but may alert the examiner to this condition. Unusual positions of the feet can indicate congenital clubfoot or other foot and ankle deformities. If the foot can be moved to the normal position with ease, the condition may just be due to intrauterine malposition.

Neurological Function

Rooting and Sucking.   Gently stroking the infant's cheek or corner of the mouth with a sterile nipple or clean finger will cause the baby to open his mouth and turn toward the stimulus. This is known as the rooting reflex. The sucking reflex can be evaluated by placing the nipple or finger in the baby's mouth and noting the strength of the sucking response. These reflexes may not be too active if the infant has eaten recently.

It is well known that during the first two months of life the newborn infant has a great need to suck and will usually suck on anything that comes in contact with his lips. Newborn infants can suck while sleeping and nonnutritive sucking can have a quieting effect on excited babies.

Grasp Reflex.   The *grasp reflex* is present at birth in both the hands and the feet (Fig. 29-7). The infant will grasp any object placed in his hands, cling briefly, and then let go. Even at birth he may be able to hold onto an adult's forefinger so securely that he can be lifted to a standing position. Although the baby cannot actually grasp with his feet, stroking the soles causes the toes to turn downward as though trying to grasp. The grasping movements are a reflex action at birth, but with practice and experience they soon become voluntary and purposeful.

By grasping the infant's hands and arms, the examiner can gently pull the infant to a sitting position. The infant will flex the elbows to resist extension (traction response). The strength of the neck muscles can be assessed by noting the amount of head lag. The normal term newborn will be able to support his head momentarily.

Moro Reflex.   The *Moro* or *startle reflex* indicates an awareness of equilibrium in the newborn (Fig.

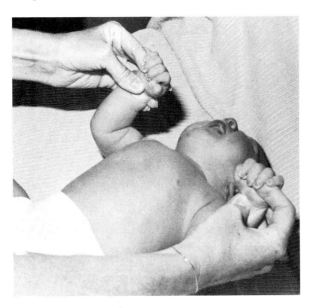

Figure 29-7. Grasp reflex.

29-8). This reflex should be elicited when the baby is lying quietly. A sudden stimulus, such as a change in position, a jarring of the crib, a jerking of the blanket or clothes, or even a loud noise (which jars his position) causes the baby to draw up his legs, bring his arms forward in an embracing motion, and usually cry. The movements should be symmetrical. If they are not, injury to the part that lags should be suspected.

The Moro reflex should be present at birth; normally it disappears by three months of age. If it cannot be elicited at birth, edema of and/or injury to the brain may be present. As the edema subsides, the reflex returns, and it should be demonstrable on the day following delivery. If frank brain damage has occurred, the reflex will be absent for several days; if the damage is not too severe, the reflex will return in three or four days. Occasionally, the reflex is present at birth but disappears over the first days. Increasing cerebral edema or slow intracranial hemorrhage then are suspected.

Tonic Neck Reflex.   When the *tonic neck reflex* is elicited, the infant assumes a "fencing" position; that is, he lies on his back with his head rotated to one side. The arm and the leg on the side to which he is facing are partially or completely extended, and the opposite arm and leg are flexed (Fig. 29-9). This reflex also disappears in a few months, since it is another manifestation of the immaturity of the newborn's nervous system.

Stepping Reflex.   The *stepping* or *dancing reflex* is another action that is present at birth but soon disappears. This reflex causes the infant to make little stepping or prancing movements when he is held upright with his feet touching a surface (Fig. 29-10). After this reflex diminishes, the infant will not attempt stepping motions until he is ready to stand and walk. However, he does exercise the leg muscles a great deal and seems to derive much enjoyment from waving and kicking his legs about.

Other Reflexes.   The next group of reflexes might be termed protective, since they are necessary and at times essential to the preservation of the newborn's safety. The *blinking reflex* occurs when the infant is subjected to a bright light. The *cough and the sneeze reflexes* clear his respiratory passages. The *yawn reflex* draws in additional oxygen. These, together with the infant's ability to cry when uncomfortable, to withdraw from painful stimuli, to resist restraint, and so on, are all defensive measures. As the baby grows and develops, these together with the other reflexes mentioned either diminish or become more highly developed according to the need. Thus, the infant's behavior patterns become more complex and highly developed.

Gestational Age.   Evaluation of gestational age may also be included in the nurse's initial examination of the newborn. This will be discussed in Chapter 38.

Behavioral Assessment

Although the newborn used to be thought of as essentially passive, we now recognize that the infant interacts actively with his environment from birth. To evaluate this interaction, a behavioral assessment can be conducted.

The Neonatal Behavioral Assessment Scale, developed by T. Berry Brazelton, includes both physical and behavioral assessment of the newborn.[16] According to Brazelton, the scale can be used both in clinical practice, as a predictive tool, and in research. Use of the scale for its intended purposes requires a trained examiner and considerable time, but some aspects of the scale and some of the findings can be useful to anyone working with newborns.

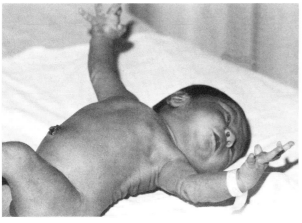
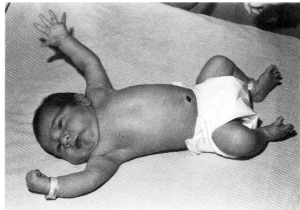

Figure 29-8. Moro reflex.

Essential to an understanding of the infant's behavior is the concept of the state of consciousness or "state." Brazelton recognizes the following six states:[17]

Sleep States

1. Deep sleep with regular breathing, eyes closed, no spontaneous activity except startles or jerky movements at quite regular intervals; external stimuli produce startles with some delay; suppression of startles is rapid, and state changes are less likely than from other states. No eye movements.

2. Light sleep with eyes closed, rapid eye movements can be observed under closed lids; low activity level, with random movements and startles or startle equivalents; movements are likely to be smoother and more monitored than in state 1; responds to internal and external stimuli with startle equivalents, often with a resulting change of state. Respirations are irregular, sucking movements occur off and on.

Awake States

3. Drowsy or semi-dozing; eyes may be open or closed, eyelids fluttering; activity level variable, with interspersed, mild startles from time to time; reactive to sensory stimuli, but response often delayed; state change after stimulation frequently noted. Movements are usually smooth.

4. Alert, with bright look; seems to focus attention on source of stimulation, such as an object to be sucked, or a visual or auditory stimulus; impinging stimuli may break through, but

with some delay in response. Motor activity is at a minimum (Fig. 29-11).

5. Eyes open; considerable motor activity, with thrusting movements of the extremities, and even a few spontaneous startles; reactive to external stimulation with increase in startles or motor activity, but discrete reactions difficult to distinguish because of general high activity level.

6. Crying; characterized by intense crying which is difficult to break through with stimulation (Fig. 29-12).

Babies vary greatly in the amount of time they spend in the various states and in the ease or difficulty with which they make the transition from one state to another. The concept of state is often helpful to parents in interacting with their baby. If they can learn to recognize the various states and the individuality of their infant, they will be better able to use the infant's timetable rather than their own in giving care and have a better understanding of when the infant will respond to them.

The Neonatal Behavioral Assessment Scale meas-

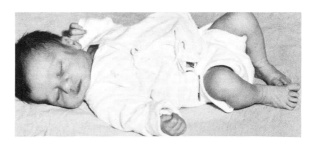

Figure 29-9. Tonic neck reflex.

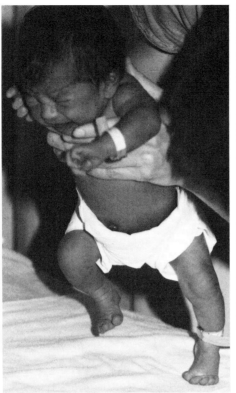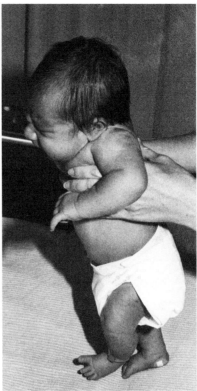

Figure 29-10. Stepping reflex.

ures a total of 27 items (see Chart). Each item is scored on a scale of 1 to 9 and is based on the infant's best rather than his average performance. The infant's state at the time any given item is tested is important. Some items require that the infant be in a certain state for valid testing.

The items can be divided into six categories:[18]

1. Habituation—how soon the neonate diminishes his responses to specific repeated stimuli
2. Orientation—how often and when he attends to auditory and visual stimuli
3. Motor maturity—how well the infant coordinates and controls motor activities
4. Variation—how often he exhibits alertness, state changes, color changes, activity, and peaks of excitement
5. Self-quieting abilities—how often, how soon, and how effectively the neonate can use his own resources to quiet and console himself when upset or distressed
6. Social behaviors—how often and how much the newborn smiles and cuddles

A better understanding of the scale may be obtained from the booklet[19] or the films prepared by Dr. Brazelton. The discussion here will be limited to a few items of particular interest.

Most parents are interested in what kinds of stimuli their infant will focus attention on. Some parents discover these things for themselves. Others need to be told that most infants will focus on a bright red ball and follow it briefly when they are in the quiet-alert state (state 4), or that the infant particularly likes to follow a moving human face or a high-pitched voice.

Many people think that all infants are cuddly and that if an infant does not cuddle when held there is either something wrong with them or with the infant. In fact, infants respond in many different ways to being cuddled. Scores on "cuddliness" range from: (1) "Actually resists being held, continuously pushing away, thrashing or stiffening" to (9) "Molds into arms and relaxes, turns toward body when held horizontally, on shoulder seems to lean forward, all of body participates and baby grasps examiner to cling to him."[20]

Infants also vary in their ability to be consoled or to console themselves. These items are scored when the infant is upset (state 6). Some babies will only

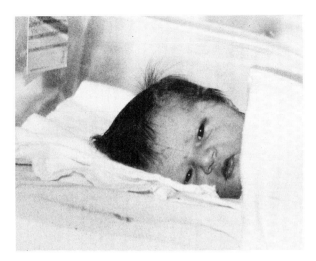

Figure 29-11. Quiet alert state.

quiet down when they are dressed and left alone. Others need restraint to help them inhibit the startle reflex. These babies are the ones that usually do best when swaddled in a blanket.

Possible self–consoling activities that are counted in the assessment are: hand to mouth efforts; sucking on fist or tongue (Fig. 29-13); or using visual or auditory stimulus from the environment to quiet self. Finding out ways in which their particular infant can console himself or be consoled can be very helpful to the parents.

Babies often smile even in the first days, but the statement is usually made that it is just a reflex or "gas." Brazelton comments that he has "seen close replicas of 'social smiles' in the newborn period" and that, although they are hard to be sure of, "they surely are the precursors of such smiling behavior and a mother reinforces them as such."[21]

BRAZELTON SCALE CRITERIA

1. Response Decrement to Light
2. Response Decrement to Rattle
3. Response Decrement to Bell
4. Response Decrement to Pinprick
5. Orientation Response—Inanimate Visual
6. Orientation Response—Inanimate Auditory
7. Orientation—Animate Visual
8. Orientation—Animate Auditory
9. Orientation—Animate-Visual and Auditory
10. Alertness
11. General Tonus
12. Motor Maturity
13. Pull-to-Sit
14. Cuddliness
15. Defensive Movements
16. Consolability with Intervention
17. Peak of Excitement
18. Rapidity of Buildup
19. Irritability (to aversive stimuli: uncover, undress, pull-to-sit, prone, pinprick, TNR, Moro, defensive reaction)
20. Activity
21. Tremulousness
22. Amount of Startle During Exam
23. Lability of Skin Color
24. Lability of States
25. Self-Quieting Activity
26. Hand to Mouth Facility
27. Smiles

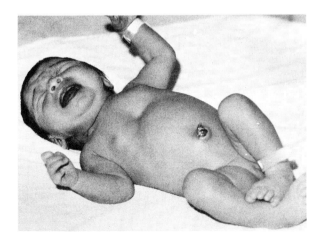

Figure 29-12. Active crying state.

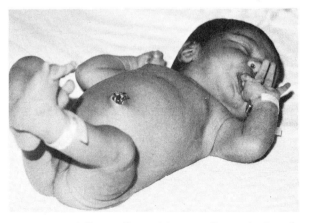

Figure 29-13. Self-consoling activity according to the Brazelton behavioral assessment scale: hand-to-mouth and sucking activity.

THE ENVIRONMENT OF THE NEWBORN

Prevention of Infection

The prevention of infection is of paramount importance in caring for the newborn. Everyone who is in contact with infants—including parents and personnel—must assume this responsibility. Staff should take special care to instruct parents so that their activities conform to the prevention of infection. The basis of "good" technique in handling the infant is thorough handwashing with an antiseptic detergent or soap. Some institutions require that the hands be scrubbed initially with a brush; others feel that detergent, water, and friction are sufficient. Whichever the procedure, meticulous handwashing is essential, whether the infant is cared for in the central or regular nursery or in a rooming-in situation. Staff should be especially careful to wash their hands before a feeding, and after a diaper change, before going from one baby to another, and after touching anything that is not clean to that baby, such as a door, or their own face or hair.

The parents will need instruction about the importance (and technique) of proper handwashing, and reinforcement should be given as necessary during the hospital stay.

As with personnel in the delivery room (see Chap 23), all nursery staff should have a preemployment physical examination and a yearly physical examination thereafter to minimize the possibility of spreading infection from the staff among the newborn. In addition, any staff member who contracts *any* infection (i.e., respiratory, gastrointestinal, skin lesions, and the like) should remain away from the nursery and contact with the newborn until the infection is gone *completely*.

If a mother shows signs of infection, particularly an elevated temperature, diarrhea or skin lesions, the infant will not be brought to her until the infection subsides. The infant who has spent some time with the mother before the symptoms were noticed may be isolated from the other babies. The importance of the precautions should be explained to the mother since she undoubtedly will find it difficult to be separated from her infant. Sometimes arrangements can be made for her to see the baby through the nursery window, but if this is not possible, the nurse should bring her frequent reports about the baby to let her know how he is eating and sleeping, and so on.

The mother who plans to breast-feed her baby should be helped to pump her breasts to ensure stimulation and a continued supply of milk. The milk is usually discarded, however, depending on the type of infection and the antibiotic used to treat it.

Babies who are delivered outside a hospital are not admitted to the regular newborn nursery. They usually are cared for in the observation nursery or with the mother in a rooming-in situation.

To further protect the infant from outside sources of infection, everyone coming in contact with the infant or his environment is required to change from his or her street clothes or wear a gown over them. For the nursery nurse, the gowns should be short-sleeved so that the hands, forearms and elbows may be given a thorough scrub or wash. A clean gown should be donned at the beginning of each shift and changed if soiled. Those coming into the patient's room when the baby is there, or into the nursery for shorter periods of time, may wear a long-sleeved cover gown over their clothes. If they are going to touch the baby, their hands and arms should be scrubbed.

Most hospitals limit the number of visitors to the maternity area and exclude visitors from the nursery proper, although sometimes exceptions are made. Children are usually excluded from the maternity unit, since various infections and particularly communicable diseases are so prevalent among them. With the increasing emphasis on the total family in maternity care, however, some hospitals are making provision for sibling visitation, usually in special rooms.

Old regulations about wearing masks and hair coverings are being changed. However, the hair should be worn short or pulled back to avoid coming in contact with the infant. Masks are no longer worn, since they must be changed every 20 to 30 minutes to be effective, and, in fact, they can become a reservoir of bacteria when not applied properly or changed regularly.

Occasionally, the mother will be instructed to wear a mask in tending the baby if she has had a recent cold or if she develops a cold when she goes home. The nurse should make certain that the mother understands the underlying principles for applying and wearing the mask and especially that she be aware of how her hands can be contaminated in adjusting and tying it. Even at home a clean mask should be worn each time the need arises, and the mother should be instructed to wash her hands each time after she adjusts it.

Hospital Set-ups for Care of The Newborn

Rooming-In

Rooming-in is a term applied to the plan of having the new infant share the mother's hospital unit so that mother and child may be cared for together. This type of arrangement has come to mean much more than caring for the mother and the infant in the same unit of space. Rather, it implies an attitude in maternal and infant care that supports parental education and is based on recognition and understanding of the needs of each mother, infant and family. Some authorities feel that the separation of mother and child (and father) results in an unnatural fragmentation of the family at an important time for building family unity.

Rooming-in often is discussed as if it were a modern innovation. Historically, however, all mothers back to Paleolithic times "roomed-in" until the central nursery was instituted during the first two decades of the 20th century. Nevertheless, rooming-in as it is practiced today does represent a departure from the concept of the traditional central nursery.

Attitudes in maternal and infant care have changed, in part because of increased insight into the needs of the mother, her baby, and the family as a unit. Rooming-in plays an important part in the family-centered approach to maternity care, for it not only provides an environment which fosters a wholesome, natural mother-child relationship from the very beginning, but it also affords unlimited opportunities for the parents to learn about the care of their baby (Fig. 29-14).

Some hospitals have special rooming-in units with adjoining nurseries and workrooms. Although this is an ideal arrangement, it is not always possible, and the benefits of rooming-in should not be denied the family because of the physical set-up of the hospital. Many hospitals allow rooming-in if the mother has a private room and keeps the baby in the room all the time. Some women are discouraged by this arrangement because of the expense of a

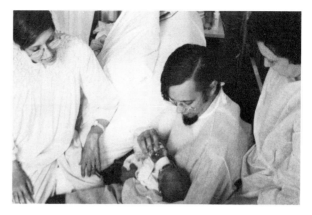

Figure 29-14. Rooming-in unit. Mother is assisting father to feed their baby as nurse observes. (Woman's Hospital Division, Hospital of the University of Pennsylvania, Philadelphia)

private room or their desire to have more contact with other people. Perhaps a good compromise is the modified program used in many hospitals which allows a mother to have her infant in the room for long periods of time and utilize the central nursery the rest of the time.

The newborn infant must be protected from sources of infection regardless of where he is cared for. The same basic principles for asepsis employed in the nursery must be followed in infant care in the rooming-in unit.

The Central Nursery System

The central or general newborn nursery on the postpartal division is designed for the care of a variable number of healthy newborn infants (Fig. 29-15). In this system the infants are brought to their mothers at certain specified times during the day—generally for feeding and/or visiting. The staff assumes the responsibility for all the care of the babies. Some type of central nursery is usually found in most hospitals.

With the emergence of the many drug-resistant organisms that abound in the hospital environment, the danger of epidemics (whenever a large aggregate of persons collect) is enhanced. Control of the physical facilities and stringent personnel policies accomplish a good deal of protection of the newborn so managed. For instance, cribs should be placed at least 2 feet apart with 3-feet-wide aisles between the cribs. Limiting the number of infants in a nursery to from 8 to 12 is also helpful. The precau-

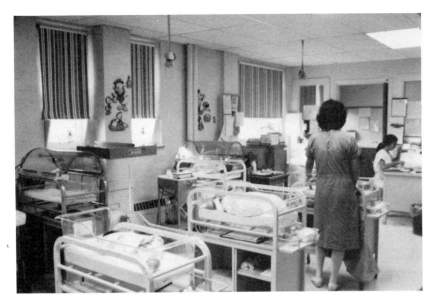

Figure 29-15. Term newborn nursery

tions previously mentioned, such as handwashing, wearing scrub clothes and following other aspects of nursery aseptic technique, afford additional protection.

The central nursery is a so-called clean nursery. But it must be understood that there is a difference in nursery technique between what is considered to be nursery clean and what is considered to be baby clean (i.e., what is clean for an individual baby). There should be no common equipment, such as a common bath table, used in providing care for the babies. There should be provisions in the nursery for individual technique to be followed. Each infant should have his own crib and general supplies, so that he can be given such care as his daily inspection bath or be diapered or dressed in his own bed. Most cribs are constructed with a built-in cabinet for the infant's own supplies (clean diapers, shirts, and linens) and a drawer to hold the containers for cotton balls, safety pins, thermometer, and so on. When such cribs are not available, improvised units for the infant's crib should be obtained so that individual-care techniques can be carried out.

If there is any evidence of a questionable infection at the time of delivery, if the infant is born on the way to the hospital, or if the infant is suspected of having an infection of the eyes, the skin, the mouth, or the gastrointestinal tract, the infant should not be admitted to the central nursery but should be kept in isolette isolation.

Observation Nursery

Maternity hospitals should have an observation nursery where infants suspected of developing an infectious condition may be kept until the presence or absence of infection is determined. When a definite diagnosis of infection is made, the infant must be transferred immediately to an isolation nursery away from the maternity division.

Aside from the fact that infants in the suspect or observation nursery must be segregated from others, and naturally require closer supervision and care because of suspected infection, their nursing care otherwise should be like that given a healthy newborn infant.

NURSING CARE OF THE NEWBORN

Care During The Transition Period

In the delivery room initial care has been given to the infant and any early problems have been dealt with (see Chap. 23). From the delivery room the infant may be taken to the recovery room and remain with the mother and father for a while, go to a transitional nursery, or be admitted directly to the regular nursery. Of course, if the infant has serious problems, a special care nursery would be indicated (see Chap. 38).

Since the day of birth is the most hazardous time for the infant, it is important that continuing observations be made during the first 24 hours. A receiving or transition nursery in the labor or nursery section provides an excellent physical environment for the extensive observations that are necessary, similar to that of recovery room care for adults. An infant whose mother has been heavily medicated during labor and delivery will be particularly in need of this recovery care. If this kind of set-up is not available, the new babies should be placed in an area of the regular nursery where they can be easily observed. Low-risk babies whose mothers had little or no medication, can probably be safely left with their mothers for a time under close supervision of a nurse in case of presence of mucus or other sudden changes in the infant's condition. If the mother plans to have rooming-in, it is often delayed until the infant is 12 to 24 hours old.

Initial Assessment and Care.   On admission of the infant to the nursery, the nursery nurse receives a report from the delivery room nurse, checks identification bands according to hospital policy, and does an initial assessment of the infant (see p. 448–449). If silver nitrate was not placed in the infant's eyes in the delivery room, it is done as soon as possible in the nursery. Also, the vitamin K injection, if ordered, may be given in the nursery (see Fig. 29-16 for injection technique).

The vital signs should be checked every half hour until they are stable or as indicated by hospital policy. Apical heart rate and respirations should each be counted for a full minute. The pulse, as noted before, varies with the infant's activity, but a persistent rate below 120 or above 150 should be reported (see p. 444).

Depending on the infant's temperature and the facilities available, he is usually placed under a radiant warmer or in an isolette, until the axillary temperature reaches about 36.6° C. (97.8 F.). Axillary temperature is preferred over rectal because it gives an indication of skin temperature rather than core body temperature and will alert the nurse to cooling of the infant before cold stress is severe (Fig. 29-17). Also, it eliminates the potential danger of perforation of the rectum with the rectal thermometer. If a radiant warmer is used, frequent checking of the skin probe is essential. If it detaches from the infant's skin, the warmer continues to radiate heat after the desired temperature is reached and the infant can become overheated. The temperature of an isolette, if it is being used to warm the baby, should be checked since it can also rise higher than expected and cause overheating.

The first bath is usually delayed until after the temperature has stabilized. The temperature should

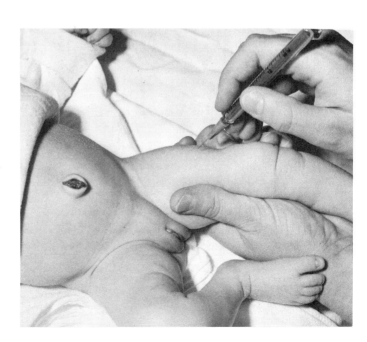

Figure 29-16. IM injection for infant.

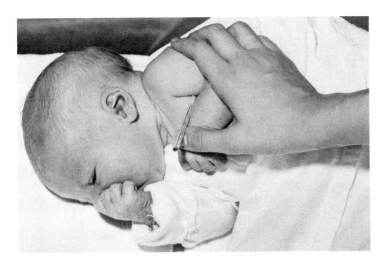

Figure 29-17. Taking axillary temperature.

be taken again following the bath and the infant placed back under the warmer if the temperature has dropped.

In a vigorous, normal infant, the cry should be lusty and should occur especially when the baby is handled or moved. If this does not happen, and the infant seems "sleepy" or depressed, it may be necessary to stimulate him to cry every hour or more frequently, depending on the degree of depression. This response may be aroused by changing his position or rubbing his back, head, or feet.

Brief tremors and twitching are not unusual in the transition period, but if they are prolonged or occur frequently, they may indicate a problem and the doctor should be notified.

Respiration and Color. The infant's color and respiratory pattern are good indices of whether or not the newborn is experiencing respiratory insufficiency. Dyspnea, rapid respiration exceeding 50 breaths per minute, and persistent cyanosis should be reported. Since mucus in the nasopharynx often causes respiratory distress, the nurse should be particularly watchful for its presence. Gagging, vomiting, breath holding, retraction of the head, choking, and cyanosis are all signs of the presence of mucus, which is particularly prone to develop in the second period of reactivity following the first sleep. Postural drainage and the technique for aspirating mucus are explained in Chapter 39.

Skin. The baby's skin should be observed for pallor and jaundice as well as cyanosis. Pressing the skin with a finger often enables clearer visualization of jaundice. The blanching that occurs with the maneuver provides a contrast that shows up the icteric color more clearly. The significance of pallor and jaundice in the first 24 hours is explained in Chapter 39.

Stools and Urine. The time of the baby's first stool and voiding should be noted, to indicate proper excretory function. It is sometimes necessary for the nurse to check with the delivery room records to see whether the infant voided or defecated at delivery.

Condition of the Cord. The cord should be checked periodically; any oozing or hemorrhage should be reported immediately, and the cord should be reclamped or retied as indicated. Oozing occurs most often between the second and the sixth hours of life and frequently is associated with crying or the passage of meconium.

Continuing Care

During the infant's hospital stay, the nurse will be responsible for providing daily care. The mother should be involved with as much of this care as possible to help her prepare for taking over the responsibility when she gets home. This is easiest if there is a rooming-in or modified rooming-in arrangement, but it is possible even with central nursery care.

It is important that the nurse assess the mother's understanding and her skill in caring for her infant. Any basic principles or procedures related to infant care that the mother finds necessary and useful should be part of the nurse's teaching plan for the mother during her hospital stay. The following principles of care can be conveyed easily to the mother (and the father when he is present).

Handling the Infant

Although small, newborns are not as fragile as they sometimes seem. They should be treated gently, of course, but firm, smooth handling will help them feel secure. There is no one right way of turning, lifting or holding a newborn, but several points should be kept in mind.

1. The head and buttocks need to be supported.
2. Babies are wiggly and can push themselves out of your grasp.
3. It is easier to pick an infant up from the supine position than from the side-lying or prone position.

A suggested way to lift a baby is to place one hand under the neck to support the head and shoulders and the other hand under the buttocks to grasp the opposite thigh (Fig. 29-18). The baby can then be lifted up to a holding position or moved from one place to another. A useful position for holding or carrying is the "football hold" (Fig. 29-19). Mothers appreciate learning about this position, because, like the nurse, they often have times when they need to hold the baby and still have one hand free.

Feelings of confidence in dressing and undressing the baby come with practice. It is helpful, when

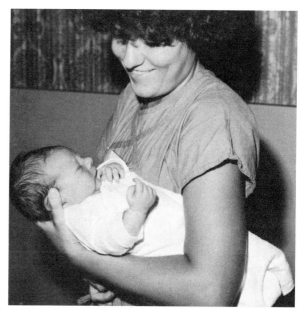

Figure 29-19. Football hold for carrying the infant.

putting on a shirt or gown, to reach through the sleeve with your fingers and pull the infant's hand through. Diapering is fairly simple if disposable diapers, fastened with tapes, are used, as they are in most hospitals. If pins are needed they should be inserted pointing toward the infant's back so there is less danger to the infant if they come open. The infant is usually wrapped snugly in a blanket (swaddling) before he is taken to his mother or placed in his crib. Some infants seem happier with their arms inside the blanket, and others like their arms free. Positioning in the crib is usually on the side with a blanket roll at the infant's back for support. This should extend from shoulder to hip. If it is behind the baby's head, it will push the head forward.

Bathing and Hygiene

The daily cleansing of the infant affords an excellent opportunity for making the observations that are necessary during the immediate postnatal period. How frequently a bath is given and what materials are used may vary from institution to institution.

Several decades ago the daily soap and water and oil baths were replaced with merely wiping off excess vernix with dry or slightly moist cotton balls. The diaper area was cleansed as necessary. However, in view of the increase in staphylococcal infections in newborn nurseries, in many centers an

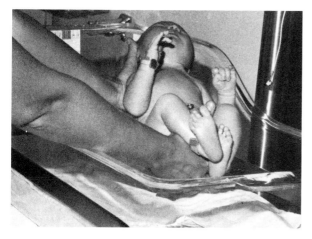

Figure 29-18. One method of lifting the baby is to place one hand under the infant's neck and the other under the buttocks.

initial sponge bath with a liquid detergent containing 3 percent hexachlorophene is used, with special attention to the cord and genital areas. It is particularly important to rinse the baby well after the use of hexachlorophene. Daily use is no longer recommended because of suggestive evidence of CNS damage following prolonged exposure.

For the remainder of the baby's stay in the hospital, a mild soap and plain warm water can be used for cleansing purposes. The use of strong soap, oil, and baby powder is discouraged by many pediatricians because of the sensitivity of the newborn's skin.

Blood is removed from the skin after the delivery, but no attempt is made to thoroughly remove the vernix caseosa unless it is stained with blood or meconium. The vernix caseosa serves to protect the skin and disappears spontaneously in about 24 hours. If it remains in the creases and folds of the skin longer than two days, it is apt to cause irritation. In this case gentle wiping usually removes it sufficiently.

Basic Principles.   Each nurse and mother will develop her own manner of bathing the newborn according to her manual dexterity, the size and the activity of the infant, and the facilities available (Fig. 29-20).

Several basic principles should be observed.
1. First, all equipment, clothing, and supplies should be assembled. Safety pins, if used, should be closed and placed out of the reach of the baby. Receptacles for soiled clothing, cotton balls, and so on should be available.
2. Second, care should be taken so that the environment is free from drafts and warm enough (i.e., 24 to 27° C. or 75 to 80° F.). The nurse should not have to interrupt the bath to close a door or a window. The water for the bath should be about 37 to 38° C. (98 to 100° F.). Water that feels warm to the elbow is approximately that temperature.
3. Third, in giving the bath the nurse should proceed from the "cleanest" areas to those that are "most soiled." Thus, the eyes are bathed first, then the face, ears, scalp, neck, upper extremities, trunk, lower extremities, and finally the buttocks and the genitals. Each of these in turn is washed, *rinsed well*, and dried.
   Particular attention should be paid to cleansing and drying the scalp and all creases at the neck, behind the ears, under the arms, the palms of the hands and between the fingers and the toes, under the knees, and in the groin, the buttocks, and the genitals.
4. Finally, *the infant never should be left alone,* even on a large work area; one hand should be kept on him at all times. If it is necessary to leave the area, even for a second, he should be taken along or placed in the crib.

Demonstration and Practice.   Each mother should have an opportunity to observe a demonstration of a sponge bath and, if at all possible, to give a bath to her infant. If there is an opportunity for only one bath, the nurse can combine the demonstration and return demonstration by discussing the bath with the mother first and then letting her give the bath with the nurse there for moral support and assistance as necessary.

The various principles enumerated above can be conveyed to the mother readily. In addition, the nurse should explore with the mother what facilities are available in the home so that the necessities can be met and undue expense and difficulty avoided. For instance, a large drainboard which can be washed and padded adequately (and is a comfortable height for handling the infant) can be utilized for the bath area. A large pan or basin does very well for the bathtub in the early weeks; it should be kept only for the baby's use. Thus, the extra expense of special equipment can be minimized.

At discharge time, the mother can be advised to give a sponge bath using a soft washcloth and mild soap until the cord has fallen off and the area is healed. After this, a tub bath can be given. The mother is also advised to wash the baby's hair when she gives the baby a sponge bath. The same soap the baby is washed with, or any brand of baby shampoo can be used. She should be told not to put any kind of baby oil in the hair, as this may predispose to "cradle cap."

A mother should not be made to feel that she has to give the baby a bath every day. Some mothers and babies enjoy the bath as a daily routine, but for those who do not, as long as the face and diaper area are washed as needed, a bath every other day may be sufficient.

Eyes.   In the daily care of the baby, no special treatment other than necessary cleansing with clean water is given the baby's eyes unless there is a

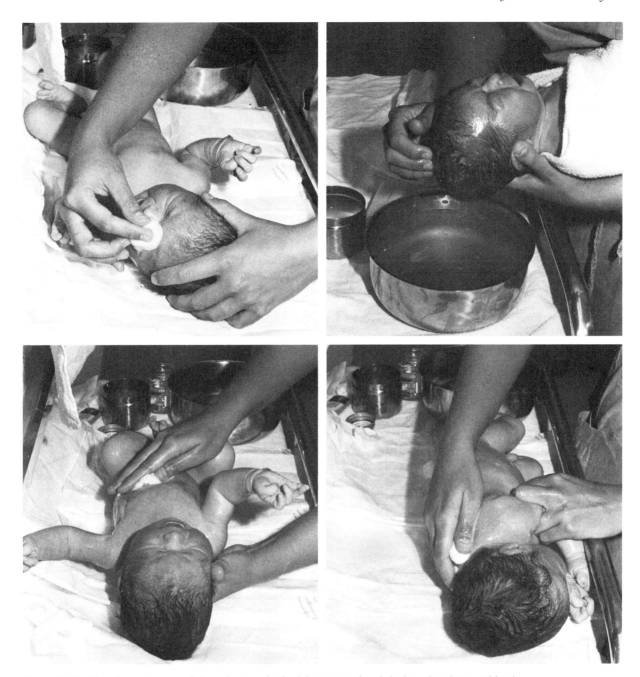

Figure 29-20. The cleanest areas of the infant are bathed first (eyes, head) before the chest and back.

discharge. Any redness, swelling, or discharge should be reported and recorded on the chart. There may be some reaction from the medication used for prophylaxis against ophthalmia neonatorum, but the physician will prescribe treatment if necessary. When cleaning the eyes, one should wipe them from the inner corner to the outer corner, using a clean cotton ball or clean area of the wash cloth for each eye.

Nose and Ears. Cotton-tipped applicators should not be used in cleaning the infant's nose or ears because of danger of injuring the delicate tissues. The nose usually does not need cleaning because the infant sneezes to clear the nasal passages. If some dried mucus does need to be removed from the nose, a small twisted piece of cotton moistened with water may be used. Only the outer ear should be cleaned. Nothing should be put inside the ear.

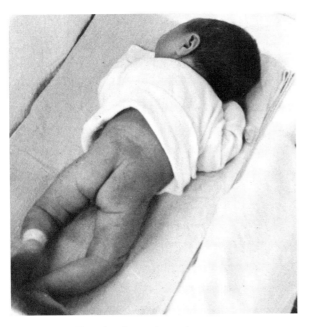

Figure 29-21. Exposing buttocks to air.

Care of the Skin

The newborn's skin is often dry and peeling within a few days after birth, and dry cracks may appear in the wrist and ankle areas. This is sometimes a cause of concern to mothers and they want to put oil or some other preparation on the skin to get rid of the dryness. They can be reassured that the flakiness and cracks will disappear in a few days and that oil and some lotions may make matters worse by causing a rash.

The skin is thin, delicate, extremely tender, and very easily irritated. Since the skin is a protective covering, breaks in its surface may initiate troublesome infection; hence skin disturbances constitute an actual threat to the baby's well-being.

The new baby does not perspire, usually, until after the first month. Warm weather or excessive clothing may cause the infant to develop prickly heat, a closely grouped pinhead-sized rash of papules and vesicles, on the face, the neck, and wherever skin surfaces touch. Fewer clothes and some control over the room temperature will help to relieve the discomfort.

Buttocks. Sometimes, despite good nursing care, the infant's buttocks become reddened and sore. A diaper rash may occur, caused by the reaction of bacteria with the urea in the urine. This in turn causes an ammonia dermatitis. The most important

prophylaxis is to keep the diaper area clean and dry. Sometimes petroleum jelly, baby oil, or a bland protective ointment, such as vitamin A and D ointment, is used to protect the area. Pastes may not be advised, because they are much more adhesive than ointments and thus create cleansing problems.

A simple treatment that is often effective is merely to expose the infant's reddened buttocks to air (Fig. 29-21) and light several times a day, using care to keep the infant covered otherwise. Air may be all that is necessary, although the use of a *lamp* treatment is more effective and at the same time provides a measure of warmth. An ordinary gooseneck lamp with a screened blub (no stronger than 40 watts) can be placed on the table so that it is a foot or more away from the infant's exposed buttocks. The light may be used for 30 minutes at a time. Because the skin is already irritated, the nurse should exercise care not to burn it further by using too strong a bulb or placing the light too close.

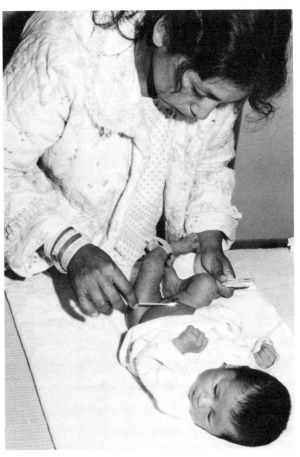

Figure 29-22. The mother can be encouraged to give cord care to her infant.

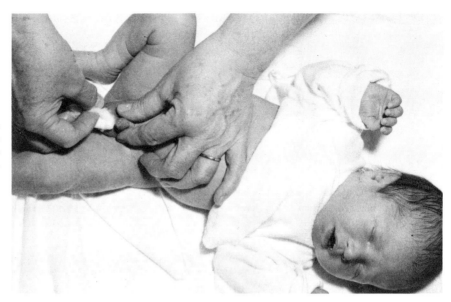

Figure 29-23. Retracting foreskin for cleansing penis (uncircumcised.) (MacDonald House, The University Hospitals of Cleveland, Cleveland, Ohio)

If the condition occurs at home, the treatment described above also is appropriate, and the mother can be so instructed. Boiling the diapers is another effective measure, since this destroys the bacteria. However, many of the detergents and conditioners used today have antibacterial agents in them, and these may be effective in washing the diapers. Care should be taken to rinse the diapers thoroughly, since the residue of the detergent in itself can be irritating. In this respect, the modern diaper services have very effective facilities; many sterilize diapers and entire layettes as part of the service.

Cord Care.   Babies do not receive a tub bath until the cord has separated, and the umbilicus has healed. A cord dressing is considered to be unnecessary since exposure to the air enhances drying of the cord.

Most physicians prefer that the base be wiped with alcohol daily to encourage drying further and to discourage the possibility of infection. In some hospitals, an antibiotic ointment is used (Fig. 29-22).

No attempt should be made to dislodge the cord before it separates completely. If there is a red inflamed area around the stump or any discharge with an odor, this condition should be recorded and reported immediately. The cord usually becomes detached from the body between the fifth and the eighth days after birth, but it may not detach until the twelfth or the fourteenth day. When the cord drops off, the umbilicus is depressed somewhat and

usually free from any evidence of inflammation. No further treatment is necessary, except to keep the part clean and dry. When inflammation is present, the physician will give specific orders for care. The cord clamp is removed in 24 hours, provided that the umbilical stump has dried sufficiently.

Cleaning the Genitalia.   In a male infant, adhesions between the prepuce and the glans penis are very common. The foreskin may be extended beyond the glans. A curdy secretion, *smegma,* may form in considerable amount and collect under the prepuce behind the glans. Also, small amounts of urine may be retained. Any of these conditions favor irritation and, if found, should be reported to the obstetrician who may perform the delicate operations of separating the adhesions, stretching the prepuce, or circumcising the baby.

If a circumcision is not done, some doctors recommend retracting the foreskin for cleaning purposes beginning a few days after birth (Fig. 29-23); others recommend waiting until further growth and development causes some separation and makes it easier to retract (see p. 454). If the foreskin is retracted, it must be replaced over the glans after cleaning or edema may occur.

In female infants, smegma may accumulate between the folds of the labia and should be carefully cleansed with moistened cotton balls using the front-to-back direction and a clean cotton ball for each stroke. When demonstrating this technique to the mother the nurse can underscore the importance of teaching a little girl to wipe herself from front to back to help prevent urinary tract infections.

Circumcision and Care

Whether or not a male infant should be circumcised is an old controversy. The procedure is said by some to promote better hygiene, prevent inflammation and infection and decrease the incidence of cancer of the penis. Others say that these advantages are also present in uncircumcised males who practice good personal hygiene. The Committee on Fetus and the Newborn of the American Academy of Pediatrics states that there are no valid medical indications for circumcision.[22] Traditional, cultural and religious factors are all involved in deciding whether or not the procedure will be done. The final decision should be made by the parents and a consent signed by one of them before the circumcision is done.

The infant should not be fed for several hours prior to being circumcised, since he will be restrained in a supine position for some time and might regurgitate (Fig. 29-24). The procedure is a sterile one, with the use of sterile gloves, instruments and drapes by the physician. Several methods have been devised, including the use of the Gomco (Yellen) clamp and the Plastibell.

Care Following Circumcision. When the newborn infant is circumcised, the main principles of postoperative care are to keep the wound clean and to observe it closely for bleeding (see Fig. 29-25). For the first 24 hours the area is covered with a sterile gauze dressing to which a liberal amount of sterile petrolatum has been added. If the circumcision is done with the Plastibell, no dressing or petrolatum (or petroleum jelly) is used.

Mothers are naturally anxious about their babies at this time, so, as soon as it is feasible after the circumcision has been done, the nurse should take the baby to his mother for a brief visit. She can be reassured that the procedure has not been very painful for her child. The infant will cry during the operation, but this is due as much to the necessary restraints as to the discomfort. It may be helpful to show her what the circumcision looks like and explain how it will look when healing, so that she can recognize any deviations from normal. With the

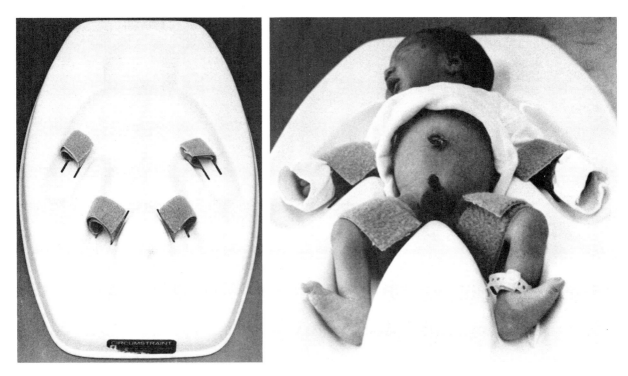

Figure 29-24. Preparation of the infant, restrained for circumcision. (*Left*) Board as used in many hospitals for circumcision. (*Right*) The infant, restrained on the board with towels, ready for circumcision.

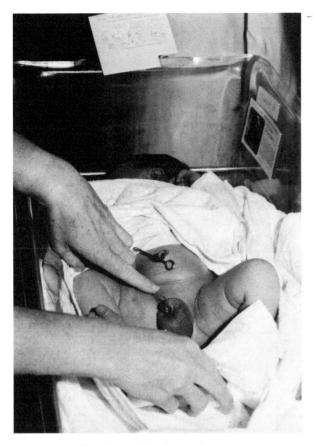

Figure 29-25. Postcircumcision inspection.

Plastibell, there will be a plastic ring and suture in place which will drop off with the foreskin in about 7 to 10 days.

Occasionally, a local anesthetic will be used, but generally the procedure is performed without it. Thus, the infant may be fed immediately after the circumcision, and both mother and baby seem to enjoy the comfort that the feeding and cuddling bring. If the infant is left in the room for an extended length of time, the nurse should go in periodically to check the circumcision for bleeding.

In changing the infant's diaper the nurse should hold his ankles with one hand so that he cannot kick against the operative area. Unless the physician orders otherwise, the circumcision dressing can be removed postoperatively when the infant voids for the first time. Cleansing must be done gently but can be accomplished as necessary with cotton balls moistened with warm tap water. A fresh sterile petrolatum dressing usually is applied to the penis each time the diaper is changed for the first day. The penis must be observed closely for bleeding,

and during the first 12 hours should be inspected every hour. It is advisable to place the infant's crib where he can be watched conveniently. Moreover, to keep all the nursing personnel alerted, some signal, such as a red tag, can be attached to the identification card on the crib. If bleeding occurs, usually it can be controlled with gentle pressure. If bleeding persists, the physician should be notified immediately.

Since the length of the maternity stay has been considerably shortened, circumcision may be done on the second or the third postnatal day or even before the baby leaves the delivery room. Sometimes the operation is performed on the day preceding or day of discharge; therefore the nurse should ascertain the physician's wishes for aftercare and make certain that the mother knows how to care for her newly circumcised infant. Generally, the care will be the same as that described.

Other Areas of Concern

Weight.   The baby should be weighed on the birth date and every day or every other day thereafter. If the infant remains in the hospital longer than five days, he should be weighed at intervals prescribed by the medical staff. His weight should be recorded accurately.

During the first few days after birth the infant may lose 5 to 10 percent of his birth weight. This is due partly to the minimal intake of nutrients and fluid and partly to the loss of excess fluid. About the time the meconium begins to disappear from his stools, the weight begins to increase, and in normal cases does so regularly until about the tenth day of life, when it may equal the birth weight. Then the baby should begin to gain from 4 to 6 ounces per week during the first five months. After this time the gain is from 2 to 4 ounces weekly. At six months of age, the baby should be double his birth weight, and he should triple it when he is a year old. This is one way to note the baby's condition and progress; when the baby is not gaining, that fact should be reported to the physician. Besides gaining regularly in weight and strength, the baby should be happy and good-natured when awake and inclined to sleep a good part of the time between feedings.

Sleeping. The baby will need rest and sleep, with as little handling as possible. If he is well and comfortable, he usually sleeps much of the time and wakes and cries when he is hungry or uncomfortable. He may sleep as much as 20 hours out of 24 (although this varies considerably from infant to infant). It is not the sound sleep of the adult; rather he moves a good deal, stretches, and at intervals awakens momentarily. Since he responds so readily to external stimuli (and this may make him restless), his clothing and coverings are important. They should be light in weight, warm but not too warm, and free from wrinkles. His position should be changed frequently when he is awake. He can be placed on either side or on his abdomen, especially when he is ready for sleep. If he is positioned on his back, someone should be present, for if the baby regurgitates, he is more likely to aspirate in this position. As he gets older and learns to roll over, he will assume the position that he likes most for sleep.

Crying. After the baby is dressed and placed in a warm crib he usually does not cry unless he is wet, hungry, ill, uncomfortable for some reason, or is moved. One learns to distinguish an infant's condition and needs from the character of his cry, which may be described as follows:

1. A loud, insistent cry with drawing up and kicking of the legs usually denotes colicky pain.
2. A fretful cry, if due to indigestion, will be accompanied by green stools and passing of gas.
3. A whining cry is noticeable when the baby is ill, premature, or very frail.
4. A fretful, hungry cry, with fingers in the mouth and flexed, tense extremities, is easily recognized.
5. A peculiar, shrill, sharp-sounding cry suggests injury, especially CNS.

Every effort should be made to recognize any deviation from the usual manner in which a baby announces his normal requirements. Moreover, this information should be conveyed to the mother, since it is essential that the mother learn to interpret her infant's cues. The newborn has only his posture and his voice at this time to inform others of his needs.

HYPERTONIC BABIES. Occasionally, the nurse will find that an infant seems to be fussy from birth. He appears very active, startles easily, cries readily and more frequently (and apparently for no reason), is alert and awake much of the time, and in general does not fit the usual pattern of activity, feeding, and sleeping described. These babies may be described as *hypertonic,* that is, they do not seem to be able to relax as well as other infants.

The parents, particularly, may find it difficult to adjust to their new baby and may experience a great deal of anxiety until they are informed (or learn by trial and error) that this is "normal behavior" for this child. Too often they assume they must be doing something "wrong," since despite their efforts, their baby remains fussy, tense, and crying. The nurse can be very helpful to the parents in giving them anticipatory guidance about their baby's behavior and helpful ways in which he can be soothed. The physician should also be informed of the nurse's observations in order to give appropriate advice to the parents.

These infants usually respond favorably to being held securely. Thus, wrapping them snugly with a receiving blanket, cuddling them securely, changing their position slowly and surely rather than quickly all help to allay undue tenseness. Rocking the baby and walking with him are particularly successful measures, but no parent can or should do this over protracted periods of time.

Any new activity or procedures should be introduced slowly to this kind of infant. For instance, when a tub bath is given for the first time, the infant should be placed very slowly in a small amount of water, and each lower extremity immersed gradually in order not to frighten or startle the infant too much. The parents should not consider an occasional evening out a luxury; rather it should be considered a necessary item in the care of their baby. These infants do place greater demands on their parents than do infants of a more placid nature, and a short time away from the baby does wonders in restoring the perspective and good humor of the parents.

Urinary Elimination. Urinary activity of the fetus is evidenced by the presence of urine in the amniotic fluid. The baby usually voids during delivery or immediately after birth, but the function may be suppressed for several hours. However, if the baby does not void within 24 hours, the condition should be reported to the physician, as retention of the urine may be due to an imperforate meatus. After the first two or three days the baby voids from 10 to 15 times a day. When the urine is concentrated, red or rusty stains on the wet diaper may be due to uric-acid crystals in the urine.

Intestinal Elimination. During fetal life the content of the intestines is made up of brownish-green tarlike material called meconium. It is composed of epithelial and epidermal cells and lanugo hair that probably were swallowed with the amniotic fluid. The dark greenish-brown color of the meconium is due to the bile pigment. During fetal life and for the first few hours after birth, the intestinal contents are sterile. Apparently, there is no peristalsis until after birth, because normally there is no discoloration of the amniotic fluid.

STOOLS. For the first five or six days, the stools gradually change from meconium to transitional stools (after which they become the regular milk stools). During this time the color of the stools changes from tarry black to a greenish black, to greenish brown, to brownish yellow, and thence to greenish yellow. The transitional stools are composed of both meconium and milk stools; hence their variation in color.

After the transitional stools the color gradually changes to a soft yellow of a smooth pasty consistency with a characteristic foul odor if the infant is formula-fed. Stools of breast-fed infants tend to be golden yellow and of mushy consistency. Most newborns pass the first stool within 12 hours of birth—nearly all have a stool in 24 hours. If an infant has not passed a stool by this time, intestinal obstruction must be considered as a possible reason for the delay, and the baby must be observed closely.

The daily number of stools on about the fifth day of life is usually four to six. As the infant grows, this number decreases to one or two each day. The type of stool of the breastfed baby may be influenced by the mother's diet. However, there may be slight variations from the normal, which may have little significance if the baby appears to be comfortable and sleeps and nurses well. If the baby's stools have a watery consistency, are of a green color, contain much mucus, and flatus is being passed, the condition may be evidence of some digestive or intestinal irritation and should be reported to the physician.

The number, color, and consistency of stools should be recorded daily on the baby's record.

Discharge from the Hospital

Discharge planning for a new mother and baby may begin in the prenatal class or clinic, when discussions are held about planning for "What happens after the baby comes?" During the hospital stay the nurse continues to assess the needs of the family in planning for care of the baby at home. Although much teaching can be done in the hospital, for some new mothers, especially the inexperienced, a referral to a community health agency may be appropriate for follow-up. Some families with financial problems may need to be referred to a family service agency.

Plans for health care follow-up of the infant should be discussed with the mother. A follow-up appointment should be made with a private physician or at a well-baby clinic. Most new mothers appreciate an opportunity to talk to the nurse regarding their concerns about taking the baby home. Taking time for such a talk is well worth the nurse's effort, since it can help make those first few days at home less frightening and more enjoyable for the new parents.

REFERENCES

1. F. A. Manning, L. Platt and M. LeMay: "Fetal breathing." In *Current Practice in Obstetric and Gynecologic Nursing*, Vol. 2. Ed. L. McNall and J. Galeener. St. Louis, C. V. Mosby, 1977.
2. H. Harned, Jr.: "Respiration and the respiratory system." In *Perinatal Physiology*. Ed. U. Stave. New York, Plenum Medical Book Co., 1978.
3. Ibid.
4. Ibid.
5. N. M. Nelson: "Respiration and circulation after birth." In *The Physiology of the Newborn Infant*, ed. 4. Ed. C. A. Smith and N. M. Nelson. Springfield, Ill., Charles C Thomas, 1976.
6. G. Honig, and M. Hruby: "Disorders of the blood and hematopoietic system." In *Neonatal-Perinatal Medicine*, ed. 2. Ed. R. D. Behrman. St. Louis, C. V. Mosby, 1977.
7. A. Hernandez, D. A. Meyer and D. Goldring: "Blood pressure in neonates." *Contemp OB/Gyn* 5:34–37, March 1975.
8. Honig and Hruby, op. cit.

9. Ibid.

10. L. Gartner and K. Lee: "Unconjugated hyperbilirubinemia." In *Neonatal-Perinatal Medicine,* ed. 2. Ed. R. D. Behrman. St. Louis, C. V. Mosby, 1977.

11. Ibid.

12. J. C. Sinclair: "Metabolic rate and temperature control." In *The Physiology of the Newborn Infant.* ed. 4. Ed. C. A. Smith and N. M. Nelson. Springfield, Ill., Charles C Thomas, 1976.

13. F. B. Roberts: *Perinatal Nursing.* New York, McGraw-Hill, 1977.

14. A. Spitzer, J. Bernstein and C. M. Edelmann, Jr.: "Diseases of the urinary tract." In *Neonatal-Perinatal Medicine,* ed. 2. Ed. R. D. Behrman. St. Louis, C. V. Mosby, 1977.

15. Nurses Association of the American College of Obstetricians and Gynecologists: "Physical asssessment of the neonate." *NAACOG Technical Bulletin No. 2,* September 1978.

16. T. B. Brazelton: *Neonatal Behavioral Assessment Scale.* Clinics in Developmental Medicine, No. 50. Philadelphia, J. B. Lippincott, 1973.

17. Ibid.

18. M. P. Erickson: "Trends in assessing the newborn and his parents." *MCN,* 3, 2:99–103, March/April 1978.

19. Brazelton, op. cit.

20. Ibid.

21. Ibid.

22. Committee on Fetus and Newborn, American Academy of Pediatrics: "Report of the ad hoc task force on circumcision." *Pediatrics* 56: 610–611, Oct. 1975.

SUGGESTED READING

Als, H., and Brazelton, T. B.: "Comprehensive neonatal assessment." *BFJ,* 2, 1:3–9, Winter 1974–1975.

Arnold, H. W. et al.: "Transition to extra-uterine life." *Am. J. Nurs.* 65, 10:77–80, Oct. 1965.

Behrman, R. E., ed.: *Neonatal-Perinatal Medicine,* ed. 2. St. Louis, C. V. Mosby, 1977.

Binzley, V.: "State: Overlooked factor in newborn nursing." *Am. J. Nurs.,* 77:102–103, Jan. 1977.

Desmond, M. et al.: "The clinical behavior of the newly born." *J. Pediatrics,* 62:307–325, March 1963.

Faber, M.: "Circumcision revisited." *BFJ,* 1, 2: 19–21, Spring 1974.

Hervada, A.: "Nursery evaluation of the newborn." *Am. J. Nurs.,* 67:1669–1671, Aug. 1967.

Nalepka, C. D.: "Understanding thermoregulation in newborns." *JOGN Nurs.,* 5, 6:17–19, Nov./Dec. 1976.

Pang, L. M. and Mellins, R. B.: "Neonatal cardiorespiratory physiology." *Anesthesiology* 43, 2:171–196, Aug. 1975.

Simkin, P. et al.: "Physiologic jaundice of the newborn." *BFJ* 6, 1:23–40, Spring 1979.

Smith, A. N.: "Physical examination of the newborn." In *Maternity Nursing Today,* ed. 2. Ed. J. P. Clausen, et al. New York, McGraw-Hill, 1977.

Smith, C. A. and Nelson, N. M., eds.: *The Physiology of the Newborn Infant,* ed. 4. Springfield, Ill., Charles C Thomas, 1976.

Stave, U., ed.: *Perinatal Physiology.* New York, Plenum Medical Book, 1978.

Williams, J. K. and Lancaster, J.: "Thermoregulation of the newborn." *MCN,* 1, 6:355–360, Nov./Dec. 1976.

Thirty

Infant Nutrition

The Newborn's Ability to Handle Food | Methods of Feeding—Making the Decision | Breast-Feeding | Artificial Feeding | Common Concerns in Infant Feeding | Nutritional Considerations During the First Year

Nutrition is very important in preserving health throughout the life cycle. It is particularly important during the rapid growing phase of infancy. The long-term effects of feeding practices in early infancy are just beginning to be recognized. According to Neumann and Jelliffe, infant feeding is more than just "nutrient refueling"; it is also a "social, psychological and educational interaction between caretaker and baby."[1]

THE NEWBORN'S ABILITY TO HANDLE FOOD

Up until the time of birth, the nutritional needs of the fetus have been met through placental circulation. One of the major physiological adaptations which the infant must make in the transition from intrauterine to extrauterine life is the change in the source of nourishment and the ability to take food into the body, digest it, and assimilate it.

Following birth, the gastrointestinal tract begins abruptly to process a rather large amount of food. At the same time the infant must begin to suck and swallow as a means of taking food into the stomach. The sucking and swallowing reflexes are already present at birth, and are normally quite strong. In fact, the swallowing reflex, as well as peristaltic movements in the stomach, becomes active during the last two months of fetal development, as noted in the bits of vernix caseosa and lanugo that are found with other debris in the meconium stool. In the delivery room, the infant will often swallow mucus or suck on anything that gets near his mouth.

Another important instinctive reaction is the rooting reflex, which enables the newborn to find food. The human infant does not have to search for its food, but it does turn toward anything that touches its cheeks or lips. This is a help in latching onto the bottle or breast.

At the time of birth, the infant's stomach is small, with a capacity of approximately 50 to 60 cc. But it can dilate considerably so that during feeding it stretches to at least three or four times its approximate capacity. Not only is it distended by the amount of food taken in (i.e., milk) but also by the amount of air swallowed as the infant sucks the milk or cries. In the act of crying, the infant tends to gulp in air.

The glandular structures in the gastric mucosa are present at birth, although shallow in comparison to those of the adult. The gastric musculature is somewhat deficient. This, plus the relatively greater length of the intestinal tract and the weakness of the abdominal musculature which serves as a supporting structure explain in part why considerable distention of the stomach is possible.

Although gastric digestion is not considered to be a factor of primary importance to the nutrition of the newborn infant, many of the findings reported by Clement Smith in his textbook could be useful in considering infant feeding schedules.[2] For example, the stomach empties more slowly in the newborn period than at any other time in life, but the distended stomach is able to adjust its content by promptly emptying some or all of its content into the duodenum. A number of the studies on gastric motility have demonstrated wide individual differences in emptying time. The major portion of the feeding usually leaves the stomach in less than three or four hours, however, in some instances, the emptying time of the infants' stomachs was more than eight hours. It was found also that the introduction of a second feeding before the stomach was empty caused portions of the first feeding to remain somewhat longer in the stomach than if the stomach was emptied before the next feeding was offered. Another important finding is that human milk leaves the stomach somewhat more rapidly than cow's milk, although a formula made of cow's milk which has been boiled leaves the stomach more rapidly than that which is fed without being boiled.

METHODS OF FEEDING—MAKING THE DECISION

The type of infant feeding to use is an important decision for the parents to make. Their ultimate choice will be influenced by a variety of factors, physical and psychologic as well as social. Ideally, the subject of infant feeding will be raised during the antepartal period, thereby providing an opportunity to guide the parents in making a decision that is most suitable for them. It is wise for the physician and the nurse to explore adequately with the mother (and the father, if necessary) mutual attitudes concerning this subject.

In the past, breast-feeding, by the mother or a "wet-nurse," was essential for the survival of the infant. This is still true to some extent in underdeveloped countries, but in most of the world modern methods of artificial feeding have offered women an alternative. Although the production of infant formulas has become a big business and the choice of artificial feeding is now safe for the infant and convenient for the mother, there are still many advantages to breast-feeding.

One should avoid being so overzealously in favor of breast-feeding that it is forced on a reluctant mother. Those women who do not want to breast-feed their infants should not be made to feel guilty about their choice. On the other hand, the nurse should not hesitate to inform expectant parents of the differences between the various milks available (including human) and of the advantages of breast-feeding to both mother and infant. Many women are uninformed about the differences in the available methods and may base their decision on how their mothers fed them or what a friend has said. For these women, information can be very useful in helping make a decision based on facts.

Advantages of Breast-Feeding

For many years, the saying "breast is best" was used in talking about the relative merits of breast or bottle feeding. At the same time reassurances were given that formula was fine for babies, too. In the past five to ten years, research studies from many disciplines have focused attention on the uniqueness of human milk and other favorable aspects of breast-feeding. Though knowledge is still incomplete, certain advantages of breast-feeding can be identified.

Biochemical/Nutritional Considerations. Contrary to the idea promoted by some commercial literature that modern formula is "almost like mother's milk," the constituents of cow's milk and human milk are dissimilar in almost every way except for water and lactose.[3] Even when the formula has been "modified" or "humanized," there are still many differences. For example, whey protein which accounts for more than 60 percent of the total protein in human milk constitutes only 20 percent of cow's milk. Even when amounts of a substance are approximately the same, absorption may be different. For instance, similar concentrations of zinc are present in both milks, but the human infant absorbs zinc more effectively from human milk because it has a different zinc binding factor than is found in cow's milk.[4] Formulas also have added substances such as emulsifiers, thickening agents, pH adjusters and antioxidants which are "not found in the original product for human infants."[5]

Immunological and Antiallergic Factors. Human milk and colostrum have been shown by many recent studies to be rich in defense factors, such as immunoglobulins, lactoferrin, enzymes, macrophages, lymphocytes, and *Lactobacillus bifidus* (a growth enhancer of lactobacilli). "These components promote a 'normal' bacterial colonization of the gastrointestinal tract and also suppress the invasiveness of certain pathogenic microorganisms. They may be of major importance to the newborn's system of defense against infection. However, further studies are needed to verify this view and to fill in some of the gaps in our knowledge."[6]

One known advantage of the immunoglobulin, secretory IgA, which is present in human milk, is the protective anti-absorptive effect it has in keeping protein molecules from passing through the intestinal walls. During the first six months of life, foreign proteins are more likely to be absorbed through the intestinal wall than they are in later life, which can lead to allergies. The protein in cow's milk is one of the most common food allergens encountered in infancy. Human milk proteins, on the other hand, are virtually non-allergic to humans.[7]

Psychological Aspects. The psychological advantages of breast-feeding are not as easily documented, and sometimes it is said that bottle-feeding and breast-feeding are interchangeable for the emotional well-being of mother and child. However, breast-feeding, by establishing a more direct and intimate biologic relationship between infant and mother, may very well influence the quality of the mother-child interaction.[8]

Other Aspects. *For the baby:* Breast milk can be safer, because it is not subject to incorrect mixing or contamination. The baby does not have to wait to eat—if mother is nearby the milk is always available and at the right temperature. The action of sucking at breast is different from sucking on a bottle, and may help the mouth and jaw to develop better.

For the mother: An early benefit is promotion of uterine involution stimulated by the release of oxytocin when the infant sucks. The mother also has the convenience of not having to prepare bottles or incur the added expense of buying formula. When a woman breast-feeds her infant, she is less likely to conceive again during the first eight to ten months of lactation. This is, of course, not as reliable as modern contraceptive measures, but can be helpful for those who cannot afford or accept artificial contraception.[9] (See References for a more complete discussion of advantages of breast-feeding.)

Choosing to Bottle-Feed

Throughout recorded history, women have sought alternatives to breast-feeding their infants. While the most popular alternative was the use of a wet-nurse, attempts at artificial feeding were widespread, as can be seen in the remains of spouted feeding pots, artificial teats, and other mechanical feeding devices. Historical writings show that women were often urged to breast-feed their own children, but many ignored these admonitions for various reasons.[11]

Women still give a variety of reasons for choosing artificial feeding. Some feel that breast-feeding is too tiring, confining, or simply distasteful; some may be afraid that it will disfigure their breasts. Others fear that they will fail at breastfeeding, especially if previous attempts to breast-feed a child were unsuccessful.

The mores and pressure of the mother's socio-economic class and peer group also are important. Bottle-feeding may be the acceptable practice in the community or neighborhood; relatives, friends, and others may be either very much for or against breast-feeding. Return to employment for the mother may be a very significant factor.

Certain conditions in both the mother and the infant also can have a bearing on the decision and outcome. Diseases and infection (i.e., syphilis, tuberculosis, heart and kidney disease, staphylococcal infections, communicable diseases) generally are contraindications for breast-feeding. Similarly, certain infections and anomalies in the infant may make nursing impossible, or at least temporarily impossible. Breast infection or painful, cracked or fissured nipples also may require that breast-feeding be discontinued temporarily. Pregnancy usually is considered to be an indication for weaning because of the physiologic strain that it places on mother.

BREAST-FEEDING

If breast-feeding is the method of choice for a new mother, the degree to which she perseveres in this endeavor is often influenced by her care in the hospital. Recent studies have shown that many breast-feeding mothers perceive nurses as being negative or neutral toward breast-feeding.[12] After returning home, many mothers encountered problems that they felt could have been prevented if they had been given more anticipatory guidance by the nurses in the hospital about possible problems.[13] In light of these findings, it seems safe to say that support from knowledgeable nursing personnel, permissive hospital policies, and anticipatory teaching can do much to make breast-feeding a pleasant and successful experience for mother and infant.

Mechanisms of Lactation

A working knowledge of how the breasts function in the lactation process can help the nurse to guide the new mother. The anatomy of the breasts and the physiology of lactation have been discussed in Chapters 26 and 28, to which the student is referred for a renewal of background understanding of the subject.

Secretion of Milk. Two major mechanisms are involved in lactation. The first of these is the secretion of milk. It is believed, that the hormone luteotrophin (prolactin, LTH, the lactogenic or mammogenic hormone) is responsible for the initiation of lactation and that the release of this hormone is enhanced by the sucking of the infant. The milk itself is secreted by the alveoli or acini cells, usually within three to four days postpartum and continuing for as long as the breasts are sufficiently emptied. Emptying the breasts frequently is also very important, especially in the early stages of lactation. Both the production of milk and the quantity produced are dependent on *frequent* and *complete* emptying of the breasts. If the breasts are not entirely emptied, and the back pressure in the alveoli is not relieved, milk secretion decreases and eventually stops.

In the early stages of lactation, milk secretion can be stimulated by having the infant nurse from both breasts at each feeding and by increasing the frequency of the feedings. Care should be taken not to tire the mother unduly. Milk production is slow in some mothers, but it can be stimulated by allowing the infant to nurse both breasts every two to three hours.

Milk-Ejection Reflex. The second mechanism involved in lactation is the milk-ejection reflex which has also been called the expulsion mechanism, the *let-down reflex* and the draught reflex. It is postulated that the mechanism works in the following way: Impulses from the baby's sucking cause release of oxytocin from the posterior portion of the pituitary. This hormone causes the contractile tissue (myoepithelial cells) around the alveoli to squeeze the milk into the larger ducts and eventually to propel it to the ducts leading to the nipples. Then the milk is removed by the compression and suction action of the baby's nursing.

The let-down reflex can be influenced profoundly by psychic factors and the emotions of the mother. For instance, some mothers find that the let-down reflex is elicited (i.e., their breasts begin to drip milk) by an infant's cry or some sound, sight, or other stimulus, that has become associated with nursing. Often they will say that they can feel their milk "come down" in anticipation of nursing. Fear, worry, pain and tension all may affect the expulsion mechanism adversely. Thus, it is particularly important for the nurse to help the mother to avoid these emotional disturbances whenever possible. A relaxed atmosphere for nursing, adequate assistance, effective pain relief, and a supportive attitude on the part of the nurse are essential components of effective nursing care for the mother who is breast-feeding.

Sometimes oxytocin is given to the mother during early lactation to facilitate the milk flow. It may be administered by injection or by a nasal spray (40 U.S.P. units per ml. of solution). This hormone assists the ejection of milk when the let-down reflex is inhibited (as in times of stress) and also is effective in facilitating the milk flow when the breasts are engorged.

Initiation of Breast-Feeding

Depending on the condition of both mother and infant, breast-feeding may be started shortly after birth, in the delivery or recovery room. The newborn usually is awake and alert for the first hour or so after birth and will often be seen trying to suck on its fist. Taking advantage of this heightened sucking reflex will give an opportunity for a successful initial breast-feeding experience.[14] Of course, if the mother has been heavily medicated or has experienced a difficult delivery, the infant may be sleepy and initial breast-feeding may have to be postponed. The Committee on Fetus and Newborn of the American Academy of Pediatrics recommends that breast-feeding begin as soon as possible after delivery.[15]

Some physicians still prefer to give the baby one or two bottles of plain water or glucose water before allowing breast-feeding to begin. The purpose of this is to help the infant regurgitate any mucus or secretions that may have been swallowed during delivery, although the same function can be served by colostrum. Another reason for using the bottle at this time is to provide an opportunity to observe the infant for any possible congenital anomalies, such as tracheoesophageal fistula. It is also felt that if such a condition exists, water will be safer than colostrum, although others argue that colostrum, because it is a physiologic secretion, is probably just as safe since it would not have the irritating effects of a foreign substance.[16] Those advocating early breast-feeding also point out that an observant nurse would be quick to detect a problem such as tracheoesophageal fistula in the initial breast-feeding sessions and would then obtain help quite readily.

Assistance with Breast-Feeding

It is important to remember that *both* mother and baby must learn how to work as a team during the breast-feeding process. Hence, practice is essential. Even though the mother has breast-fed before, there is a wide range of nursing behavior among infants, and the experience of breast-feeding each infant can be somewhat "new." The mother will need to learn how to handle the infant appropriately, how to interpret cues of hunger and satiety, and how to help the infant to grasp the nipple and to withdraw the milk successfully. The infant, in turn, must learn to associate the nipple with food and to coordinate grasping of the nipple with sucking and swallowing in such a way as to get food successfully. No wonder that mother and baby often take a few days to become adept at this process!

An interested and experienced nurse should be immediately available to mothers in their first experiences with their new babies. Maternity nurses in the hospital can play a major role in facilitating the mothers' efforts to breast-feed their babies (Fig. 30-1).

Many of the problems associated with unsuccessful breast-feeding experiences can be prevented or solved through purposeful nursing action. Nurses need to accept the responsibility of helping mothers gain the knowledge and skill necessary to successfully breastfeed their babies.[17]

Preparing the mother *before* the actual breast-feeding experience plays a large part in giving effective care. This includes instructions about "hand-washing," sterile technique procedures and other rituals associated with the feeding of the infant in the hospital. If these tasks have to be carried out after the infant is brought to the mother for feeding, the delay can be frustrating and stress-producing for both mother and baby.

Whenever it is indicated, the mother should be informed about the feeding reflexes of her infant (see p. 475). During the actual nursing period the nurse can reinforce this information (as necessary) and *show* the mother how to elicit these responses. It is essential that the mother be able to evoke these reflexes herself, since she ultimately must assume total responsibility. Too often the nurse takes over these aspects, and the mother does not get sufficient practice to acquire any skill during these first days in the hospital. It is not easy to "stand by" and watch the inexperienced mother trying to breast-feed her baby without offering too much interference. But it is necessary to be careful not to disrupt the learning process.

Whether the first nursing is done in the delivery room, recovery room or in the patient's room later, the nurse who assists the mother should record the type of instruction given and the response of the mother and infant to the experience.

Positioning

Assisting the mother to experiment with various positions during breast-feeding is another important facet of care. The mother is sometimes asked whether she wants to nurse the baby sitting up or lying down. An inexperienced mother may be unaware of the options and should be given an opportunity to try various positions, while help is available. If the mother is shown only one position,

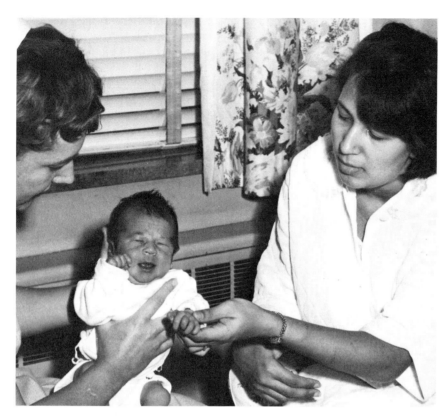

Figure 30-1. The nurse demonstrates methods of handling the baby prior to feeding.

she may think there is only one "right" way to do it.

The best positions for any given mother and infant depend on several factors, including the size and shape of the breast, the size of the infant, and the condition of the mother, who may have a sore perineum or tender incisional area from a cesarean section. Varying the nursing positions from one feeding to the next can be helpful because it changes the position of the infant's mouth on the nipple.

This allows the breast to empty more completely and prevents the nipples from becoming tender and the ducts from becoming plugged.[18]

To nurse satisfactorily, the infant needs to be held properly by the mother. Although some mothers seem to know how to support a baby at the breast, many are awkward at first and need definite instructions. The following are some helpful teaching points:

1. The mother and baby must be comfortable.

Comparative Data on Relative Components in Human Milk, Cow's milk, and Evaporated Cow's Milk in Normal Dilution

	Normal Dilution		Approximate Percentage Composition in Normal Dilution (Gm. per 100 ml.			
Type of Milk	Ratio	Cal./Oz.	Protein	Fat	CHO	Minerals
Human Milk, average	undiluted	20	1.2	3.8	7.0	0.21
Cow's Milk, market average	undiluted	20	3.3	3.7	4.8	0.72
Cow's Milk, evaporated (many brands)	1:1	22	3.8	4.0	5.4	0.8
Commercial Premodified Milks:						
Infant Formula, Baker	1:1	20	2.2	3.3	7.0	0.6
Bremil with Iron, Borden	1:1	20	1.5	3.5	7.0	0.5
Modilac, Gerber	1:1	20	2.2	2.7	7.8	0.4
Enfamil, Mead	1:1	20	1.5	3.7	7.0	0.3
Similac with Iron, Ross	1:1	20	1.8	3.4	6.6	0.4
SMA S-26, Wyeth	1:1	20	1.5	3.6	7.2	0.25

Source: Adapted from Vaughan V. C., III, M.D., and McKay, R. J., M.D. (eds.): *Nelson Textbook of Pediatrics,* ed. 10, Philadelphia, W. B. Saunders Co.

2. The baby should be at the level of the breast so its weight does not pull on the breast.

3. The baby must be able to grasp the nipple and most of the areola. If only the nipple is grasped, the baby will not be able to draw out the milk, because the milk sinuses will not be compressed. Possible damage to the nipple may occur along with pain to the mother.

If the mother is lying down (Fig. 30-2), she should be on her side with her arm raised and her head comfortably supported. The baby lies on his side, flat on the bed or supported so that he can grasp the breast easily. Tucking the baby's feet close to the mother's body will help give him room to breathe. If the mother prefers to sit up to nurse, she may be most comfortable in a chair, with a stool to support her feet, if necessary. If she stays in bed, the high Fowler's position is probably best so she can lean over slightly, toward the infant on her lap. It is often helpful to place a pillow under the arm that is supporting the infant to reduce the tension on the muscles (Fig. 30-3) or to place a pillow under the baby to raise him to a sufficient height to reach the breast easily. An alternate position for the baby is facing the breast with its body supported on a pillow along the mother's side and under her arm

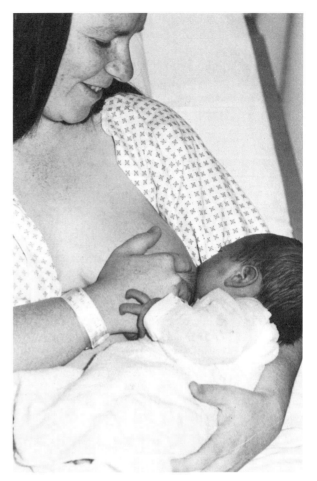

Figure 30-3. The mother may prefer to assume a sitting position when nursing her infant.

in the "football hold." This is especially helpful for the mother who has delivered by cesarean section, or the mother who wants to nurse twins simultaneously.

The nurse may have to work with the mother a bit to be sure that she is comfortable. Often mothers in their eagerness to get the baby on the breast become very tense and assume quite uncomfortable positions (although they assure the nurse that they are "comfortable"). Patience and gentle reminding on the part of the nurse encourages these mothers to relax more readily.

Orientation of Infant

After being placed beside the mother, the baby needs to be allowed a little time to become accustomed to the new environment and to hunt for the nipple. The baby should not be forced to nurse

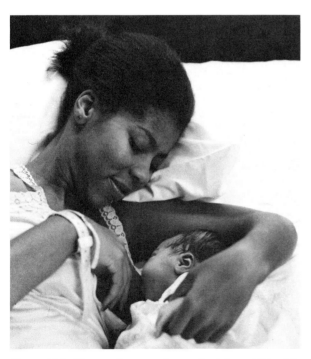

Figure 30-2. The mother may breast-feed her child while lying down.

immediately, especially if he is hesitant or shows disinclination. If the rooting reflex is well developed (and as he smells the milk), the baby will turn toward the nipple or any object that brushes the cheek. Thus, if the mother or the nurse touches his cheek gently with the nipple, he will turn toward it, open his mouth and grasp it.

The mother can help the baby grasp the nipple by making a V with two fingers of her free hand, placing one finger on the upper edge of the areola and the other on the lower edge, while shaping the breast to better correspond to the shape of the infant's mouth. Sucking usually follows closely thereafter. If the infant seems to have some difficulty in finding and grasping the nipple, although he seems to be eager, the mother or nurse can gently cup a hand around the baby's head and guide him to the nipple.

When the mother assumes the sitting position, the infant's head can be held in the bend of the mother's arm while she guides the infant toward the breast by moving her arm. Care should be taken, however, not to touch his cheek or to force his head, since he will only turn away and resist the pressure. In addition, he may cry, and a crying baby tends not to grasp a nipple successfully even though he may be hungry.

Sucking Behavior of Infant

Babies exhibit a wide variety of sucking behaviors. Some, after finding the nipple, suck vigorously without stopping until they are satisfied. Others may suck vigorously for a time, appear to sleep or to rest and then resume sucking. Still others mouth the nipple before actually sucking, but eventually nurse well. Others seem rather disinterested in the whole thing and dawdle throughout the nursing period. When the milk comes in, however, a change usually is noted, and even these infants begin to nurse more in earnest.

The important point here is that individual differences do exist in infants, apparently from birth; hence care must be taken to allow for these differences. To try to force the infant into a style or speed that is not natural for him will only result in screaming, resistance and refusal; the nursing period should be adapted to the infant and not the infant to the nursing period.

Mothers, especially, are appreciative of learning about this; often they think there is "a way to nurse"

and do not realize that infants have different eating behaviors. Giving mothers anticipatory guidance and instruction in this aspect of nursing a baby is a very important component in nursing care.

If the infant is to suck effectively, he must place the nipple well back in his mouth, close his lips tightly around the areola, and squeeze the nipple against his palate with his tongue. He then can compress the lactiferous sinuses behind the areola and draw the milk into his mouth by sucking. He empties the breast through a combination of compression and suction. As he nurses, he moves his jaws up and down to compress and empty the sinuses; his tongue, as it draws the nipple back against the palate, suctions the milk from the nipple. Swallowing occurs when enough milk has been obtained to induce the reflex. This activity is carried on rhythmically, interspaced with periods of rest, until the infant is satisfied.

Sometimes the let-down reflex is so active that the milk literally streams, and the baby not only does not have to suck very hard but may have difficulty in swallowing fast enough to keep up with the stream. Placing the baby in a more upright position sometimes helps to prevent choking in these cases. He may have to nurse a bit, stop, and then continue as he learns to cope with the increased stream.

When assisting the mother, the nurse should be sure that the baby has the nipple on top of his tongue and that enough of the areola is in his mouth to prevent damage to the nipple. If he has a good grasp, his jaws will move up and down regularly, and sucking and swallowing movements can be seen in his cheeks and throat. If his grasp is poor, sucking and swallowing may be infrequent/or absent, although his jaws may continue to move. If the breast tissue seems to press against the infant's nose and thus obstructs his breathing, the nurse can instruct the mother to take her forefinger and gently compress the tissue so that the breast no longer impinges on the infant's nose (Fig. 30-4). Care should be taken not to pull the nipple away from the infant in this maneuver.

Usually, getting the nipple in his mouth and tasting the milk seem to increase the baby's interest and ability to nurse. If the infant does not seem too interested or adept, moistening the nipple by expressing a few drops of colostrum or milk often encourages sucking.

Occasionally, a breast shield may be used to start

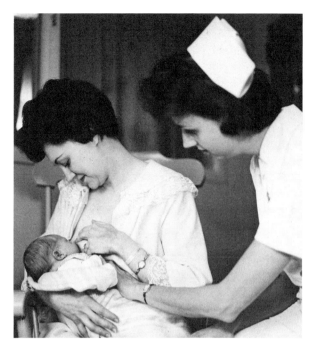

Figure 30-4. The nurse instructs the mother in the techniques of breast-feeding.

the infant nursing if for some reason he cannot grasp the nipple. Continued use of this appliance is unwise, since the breasts cannot be emptied because the lacteal sinuses are not compressed during the nursing. The shield can be useful during the first few minutes of nursing to draw the nipples out if they are flattened by engorgement or inversion. Usually, however, even inverted nipples become prominent if the alveolar area is compressed gently by the fingers before nursing; they generally evert more when the infant sucks.

Sometimes a baby will be sleepy and difficult to arouse. If, the mother unwraps him, plays with his hands, sings to him or uses some other type of loving stimulation it may be enough to awaken him. If it does not, the mother should be reassured that the baby will nurse when he is hungry. The nurse should then make sure that the baby is brought to the mother as soon as he awakens and is not given any feeding in the nursery. If possible, the infant should be left at the mother's bedside, so that she is available when the baby is ready to eat.

Once the infant is sucking well, the mother should be reminded to break the suction before removing him from the breast. Failure to do this can result in pain or trauma to the nipple. To break the suction, a clean little finger can be placed in the

corner of the infant's mouth or the infant's chin can be pulled down. Sometimes the mother needs to pull away a little at the same time so the infant does not grasp the nipple again.

The mother may also inquire about bubbling or burping the infant. This may be done when she changes breasts and at the end of the feeding period. If the infant was crying hard before the feeding, she may want to bubble him before beginning. For the infant who has difficulty getting started, it might be better to bubble him only at the end of the feeding. Breast-fed babies tend not to swallow as much air as bottle-fed infants, hence the need for bubbling usually does not present much of a problem. (For techniques see p. 497.)

Giving Support and Supervision

Once the infant has taken the breast without difficulty and has been sucking well for several minutes, the nurse probably does not need to remain in constant attendance at the bedside. The mother needs some opportunity to feel that she can manage on her own. Letting her have reasonable periods of managing breast-feeding by herself will help to instill some confidence. However, she should never be left without adequate instruction and reassurance. The nurse might find something else to do in the room or can place a call-bell within easy reach so that the mother can ring for help if need be. The nurse should make a point of looking in occasionally to observe the progress. The reassurance that the nurse is readily available may be all the encouragement the mother needs.

Since some infants do not nurse well during the first few days, the nurse will want to remind the mother that the first week is a time of learning for both the nursing mother and the child. Many mothers feel that all infants are born knowing how to suck and that if their infant does not latch on immediately, it must be due to something the mother is doing wrong. Some mothers even have a feeling of being rejected, stating, "The baby doesn't like me," or "The baby doesn't want my milk." Actually, taking milk from the breast is more than just a simple act of sucking, and some infants do need help in learning how. If the mother is helped to understand this, she will be less inclined to blame herself and more able to enjoy the nursing experience.

Because hospital stays are so short, there is less

time available to provide professional assistance to the new mother. Most women still need support after leaving the hospital. In some cases the father fills this need, but in others another support person is needed. In the past, information and positive feelings about breast-feeding were passed from mother to daughter. However, since breast-feeding has not been a universal practice recently, grandmothers or other relatives may not have breast-feeding experiences to relate. Also, in our mobile society and with the trend toward nuclear families, female family members are not always available to give support to the new mother. To fill this void, nursing mothers' groups have been started across the country. One particularly popular group is La Leche League, International, which holds classes about breast-feeding for women either before or after the baby is born. This organization also publishes a book about breast-feeding (*The Womanly Art of Breast Feeding*) along with other pamphlets, including one called "How the Nurse Can Help the Breast-Feeding Mother." In many communities there are 24-hour phone numbers that nursing mothers may call if they are having problems with breast-feeding.

The mother may also be referred to a public health agency if necessary. Some hospitals are now encouraging mothers to call the nursery or obstetric unit if they need support or help with problems. While many mothers are reluctant to call, they welcome the chance to ask questions if the nurse makes the call or a home visit. Some hospitals and some private doctors are hiring nurses to make follow-up visits after the woman leaves the hospital.

Schedule

A self-regulatory or self-demand schedule is the usual accepted practice today, especially for breast-fed babies; that is, the baby is fed when he indicates hunger by crying and body posture. The infant cries when he is hungry because actual contractions in his stomach cause him pain. If he is fed when he cries and is experiencing pain, he learns to associate food with the relief of pain. Thus food (and the mother who supplies it) become pleasant factors in his life. If, on the other hand, he is made to wait until "time" for feeding, he may not nurse well because he is exhausted from crying or has lost his feeling of hunger. Similarly, if a baby is "sleepy" and not allowed to wake up sufficiently by himself,

he also will not nurse well and will soon resent efforts made to wake him up. Slapping the soles of his feet, spanking his bottom and the like generally are not effective.

Problems of this type can often be avoided in a rooming-in situation, because with the mother and baby together most of the time, the mother knows when the infant is awake for a feeding. She also has the opportunity to learn to recognize the cry and behavior which indicate that her baby is hungry.

Most breast-fed babies will want to nurse every two to three hours at first. This is helpful in stimulating milk production and in satisfying the infant's sucking needs. The nursing pattern will vary greatly in the early weeks of life. Each time the infant has a growth spurt he will want to nurse more frequently for a few days until the supply catches up with his increased demand. The mother will be encouraged to know that her baby will gradually go longer between feedings and that his eating pattern will become less varied.[19]

Length of Nursing Time

In the early stages of breast-feeding, some authorities suggest that the sucking time be limited and then gradually increased each day as a means of preventing sore nipples. Whitley[20] found that of the women who restricted nursing time, fewer developed sore nipples while in the hospital, but more developed soreness at home. If the time limitation is drastic, such as starting with one minute on each breast at each feeding and increasing by one minute each day, the let-down reflex will not have a chance to function before the baby is removed from the breast. Another disadvantage is that the mother becomes too involved in clock watching to have a pleasant, relaxed time with her baby.

It is best to offer both breasts at each feeding to provide maximum stimulation for the mother and an adequate supply of milk for the infant. If initial sucking time is going to be limited, five to seven minutes on each side for the first day's feedings is probably reasonable. This allows time for the let-down reflex to occur and the ducts to be emptied. The time can then be gradually increased up to 10 to 15 minutes on the first breast and as long as the infant desires on the second. The condition of the mother's nipples should be considered and the time shortened if there are problems.

When the breasts are full and the let-down reflex

functioning well, the baby usually gets most of the milk in the first five to ten minutes of sucking. Therefore, the mother need not worry that the baby is not getting enough milk if she has to limit nursing time for a short period due to nipple soreness. Nursing should begin on the side used last at the previous feeding. A safety pin on the bra strap will help the mother remember which breast to start with.

Not Enough Milk

Many mothers worry that they will not have enough milk. The mother can be assured that the baby is probably getting an adequate amount of milk if he is wetting four to six diapers a day, sleeping fairly well and gaining weight at a steady rate. The wet diapers may be the best guide, because "colicky" babies cry for reasons other than hunger and usually gain well, and some breast babies are slow weight gainers even when the milk supply is adequate.

If mother thinks her baby is not getting enough milk, putting the baby to breast more often will usually increase the supply. The concept of supply and demand, that the more milk the baby takes from the breast, the more the mother will produce, is important for the mother to remember. Sometimes women mistakenly think that they can "save" their milk and have more for the next feeding if they give the baby a bottle at one feeding.

Some mothers fear that they are losing their milk at the time when engorgement subsides because their breasts go back to a more normal size and feel less full. An explanation that this might happen and that it is just the swelling that has gone down, not the milk supply, would help prevent worry.

If the mother's breasts seem full but the infant does not seem to be getting enough, there could be a problem with the let-down reflex. The mother may need to lie down, have a warm drink, or find some other way to relax before the feeding time. Getting more rest and increasing fluid and protein intake may also help increase the milk supply.

Supplementary or Complementary Feedings

A bottle given instead of a breast-feeding is called a supplementary feeding, while one given in addition to the breast-feeding is called complementary (Fig. 30-5).

This subject has long been controversial. Some

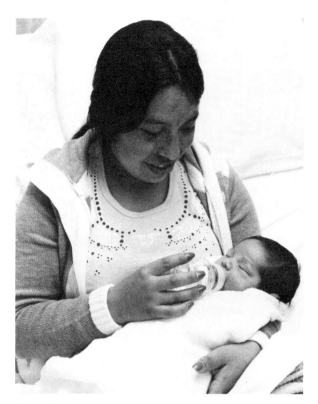

Figure 30-5. Supplemental feeding.

physicians (and mothers) feel that giving the infant any artificial feedings diminishes the success of breast-feeding and is extremely detrimental to establishing and maintaining lactation (see References). Others feel that there are legitimate indications for an occasional artificial feeding. A variety of feedings may be used (i.e., plain water, glucose water, dilute formula, full-strength formula). It is sometimes suggested that these be given by spoon or dropper to avoid the use of a rubber nipple.

If the mother is to use supplemental or complementary feedings when she returns home, the nurse will want to be sure that she understands how to prepare these feedings, the kind and the amount of feedings, and the indications for their use.

Care of the Nipples

To facilitate breast-feeding, it is important to discuss nipple care with the new mother. Cleanliness is important in breast-feeding, but it is the hands that need washing, not the nipples. There is a natural antisepsis provided in the oils secreted by the nipple and by enzymes in the milk.[22] Washing the breasts with plain water at the time of the daily bath or shower is thought to be enough. The use of soap should be avoided, because it is drying and can lead to cracking. There are many commercial nipple ointments or creams available, but hydrous lanolin has also been found to be soothing to tender nipples. Whatever is used should be safe for mother and baby and not have to be washed off before nursing. The nipples should be dried and the ointment or cream applied lightly so air circulation will not be obstructed. Keeping the nipples dry is another important aspect of their care. Air drying after each nursing period and leaving the bra flaps down for 15 to 30 minutes several times a day is suggested.[23] Also, plastic liners of any kind in the bra should be removed, because they hold the moisture in. In case of some milk leakage, especially in the first days after the milk comes in, something absorbent, such as a breast pad or a clean, folded man's handkerchief, can be helpful to keep the nipple drier and prevent the outer clothing from getting wet. They should, of course, be changed frequently when they get damp.

Common Concerns and Problems of Nursing Mothers

Painful Nipples

Nipple pain is frequently a reason mothers give for discontinuing breastfeeding. Although it may not be possible to completely prevent or eliminate this problem, it can be minimized with good care. Measures to prevent nipple trauma include:

1. Make sure most of the areola is in the infant's mouth so that he does not just chew on the nipple.
2. Change nursing positions with each feeding so that different areas of the nipple are subjected to the greatest stress from sucking.
3. Do not allow the breasts to become engorged so that the infant has difficulty grasping the breast.
4. Feed the infant on demand so that he does not become overly hungry, causing him to suck the nipple too vigorously.
5. Start each feeding on alternate breasts so that both breasts are subjected to the vigorous sucking that occurs at the beginning of the feeding.
6. Limit sucking time as necessary.

The mother should also avoid allowing the infant to suck on empty ducts. Before the let-down reflex is established, she can manually express a few drops of colostrum or milk to fill the ducts prior to allowing the baby to begin nursing.

The mother can probably benefit from some anticipatory guidance about nipple soreness. She needs to know that it is not unusual and is usually self-limiting. The discomfort is often most noticeable as the baby begins to suck, but diminishes rapidly as the let-down reflex occurs. The discomfort with the first few sucks can last for several days or weeks and does not mean that there is anything wrong.

It is possible, of course, for the nipples to develop fissures, erosions or blisters, which can serve as entryways for bacteria and possible infection. If any of these do develop, the nurse should check with the mother to be sure she is carrying out proper nipple care. The nipples may be exposed to a lamp with a 40-watt bulb for 15 to 20 minutes. Grassley and Davis also suggest that an application of cold tea to the nipples can aid healing because of the tannic acid it contains.[24] If mastitis or an abscess develops, the physician should be consulted. Since these problems usually occur after the woman has left the hospital, she should be given some guidance prior to discharge and instructed to observe her breasts for signs of infection. Antibiotics are usually the treatment of choice. Many physicians now feel that it is best for the woman to continue breastfeeding even when these difficulties develop.[25]

Engorgement

The mechanism underlying engorgement has been discussed in Chapter 26. The discussion in this chapter will center on means of relieving engorgement.

The major means of treating breast engorgement is to relieve the symptoms by removing the milk. While lactation is being established, the let-down reflex is often inefficient and milk is not being moved consistently from the alveoli to the sinuses where the baby can obtain it. Murdaugh and Miller suggest that the breasts be massaged before nursing, especially if they are engorged, in order to open the lacteal ducts and relieve breast tightness by increasing circulation, thus making the breast softer and the nipple area easier to grasp. This prefeeding massage is done by placing both hands at the upper part of the breast near the clavicle. With continuous downward pressure the fingers move out and around on opposite sides of the breast until they encircle it, then slide smoothly over the tip. Some lubrication, such as lotion, should probably be used for this procedure. When the breasts begin to soften, the infant can be placed at the breast.[26]

Another aid to empty the breast and further relieve engorgement is alternate massage. To do this, the infant's sucking movements should be observed during nursing. When they become short and choppy instead of long and rhythmic, it indicates that the milk is no longer flowing as freely. At this time the mother can alternately massage different areas of the breast, at the same time allowing the baby to nurse to remove the milk that is brought down by the massaging. This is done without removing the baby from the breast.[27]

Expression of Milk

There are some instances in which the mother wishes to breast-feed, but for certain reasons the infant cannot be "put to breast." There are also situations in which the breast-fed infant is not able to empty the breast completely. As such times it becomes necessary to empty the breasts of milk through artificial means. Otherwise, if this condition is allowed to persist for several days, lacteal secretion is inhibited, and the future milk supply may be jeopardized. Before attempting to empty the breast by hand or pump, the mother may find it helpful to use measures to facilitate the let-down reflex, such as taking a warm shower, having a warm drink, or gently massaging the breasts.[28]

Manual Expression It is helpful if a woman can learn this technique before the baby is born, but it can be taught afterward if necessary. The mother should have the opportunity to try it in the hospital where she can have guided practice under the supervision of the nurse, so that she will be able to do it with more confidence when she returns home.

A sterile glass or wide-mouthed container is to be in readiness before beginning, and if the milk is to be fed to the infant, a sterile bottle and cap also will be needed. It may be desirable first to massage the breast for a few seconds to stimulate the flow of milk, as described in the section on engorgement.

The hands of the person expressing the milk are washed thoroughly with warm water and soap and dried on a clean towel. Since the daily care of the breast is designed to maintain cleanliness, the same cleansing ritual required before putting the baby to breast would be utilized here.

1. One hand is used to support the breast and to express the milk; the other, to hold the container which will receive the milk. Although some authorities advocate that the right hand be used to milk the left breast, the decision as to which hand is used should depend on how the mother can accomplish this with the greatest ease.

2. The forefinger is placed below and the thumb above the outer edge of the areola. The first action is pressure toward the chest wall and the second is movement of the finger and thumb toward each other. The forefinger is to be kept straight so that pressure can be exerted between the middle of this finger and the ball of the thumb. As the finger and thumb are alternately compressed and released, with the area of the collecting sinuses between them, milk is forced out in a stream (Figs. 30-6 and 30-7). It is of paramount importance to avoid pinching and possibly bruising the breast tissue.

3. The fingers should not slide forward on the areola or the nipple during the milking process. However, they must be moved in clockwise fashion around the areola, each time compressing and releasing the fingers on that area, so that all the collecting sinuses may be emptied.

Many authorities advocate this method of emptying the breasts rather than using the breast pump, because the action more nearly simulates the action of the infant's jaws as he nurses. Furthermore, since no mechanical equipment is required, it is a method which can be readily used when necessary after discharge from the hospital.

Electric Pump Expression. When an electric pump is used, there is always the potential danger of traumatizing the breast tissue. This was particularly true of the older style electric pumps that were originally designed for other purposes and then modified for use as a breast pump. The more recently introduced Egnell electric breast pump was specifically designed for pumping the breast and has a physiological sucking action which decreases the danger of trauma. Mothers using the pump have found it efficient and easy to use.

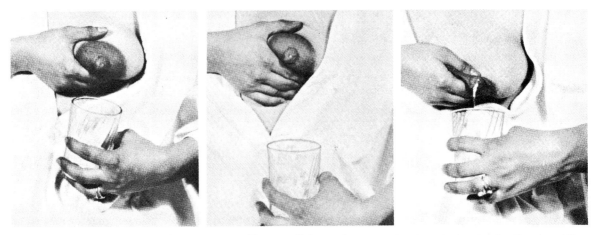

Figure 30-6. (Left) First position in the expression of breast milk from a large, pendant breast, showing the thumb and fingers properly placed and pressing backward. *(Center)* First position, showing the thumb and finger pressed deeply into the breast, at the same time compressing the breast well behind the nipple. This deeper pressure is necessary in a round, virginal-shaped breast. *(Right)* Second position, showing compression of the breast between the thumb and fingers, well behind the nipple, and the milk coming in a stream. Care is exercised to avoid pinching or bruising the breast tissue.

Before using any pump, the mother should be given explanations about why it is used, how it works, and how to use it. If this information is not offered, the mother may experience fear and anxiety which could retard the flow of milk. The nurse should stay with the mother and assist her the first few times until she feels confident to use the pump alone.

It takes approximately 5 to 12 minutes to empty a breast completely, depending on the stage of lactation, but pumping should be stopped as soon as milk ceases to flow. A breast should never be pumped longer than 10 minutes at any one time. If the mother experiences back or chest pain, an indication that the breast is dry, the pumping should be stopped immediately.

The breast milk obtained is measured and the amount recorded. When only one breast is pumped at a time, the record should indicate whether it was the right or the left breast, so that the next time the

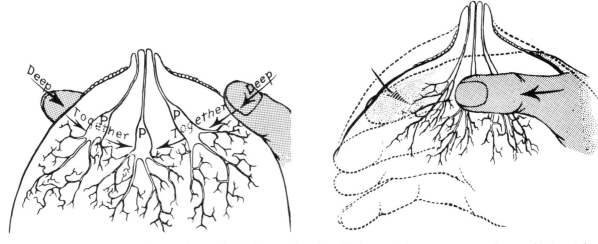

Figure 30-7. (Left) Diagram showing the method of expressing the milk from the breast, as the mother would view it from above, by compressing the milk pockets between the thumb and forefinger. The three unused fingers are used to support the breast. This represents the second or "together" motion. *(Right)* Illustrating the movements needed to force milk out of the little pockets (P) in which it collects. Place a finger and thumb on opposite sides of the nipple at "Deep." Press deeply into the breast in the direction of the black arrows. Then compress the breast together in direction of the arrows toward center point "P." This will force the milk out of the ducts in streams. "Deep" and "together" express in two words the motions required. (After U. C. Moore, *Nutrition of Mother and Child.*)

other breast can be pumped. If the milk is to be fed to the infant, it can be poured into a sterile nursing bottle, labeled with the infant's name, the time and the date and refrigerated immediately.

The electric breast pump may be used for more than one mother and thus should be washed with soap or detergent each time that it is used. In addition, certain removable parts, such as the breast-pump bottle and cap, the breast funnel and the rubber connection tubing, must be washed thoroughly, wrapped and autoclaved immediately after use.

Hand-Pump Expression. The most common type of manual breast pump is the one that looks a little like a bicycle horn, with a glass cone and a rubber bulb. To minimize pain and nipple damage, which may occur if the hand pump is used improperly, the inside of the cone should first be lubricated with warm water and the bulb compressed half-way before the cone is placed on the breast and the bulb released to create suction. The bulb is alternately compressed and released to extract the milk. This pump is not too effective and the hand action can be tiring for the mother, but it is probably the least expensive.

There are two newer nonelectric pumps on the market. One is the "Loyd-B" hand pump which operates with a trigger action that creates a vacuum that can be controlled by the mother. The other is the "Ora ' Lac" pump which operates by suction from a tube which the mother puts in her mouth.[29]

Hygiene Of The Nursing Mother

Rest

Rest is one of the most important considerations for the lactating mother. The detrimental effects of fatigue and worry already have been discussed. In the hospital the nurse is able to act as a buffer between the mother and some of these problems. In addition, the mother is relieved of household responsibilities and is able to have meals served to her. When she leaves the hospital, she no longer has this somewhat protected environment. Thus, it is important for the nurse to make sure that the parents understand the importance of rest and that they have made adequate plans to provide for it. If it is at all possible, the mother should have help at home.

Her main energies then can be directed to the care of the infant and other family members. House-keeping chores will have to be simplified and the mother's activity restricted so that she will get sufficient rest. Since her sleep will be broken at night, naps during the day become particularly *essential*—they should not be considered a luxury. Without adequate rest, the milk supply soon will be reduced to a dribble. If heretofore the woman has been very active, she may need special help to realize the importance of naps and rest periods. It is helpful, also, if visitors (including relatives) are restricted at first. They can become fatiguing to the mother, and they may be a source of potential infection to the newborn.

Diet

The daily diet of the lactating mother should be similar to that recommended during pregnancy (see Chap. 19) except that, according to the Food and Nutrition Board of the National Research Council, the need for calories, vitamin A, vitamin C, niacin, riboflavin, and iodine are greater than during pregnancy. It is hoped that the new mother has become more aware of good nutrition during her pregnancy and will be able to incorporate the proper foods into her diet to meet these increased needs. The nurse should discuss the recommendations with her, assess her knowledge, and give instruction as necessary.

If the mother's diet was adequate in pregnancy, then additions rather than changes are all that will be necessary. Often nursing mothers, not realizing that their nutritional needs increase even over the needs of pregnancy, try to go back to their pre-pregnant diet.

Individual caloric needs will vary with the body size of the woman and with the quantity of breast milk produced. Since it is difficult to determine exactly how much milk is being produced, a calorie intake of 800 to 1000 calories over that recommended for a nonpregnant woman is usually suggested. The mother's weight is one of the best criteria in determining adequate caloric intake—it should remain stationary. Wide fluctuations will require that the diet be adjusted, most likely in the amount of carbohydrates and fats consumed, assuming that protein intake is adequate.

The value of protein in the diet should be stressed. The efficiency of converting the dietary protein into milk protein is about 75 percent, so that about three-fourths of the extra protein taken in by the lactating woman is secreted in the milk she makes.[30]

Increasing the milk intake to at least 1½ quarts daily will meet the additional protein, thiamin, riboflavin, calcium, phosphorus and niacin needs. Supplementing the citrus fruit recommendations in pregnancy with generous servings of other fruits and vegetables will meet the vitamin C requirements. To further ensure optimum vitamin and mineral intake, many physicians will prescribe that the vitamin supplement capsules taken during pregnancy be continued.

A high fluid intake also is necessary for milk production. Between 2,500 and 3,000 ml. is recommended for the mother engaged in usual activity under pleasant environmental conditions. More may be required in hot weather or with physical exertion. This fluid intake should include a good deal of water as well as other beverages. Many mothers find that taking a beverage prior to nursing facilitates the letdown reflex. Concentrated urine or constipation may be indications of inadequate fluid intake.

Mothers have often heard that there are foods, such as chocolate and cabbage, that should be avoided during lactation. While some babies are bothered by certain things their mothers eat, this is not universally true. Most mothers can eat any nutritious food without causing the baby any distress. If the mother, herself, is bothered by a particular food, she would be wise to avoid it because it could also have an effect on the baby. Eating large quantities of some foods, such as chocolate, seems to upset many babies, so moderation should be the rule. Also, some babies seem to have more sensitive taste buds and object to flavors that come through in the milk.

Drugs

Most drugs ingested by the mother while she is lactating are secreted in the milk, but in varying amounts and with differing effects on the infant. Concentration of the drug in the breast milk depends on several factors, including the concentration in the mother's blood, the lipid solubility of the drug, the degree of ionization, and the composition of the milk. Usually the amount of drug in the milk is small, but the cumulative effect over a 24-hour period may give the infant a fairly large dose. Some drugs seem to have highest concentrations shortly after they are ingested; therefore, taking them after breast-feeding rather than before might help to minimize the infant's exposure.[31] Delayed excretion or inactivation of drugs due to the immaturity of the infant's renal and hepatic function can be a factor in the concentration of the drug in the infant's body. Decreased renal function in the mother can also lead to increased concentrations of drugs in the milk.

Interpreting the data concerning concentration of drugs in breast milk is hampered by the fragmentary and contradictory nature of the information available. Most drug companies state in their inserts that "Safety in pregnancy and lactation has not been established and the benefits of the drug must be weighed against possible risks." When drugs are prescribed for a nursing mother, she should remind the physician that she is breast-feeding. If she is taking drugs for a chronic condition, she should discuss their possible effects with the physician during pregnancy, before she decides on the method of feeding her infant.

Drugs which have been shown to have adverse effects on some infants should be avoided (Table 30-1).[32, 33, 34] If any of these drugs are given to the mother, the infant should be kept under close observation.

Contaminants in Breast Milk

Ever since investigators first discovered DDT in breast milk in the 1950s, people have been asking if breast milk is still safe for babies. A variety of contaminants are now known to be present in breast milk, including DDT, pesticides, and other chemicals. Pesticides are stored in body fat from whence they are mobilized and enter into milk fat. Toxic chemicals, such as PCB (polychlorinated biphenyls) and PBB (polybrominated biphenyls), have also been detected in human milk. None of these substances have yet been shown to have damaging effects on human infants as a result of ingestion from mother's milk, but newborn rats were shown to have a higher mortality rate when their lactating mothers were heavily dosed with DDT.[10] Lead, another contaminant of human milk, is found in larger amounts in other forms of milk. More research is needed to determine the possible long-term effects of contaminated breast milk. The benefits of breast-feeding still seem to outweigh the possible dangers in most cases. Excessive exposure to contaminants should prompt mothers to have

TABLE 30-1
DRUGS IN BREAST MILK

Drug	Reference	Effect on Infant
Anticoagulants	(1, 2, 3)	Could cause hemorrhage; avoid or closely monitor infant
Anti-infective Drugs		
Chloramphenicol	(2)	Could harm infant bone marrow
Erythromycin	(1)	High concentration in breast milk, may cause sensitization
Isoniazid and Kanamycin	(3)	Observe infant for signs of toxicity
Penicillin	(1)	May cause sensitization in later life
Streptomycin	(1)	Nephrotoxicity
Sulfa Drugs	(3)	Have caused skin rashes
Sulfisoxazole (Gantrisin)	(3)	Avoid for first two weeks of life, may cause kernicterus
Sulfanilamide Vag Cream	(1)	May cause jaundice
		Any antimicrobial in breast milk could alter the bacterial content and normal flora of the infant's intestinal tract, and affect development of the immune system (2)
Anti-thyroid Drugs		
Iodides	(2)	Could cause hypothyroidism or goiter
Propylthiouricil	(2)	Could inhibit activity of infant thyroid
Radioactive Iodine	(2)	
Diagnostic amount		Safety not known
Therapeutic amount		Should stop nursing—amount in breast milk sufficient to destroy infant's thyroid
Barbiturates	(1, 2)	Effects controversial; have effect on infant's liver enzymes
Corticosteroids	(2)	If necessary for mother to take, should advise against breast-feeding; could suppress growth or have other untoward effects
Diuretics		
Chlorothiazide	(2)	Thrombocytopenia
Oral Contraceptives	(1, 2)	No harm documented, long-term effects not studied. May reduce milk production
Other Prescription Drugs		
Atropine	(1, 2)	Infant very sensitive. Should avoid. Could cause drowsiness, urinary retention, tachycardia, respiratory symptoms
Reserpine	(1, 2)	Lethargy, diarrhea and nasal congestion; excessive milk flow
Valium	(1, 3)	Nursing not recommended. Lethargy, weight loss, hyperbilirubinemia
Nonprescription Drugs		
Acetaminophen (Tylenol)		No known effects
Alcohol	(2)	Concentration about equal to mother's blood—apparently not harmful in moderate amounts
Aspirin	(2)	Can produce bleeding tendency, risk probably minimal if taken just after nursing and infant's vitamin K adequate
Bromides (found in Bromo-Seltzer and over-the-counter sleeping aids)	(1)	Drowsiness and rash
Caffeine (found in beverages or analgesics)	(2)	Reaches detectable level, probably no effect on infant
Ergot (found in preparations for migraine headaches)	(1)	Vomiting, diarrhea, weak pulse, unstable blood pressure
Laxatives (with cascarra or senna)	(1)	May cause diarrhea
Nicotine (in cigarettes)	(3)	In moderation, no effect

1. Rothermel, Paula C. and Myron Faber: "Drugs in breast milk—A consumer's guide," pp. 76–88.
2. *The Medical Letter*, March 15, 1974.
3. O'Brien, T. E. "Excretion of drugs in human milk," *Amer. J. Hosp. Pharm.*

their milk analyzed to aid them in making a decision about the method of feeding. Nurses should join with others in attempts to rid the environment of pollutants as a more permanent solution to the problem.

Weaning

When it comes to initiating breast-feeding, many mothers receive advice and counseling. However, frequently, little is said about how or when they should stop nursing. Although stopping abruptly at a time set by the physician has sometimes been the accepted method of weaning, this can be very uncomfortable and distressing to both mother and baby. Most recent professional advice advocates that the infant be weaned slowly at a time chosen by either mother or infant. The mother should be helped, from the beginning, to feel comfortable with any length of time she chooses, even if it is considerably longer or shorter than usual.

The mother can begin to wean her infant by omitting either the feeding the infant is least interested in or the one that is least convenient for her. Parsons[35] suggests substituting the feeding with another comforting experience that the baby enjoys, such as rocking, singing or sucking on a pacifier. Anywhere from a week to a month later, when both mother and baby are ready, another feeding may be dropped. This can be continued with periodic omissions until the child is completely off the breast. Additional omissions should be avoided when there are stressful situations in the family, such as illness, traveling or guests. The child can be weaned to a cup or to a bottle depending on age and sucking needs.

Weaning is as likely to be traumatic to the mother as it is to the baby, especially if nursing has been a satisfying experience. Support from the father or another significant person may help guide her through this difficult time.

Sudden weaning is seldom necessary since the mother can express milk for a short time if she and the baby must be separated because of illness or absence for some other reason. If it does become necessary, a good supportive bra and mild analgesics for discomfort will probably be helpful for the mother. Breast-drying medications used during the early puerperium do not stop established lactation.

ARTIFICIAL FEEDING

The mother who chooses to bottle-feed her infant may have as many concerns about feeding as the breast-feeding mother, especially if this is her first child. Depending on what she has heard about the comparison between breast milk and formula, she may feel a little uncertain about her choice and become defensive if questioned. She may also have heard about formulas disagreeing with some infants or causing allergies so that it becomes necessary to switch from one formula to another. By keeping up-to-date on the latest information about infant nutrition, the nurse can help allay the mother's fears about the adequacy of formulas, instruct her in safe preparation, and give guidance about when to seek medical assistance.

Comparison of Formulas

In today's hospital nursery the infant will probably receive ready-to-feed formula in a disposable bottle. However, since formula in disposable bottles is expensive, one of the other packaging methods will be recommended once the baby is ready to go home. Formula is available in various sized cans in ready-to-use, concentrated or powdered form.

The model usually used in planning a formula is human milk. Companies that manufacture formula are continually adjusting their formulas to match each new discovery concerning the composition of human milk.

To provide adequate nutrition for an infant, a formula must meet the following criteria: it must have an appropriate distribution of calories from protein, fat and carbohydrate; it must meet the infant's need for water, energy, vitamins and minerals; and it must be readily digestible. Recommended standards for calories, protein, fat, vitamins and minerals in formulas have been published by the Committee on Nutrition of the American Academy of Pediatrics.[36]

Cow's milk has more protein, sodium, calcium and less carbohydrate than human milk, but is about the same in fat, calories and the ratio of water to solids. The protein of cow's milk is quite different from human milk and contains much more casein and less whey protein. The approximate whey/casein ratios are: 20:80 in cow's milk and 60:40 in human milk. The increased casein leads to a tougher curd which is more difficult to digest. Boiling or pasteurizing fresh milk, and using the process employed in making evaporated milk, will soften the curd and make it more digestible. Adding water to the milk also softens the curd and dilutes the composition, bringing it closer to human milk. However, since the dilution lowers the proportion of carbohydrate, corn syrup or dextro-maltose is usually added.

Before commercially prepared formulas became widely available, evaporated milk formulas were most commonly used. They are still less expensive than the commercial formulas and are in use in many areas. Evaporated milk contains adequate amounts of vitamins A, B and K and is usually fortified with vitamin D, but along with fresh whole milk, it fails to meet current recommendations for vitamin C, vitamin E and essential fatty acids.

Many ingredients and processes are used in an effort to make commercial formulas meet the recommended nutritional standards and come as close as possible to human milk. Most of the formulas, such as Similac and Enfamil, use a nonfat cow's milk base with added vegetable oil and carbohydrate. Another group, called "humanized" formulas, attempts to duplicate the 60:40 whey/casein ratio by using dialyzed whey. The dialysis removes electrolytes, bringing the formula closer to the low electrolyte human milk. An example of this type is SMA.

Some infants are not able to tolerate formulas based on cow's milk. Many formulas have been developed to try to meet the nutritional needs of these infants. Some of these, such as meat-based formulas, may be difficult for the mother to accept since they do not look like milk. Soybean-derived products are commonly used as the protein source in these artificial formulas. Soy protein isolate has a lower biologic value than casein and whey, so slightly larger amounts are needed to meet the infant's needs.

Sometimes an infant will be given milk other than a formula. In our weight-conscious society it might seem that *nonfat milk* would be a good choice for an infant who was gaining weight too rapidly. Or nonfat dry milk may seem desirable for economic reasons. But nonfat milk is not recommended for infants under one year because it provides an excessive intake of protein with inadequate calories. In order to meet energy requirements and growth needs, body fat is mobilized. The infant may look

healthy but have little reserve for illness. Nonfat milk also lacks an adequate content of iron, ascorbic acid and essential fatty acids. *Low-fat* (2 percent) milk is midway between nonfat and whole milk in fat content, but probably would not meet all the infant's energy needs.[37]

Commercial milk substitutes such as filled milk or imitation milk are also available. *Filled milks* consist of a combination of true milk solids and a nonmilk fat. They usually have all the nutrients of regular milk but may have more carbohydrate. Depending on which nonmilk fat is used, one or more of the essential fatty acids may be missing along with the fortified vitamins that are usually found in regular milk. Thus they usually are not recommended for infants. *Imitation milk* is available in a few states. Although it may be cheaper than regular milk, it is also nutritionally inferior and should not be given to infants or children as a substitute for milk.[38]

Feeding in the Hospital

Most hospitals have a routine for when the bottle-fed baby will receive the first water feeding and when the formula feedings will start. In some it is the rule that the first water is given by the nurse in the nursery. Other hospitals are more permissive and allow the mother to give the first water. If this is the case, the nurse should show the mother how to use the bulb syringe since the water often causes the infant to bring up mucus. The nurse should also stay nearby to observe the infant's responses to the water.

The first feeding experiences can be very important for mother and infant. The mother begins to learn how the infant communicates his wants and needs, while the infant, besides learning to coordinate his feeding behaviors, begins to find out how the discomfort from hunger is relieved and who provides the relief. The nurse can help the mother and infant with these tasks by being available during initial feeding periods to observe their behaviors, assess the interaction and intervene with suggestions or demonstrations as necessary. When intervening, the nurse should be careful not to make the mother feel as though she is incompetent or inadequate.

Before feeding begins, the mother should be helped to get into a comfortable position. She may want to sit up in a chair instead of in the bed.

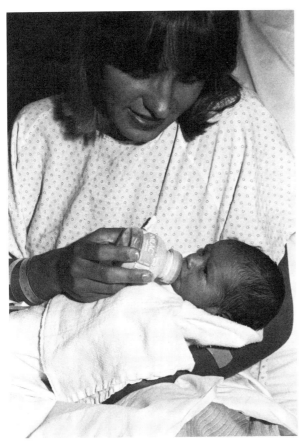

Figure 30-8. When bottle-feeding her infant, the mother tilts the bottle in such a way that the nipple is filled with milk.

Holding the baby in a semireclining position will allow any air that is swallowed to rise to the top of the infant's stomach where it is more easily expelled. To minimize the amount of air swallowed, the bottle should be tilted enough to keep the nipple filled with milk (Fig. 30-8).

The mother may need some help in getting the infant started on the bottle. If the infant does not open his mouth readily, gently stroking the lips with the nipple might help. Some babies elevate their tongue when opening their mouths and an inexperienced mother may not recognize that the nipple is under the tongue. Having the baby open his mouth wide enough so that the tongue can be seen usually helps in placing the nipple in the right position. Also, care should be taken that the nipple is not pushed too far into the mouth where it may cause gagging if it strikes the soft palate.

As the baby sucks, air bubbles rise in the bottle,

indicating that the baby is getting milk. If air bubbles do not appear, the nipple should be checked to see it the hole is clogged or too small. If the milk is coming too fast the nipple holes may be too large. Nipple holes can be checked by holding the bottle upside down. The milk should drop freely, but not run in a stream. If milk is coming at the right speed a feeding should take 15 to 20 minutes. If it takes much longer the infant may get too tired, but if it is much shorter the infant may not meet his sucking needs.

Babies have many different feeding behaviors, some of which may not correspond to the mother's expectations. Identifying the infant's individual behavior patterns and interpreting the baby's individuality to the mother can help to avert potential problems.[39]

If the mother is concerned that the baby is not taking enough milk, it may help her to know that babies are often sleepy the first few days but that they are born with reserves of fat and water and do not really need too many calories until the second or third day.[40] The bottle-fed baby, like the breast-fed baby, should have the opportunity to be on a self-demand schedule. Some babies get hungry more frequently than every four hours and some will want to wait longer than that between some feedings.

Before the mother and baby leave the hospital, the mother should be given some anticipatory guidance in how much formula the infant may take and how to prepare it.

According to the Recommended Dietary Allowances established by the Food and Nutrition Board of the National Academy of Sciences in 1973, infants from birth to five months need approximately 117 calories/kg (51 calories/lb.) each day. From six months to a year the need decreases to 108 calories/kg. (47 calories/lb.).[41] Using this as a guide, the nurse can help the mother calculate the infant's daily caloric needs. Most formula contains 20 calories per ounce, so a 7-pound baby would need about 17½ ounces a day, or a little less than 3 ounces at each of six feedings. As the infant grows, he will increase his consumption. At times of particularly fast growth, he will want to eat more at each feeding or more frequently. Again, the reminder should be given that each baby is an individual and that babies of the same age and weight may have different needs.

Preparation of Formula at Home

Bottles and Nipples

With the wide variety of bottles and nipples available on the market, selection depends on the parents' preference. Some will prefer glass bottles with plastic nipple caps; others will opt for the boilable plastic bottles which are nonbreakable. Then there are the kits that have a hollow plastic holder in which a disposable plastic bag containing the milk is suspended. Supposedly less air will be swallowed with this method because the bag collapses rather than filling with air when the milk is sucked out. However, the infant can still swallow air around the nipple.

Nipples also come in several shapes and sizes. One supposedly resembles the mother's breast in looks; another (Nuk) is supposed to elicit sucking responses more like the breast. The number of bottles and nipples needed will depend on the method of preparation. (For examples of bottles and nipples available, see Fig. 30-9.)

Methods of Preparation

Strict sterilization procedures for preparing formulas have been considered a must in the past. Some recent studies have shown that formulas that are prepared at home and sterilized are frequently contaminated.[42] Many physicians are no longer insisting that bottles or formulas be sterilized if there is an uncontaminated water source and good refrigeration, and if hands and equipment are cleaned properly, since this clean technique is proving to be as safe as sterilization. There was no higher incidence of illness or infection when infants were fed formula prepared by the clean technique than when infants were fed formula prepared by terminal sterilization.[43]

Points common to all methods of preparation are:

1. Hands should be washed well before starting.
2. If canned milk is used, the top of the can should be washed with soap and water using friction and then rinsed thoroughly. Hot water can be poured over the top just before opening.
3. All equipment should be washed thoroughly

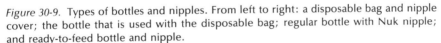

Figure 30-9. Types of bottles and nipples. From left to right: a disposable bag and nipple cover; the bottle that is used with the disposable bag; regular bottle with Nuk nipple; and ready-to-feed bottle and nipple.

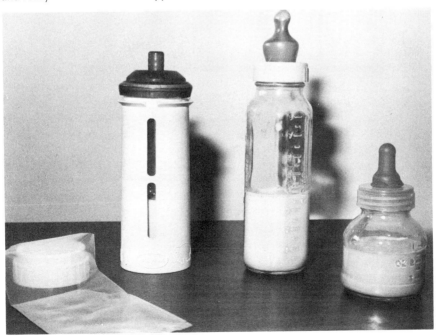

in warm soapy water. A bottle and nipple brush should be used and water should be squeezed through the nipple to make sure no milk particles or residue remain. Rinse thoroughly so all soap or detergent is gone.

4. Opened cans of formula or milk should be covered with fresh foil or plastic wrap, placed in the refrigerator and used within 48 hours.

One Bottle Method.   This is the method recommended in the pamphlet, *Infant Care,* put out by the Children's Bureau of HEW.[44] According to these recommendations, a concentrated prepared infant formula is poured directly into the bottle once the four steps mentioned above are carried out. One-half the total amount of formula desired is measured according to the markings on the bottle. For example, if 4 ounces of formula is needed, 2 ounces of concentrated formula would be used. Assuming a safe water supply, an equal amount of fresh tap water is added. The bottle should be fed to the infant within 30 minutes of the time it is made. If it is not used within an hour, it should be discarded.

Clean Method.   The major difference between this "clean" method and the "one bottle method" is that the whole day's formula is prepared at one time with the clean method. The bottles should be refrigerated immediately after preparation.

Since some physicians still recommend sterilization and since some people still live under conditions where sterilization is necessary, the aseptic method and terminal sterilization are included.

Aseptic Method.   In this method, the bottles, nipples, nipple caps, and equipment used in making the formula are sterilized before the formula is prepared. The mother will need a glass or enamel pitcher in which to mix the formula, a measuring cup, measuring spoons, tablespoon (to mix the formula), funnel (depending on the size of the bottle mouth), can opener (if canned milk is used) and some kind of tongs that can be sterilized. The tongs will be used as a forceps to handle the equipment. These items, together with the bottles, caps, and nipples are placed in a large pan or sterilizer half full of water and boiled vigorously for ten minutes. The equipment and the bottles, nipples, and so on, may be done separately if the sterilizer cannot accommodate such a large load. Care should be taken to

place the forceps in such a way that the handles can be reached easily after sterilization. If the mother must reach into the water for them, the water will become contaminated as will the materials being sterilized. After sterilization the formula is made according to directions. A specific amount of the formula is put into each bottle. The bottles are then nippled, capped and refrigerated.

Terminal Sterilization.   In this method, the formula is prepared under a clean but not aseptic technique. The equipment, bottles, nipples, and nipple caps are washed thoroughly but are not sterilized. The formula is prepared and poured into the bottles, and the nipples and the caps are applied loosely. They then are placed in the sterilizer, covered with a tight-fitting lid and sterilized by having the water boil rapidly in the bottom of the sterilizer for 25 minutes. In this method, formula, bottles, nipples, and protectors are all sterilized in one operation. Before the formula is refrigerated, the screw collar should be made secure.

COMMON CONCERNS IN INFANT FEEDING

There are several topics related to infant feeding that are of concern to the new mother regardless of the method of feeding.

Hunger.   The mother may wonder how she can tell if her infant is getting enough to eat. She can be told that most babies when awakened from sleep by hunger "pains" will fuss and cry and make sucking movements with their mouths, but that at first the infant may have difficulty distinguishing between hunger and other discomforts. If the baby awakens a short time after a feeding, the mother should try other comfort measures such as holding, changing the diaper, and bubbling, before assuming he is hungry. Occasionally a baby appears hungry, when in reality he is only thirsty and will be satisfied with a small amount of water. If he is obviously hungry and crying, and refuses water with apparent disgust, and when a feeding is offered, seizes the nipple ravenously and nurses with great vigor, he may need to eat more frequently for a while if he is breast-fed, or be offered more in his bottle at each feeding.

Bubbling (Burping). After five minutes or so, or in the middle and at the end of each feeding, the infant should be held in an upright position and his back *gently* patted or stroked (Fig. 30–10). Pounding the baby on the back vigorously is neither effective for bubbling him nor conducive to his well-being. The change in position (from semireclining to upright) is an important factor in eliciting a bubble. Often holding the infant upright and pressing him against the breast is all that is necessary.

An alternate position is for the mother to sit the infant up on her lap, with his chest resting on her hand and his chin supported by her thumb and index finger, while she pats him with her other hand. A third position is to place the infant prone over her knees. The last two positions are sometimes preferred by nurses in the newborn nursery, because they keep the infant away from the nurse's face and hair (Figs. 30–11 and 30–12).

Because the new infant's gastrointestinal tract is labile, milk may be eructated with the gas bubbles. A diaper is usually kept in front of the infant while he is being bubbled, in case this occurs (Fig. 30–10).

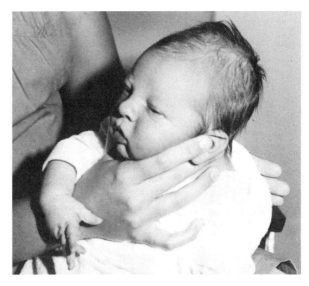

Figure 30-11. When bubbling the infant in the nursery, the nurse sits the infant up in her lap, with his chest resting on her hand and his chin supported by her thumb and index finger.

If there is doubt about whether or not the infant has brought up all the air when he is placed in his crib, putting him on his right side or in a prone position will help bring up the air and also prevent the infant from choking on any milk that might be regurgitated with the air.

Regurgitation. Regurgitation, which is merely an overflow and often occurs after nursing, should not be confused with vomiting, which may occur at any time, is accompanied by other symptoms, and usually involves a more complete emptying of the

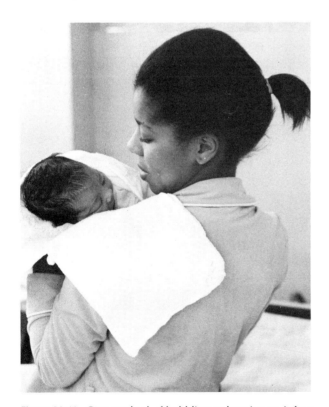

Figure 30-10. One method of bubbling or burping an infant is to place him in an upright position over the shoulder where he can be pressed gently against the breast.

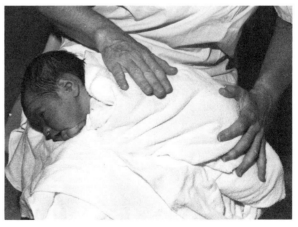

Figure 30-12. For an alternate method of bubbling, the infant is placed over the knees while his back is gently rubbed.

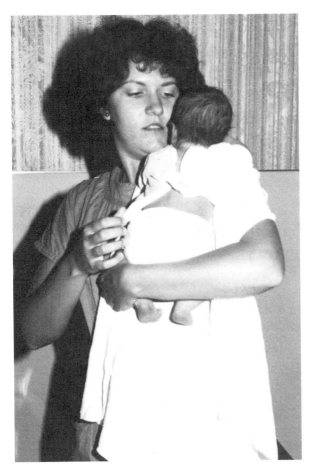

Figure 30-13. A blanket is used over the nurse's uniform as she holds the baby for burping.

stomach. This regurgitation is the means of relieving the distended stomach and usually indicates that the baby either has taken too much food or has taken it too rapidly.

Hiccups.   Some mothers need reassurance that hiccups are not unusual for infants and really do not seem to bother them. If the mother is disturbed, she can try giving the infant a few sips of water, but the hiccups go away by themselves without treatment.

Constipation.   This is almost nonexistent in breast-fed babies and uncommon in those fed prepared formulas, but mothers frequently express a concern about possible constipation. Many parents believe that an infant is constipated if he misses having a bowel movement one day. The nurse can explain that it is quality not quantity of the stool that indicates the presence of constipation. An infant is considered to be constipated when the stools are hard, formed and difficult to pass.

NUTRITIONAL CONSIDERATIONS DURING THE FIRST YEAR

Diets for infants are sometimes based on temporary scientific fashions or local customs. Long-term effects of infant diets are not known. Standards for formulas and baby foods are based on infant growth, but it is not known whether a diet that is optimum for growth in infancy will offer freedom from allergy, obesity, arterial disease or cancer later in adult life.

During the first year of life the infant's growth exceeds that of any future period. In the first four months, he usually doubles his birth weight and may triple it by one year. Watching the infant grow is pleasing to the parents and they often see the chubbiness of the infant as evidence of good health and their good parenting. This attitude can lead to overfeeding.

The infant's caloric needs per unit of body weight are relatively constant during the first year. This is because as he becomes more physically active from the fourth month on, his rate of growth is slowing down and energy is relocated from growth to activity.

INTRODUCTION OF SOLID FOODS

The time for adding solid foods is an area where recommendations in the literature and actual practice often differ markedly. Although an adequate amount of all essential nutrients can be provided during the first six months without the addition of solids, many babies in the United States are receiving solid foods before they are a month old.[45] This early feeding often occurs because the parents request it, thinking it will help the baby sleep through the night or considering it a sign that he is more advanced than infants who are "only taking milk."

There are many reasons suggested for delaying the introduction of solids until the infant is four to six months old. First, the baby is not developmentally ready to deal with nonliquid foods until about the end of the third month, and his tongue will usually push them out of the mouth. Also, the large protein molecules from the foods may pass through the mucosa of the infants immature gastrointestinal tract and become antigens, sensitizing the infant and causing allergic reactions. After six months the GI system is more mature and the infant's antibody production has reached a more desirable level. Other drawbacks to early feeding of solids are: the potential for not supplying the infant's nutritional needs, the relatively high cost of the food, and the possibility of overfeeding.

Infantile obesity has become a growing concern in recent years because of its possible relation to adult obesity. Growth during infancy is mostly due to cell hyperplasia (tissue growth involving increases in the number of cells). It is felt that the obese infant will have more fat cells than normal throughout life and therefore be more prone to continuing obesity.[46]

Some suggestions for avoiding infant obesity are:
1. Help parents use factors other than weight gain to evaluate their role as parents.
2. Help mothers discover the infant's satiety behavior and avoid encouraging the infant to get down the last drop or bite.
3. Encourage practices which promote more physical activities in infants.
4. Avoid early introduction of solids.

Nutritional Supplements

Vitamins. Woodruff states that since both breast milk and prepared formulas contain adequate vitamins for normal infants, routine supplementation should be abandoned.[47] However, some sources still recommend a vitamin D supplement for breast-fed babies. If the infant is on a formula made of fresh or evaporated cow's milk, then a vitamin C supplement might be necessary.

Iron Iron deficiency anemia is currently the most common specific nutritional deficiency encountered. Infants and children between the ages of 6 and 30 months, especially those from lower socioeconomic groups, are particularly vulnerable. Breast-fed infants rarely have iron deficiency anemia and it is now recommended that formulas be fortified with iron at a level of 10 to 12 mg. per liter. Infant cereal has been fortified with iron for a long time, but the form of iron used was recently found to be poorly absorbed and has now been changed to a more absorbable form in most cereals.

These sources of iron would probably be adequate, but they may not continue to be available to the infant as he grows older. By the age of six months many infants are switched to fresh cow's milk. This causes two problems. First, it is low in iron. Second, there is increasing evidence that drinking fresh cow's milk during infancy is associated with occult blood loss from the intestine resulting in iron deficiency anemia. The latter is less likely if the milk is boiled. Prepared formulas fortified with iron are recommended for the nonbreast-fed baby for the first 12 months of life.[48]

REFERENCES

1. C. C. Neumann and D. B. Jelliffe: "Forward." Symposium on Nutrition in Pediatrics. *Pediatric Clinics of North America,* 24,1:1, February 77.
2. C. Smith and N. Nelson: *The Physiology of the Newborn Infant.* Springfield, Ill., Charles C Thomas, 1979.
3. D. B. Jelliffe and E. F. P. Jelliffe: "Current concepts in nutrition, Breast is best: Modern meanings." *New England J. Med.* 912–915, October 27, 1977.
4. Ibid.
5. Ibid.
6. K. E. Grams: "Breast feeding: A means of imparting immunity?" *MCN* 3,6:340–344, Nov./Dec. 1978.
7. M. Gunther: "The value of breast feeding." In *Early Nutrition and Later Development,* Chicago, Yearbook Medical Publishers, 1976.
8. Jelliffe and Jelliffe, op. cit.
9. Gunther, op. cit.
10. J. S. Doucette: "Is breast feeding still safe for babies?" *MCN* 3,6:345–346, Nov./Dec. 1978.
11. A. Gerard: *Please Breast-feed Your Baby.* New York, Hawthorn Books, 1970, Chap. 7.
12. B. Lawson: "Perception of degrees of support for the breast-feeding mother." *BFJ,* 3:2, Summer 1976.
13. N. W. Johnson: "Breast feeding at one hour of age." *MCN,* 121:12–16, Jan./Feb. 1976.
14. Ibid.
15. Committee on Fetus and Newborn: *Hospital Care of Newborn Infants,* 6th ed. Illinois, American Academy of Pediatrics, 1977, p. 73.

16. B. A. Countryman: "Hospital care of the breastfed newborn." *AJN* 71:2365–2367, Dec. 1971.

17. Sister M. C. Iffrig: "Nursing care and success in breast feeding." *Nursing Clinics North America*, 3:353, June 1968.

18. M. G. Nichols: "Effective help for the nursing mother." *JOGN*, 7,2:22–30, March/April 1978.

19. Doris Haire and John Haire: "The nurse's contribution to successful breast-feeding," and "The medical value of breast-feeding." *Implementing Family Centered Maternity Care with a Central Nursery*, New Jersey, ICEA.

20. N. Whitley: "Preparation for breastfeeding." *JOGN* 7,3:44–48, May/June 1978.

21. Nichols, op. cit.

22. Ibid.

23. Ibid.

24. J. Grassley and K. Davis: "Common concerns of mothers who breastfeed." *MCN*, 3,6: 347–351, Nov./Dec. 1978.

25. B. L. Nichols and V. N. Nichols: "The biologic basis of lactation." *Comprehensive Therapy*, 4,10:63–70, Oct. 1978.

26. Sister A. Murdaugh and L. E. Miller: "Helping the breast-feeding mother." *Am. J. Nurs.*, 72:1420–1423, Aug. 1972.

27. Ibid.

28. Nichols, op. cit.

29. Ibid.

30. R. MacKeith and C. Wood: *Infant feeding and feeding difficulties*. Edinburgh, Churchill Livingstone, 1977.

31. M. G. Horning, et al.: "Identification and quantification of drugs and drug metabolites in human breast milk using GC-MS-COM methods." in *Modern Problems in Paediatrics—Milk and Lactation*, 15:73–79, Basel, S. Korger, 1975.

32. B. S. Rothermel and M. M. Faber: "Drugs in breastmilk—A consumer's guide." *BFJ*, 2,3: 76–88, Summer 1975.

33. "Drugs in breastmilk." *Medical Letter on Drugs and Therapeutics*, 16:6, March 15, 1974.

34. T. E. O'Brien: "Excretion of drugs in human milk." *Am. J. Hosp. Pharm.*, 31:844.

35. L. J. Parsons: "Weaning from the breast." *JOGN*, 7,3:12–15, May/June 1978.

36. American Academy of Pediatrics, Committee on Nutrition. "Commentary on breast feeding and infant formulas, including proposed standards for formulas." *Pediatrics*, 57:278–285, Feb. 1976.

37. C. Woodruff: "The science of infant nutrition and the art of infant feeding." *JAMA*, 240,7:657–661, August 18, 1978.

38. M. S. Brown and M. A. Murphy: *Ambulatory Pediatrics for Nurses*. New York, McGraw-Hill, 1975.

39. M. C. Scahill: "Helping the mother solve problems with feeding her infant." *JOGN*, 4,2: 51–54, March/April 1975.

40. Woodruff, op. cit.

41. J. Slattery: "Nutrition for the normal healthy infant." *MCN* 2,2:105–112, March/April 1977.

42. V. Kendall and Kusakcroglu: "A study of preparation of infant formulas." *Am. J. Dis. Child* 122:215, 1971.

43. T. Hargrove and C. Hargrove: "Formula preparation and infant illness." *Clin. Pediatrics*, 13:1057, 1974.

44. Children's Bureau, U.S. Dept. of Health, Education, and Welfare. *Infant Care*. Washington, D. C., U.S. Government Printing Office, 1973, p. 11.

45. T. A. Anderson and S. Fomon: "Beikost." In *Infant Nutrition*, 2nd ed. Philadelphia, W. B. Saunders, 1974.

46. E. Parham: "The effect of early feeding on the development of obesity." *JOGN* 3,3:58–61, May/June 1975.

47. Woodruff, op. cit.

48. Ibid.

Assessment and Management of Maternal Disorders

Complications of Pregnancy
Concurrent Diseases in Pregnancy
Complications of Labor
Operative Obstetrics
Postpartal Complications

Thirty-One

Complications of Pregnancy

Hemorrhagic Complications of Early Pregnancy /
Hyperemesis Gravidarum / Hemorrhagic Complications
of Late Pregnancy / The Hypertensive Disorders of
Pregnancy

From a biologic point of view childbearing is considered to be a normal process. Nevertheless, the borderline between health and illness is less distinct in this time because of the numerous physiologic changes that occur during the course of pregnancy. The importance of early and continued health supervision during pregnancy for the total well-being of the mother and her infant is paramount, for such preventive care makes possible the early detection of warning signals of potential pathologic conditions. Serious problems can be averted or controlled by prompt treatment.

Certain "common complaints" are experienced by most expectant mothers to some degree. These are the so-called minor discomforts of pregnancy, which in themselves are not serious but detract from the mother's feeling of well-being. Since these discomforts are usually related to physiologic changes occurring within the mother's body and are not in themselves pathologic, they have been included in the chapter on antepartal care (see Chapter 20).

Certain complications of pregnancy may seriously jeopardize the health of both the mother and her unborn infant. Although dramatic progress has been made in reducing maternal and perinatal morbidity and mortality, some problems remain unsolved.

Despite expanding social programs, a great many underprivileged women receive inadequate or no prenatal care. These women, in contrast to those with optimal care, have an increased rate of complications, morbidity, and mortality, both maternal and perinatal.

Pregnancy-related maternal disorders are divided into two broad categories: complications related to the pregnancy itself and not seen at other times, and diseases which are not pregnancy-related but occur coincidentally. The latter may arise in the nonpregnant patient as well, but when they occur during pregnancy they may complicate the pregnancy and influence its course or may be aggravated by the pregnancy. Such conditions are considered in Chapter 32.

There are only a few major complications that result from pregnancy, but these may present serious health hazards. These complications, which will be considered here, include: 1) hemorrhagic conditions of early pregnancy (abortion, ectopic pregnancy and hydatidiform mole), 2) hyperemesis gravidarum, 3) hemorrhagic complications of placental origin in late pregnancy (placenta previa and abruptio placentae), and 4) hypertensive disorders of pregnancy, formerly called *toxemia* (preeclampsia and eclampsia).

HEMORRHAGIC COMPLICATIONS OF EARLY PREGNANCY

The causes of bleeding in pregnancy are usually considered in relation to the stage of gestation in which they are most likely to cause complications. Frequent causes of bleeding during the first half of pregnancy are abortion, ectopic pregnancy, and hydatidiform mole. Although hydatidiform mole is a less common cause (it occurs once in about 2,000 pregnancies), it is nevertheless important, because uterine bleeding is its outstanding symptom. The two most common causes of hemorrhage in the latter half of pregnancy are placenta previa and abruptio placentae.

Abortion

Definitions

Abortion is the termination of pregnancy at any time before the fetus has attained a stage of viability, that is, before it is capable of extrauterine existence. The term *miscarriage* is commonly used by lay persons to denote an abortion that has occurred spontaneously rather than one which has been induced. Since *abortion* is the accepted medical term for either, this point should be clarified in discussions with patients to avoid confusion or misinterpretation. In medical parlance the word miscarriage is rarely employed.

It is customary to use the weight of the fetus as an important criterion in abortion. Infants weighing 1,000 gm. (2 lb., 3 oz.) or less at birth possess little chance for survival, whereas those above this weight have a substantial chance of living. Thus some authorities regard a pregnancy that terminates when the fetus weighs 1,000 gm (about 28 weeks of gestation) or less as an abortion. On the other hand, a small percentage of infants weighing 1,000 gm. or less do survive. Modern advances in the management and care of preterm infants have made it possible for smaller and smaller infants to survive, so fetuses weighing only 800 to 900 gm. (1 lb., 13 oz. to 2 lb.) may live. For this reason many authorities now maintain that fetal weight of 1,000 gm. or less but more than 500 gm. is classified as *immature,* and that fetal weight of 500 gm. (about 20 weeks of gestation) or less constitutes an *abortion*. In many states a birth certificate is prepared for any pregnancy terminating beyond the twentieth week of gestation or when the fetus weighs 500 gm. or more. It is obvious, therefore, that how the termination of pregnancy is classified in different hospitals will depend wholly on the interpretation to which they subscribe.

A preterm infant is one born after the stage of viability has been reached but before it has the same chance for survival as a full-term infant. By general consensus, an infant which weighs 2,500 gm. or less at birth is termed *preterm;* one which weighs 2,501 gm. (5½ lb.) or more is regarded as *full term.*

It is well to remember that preterm labor does not refer to abortion. *Preterm labor* is the termination of pregnancy after the fetus is viable but before it has attained full term. Although the cause of many preterm labors cannot be explained, the condition can be brought on by maternal diseases, such as chronic hypertensive vascular disease, abruptio placentae, placenta previa, untreated syphilis or a mechanical defect in the cervix.

Types of Abortions

The term abortion includes many varieties of termination of pregnancy prior to viability but may be subdivided into two main groups: spontaneous and induced.

Spontaneous abortion is one in which the process starts of its own accord through natural causes.

Induced abortion is one which is artificially induced whether for therapeutic or other reasons. Induced abortion has been considered in Chapter 13.

Threatened Abortion. An abortion is regarded as threatened if vaginal bleeding or spotting occurs in early pregnancy. This may or may not be associated with mild cramps. The cervix is closed. The process has presumably started but may abate.

Inevitable Abortion. Inevitable abortion is so called because the process has gone so far that termination of the pregnancy cannot be prevented. Bleeding is copious, and the pains are more severe. The membranes may or may not have ruptured, and the cervical canal is dilating.

Incomplete Abortion. An incomplete abortion is one in which part of the products of conception has been passed, but part (usually the placenta) is retained in the uterus. Bleeding usually persists until the retained products of conception have been passed.

Complete Abortion. Complete abortion is the expulsion of all the products of conception.

Missed Abortion. In a missed abortion the fetus dies in the uterus but is retained. The term is generally restricted to cases in which two months or more elapse between fetal death and expulsion. During this period the fetus undergoes marked degenerative changes. Of these, maceration, or general softening, is the most common. Occasionally it dries up into a leatherlike structure (mummification), and very rarely it is converted into stony material (lithopedion formation). Symptoms, except for amenorrhea, are usually lacking, but occasionally such patients complain of malaise, headache and anorexia. Hypofibrinogenemia, a hemorrhagic complication, may result (see p. 516).

Habitual Abortion. This term indicates a condition in which spontaneous abortion occurs in successive pregnancies (three or more). This is a most distressing condition, some women having six or eight spontaneous abortions.

Criminal Abortion. Criminal, or perhaps better stated, extra-hospital (or extra-clinic) abortion is the termination of pregnancy outside of appropriate medical facilities, generally by nonphysician abortionists, regardless of the validity of the indication. The frequency of such abortions is not precisely known but has dropped precipitously in the United States following the Supreme Court decision of 1973. In years past, estimates ranged from 200,000 to 1,200,000 per year in the United States. In most urban areas, abortions were responsible for the majority of maternal deaths, with estimates of 800 to 5,000 abortion deaths per year.

Attempts at producing abortion are generally made by the ingestion of drugs such as quinine or castor oil, which usually do nothing or, if taken in sufficient quantities to produce an abortion, place the woman in serious jeopardy.

Another common approach involves the placement of a foreign body, such as a urethral catheter, into the uterus with or without the instillation of toxic substances. Severe infection, often with shock and renal failure, is a common consequence of such crude efforts at pregnancy termination. Patients so affected surely are some of the most critically ill the nurse may ever have to care for and, unfortunately, they sometimes succumb in spite of the best efforts of all concerned.

Manifestations and Causes

Clinical Picture. About 75 percent of all spontaneous abortions occur during the second and the third months of pregnancy, that is, before the twelfth week. The condition is very common; it is estimated that about one pregnancy in every ten terminates in spontaneous abortion. Almost invariably the first symptom is bleeding due to the separation of the fertilized ovum from its uterine attachment. The bleeding is often slight at the beginning and may persist for days before uterine cramps occur; or the bleeding may be followed at once by cramps. Occasionally the bleeding is torrential, leaving the patient in shock. The uterine contractions bring about softening and dilatation of the cervix and either complete or incomplete expulsion of the products of conception.

Causes. What causes all these spontaneous abortions—so tragic and shattering to so many women? If the evidence is reviewed with some perspective and with full fairness to all concerned, it is the inevitable conclusion that most of these abortions, far from being tragedies, are blessings in disguise, for they are Nature's beneficent way of extinguishing imperfect embryos. Indeed, careful microscopic study of the material passed in these cases shows that the most common cause of spontaneous abortion is an inherent defect in the products of conception. This defect may express itself in an abnormal embryo, an abnormal *trophoblast* or both abnormalities.

In early abortions, 80 percent are associated with some defect of the embryo or trophoblast which is either incompatible with life or would result in a grossly deformed child. The incidence of abnormalities after the second month is somewhat lower but not less than 50 percent. Whether the germ plasm of the spermatozoon or the ovum is at fault in these cases, it is usually difficult, if not impossible, to say.

Abortions of this sort are obviously not preventable and, although often bitterly disappointing to the parents, serve a useful purpose.

Spontaneous abortions may result from causes other than defects in the products of conception. Severe acute infections, such as pneumonia, pyelitis and typhoid fever, often lead to abortion. Occasionally, abnormalities of the generative tract, such as a congenitally short cervix or uterine malformations, produce the accident. Retroposition of the uterus rarely causes abortion, as was formerly believed. Many women tend to explain abortion as a result of an injury or excessive activity. Women exhibit the greatest variation in this respect. In some the pregnancy may go blithely on despite falls from second-story windows and automobile accidents severe enough to fracture the pelvis. In others a trivial fall, anxiety or overfatigue may appear to be related to abortion, but there is obviously no way to determine a cause-and-effect relationship.

Management

The severity of the symptoms manifested in threatened abortion will determine the treatment prescribed. If the patient is having only slight vaginal bleeding or even spotting, without pain, she should be advised to stay in bed, eat a light well-balanced diet, and avoid straining at bowel evacuation and using cathartics. If she appears to be apprehensive, a mild sedative may be given. Some physicians do not restrict activity, based on the concept that the uterus is well insulated from outside influences.

Uniformly the patient should be advised to save all perineal pads, as well as all tissue and clots passed, for inspection. In cases where bedrest has been prescribed, if the bleeding disappears within 48 hours, the woman may get out of bed but should limit her activities for the next several days. Coitus should be avoided for two weeks following the last evidence of bleeding.

In cases in which pain accompanies the vaginal bleeding, the prognosis for saving the pregnancy is poor. Usually bleeding is observed first, and a few hours, sometimes days later, uterine contractions ensue. When the pain and the bleeding increase, the patient should be hospitalized, if this has not already been done.

If the abortion is incomplete, ordinarily efforts are made to aid the uterus in emptying its contents.

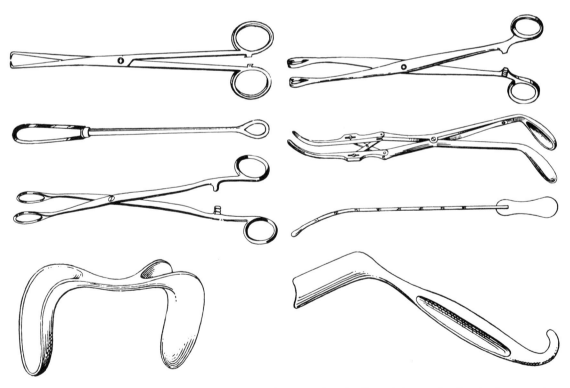

Figure 31-1. (Left, top to bottom) Bullet forceps used in grasping the lips of the cervix. Sims's sharp curet, a scraper or spoonlike instrument for removing matter from the walls of the uterus. Sponge holder. Sims's speculum for inserting into the vaginal canal so as to expose the cervix to view. *(Right, top to bottom)* Placental forceps with heart-shaped jaws. Modified Goodell-Ellinger dilator used for enlarging the canal of the cervix. Uterine sound. Schroeder vaginal retractor for drawing back the vulvar or vaginal walls during an operation.

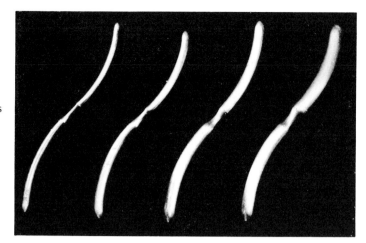

Figure 31-2. Hegar dilators of graduated diameters from 5 to 12 mm. Larger sizes are also used.

Oxytocin may be administered, but if this is ineffectual, surgical removal of the retained products of conception should be done promptly. Active bleeding may make this urgently necessary. Many times the tissue lies loose in the cervical canal and can simply be lifted out with ovum forceps; otherwise, curettage of the uterine cavity must be done. The instruments commonly used in completing an incomplete abortion are shown in Figures 31-1 and 31-2. The suction curet may also be used.

If evidence of infection is present (fever, foul discharge, or suspicious history of criminal abortion), evacuation of the uterus should be delayed only long enough to obtain appropriate studies (especially smears and cultures) and to initiate antibiotic therapy. Such prompt and aggressive management of the patient with an infected abortion will effectively reduce the incidence of more serious complications such as septic shock, thrombophlebitis, and renal failure, and will reduce morbidity and hospital stay as well.

Nurse's Responsibilities in Abortion Cases

Bleeding in the first half of pregnancy, no matter how slight, always must be considered as threatened abortion. The patient must be put to bed and the physician notified. An episode of this nature is indeed distressing to the expectant mother, many times alarming. The nurse should bear in mind that although it is important to give emotional support, the patient should never be reassured that "everything will be all right," because in fact the patient may lose this pregnancy.

Perineal pads and all tissue and blood clots passed by the patient should be saved. The physician will wish to examine these to determine the amount of bleeding and (when tissue has been passed) to examine the products of conception to ascertain whether or not the abortion is complete.

If bleeding is so copious as to be alarming, elevate the foot of the bed (shock position) while awaiting the physician. If surgical completion of the abortion is to be carried out, the same aseptic regimen is carried out as for delivery.

All cases of abortion carried out in nonmedical hands must be regarded as potentially infected, and strict antiseptic precautions must be carried out to prevent spread of infection to others. In caring for a woman who has had such an abortion recently, or one whose history is suspicious, it is important not to reflect a judgmental attitude or pass moral judgments. In such situations, it is best to direct concern to the gravity of the patient's illness. Occasionally circumstances make it possible for the nurse to be of definite educational help both to her patients and to the public.

Incompetent Cervical Os

A mechanical defect in the cervix, incompetent cervical os, has gained recognition as a cause of late habitual abortion or preterm labor. When repeated termination of pregnancy in the second trimester is due to an anatomical factor such as this, surgical treatment may make it possible to save the fetus.

Shirodkar Technique. One type of treatment used to prevent relaxation and dilatation of the cervix when it is incompetent is the modified Shirodkar technique. In this, the vaginal mucous membrane is elevated and a narrow strip of some material such as Mersilene is carried around the internal os of the cervix and tied. Then the vaginal mucosa is restored to its original position and sutured. The procedure may be done between pregnancies, if the diagnosis is clearly established, or during pregnancy. When done during pregnancy, it is usually elected to wait until the early part of the second trimester (12 to 14 weeks) to avoid the possibility of having to remove the suture if a spontaneous first trimester abortion occurs.

Postoperatively, the main concerns are rupture of the membranes and uterine contractions. If the membranes rupture, the suture must be removed and the uterus emptied because of the risk of infection. If contractions ensue, an effort to control the contractions is in order, and the most effective means for such control is intravenous alcohol. Attempts to control contractions should not be persistent if they are not effective promptly, since there is a risk of uterine rupture.

Decisions regarding the type of delivery a patient is to have are generally based on the position of the suture when the patient reaches term or labor begins. If the suture is in good position, with the cervical closure maintained, cesarean section may be elected to preserve the suture for future pregnancies. If the suture has loosened or rolled down on the cervix, it is not adequate for subsequent pregnancies. In that case, it is removed when labor begins and vaginal delivery is permitted.

McDonald Technique. Another more simple procedure used to treat the incompetent cervix is that devised by McDonald. This involves placing a nonabsorbable suture such as No. 1 nylon around the cervix high on the cervical mucosa. The McDonald procedure is usually carried out during pregnancy when premature dilatation of the cervix is detected or electively in the fourth month. The suture is easily removed near term to allow spontaneous delivery.

Ectopic Pregnancy

An ectopic pregnancy is any gestation located outside the uterine cavity. The majority of ectopic pregnancies are tubal gestations. Other types, which make up about 5 percent of all ectopic pregnancies, are interstitial (in the interstitial portion of the tube), cornual (in a rudimentary horn of a uterus), cervical, abdominal and ovarian gestations.

About once in every 300 pregnancies the fertilized ovum, instead of traversing the length of the fallopian tube to reach the uterine cavity, becomes implanted within the wall of the fallopian tube. This condition is known as "ectopic pregnancy" (literally, a pregnancy which is out of place) or as "tubal pregnancy" or "extrauterine pregnancy" (Fig. 31-3). Since the wall of the tube is not sufficiently elastic to allow the fertilized ovum to grow and develop there, rupture of the tubal wall is the inevitable result. Rupture most frequently occurs into the tubal lumen with the passage of the products of conception, together with much blood, out the fimbriated end of the tube and into the peritoneal cavity—so-called tubal abortion. Or rupture may occur through the peritoneal surface of the tube directly into the peritoneal cavity; and, again, there is an outpouring of blood into the abdomen from vessels at the site of rupture. In either case, rupture usually occurs within the first 12 weeks.

Occasionally an ectopic pregnancy may develop in that portion of the tube which passes through the uterine wall, a type known as "interstitial pregnancy." In very rare instances, the products of conception, after rupturing through the tubal wall, may become implanted on the peritoneum and develop to full term in the peritoneal cavity. This extraordinary occurrence is known as "abdominal pregnancy." Surprisingly, living infants have been delivered in such cases by means of abdominal incision.

Tubal ectopic pregnancy may be caused by any condition which narrows the tube or brings about some constriction within it. Under such circumstances the tubal lumen is large enough to allow spermatozoa to ascend the tube but not big enough to permit the downward passage of the fertilized ovum. Among the conditions which may produce such a narrowing of the fallopian tube are 1) previous

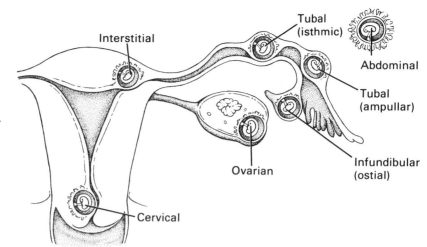

Figure 31-3. Sites of ectopic pregnancy.

inflammatory processes involving the tubal mucosa and producing partial agglutination of opposing surfaces, such as gonorrheal salpingitis; 2) previous inflammatory processes of the external peritoneal surfaces of the tube, causing kinking, such as puerperal and postabortal infections; and 3) developmental defects resulting in a segmental narrowing of the tubes.

Manifestations. In cases of ectopic gestation the woman exhibits the usual early symptoms of pregnancy and, as a rule, regards herself as being normally pregnant. After missing one or two periods, however, she suddenly experiences knifelike pain, often of extreme severity, in one of the lower quadrants. This is usually associated with slight vaginal bleeding, commonly referred to as "spotting." Depending on the amount of blood which has escaped into the peritoneal cavity, she may or may not undergo a fainting attack and show symptoms of shock.

Ectopic pregnancy is a grave complication of pregnancy and is a significant cause of maternal death. Moreover, if a woman has had one ectopic pregnancy, she is more likely to have another such accident in a subsequent pregnancy.

Management. In the vast majority of cases the tube has already ruptured and the fetus is dead when the patient is first seen by the physician. It is the rupture which produces the acute clinical picture. The treatment is to remove the tube and replace blood as necessary. Occasionally the ovary must be removed with the tube. Under certain circumstances in which subsequent fertility must be maintained, the tube may be preserved by removing the products of conception from the tube, either through a linear incision (salpingostomy) or by milking the conceptus out of the tubal lumen by external pressure applied with the fingers. This approach is applicable if the contralateral tube is badly diseased or has been previously removed and it is the patient's wish to preserve fertility.

Nursing Intervention. During the transportation of such a patient to the hospital or in the interval when the patient is awaiting operation, the nurse can be of immeasurable assistance in combating the shock that is frequently present. An intravenous infusion should be maintained so that blood or plasma expanders can be administered as needed and the patient's vital signs should be monitored and recorded.

Hydatidiform Mole

Hydatidiform mole is a benign neoplasm of the chorion in which the chorionic villi degenerate and become transparent vesicles containing clear, viscid fluid. The vesicles have a grapelike appearance and are arranged in clusters involving all or part of the decidual lining of the uterus (Fig. 31-4). Although there is usually no embryo present, occasionally

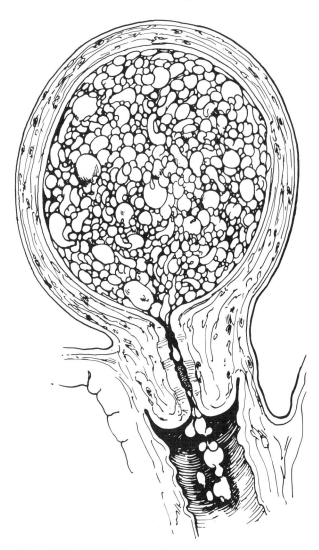

Figure 31-4. Hydatidiform mole.

there may be a fetus and only part of the placenta involved. Hydatidiform mole is rather an uncommon condition, occurring about once in every 2,000 pregnancies.

The pregnancy appears to be normal at first, although in about 50 percent of cases the uterus enlarges more rapidly than a normal pregnancy, and is larger than expected for the duration of pregnancy by dates. Then bleeding, a usual symptom varying from spotting to heavy bleeding, occurs, so that one might suspect threatened or inevitable abortion. If the patient does not abort, the uterus enlarges rapidly, and profuse hemorrhage may occur, at which time these vesicles may be evident in the vaginal discharge. Vomiting in rather severe form may appear early. Preeclampsia, a

complication which does not usually occur until the later months of pregnancy, may appear early in the second trimester.

Management. The treatment consists of emptying the uterus. The approach used for evacuating the uterine contents varies, depending on the size of the uterus at the time molar pregnancy is diagnosed. If the uterus is less than the size of a ten-week gestation, dilatation of the cervix, followed by curettage, either by curet or suction, is the usual procedure. This must be carried out with great care to avoid injury to the uterine wall, which is weakened and spongy due to the growth of the mole. If uterine size is larger, labor is stimulated with a continuous oxytocin infusion. After a portion of the uterine contents have been expelled, curettage is carried out to evacuate uterine contents completely.

The tissue obtained must be carefully evaluated by the pathologist, because, while a mole is a benign process, choriocarcinoma, an extremely malignant tumor, sometimes complicates the picture. For this reason also, follow-up care is very important in cases of molar pregnancy.

HYPEREMESIS GRAVIDARUM

A mild degree of nausea and vomiting, morning sickness, is the most common complaint of women in the first trimester of pregnancy. This manifestation is considered in the realm of a minor discomfort rather than a complication, and it usually responds to measures discussed in Chapter 20. It is uncommon today for this mild form of nausea and vomiting to progress to such a serious extent that it produces systemic effects (i.e., marked loss of weight and acetonuria), but when it becomes thus exaggerated, the condition is *hyperemesis gravidarum,* sometimes called pernicious vomiting.

Because even the gravest case of hyperemesis starts originally as a simple form of nausea, all cases of nausea and vomiting should be treated with proper understanding and judgment, and none should be regarded casually. When simple remedies do not prove to be effective, and symptoms of hyperemesis appear to be imminent, the patient should be hospitalized for more intensive treatment. Appropriate measures should be taken to rule out other disease such as cholecystitis, hepatitis, peptic ulcer and gastroenteritis. At the present time less than 1 pregnant woman in 500 has to be admitted to the hospital because of this complication of pregnancy, and, indeed, grave cases of hyperemesis gravidarum are becoming rare. The recovery of those who are admitted to the hospital is usually rapid.

Causes and Manifestations

Cause. It is currently recognized that during pregnancy there are certain organic processes that are basic to all cases of vomiting, regardless of whether the symptoms are mild or severe. The endocrine and metabolic changes of normal gestation, fragments of chorionic villi entering the maternal circulation and the diminished motility of the stomach might well give rise to clinical symptoms.

It has long been thought that hyperemesis gravidarum is in large measure a *neurosis*. The term "neurosis," it will be recalled, is employed very loosely to designate a large array of conditions in which symptoms occur without demonstrable pathologic explanation, the symptoms being due, it is thought, to a disturbance of the patient's psyche. As many examples show (quite apart from pregnancy), nausea is often psychic in origin. For instance, a repellent sight, an obnoxious odor or the mere recollection of such a sight or odor may give rise to nausea and even vomiting. Our general use of the adjective "nauseating" to describe a repulsive object is further acknowledgment that an upset mind may produce an upset stomach.

Clinical Picture. The clinical picture of the patient suffering from pernicious vomiting varies in relation to the severity and the duration of the condition. In any event, the condition begins with a typical picture of morning sickness. The patient experiences a feeling of nausea which may be most pronounced on arising in the morning but may occur at other times of the day. With the majority of these patients this pattern persists for a few weeks and then suddenly ceases.

A small number of patients who have "morning sickness" develop persistent vomiting which lasts for four to eight weeks or longer. These patients vomit several times a day and may be unable to retain any liquid or solid foods, with the result that marked symptoms of dehydration and starvation occur. *Dehydration* is pronounced, as evidenced by a diminished output of urine and a dryness of the skin.

Starvation, which is regularly present, manifests itself in a number of ways. Weight loss may vary from 5 pounds to as much as 20 or 30 pounds. This is tantamount to saying that the digestion and the absorption of carbohydrates and other nutrients have been so inadequate that the body has been forced to burn its reserve stores of fat in order to maintain body heat and energy. When fat is burned without carbohydrates being present, the process of combustion does not go on to completion. Consequently, certain incompletely burned products of fat metabolism make their appearance in the blood and the urine. The presence of acetone and diacetic acid in the urine in hyperemesis is common. In severe cases considerable changes associated with starvation and dehydration become evident in the blood chemistry. There is a definite increase in the nonprotein nitrogen, uric acid and urea, a moderate decrease in the chlorides and little alteration in the carbon dioxide combining power. Then, too, vitamin starvation is regularly present, and in extreme cases, when marked vitamin B deficiency exists, polyneuritis occasionally develops and disturbances of the peripheral nerves result.

The severe type of vomiting may occur in either acute or chronic form. With prompt, persistent and intelligent therapy, the prognosis of hyperemesis is excellent.

Management and Nursing Care

The principles underlying the treatment of hyperemesis gravidarum are as follows: 1) rule out other underlying causes of nausea and vomiting, principally hepatitis, by appropriate diagnostic measures; 2) combat the dehydration by liberal administration of parenteral fluids; 3) combat the starvation by administration of glucose intravenously and thiamine chloride subcutaneously and, if necessary, by feeding a high-caloric, high-vitamin fluid diet through a nasal tube; 4) combat the emotional component with sedatives, supportive measures and an understanding attitude.

Although it may be necessary on occasion to treat cases of hyperemesis in the home, hospitalization is urgently desirable, because isolation from relatives, change of atmosphere and better facilities for intravenous medication confer unusual benefits in this condition. During the first 24 hours in the hospital it is customary to withhold all food and fluids by mouth in order to give the gastrointestinal tract complete rest. Glucose solution, usually in 10 percent concentration, is administered intravenously and, in addition, normal saline solution intravenously. The total fluid intake should approximate or exceed 3,000 ml. in the 24 hours. The nurse must keep a careful record of the exact quantity of fluids given, the amount of urine excreted and the quantity of the vomitus. Sedation is accomplished either by hypodermically administered barbiturates or by the rectal instillation of some barbiturate drug such as sodium amobarbital, 3 grains (0.2 gm.) every 6 hours. Thiamine hydrochloride, 50 mg. daily hypodermically, supplies the most urgent vitamin needs during the first 24 hours.

After such a regimen for 24 hours, dry toast, crackers or cereal is given by mouth in small quantities every two or three hours. Fluids are given on alternate hours in small amounts (not over 100 ml. at a time); hot tea and ginger ale usually are tolerated better than plain water. If no vomiting occurs, the amounts and the variety of the food are increased gradually until the patient is on a regular soft, high-vitamin diet. The intravenous administration of fluids may have to be continued for several days, depending on the oral intake.

The success of the treatment will depend in large measure on the tact, the understanding and the attitude of the nurse. Although optimism must be the keynote of the nurse's approach to the patient, this must be coupled with a plainly avowed determination to conquer the complication. Not a few of these patients are in psychologic conflict because of family, financial or social difficulties, and many are averse to the whole idea of pregnancy. If one can only get to the root of these difficulties in a tactful, empathic way, and help the patient to become reconciled to becoming a mother, a great deal will have been accomplished.

The nurse must exercise great care in preparing and serving trays for patients suffering from hyperemesis. The portions should be extremely small and attractively arranged. Cold liquids such as ginger ale or lemonade must be ice-cold; and hot foods, such as soups, cocoa and tea, must be steaming hot, since lukewarm liquids may be nauseating. It is best not to discuss food with the patient, even when serving the tray, but simply to assume that she will enjoy it and talk about other matters. At all times keep the emesis basin out of view, since the sight of it may start vomiting. Likewise, the smell of food may be nauseating; accordingly, the patient's room should be kept well aired and should be as far from the food preparation area as possible.

If vomiting continues despite these measures, as it rarely does, the physician may institute nasal feeding. A small rubber tube (Levin tube) is inserted through a nostril and on down into the stomach. The tube is strapped to the patient's cheek, connected with an overhanging bottle and left in place. By this means, large amounts of vitamin-rich liquid foods may be administered. The secret of success with nasal feeding lies in very slow but constant introduction of food into the stomach. The apparatus should be so arranged that the number of drops per minute passing through the tube can be counted. This should not exceed 50 per minute. Even this slow rate, it may be noted, yields about 200 ml. per hour.

Even the most severe cases of hyperemesis will usually respond favorably to the treatment described if patience and persistence are exercised; but, in extremely rare instances, the patient may continue to vomit despite all efforts, and such grave signs may develop that the physician is forced to the conclusion that continuation of pregnancy will be at the cost of the woman's life.

HEMORRHAGIC COMPLICATIONS OF LATE PREGNANCY

Placenta Previa

Although abortion is the most frequent cause of bleeding early in pregnancy, the most common cause during the later months is placenta previa. In this condition the placenta is attached to the lower uterine segment (instead of high up in the uterus as usual) and either wholly or in part covers the region of the cervix. There are three types, differentiated according to the degree to which the condition is present (Figs. 31-5 and 31-6):

1. *Total placenta previa,* in which the placenta completely covers the internal os;
2. *Partial placenta previa,* in which the placenta partially covers the internal os;
3. *Low implantation of placenta,* in which the placenta encroaches on the region of internal os, so that it can be palpated by the physician on

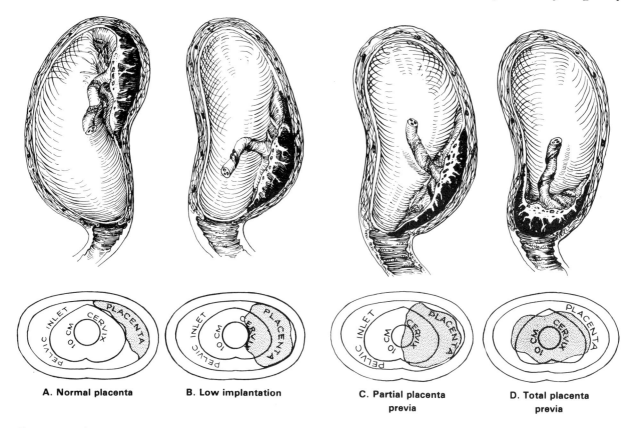

A. Normal placenta   **B. Low implantation**   **C. Partial placenta previa**   **D. Total placenta previa**

Figure 31-5. Placenta previa. (Reproduced with permission, from Benson, R. C.: Handbook of Obstetrics and Gynecology, 6th ed. Copyright 1977 by Lange Medical Publications, Los Altos, California.)

digital exploration about the cervix, but does not extend beyond the margin of the internal os.

Painless vaginal bleeding during the second half of pregnancy is the main symptom of placenta previa. Indeed, a diagnosis of placenta previa should be seriously considered and ruled out whenever there is painless bleeding in the last trimester.

The bleeding usually occurs after the seventh month. It may begin as mere "spotting," or it may start with profuse hemorrhage. The patient may awaken in the middle of the night to find herself in a pool of blood. The bleeding is caused by separation of the placenta as the result of changes which take place in the lower uterine segment during the later months. This separation opens up the underlying blood sinuses of the uterus from which the bleeding occurs.

Fortunately, placenta previa is not a very common condition, occuring about once in every 200 deliveries. It occurs much more frequently in multiparae than in primigravidae. Placenta previa always must be regarded as a grave complication of pregnancy. Until recent years it was associated with a maternal mortality of approximately 10 percent. Modern methods of management, plus the more liberal use of blood transfusion, have reduced this figure considerably. The outlook for the baby is always dubious, not only because the placental separation interferes with the infant's oxygen supply, but also because many of the babies are very premature when delivery must necessarily take place.

Diagnosis and Management

The presence of a placenta previa causes two main problems for the mother: bleeding and obstruction of the birth canal. For the baby, the most significant concern is prematurity. These problems provide the guides to treatment.

Conservative Management. Conservative management is in order when the fetus is premature (by weight or dates) and the bleeding is not excessive.

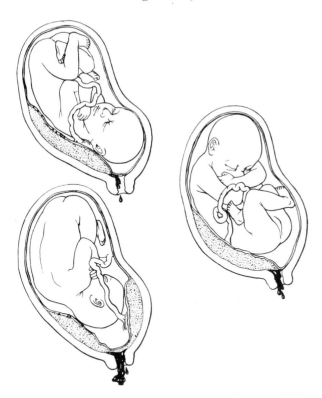

Figure 31-6. Placenta previa. *(Top)* Low implantation. *(Middle)* Partial placenta previa. *(Bottom)* Central (complete) placenta previa.

The natural history of placenta previa is such that uncontrolled bleeding is not likely to occur with the first episode. There may be, in fact, several episodes of bleeding, starting early in the third trimester, before there is sufficient bleeding to force the obstetrician to intervene and terminate the pregnancy. Thus, under such circumstances, bedrest and observation will often result in cessation of the bleeding and provide valuable days for the maturation of the fetus.

It is important that the obstetrician rule out other causes of bleeding under these circumstances. A speculum examination of the vagina is generally done to rule out other sources of bleeding such as cervicitis and cervical polyps. The examiner will *not,* however, insert a finger through the cervix under these circumstances, since such a maneuver might well precipitate bleeding and therefore the delivery of a premature infant.

Cervical manipulation must be postponed, if a course of expectancy appears reasonable, to allow additional time for fetal maturation. In any case, a more complete examination should never be carried out unless all preparations have been made for immediate cesarean section. Other techniques of placental localization are useful to confirm the diagnosis. Such measures as isotope scans, amniography and soft tissue abdominal x-rays have been utilized with varying degrees of success. These have been largely supplanted by sonography (Fig. 31-7). Placental localization by ultrasound "B" scanning offers 95 percent accuracy and should be used when available. When the placenta is found to be normally located and thus a diagnosis of placenta previa is not substantiated, the physician may elect, in the absence of bleeding, to discharge the mother from the hospital with the admonition that she is to report promptly at the first sign of recurrence of bleeding.

When the diagnosis is confirmed, in general, the patient should remain hospitalized at bedrest. Further bleeding must be carefully observed and recorded, and all perineal pads saved to allow a reasonable assessment of the amount of additional blood loss. The fetal heart tones should be monitored at frequent intervals until the bleeding has subsided completely, and the uterus should be palpated periodically to detect contractions suggesting onset of labor. Any increase in uterine activity or bleeding should be reported promptly.

Active Management. An active approach is indicated if the fetus is at term by size and dates, if labor has begun, or if bleeding is sufficient to threaten the mother. Then, the patient is taken to the operating room where a "double setup" examination is usually performed. This means that everything is prepared for an immediate cesarean section, should the examination confirm the diagnosis. This precaution is necessary, since digital examination of the cervix might precipitate increased bleeding.

In all instances of total and partial placenta previa, and in most instances of low implantation of the placenta, cesarean section is the approach of choice for delivery. In an occasional case of low implantation, especially if the baby is small and the cervix is already partially dilated, the obstetrician may elect to rupture the membranes in the hope that the presenting part may enter the pelvis and control the bleeding by compressing the area of placenta which has separated. If this does occur, vaginal delivery may sometimes be accomplished. By and large cesarean section is the procedure of choice as it is generally associated with a better fetal survival.

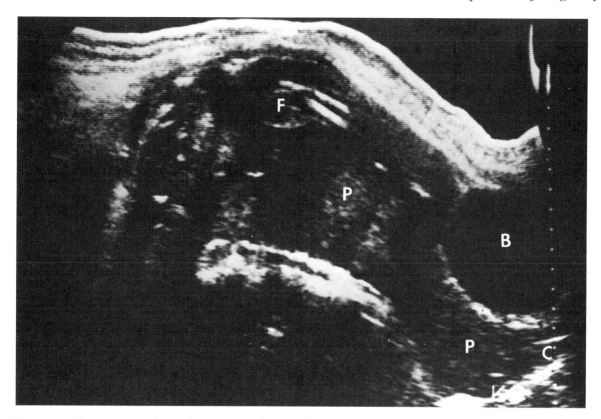

Figure 31-7. Ultrasonogram of 25 weeks' gestation, showing placenta previa. Placenta (P) lying posteriorly and completely covering cervix (C) with bladder (B) anterior. Fetal echoes (F) are seen in the upper part of the uterus.

NURSING INTERVENTION. Bleeding, shock and infection are the main dangers. Before the arrival of the physician, the nurse should keep a solicitous eye on the amount of bleeding and the pulse rate and watch for signs of oncoming shock (pallor, increased pulse rate, cold extremities, and so on). Should the bleeding be profuse, elevation of the foot of the bed and application of external heat may forestall shock. In determining the amount of bleeding, the patient should be instructed to report if she feels any fluid escaping from the vulva. The nurse, in turn, should inspect the pad or bed frequently for hemorrhage.

Abruptio Placentae

Abruptio placentae (meaning that the placenta is torn from its bed) is a complication of the last half of pregnancy, in which a normally located placenta undergoes separation from its uterine attachment. The condition is frequently called "premature separation of the normally implanted placenta"; other synonymous terms such as *accidental hemorrhage*

(meaning that it takes place unexpectedly) and *ablatio placentae* (ablatio means a carrying away) are sometimes used. Bleeding may be apparent, in which case it is called *external hemorrhage,* or concealed, in which case it is called *concealed hemorrhage.* If a separation occurs at the margin, the blood is apt to lift the membranes and trickle down to the cervical os and thus escape externally. If the placenta begins to separate centrally, a huge amount of blood may be stored behind the placenta before any of it becomes evident (Fig. 31-8). Although the precise cause of the condition is not known, it is frequently encountered in association with cases of hypertensive disorder of pregnancy (toxemia).

Premature separation of the normally implanted placenta is characterized not only by bleeding beneath the placenta but also by pain. The pain is produced by the accumulation of blood behind the placenta, with subsequent distention of the uterus. The uterus also enlarges in size as the result of the accumulated blood and becomes distinctly tender and exceedingly firm. Because of the almost woody hardness of the uterine wall, fetal parts may be

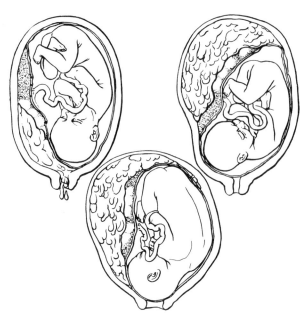

Figure 31-8. Abruptio placentae at various separation sites.

difficult to palpate. Shock is often out of proportion to blood loss, as manifested by a rapid pulse, dyspnea, yawning, restlessness, pallor, syncope, and cold, clammy perspiration.

Management

Treatment is dependent upon the condition of the fetus and the mother at the time the diagnosis is made. If the fetus is alive, prompt delivery is in order and should be by cesarean section, unless vaginal delivery can be accomplished promptly. If the fetus has already succumbed, this is usually an indication of an extensive placental separation. The complications of abruptio placentae to be described subsequently are all time-related and occur with greater frequency with more extensive separation. Therefore, although a vaginal delivery is desirable with a dead baby, one should not persist for too long.

Further Complications. Hemorrhagic shock is a common complication and demands vigorous treatment with blood replacement and control of the bleeding by emptying the uterus in the most expeditious manner. Occasionally, with a severe abruption, a coagulation defect, *hypofibrinogenemia,* develops. This complication is also seen with other entities such as amniotic fluid embolus, prolonged retention of a dead fetus, and septic abortion. It is

brought about by the entry into the circulation of thromboplastin from the uterus and placenta, which causes small fibrin clots in the capillaries and consumes fibrinogen, leaving the patient with non-clotting blood. Treatment involves the use of blood and fibrinogen replacement and termination of the pregnancy. Also, in severe abruptions, when coagulation is impaired, there is extensive bleeding into the uterine muscle, producing the so-called Couvelaire uterus. Such a uterus occasionally does not contract well after delivery, causing further bleeding and even necessitating hysterectomy. Finally, *renal failure* may result, either on the basis of acute tubular necrosis or bilateral cortical necrosis. In the latter case, the outlook is grave.

Mistaken Diagnosis of Hemorrhage

A false alarm concerning hemorrhage is sometimes due to a normal "show" at the beginning of labor. It simply means that dilatation of the cervix has begun, causing slight bleeding. No treatment is required. However, the nurse should reassure the patient and watch to determine whether or not the bleeding which is present is more than the normal show.

THE HYPERTENSIVE DISORDERS OF PREGNANCY

A condition that is characterized by hypertension and is peculiar to pregnancy is sometimes encountered during gestation or early in the puerperium. Until recently, *toxemia* was the term used to describe this syndrome, which is characterized by one or more of the following signs: hypertension, edema, proteinuria, and in severe cases, convulsions and coma. The term "toxemia of pregnancy" was coined when it was believed that the condition was caused by toxins derived from the products of conception circulating in the blood. Because this theory is no longer tenable, the term toxemia has fallen into disfavor, although it is still used in common parlance. The terms *preeclampsia* and *eclampsia* are used to describe pregnancy-induced or aggravated hypertension, usually associated with edema and/or proteinuria. Preeclampsia and eclampsia represent one and the same process, but the term *eclampsia* is used when the patient's clinical course has advanced to generalized convulsions and/or coma. The hypertensive disorders of pregnancy include other conditions associated with hypertension, which present concomitantly with pregnancy but have not arisen de novo as a result of pregnancy. They are included because their clinical course may be aggravated by the pregnancy and the patient may develop a superimposed preeclampsia or eclampsia.

Hypertensive disorders of pregnancy are a very common complication, being seen in 6 or 7 percent of all gravidae. They rank among the three major complications (hemorrhage and puerperal infection being the other two) responsible for the vast majority of maternal deaths and account for some 250 maternal deaths in the United States each year. As a cause of fetal death they are even more important. It can be estimated conservatively that at least 25,000 stillbirths and neonatal deaths occur each year in the United States from hypertensive diseases of pregnancy, and those newborns who survive may suffer impairments which affect the quality of their lives. The great majority of perinatal deaths are related to prematurity.

The huge toll of maternal and infant lives taken by hypertensive disorders of pregnancy is in large measure preventable. Proper antepartal supervision, particularly the early detection of signs and symptoms of incipient preeclampsia, and appropriate treatment will arrest many cases and so ameliorate others that the outcome for baby and mother is usually satisfactory. The nurse is often the first to encounter the early signs and symptoms, not only in the hospital's outpatient department, but also on home visits, and their detection is of utmost importance so that treatment may be instituted at the earliest possible moment.

Classification

A number of classifications have been proposed to categorize the various forms of hypertensive disorders of pregnancy. Because of changing concepts and the complexity of these conditions, a standard and uniformly acceptable classification has not yet been devised. That which has recently been proposed by Welt and Crenshaw (see Suggested Reading) is reproduced here in modified form for purposes of discussion and clarification.

I. *Pregnancy-associated hypertensive diseases*
   A. Preeclampsia and eclampsia
   B. Gestational hypertension
   C. Superimposed preeclampsia and eclampsia
II. *Concurrent hypertension and pregnancy*
III. *Hypertensive diathesis*

The term *pregnancy-associated hypertensive diseases* covers those specific conditions that develop as a direct result of pregnancy. *Preeclampsia* is characterized by hypertension with edema or proteinuria or both. When the preeclampsic patient develops convulsions or coma, unrelated to other cerebral conditions, the term *eclampsia* is used. If hypertension develops without edema or proteinuria during pregnancy, or in the first ten postpartum days, it is described as *gestational hypertension*. The term *superimposed preeclampsia and eclampsia* is used when the patient who already has underlying hypertensive vascular or renal disease develops preeclampsia and eclampsia, heralded by a significant rise in blood pressure with edema and/or proteinuria.

The term *concurrent hypertension and pregnancy* is used when the two separate conditions, pregnancy and hypertensive disease, are present in the same patient at the same time, but a causal relationship is not evident. *Hypertensive diathesis* refers to a predisposition to hypertension as a result of physiologic stress. The hypertension may be manifest in pregnancy for the first time as preeclampsia, eclampsia or gestational hypertension.

This classification is designed to cover all of the contingencies associated with hypertensive disorders in pregnancy. No doubt, as these various conditions are better understood, new classifications will be proposed. For purposes of discussion, it is useful to consider hypertensive disorders in pregnancy in two broad categories: 1) those disorders that occur only in pregnancy, namely preeclampsia and eclampsia, and 2) hypertensive disorders not confined to pregnancy but which may exist during pregnancy and may be complicated by superimposed preeclampsia or eclampsia. The latter include essential hypertension and various forms of renal disease.

Preeclampsia

Preeclampsia is characterized by elevation in blood pressure, proteinuria and/or edema in a gravida after the twentieth week of pregnancy who previously has been normal in these respects. It is a forerunner or prodromal stage of eclampsia; in other words, unless the preeclamptic process is checked by treatment or by delivery it is likely that eclampsia (convulsions and/or coma) will ensue. The rise in blood pressure may occur suddenly, or it may be gradual and insidious.

The criteria for hypertension which are applied include:

1. a systolic blood pressure of 140 mm Hg or more, or an elevation of 30 mm Hg or more above the previously observed levels;
2. a diastolic pressure of 90 mm Hg or more or an elevation of 15 mm Hg or more above that previously observed;
3. observation of the abnormal blood pressure on two occasions or more at least six hours apart, as a single reading may be misleading.

The earliest warning signal of preeclampsia is *sudden development of hypertension.* Accordingly, the importance of frequent and regular blood pressure readings during pregnancy cannot be emphasized too strongly. The absolute blood pressure level is probably of less significance than the relationship it bears to previous determinations and the time in gestation when these determinations were recorded. The normal patient often exhibits a lower than normal blood pressue in the mid-trimester of pregnancy, and hence a baseline reading in mid-pregnancy may be misleading. For example, a pressure of 120/80 may actually indicate hypertension in a patient whose mid-pregnancy pressure has been running in the 100/70 range.

The next most constant sign of preeclampsia is *sudden excessive weight gain.* If cases of preeclampsia are studied from the viewpoint of fluid intake and output, it is at once apparent that these sudden gains in weight are due entirely to an accumulation of water in the tissues. Such weight gains represent occult edema and almost always precede the visible face and finger edema which is so characteristic of the advanced stages of the disease. From what has been said, it is apparent that scales are essential equipment for good antepartal care. Weight gain of 1 pound a week or so may be regarded as normal. Sudden gains of more than 2 pounds a week should be viewed with suspicion; gains of more than 3 pounds, with alarm. Weight increases of the latter magnitude call for more frequent blood pressure determinations, and if these latter are also abnormal, hospitalization with intensive treatment is indicated. In investigating suspected edema, it is well to ask the patient if her wedding ring is becoming tight, since finger and facial edema is a more valuable sign of preeclampsia than is swelling of the ankles. In the facies of a patient with outspoken preeclampsia, the eyelids are swollen, and, associated with the edema, marked coarseness of the features develops (Fig. 31-9).

The sudden appearance of *protein in the urine,* with or without other findings, always should be regarded as a sign of preeclampsia. A complete urinalysis, including a microscopic examination, will help to exclude infection as a cause of proteinuria. Usually it develops later than the hypertension and the gain in weight and for this very reason must be regarded as a serious omen when superimposed on these other two findings.

But the very essence of preeclampsia is the lightninglike fulminance with which it strikes. Although the above physical signs of preeclampsia usually give the physician ample time to institute preventive treatment, it sometimes happens that these derangements develop between visits to the office or the clinic, even if they are only a week apart. For this reason it is imperative that all expectant mothers be informed, both orally and by some form of printed slip or booklet, about certain danger signals which they themselves may recognize.

The following symptoms demand immediate report to the physician:

1. severe, continuous headache
2. swelling of the face or the fingers
3. dimness or blurring of vision
4. persistent vomiting.
5. decrease in the amount of urine excreted
6. epigastric pain (a late symptom)

It should be emphasized that the three early and important signs of preeclampsia, namely, hypertension, weight gain and proteinuria, are changes of which the patient is usually unaware. All three may be present in substantial degree, and yet she may feel quite well. Only by regular and careful antepartal examination can these warning signs be detected. By the time the preeclamptic patient has developed symptoms and signs which she herself can detect (such as headache, blurred vision, puffiness of the eyelids and the fingers), she is usually in an advanced stage of the disease, and much valuable time has been lost.

Headache is rarely observed in the milder cases but is encountered with increasing frequency in the most severe grades. In general, patients who actually develop eclampsia often have a severe headache as a forerunner of the first convulsion. The visual disturbances range from a slight blurring of vision to various degrees of temporary blindness. Although convulsions are less likely to occur in cases of mild preeclampsia, the possibility cannot be entirely eliminated. Patients with severe preeclampsia should always be considered as being on the verge of having a convulsion.

The Roll Over Test. Recently a simple office procedure, the *roll over test,* has been proposed to identify patients who are at risk of developing preeclampsia. This can be carried out as an office procedure and is utilized for screening of patients between the twenty-eighth to thirty-second week of pregnancy.

The patient is placed in a lateral recumbent position and diastolic blood pressures are recorded for a minimum of 15 minutes, or until the blood pressure has become stable. The patient is then rolled over onto her back and blood pressure recordings are repeated at one and five minutes.

The roll over test is positive when an increase in diastolic blood pressure of 20 mm Hg or more is observed. Dr. Normal Gant, who devised this imaginative approach, has reported that patients who demonstrate a positive roll over test develop pregnancy-induced hypertension in greater than 90 percent of cases. Conversely, the patient with a negative roll over test has a greater than 90 percent chance of remaining normotensive throughout the remainder of the pregnancy.

The test offers promise of identifying patients at risk up to three months prior to the development of pregnancy-induced hypertension, and a positive test alerts the health care provider so that steps may be taken to delay the onset of the disease and modify its severity.

Management

Prophylaxis is most important in the prevention and control of preeclampsia. Since in its early stages preeclampsia rarely gives rise to signs or symptoms which the patient herself will notice, the early detection of this disease demands meticulous antepartal supervision. Rapid weight gain or an upward trend in blood pressure, although still in the "normal" range, are danger signals. Every pregnant woman should be examined every week during the

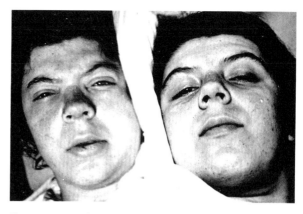

Figure 31-9. (*Left*) Facies in preeclampsia. Note edema of eyelids and facial skin and general coarsening of features. (*Right*) Same patient ten days after delivery.

last month of pregnancy and every two weeks during the two previous months. Prophylaxis of the disease lies in reduction of sodium intake and good dietary management. Finger edema is a frequent forerunner of preeclampsia, which may precede the hypertension by several weeks and is a valuable warning sign.

Ambulatory Patient. When the patient's symptoms are mild (i.e., there is minor elevation of blood pressure with minimal or no signs of edema and proteinuria), treatment may be instituted at home in the hope that symptoms will abate. During this period the patient should be examined at least twice a week, and she should be given a strict regimen to follow, as well as careful instructions about symptoms to report promptly.

1. The patient's activities should be restricted, and she should understand that bedrest during the greater part of the day is most desirable.
2. Sedative drugs, such as phenobarbital, may be prescribed to encourage rest and relaxation.
3. Of major importance is a low-salt diet. Therefore, the patient should be instructed so that she understands which foods have appreciable sodium content and therefore must be excluded from her diet, in addition to the fact that no salt may be added to her food in the kitchen or at the table.
4. The diet should be well balanced. It should contain ample protein, particularly lean meat, fish and eggs.
5. Carbonated beverages should be avoided because of their sodium content.

The restriction of sodium in the diet of the preeclamptic patient is directed at reducing the edema. Even in normal nonpregnant persons an increased intake of sodium chloride causes water retention. Pregnant women, particularly gravidae suffering from preeclampsia, show a marked tendency to retain sodium, and there is reason to believe that this tendency of the tissues to retain sodium is closely correlated with their tendency to hold water. To superimpose still more sodium in the diet on this already existing sodium and water retention is obviously unwise.

Although in the past some have suggested that routine therapy with thiazide diuretics would prevent preeclampsia, in a group of high-risk patients it has now been clearly established that this is not true. The value of diuretic therapy has been questioned because it has been shown to decrease both placental and renal clearance.

Hospital Patient. In the event that the patient's condition does not respond promptly to restricted activity at home, she should be hospitalized without delay. Hospitalization becomes mandatory if proteinuria appears. A systematic method of study should be instituted upon admission to the hospital.

1. A general physical examination and history should be obtained promptly, followed by constant vigilance for the development of such symptoms as headache, visual disturbances and edema of the fingers and the eyelids.
2. Body weight should be obtained on admission and daily thereafter.
3. Blood pressure readings should be taken every four hours except between midnight and morning, unless the midnight blood pressure has risen.
4. Daily fluid intake and output records should be kept, and urine specimens sent to the laboratory daily for analysis for protein and casts.
5. Retinal examination is always included as part of the admission physical examination and is done every two to three days thereafter, depending on the findings.
6. Once the patient is admitted to the hospital, complete bedrest is essential.

MAGNESIUM SULFATE. When severe preeclampsia develops, immediate and intensive therapy is imperative. Sedation is of major importance to forestall convulsions. The dosage of drugs employed should be regulated so that they produce drowsiness and sleep, from which the patient can be easily awakened, and also suppress the hyperactive reflexes of the patient. The drug most often used as a sedative and an anticonvulsant under these circumstances is magnesium sulfate. In addition to being an excellent anticonvulsant, magnesium causes vasodilatation and, therefore, is also effective in lowering blood pressure.

For rapid action, an IV dose of 20 to 30 ml. of a 10 percent solution (2 to 3 gm.) is used. Very often the drug is given intramuscularly in doses of 10 to 20 ml. of a 50 percent solution (5 to 10 gm.). The dose is divided, half given into each buttock, and often 1 to 2 ml. of 1 percent procaine is added to the injection to minimize discomfort.

A repeat dose of magnesium sulfate should not be given unless the reflexes and respiratory rate have been checked, since it depresses both. The antidote is calcium, and an ampul of calcium gluconate should always be readily available when magnesium is being administered.

For nursing protocol for the administration of magnesium sulfate see the chart on page 522.

OTHER SEDATIVES. Barbiturates can also be used, the dose being larger (60 to 120 mg. every four to six hours) than for mild cases and the route of administration parenteral. If the patient is in labor, it is well to avoid barbiturates because of their depressant effect on the fetus. Although many use morphine in the management of severe preeclampsia, it would seem best reserved for the patient who has the added stimulus of pain (i.e., labor). Minimizing this stimulus will certainly reduce the likelihood of a seizure.

Another drug which is an effective anticonvulsant is diazepam (Valium) in 5- to 10-mg. doses intramuscularly or, if the situation warrants, intravenously.

Diazepam is usually reserved for severe cases and is discussed further in the management of eclampsia.

ANTIHYPERTENSIVE DRUGS. Agents which reduce peripheral blood pressure find occasional use in the treatment of the patient with extreme degrees of hypertension. Opinions differ as to their general effectiveness, largely because they are known to decrease placental perfusion and hence may have an untoward effect on the fetus. Nevertheless they are sometimes prescribed in cases of severe preeclampsia and eclampsia when the diastolic blood pressure exceeds 100 mm Hg. They are used as a temporary measure to reduce blood pressure and thus decrease the possibility of a cerebrovascular accident. They have also been found to improve kidney function and are associated with some improvement in cardiac output. The most widely used antihypertensive agent at present is hydralazine (Apresoline). This is given intravenously in a dose of 60 to 100 mg. in a slow drip. The use of these agents has not been shown in careful studies to improve either fetal or maternal survival, and their long-term use in preeclampsia is generally not recommended.

DELIVERY. The treatments which have been discussed are useful only as temporary measures. The only definitive cure for preeclampsia is delivery. Careful medical judgment must be exercised in deciding how long a pregnancy should be continued when preeclampsia has supervened. This is a particularly difficult decision when the preeclampsia has developed early in the last trimester, as a premature infant may not survive extrauterine life. Monitoring fetal well-being with serial serum or urinary estriol levels may be of considerable value. If the estriol levels remain stable, continued expectancy with concomitant treatment is appropriate to allow further in utero maturation. In some circumstances evaluation of placental function with a weekly oxytocin challenge test (OCT) is recommended (see Chapter 37). If the OCT is positive, the pregnancy should not be allowed to continue.

Despite all efforts, the condition may persist to a marked degree, and in that event induction of labor may become necessary for the welfare of mother and infant. In some instances, especially when preeclampsia is severe and fulminating and conditions for induction of labor are not favorable, cesarean section may be the procedure of choice.

Postpartum. The signs and symptoms of preeclampsia usually abate rapidly after delivery, but the danger of convulsions does not pass until 48 hours have elapsed postpartum. Therefore, continuation of sedation throughout this interval is indicated. In the majority of cases the elevated blood pressure as well as the other derangements have returned to normal within ten days or two weeks. In about 30 percent of cases, however, the hypertension shows a tendency either to persist indefinitely or to recur

in subsequent pregnancies. For this reason prolonged follow-up of these patients is highly important.

Nursing Management

The nurse's responsibility in the detection and care of cases of preeclampsia is manifold. Since this complication of pregnancy is common and may occur antepartally, intrapartally or postpartally, it is important for the nurse to observe all maternity patients closely for the first indication of early symptoms, and report any evidence pointing to an aggravation of the process. The early symptoms and the manifestations related to more severe preeclampsia, such as persistent headache, blurred vision, spots or flashes of light before the eyes, epigastric pain, vomiting, torpor or muscular twitchings, are all vastly important. Data collected in relation to these symptoms in addition to an accurate record of weight gain, fluid intake and elimination, diet and attitudes and behavior, when it is accurately recorded, can assist the physician in evaluating the symptoms and planning the course of therapy.

In setting the therapeutic atmosphere, the nurse should see that the environment is as comfortable and pleasant as possible. The patient should be in a single room, free from the stimuli of noise, strong lights and the presence of unnecessary equipment which might frighten her. The nurse must protect the patient from needless traffic into the room; otherwise, the coming and going of personnel to the bedside may be so constant that it could interfere with the efficacy of the treatment being carried out. Every effort should be exerted to relieve the patient's anxiety, which sometimes is brought about by apprehension regarding her illness or may be due to concern for the welfare of her family at home.

Regardless of the severity of the preeclampsia, certain responsibilities are carried out by the nurse. Medications ordered must be administered promptly, the prescribed diet should be supervised, a careful record of intake and elimination kept, blood pressure readings and basal weights taken, specimens collected and labeled accurately, and observations of slight symptoms or change in condition should be reported immediately, both orally and on the patient's record.

Since rest is a major consideration in the care of this patient, the nurse should plan a schedule of

(*Text cont. on page 524.*)

NURSING PROTOCOL FOR ADMINISTRATION OF MAGNESIUM SULFATE★

Preparation of the Mg SO$_4$ as ordered:

Loading Dose

Mg SO$_4$ 2–4 gms. (10% solution) IV stat (by soluset)
a. 2–4 gms. of Mg SO$_4$ in 20–40 ml. of a 10% solution.
b. Add ordered gms. of Mg SO$_4$ to soluset fill to 100 ml. with IV fluid
c. Infuse Mg SO$_4$ over a 30 minute period by soluset.

Maintenance Dose

Mg So$_4$ 5 gms. (50% solution) IM immediately following loading dose and then every 4 hours
a. 5 gms. of Mg SO$_4$ in 10 ml. of a 50% solution
b. Divide 5 gms. (10 ml.) into 2 syringes of 5 ml. each
c. Add .25 ml. of Procaine 1% to each 5 ml. of Mg SO$_4$ in the syringe

OR

Mg SO$_4$ 1 gm. (10% solution) IV by IMED

a. 1 gm. of Mg SO$_4$ in 10 ml. of a 10% solution
b. Add 5 gms. of Mg SO$_4$ in 50 ml. to 250 ml. of D$_5$PSS
c. Infuse Mg So$_4$ at 50 ml. per hour by IMED to give Mg SO$_4$ 1 gm. per hour.

Nursing Assessment of patient receiving magnesium sulfate

1. Detection of the signs of magnesium intoxication
   a. Early signs mother may experience and *you* recognize are:
      1. hot all over   3. thirsty   5. depression of reflexes   7. flaccidity
      2. flushing   4. sweating   6. hypotension
   b. Later signs of hypermagnesemia:
      1. CNS depression   3. Circulatory collapse
      2. Respiratory paralysis

2. Deep tendon reflexes should be checked hourly if the patient is receiving continuous IV infusion or before each dose of intermittent therapy is administered. Disappearance of the patellar reflex is one of the most important clinical signs to detect increasing hypermagnesemia. However, if the patient has received regional anesthesia (epidural) you will have to test the biceps or radial reflex.

3. CNS depression is at first characterized by anxiety. This changes to drowsiness, lethargy, slight slurring of speech, ataxic gait and a tendency to fall sideward while standing erect. Constantly evaluate patient's orientation to person, place and time.

4. Intake and output of the patient are monitored carefully. Specific gravity should be obtained. Urine should be observed for color and volume. The volume should be 30 ml. or more/hour; if not, the next dose of Mg SO$_4$ should be held.

5. If the patient is receiving an IV infusion, BP and TPR should be evaluated at least every 15 to 30 minutes. For patient on intermittent therapy of Mg SO$_4$, a BP and TPR should be taken before and after each administration.

6. Do not administer Mg SO$_4$ if the patient respirations are less than 12 to 14 per minute or there is a drop in pulse rate, blood pressure or FHR or any other sign of fetal distress.

7. a. Complaints the patient may have are: headache, malaise, nausea and vomiting. The nurse must assess whether these signs are due to progression of toxemia or drug therapy.
   b. Another complaint that the mother may have if she is receiving Mg SO$_4$ intramuscularly is pain at the site of the injection.

8. Calcium gluconate (10% solution) is kept at the patient's bedside:
   a. This is the antidote for magnesium intoxication (usually reverses respiratory depression and heart block). The dosage should be 5 to 10 m. Eq. (10 to 20 ml.) given intravenously over a three-minute period.

Testing Deep Tendon Reflexes

1. As outlined above, deep tendon reflexes should be tested hourly.
   a. Absence of or decrease in the patellar reflex indicates that a toxic blood level (7 to 10 mg/liter of Mg) has been reached.
   b. The reflexes that are tested besides the patellar reflex (knee jerk) are the biceps and radial reflexes. These reflexes are tested by striking the tendon and watching for contraction of the appropriate muscle. The muscle need not contract forcefully enough to move the limb but must simply contract.
   c. These reflexes are difficult to elicit when the patient is tense, so relaxation is important for proper testing.
   d. Reflexes are compared from one side of the corresponding side and expressed with an arbitrary scale.

   > 0 = Reflex absent
   > +1 = Reflex hypoactive
   > +2 = Normal reflex
   > +3 = Reflex hyperactive
   > +4 = Clonus

2. In testing a muscle reflex, it is actually the tendon that is stimulated; the reflex is involuntary. A sensory impulse is initiated when a stimulus is applied to the tendon and in return a motor response is elicited.
   a. When testing reflexes on a patient who has recently received an epidural or spinal anesthesia, motor responses will be diminished. An accurate response will not be elicited if the knee jerk is used. The biceps or radial reflex will have to be used.

3. *Knee jerk reflex or patellar tendon reflex:*
   a. The knee should be positioned halfway between the longest and shortest positions.
   b. Support is given under the knee with the foot off the bed (45° angle).
   c. Patellar tendon is struck (tapped) just below the patella and the quadriceps muscle group should be observed for contraction (slight movement). The lower leg should extend in response.

4. *Biceps reflex:*
   a. The forearm should be resting on the patient's trunk.
   b. Place your thumb firmly on the patient's biceps tendon (antecubital space) and strike the thumbnail briskly with reflex hammer.
   c. The biceps muscle will respond by slight movement. The lower arm should flex in response.

5. *Radial reflex:*
   a. The patient's hand and forearm should be resting on the patient's trunk. Place a finger over the tendon and gently tap your finger with the reflex hammer.
   b. The brachioradial tendon is located on the lateral surface of the lower end of the radius. It is often difficult to feel this tendon. If the tendon cannot be felt, tap the lateral suface of the lower end of the radius. The brachioradial muscle will respond by a slight movement. The response consists of the hand jerking.

6. For relaxation:
   a. If the patient is having difficulty relaxing, two techniques can be tried:
      1) Testing the knee jerk—have patient lock her fingers together and pull in the opposite directions (monkey grip). This technique will help the patient relax her leg by having her concentrate on a physical activity.
      2) Testing the biceps or radial reflexes—have the patient bite down hard. This technique will help patient relax her arm by having her concentrate on doing something else.
   b. If it is necessary to try either of these techniques while testing the reflexes, it is likely that the reflexes are slightly depressed.
   c. *Clonus* is the sudden stretching of a hypertonic muscle, producing reflex contraction. If the stretch is maintained during subsequent relaxation, further reflex contraction occurs and this may continue almost indefinitely, unless the stretch stimulus is released. It is demonstrated by dorsiflexion of the foot or by sharply moving the patella downwards, but it may be present at any joint. Clonus represents an increase in reflex excitability and may be present in a very tense patient.

* *Used at the Hospital of the University of Pennsylvania.*

activities so that the patient is disturbed as little as possible. Medications, treatments and nursing procedures should be administered at the same time as far as the physician's orders will permit, but always with the thought in mind that only as much as will not overtire the patient should be planned for any one time. When any treatment is ordered, the procedure is best carried out after sedation has been administered. Before heavy sedation is initiated, any removable dentures or eyeglasses should be stored in a secure place. If the patient is not in labor, the nurse must be alert to watch for signs of labor, particularly after sedation has been given. Any time an intravenous fluid is administered, if the physician has not specified the rate at which the fluid is to flow, it should be given slowly.

The nurse should see that the equipment necessary for the safe and efficient care of the patient is immediately available and in good working order. A padded mouth gag should always be ready for use at the bedside to prevent the patient from biting her tongue if a convulsion develops. Trays for catheterization equipment and for the administration of special medications constitute part of the necessary equipment. Since water retention plays such a large role in the disease, and urinary output is likely to be diminished, an indwelling bladder catheter may be ordered to ensure accuracy in obtaining output from the kidneys. Since the urinary output must be watched carefully, it is imperative to see that the retention catheter is draining properly at all times. In severe cases suction apparatus should be readily available for aspirating mucus, as well as equipment for administering oxygen, should symptoms such as cyanosis or depressed respiration indicate the need.

Eclampsia

Clinical Picture

As indicated, the development of eclampsia is almost always preceded by the signs and symptoms of preeclampsia. A preeclamptic patient, who may have been conversing with you a moment before, is seen to roll her eyes to one side and stare fixedly into space. Immediately, twitching of the facial muscles ensues. This is the *stage of invasion* of the convulsion and lasts only a few seconds.

The whole body then becomes rigid in a generalized muscular contraction; the face is distorted,

the eyes protrude, the arms are flexed, the hands are clenched and the legs are inverted. Since all the muscles of the body are now in a state of tonic contraction, this phase may be regarded as the *stage of contraction;* it lasts 15 or 20 seconds.

Suddenly the jaws begin to open and close violently, and forthwith the eyelids also. The other facial muscles and then all the muscles of the body alternately contract and relax in rapid succession. So forceful are the muscular movements that the patient may throw herself out of bed, and almost invariably, unless protected, the tongue is bitten by the violent jaw action. Foam, often blood-tinged, exudes from the mouth; the face is congested and purple, and the eyes are bloodshot. Few pictures which the nurse is called upon to witness are so horrible. This phase in which the muscles alternately contract and relax is called the *stage of convulsion;* it may last a minute or so. Gradually the muscular movements become milder and farther apart, and finally the patient lies motionless.

Throughout the seizure the diaphragm has been fixed with respiration halted. Still no breathing occurs. For a few seconds the woman appears to be dying from respiratory arrest, but just when this outcome seems almost inevitable, she takes a long, deep, stertorous inhalation, and breathing is resumed. Then coma ensues. The patient will remember nothing whatsoever of the convulsion or, in all probability, events immediately before and afterward.

The coma may last from a few minutes to several hours, and the patient may then become conscious; or the coma may be succeeded by another convulsion. The convulsions may recur during coma, they may recur only after an interval of consciousness, or they may never recur at all. In the average case, from five to ten convulsions occur at longer or shorter intervals, but as many as 20 are not uncommon. Convulsions may start before the onset of labor (antepartum), during labor (intrapartum) or anytime within the first 48 hours after delivery (postpartum). About a fifth of the cases develop postpartally.

Upon physical examination, the findings of eclampsia are similar to those in preeclampsia, but exaggerated. Thus, the systolic blood pressure usually ranges around 180 mm. Hg and sometimes exceeds 200 mm. Hg. Proteinuria is frequently extreme, from 10 to 20 gm. per liter. Edema may be marked but sometimes is absent. Oliguria, or suppression of urinary excretion, is common and may amount to complete anuria. Fever is present in about half the cases.

In favorable cases the convulsions cease, the coma lessens, and urinary output increases. However, it sometimes requires one or two days for clear consciousness to be regained. During this period eclamptic patients are often in an obstreperous, resistant mood and may be exceedingly difficult to manage. A few develop actual psychoses. In unfavorable cases the coma deepens, urinary excretion diminishes, the pulse becomes more rapid, the temperature rises, and edema of the lungs develops. The last is a serious symptom and usually is interpreted as a sign of cardiovascular failure. Edema of the lungs is readily recognizable by the noisy, gurgling respiration and by the large quantity of frothy mucus which exudes from the mouth and the nose. Toward the end, convulsions cease altogether, and the final picture is one of vascular collapse, with falling blood pressure and overwhelming edema of the lungs.

Like preeclampsia, eclampsia is a disease of young primigravidae, the majority of cases occurring in first pregnancies. It is more likely to occur as full term approaches and is rarely seen prior to the last three months. Eclampsia is particularly likely to develop in twin gestations, the likelihood being about four times that in single pregnancies.

Prognosis

Eclampsia is one of the gravest complications of pregnancy; the maternal mortality in different localities and in different hospitals ranges from 5 to 15 percent. The outlook for the baby is particularly grave, the fetal mortality being about 20 percent. Although it is difficult in a given case to forecast the outcome, the following are unfavorable signs: oliguria; prolonged coma; a sustained pulse rate over 120; temperature over 39.5 C. (103° F.); more than ten convulsions; 10 or more gm. of protein per liter in the urine; systolic blood pressure of more than 200; edema of lungs. If none of these signs is present, the outlook for recovery is good; if two or more are present, the prognosis is definitely serious.

Even though the patient survives, she may not escape unscathed from the attack but sometimes continues to have high blood pressure indefinitely. This applies to both preeclampsia and eclampsia.

Indeed, about 10 percent of all preeclamptic and 5 percent of all eclamptic patients are left with chronic, permanent hypertension. It is even more important to note that a still larger percentage of these women (about 50 percent of preeclamptics and 30 percent of eclamptics) again develop hypertensive toxemia in any subsequent pregnancies. This is known as "recurrent" or "repeat" toxemia. These facts make it plain that careful, prolonged follow-up of those mothers who have suffered from preeclampsia or eclampsia is imperative. Moreover, the prognosis for future pregnancies must be guarded, although, as the figures indicate, such patients stand at least an even chance of going through subsequent pregnancies satisfactorily.

Principles of Management

Since the cause of eclampsia is not known, there can be no "specific" therapy, and treatment must necessarily be empirical, which means utilization of those therapeutic measures which have yielded the best results in other cases. Empirical treatment is thus based on experience. Since the experience of different physicians and different hospitals varies considerably, the type of therapy employed from clinic to clinic differs somewhat in respect to the drugs used and in other details. However, the general principles followed are almost identical everywhere. These are enumerated as follows:

1. *Prevention.* Let it be emphasized again that eclampsia is largely (but not entirely) a preventable disease. Vigilant antepartal care and the early detection and treatment of preeclampsia will do more to reduce deaths from eclampsia than the most intensive treatment after convulsions have started.

2. *Termination of Pregnancy.* Although the precise cause of preeclampsia and eclampsia is not known, it is quite clear that since they occur in pregnancy, the one sure "cure" is to render the patient nonpregnant. In almost all instances of eclampsia, efforts to effect delivery should be undertaken as soon as the patient is stabilized. This involves control of seizures as well as hyperreflexia, by adequate doses of anticonvulsants and the initiation of diuresis. It is often helpful to monitor central venous pressure in addition to urinary output in an attempt to optimize fluid balance.

   Efforts to accomplish delivery before the patient is stabilized may result in increased maternal morbidity and mortality. The method of delivery should be by the most expeditious route. Prolonged attempts at induction in the face of an unripe cervix are not indicated; however, the possibility of vaginal delivery should not be discounted even at early gestational age since for unexplained reasons the cervix often quickly becomes favorable for induction. Occasionally the obstetrician is faced with the dilemma of an eclamptic with an immature fetus. Although it is tempting to try to prolong the pregnancy in the interest of bringing about greater fetal maturity, such attempts are generally unsuccessful, with impaired placental function and failure of the fetus to prosper.

3. *Sedation*. The purpose of administering sedative drugs is to depress the activity of the brain cells and thereby stop convulsions. The drugs most commonly employed are described below:

MAGNESIUM SULFATE.	This drug is an excellent central nervous system depressant, and therefore anticonvulsant, and also a smooth muscle relaxant which causes dilatation of peripheral blood vessels and thereby reduces blood pressure. For these reasons it is probably the most common drug used in eclamptic patients. The routes of administration, doses and precautions have already been discussed. Since the situation with the eclamptic patient is so urgent, the drug is most often given intravenously, at least initially.
BARBITURATES.	Rapid-acting drugs, such as intravenous sodium amobarbital (Amytal) (0.3 to 0.6 gm.), are often used to control the seizure, while subcutaneous doses of sodium phenobarbital (0.1 to 0.3 gm.) may be used subsequently. Intravenous barbiturates must be used with great caution, as they sometimes produce a sudden fall in blood

pressure, compromising placental function.

DIAZEPAM {VALIUM}.	Intravenous diazepam is widely used for seizure control. Generally 40 mg. is diluted in 500 cc. of 5 percent dextrose in water, and this is administered at a rate of 30 drops per minute. Diazepam can cause neonatal depression if more than 30 mg. are used within 15 to 20 hours before delivery. For this reason magnesium sulfate remains the sedative drug of choice.

4. *Protection of Patient from Self-Injury*. The eclamptic patient must never be left alone for a second. When in the throes of a convulsion, she may crash her head against a bedpost or throw herself onto the floor; or she may bite her tongue violently. To prevent the latter injury, some device should be kept within easy reach which can be inserted between the jaws at the very onset of a convulsion. A piece of heavy rubber tubing, a rolled towel or a padded clothespin is often employed. The nurse must take care in inserting it not to injure the patient (lips, gums, teeth) and not to allow her own fingers to be bitten.

Eclamptic patients must never be given fluids by mouth unless thoroughly conscious. Failure to adhere to this rule may result in aspiration of the fluid and consequent pneumonia.

5. *Protection of Patient from Extraneous Stimuli*. A loud noise, a bright light, a jarring of the bed, a draft—indeed, the slightest irritation—may be enough to precipitate a convulsion.

Nurse's Responsibilities in Eclampsia

The nurse's responsibilities in the management of a patient with eclampsia are serious. Some of them have already been mentioned in the discussion of treatment. Although eclampsia usually is regarded as the climax to a mounting preeclampsia which has been present, the nurse must remember that it is occasionally observed as a fulminating case in an apparently normal woman who may develop severe symptoms in the span of 24 hours. In the event that eclampsia occurs, the highest quality of nursing care is necessary. The attack may come on at any time, even when the patient is sleeping.

During the seizure it is necessary to protect the patient from self-injury. Never leave the patient for an instant unless someone is actually at the bedside to relieve you. Gentle restraint should be used to guide the patient's movements whenever necessary to prevent her from throwing herself against the head of the bed or out of it. Canvas sides, as well as pads at the head and the foot of the bed, are helpful. The padded mouth gag should be inserted between the upper and lower teeth at the onset of a convulsion to prevent the tongue from being bitten.

Regardless of the fact that the nurse is exceedingly "busy" with the patient during a seizure, she should make careful and complete observations of the duration and the character of each convulsion, the depth and duration of coma, the quality and the rate of pulse and respiration and the degree of cyanosis. A careful record should be kept so that this information can be used by the physician in treating the patient.

During the coma which follows, care must be taken to see that the patient does not aspirate. It is understood, of course, that one never gives an eclamptic patient fluids by mouth unless it is certain she is fully conscious. The position of the patient in bed should be such that it promotes drainage of secretions and the maintenance of a clear airway. It may be necessary to raise the foot of the bed of the comatose patient a few inches to promote drainage of secretions from the respiratory passage. When this measure must be resorted to, it is particularly important to watch for signs of pulmonary edema, which would be aggravated by this position. The head of the bed may need to be elevated to relieve dyspnea.

The patient should be protected from extraneous stimuli. Light in the room should be eliminated except for a small lamp, so shaded that none of the light falls on the patient. Although the room should be darkened, the light should be sufficient to permit observations of changes in condition, such as cyanosis or twitchings. A flashlight, directed well away from the patient's face, may be used during catheterization and during the physician's examinations. Sudden noises, such as the slamming of a door or the clatter of a tray as it is placed on a table, and jarring of the bed must be avoided, because they are often sufficient stimuli to send the patient into convulsions. Only absolutely necessary conversation should be carried on in the room, and this should be in the lowest tones possible.

The fetal heart tones should be checked as often as time will permit. Also, the nurse must watch for signs of labor. In eclampsia this may proceed with few external signs, and occasionally such a patient gives birth beneath the sheets before anyone knows that the process is under way. Be suspicious when the patient grunts or groans or moves about at regular intervals, every five minutes or so. If this occurs, feel the consistency of the uterus, watch for "show" and bulging and report your observations to the physician. Convulsions which occur during labor may speed up this process, and more rapid preparation for delivery should be made. During the delivery, the same atmosphere of quiet should be maintained, and glaring lights should be kept away from the patient's face.

Throughout the care of the eclamptic patient a careful account of fluid intake and output should be recorded, along with all the other observations and pertinent data. And, since further complications of pregnancy may occur in eclampsia, the patient should be observed for signs and symptoms of cerebral hemorrhage, abruptio placentae, pulmonary edema and cardiac failure.

Concurrent Hypertension and Pregnancy

As the name implies, this is a process in which high blood pressure is present before pregnancy. Difficulty is encountered in establishing such a diagnosis, because many women are not seen between pregnancies and blood pressures are, therefore, not recorded. Also, there is normally a decrease in blood pressure during the second trimester which could mask a preexisting hypertension, if the patient does not report for care until the fourth or fifth month of gestation. The diagnosis is justified if hypertension is detected prior to the twenty-fourth week of gestation. Most often patients with chronic hypertension are multiparae and commonly over the age of 30.

At least 75 percent of such patients are able to complete their pregnancies successfully, with no significant change in the status of their hypertension. Fifteen percent develop superimposed preeclampsia, an occurrence which carries an ominous fetal prognosis (20 percent mortality), and even an increase in maternal mortality.

The treatment, then, for the majority of those patients with chronic hypertension is no different from treatment for the nonpregnant patient. It includes salt restriction, restricted activities, and sedation. The pregnancy is allowed to run its normal course under such circumstances, unless the pregnancy aggravates the already existing hypertension. When the gravida with this chronic process develops a further elevation of blood pressure, significant proteinuria or edema, the condition is called *superimposed preeclampsia*.

In the case of superimposed preeclampsia, after 24 to 48 hours of intensive medical therapy, pregnancy termination is generally indicated. Even though the fetus may be preterm, its chances for survival under these circumstances are generally better outside the uterus.

In a small number of patients the hypertension will be so severe, with evidence of kidney involvement, severe retinal changes, or cardiac involvement, that therapeutic abortion might be considered if the patient comes to medical attention in the first trimester. It is also well to consider the advisability of postpartum tubal ligation in this group of patients who are generally older, with established families, and for whom additional pregnancies may represent a serious health hazard. This, of course, can only be a recommendation, the final decision resting with the patient and her mate.

SUGGESTED READING

Cavanah, D. and O'Connor, R. C. F.: "Eclamptogenic toxemia." In *Obstretic Emergencies*, ed. 2. Cavanagh, D., Woods, R. F. and O'Connor, T. C. F., eds. Hagerstown, Md., Harper & Row, 1978, pp. 105–132.

Gant, N. F., Worley, R. J., Cunningham, G. and Whalley, P. F.: "Clinical management of pregnancy induced hypertension." *Clin. Obstet. Gynecol.* 21: 397, 1979.

Welt, S. I. and Grenshaw, M. C.: "Concurrent hypertension and pregnancy." *Clin. Obstet. Gynecol.* 21: 619, 1979.

Wingate, M. B., Iffy, L., Kelly, J. V. and Birnbaum, S.: "Diseases specific to pregnancy." In *Gynecology and Obstetrics, The health care of women*, ed. 2. Romney et al., ed. New York, McGraw-Hill, 1980, pp. 718–776.

Woods, R. E. and Cavanagh, D.: "Hemorrhage in early pregnancy." In *Obstetric Emergencies*. ed. 2. Cavanagh, D., Woods, R. F. and O'Connor, T. C. F., eds. Hagerstown, Md., Harper & Row, 1978, pp. 133–176.

Thirty-Two

Concurrent Diseases in Pregnancy

Hematologic Disorders | Heart Disease | Diabetes Mellitus | Disturbances in Thyroid Function | Renal Disease | Infectious Diseases

It has been said wisely that the pregnant woman can have any disease which her nonpregnant counterpart can have except for infertility. One must be aware that many disease states are modified by the physiologic changes of pregnancy. Pregnancy may alter the classic clinical picture of a disease state and, indeed, some of the normal physiologic changes of pregnancy mimic disease. Therapeutic approaches must be altered in some cases, especially with regard to possible effects on the fetus. For most coincidental diseases, the effects of pregnancy on the disease and of the disease on pregnancy are negligible and do not influence the management of either. Some diseases, however, have profound fetal effects, as discussed in Chapter 36; others have a predominantly maternal effect; and some, such as diabetes, affect both. The more common diseases in the latter two categories will be discussed in this chapter.

HEMATOLOGIC DISORDERS

Iron Deficiency Anemia

Iron deficiency anemia is the most common hematologic disorder in pregnancy. Because of the expanded blood volume there is an element of hemodilution with a resultant fall in hemoglobin concentration unless the need is met by augmented hematopoiesis. There is, in addition, the fetal requirement for iron to contend with. Since many women have depleted iron stores as a result of regular menstrual blood loss, these added demands often result in the total depletion of storage iron and the development of overt anemia. The socio-economically deprived patient with poor general nutrition is more susceptible to this condition.

In most patients with mild to moderate anemia, the signs and symptoms are few and often indistinguishable from the normal symptoms of pregnancy. Such patients are detected by frequent antepartum hemoglobin or hematocrit determinations. Severely anemic patients are symptomatic and in the most severe cases can even develop heart failure as a result of the anemia.

Treatment for mild to moderate cases consists of iron-rich diet and an oral iron compound such as ferrous sulfate or gluconate. Similar recommendations hold for the nonanemic gravida as prophylaxis. It has been estimated that the pregnant patient requires 3 to 5 mg. of iron/day to supply the needs of mother and fetus, with demands for iron increasing in the last five months of pregnancy to as much as 3 to 7.5 mg./day. Thus, oral iron supplementary therapy is recommended throughout pregnancy,

529

but especially in the latter half. Ferrous sulfate, 200 mg., or ferrous gluconate 320 mg. three times a day satisfies this need. Injectable iron therapy is rarely required since absorption is generally not a limiting factor. More often a failure to respond to oral iron therapy is the result of failure to take the medication (iron tends to produce gastrointestinal symptoms) or a concurrent folic acid deficiency.

Folic Acid Deficiency

Folic acid deficiency can produce severe anemia of the megaloblastic type in pregnancy. Megaloblastic anemia is much less common than iron deficiency anemia, occurring in less than 3 percent of gravidae. In its full-blown form there is also a reduction in white cells and platelets and is usually associated with glossitis and a sore tongue.

Treatment consists of oral folic acid and diet. Prevention is achieved by the inclusion of folic acid in prenatal vitamin-mineral supplements.

Hemoglobinopathies

Hemoglobinopathies present special problems in pregnancy. Sickle cell trait, although not considered a disease, does predispose to urinary tract infection. The genetic implications should be explained to the patient after the father's hemoglobin pattern is evaluated. Sickle cell-C disease is generally innocuous in the nonpregnant woman, producing, at worst, a mild anemia. During pregnancy, however, life-threatening hemolytic crisis can occur. Sickle cell anemia (S-S disease) is generally manifest before childbearing and in contrast to sickle cell-C disease, crises occur in the nonpregnant state as well.

One must consider not only the impact of pregnancy in precipitating crises, but also the genetic outlook and the fact that patients with S-S disease have a limited life expectancy. Childbearing might well be limited or even avoided completely after appropriate counseling of these patients.

Treatment in the case of sickle trait consists of looking for and treating urinary tract infection, while in the case of S-C and S-S disease more drastic measures may be necessary. Folic acid supplements are indicated because of the rapid turnover of red cells. In the instance of patients with previous crises or the occurrence of crises during pregnancy, multiple transfusions are sometimes used to suppress the patient's marrow from forming the abnormal cells, at the same time permitting her to exist on transfused cells during the period of risk (pregnancy and the puerperium).

HEART DISEASE

Although rheumatic heart disease has for some time been the most common type of heart disease in pregnancy, recognition of the role of streptococcal infection and its appropriate therapy has reduced the frequency of rheumatic fever and its cardiac consequences. Still another dimension has been added by cardiac surgeons, as there are now appearing surgically treated patients, even some with valve replacements.

For most types of heart disease, the major threat imposed by pregnancy is that the increasing blood volume will precipitate congestive heart failure. With appropriate therapy and restriction of activities, however, most patients can tolerate that stress and carry a pregnancy to a successful conclusion. The exception might be that individual falling into functional class IV (symptomatic at rest) in the first trimester, especially if she does not have a surgically correctable lesion. It is now the very rare cardiac patient who should be considered for therapeutic abortion on medical grounds.

Appropriate therapy demands close cooperation between the obstetrician and cardiologist, with the nurse playing a major role by coordinating information for the patient as well as providing day-to-day patient supervision. Treatment is governed to a considerable extent by the functional capacity of the patient, and rest is one of the most important ingredients with bedrest being necessary in some advanced cases. Digitalis, diuretics and salt restriction may all be required, depending upon the severity. In the case of valvular lesions, penicillin prophylaxis is recommended during labor and at delivery to prevent bacterial endocarditis to which patients with valvular lesions are susceptible.

As for all patients with heart disease, any respiratory infection can be devastating and consequently patients should avoid any predisposing situation and report even a sore throat or cold to the nurse and/or physician. The patient with heart disease who develops a cough should be examined forthwith, as coughing is one of the early symptoms of pulmonary congestion and cardiac failure.

Since the onset of heart failure may be insidious, it behooves the nurse to be alert to the signs and symptoms of this problem. These might include inability to carry on normal activities, increased dyspnea on exertion and paroxysmal nocturnal dyspnea, tachycardia, palpitations and cough, especially if blood or rusty sputum is evident.

Very special problems are presented by the patients with valve prostheses, since they require anticoagulant therapy. Sodium warfarin (Coumadin) and related drugs are contraindicated because they cross the placenta; this requires changing such patients to heparin therapy for the duration of pregnancy.

DIABETES MELLITUS

Diabetes mellitus illustrates well the interplay between the altered physiology of pregnancy and the pathophysiology of disease. In contrast to the majority of disease states which do not alter or are not affected by pregnancy, there is a significant change in the course of diabetes when pregnancy supervenes, and diabetes has a profound effect on the course of pregnancy as well as on the fetus. In addition to participating in the regular medical and prenatal care of the diabetic gravida, the nurse can serve a very important counseling role. Care is a team effort and must involve cooperation among obstetrician, internist, pediatrician, nurse and nutritionist.

In recent years, the number of pregnant diabetics has increased, partly because with modern mangement, diabetics are now able to conceive and maintain pregnancies, and partly because there is presently an increased recognition of the milder forms of gestational diabetes.

During the course of normal pregnancy, glucose may appear in the urine, with blood sugars as low as 100 mg., because of a lowered renal threshold to glucose excretion. Nevertheless, although the presence of glucose in the urine does not necessarily indicate high glucose blood levels, any patient exhibiting glucosuria should be suspected of having diabetes, and the diagnosis should be established or ruled out by evaluation of glucose blood levels. A fasting blood glucose of over 130 mg. is almost invariably associated with diabetes. However, if a woman has already been identified as being diabetic prior to pregnancy, then diagnostic glucose tolerance tests are not required.

On the other hand, there are large numbers of patients in whom gestational diabetes might be suspected on the basis of the following:
1. previous large babies
2. family history of diabetes
3. glucosuria
4. obesity
5. unexplained pregnancy wastage

In these patients the appropriate screening test is a two-hour postprandial blood sugar. Fasting blood sugars are not adequate since the fasting sugar is normally reduced in pregnancy in the first trimester. When a normal value is obtained initially, the patient should be screened for diabetes again in the second and third trimesters. Abnormal values indicate the need for a full glucose tolerance test.

A special diagnostic problem occurs when a patient is not suspected of being diabetic until after delivery, as might be the case if she delivered an unusually large baby or an unexplained stillborn. Since the diabetogenic effects of pregnancy disappear quickly following delivery, a normal glucose tolerance test 48 to 72 hours postpartum is not necessarily reassuring. The so-called steroid enforced glucose tolerance test in which cortisone is administered prior to the testing may bring out the abnormality.

Classification A number of confusing terms have been applied and definitions are in order: Prediabetes and latent diabetes are terms which pertain to that period of time prior to the establishment of the diagnosis. Gestational diabetes designates those patients in whom during pregnancy diabetes is first diagnosed and often becomes undetectable following delivery.

The most universally used classification of diabetes is that by White, which is as follows:

CLASS A—glucose tolerance test diabetes
CLASS B—onset: over age 20
        duration: 0–9 years
        vascular disease: 0
CLASS C—onset: age 10–19
        duration: 10–19 years
        vascular disease: 0
CLASS D—onset: under age 10
        duration: 20+ years
        vascular disease: calcification in legs, retinitis
CLASS E—patients with calcified pelvic vessels
CLASS F—patients with nephritis

Although this classification has some pitfalls in that duration of disease and vascular disease are not always absolutely parallel, in general perinatal wastage is a function of the class. The wastage is invariably greater in Classes D, E, and F, those patients with vascular disease, and less in Classes A, B, and C. It should also be noted that mothers with significant vascular involvement have small rather than large-for-date babies.

Management

Careful medical management of the pregnant diabetic woman is the key to a successful outcome. The initial evaluation should include examination of the optic fundi for detection of vascular disease, and also urine analysis and culture to detect asymptomatic bacilluria, a precursor to overt pyelonephritis, to which the diabetic is especially prone.

Diet.   Diet is of paramount importance, and the nurse must be prepared to assist the patient in this area. The caloric requirement for the normal-weight patient is approximately 2,200 calories with 1 to 1.5 gm. of protein per kg. of body weight. In the case of many gestational diabetics who are overweight, total calories must be reduced to control blood sugar. It is difficult to go below 1,500 calories and still maintain adequate protein intake and a palatable formulation. Standard diabetic diets tend to lack the protein needed in pregnancy. Occasionally one needs to increase carbohydrate and total calories because of the patient's activities, or in some cases of juvenile diabetes, the large amount of glucose lost in the urine. Food costs and ethnic dietary habits must also be considered when making such recommendations.

Preeclampsia and hydramnios both occur relatively frequently in diabetic pregnant patients. These serious complications should be kept in mind and watched for throughout the entire course of prenatal care.

Insulin.   Although diet alone may control many gestational diabetics, if the two-hour postprandial sugar exceeds 150 to 160 mg. percent, despite the diet, insulin therapy is indicated. Although occasionally used, the oral hypoglycemics are not cleared for use in pregnancy. Progressive insulin resistance is characteristic of pregnancy and it is not unusual for insulin requirements to increase as much as fourfold. This commonly necessitates the use of evening as well as morning doses of insulin to achieve good control. Although in the majority of patients, insulin requirements increase as pregnancy progresses, about 35 percent require the same dose or less. This variability highlights further the importance of meticulous management of insulin needs during the prenatal course.

Obstetrical Considerations.   Obstetrical management involves evaluating fetal well-being and determining the timing and method of delivery. Since the major target of diabetes is the small blood vessels, it is not surprising that the placenta may also be involved and therefore placental insufficiency and even fetal death may occur. This result is far less common in gestational than prepregnancy diabetics and is the basis for the common practice of delivering diabetic patients three to four weeks prior to the expected date of confinement. This is not, however, always necessary if one can identify the fetus at risk by another type of technique such as serial 24-hour urinary estriol determinations (see Chapter 36).

In those patients with no evidence of fetal compromise and who are otherwise stable (good diabetic control, absence of toxemia and no significant hydramnios), pregnancy may be allowed to go to term, with careful surveillance. The method of delivery is a matter of obstetric judgment at the time. Early deliveries are carried out more often by cesarean section because the cervix is not prepared for induction, and even at term there is an increased need for section because of the mechanical problems created by the fetal macrosoma.

During vaginal deliveries fetal size may cause problems in the form of shoulder dystocia.

Newborns of diabetic mothers show a high incidence of congenital anomalies, reported as high as 8 percent. They also display a greater incidence of respiratory distress syndrome and neonatal hyperbilirubinemia.

The problems of the diabetic offspring are discussed in detail in Chapter 36. However, it is important to realize that even under the best of circumstances the perinatal mortality is two to three times that in the nondiabetic, and pregnancy is a very major undertaking for the diabetic and her family.

DISTURBANCES IN THYROID FUNCTION

Hyperthyroidism is probably the second most significant endocrinopathy in pregnancy, second only to diabetes mellitus. Although a woman with uncontrolled hyperthyroidism is likely to be anovulatory and thus unable to conceive, many with milder disease do conceive, and some patients with hyperthyroidism are first diagnosed as such during pregnancy. If the condition is uncontrolled during pregnancy, spontaneous abortion and premature labor are common. Diagnosis may be somewhat of a problem in milder cases since some thyroid enlargement and confusing hyperdynamic symptoms occur in normal pregnancy. Laboratory studies may also be confusing since there is increased protein binding of thyroid hormone in pregnancy resulting in higher values for studies such as the protein bound iodine and total T_4, with lower T_3 uptake. Multiple studies and newer methods, however, can overcome the confusion.

Once-popular surgical treatment (subtotal thyroidectomy) has been replaced by medical approaches except in special cases (reaction to the antithyroid drugs, unusually large dosage requirements, etc.). The problem with medical therapy is that the antithyroid drugs do cross the placenta and if doses are excessive the fetal thyroid can be suppressed, leading to fetal goiter or even cretinism. This is best avoided if the level of control is maintained at high normal levels, although some have suggested that therapy with methimazole (Tapazole) or propylthiouracil be combined with thyroid extract to avoid that problem.

Patients with exophthalmic goiter produce a substance called LATS (long acting thyroid stimulator), which is a gamma-g globulin. This does cross the placenta and if present can cause hyperthyroidism in the newborn.

Hypothyroidism and parathyroid disorders are reported in pregnancy but are rare. Adrenal, pituitary, and ovarian disorders generally result in infertility.

RENAL DISEASE

Almost all forms of acute and chronic renal disease have been reported in association with pregnancy. Not infrequently, specific diagnosis is difficult during pregnancy since proteinuria and hypertension may mimic preeclampsia, and also because definitive studies such as renal biopsy and intravenous urography are contraindicated. Chronic renal disease, especially if accompanied by hypertension, may be associated with fetal growth retardation and increased perinatal mortality.

The most common renal problem in pregnancy is urinary tract infection. Anatomical changes as well as hormonal effects cause narrowing of the lower ureter with dilatation of the upper ureter and renal pelvis. These changes result in delayed emptying and an increased risk of infection. The risk increases as pregnancy progresses and continues into the puerperium.

Symptoms include chills, fever, frequency, dysuria and pain in the area of the kidneys. Severity may vary from extremely mild to extremely toxic, with nausea, vomiting and abnormal distension. Uterine irritability is an important complication of pyelonephritis. The correlation is sufficiently common that is is wise to look for urinary tract infection in any patient with premature labor.

In order to treat the patient adequately, a carefully collected midstream clean catch urine specimen must be obtained. To assure an adequate specimen the nurse should instruct the patient as to the proper method of collecting the sample. An examination of the urinary sediment as well as a culture and antibiotic sensitivity studies should be carried out. In addition to the selection of an appropriate antibiotic, it is imperative that a good fluid intake be maintained, parenterally if necessary. Antimicrobial therapy should be continued for seven to ten days even if the response is good, and the urine should be recultured once therapy is stopped. Recurrences are common, causing some authorities to recommend long-term suppressive antimicrobial therapy.

Asymptomatic bacteriuria in pregnancy is significant because of its high association with subsequent pyelonephritis and consequently should be treated. Association with other obstetrical problems such as prematurity has been suggested, but it is likely that these are simply coincidental findings in a group of high-risk patients.

INFECTIOUS DISEASES

Although most infectious diseases have no established specific ill effects on mother or baby, there are those that produce profound effects. Diseases with particular fetal effects are discussed in Chapter 36.

The Common Cold. Susceptibility to acute upper respiratory infections is apparently greater during pregnancy. Therefore, the pregnant woman should make every effort to avoid contacts with these infections. When she does acquire a cold, prompt medical attention is usually desirable, because the common cold often precedes more serious conditions affecting the upper respiratory tract. Prescribed medication should be used in preference to the various antihistamine drugs obtainable without a prescription. Rest in bed helps the individual and aids in checking the spread of the disease.

Influenza. Although the pregnant woman is not more likely to contract influenza, she is more prone to the development of complicating pneumonia, especially if she is in the third trimester during which time the diaphragm is elevated and respiration compromised.

The development of pneumonia represents a serious threat to the gravida. In the face of an epidemic involving a specific strain of influenza virus, immunization with a killed or attenuated virus vaccine is indicated. Nonspecific polyvalent vaccines are probably ineffectual.

Measles. Ill effects are not commonly noted in pregnancy, but pregnant women who contract measles are said to be more likely to have premature labors. No other definite effects are reported, although eruptions have been noted on infants at birth.

Typhoid Fever. Typhoid fever, which is now relatively rare in the United States, may cause serious complications in pregnancy, resulting in abortion, prematurity and infant mortality. Immunization is not contraindicated during pregnancy, and antityphoid vaccine should be administered when necessary.

Tuberculosis. The average case of tuberculosis in itself has only a slight effect on the course of pregnancy, since it rarely predisposes to abortion, premature labor or even stillbirth. (Fortunately, the disease is seldom acquired congenitally, although a small number of authentic cases have been reported in which, in addition to a tuberculous condition of the placenta, tubercle bacilli were found in the cord blood, together with tuberculous lesions in the baby.)

Medical opinions differ, but the consensus is that pregnancy does not exert an adverse effect on tuberculosis. Some authorities think that this disease becomes aggravated by pregnancy and that only a patient in an arrested case should consider becoming pregnant. Pregnancy is undertaken with some risk, for although a tuberculous lesion may remain latent for an indefinite time, provided that the natural resistance is not overtaxed, it must be noted that pregnancy is one of the factors often responsible for overtaxing the resistance sufficiently to convert a latent, inactive lesion into an active one. Maintenance of proper nutrition will do much to prevent activity in a latent focus. Other authorities deny that the tuberculosis is necessarily aggravated by pregnancy, basing this belief on statistics of a large series of tuberculous patients who have progressed satisfactorily in pregnancy.

Treatment with modern antituberculosis drugs, streptomycin, isoniazid (INH), and para-amino-salicylic acid (PAS), has completely altered management in general, as well as during pregnancy. New advanced cases are rare and a majority of patients are managed as outpatients. Treatment of active cases generally consists of streptomycin, 1.0 gm. daily for three to four weeks, then 1.0 gm. twice weekly. Isoniazid, 300 mg., and para-aminosalicylic acid, 12.0 gm. daily, are given in divided doses. No deleterious effects of these agents on the mother or the infant have been reported.

Labor and delivery are conducted in a normal fashion, avoiding inhalation anesthesia, and mother and baby are separated if disease is active. Breast-feeding is unwise even when the disease is inactive. Some authorities recommend INH therapy on the third trimester and puerperium for the inactive patient who has had active disease within two years of pregnancy.

Poliomyelitis This disease generally does not complicate pregnancy or delivery, except in the very unusual cases in which respiratory paralysis develops; in these rare cases cesarean section has given satisfactory results. Fortunately, the disease has virtually disappeared as a result of immunization.

Viral Hepatitis

The hepatitis viruses (hepatitis A and B) are the most common causes of liver disease in pregnancy. Anorexia, nausea and vomiting are the most characteristic symptoms of hepatitis. Since 75 percent of affected patients do not exhibit clinical jaundice, the diagnosis may be missed or delayed in patients exhibiting the nausea and vomiting characteristic of pregnancy, or cases may be misdiagnosed as hyperemesis gravidarum. In contrast to the latter, in hepatitis the liver is characteristically enlarged and tender and bilirubin levels rise as high as 25 mg. %. When nausea and vomiting persist unabated in pregnancy, hepatitis should be considered and ruled out.

Hepatitis is associated with an increased incidence of abortion, premature labor and stillbirth. Maternal mortality from viral hepatitis varies, and has been reported at from 1 percent to 17 percent. Its course is substantially influenced by the nutritional status of the patient, and hence maternal mortality is higher in the less developed regions of the world. Prompt diagnosis and treatment with bedrest, good nutrition and intravenous therapy generally result in a favorable maternal outcome.

The fetus may acquire the virus in utero or during delivery, and the newborn may develop active hepatitis or a carrier state. Prompt treatment of the newborn with hyperimmune gammaglobulin has been recommended. Since hepatitis B surface antigen has been detected in breast milk, and since the virus is present in maternal serum and could be transmitted from excoriations around the nipple, breast-feeding should be avoided.

Syphilis

In the past the major hazard of syphilis in pregnancy was the occurrence of intrauterine infection and late abortion or stillbirth. Congenital syphilis has now been reduced nearly to the point of elimination. The antenatal blood test for syphilis is required by law and, except for the instances in which prenatal care is nonexistent, maternal syphilis should be detected and adequately treated, thereby protecting the fetus.

Syphilis can occur at any stage during pregnancy. The primary and secondary stages are usually apparent because of their lesions. In latent syphilis, the diagnosis is based upon a positive serology; the most difficult problem occurs when the serology is repeatedly positive and the patient denies a history. Biologic false positives do occur in a number of circumstances, but, fortunately, new, more specific tests are now available which can be used in the questionable case.

Treatment is indicated in the following circumstances:

1. When a diagnosis of early syphilis is made, regardless of stage.
2. When late symptomatic syphilis is discovered.
3. When latent syphilis is diagnosed by repeated positive serologic tests and the patient's history corroborates the diagnosis, and when there has been either inadequate or no treatment.
4. When the diagnosis is made by repeated positive tests, even though the history does not confirm, and when either the more specific tests are not available or there is not time for adequate therapy. Retreatment in subsequent pregnancies is necessary if there is any doubt about the adequacy of previous therapy.

The treatment consists of a course of penicillin in the total dose of 6 million units (12 million for neurosyphilis), or a suitable substitute if penicillin allergy exists. Both mother and baby should be carefully followed by serologic tests postpartum. It is important to know that even the unaffected baby will have a positive test because the mother's test is positive; however the titer in the baby will be lower than that of the mother and will become negative within three months.

Gonorrhea

Gonorrhea is of special concern in maternity care because of the consequences to the mother at the time of labor and during the puerperium, as well as the risk of permanent injury to the baby's eyes at the time of birth.

The disease is caused by *Neisseria gonorrhoeae,* an organism which may attack the mucous membrane but most commonly affects the mucosa of the lower genital tract. The endocervical glands and urethra are common foci, but for complete detection, the anus and oropharynx should be cultured.

Gonorrhea is spread by sexual contact and in the majority of women remains asymptomatic except for a nonspecific vaginal discharge. This is particularly the case in pregnancy, in which the normal route of spread through the endometrial cavity to the tubes is occluded by the pregnancy. The rate of asymptomatic carriers in pregnancy is reported to be as high as 5 to 10 percent in many clinics.

Although gonorrhea causes few problems for the patient during pregnancy, it can produce serious puerperal infection if present in the cervix at the time of delivery. Routine gonorrhea cultures are recommended during pregnancy. Gram-stained smears are suggestive but not conclusive in women.

The treatment of asymptomatic gonorrhea involves a single injection of 4.8 million units of procaine penicillin preceded by 1.0 gm. of probenecid to produce the high level of penicillin needed to eradicate the increasingly resistant gonococcus. Cure should be proven by reculture, although reinfection is possible and should be watched for. Sexual partners should be evaluated and treated appropriately.

The organism can infect the infant's eyes at birth, and if prophylactic treatment of the eyes is not adequate, blindness may result.

SUGGESTED READING

Burrow, G. W.: "The thyroid gland and reproduction." In *Reproductive Endocrinology*. Eds.: S. Yen and R. B. Jaffe. Philadelphia, W. B. Saunders, 1978, pp. 373–387.

Gabbe, S. G.: "Diabetes in pregnancy: Clinical controversies." *Clin. Obstet. Gynecol.* 21:443, 1978.

Gabbe, S. G. and Hagerman, D. D.: "Clinical application of estrial analysis." *Clin. Obstet. Gynecol.* 21:353, 1978.

Marchant, D. J.: "Urinary tract infections in pregnancy." *Clin. Obstet. Gynecol.* 21:921, 1978.

Rovinsky, J. J.: "Diseases complicating pregnancy." In *Gynecology and Obstetrics, The Health Care of Women*. Eds.: S. Romney et al. New York, McGraw-Hill, 1975, pp. 777–866.

Sever, J. L.: "Viral infections in pregnancy." *Clin. Obstet. Gynecol.* 21:477, 1978.

Ueland, K.: "Cardiovascular diseases complicating pregnancy." *Clin. Obstet. Gynecol.* 21:429, 1978.

Wiesner, P. J. and Tyler, C. W., eds.: "Venereal disease in obstetrics and gynecology." *Clin. Obstet. Gynecol.* 18, 1975.

Thirty-Three

Complications of Labor

*Dystocia Due to Abnormalities of Labor Mechanics /
Hemorrhagic Complications / Prolapse of the Umbilical
Cord / Amniotic Fluid Embolism / Multiple Pregnancy*

A complicated labor requires sensitive and astute nursing care, for it represents a period of great stress for the laboring woman, her partner, nurses and physicians. The principles of nursing care during normal labor (see Chapter 23) also apply when the labor is complicated, with certain modifications depending upon the nature of the problems. The nurse's ability to use clinical judgment is crucial, as the nursing diagnoses and care deriving from such judgments may be of life-saving significance for both the mother and the infant. Assessment skills including observation, interviewing and physical examination provide important data on the nature and extent of the problem. Reporting, recording and professional intercommunication promote accurate decision making and implementation of appropriate treatment. Physical and emotional supportive measures assist the mother and father to understand and cope with the unusual events in the labor experience, which is often prolonged and painful.

DYSTOCIA DUE TO ABNORMALITIES OF LABOR MECHANICS

Dystocia, or difficult labor, can result from abnormalities in the machinery of labor. When there is cessation or delay of progress in the labor process due to such abnormalities, it is termed *mechanical dystocia* and may be caused by one or a combination of these three major conditions:

1. Uterine dysfunction, subnormal or abnormal uterine forces that are not adequate to overcome the natural resistance which the maternal soft parts and bony pelvis present to the passage of the baby through the birth canal.
2. Faulty fetal presentation or developmental anomalies of the type which prevent entrance to or passage of the baby through the birth canal.
3. Variations in the size or shape of the bony pelvis which create an obstacle to the entrance or descent of the baby.

Frequently two or more of these conditions occur together, for faulty fetal presentation or a contracted maternal pelvis are often associated with uterine dysfunction. Or a contracted pelvis may cause an abnormal fetal presentation.

To further understand the nature of these problems, the process of labor can be thought of as divided into three components, each of which must be normal for progress to be made and birth to occur. These components may be described as the *forces* of labor, the *passenger* and the *passage.* The *forces,* including uterine contractions with the addition of maternal "bearing down" during the second stage, must be of adequate strength with coordination of muscle activity. These forces propel

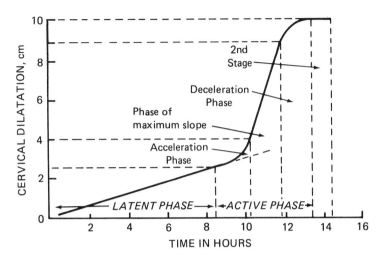

Figure 33-1. A composite Friedman labor curve based on 500 multiparas. (From Friedman, E.: "Primigravid labor, *Obstetrics and Gynecology* 6:569.)

an irregular object, the infant or *passenger,* through the birth canal or *passage.* The *passenger* must be of appropriate size and shape, and able to undergo the necessary maneuvers to pass through the different dimensions of the birth canal. The *passage* must also be of normal size and configuration, not presenting any undue obstacles to the descent, rotations and expulsion of the baby.

Thus, when nature tries to propel the fetus through the birth canal and fails to do so, there can be one of three causes for the failure: the forces are inadequate (uterine dysfunction [inertia]); the position of the infant is at fault; or the size of the infant and that of the birth canal are disproportionate.

Uterine Dysfunction

Definition

When the stages of labor are described diagrammatically by plotting elapsed labor time on the abscissa and cervical dilatation on the ordinate of a graph, an S-shaped curve results (Fig. 33-1). The first stage of labor is divided into a latent and an active phase. Normally, the *latent phase* is a period of some effacement and slow dilatation of the cervix, lasting perhaps an average of eight and one-half hours in a nullipara. About a 4 cm. dilatation is accomplished in this stage.[1,2] This latent phase has also been called *prodromal labor.*[3] The *active phase* or clinically apparent labor is briefer and consists, according to Freidman, of an acceleration phase, a phase of maximum slope, and a deceleration phase, before full dilatation is accomplished. This phase of

labor lasts approximately three and one-half to four hours in the primigravid patient.[4] Hendricks and his associates describe slightly different curves in normal labor (Fig. 33-2). They found in normal active labor that there is a rather constant active acceleration phase without the *deceleration* described by Freidman. Also, these investigators found that cervical dilatation progressed at about the same rate in both nulliparae and multiparae after 4 cm. dilatation was reached.[5] Despite these divergent points of view, any significant prolongation of any of the phases described by Friedman or any significant variation from the curves presented by Hendricks and associates constitutes uterine dysfunction.[6]

Etiological Factors

When there is failure to progress despite the presence of uterine contractions, one of the first factors to consider is whether or not the patient is actually in labor. It is not unusual for a woman in late pregnancy to experience Braxton-Hicks contractions that are so strong and regular that they can easily be mistaken for true labor. Progressive cervical changes must be present to signify true labor, as effective contractions gradually accomplish effacement and dilatation. Appearance of bloody show assists in the diagnosis of labor, particularly when it accompanies cervical changes. Without these other signs to confirm labor, uncomfortable uterine contractions signify false labor. For the diagnosis of dystocia, cervical changes must have occurred and progressed, only to have continued progression in effacement and dilatation slowed or halted at some point.

The chief factors associated with uterine dysfunction are injudicious use of analgesia (i.e., excessive or too early admininstration of the drugs), minor degrees of pelvic contraction, and fetal malposition of even a small degree, such as a slight extension of the head as seen in some occiput posterior positions. Similarly, postmaturity and a large infant have been found to be significantly related to dysfunctional labor. These conditions may occur singly or in combination in cases of dysfunction.

Other factors that are associated with this condition include overdistension of the uterus, grand multiparity, excessive cervical rigidity and maternal age. The latter group of factors has been shown to play an etiological role although not such an important one as was once believed. The cause is often unknown. Considering the possible role of cortical steroids in the initiation of labor, and their relation to stress states, the effects of emotional factors in dystocia cannot be overlooked when no other cause is apparent. More research at the cellular level will have to be done to obtain increased definitive knowledge concerning the etiologic factors in this condition.

Complications

The complications of uterine dysfunction are unfortunate for both mother and infant. Fetal injury and death are the most serious outcomes of this disorder. For the mother, exhaustion and dehydration may occur if labor is allowed to become too prolonged. Elevation of the maternal temperature and pulse are the clinical signs that herald the onset of secondary complications. Acetonuria is another sign of exhaustion and dehydration. These symptoms are to be reported immediately. Generally, in patients having dysfunctional labor, supportive intravenous therapy and electrolyte replacement are instituted before this syndrome occurs.

Intrauterine infection is another common maternal complication in these types of labor; broad-spectrum antibiotics are the usual choice of treatment. It is particularly important not to allow intrauterine infection to occur, since it contributes heavily to the increased perinatal mortality.

Dysfunctional labor appears to have some long-term consequences. Research has indicated that difficult labors and deliveries may have a deleterious effect on future childbearing.[7] Apparently, the more

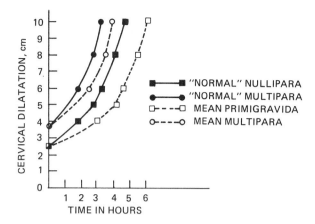

Figure 33-2. Cervical dilatation in normal nulliparous and multiparous women after the onset of true labor. (From Hendricks, Brenner, and Kraus: *Am. J. Obstet. Gynecol.* 106:1065, 1970.)

difficult the labor and delivery, the less inclination there is to have future children. In addition, the fear and anxiety that are engendered by a complicated childbirth become a special concern of the health team if these patients do have subsequent children.

Fortunately, there have been several significant advances in the treatment of uterine dysfunction in the past decade. First, it is now realized that undue prolongation of labor contributes to perinatal mortality. Second, the judicious use of dilute intravenous oxytocin in the treatment of some types of uterine dysfunction has been introduced. Third, cesarean sections are used more frequently to effect delivery in place of the difficult midforceps delivery when oxytocin fails or is inappropriate for use.[8]

Types of Uterine Dysfunction

Several groups of investigators have contributed to our understanding of the problem of uterine dysfunction. Larks described the stimulus of a contraction as starting in one cornu, followed several milliseconds later in the other cornu, with the contraction waves then joining and sweeping down over the fundus and upper segment, thus pulling up the isthmus and cervix.[9] Caldeyro-Barcia and associates in Montevideo furthered the work of Reynolds by determining that the pressure of a contraction necessary to dilate the cervix is at least 15 mm. Hg[10,11]. Finally, Hendricks and his co-workers found that a normal uterine contraction may exert as much as 60 mm. Hg.[12] Thus, contractions have come to be described in terms of

Montevideo units, which are the product of contraction intensity and frequency per 10 minutes. Optimal results are achieved in labor with a frequency of about 22 contractions per hour together with 50 to 60 mm. Hg amniotic pressures (140 to 180 Montevideo units).[13]

Uterine dysfunction has been classified according to two types: *hypertonic* and *hypotonic*. In the former there is incoordinate uterine action; in the latter there is coordinate activity but the intensity is not strong enough (less than 15 mm. Hg) to produce dilatation.

Hypertonic Dysfunction

Hypertonic dysfunction generally comes at the onset of labor. The gradient of the contraction is distorted, perhaps by contraction of the midsegment with more force than the fundus or perhaps by complete asynchronism of the electrical impulses originating in each cornu. There is constant tension in the muscle but the contractions are of poor quality.

Friedman has a somewhat different classification of dysfunction which uses length of the phases of labor rather than the quality of the contractions. However, his *prolonged latent phase* occurs during the onset and first part of labor and hence is associated with hypertonic dysfunction. By definition, the latent phase is prolonged if it lasts longer than 20 hours in the primigravida and 14 hours in the multigravida. In practice, however, the diagnosis should be suspected and treatment instituted long before these time intervals have elapsed. Treatment is the same as for hypertonic dysfunction.[14]

Although the contractions in this type of dysfunction are ineffectual in accomplishing dilatation, they are extremely painful and have been described as "colicky."

It is particularly important to help mothers with this type of labor to distinguish between the anticipation of pain and the actual pain (see Chapter 23), for as labor wears on, and no progress is made, the mother's strength and ability to cope with the contractions diminish, and hence the pain seems to be intensified. The anxiety and fear which are generated can easily lead to panic, which is detrimental to resumption of a successful labor course.

It is of paramount importance for the nurse to be able to accurately evaluate the intensity of labor contractions without relying exclusively on the electric monitor. At the height of an efficient uterine contraction it is impossible to indent the uterine wall with one's fingertips, and during a fairly good contraction it may be possible to cause some slight indentation; but if the uterine wall can be indented easily at the height of a contraction, it is a poor one. In evaluating the intensity of a labor contraction, reliance should be placed on tactile examination and data from the electronic monitor and not on the amount of "complaining" done by the patient about her pain.

Management   Treatment for this type of dysfunctional labor generally consists of rest and fluids. When medication is indicated to produce the needed rest and relaxation, an injection of 10 to 15 mg. of morphine may be prescribed, because it usually stops the abnormal contractions. In addition, a 0.1- to 0.2-gm. dose of a short-acting barbiturate may be administered. Intravenous fluids are utilized to maintain hydration and electrolyte balance, and in most instances normal labor resumes when the patient awakens.

Oxytocin is contraindicated in treating this type of dysfunction. With the uterus in a constant state of increased muscle tone, oxytocin presents the danger of causing an even greater resting tension, which might interfere with fetal oxygenation. Moreover, it does not correct the uncoordinated action of the two segments, which underlies this problem.

Occasionally the contractions remain uncoordinated and ineffective even after the patient has had a good rest. In these cases, cesarean section employed if the fetal heart rate becomes abnormal.[15] Thus the nurse needs to be particularly attentive to the mother's progress.

Complications.   Fetal distress tends to appear quite early in labor when there is hypertonic dysfunction. Fetal heart rate must be carefully monitored, and other signs of distress, such as meconium-stained amniotic fluid, noted. Occasionally in cases of hypertonic dysfunction, membranes will have been ruptured 24 hours or more without effective labor. In this situation, bacteria are likely to ascend into the uterus and give rise to infection. This is *intrapartal infection* and is a serious complication. It is signaled by a rise in temperature, often in association with a chill.

Because of the danger of intrapartal infection, it is customary to take temperatures every two hours in patients whose labors have lasted more than 24 hours or who have ruptured membranes. Even an elevation of half a degree should be reported at once to the physician. Intrapartal infection is much more likely to occur if the membranes have been ruptured for a long time. As previously stated, treatment is usually in the form of antibiotics. Cesarean section is resorted to if fetal distress occurs.

Hypotonic Dysfunction

After the onset of true labor, contractions in hypotonic dysfunction decrease in strength and the tone of the uterine muscles is less than usual. Minimum uterine tension during the resting stage is about 8 to 12 mm. Hg in the normally functioning uterus, while normal labor contractions reach an intrauterine pressure of 50 to 60 mm. Hg at acme. These values are reduced in hypotonic dysfunction, and contractions are not strong enough to affect dilatation. Contractions may become farther apart and irregular.

Dysfunction often is nature's protection against pelvic contraction and abnormal fetal position, and signifies the need for careful assessment for these factors. Thorough vaginal examination to determine position of the presenting part, dimensions of the pelvis, and state of the cervix will usually be done by the obstetrician. The cervix will be at least 3 cm. dilated if the diagnosis of hypotonic dysfunction in the active phase of labor is correct. X-ray pelvimetry is often done for accurate measurement of the pelvis and to confirm abnormal fetal position or abnormalities of development.

This condition usually occurs in the accelerated or active phase, or even during the second stage of labor; the contractions become infrequent and of

TABLE 33-1
CRITERIA FOR DIFFERENTIATING DYSFUNCTIONAL LABOR

Criteria	Hypertonic	Hypotonic
Phase of Labor	Latent	Active
Symptoms	Painful	Painless
Fetal Distress	Early	Late
Medication:		
Oxytocin	Unfavorable reaction	Favorable reaction
Sedation	Helpful	Little value

Modified from Pritchard, J. A. and P. C. McDonald: *Williams Obstetrics,* ed. 15. New York, Appleton-Century Crofts, 1976, p. 659.

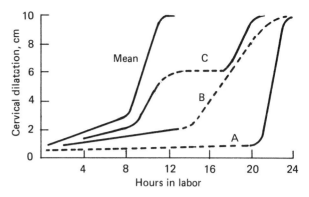

Figure 33-3. The major labor aberrations shown in comparison with the mean cervical dilatation time curve for nulliparae. (*a*) prolonged latent phase; (*b*) protracted active phase dilatation; (*c*) secondary arrest of dilatation. (From Friedman, E.: *Greenhill Obstetrics,* ed. 13.)

poor quality, and the uterus is easily indentable at the acme of a contraction.

Friedman describes two types of dysfunction that can occur at this time. *Active phase dysfunction* is recognized by a maximum slope phase of less than 1.2 cm. of dilatation per hour in the primigravid patient or less than 1.5 cm. in the multigravida (Fig. 33-3). The majority of these patients, with supportive fluids, reassurance and *minimum* sedation go on to dilate fully although more slowly than is optimal. However, about 10 percent will develop the most serious dysfunction, *secondary arrest dysfunction.* This occurs when there is no cervical dilatation for two or more hours in the active phase of labor. Cephalopelvic disproportion is suspected in these cases.[16]

Treatment. Early and accurate diagnosis of hypotonic dysfunction is a major factor in reducing fetal death and injury. If a marked degree of disproportion exists or if there is an uncorrectable malposition, then cesarean section will be employed to effect delivery. If these conditions are not present, stimulation of labor is generally the treatment of choice rather than "watchful waiting" for more effective labor to resume spontaneously. The main reason for this is the increased perinatal loss and injury which accompany unduly prolonged first or second stages of labor.

If membranes are intact, initial treatment may include artificial rupture. This procedure alone may stimulate effective labor contractions.

Oxytocin augmentation, however, is usually resorted to when strong, regular contractions with progressive effacement and dilatation or fetal descent fail to occur, or if membranes are already ruptured. Ten units of oxytocin are mixed with 1,000 ml. of 5 percent glucose in a balanced salt solution or water for controlled intravenous drip. Initially the infusion is begun at a flow of 2 mU. oxytocin per minute. This amount will not initiate tetanic contractions in true hypotonic dysfunction unless there is hypersensitivity to the drug. Contractions and fetal heart rate are carefully evaluated, and if no problems develop, the infusion can be gradually increased up to 20 mU. oxytocin. Flows above this rate are rarely necessary, for if effective contractions are not initiated by this dosage of oxytocin, greater amounts are also unlikely to do so and present serious dangers to both the baby and the mother.

A constant infusion pump is often used to administer oxytocin, as this method enhances the precision of dosage. The *Harvard pump* or *Ivac peristaltic pump* are two types in common use. The oxytocin solution in a separate bottle flows into a syringe mounted on the pump, which delivers an exact amount of solution depending on the drip rate set. This solution can be piggybacked into a plain glucose infusion, if the two-bottle set-up is used. Although the pump method allows more precise regulation of the oxytocin flow than simply adjusting clamps attached to the intravenous tubing, both approaches require constant and careful monitoring. Clamps can slip and the pump can malfunction. The dangers of an excessive dosage of oxytocin include uterine tetany with resultant fetal hypoxia, or rupture of the uterus with fetal anoxia and maternal hemorrhage and shock.

Oxytocin stimulation is contraindicated in cases of fetal-pelvic disproportion, overdistension of the uterus, and great parity (para 5 and over). Signs of fetal distress must be carefully watched for, and the infusion immediately slowed or stopped if these occur. Use of external or internal monitors is often mandatory when oxytocin stimulation of labor is employed. With internal monitoring, the strength of contractions as well as continual rate of the fetal heart may be constantly evaluated.

Occasionally intramuscular or buccal oxytocin is used, but these methods do not allow accurate control of blood levels, either to accomplish effective contractions or to avoid dangers of excessive dosage.

Sparteine sulfate (Tocosamine) sometimes is used as an alternative to oxytocin to stimulate labor. It is given in repeated doses until satisfactory uterine action is achieved; however, there are limits to the total dosage that can be used and it is not as safe or effective as oxytocin.

Complications. Untreated hypotonic uterine dysfunction exposes the mother to the dangers of exhaustion, dehydration, and intrapartum infection. Signs of fetal distress often do not appear until intrapartum infection has developed. While treatment of intrauterine infections with antibiotics offers protection to the mother, this is of little value to the fetus. Nursing observations include assessment of the mother for signs of infection, as previously discussed.

Nursing Care

In addition to observing and reporting the maternal and fetal conditions as noted above, nursing care includes offering explanations to the parents and providing emotional support.

Psychosocial support. Labors of this type are extremely discouraging for the mother and the father. The diagnostic procedures as well as the therapy will take a certain amount of time, and carrying out these measures will require patience and waiting on the part of everyone concerned.

It is essential that the couple know and understand this fact. The physician and the nurse need to spend sufficient time with the parents to explain what is happening in depth and in terms that are appropriate for them. It is very possible that repeated reinforcement of the explanations, progress, and so on will be needed. Feedback from the parents should be encouraged, so that their level of understanding and acceptance can be ascertained. The normal tension and anxiety found in any labor certainly will be intensified, and it is important that it not be compounded by fantasy or misunderstanding.

Since dysfunctional labor is so variable, it is often impossible (and unwise) to give the parents any definite reassurances as to when effective labor will commence. Yet some kind of boundaries must be placed on when this ineffective phase will end and progress will begin, so that the mother will have some goal to look forward to and to work for. Therefore, it is important to reassure the patient, reminding her that her case is not unique (patients think after many hours that theirs is the longest labor in obstetric history), that certain specific measures are known and can be taken to help effective labor to begin, and that competent medical and nursing care will be given throughout labor.

An explanation of the plan for treatment will enable the parents to anticipate more realistically what is in store and therefore reassures them that certain definite measures are available and are being employed.

Comfort Measures. In addition, all the comfort measures which promote relaxation should be utilized. Sponge baths, various positioning, soothing backrubs, clean, dry linen, quiet conversation, reading or other diversionary activities as well as a quiet restful environment are all appropriate. However, isolating the patient in a dark room on the premise that she needs sleep or rest only contributes to her fear unless she is actually sleeping, and then frequent observations are needed to see when she awakens. Human contact is one of the most important items of "treatment" in cases of complicated labor and should never be neglected. The presence of the same person, nurse and/or physician, is very helpful for the reasons already mentioned in Chapter 23. Coaching the mother in breathing patterns and relaxation techniques also will conserve her strength.

The physician may want the patient to have fluids by mouth, or may order intravenous infusions to maintain hydration and electrolyte balance. A total of 2,000 ml. or more of intravenous fluid may be given in 24 hours.

Oxytocin Monitoring. If oxytocin stimulation of labor is used, the patient must have someone in attendance at all times during the infusion. Uterine contractions and fetal heart tones are to be monitored continuously. Maternal blood pressure and pulse are checked every half hour. As the physician specifies the dosage, the nurse (or other attendant) ascertains that the infusion is running at the prescribed drops per minute and reports any maternal or fetal aberrations immediately. Many institutions have an "Oxytocin Record" or a "Pitocin Sheet" which provides space for recording times, amount and frequency of the oxytocin given, fetal heart tones, maternal blood pressure and pulse, frequency, intensity and length of contractions, and other relevant comments. This type of sheet gives an easily accessible record of the patient's progress during the infusion.

Recording and reporting the physiologic signs and symptoms cannot be stressed enough during these infusions. However, supportive care is also to be maintained. Adequate explanation and reassurance can be given, and since the nurse will be with the mother continuously this time can be utilized to good advantage to establish a relationship of

NURSING CARE PRIORITIES FOR PATIENTS WITH DYSFUNCTIONAL LABOR*

Assessment	Intervention	Evaluation
Monitor level of fatigue and ability to cope with pain	Stay with patient or have partner stay continually. Help patient relax between contractions. Record and report behavior.	Patient works with contraction Exhaustion avoided Panic and discouragement alleviated
	Assist as needed with effleurage, concentration and/or distraction for pain management. Reassure, explain labor progress and support as indicated. Provide quiet environment.	
Determine hydration level	Monitor intravenous fluids for infiltration. Check condition of lips, skin for dryness.	Dehydration avoided
Bladder hygiene	Encourage patient to void frequently. Catheterize as necessary.	Bladder distention avoided
Vital signs	TPR and BP of 2° or more frequently as indicated	Secondary infection avoided/alleviated
Monitor oxytocin and/or antibiotics if necessary	Record all contractions and FHR; report as necessary; give and record administration of antibiotics if indicated.	Labor progress Tetanic contractions avoided, fetal distress avoided

*In addition to nursing care for normal labor, with these priorities to be considered uppermost.

rapport. While the infusion will stimulate contractions (and therefore, discomfort), the mother and her partner often look upon this treatment optimistically, for it marks the end of a desultory, ineffective period in labor and brings with it promise of termination of a difficult time. This positive attitude can be especially reinforced if the nurse provides explanation and assurance.

Abnormal Fetal Positions

Persistent Occiput Posterior Positions

The fetal head usually enters the pelvis inlet transversely and therefore must traverse an arc of 90° in the process of internal rotation to the direct occiput anterior position. (See Fig. 7-3, p. 70).

In about a quarter of all labors, however, the head enters the pelvis with the occiput directed diagonally posterior, that is, in either the R.O.P. or the L.O.P. position. Under these circumstances the head must rotate through an arc of 135° in the process of internal rotation.

With good contractions, adequate flexion and a baby of average size, the great majority of these cases of occiput posterior position undergo spontaneous rotation through the 135° arc as soon as the head reaches the pelvic floor. This is a normal mechanism of labor. It must be remembered, however, that labor is usually prolonged, and the mother has a great deal of discomfort in her back as the baby's head impinges against the sacrum in the course of rotating.

Nursing intervention is aimed at relieving the back pain as much as possible. Sacral pressure, backrubs and frequent change of position from side to side can be helpful, and they should be employed to the degree that seems to be well-tolerated by the patient.

In a majority of cases, however (perhaps 5 percent), these favorable circumstances do not exist, and rotation may be incomplete or may not take place at all. If rotation is incomplete, the head becomes arrested in the transverse position, a condition known as *transverse arrest*. If anterior rotation does not take place at all, the occiput usually rotates to the direct occiput posterior position, a condition known as *persistent occiput posterior*. Both transverse arrest and persistent occiput posterior position represent deviations from the normal mechanisms of labor.

Some controversy persists in the management of persistent occiput posterior. When labor progresses, although first and second stages tend to be prolonged in primigravidas, management is the same as for occiput anterior positions and results in no increased risk to the fetus. Premature operative intervention, particularly if the station is high, seems contraindicated. Forceps rotation on the perineum is appropriate to reduce lacerations if this can be easily accomplished.[17]

Sometimes the mechanical problem associated with abnormal uterine action is an abnormal position of the presenting head. Hence, these conditions of posterior or transverse arrest of the occiput appear to have, in some cases, an adverse effect on uterine behavior. Here the malposition is the cause rather than the effect of uterine inefficiency. This conclusion can be verified by the following findings. 1) When the fetal head is rotated or rotates spontaneously, uterine action improves. 2) Oxytocin therapy for dysfunction associated with an occipitoposterior position does not cause the infant's head to rotate.

It should be remembered that the uterus of the multigravid patient usually reacts to mechanical obstruction by becoming more active and ultimately rupturing itself. On the other hand, when the primigravid uterus encounters resistance it nearly always responds by inertia or incoordinate behavior. It is imperative, then, that the obstetrician rule out mechanical obstruction before deciding that labor is prolonged due to idiopathic faulty uterine action. Since disproportion may be slight and therefore easily overlooked, only the most careful observation and study can disclose the important association between faulty uterine action and smallness of the pelvis or large size of the baby. The nurse can make an important contribution in this diagnosis by her continuous and critical observations of the character and frequency of the contractions, the amount of the mother's discomfort, her vital signs and general condition, and the fetal heart rate.

Breech Presentations

The breech is the presenting part in 3 to 4 percent of deliveries and is more common when the baby is premature or there is multiple gestation. The reasons for breech presentations are not always apparent, although associated factors include great parity, twinning, hydramnios, hydrocephalus, and placenta previa. Recent studies indicate no positive correlation between breech presentation and contracted pelvis.

Possible Complications. There is no significantly increased danger for the life of the mother in breech presentations, although there is increased incidence of lacerations of the birth canal, episiotomy extensions, cesarean sections, and postpartum infections. Labor is not prolonged, contrary to previous belief.[18]

For the infant, however, there is considerably increased risk of both death and injury in comparison to vertex presentations. Uncorrected perinatal loss is about 12 percent in the United States, and when corrected for congenital anomalies and maternal disease, fetal loss is still three times higher in single breech than in vertex. Traumatic morbidity is 12 times higher, including fractures, dislocations, and peripheral nerve injuries.[19] Although pulmonary morbidity (pneumonitis, atelectasis, or respiratory distress syndrome) occurs with similar frequency in both breech and vertex, brain damage from asphyxia resulting in neurological abnormalities at one year is increased in breech infants.[20]

The major cause of perinatal death is trauma sustained in delivery. Tentorial tears and subsequent intracranial hemorrhage are twice as common in breech presentations as they are in cephalic presentations. The symptoms and nursing care associated with these conditions are discussed in Chapter 39. Lesions of the spinal cord and extrusion of the medulla into the foramen magnum also account for a large portion of deaths. In footling presentations (Fig.33-4C), prolapse of the umbilical cord is common. Even in the most skilled hands, and considering only full-term infants, about 1 breech infant in 15 succumbs as the result of delivery.

Unrecognized fetopelvic disproportion is the primary cause of the increase in perinatal mortality and morbidity in breech deliveries. Recommendations for medical management to reduce these complications include accurate x-ray pelvimetry, at least mean normal pelvic measurements and fetal size to permit trial labor, constant monitoring of fetal heart rate for signs of asphyxia, and cesarean section for estimated fetal size of above 8.5 pounds, minimal fetopelvic disproportion, failure to progress in labor, and signs of fetal distress.[21]

Classification. Breech presentations are classified as follows:

1. *Complete:* the buttocks present with the feet and legs flexed on the thighs and the thighs flexed on the abdomen (Fig. 33-4A).
2. *Frank:* the buttocks present with the hips flexed and the legs extended against the abdomen and chest (Fig. 33-4B). This is the most common type of breech presentation.
3. *Incomplete:* one or both feet or the knees extend below the buttocks (Fig. 33-4C). This type of presentation is also known as a single or double footling breech (Fig. 33-5).
4. *Compound:* the buttocks present together with another part such as a hand.

Mechanism of Labor in Breech Delivery

If the powers, passage and passenger are of adequate capacity and functioning properly, delivery in a breech presentation will progress at about the same rate as in vertex presentations. Descent will be slower initially in the case of a breech but among patients with similar parity, dilatation and effacement are approximately the same for breech and

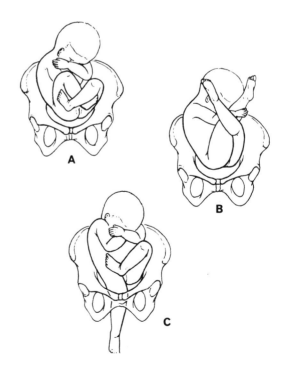

Figure 33-4. Breech presentation may be (A) complete breech, (B) frank breech, and (C) an incomplete or footling breech.

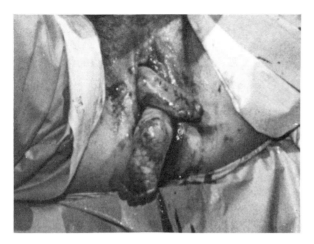

Figure 33-5. Double footling breech. (From the film *Human Birth,* published by J. B. Lippincott Co., Philadelphia.)

vertex presentations. Whether spontaneous or assisted, the delivery of the fetus is most efficiently accomplished when the largest planes of the fetus descend into the largest planes of the pelvis. The mechanism of delivery is as follows:

1. *Descent* of the breech basilic diameter through the pelvic inlet usually occurs in the oblique plane with the fetal anterior hip leading (Fig. 33-6A).
2. *Internal rotation* toward the AP plane of the pelvis occurs as pelvic muscle resistance is met and the posterior hip then descends as *lateral flexion* of the fetal back occurs (Fig. 33-6B).
3. *Delivery and external rotation* of the hips to the lateral back-up position occur as the bisacromial plane of the shoulders enter the pelvis in the oblique maternal plane (Fig. 33-6C).
4. The descending shoulders are delivered after the arms in the AP plane (Fig. 33-6D). The anterior shoulder descends to behind the symphysis and the posterior shoulder descends into the hollow of the sacrum with resultant *lateral flexion* (Fig. 33-6E). In a spontaneous delivery, the posterior shoulder and arm may be delivered next, which allows the body to drop posteriorly and the anterior shoulder to be delivered from behind the symphysis. Next the flexed head descends, internally rotates to the AP plane (Fig. 33-6F) and is delivered by flexion (Fig. 33-6G). The obstetrician may assist this by slightly extending the infant's body to allow easier flexion of the head.[22]

Delivery

There is becoming more of a consensus that cesarean section should be used liberally, especially if there is dysfunctional labor, prematurity, or small pelvis[23,24] since the perinatal mortality and morbidity is so high in this kind of presentation. In those instances when delivery is attempted vaginally, especially in the primigravida, it is often necessary for the physician to perform a partial or complete breech extraction.

Selection of a Delivery Method. Occasionally there is no choice of delivery method if the patient arrives in the labor suite when delivery is imminent. Thus physicians need to be skilled in atraumatic vaginal delivery techniques. Cesarean section will be utilized for such conditions as acute fetal distress, abruptio placentae, placenta previa, cord prolapse, dysfunctional labor and those conditions directly related to the breech presentation.[25]

Vaginal Delivery. Several scoring systems are utilized to evaluate the feasibility of vaginal delivery in breech presentations. The Zatuchni-Andros system and its modifications are used extensively (Table 33-2). These systems give an estimate of whether the shoulders and head can traverse the pelvis without undue delay when the fetus is maintained in the most advantageous position. Some investigators have reported the effectiveness of low scores in predicting infants at risk for mortality and morbidity, prolonged labor, and eventual cesarean section. A score of three or less will justify a section. A score of four will require further observation and subsequent evaluation. A score of five will hopefully result in a successful vaginal delivery. Unfortunately, serious fetal morbidity, mortality, and low Apgar scores are found with vaginal delivery of patients with high Zatuchni-Andros scores in whom CPD is not a problem. Moreover, dysfunctional labor and resuscitation of the infant frequently accompany vaginal delivery. Thus, in many tertiary care centers, breech presentation is an indication for cesarean section in term or near term primigravidae, in multiparae with a fetus estimated at 7½ lbs. when labor is desultory or when complications are apparent.[26] [27,28]

Vaginal delivery has been classified according to the amount of professional assistance that is required to effect delivery.

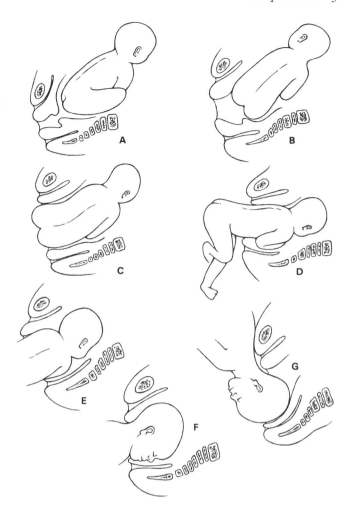

Figure 33-6. Movements of the breech-presenting fetus during labor and delivery.

A *spontaneous breech delivery* is one in which the mother essentially delivers herself in a more or less emergency situation (i.e., en route to the hospital) or is found in the labor room with her infant delivered. This latter case indicates sheer neglect on the part of the staff. This type of delivery is often found with premature labor.

An *assisted breech delivery* requires minimal intervention from the physician. The mother may be a multipara in strong labor who has made optimal

TABLE 33-2
ZATUCHNI-ANDROS PROGNOSTIC INDEX*

	Points		
	0	*1*	*2*
Parity	Primigravida	Multipara	
Gestational age	39 weeks or more	38 weeks	37 weeks or less
Estimated fetal weight	8 pounds (3630 gm.)	7–7 15/16 pounds (3629–3176 gm.)	< 7 pounds (3173 gm.)
Previous breech†	0	1	2 or more
Dilation‡	2 cm.	3 cm.	4 cm. of more
Station‡	−3 or higher	−2	−1 or lower

   * Zatuchni G. I., Andros, G. J.: "Prognostic index for vaginal delivery in breech presentation." *Am. J. Obstet. Gynecol.* 98: 854, 1967.
   † Greater than 2500 gm.
   ‡ Determined by vaginal examination on admission.

progress. Her infant may be smaller than average.

Partial breech extraction requires the assistance of the physician with delivery of the shoulders and head (Fig. 33-7).

The following steps are usually performed:

1. The cord is extracted to prevent compression as soon as the umbilicus appears, after the feet and legs have been delivered. If there is a short cord or nuchal cord, it is doubly clamped and cut.
2. After delivery of the cord, a deep *mediolateral* episiotomy is done to prevent tearing and to minimize perineal resistance. A midline episiotomy is contraindicated in a breech extraction because of the danger of extension into surrounding structures.
3. The infant's trunk is wrapped in a towel to provide warmth and prevent slippage when traction is applied. Traction together with slight rotation results in the bisacromial diameter of the infant coming into the AP plane of the maternal pelvis. The posterior shoulder can then be delivered by inserting two fingers into the vagina and elevating the fetus upward toward the mother's inguinal area. The posterior shoulder then rests on the perineum, the arm and hand are delivered and the anterior arm can be extracted with the fingers. If the infant has an arm extended above the head, it can be passed downward across the chest by passing two fingers over the shoulder. Rough traction on the arm is to be avoided since neurological damage can result.
4. The aftercoming head may be delivered by application of the Piper forceps (Chapter 34) or by the Mauriceau-Smellie-Veit or the Bracht maneuvers.
   a. In the Mauriceau-Smellie-Veit maneuver, the fetus is placed astride the physician's left arm. Two fingers of the left hand are placed firmly over the mandibles to flex the head. The right hand is placed over the back, with the fingers over the shoulders to guide the shoulders and head. The torso is elevated slowly with flexion of the head maintained by the maxillary pressure. Suprapubic pressure is applied by an assistant during these maneuvers to aid the descent of the head into the pelvis and eventually with the suprapubic and maxillary pressure, the occiput is delivered (Fig. 33-8).[29]
   b. In the Bracht maneuver, the back is gently arched toward the mother's abdomen when the scapulas are seen. The arms then tend to deliver spontaneously. Suprapubic pressure is applied to assist descent of the head into the pelvis and the suspended body continues to be brought *slowly* to the mother's abdomen. The face and occiput should then deliver spontaneously. This maneuver requires no intravaginal invasion or traction and hence is often preferred. However, if the infant is not in the right position or tries to breathe before the head is delivered, or the mother cannot work with the operators, this is not the maneuver of choice.

A *complete breech extraction* also may be called "decomposing" or "breaking up" a breech or a total breech extraction. As the name implies, the small parts are rearranged so that labor resumes and progress can be made. Decomposition may be effected in a frank breech by bringing the legs down for traction by means of *Pinard's* maneuver. Here the physician's hand is inserted into the vagina and the thigh is abducted, which causes the knee to flex. The foot is grasped and delivered (see Fig. 34-6). Traction is applied downward and if the buttocks descend, delivery can proceed as previously described. If the breech does not descend, the other foot may be extracted.[30]

Anesthesia. Many physicians prefer local or pudendal anesthesia since it does not interfere with labor and allows the mother to participate actively. Epidural anesthesia is also preferred for these reasons and also because it permits comfortable intravaginal manipulation and extraction. Some physicians prefer a general anesthetic such as halothane if the breech must be decomposed, since these agents inhibit uterine contractions and intravaginal manipulation is easier. Both conduction and general anesthesia have been used successfully for cesarean section.

Nursing Care

The nurse will want to be extremely meticulous in her monitoring of the mother. This means not just relying on electronic equipment, but also frequent physical checks, comfort measures and explanations to the parents.

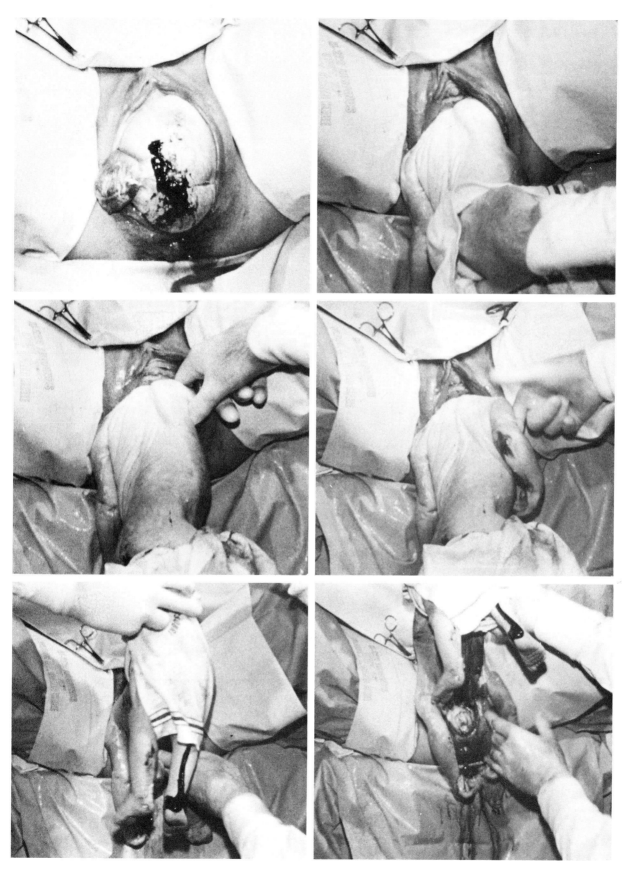

Figure 33-7. Partial breech extraction. (From the film *Human Birth*, published by J. B. Lippincott Co., Philadelphia.)

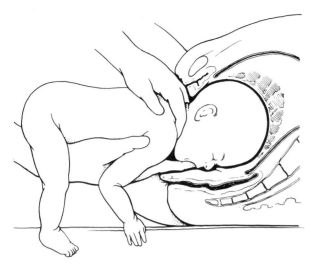

Figure 33-8. Mauriceau maneuver for extracting head in breech delivery.

In breech presentation the infant often passes meconium from the rectum during the course of labor, and after the membranes are ruptured, and the liquor amnii has escaped, the nurse may find the black, tar-colored material coming from the patient's vagina. She needs to ascertain that the presentation is, in fact, a breech, for if such a phenomenon occurred in a vertex presentation, it would be an indication of probable fetal distress.

Explanation and appropriate reassurance are important for mothers who have breech presentations, as they are for any patient having an abnormal presentation or complicated labor of any type. Many patients are steeped in old wives' folklore of the fearfulness of a breech birth and become exceedingly anxious and terrified as soon as they find out (or overhear) that theirs is this type of presentation; the same is often true of their partners, and the anxiety and fear that are communicated between them can impede the patient's working effectively with her labor. With modern obstetric techniques and knowledge, labor need not be prolonged or exceptionally painful.

Shoulder, Face, and Brow Presentations

In shoulder presentations the infant lies crosswise in the uterus instead of longitudinally (see Fig. 21-2). This complication occurs about once in every 300 cases and is seen most often in multiparae. Not

infrequently an arm prolapses into the vagina, making the problem of delivery even more difficult.

Shoulder presentation is a serious complication, with a slightly increased maternal mortality rate and an extremely high perinatal mortality with vaginal delivery—about 30 percent for term infants. External version in late pregnancy or early labor is occasionally successful, especially in multiparae, in converting the shoulder to a longitudinal lie. Internal podalic version and extraction is a very hazardous procedure (see Chapter 34), the second most common cause of rupture of the uterus, and associated with high perinatal mortality. Its use is justified only in carefully selected cases. Virtually all transverse presentations should be delivered by cesarean section, which reduces perinatal mortality to about 4 percent.

Face presentations are seen in about one out of 600 patients. Factors that favor extension of the head and prevent flexion are implicated in these presentations, a contracted pelvis being paramount among these. These infants may deliver spontaneously if labor is effective and the pelvis is adequate. The face will come through the vulva with the chin anterior. However, if there is indication that the pelvis is contracted or that there is fetal distress, cesarean section is employed for delivery. As edema of the scalp is common in vertex presentations; facial edema is often present to the extent that the landmarks resemble a breech presentation. The edema and purplish discoloration disappear within a few days but the infant's appearance gives the parents a great deal of concern. The nurse can be very helpful in reassuring the parents that the condition is temporary and will resolve without sequelae.

Brow presentations are somewhat more rare than the other malpresentations. They are impossible to deliver as long as the brow presentation persists since the largest diameter of the fetal head, the occipitomental, presents. They are, however, an unstable presentation, and often spontaneously covert to an occiput or face presentation. The same etiological factors that underlie a face presentation pertain here. The principles of treatment are the same as for face presentations. If the labor is progressing and it is not unduly vigorous and there is no fetal distress in the closely monitored infant, no intervention is necessary. If labor does become tumultuous or more likely desultory, then prompt cesarean section is indicated.[31]

Cephalopelvic Disproportion

Contracted Pelvis

Disproportion between the size of the infant and that of the birth canal (commonly spoken of as cephalopelvic disproportion) is caused most frequently by contracted pelvis. The pelvis may be contracted at the inlet, the midpelvis or the outlet. In the case of inlet contraction, the anteroposterior diameter of the inlet is shortened to 10 cm. or less, or the greatest transverse diameter is 12 cm. or less. The sacrum is broader and less concave from side to side, thinner from behind forward and shorter from above downward.

Inlet contraction is most often due to rickets, a fact indicating how much good may be accomplished by the prevention of rickets in infants and children through an adequate intake of vitamin D. Contracted pelvis due to rickets has been found to be more common among black peoples than among whites.

In midpelvic contraction, the distance between the ischial spines is diminished; it is often found in conjunction with outlet contraction. In outlet contraction, the angle formed by the pubic rami is narrow, and the ischial tuberosities are close together; it thus resembles a male pelvis insofar as the outlet is concerned. This type of pelvic contraction occurs with equal frequency in white and black peoples, but its cause is not known. It is not only likely to hinder the egress of the infant at the outlet but also may be responsible for deep lacerations, since the narrow pubic rami tend to push the infant's head posteriorly in the direction of the rectum.

One purpose of antepartal care is to detect pelvic contraction during pregnancy, so that—long before labor begins—some intelligent decision can be reached about how best to deliver the infant. Of course, in a case of extreme pelvic contraction, cesarean section is obligatory. But all gradients of contracted pelvis are encountered, and, depending on the size of the infant and other factors, many patients with moderate degrees of the condition can be delivered vaginally with care.

In doubtful cases, the physician may give the patient a "trial labor," that is, four to six hours of labor to ascertain whether or not with adequate contractions the head will pass through the pelvis. For these patients labor may be even more anxiety-provoking than usual (depending in part on the extent and the depth of supportive antepartal counseling), and if cesarean section is the ultimate outcome, there may be a great deal of disappointment and perhaps even a feeling of failure. The warm empathic attitude of the nurse is particularly needed with these patients. Frequent reports on the progress of labor should not be overlooked when the progress is favorable; if it is not, then explanation and anticipatory guidance regarding cesarean section may be given. The health team does the patient a disservice in avoiding the subject if progress is not made in labor.

Oversized Baby

Excessive size of the infant is not commonly a cause of serious dystocia unless the fetus weighs over 4,500 gm. (10 pounds). About 1 infant in 138 will fall into this class. The trauma associated with the passage of such huge infants through the birth canal causes a decided increase in fetal mortality; this has been estimated as 13 percent (almost 1 in 7), in contrast with the usual death rate of 4 percent for normal-size infants. Uterine dysfunction is frequent in labors with excessive-size infants because the head becomes not only larger but harder and less malleable with increasing weight. Even though these infants are born alive, they often do poorly in the first few days because of a variety of conditions.

Excessive size of the fetus is usually due to maternal diabetes, large size of one or both parents, or multiparity. Postmaturity due to prolonged gestation is not thought to be an important cause of excessive-size infants. Tremendously large infants, weighing over 13 pounds, are extremely rare, and almost all are born dead. Most oversized babies are boys. Although studies have shown a relationship between maternal diet and growth and survival of the fetus, it is doubtful that strict regulation of diet during pregnancy can significantly reduce excessive growth of the infant. However, large women who are heavy may tend to have excessive weight gain during pregnancy and also larger babies, and in this way weight gain is associated with large babies.

Shoulder Dystocia. One serious complication of an oversized infant is shoulder dystocia. After the head has passed through the pelvic canal, the infant's unusually large shoulders may arrest at either the pelvic brim or the outlet. The incidence of shoulder dystocia is 1.7 percent in infants over 4,000 gm., with mortality of about 16 percent. The time between delivery of the head and delivery of the body must be short to ensure an uncompromised fetus: A large mediolateral episiotomy and adequate anesthesia are mandatory. The infant's nose and mouth are cleared. Then, without using force, the physician sweeps the posterior arm across the chest and delivers it. The shoulder girdle is then rotated into one of the oblique pelvis diameters. At this time the anterior shoulder can usually be delivered. Care must be taken not to apply vigorous traction on the head or neck or to excessively rotate the body. Occasionally deliberate fracture of the clavicle is necessary to save the infant's life.[32]

Hydrocephalus

Hydrocephalus, or an excessive accumulation of cerebrospinal fluid in the ventricles of the brain with consequent enlargement of the cranium, is encountered in approximately 1 fetus in 2,000 and accounts for some 12 percent of all malformations at birth. Associated defects are common, spina bifida being present in about one-third of the cases. Varying degrees of cranial enlargement are produced, and not infrequently the circumference of the head exceeds 50 cm., sometimes reaching 80 cm. The amount of fluid present is usually between 500 and 1,500 ml., but as much as 5 liters has been reported. Since the distended cranium is too large to fit into the pelvic inlet, breech presentations are exceedingly common, being observed in about one-third of such cases.

Whatever the presentation, gross disproportion between the size of the head and that of the pelvis is the rule, and serious dystocia is the usual consequence. This is a tragic and serious complication of labor, with diagnosis based on nography and x-ray.

The obstetrician will find it necessary, as a rule, to puncture the cranial vault and aspirate as much of the cerebrospinal fluid as may be necessary to permit delivery. This procedure in itself does not injure the child. Nevertheless, fetal mortality is as high as 70 percent (this percentage includes very mild forms of the disease).

Births of this type are a terrible tragedy for all concerned; the mother must undergo a difficult labor at great risk to herself, the father will suffer with her, the fetus may expire, and the physician and the nurse must cope with a grave crisis with a poor prognosis. It is often difficult to describe the emotional climate at this time; perhaps it is impossible if one has not experienced a similar loss or disappointment. A state of emotional shock prevails, in which disbelief, noncomprehension and, sometimes, denial prevail. This is a situation in which the nurse will be called on to exercise nursing skill to the utmost, not only during labor but after the delivery, and particularly if there is an obvious abnormality, or if a fetal demise occurs. The components of care that are useful in helping the parents in such a crisis are discussed fully in Chapter 39.

HEMORRHAGIC COMPLICATIONS

Hemorrhage is probably a more important cause of maternal death in the United States than statistics

NURSING CARE PRIORITIES IN ABNORMAL PRESENTATIONS

Assessment	Intervention	Evaluation
Meticulous attention to the status of the mother and infant.	Remain with patient. Check electronic monitor frequently for signs of uterine contractions and fetal distress.	Labor progress; fetus uncompromised
Comfort measures	Frequent backrubs, linen change, oral hygiene as tolerated. Sacral pressure as appropriate in back labors	Patient relatively comfortable
Orientation to continuing labor	Reassurance and explanation as indicated	Discouragement/panic alleviated
Determine hydration level	Monitor IV if present. Check skin and lips for dryness.	Dehydration avoided
Bladder hygiene	Encourage frequent voiding. Catheterize as necessary.	Bladder undistended

indicate, because national vital statistics are based only on the *immediate* cause of death. A woman who hemorrhaged after labor, contracted postpartum infection, and died would be classified as a death due to infection, although hemorrhage was the real underlying cause. The major causes of hemorrhage associated with childbearing are placenta previa and abruptio (see Chapter 31) and uterine atony.

Postpartum Hemorrhage

Hemorrhage during the postpartum period is the most common cause of serious blood loss associated with pregnancy, and it causes about one-fourth of all maternal deaths from hemorrhagic complications. The debilitation and lowered resistance which often accompany it are related to postpartum infections, another leading cause of maternal death. To a large extent, death from postpartum hemorrhage is preventable if the condition is diagnosed early and treated aggressively.

Definition and Incidence

Postpartum hemorrhage is commonly defined as loss of more than 500 cc. of blood during the first 24 hours after giving birth. However, ordinary blood loss following vaginal delivery frequently is more than 500 cc. by accurate measurement. Most obstetricians estimate the amount of bleeding at delivery, and studies show that estimated blood loss is usually only about one-half of actual loss. Therfore, an *estimated* blood loss over 500 cc. serves to alert the nurse and physician that the patient has bled excessively and is in danger of postpartum hemorrhage.

Bleeding of this degree occurs once in every 20 or 30 cases despite the most skilled care. Hemorrhages of 1,000 cc. and over are encountered once in about every 75 cases, whereas blood losses of even 1,500 and 2,000 cc. are encountered less frequently. Postpartum hemorrhage is a fairly common complication of labor. Moreover, it is one with which the nurse must be intimately familiar, as nurses are expected to assume an important role in the prevention and treatment of the condition.

Causes

In order of frequency, the three immediate causes of postpartum hemorrhage are:

1. Uterine atony.
2. Lacerations of the perineum, the vagina and the cervix.
3. Retained placental fragments.

Clotting defects, uterine tumors and infections, as well as obstetrical accidents such as inversion of the uterus, can also be classified as causes, but they are less common and are of a more indirect nature.

Uterine Atony. Uterine atony is by far the most common cause of postpartum hemorrhage. The uterus contains huge blood vessels within the interstices of its muscle fibers, and those at the placental site are open and gaping. It is essential that the muscle fibers contract down tightly on these arteries and veins if bleeding is to be controlled. They must *stay* contracted down, because relaxation for only a few seconds will give rise to sudden, profuse hemorrhage. They must stay *tightly* contracted down, because continuous, slight relaxation gives rise to continuous oozing of blood, one of the most treacherous forms of postpartum hemorrhage.

In a study of 56 maternal deaths from pregnancy-related hemorrhage over a nine-year period in California, 19 were due to uterine atony. The majority of these women died within four hours of delivery, possibly before the seriousness of their bleeding was recognized. Generally, these patients were older multiparae with spontaneous term deliveries; most of their deaths were avoidable had the hemorrhage been diagnosed earlier and adequate blood and fibrinogen replacement been instituted in time. Most of their babies survived.[33]

Lacerations. Lacerations of the perineum, the vagina and the cervix are naturally more common after operative delivery. Tears of the cervix are particularly likely to cause serious hemorrhage. Bright red arterial bleeding in the presence of a hard, firmly contracted uterus (no uterine atony) suggests hemorrhage from a cervical laceration. The physician will establish the diagnosis by actual inspection of the cervix (retractors are necessary) and, after locating the source of bleeding, will repair the laceration.

Perineal and vaginal tears also contribute to postpartal blood loss. In addition, perineal tears may do great damage in destroying the integrity of the perineum and in weakening the supports of the uterus, the bladder and the rectum. Unless these lacerations are repaired properly, the resultant weakness, as the years go by, may cause prolapse of the uterus, cystocele (a pouching downward of the bladder) or rectocele (a pouching forward of the rectum). These conditions, which originate from perineal lacerations at childbirth, give rise to many discomforts and often necessitate operative treatment.

Lacerations of the birth canal sometimes occur during the process of normal delivery, and may be unavoidable even in the most skilled hands.

Retained Placental Fragments. Small, partially separated fragments of placenta may cause postpartum hemorrhage by interfering with proper uterine contraction. Careful inspection of the placenta to determine whether a piece is missing should be routinely carried out at delivery. If a portion is missing, exploration of the uterus is indicated to remove the placental fragment. In the case of continued postpartum bleeding, retention of placental fragments is generally ruled out by manual exploration. However, this is rarely a cause of immediate postpartum hemorrhage, and is more commonly implicated in late hemorrhage in which profuse bleeding occurs suddenly a week or more after delivery.

Predisposing Factors

There are certain factors which predispose to postpartum hemorrhage, so that to a certain extent it may be anticipated in advance. Among these, one of the most important is the size of the infant. With a 9-pound infant, the chances of postpartum hemorrhage are five times as great as they are with a 5-pound infant. Excessive bleeding is twice as common in twin pregnancy. Hydramnios (excessive amount of amniotic fluid) is another predisposing factor. It has been shown, however, that with the careful use of oxytocin in the placental stage and special care to achieve effective contraction in this stage, the incidence of hemorrhage due to overdistention can be reduced considerably.

Operative delivery with deep general anesthesia, prolonged labor with maternal exhaustion, and mismanagement of the third stage of labor greatly increase the likelihood of this complication. Other conditions in which postpartum hemorrhage is extremely frequent are high parity and premature separation of the placenta.

It should be noted also that a small woman withstands blood loss less well than a woman of average size or larger. An average-sized, relatively healthy mother can lose up to 1 percent of her blood volume without immediate crises. It is not difficult to relate body weight to blood volume since 1 mm. of blood equals 1 gm. Therefore, if a woman loses 1 percent of her body weight through blood loss, she is considered to have a hemorrhage.[34]

Hemorrhage and Shock

During any stage of pregnancy, hemorrhage poses a severe threat to the mother. This is especially true of postpartal hemorrhage, since the shock that accompanies the blood loss is often out of proportion to the amount lost.

Pathophysiology of Shock. When hemorrhaging occurs, the body activates certain compensatory mechanisms. The adrenals release catecholamines which cause the arterioles and venules of the skin, liver, gastrointestinal tract, lungs and kidneys to constrict. This diverts blood to the brain and heart. When shock persists, cellular oxygenation continues to be reduced, which results in accumulation of lactic acid and consequent acidosis. Serum acidosis in turn causes arteriole vasodilatation, but venule vasoconstriction persists. Thus, a downward spiral is established in which the decreased perfusion, increased tissue acidosis and anoxia, edema and blood pooling further decrease perfusion of the tissues. Eventually cellular death occurs and the patient dies.[35]

Clinical Picture. Excessive bleeding may occur prior to the birth of the placenta, but it is seen more commonly thereafter. Although it is occasionally torrential in character, the most common type is a continuous trickle—minute by minute. These small constant trickles are not alarming in appearance; consequently, no one may become concerned and no action may be taken.

Such hemorrhages are particularly treacherous for this reason. The condition and size of the patient determines the amount of blood loss which can be tolerated, with exhaustion from prolonged labor or antecedent anemia or chronic disease reducing the ability of the body to compensate. When hemorrhage has been profuse enough, the pulse becomes rapid and thready, the skin pallid and clammy; chills and disturbed vision occur. As shock deepens air hunger develops, with restlessness and sweating; then unconsciousness and death may follow. The pulse and blood pressure may not change significantly until large amounts of blood have been lost; then the vascular mechanism fails and shock ensues. Vascular collapse may lead to death when intravenous infusion cannot be maintained for blood replacement. Cardiac arrest may also occur at this point.

Treatment

If one suspects that a woman may be hemorrhaging, it is important that the nurse remain with her constantly. The fundus should be checked immediately. The physician will need to be notified and the emergency equipment made easily accessible, including intravenous fluid packs, tubing and large bore (#18) needles, oxygen equipment, retention catheter, suction, blood pressure and CVP apparatus. Signs of shock are to be monitored through the appropriate vital signs, skin, urinary output and level of consciousness (Fig. 33-9 and Table 33-3).[36]

The physician will ascertain the reason for the hemorrhage. If it is the result of vaginal or uterine injuries or retained placental fragments, the patient will be returned to the delivery room for repair or uterine evacuation. However, it is far more likely that uterine atony is to blame and the nurse plays a key role in managing this condition.

Massaging the Fundus. The uterus should be grasped immediately and massaged gently but firmly. The lower uterine segment is supported with the edge of the hand a little above the mother's symphysis, while the fundus is massaged with the other (Fig. 33-10). Thus the uterus is cupped between the two hands and is supported as it is massaged. Massage is to be continued until the uterus assumes a woody hardness; if the slightest relaxation occurs, the massage must be reinstituted. In many cases the uterus stays contracted most of the time but occasionally it relaxes; it is therefore obligatory to keep a hand on the fundus constantly for a full hour after bleeding has subsided. When the uterus is well contracted, care should be taken to *avoid overmassage,* because such practice contributes to muscle fatigue, which in turn further encourages uterine relaxation and excessive bleeding.

It must be remembered that relaxation sometimes occurs two or more hours after delivery; in these cases the uterus may balloon with blood, with very little escaping externally. Accordingly, the consistency, size and height of the uterus should be checked frequently until several hours have elapsed. Ordinarily, the height of the fundus after delivery will be about at the level of the umbilicus. If the uterus becomes distended with blood, or if the bladder becomes full and presses upward against the uterus, causing it to rise in the abdomen, then the fundus can be palpated several centimeters above the umbilicus. The nurse must make absolutely certain that

TABLE 33-3
SYMPTOMS OF SHOCK*

	Mild	Moderate	Severe	Irreversible
Respirations	Rapid, deep	Rapid, becoming shallow	Rapid, shallow, may be irregular	Irregular, or barely perceptible
Pulse	Rapid, tone normal	Rapid, tone may be normal but is becoming weaker	Very rapid, easily collapsible, may be irregular	Irregular apical pulse
Blood pressure	Normal or hypertensive	60 to 90 mm. Hg systolic	Below 60 mm. Hg systolic	None palpable
Skin	Cool and pale	Cool, pale, moist, knees cyanotic	Cold, clammy, cyanosis of lips and fingernails	Cold, clammy, cyanotic
Urine output	No change	Decreasing to 10 to 22 cc./hr. (adult)	Oliguric (less than 10 cc.) to anuria	Anuric
Level of consciousness	Alert, oriented, diffuse anxiety	Oriented, mental cloudiness or increasing restlessness	Lethargy, reacts to noxious stimuli, comatose	Does not respond to noxious stimuli
CVP	May be normal	3 cm. H²O	0 to 3 cm. H²O	

*From Royce, J. A.: "Shock: Emergency nursing implications." *Nurs. Clin. North Am.* 8:377, 1973; Wagner, M. M.: Clinical Nursing Specialist, University of Iowa Hospitals and Clinics.

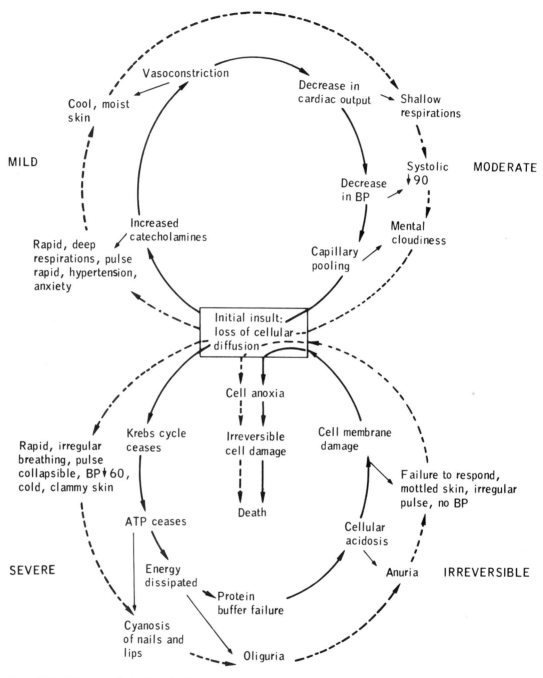

Figure 33-9. Diagram of physiologic alterations in shock in relation to symptoms. (From Royce, J. A.: 1973, *Nurs. Clin. N. Am.* 8:377.)

the uterus is in fact being massaged, not a roll of abdominal fat or a distended bladder. When properly contracted, the uterus should feel like a small-to-large hard apple.

Frequently, a big, boggy, relaxed uterus is difficult to outline through the abdominal wall, and it may be necessary to push the hand well posteriorly

toward the region of the sacral promontory to reach it. The very fact that the uterus is hard to identify usually means that it is relaxed.

Allaying Anxiety.   The frequent massage and deep palpation are often painful to the mother; at best they are disturbing, since they come at a time when she wants nothing more than to rest and sleep after her great effort. If she is awake and alert, then the continued attention and scrutiny may increase her anxiety. It must be remembered that apprehension is a natural concomitant of hemorrhage and shock. Quick and efficient nursing observations and appropriate explanation and reassurance help allay the concerns of both the mother and her partner.

This aspect of nursing care may be difficult to implement. If the mother or the father expresses concern and questions the activity by asking "What's wrong?", then the nurse can say simply, "The uterus has a tendency to relax, and must be massaged so that it will contract down as it should." Usually, such a statement will suffice. This will indicate the reason for the continued activity without associating hemorrhage and its fearsome consequences with the actions of the attendants. If the mother drifts off to sleep between the nurse's observations, then the nurse can gently rouse her by speaking her name before commencing massage, so that the mother is not awakened abruptly to the painful sensation of someone squeezing her abdomen.

Other Aspects of Care. Vital signs will be required every 5 to 15 minutes, and any variation, however slight, is to be reported immediately. Skin condition, level of consciousness, and urinary output are also monitored.

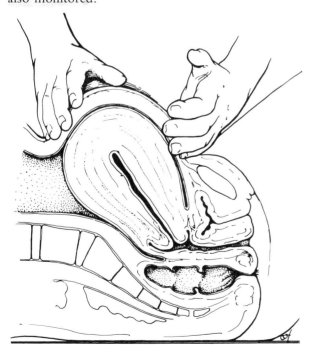

Figure 33-10. Massaging the uterus.

One way that the nurse can keep a more accurate account of the blood loss is to keep a perineal pad count. A record is kept of the number of pads saturated, how fully they are saturated, and the time it took for the saturation to occur. Thus, the nurse's notes might read: "Two pads ¾ saturated in 20 minutes." This type of report is more helpful to the physician than a more general, vague statement like, "Saturating perineal pads quickly."

If the bleeding occurs prior to delivery of the placenta, the physician may find it necessary to extract the placenta manually. (A change of gloves as well as gown may be called for to ensure strict asepsis, since the uterine cavity is to be invaded.) Oxytocics will invariably be requested, ergonovine or oxytocin or both intramuscularly. One or the other of these may be given intravenously.

It is necessary that there be *fluid replacement* for serious hemorrhage to combat hypovolemia. Pritchard recommends two general guidelines: First, lactated Ringer's solution and whole blood are given in amount and proportion to maintain a urine flow of at least 30 ml. per hour and preferably 60 ml. per hour (1 ml. per minute). In addition, the hematocrit is maintained at 30 percent or slightly higher. Second, if initial vigorous fluid replacement therapy does not maintain or restore the urine flow, then the central venous pressure (CVP) is monitored and fluids adjusted accordingly.[37]

CENTRAL VENOUS PRESSURE. *CVP readings* measure the contractility of the heart and the adequacy of the blood volume. The normal range is between 6 and 12 mm. H_2O. Falling values indicate hypovolemia and rising values indicate impaired contractility. To institute this type of monitoring, a catheter is inserted into a large antecubital vein in the forearm and threaded into the right atrium of the heart (Fig. 33-11). The data obtained provide a more precise estimate of the amount of fluid replacement necessary to combat shock.[38]

Since *blood transfusion* plays an important role in preventing serious shock, the blood groups of *all* maternity patients should be known before labor and crossmatched blood should be available for those in whom hemorrhage is anticipated or appears imminent. Seeing that the bloodtyping is carried out, ordering and calling for the cross match and the blood to be sent to the unit are usually responsibilities of the nurse. Time is of the essence for these patients; therefore the nurse must preplan and establish priorities with rapidity.

If oxytocin therapy fails to stop the bleeding, the

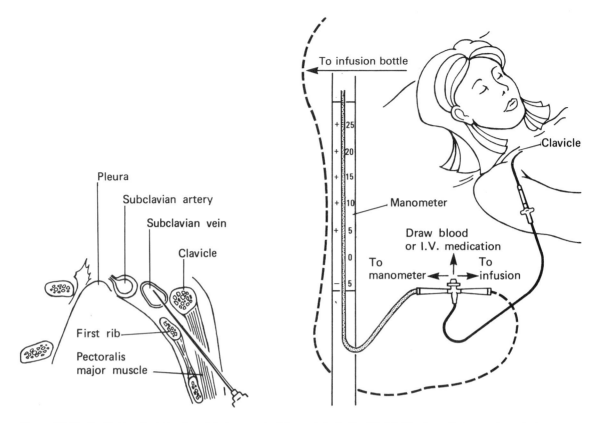

Figure 33-11. (*Left*) Needle introduced between clavicle and first rib. (*Right*) Plastic catheter and central venous pressure setup in place. (B-D: From Malinak, et al.: *Am. J. Obst. Gynecol.* 92:447, 1965.)

physician probably will carry out bimanual compression of the uterus. This provides the most efficient means of compressing the site of bleeding. Packing the uterus with gauze, a procedure once considered valuable to promote hemostasis in such cases, is seldom utilized today. It is considered by many authorities (e.g., Hellman, Cosgrove, Leff and Berkeley) to be inadequate and conducive to infection. If shock threatens, the right hip is elevated, external heat is applied, and preparations for blood transfusion and fluid replacement are made. An airway may be inserted.

In the handling of a case of postpartum hemorrhage, the nurse often assumes the important tasks of massaging the uterus, giving oxytocics, helping with the infusions and caring for the infant. The nurse must be prepared to act quickly and efficiently if the lives of these mothers are to be saved.

If postpartal hemorrhage occurs after the physician has left, the nurse gently grasps the uterus at once, pressing out as much blood as possible, and begins gentle, but vigorous, massage, sending word, of course, to the physician. If massage fails

to stop the bleeding, the physician usually will not object if the nurse gives the patient an intramuscular injection of ergonovine or oxytocin. If possible, this arrangement should be understood beforehand.

Late Postpartum Hemorrhage

Occasionally, postpartum hemorrhage may occur later than the first day following delivery. These late postpartum hemorrhages may take place any time between the second day and sixth week and are usually sudden in onset and may be so massive as to produce shock. Late postpartum hemorrhage is fortunately uncommon, occurring perhaps once in 1,000 cases.

While this condition is relatively uncommon, it is most dangerous because the mother will usually be home, often alone, and without professional attendance. Thus, if the hemorrhage is massive, she may be in immediate danger. Even if the bleeding is not great, there is still considerable difficulty getting medical assistance, and all of this can produce a great deal of anxiety and fatigue.

Arrangements must be made for the care of the infant even if the mother is to be seen only for a short while in the emergency room. Partners must be contacted, transportation arranged, and often myriads of other details worked through so that the mother can receive medical attention. This is why it is so important that the mother know where she can readily contact her physician should she need him in an emergency. Moreover, it becomes clearer why the mother should have help in the person of someone who is readily available and responsible for the first weeks of the puerperium.

Factors which most often cause these late hemorrhages are retention of placental fragments, recurrent bleeding from lacerations or episiotomy and subinvolution of the placental site. The latter condition is especially interesting because as yet the pathogenesis is unknown. The regeneration of the placental site takes longer than the rest of the uterus. It is accomplished in about six weeks as compared with about 21 days for the rest of the endometrium. The regeneration of the placental site begins from the remains of the epithelial glands; if these are not viable, then regeneration must occur from the spread of the surrounding epithelial tissue in the rest of the uterus. Until the site is firmly epithelialized, sloughing of clots may cause bleeding. Certain factors have been found to be associated with clot sloughing and hemorrhage, among them low grade fever, a history of abortion or uterine bleeding during pregnancy, hormonal influences, and the absence of breast-feeding. Often, however, none of these factors are found to be present; and the reason for the subinvolution remains a mystery. The physician will probably want to examine the patient and then carry out instrumental dilatation of the cervix at which time any placental fragments that are present will be removed with a curet or ovum forceps and any lacerations or incisions repaired.

Use of ultrasonic scanning of the uterus to detect the presence of retained products of conception, thus avoiding unnecessary curettage, has been suggested.[39]

If the mother must return to the hospital, this will no doubt upset to some degree the beginning relationship with the newborn. If the mother is nursing her infant and it is within a two-week period after delivery, the physician often can arrange to have the mother room-in with her infant for the short one- or two-day hospital stay. If the mother is bottle-feeding, then relatives, husband or "mother's helpers" can help in the interim until the mother's return. The nurse will want to remember that much of the mother's apparent anxiety and/or desire to return home as quickly as possible arises from these often abrupt and temporary arrangements that she has had to make. Understanding and counseling the mother to help her get adequate rest upon her return home is one of the helpful measures that the nurse can offer.

Rupture of the Uterus

Rupture of the uterus is fortunately a rare complication, occurring about once in every 2,000 pregnancies. It constitutes one of the gravest accidents in obstetrics, however, since the mortality rate for the infant is 50 percent to 75 percent and virtually all untreated mothers succumb to hypovolemia from hemorrhage or, less often, to infection. In this condition, the uterus simply bursts because the strain placed upon its musculature is more than it can withstand. Uterine rupture may occur in pregnancy but is far more frequent in labor.[40]

While the incidence has not changed to any degree in the last several decades, the etiology has changed, and the outcome has improved significantly. Today, the most common cause is attributed to rupture of the scar from a previous cesarean section. So great is this condition indited that the dictum "once a cesarean, always a cesarean" continues to be valid.[41] The second most common etiological agent is felt to be injudicious stimulation of labor with oxytocin. Other contributing factors include previous surgery involving the myometrium, prolonged and/or obstructed labor, certain faulty positions and/or fetal abnormalities, multiparity, excessive fetal size, and traumatic delivery, such as version and extraction or injudicious use of forceps.[42]

When rupture occurs, the patient complains of a severe, sudden, lacerating pain during a strong labor contraction. The rupture may be complete or incomplete; pain and abdominal tenderness are usually present in both cases. If there is complete rupture, regular contractions cease, since the torn muscle can no longer contract. There is an outpouring of blood into the abdominal cavity and sometimes into the vagina. The uterus may be palpated abdominally as a hard mass lying alongside the fetus. The patient soon exhibits signs of shock.

If the rupture is incomplete, the contractions may continue, and the signs of shock may be delayed, since the blood loss is slower. As soon as the diagnosis of rupture of the uterus is made, rapid preparations for an abdominal operation should ensue, since hysterectomy is the usual treatment. In addition, antibiotics are administered to combat infection, and blood transfusions and fluids are given to replace blood loss and to alleviate shock.

Since this accident gravely compromises the lives of both the infant and the mother, prevention, early diagnosis, prompt treatment, blood transfusions and antibiotics are essential components in improving the prognosis.

The nursing care will be essentially that for any complicated delivery and postpartum hemorrhage and shock. Whenever possible it is advisable to have the nurse who has been attending the mother during labor remain with her until the anesthetic for the cesarean section is given. This will provide some measure of continuity of care and help in reassurance and comfort of the parents.

Inversion of Uterus

Inversion of the uterus is a highly fatal accident of labor in which, after the birth of the infant, the uterus turns inside out. Shock is profound, and hemorrhage may occur, which if not treated quickly will cause the death of the mother.

There are two common causes of this accident, both of which are preventable: 1) pulling on the umbilical cord and 2) trying to express the placenta when the uterus is relaxed. In the former case, the traction on the attached placenta simply pulls the uterus inside out, while in the latter, the hand pushes the relaxed muscular sac inside out. Thus, the umbilical cord should never have strenuous traction applied nor should the uterus be pushed downward unless it is firmly contracted.

It is imperative that several steps in treatment be taken promptly and simultaneously: 1) Two intravenous infusions systems are instituted, one with lactated Ringer's solution and one with whole blood. These are given promptly to refill the intravascular compartment and support cardiac output. 2) An anesthesiologist gives a general anesthesia, usually halothane, to relax the uterus. The placenta is left in place until the infusions are operational and uterine relaxation has been accomplished. If the placenta is removed prematurely, hemorrhage is only increased. Attempts are then made to replace the uterus in the vagina by placing the palm of the hand on the center of the fundus with the fingers

extended to identify the cervical margins. The fundus is then pushed up through the cervix. When the uterus is returned to its normal shape, anesthesia is discontinued and oxytocin is begun to help the uterus remain contracted. Bimanual compression also aids in this. The uterus is then monitored transvaginally until normal tone is assured.

If the uterus cannot be replaced from below because of a constriction ring, a laparotomy is performed so that the uterus can be pulled up simultaneously from above and pushed up from below. The constriction ring may be incised. A traction suture in the fundus aids in repositioning. Treatment continues as previously described. Subsequent inversion is unlikely.[43]

Disorders of Placental Attachment

Other important causes of bleeding associated with pregnancy and labor are placenta previa and abruptio placentae. These have been discussed previously as complications of pregnancy in Chapter 31. However, at times the first signs of these problems occur during labor, and the nurse in the delivery suite must be familiar with their diagnosis and management.

The cardinal sign of *placenta previa* is painless, bright red vaginal bleeding. If partial separation occurs after the onset of labor, contractions may confuse the situation; identification depends upon accurately assessing the extent of vaginal bleeding. Overt hemorrhage with huge blood loss is not difficult to diagnose, but it requires fine judgment to decide when bloody vaginal discharge ceases to be heavy "show" and becomes potential hemorrhage. It is wise to report any vaginal bleeding which the nurse believes is excessive to the physician and to refrain from digital examination of these patients.

Abruptio placentae can be a true obstetrical emergency if the area of separation is extensive. The signs that alert the delivery room nurse to this complication include a hypertonic uterus which does not relax well between contractions, an area of extreme sensitivity when the uterus is palpated, sudden sharp and persistent uterine pain, and symptoms and signs of shock which seem greater than the observable blood loss would indicate. An extremely hard, boardlike uterus which cannot be indented and which does not relax indicates a severe degree of placental separation and bleeding.

Marginal sinus rupture was formerly treated as a separate clinical entity, but now is felt to be a mild type of abruptio placentae in which slight separation occurs at the edge of the placenta. The marginal sinus is located under the edge of the placenta, and is one of the large maternal sinuses bathing the placental villi. If the placenta separates at a point along its margin, this maternal sinus is disrupted and bleeding occurs. There is usually no increased pain or uterine tension, and the amount of vaginal bleeding may vary considerably. If the area of separation is small, as it usually is in marginal sinus rupture, there is no danger of hypoxia to the fetus and generally no changes in fetal heart rate. When there is excessive vaginal bleeding during labor, and placenta previa and abruptio have been ruled out, the most probable cause is a small marginal separation of the placenta.[44] Nursing Care is the same as for other hemorrhage conditions.

PROLAPSE OF UMBILICAL CORD

In the course of labor, the cord prolapses in front of the presenting part about once in every 400 cases. It is a grave complication for the fetus, since the cord is then compressed between the presenting part and the bony pelvis, and the fetal circulation is shut off (Fig. 33-12). Any factor which prevents proper adaptation of the presenting part to the maternal pelvis predisposes to prolapse of the cord. The accident occurs more commonly in shoulder and footling breech presentations, and less often with frank breeches and multiple pregnancy. In cephalic presentations, it rarely occurs unless there is pelvic contraction or excessive development of the fetus. There is an increased incidence with prematurity, probably because the small fetus is poorly fitted to the pelvic inlet.

Prolapse frequently occurs following rupture of the membranes when the head, the breech or the shoulder is not sufficiently down in the pelvis to prevent the cord from being washed past it in the sudden gush of amniotic fluid. After the membranes rupture, the cord comes down, and it may be either a concealed or an apparent prolapse. In the latter instance, the diagnosis is made when the cord is seen; but when the cord is not visible, the correct diagnosis is made when the patient is examined and the cord is felt or examination of the fetal heart reveals distress due to pressure on the cord. This is why it *must* be a routine practice to listen to the fetal heart sounds immediately after the membranes rupture and again in about 5 to 10 minutes. When fetal heart rate is monitored internally, a character-

---

NURSING CARE PRIORITIES IN POSTPARTUM HEMORRHAGIC COMPLICATION

Assessment	Intervention	Evaluation
Status of fundus	Hold fundus; massage gently until firm (not continuously); express clots as needed.	Bleeding controlled
Amount of flow	Pad count: amount saturated in amount of time	
Vital signs a. TPR., BP b. Skin c. Urine output d. Level of consciousness	Check q 5–15 min. Record and report. Provide warmth with clean, dry, warm blankets. Record, report accurately; maintain @ 30–60 ml./hr. Check frequently, speak to patient to ascertain if she is oriented; reassurance as indicated to couple.	Profound shock avoided
4. Monitor intravenous/oxytocin	Check frequently to be sure needle is in place, uterus contracted.	Uterus contracts and patient hydrated
5. Monitor CVP if necessary	Maintain approximately 6–12 mm H$_2$O. Record, report as indicated.	Blood volume more precisely ascertained
6. Type and cross match	Order if indicated; follow through with lab.	In readiness if continued hemorrhage

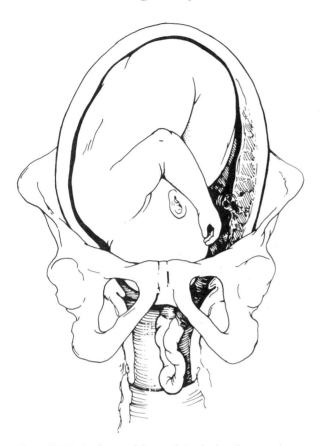

Figure 33-12. Prolapse of the cord. As the head comes down, the compression of the cord between the fetal skull and the pelvic brim will shut off its circulation completely.

istic slowing of the fetal heart with onset early during the contraction and persistence of bradycardia beyond the end of contraction are suggestive of cord compression.

The immediate treatment of cord prolapse is to minimize the pressure of the presenting part upon the cord and the resultant impaired umbilical circulation. The head of the bed or table should be lowered, or the patient placed in a knee-chest position to raise the level of the hips above the shoulders and allow the presenting part to gravitate away from the pelvis. Additionally, the presenting part may be pushed upward by pressure from a sterile gloved hand in the vagina.

The physician and other staff must be notified at once so emergency procedures can be instituted. No attempt should be made to reposition the cord, and with a live baby near term the goal of therapy is to effect delivery as soon as possible. If dilatation is incomplete, immediate cesarean section yields the best results for fetal salvage. In occasional carefully

selected cases, prolapsed cord in vertex presentations with nearly complete dilatation can be delivered with minimal trauma to mother and infant using vacuum extraction.

Perinatal mortality with cord prolapse, which is usually about 26 percent, can be reduced to 5 to 10 percent when delivery is accomplished within one-half hour after diagnosis. More frequent vaginal examinations, checking fetal heart after rupture of membranes, and active rapid treatment combine to reduce mortality.

This particular complication is not painful for the mother; however, it can be very frightening, for many patients realize it can result in their infant's death. Also whether they realize the grave implications or not, the various antic positions and quickened responses of the attendants give them an indication that all is not well. Therefore, again, the calmness, warmth and efficiency of the nurse can do much to reassure the patient that all possible measures are being taken to bring the situation under control.

It goes without saying that these patients never should be left unattended, and their partners, if they are present, should be treated with consideration. It is difficult, when any crises occur, to deal with the relatives of the patient with appropriate thoughtfulness, since most of the energy is directed toward meeting the pressing (and often lifesaving) demands of the situation. However, it must be remembered that the patient and her family are considered as a unit, and a few moments usually can be found to provide essential information.

AMNIOTIC FLUID EMBOLISM

At any time after the membranes have ruptured there is a possibility that amniotic fluid may enter the gaping venous sinuses of the placental site as well as the veins in the cervix, be drawn into the general circulation and in this way reach the pulmonary capillaries. Since the amniotic fluid invariably contains small particles of matter, such as vernix caseosa, lanugo and sometimes meconium, multiple tiny emboli may reach the lungs in this manner and cause occlusion of the pulmonary capillaries. This complication, amniotic fluid embolism, is almost invariably fatal and, as a rule, causes the death of the mother within one or two hours.

Fortunately, this tragic condition is rare, occurring only once in many thousand labors.

The clinical characteristics of the condition are sudden dyspnea, cyanosis, pulmonary edema, profound shock and uterine relaxation with hemorrhage. A highly important feature of amniotic fluid embolism is a diminution in the fibrinogen content of the blood, or hypofibrinogenemia. The mechanism is similar to, if not identical with, that which occurs in abruptio placentae and missed abortion, as described in Chapter 31.

The treatment consists of oxygen therapy, blood transfusion and the intravenous administration of fibrinogen, but, as indicated, this is usually futile.

MULTIPLE PREGNANCY

When two or more embryos develop in the uterus at the same time, the condition is known as multiple pregnancy. Multiple pregnancies account for about 2 percent to 3 percent of all viable births. The frequency of identical (monozygotic or one-egg) twins is apparently relatively constant throughout the world at about 1 set in every 250 pregnancies. Moreover, their appearance is largely independent of race, heredity, maternal age, parity, infertility drugs and environmental factors. On the other hand, fraternal (dizygotic, two-egg) twins are influenced by these factors. Their incidence in the white race is about 1 set in 95 and in the black race one set in 78. Twinning among orientals is less common. Women who were themselves a dizygotic twin tend to have more multiple pregnancies. Similarly, increased age, parity, endogenous gonadotropin, and taking infertility drugs also increases the probability of multiple pregnancy.[45]

Types of Twins

Twins may be identical (monozygotic) or fraternal (dizygotic). Identical twins *are* identical because they come from a single egg; hence they are called "single-ovum twins." Fertilization takes place in the usual way, by a single spermatozoon, but then, very early in the ovum's development, it divides into two identical parts instead of continuing as a single individual. Such twins are always of the same sex and show close physical and mental resemblances. Nonidentical or fraternal twins result from the fertilization of two ova by two spermatozoa and are therefore *double-ovum twins* (Fig. 33-13). Such twins, according to chance, may be of the same sex or of opposite sexes; and the likelihood of their resembling each other is no greater than that of any brother and sister.

Basically, two types of placentae exist in twins, those with monochorial (one chorion) and those with dichorial (two chorions) membranes. Also, the placentae may be fused, separate or a single disk and there may be one or two amnions. Each fetus usually has its own umbilical cord, however. The possible combinations thus include:

1. Monozygotic (identical)

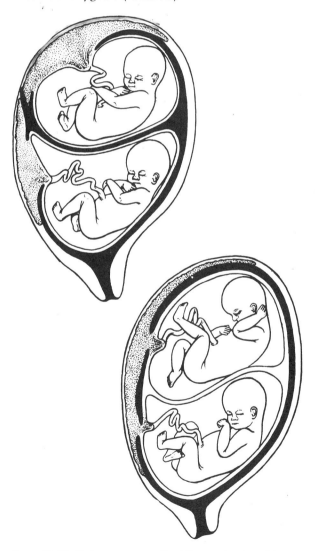

Figure 33-13. Twin pregnancy. (*Top*) Fraternal twins with two placentas, two amnions, two chorions. (*Bottom*) Identical twins with one placenta, one chorion, two amnions.

a. Diamniotic monochorionic (two amnions, one chorion). Common.
b. Diamniotic dichorionic (two amnions, two chorions). 30 percent.
c. Monoamniotic monochorionic (one amnion, one chorion). Very rare.
2. Dizygotic (fraternal or nonidentical)
   a. Diamniotic dichorionic (two amnions, two chorions).

Examination of the fetal membranes is used to assist in diagnosing the zygosity of twins but is not always accurate. Only monozygotic twins can have a single chorion, so this establishes identical twinning. Two chorions are always present in dizygotic twins, but are also the placentation of about 30 percent of monozygotic twins. If the sexes are different, the twins are obviously fraternal; but if twins are the same sex and dichorionic, the diagnosis is uncertain.[46] The usual twin placentations are shown in Figure 33-14. In the United States, 33 percent of twins are identical.

Diagnosis

Twins are suspected whenever uterine size is greater than ordinarily expected for any point in pregnancy. In addition, the palpation of three or four large parts in the uterus, the appearance of two fetal heart tones, of differing frequency, and the history of twins "running in the family" all serve to alert the obstetrician and nurse to the possibility of a multiple pregnancy. Sonography can confirm the diagnosis.

Twins are likely to be born about two weeks before the calculated date of delivery. Even though pregnancy goes to full term, twins are usually smaller than single infants by nearly 1 pound; however, the outlook for such infants, provided that the pregnancy continues into the last month, is almost as good as that for single infants.

Pathophysiology of Multiple Pregnancy

Several high-risk conditions are associated with multiple pregnancy. These include premature delivery (50 percent), hemorrhage (20 percent), hypertensive disorders preeclampsia and eclampsia (25 percent), abnormal presentation and position (10 percent), hydramnios (7 percent) and uterine dysfunction (10 percent). Cord compression and entanglement, intrauterine growth retardation and operative delivery also contribute to morbidity and mortality. In addition, monozygotic twins are less hardy than dizygotic twins. Weight differences are more pronounced, and they have a higher incidence of congenital anomalies and neonatal mortality.

Some of these problems may be due to the monochorionic placenta which is thought to be less competent than the dichorionic variety. The problems center on placental vascular disorders.

The most serious of these is the shunting of blood due to vascular anastamosis which results in a twin-to-twin transfusion syndrome (intrauterine parabiosis). The anastamosis may be artery-to-artery, artery-to-vein, or vein-to-vein. An artery-to-vein anastamosis is the most serious and accounts for the disparity in size and appearance seen in these supposedly identical infants. The *doner* twin will be pallid, anemic, dehydrated, growth retarded and hypovolemic. Hydrops and cardiac decompensation may be present as well as polyhydramnios. In contrast, the *recipient* twin appears healthy, large by contrast and ruddy. However, this appearance is due to edema, plethora and hypertension. Kernicterus, ascites, glomerular-tubal hypertrophy, enlarged heart and liver and/or congenital heart anomalies may be accompaniments. Fetal polyuria and hydramnios may also be present. These infants are at great risk for death in the first 24 hours of life.[47,48]

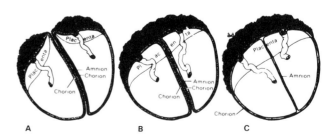

Figure 33-14. Single- and double-ovum twin differences. *A* and *B,* double-ovum twins; there are two chorions; in *B* the two placentas have fused. *C,* single-ovum twins; there is only one chorion and one placenta.

A   B   C

Management of Multiple Pregnancy

Antenatally, the mother will be monitored carefully. She will be asked to see the obstetrician at least every two weeks in the second trimester and every week in the third trimester. Diet is regulated to allow for adequate weight gain (as much as 35 to 40 lbs. above the ideal nonpregnant weight). Protein intake is supervised and iron and folic acid supplements are prescribed. Rest periods on the side are also required, although the efficacy of complete bedrest in the absence of complications is questioned.[49]

The latter weeks of a twin pregnancy are likely to be associated with heaviness of the lower abdomen, back pains and swelling of the feet and the ankles. Abdominal distention makes sleeping difficult, and therefore the physician may prescribe a hypnotic. A well-fitting maternity girdle will make daytime more comfortable. Because of the excessive abdominal size, the patient may find that frequent small feedings are more suitable than the usual three larger meals a day. The nurse can be very helpful in giving the mother anticipatory guidance regarding these matters during the antepartal period.

Travel will be curtailed, since labor may begin at any time without warning, and delivery in strange surroundings may be hazardous.

A spontaneous delivery is particularly desired in instances of twins, since this type of delivery results in less blood loss and maternal morbidity and a greater likelihood of healthy, undamaged infants.

Delivery

The patient is requested to come to the hospital at the first sign of labor. If there is any suspicion of labor, she is kept in the labor and delivery area. A local or pudendal block is preferred to minimize the effect of anesthetic on the infants. However, general anesthesia may be required if the delivery of the second twin requires operative intervention.

The first twin is delivered either by vertex or assisted breech delivery. If the first infant is transverse, an external version is utilized to bring about a deliverable presentation.

If the twins are monozygotic, the first infant's cord must be clamped to prevent the second twin from bleeding through it. The cords should be labeled. The position of the second twin is ascer-

tained and it is brought into position by a combination of vaginal and abdominal manipulation. If there is a second sac, it is carefully ruptured to allow a slow loss of fluid and guard against cord prolapse. A spontaneous or a prophylactic forceps vertex delivery is preferred. If the breech presents, then the physician may have to assist in the extraction. If descent does not come about, then a version and extraction may be required. These require astute management on the part of both the obstetrician and the anesthesiologist.

After delivery of the second twin, 1 ml. oxytocin is given intraveneously. The uterus is not massaged until after the placenta(s) separate, then massage is continued until the uterus remains hard and contracted (15 to 30 minutes); 1 ml. of Ergonovine is given after the placenta separates if the mother's condition does not contraindicate it.

As with any delivery, the nurse will have the responsibility of supportive care for the patient as well as assisting the physician in whatever activities are indicated. Since these infants are apt to be small, oxygen and/or resuscitative measures may be necessary. The care will be similar to that for the premature baby (see Chapter 38). Any supplies and/or equipment that may be needed (resuscitator, oxygen apparatus, etc.) should be procured early in the delivery and kept in readiness (but out of the patient's sight, if possible). Maternal vital signs as well as the fetal heart rate should be checked frequently.

Postpartum

When there is a twin birth, there is frequently a decided psychologic and economic (albeit somewhat delayed) shock to the parents. Emotionally, one additional child may be desired and acceptable; two may impose a burden, particularly if this pregnancy was to be "the last." The parents may wonder if they can manage the care of two newborn infants simultaneously. Problems may be compounded in feeding, especially if the mother wants to nurse her infant. In addition, two of everything must be provided, instead of one, and this additional cost may put a strain on the budget. In terms of long-range planning, the present housing may be inadequate, especially if the children are of different sexes and eventually will require separate rooms. The cost entailed in additional construction and/or new housing is considerable. None of these problems is insurmountable but resolution takes time and effort.

Some parents need an understanding and empathic person to help them over the initial adjustment period. In some cases they may need the help of a social worker or a public health nurse to plan for the unexpected new baby. Many parents seem to adjust nicely through being able to ventilate their concerns. If the twins are undiagnosed, that is, not discovered until labor, then these problems are compounded.

The parents will also benefit from any assistance or advice that helps them simplify their household schedule. The mother will need to have adequate rest and additional help, if it can be afforded. Household chores and responsibilities need to be as simple and flexible as possible. If at all possible, the father should be an active participant in the home and child care responsibilities.

If the babies must remain in the hospital, there may be problems in bonding and sibling rivalry. The parents may need help in working out a schedule of visiting the infants that allows the mother to recover her strength and yet provides some communication with the infants. Anticipatory guidance of the other children can be helpful in preventing intense sibling rivalry. All of these contingencies require astute discharge planning on the part of the physician and the nursing staff.

REFERENCES

1. E. A. Friedman: *Labor, Evaluation and Management.* New York, Appleton-Century-Crofts, 1978.
2. K. R. Niswander: *Obstetric and Gynecologic Disorders.* Flushing, New York, Medical Examination Publishing Company, 1975.
3. J. A. Pritchard and P. C. McDonald: *Williams Obstetrics,* ed. 15. New York, Appleton-Century-Crofts, 1976.
4. Friedman, op. cit.
5. C. H. Hendricks et al.: "The normal cervical dilatation patterns in late pregnancy and labor." *Am. J. Obstet. Gynecol.* 106: 1065, 1970.
6. Pritchard and McDonald, op. cit.
7. C. M. Steer: "Effect of type of delivery on future childbearing." *Am. J. Obstet. Gynecol.* 60: 395, 1950.
8. Pritchard and McDonald, op. cit.
9. S. D. Larks: *Electrohysterography.* Springfield, Ill., Charles C Thomas, 1960.
10. Pritchard and McDonald, op. cit.
11. R. Caldeyro-Barcia et al.: "A better understanding of uterine contractility through simultaneous recording with an internal and seven channel external method." *Surg. Obstet. Gynecol.* 91: 641, 1950.
12. Pritchard and McDonald, op. cit.
13. R. G. Douglas and W. B. Stromme: *Operative Obstetrics,* ed. 3. New York, Appleton-Century-Crofts, 1976.
14. Friedman, op. cit.
15. Pritchard and McDonald, op. cit.
16. Friedman, op. cit.
17. R. D. Phillips and M. Freeman: "The management of the persistent occiput posterior position." *Amer. J. Obstet-Gynecol.* 43: 171, Feb. 1974.
18. Pritchard and McDonald, op. cit.
19. J. J. Rovinsky et al.: "Management of breech presentation at term." *Amer. J. Obstet.-Gynecol.* 115: 497–513, Feb. 15, 1973.
20. W. L. Benson et al.: "Management delivery in the primigravida." *Amer. J. Obstet.-Gynecol.* 40: 417–428, 1972.
21. Rovinsky et al., op. cit.
22. W. E. Brenner: "Breech presentation." In Makowski, E. L., ed.: *Clinical Obstetrics and Gynecology.* New York, Harper & Row, 21: 2 June 1978, 511: 31.
23. Ibid.
24. Pritchard and McDonald, op. cit.
25. Brenner, op. cit.
26. Ibid.
27. W. E. Brenner et al.: "The characteristics and perils of breech presentation." *Am. J. Obstet. Gynecol.* 118: 700, 1974.
28. Pritchard and McDonald, op. cit.
29. Brenner et al., op. cit.
30. Ibid.
31. Pritchard and McDonald, op. cit.
32. Ibid.
33. H. Hammond: "Death from obstetrical hemorrhage." *Calif. Med.* 117: 16–20, Aug. 1972.
34. Douglas and Stromme, op. cit.
35. J. A. Royce: "Shock, emergency nursing implications." *Nurs. Clin. North Am.* 8: 377, 1973.
36. Ibid.
37. Pritchard and McDonald, op. cit.
38. Douglas and Stromme, op. cit.

39. J. Malvern et al.: "Ultrasonic scanning of the puerperal uterus following secondary postpartum hemorrhage." *J. Obstet. Gynecol. Br. Comm.* 80: 320–324, April 1973.

40. Pritchard and McDonald, op. cit.

41. T. Klein and J. H. O'Leary: "Rupture of the gravid uterus." *J. Reproductive Med.*, 6: 43–47, May 1971.

42. Douglas and Stromme, op. cit.

43. Pritchard and McDonald, op. cit.

44. Y. Robello: "Placenta previa, placenta abruptio." Paper read at the National Symposium of Perinatal Nursing, San Francisco, California, June 7–10, 1978.

45. K. Benirschke and K. K. Chung: "Multiple pregnancy, Part 1." *New Eng. J. Med.* 288: 1276–1284, June 14, 1973.

46. Ibid.

47. Ibid.

48. Pritchard and McDonald, op. cit.

49. Ibid.

Thirty-Four

Operative Obstetrics

Repair of Lacerations | Forceps | Vacuum Extraction |
Version | Cesarean Section | Destructive Operations |
Induction of Labor

A number of special procedures which the physician may use to assist the mother in labor and delivery come under the heading of operative obstetrics. These include repair of lacerations, the application of forceps or vacuum extractor, destructive operations on the fetus, version, cesarean section, and induction of labor.

REPAIR OF LACERATIONS

Except for clamping and cutting the umbilical cord, episiotomy is the most common operative procedure performed in obstetrics. In view of the fact that this incision of the perineum, made to facilitate delivery, is employed almost routinely in primigravidaes, the procedure has been discussed in the section on the conduct of normal labor (see Chapter 23).

Lacerations of the perineum and the vagina which occur in the process of delivery have also been discussed previously, because some tears are unavoidable, even in the most skilled hands. The suturing of spontaneous perineal lacerations is similar to that employed for the repair of an episiotomy incision, also considered in the section on the

conduct of normal labor, but may be more difficult because such tears often are irregular in shape with ragged, bruised edges.

FORCEPS

Some of the common types of obstetric forceps are illustrated in Figure 34-1. The instrument consists of two steel parts which cross each other like a pair of scissors and lock at the intersection. The lock may be of a sliding type, as in the first three types shown, or a screw type, as in the Tarnier instrument.

Each part consists of a handle, a lock, a shank, and a blade; the blade is the curved portion designed for application to the sides of the baby's head. The blades of most forceps (the Tucker McLane is an exception) have a large opening or window (fenestrum) to give a better grip on the baby's head, and usually consist of two curves: a cephalic curve, which conforms to the shape of the baby's head, and a pelvic curve, to follow the curve of the birth canal. Axis-traction forceps, such as the Tarnier, have a mechanism attached below which permits the pulling to be done more directly in the axis of the birth canal. An axis-traction handle is also available for use on standard forceps.

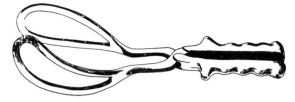

A. Simpson forceps

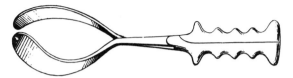

B. Tucker McLane forceps

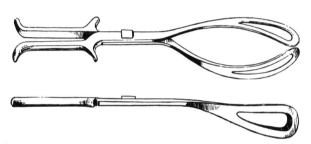

C. Kielland forceps (*top*) Front view, (*bottom*) side view

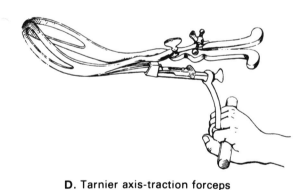

D. Tarnier axis-traction forceps

Figure 34-1. Types of Forceps.

The two blades of the forceps are designated as right and left. The left blade is the one which is introduced into the vagina on the patient's left side; the right blade goes in on the right side. If the nurse anticipates assisting the obstetrician, it is helpful to articulate and disarticulate the forceps to be able to know which blade is which.

Reasons for Forceps Delivery. It may become necessary to deliver the baby by forceps for reasons related to the mother's welfare (maternal indications), or because of conditions associated with the baby's condition (fetal indications). Maternal indications include inability of the mother to push after full dilatation of the cervix, because of conduction anesthesia, exhaustion, heart disease or any condition affecting the mother which is likely to be improved by delivery.

The chief fetal indications for forceps delivery are fetal distress, as suggested by a slow, irregular fetal heart and, in general, conditions which would potentially cause fetal distress such as placental abruption or prolapsed umbilical cord.

Many obstetricians, however, deem it desirable to deliver almost all primigravidae with forceps electively, in the belief that the operation spares the mother many minutes of bearing-down efforts and relieves pressure on the baby's head. This is usually referred to as "elective forceps."

Forceps delivery is never attempted unless the cervix is completely dilated and the vertex is engaged (i.e., the greatest biparietal diameter of the fetal head is at, or has already traversed, the pelvic inlet). Usually, but not always, when engagement has occurred, the vertex is at or below the ischial spines.

Types of Forceps Deliveries. In the vast majority of instances today, the forceps delivery is carried out at a time when the fetal head is on the perineal floor (visible or almost so) and internal rotation may have already occurred, so that the fetal head lies in a direct anteroposterior position. This is called *low forceps,* or "outlet forceps." When the head is higher in the pelvis but engaged, its greatest diameter having passed the inlet, the operation is called *midforceps.* If the head has not yet engaged, the procedure is known as *high forceps.* High-forceps delivery is an exceedingly difficult and dangerous operation for both mother and baby and is rarely done. Increasingly, cesarean section is preferred to a potentially difficult midforceps delivery.

After a decision is made to use forceps, the obstetrician will select the type of instrument to be used. Several pairs of the generally approved forceps, each encased in suitable wrappings, are autoclaved and kept in the delivery room for immediate use. The other instruments needed for a forceps delivery are the same as those required for a spontaneous delivery, plus those necessary for repair.

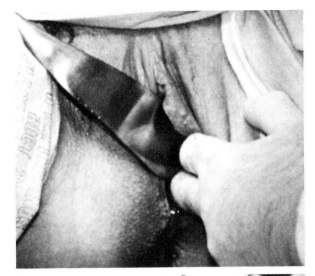

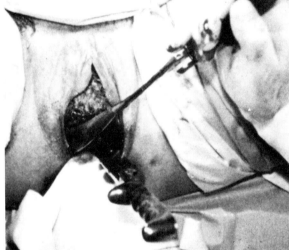

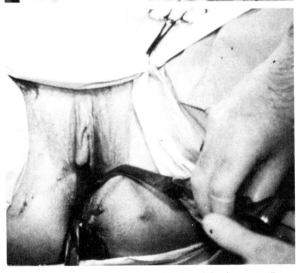

Figure 34-2. Insertion of the two blades of the forceps. (From the film *Human Birth*, published by J. B. Lippincott Co., Philadelphia.)

Procedure. Anesthesia is recommended, but in low–forceps deliveries it may be light, and in most institutions this type of operation is performed successfully under pudendal block anesthesia. The patient is placed in the lithotomy position and prepared and draped in the usual fashion. For a midforceps delivery the bladder should be emptied by catheterization.

After checking the exact position of the fetal head by vaginal examination, the physician introduces

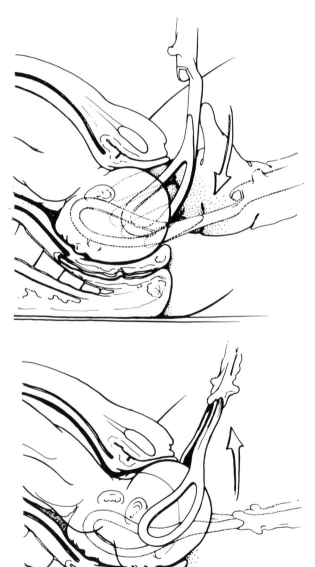

Figure 34-3. (*Top*) Insertion of forceps blade and (*Bottom*) applied forceps and direction of traction.

two or more fingers of one hand into the left side of the vagina; these fingers guide the left blade into place and at the same time protect the maternal soft parts (vagina, cervix) from injury. The other hand is used to introduce the left blade of the forceps into the left side of the vagina, gently insinuating it between the baby's head and the fingers of the hand (Fig. 34-2). The same procedure is carried out on the right side, and then the blades are articulated. Traction is not continuous but intermittent (Fig. 34-3); and between traction, the blades are partially disarticulated in order to release pressure on the fetal head. Episiotomy is routine nowadays in these cases.

Piper forceps for breech delivery. The Piper forceps have been designed to assist in the delivery of the after-coming head in breech presentations (Fig. 34-4). They are applied after the shoulders have been delivered and the head has been brought into the pelvis by gentle traction combined with suprapubic pressure. Suspension of the body and arms with a towel facilitates application of the blades. The left blade is introduced in an upward direction along the fetal head on the left side, and the right blade is then applied in similar fashion. The forceps are locked in place, and their position on the head is confirmed by palpation. An episiotomy is made and, as traction is applied, the chin, mouth and nose emerge over the perineum. The Piper forceps are often used electively as a substitute for the Mauriceau maneuver, or when the Mauriceau maneuver for delivery of the fetal head has failed (see Chapter 33).

VACUUM EXTRACTION

Occasionally, an instrument known as the vacuum extractor is used in place of the forceps. The vacuum extractor consists of a metal cup that is applied to the fetal head and tightly affixed there by creating a vacuum in the cup through withdrawal of the air by a pump (Fig. 34-5). Cups are supplied in various sizes. The largest cup which can be applied with ease is selected for use. Vacuum is built up slowly, and the suction creates an artificial caput within the cup, providing a firm attachment to the fetal scalp. Traction can then be exerted by means of a short chain attached to the cup, with a handle at its far end.

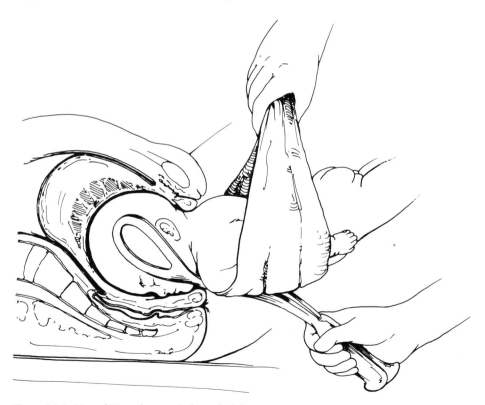

Figure 34-4. Use of Piper forceps in breech delivery.

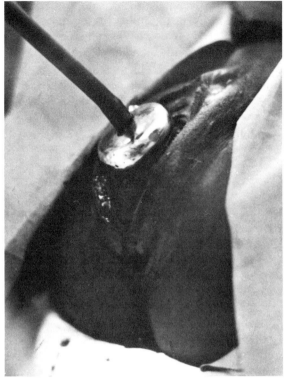

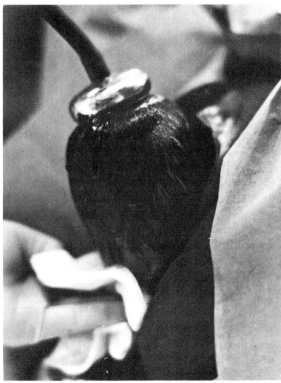

Figure 34-5. Application of the vacuum extractor and delivery of the fetal head.

VERSION

Version consists of turning the baby in the uterus from an undesirable to a desirable position. There are two types of version: external, and internal.

External Version.   This is an operation designed to change a breech presentation into a vertex presentation by external manipulation of the fetus through the abdominal and the uterine walls. It is attempted in the hope of averting the difficulties of a subsequent breech delivery. Obstetricians find the procedure most successful when done about a month before full term; it often fails, however, either because it proves to be impossible to turn the fetus around, or because the fetus returns to its original position within a few hours. Some obstetricians disapprove of it altogether.

Internal Version.   Sometimes called internal podalic version, this is a maneuver designed to change whatever presentation may exist by converting it into a breech presentation (see Fig. 34-6).

With cervical dilatation complete, the whole hand of the operator is introduced high into the uterus, one or both feet are grasped and pulled downward in the direction of the birth canal. With the external hand, the obstetrician may expedite the turning by pushing the head upward. The version is followed by breech extraction.

Figure 34-6. Internal podalic version.

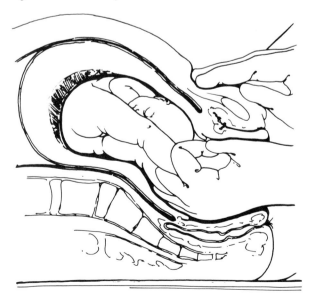

Internal version is most useful in cases of multiple pregnancy in which the birth of the second twin is delayed or when the second twin is in a transverse lie. It is now almost never used in other circumstances.

CESAREAN SECTION

Cesarean section is the removal of the infant from the uterus through an incision made in the abdominal wall and the uterus.

The main indications for cesarean section fall into five groups:

1. Disproportion between the size of the fetus and that of the bony birth canal—that is, contracted pelvis (p. 551), tumor blocking birth canal, etc.
2. Certain cases in which the patient has had a previous cesarean section, the operation being done because of the fear that the uterus will rupture in labor.
3. Certain cases of very severe preeclampsia or eclampsia.
4. Certain cases of placenta previa and premature separation of the normally implanted placenta.
5. Fetal distress, actual or pending.

When a cesarean section is done prior to the onset of labor, as the result of a prearranged plan, it is called *elective* cesarean section (as with elective low forceps, the obstetrician is not forced to perform the operation immediately, but elects to do it as the best procedure for mother and baby).

Prematurity is the most common fetal complication of elective cesarean section, occurring because the duration of gestation is misjudged. This can now be avoided by evaluating fetal maturity preoperatively through determination of amniotic fluid L-S (lecithin-sphingomyelin) ratio (see Chapter 36).

Main Types of Cesarean Section

Although there are four types of cesarean section, the lower segment section is usually the operation of choice. In this operation, the uterus is entered through an incision in the lower segment. Other types of cesarean section include the classical cesarean section, in which the incision is made directly into the wall of the body of the uterus; the extra-

peritoneal cesarean section, in which the operation is arranged anatomically, such that the incision is made into the uterus without entering the peritoneal cavity; and cesarean-hysterectomy, which involves a cesarean section of any variety followed by removal of the uterus.

The Low Segment Cesarean Section. This procedure is usually the operation of choice for a number of important reasons. Since the incision is made in the lower segment of the uterus, which is its thinnest portion, there is minimal blood loss, and the incision is easy to repair. The lower segment is also the area of least uterine activity, and thus the possibility of rupture of the scar in a subsequent pregnancy is lessened. Since the incision can be properly peritonealized, the operation is associated with a lower incidence of postoperative infection.

The initial incision (the abdominal cavity having been opened) is made transversely across the uterine peritoneum, where it is attached loosely just above the bladder. The lower peritoneal flap and the bladder are now dissected from the uterus, and the uterine muscle is incised either vertically or transversely. The membranes are ruptured, and the baby is delivered (Fig. 34-7). After the placenta has been extracted (Fig. 34-8) and the uterine incision sutured, the lower flap is imbricated over the uterine incision. This two-flap arrangement seals off the uterine incision and is believed to prevent the egress of infectious lochia into the peritoneal cavity.

Classical Cesarean Section. A vertical incision is made directly into the wall of the body of the uterus; the baby and the placenta are extracted, and the incision is closed by three layers of absorbable sutures. Thus, this approach requires traversing the full thickness of the uterine corpus. It is still recommended in certain circumstances. It is particularly useful when the bladder and lower segment are involved in extension adhesions resulting from a previous cesarean section, and occasionally is selected when the fetus is in a transverse lie or when there is an anterior placenta previa.

Extraperitoneal Cesarean Section. By appropriate dissection of the tissues around the bladder, access to the lower uterine segment is secured without entering the peritoneal cavity. The baby is delivered through an incision in the lower uterine segment. Since the entire operation is done outside the peri-

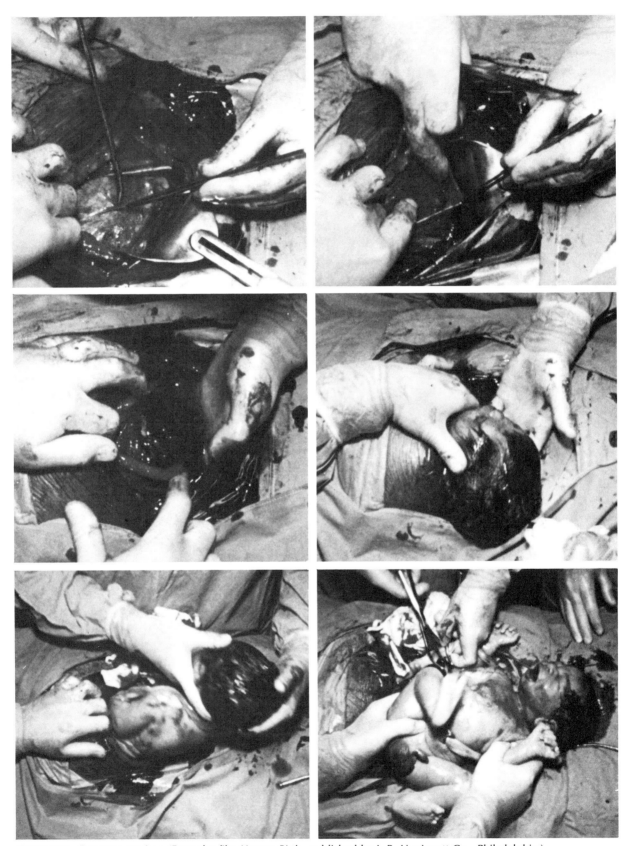

Figure 34-7. Cesarean section. (From the film *Human Birth*, published by J. B. Lippincott Co., Philadelphia.)

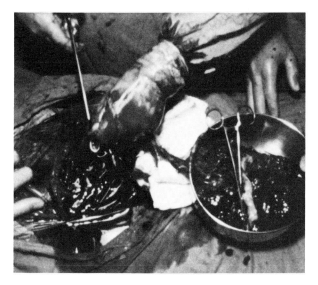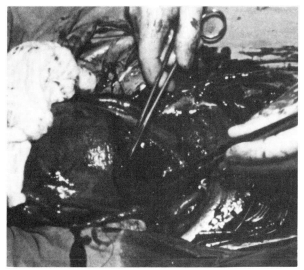

Figure 34-8. Extracting the placenta in cesarean section. (From the film *Human Birth,* published by J. B. Lippincott Co., Philadelphia.)

toneal cavity, neither spill of infected amniotic fluid nor subsequent seepage of pus from the uterus can reach the peritoneal surfaces. This approach was used extensively in the preantibiotic era, but is rarely employed today.

Cesarean Section–Hysterectomy. (Porro's operation). This operation comprises cesarean section followed by removal of the uterus. It may be necessary in certain cases of *premature separation of the placenta,* in patients with multiple *fibroid tumors of the uterus,* and in some circumstances is done electively for sterilization purposes.

Preparation

Preparations for cesarean sections are similar to those for any other abdominal operation, except that in these cases it includes preparations for the care of the infant. An elective cesarean section allows ample time for a physical examination, routine laboratory studies, typing and crossmatching blood, and other customary procedures. However, if there is an emergency, or if labor has started, then such preparations must be made with expediency. In any event, the usual hospital procedure should be followed.

Nursing Management

Preoperative Preparation. When the patient is admitted for an elective cesarean section, nursing care which is routine for any waiting mother (e.g.,

checking fetal heart tones and being alert to prodromal signs of labor) is employed. A short time before the operation the abdomen is shaved, beginning at the level of the xiphoid cartilage and extending out to the far sides and down to the pubic area. A retention catheter is inserted to ensure that the bladder remains empty during the operation and attached to a constant drainage system. One should make certain that the catheter is draining properly before the procedure.

The preoperative medication usually ordered is atropine. The use of narcotic drugs prior to delivery is avoided because of their depressant effect on the infant, but these medications should be readily available. Oxytocic drugs (e.g., oxytocin and ergonovine) should be ready in the operating room· so that they can be administered promptly on the verbal order of the obstetrician when the infant is born.

Preparation for Infant. In addition to the preparation of the operating room for the surgical procedure, preparation for the care of the infant must be accomplished. There must be a warm crib and equipment for the resuscitation of the infant. An infant resuscitator, equipped with heat, suction, oxygen (open mask and positive-pressure), and an adjustable frame to permit the proper positioning of the infant is most useful. A competent person should be present at cesarean section to give the infant initial care and to resuscitate, if necessary. This person may be an experienced nurse, but in many hospitals today it is customary to have a pediatrician at hand to take over the care of the infant as soon as it is born and thus free the obstetrician to devote full attention to the mother.

Postoperative Management

Usually postoperative care is the same as that following any abdominal surgery. It is well to remember that the patient who has had a cesarean section has had both an abdominal operation and a delivery.

Assessing for Hemorrhage. As with any delivery, the patient must be watched for hemorrhage by frequently inspecting the perineal pad and checking the fundus. If the abdominal dressings are bulky, it may be difficult to palpate the fundus to see if the uterus is well contracted, but if the dressings are not massive, and do not extend above the level of the umbilicus, the nurse may feel the consistency of the fundus. Oxytocics may be ordered to keep the uterus contracted and to control bleeding. The vital signs should be checked regularly until they have stabilized, and if there is any indication of shock or hemorrhage, it should be reported promptly. Although there may be no visible signs of external hemorrhage, one would suspect internal hemorrhage if the pulse rate becomes accelerated, the respiration increases in rate, or the blood pressure falls, bearing in mind, of course, that the drop in blood pressure could be due to the effects of some types of anesthetic drugs.

Input and Output. If the retention catheter is to remain in place until the following morning, it should remain attached to "constant drainage" and should be watched to see that it drains freely. Intravenous fluids are usually administered during the first 24 hours, although small amounts of fluids may be given by mouth after nausea has subsided. A record of the mother's intake and elimination is kept for the first several days or until the need is no longer indicated.

Comfort and Respiratory Function. Sedative drugs should be used to keep the mother comfortable and encourage her to rest. Her position in bed during the early postoperative hours may be dictated by the type of anesthesia that she received. She should be encouraged to turn from side to side every hour. Deep breathing and coughing should

---

NURSING MANAGEMENT FOLLOWING CESAREAN SECTION

Assessing for Hemorrhage

1. Inspect perineal pads frequently.
2. Palpate fundus to see if uterus is contracted.
3. Administer oxytocin if prescribed, to contract uterus and control bleeding.
4. Check vital signs regularly until stabilized. Signs of internal hemorrhage:
   Accelerated pulse rate
   Increased rate of respiration
   Fall in blood pressure (due in some cases to effects of anesthetic)

Monitoring Intake and Output

1. Check to see that retention catheter (if left in place) is draining freely.
2. Attend to IV therapy—usually given during first 24 hours postop.
3. Record intake and output for several days postop or as indicated.

Assuring Adequate Respiratory Function

1. Encourage deep breathing and coughing.
2. Encourage mother to turn from side to side every hour.

Attending to Comfort Measures

1. Give sedative medication as prescribed.
2. Position as indicated by the type of anesthetic.

Providing General Postoperative Care

1. Give daily breast care and perineal care.
2. Relieve breast engorgement and afterpains.

---

also be encouraged to promote good ventilation. Today most mothers delivered by cesarean section are allowed early ambulation. It is felt that this contributes considerably to maintaining good bladder and intestinal function.

Psychosocial Considerations. When the cesarean is carried out under conduction anesthesia, the mother has the satisfaction of being able to see her newborn shortly after delivery. In some centers, arrangements can be made to have the father present at the delivery to provide added support (see Chapter

25). Under other circumstances, the father should be permitted to visit as soon as it is feasible. The mother will be anxious to see her infant, too, and it should be brought to her as soon as she is able to see it. The nurse should remain with the mother while she has her infant with her.

General Postpartum Care.   The general care of the mother will be similar to that given any postoperative or postpartal patient. Daily breast care and perineal care are carried out per routine. The mother may have the afterpains, engorgement of the breasts, and the emotional reactions which often accompany a normal delivery.

DESTRUCTIVE OPERATIONS

Destructive operations (designed for the most part to reduce the size of the baby's head and thus to expedite delivery) are rarely done in modern obstetrics. Even in large maternity hospitals many years may pass without a single destructive operation. This salutary state of affairs is attributable in part to the widespread extension of prenatal care, in part to better management of women in labor, and in part to the availability of cesarean section, which makes it safe to effect abdominal delivery even in neglected cases. In the event that a destructive operation is necessary, the obstetrician will choose the necessary instruments.

INDUCTION OF LABOR

Induction of labor means the artificial bringing on of labor after the period of viability. Induction of labor is indicated when continuation of pregnancy would affect maternal health or when there are conditions in the mother which would affect fetal well-being. Complications of pregnancy which may require induction include hypertensive disease of pregnancy, diabetes, hemolytic disease, and postmaternity (see Chapter 31, Complications of Pregnancy).

Since it was believed that the intestinal peristalsis produced by a cathartic is somehow transferred to the uterus, with the consequent initiation of uterine contractions, castor oil has long been employed to induce labor. It was often followed by the administration of a hot soapsuds enema. While this is a harmless approach, it is at the very least uncomfortable and it usually fails.

Oxytocin Induction

An efficient and safe method for the induction of labor is the administration of oxytocin by intravenous drip. The properties of this oxytocic agent and its use in the third stage of labor have already been discussed.

Rate of Administration   Since oxytocin has dangerous potentialities when administered to a pregnant woman, the dosage used is always extremely small. Administration by intravenous drip assures a uniform, although infinitesimal, concentration of the agent in the bloodstream. The amount of oxytocin being administered can be readily controlled and is governed by the response of the uterus. Oxytocin has also been administered intramuscularly, but this approach is no longer recommended. Since the response of a given patient is not predictable, there is no way to select an appropriate intramuscular dose.

For the intravenous administration of oxytocin, the physician will usually ask for a flask containing 500 ml. of 5 percent glucose to which will be added the quantity of oxytocin indicated. The intravenous equipment is set up as usual so that the number of drops flowing per minute can be closely observed in the observation tube. This is extremely important, and the physician will specify the precise number of drops per minute. Initially, the drip should be run very slowly—4 to 5 drops per minute. The rate of administration should be increased gradually thereafter, always being governed by the response of the patient. To avoid a sudden infusion of oxytocin during placement of the intravenous, a piggyback system is usually recommended (Fig. 34-9). After an infusion of 5 percent D+W is running, the solution containing the pitocin is introduced for a second intravenous setup by placing the needle into the rubber adaptor of the infusion already in place. The amount of pitocin delivered can then be regulated—increased, decreased, or discontinued—without interfering with the continuity of the IV delivery system. Oxytocin administration can also be very accurately controlled with the use of a constant infusion pump.

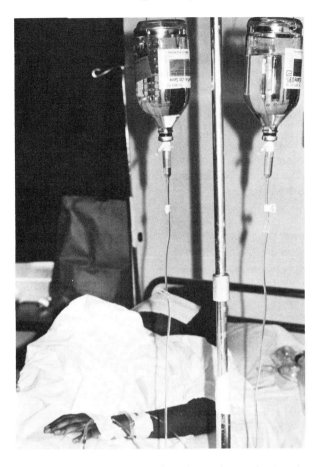

Figure 34-9. Administration of pit drip with piggyback technique.

Precautions   The administration of oxytocin to a gravida carries certain hazards, and it is obligatory for her safety and that of the baby that a physician or a nurse be in constant bedside attendance to make certain that the number of drops flowing per minute does not change and to watch for certain untoward effects.

1. The observer must check the rate of flow of the oxytocin solution at frequent intervals to make certain that it remains constant.
2. The duration and the intensity of each uterine contraction must be watched closely and recorded.
3. Any contraction lasting over 90 seconds indicates that the quantity of solution is too great, and the rate of flow should either be decreased or tentatively discontinued altogether.
4. Furthermore, the fetal heart rate should be counted and recorded. In many hospitals con-

tinuous electronic fetal monitoring is used routinely when oxytocin is administered.

5. The fetal heart tones should return to their normal rate and rhythm within 15 seconds or so after the termination of a contraction, any persistence of fetal bradycardia is an indication for discontinuation of the oxytocin drip.
6. If any abnormality in the uterine contractions or the fetal heart tones is observed, the solution should be turned off *immediately* and the findings reported to the physician. The major advantage of the oxytocin drip is that it may be discontinued immediately in the event that untoward effects should be observed—an obvious safety factor.

Some obstetrical units have found it helpful to utilize a protocol for oxytocin induction or augmentation of labor. One such protocol is outlined on next page.

Artificial Rupture of the Membranes

Amniotomy, or artificial rupture of the membranes, is a common method of enhancing labor. Amniotomy has also been used to induce labor. When the patient is near term and the cervix is favorable, it is almost always followed by labor within a few hours.

The membranes serve as a barrier against bacterial invasion. For this reason, once this barrier has been eliminated by amniotomy, delivery should be accomplished expeditiously. Many obstetricians, now feel that the primary use of amniotomy for labor induction is tantamount to burning one's bridges and that the procedure should be delayed until after the initiation of good contractions with intravenous pitocin.

Amniotomy is accomplished after placing the patient in the lithotomy position and carrying out antiseptic preparation of the vulva. The first two fingers of one hand are inserted into the cervix until the membranes are encountered. A long hook, similar to one blade of a disarticulated vulsellum tenaculum, or an Allis clamp, is inserted into the vagina, and the membranes are simply hooked and torn by the tip of the sharp instrument. As much fluid as possible is allowed to drain. The quality of the fluid should be noted. Normally, it is watery-clear.

Fetal heart tones should be checked immediately after amniotomy; extra care should be exercised, as there is an increased possibility of cord prolapse.

PROTOCOL FOR PITOCIN (OXYTOCIN) INDUCTION AND AUGMENTATION*

Physician Responsibility:

1. The physician will evaluate the patient and determine if patient is to be started on intravenous pitocin.

2. The physician will obtain at least a 10-minute baseline monitor strip of uterine contractions and fetal heart rate, using an external system if membranes are intact.

3. The physician will write on patient's order sheet that pitocin is to be started at 0.2 mU/minute or at a level to be determined by the physician and may progress to 10 mU/minute using the increments listed below. The pitocin infusion may be increased every 15 to 20 minutes.

TABLE I

Pitocin infusion starts at	0.2 mU/minute
then increases to	0.4 mU/minute
	1 mU/minute
	2 mU/minute
	4 mU/minute
	8 mU/minute
hold at	10 mU/minute

4. The physician will evaluate the patient when the dosage of pitocin reaches 10 mU/minute. If continuation of pitocin is needed, the physician will write on patient's order sheet that the pitocin infusion be increased every 15 to 20 minutes until a dose of 20 mU/minute is reached. The following dose schedule should be used:

TABLE II

Pitocin infusion continued	12 mU/minute
	16 mU/minute
hold at	20 mU/minute

5. The resident physician will consult with the Chief Resident when pitocin infusion has reached 20 mU/minute.

6. The physician must be present on the Labor and Delivery Floor while pitocin is being infused. (At least one physician is present at all times.)

7. The physician will frequently observe the patient's progress, at least hourly or more often if indicated.

Nursing Responsibilities:

1. Prepare the pitocin solution:
   a. 5 units of pitocin are added to 250 ml. of normal saline, 0.9%. solution. This yields a solution with a concentration of 20 milliunits of pitocin per ml. TO BE USED WITH HARVARD PUMP.
   OR
   b. Add 2.5 units of pitocin to 500 ml. of normal saline, 0.9% solution. This yields a solution with a concentration of 5 milliunits of pitocin per ml. TO BE USED WITH IMED OR CONSTANT INFUSION (2620 HARVARD) PUMP.

2. Take infusion pump to bedside.

3. Assemble infusion pump with pitocin solution.

4. Set infusion pump to correspond to the pitocin dosage which was ordered.

5. Start pitocin infusion (secondary line) by inserting needle into the connector most proximal to the primary line. Be sure to keep primary line running at a slow rate.

6. Turn on pitocin infusion pump at set rate.

7. Observe contraction pattern and fetal heart rate on the monitor. If no abnormalities are noted, in 15 to 20 minutes, increase the pitocin infusion according to Table I so that the uterine contractions are observed every 2 to 3 minutes and last approximately 60 seconds.

PROTOCOL FOR PITOCIN (OXYTOCIN) INDUCTION AND AUGMENTATION*

8. Once a regular contraction pattern is established, hold the pitocin infusion at that rate or decrease the infusion rate and determine if a regular contraction pattern will still be sustained.

9. If at any time a question arises as to 1) the possibility of hyperstimulation (less than 2 minutes between contractions or contractions lasting longer than 60 seconds); 2) an abnormal fetal heart rate pattern, the nurse will immediately:
    a. Turn off pitocin infusion
    b. Turn patient on left side
    c. Start oxygen by mask at 6 to 8 liters per minute
    d. Notify physician

10. Notify the physician if the contraction pattern slows and labor is not well established.

11. Check the pitocin infusion bottle as to amount being absorbed and the rate of infusion, at least every ½ hour.

12. Remember that all patients receiving intravenous pitocin must be continuously observed by a qualified member of the nursing staff who is under the direct supervision of a registered nurse.

13. Continuously assess the patient's progress both physically and emotionally as well as by the monitor tracings.
    Remember, the patient and not the monitor is being treated.

14. Notify the physician when 10 mU/minute of pitocin is reached so that an evaluation of the patient may be made by the physician.

15. Carry out the written prescription for pitocin infusion, if it is to be continued to 20 mU/minute, according to Table II.

16. Take vital signs and fetal heart rate every 15 minutes and record these on the intrapartum flow sheet as well as on the monitor strip.

17. Record the characteristics of the contraction pattern every 15 minutes on the intrapartum flow sheet. These observations include palpation of the intensity of the uterine contraction and their frequency at least every ½ hour.

REMEMBER: IF IN DOUBT AT ANY TIME ABOUT THE RESPONSE OF THE PATIENT OR FETUS TO PITOCIN, TURN THE PITOCIN INFUSION OFF AND NOTIFY THE PHYSICIAN IMMEDIATELY.

Chart Notations:

Intrapartum Flow Sheet

1. Dosage of pitocin, the name and amount of the solution

2. Rate of the flow of pitocin increased, held or decreased

3. Contraction pattern every 15 minutes

4. Vital signs and fetal heart rate every 15 minutes

5. Vaginal exams and results done by the physician

6. Adjustments to the monitor

Nurses Record

1. Intake
    a. Oral
    b. Intravenous

2. Output
    a. Urine
    b. Vomitus
    c. Other

3. 8-hour summary of intake and output

PROTOCOL FOR PITOCIN (OXYTOCIN) INDUCTION AND AUGMENTATION*

4. Vaginal exams and results done by the physician

5. Treatments

6. Nursing care
   a. Physical
   b. Emotional
   c. Teaching

Monitor Tracings

1. Dosage of pitocin and time started

2. Time and the dosage of pitocin when increased, held or decreased

3. Vital signs every 15 minutes and the time

4. Exams and procedures by physician and the time

5. Any movement or changes to the patient or monitor that may interfere with recording of the tracing

* Hospital of the University of Pennsylvania: Department of Nursing; Department of Obstetrics and Gynecology.

SUGGESTED READING

Prichard, J. A., and Macdonald, P. C.: Williams Obstetrics, ed. 5., New York, Appleton-Century-Crofts, 1976.

Willson, S. R., and Carrington, E. R., Obstetrics and Gynecology, ed. 6, St. Louis, C. V. Mosby, 1979.

Thirty-Five

Postpartal Complications

Postpartum Infections of the Genital Tract | Pulmonary Embolism | Subinvolution of the Uterus | Vulvar Hematomas | Mastitis | Urinary Tract Infection | Other Complications

The postpartal period is a time of increased physiologic stress, as well as a phase of major psychological transition. During this time the woman's body is more vulnerable because of the energy depletion and fatigue of late pregnancy and labor, the tissue trauma of delivery, and the blood loss and propensity for anemia which frequently occurs. Most women recover from the stresses of pregnancy and childbirth without significant complications. When postpartal complications do occur, the most common are *infection* involving the genital tract, urinary system and breasts; *hemorrhage,* immediate or delayed; *embolic clotting disorders;* and *uterine subinvolution.* The potentially critical nature of many postpartal complications, the associated pain and procedures, medications, frequent need to be isolated or removed from the maternity unit, and emotionally disruptive effects of the physiologic malfunction can interfere with the maternal-infant bonding process. Nursing care must minimize physical separation of mother and infant and encourage attachment through such means as frequent discussions about the baby's behavior and characteristics, pictures, and so forth. Prompt diagnosis and treatment of postpartal complications to reduce their dysfunctional effects are also important.

POSTPARTUM INFECTIONS OF THE GENITAL TRACT

When inflammatory processes develop in the birth canal postpartally, as a result of bacterial invasion of these highly vulnerable areas, the condition is known as puerperal infection. It is really a postpartal wound infection of the birth canal, usually of the endometrium. As is true of other wound infections, the condition often remains localized but may extend along various pathways to produce diverse clinical pictures. Febrile reactions of more or less severity are the rule, and the outcome varies according to the portal of entry, the type, the number and the virulence of the invading organisms, the reaction of the tissues and the general resistance of the patient. Puerperal infection is one of the most common causes of death in childbearing.

Febrile morbidity in the postpartum period is defined as a temperature elevation of 38°C. (100.4°F.) or more occurring after the first 24 hours postpartum on two or more occasions that are not within the same 24 hours.[1] Low-grade temperature elevations postpartally are not uncommon, and have been attributed to such factors as dehydration, infusion of fetal protein, breast engorgement, and respiratory infection. However, the endometrial cavity is the site of significant anaerobic bacterial growth in the immediate postpartal period, and probably most women with temperature elevations in the first 24 hours do have genital tract infections. When delivery has occurred vaginally, the spontaneous clearance of necrotic decidua and blood from the uterine cavity is adequate to remove bacteria in most cases. The transient temperature elevation seen in the first 24 hours after delivery represents this process. When the delivery has been by cesarean section, there is a much higher risk of postpartum infection, with the risk of death 26 times greater than from vaginal delivery.[2] Figures 35-1 and 35-2 show febrile patterns of transient temperature elevation in the first 24 hours and clinically significant postpartum infection.

Causative Factors

The most common organisms causing postpartum infections are anaerobic nonhemolytic streptococci, coliform bacteria, bacteroides, and staphylococci. There is reduced incidence of beta-hemolytic streptococcal infection due to improvements in obstetrical care and aseptic technique. Multiple bacterial pathogens are present in the cervix and lower uterine segment during pregnancy and for a short time after delivery. Generally, such organisms harbored in the female genital tract do not cause infections, but the trauma of birth and alteration of immunologic function and resistance caused by fatigue and stress make the postpartal woman more susceptible. Hem-

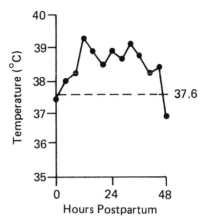

Figure 35-2. The pattern of fever (>38.4 C) in the first 24 hours postpartum following either spontaneous vaginal delivery or cesarean section. (Source for Figures 35-1 and 35-2: Filker, R. and Monif, G. R. G.: "The Significance of temperature during the first 24 hours postpartum." *Obstet. & Gynecol.,* 53, 3:358–361, March 1979.)

orrhage and anemia also predispose to postpartal infection.

Endogenous infections are caused by bacteria in the genital tract which enter and colonize wounds in the perineum, vagina, cervix, or endometrium at the site of placental attachment. Existing infections in other organs or septicemia may also be a cause. Exogenous infections are caused by introduction of organisms into the genital tract. Nurses, physicians and other personnel are the most frequent source of exogenous infections.

Although attending personnel wear gloves, the hands and the instruments used may become contaminated by pathogenic bacteria as the result of droplet infection from the nasopharynx. Even in modern obstetrics, this is a very common mode of infection, and unless the utmost vigilance is used in masking all attendants in the delivery room (both nose and mouth) and in excluding all persons suffering or recovering from an upper respiratory infection, it is a constant source of danger.

Although a less common means of transfer today than a few decades ago, careless physicians and nurses have been known to carry bacteria to the parturient from countless extraneous contacts—from other cases of puerperal infection, from suppurative postoperative wounds, from cases of sloughing carcinoma, from patients with scarlet fever, from infants with impetigo neonatorum, and from umbilical infections of the newborn. The physician and nurse, themselves, may have an infection such as an infected hangnail or furuncle.

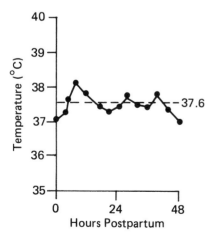

Figure 35-1. The pattern of resolving postpartum fever (single spike) following spontaneous vaginal delivery.

Coitus late in pregnancy may introduce extraneous organisms to the birth canal or carry upward bacteria already present on the vulva or in the lower vagina. However, there is little risk unless the membranes are ruptured, in which case coitus should be avoided.

During the second stage of labor, the chances of fecal matter being transferred to the vagina are great, another source of introducing coliform bacteria.

In addition to traumatic labor and postpartal hemorrhage, other factors are prolonged labor, prolonged rupture of the membranes, retention of placental tissue, and retained blood clots.

Types of Genital Tract Infection

Genital tract (puerperal) infection can be divided into two main types: 1) *local lesion processes* and 2) *extensions of the original lesion process.* When a lesion of the vulva, the perineum, the vagina, the cervix or the endometrium becomes infected, the infection may remain localized in these wounds. However, the original inflammatory process may extend along the veins (the most common way) and cause thrombophlebitis and pyemia, or through the lymph vessels to cause peritonitis and pelvic cellulitis.

Lesions of the Perineum, the Vulva and the Vagina

These lesions are highly vulnerable areas for bacterial invasion in the early puerperium. The most common is a localized infection of a repaired perineal laceration or episiotomy wound.

The usual symptoms are elevation of temperature, pain and sensation of heat in the affected area and burning on urination. The area involved becomes red and edematous, and there is profuse seropurulent discharge. If a wound of the vulva becomes infected, the entire vulva may become edematous and ulcerated. Infections involving the perineum, the vulva and the vagina cause the patient considerable discomfort and alarm.

These local inflammatory processes seldom cause severe physical reactions, provided that good drainage is established and the patient's temperature remains below 38.4°C. (101°F.). To promote good drainage, all stitches may be removed to lay open the surface. Because the drainage itself is a source of irritation and contamination, the wound must be kept clean and the perineal pads changed frequently. Care must be exercised in cleansing the wound to see that none of the solution runs into the vagina.

Treatments by such means as sitz baths or the perineal heat lamp are generally used for the relief of pain. Antibiotics are prescribed to combat the infection. If drainage is impaired, the patient not only will have more pain but also may have a chill, followed by a sudden elevation of temperature.

Endometritis

This is a localized infection of the lining membrane of the uterus. Bacteria invade the lesion, usually the placental site, and may spread to involve the entire endometrium.

When endometritis develops, it is usually manifest about 48 to 72 hours after delivery. In the milder forms the patient may have no complaints or symptoms other than a rise in temperature to about 38.4°C. (101°F.) which persists for several days and then subsides. On the other hand, the more virulent infections are often ushered in by chills and high fever, with a comparable rise in pulse rate. In the majority of severe cases the patient experiences a chilly sensation, or actual chills, at the onset and often complains of malaise, loss of appetite, headache, backache and general discomfort.

It is not unusual for the patient to have severe and prolonged after-pains. The uterus is usually large and is extremely tender when palpated abdominally. The lochial discharge may be decreased in amount and distinguished from normal lochia by its dark brown appearance and foul odor. In some cases, particularly those caused by the hemolytic streptococcus, the lochia may be odorless.

If the infection remains localized in the endometrium, it is usually over in about a week or 10 days. But when extension of the infection occurs to cause peritonitis, pelvic thrombophlebitis or cellulitis, the disease may persist for many weeks, often with dramatic temperature curves and repeated chills.

Treatment depends on the severity of the condition. Mild cases with temperature under 100°F. and no chills are best handled by simple measures. Fowler's position facilitates lochial drainage. Ergonovine four times daily for two days promotes uterine tone, and forced fluids provide additional support. The lochia is cultured and the patient is treated with the appropriate antibiotic. Isolation is desirable to protect other patients and to afford the mother greater rest. In this group it is unnecessary to discontinue breast-feeding.

In severe cases, breast-feeding is discontinued not only because it exhausts the mother but also because it is usually futile in the presence of high fever.

Pelvic Cellulitis, or Parametritis

This is an infection which extends along the lymphatics to reach the loose connective tissue surrounding the uterus. It may follow an infected cervical laceration, endometritis or pelvic thrombophlebitis. The patient will have a persistent fever and marked pain and tenderness over the affected area. The problem is usually unilateral but may involve both sides of the abdomen. As the process develops, the swelling becomes very hard and finally either undergoes resolution or results in the formation of a pelvic abscess. If the latter occurs, as the abscess comes to a point, the skin above becomes red, edematous and tender. Recovery is usually prompt after the abscess is opened.

Thrombophlebitis

This is an infection of the vascular endothelium with clot formation attached to the vessel wall. It may be of two types: pelvic thrombophlebitis, an inflammatory process involving the ovarian and the uterine veins, or femoral thrombophlebitis, in which the femoral, the popliteal or the saphenous vein is involved. Early ambulation may be a factor in preventing this complication.

Femoral Thrombophlebitis. This condition presents a special group of signs and symptoms. It is a disease of the puerperium characterized by pain, fever and swelling in the affected leg. These symptoms are due to the formation of a clot in the veins of the leg itself, which interferes with the return circulation of the blood. When this condition develops, it usually appears about 10 days after labor, although it may manifest itself as late as the twentieth day. As in all acute febrile diseases occurring after labor, the secretion of milk may cease.

The disease is ushered in with malaise, chilliness and fever, which are soon followed by stiffness and pain in the affected part. If it is in the leg, the pain may begin in the groin or the hip and extend downward, or it may commence in the calf of the leg and extend upward. In about 24 hours the leg begins to swell, and although the pain then lessens slightly, it is always present and may be severe enough to prevent sleep. The skin over the swollen area is shiny white in color.

The acute symptoms last from a few days to a week, after which the pain gradually subsides, and the patient slowly improves.

The course of the disease covers a period of four to six weeks. The affected leg is slow to return to its normal size and may remain permanently enlarged and troublesome.

The prognosis is usually favorable. However, in some of the very severe cases, abscesses may form and the disease may become critical and produce fatality. Since the clot tends to be attached to the vessel wall somewhat loosely, there is a tendency for the clot to dislodge and produce a pulmonary embolism which also is fatal in the majority of cases.

Treatment of femoral thrombophlebitis consists of rest, elevation of the affected leg, and analgesics as indicated for pain. Anticoagulants, such as heparin and dicumarol, may be prescribed to prevent further formation of thrombi. Antimicrobial drugs may be used in cases where more generalized infection is known or suspected. A "cradle" is used to keep the pressure of the bedclothes off the affected part. Heat or icebags may be used along the course of the affected vessels.

Surgical treatment may be indicated in some severe and/or nonresponding cases and consists of incision of the affected vessel, removal of the clot, and repair of the vessel. Ligation of the major vessels is sometimes resorted to as a preventive measure for pulmonary embolism.

Under no circumstances should anyone rub or massage the affected part. The leg should be handled with the utmost care when one is changing dressings, applying a bandage, making the bed or giving a bath.

Pelvic Thrombophlebitis. This is a severe complication in the puerperium. The onset usually occurs about the second week following delivery with severe repeated chills and dramatic swings in temperature. The infection is usually caused by anaerobic streptococci, and although it is difficult to obtain a positive blood culture, bacteria are present in the bloodstream during chills. Antimicrobial therapy is used and is effective in treating most strains of this organism; as long as the chills and the fever persist, blood transfusions may be given. Heparin and dicumarol may be prescribed to prevent the formation of more thrombi. A further problem is likely to arise with metastatic pulmonary complications, such as lung abscesses or pneumonia.

These patients are often depressed, discouraged and feel physically unwell. Breast-feeding may have been interrupted and the significant emotional and physiologic changes following childbirth may be compounded by the illness.

Astute nursing care at this time is particularly essential. Accurate observing, recording and reporting, and paying particular attention to details of the physical care aspects are extremely important in helping to resolve the disorder and to prevent further complications. Supportive care to help the mother (and family) work through the depression and discouragement is another crucial aspect of care. The principles outlined in the discussion of grief are appropriate here. (See Chap. 39.)

Peritonitis

Peritonitis is an infection, either generalized or local, of the peritoneum. Usually the infection reaches the peritoneum from the endometrium by traveling via the lymphatic vessels; but peritonitis may result also from the extension of thrombophlebitis or parametritis.

The clinical course of pelvic peritonitis resembles that of surgical peritonitis. The patient has a high fever, rapid pulse and, in general, has the appearance of being profoundly ill. She is usually restless and sleepless and has constant and severe abdominal pain. Hiccups, nausea and vomiting, which is sometimes fecal and projectile, may be present.

Antimicrobial therapy is given to combat the infection, while analgesic drugs are prescribed for discomfort and mild sedative drugs to relieve the restlessness and apprehension. If there is intestinal involvement, oral feedings are withheld until normal intestinal function is restored; meanwhile, fluids are administered intravenously. Blood transfusions and oxygen therapy may be indicated for supportive treatment. The record of intake and output must be kept.

Signs and Symptoms

It is very important that the nurse recognize and report early signs and symptoms of postpartal genital tract infection so that proper treatment may be instituted without delay. When such puerperal infection develops, one of the first symptoms usually seen is a rise in temperature. Although temperature elevations in the puerperium may be caused by upper respiratory infections, urinary tract infections and the like, the majority are due to genital tract infection.

The symptoms may vary, depending on the location and the extent of the infectious process, the type and the virulence of the invading organisms and the general resistance of the patient. The affected area is usually painful, reddened and edematous and the source of profuse discharge. The patient may complain of malaise, headache and general discomfort. As mentioned above, the temperature is elevated, and in the more severe infections, chills and fever may occur.

In its typical form each of the clinical types of puerperal infection presents a very characteristic set of signs and symptoms, although occasionally one form of the disease is combined with another. The distinctions between these different types of infections are important, because the clinical course, the treatment and the prognosis depend on the particular form of infection (Table 35-1).

Management

The use of antimicrobial therapy provides highly effective treatment and has vastly improved the prognosis of puerperal infection. These drugs are effective in combating most of these infections, but, nevertheless, the management and the care of patients with puerperal infections are highly important and demand the utmost in skill. Penicillin is effective against the hemolytic streptococcus, the clostridium bacillus and the staphylococcus. Since penicillin is not effective against the colon bacillus and certain strains of staphylococci, a broad-spectrum antibiotic (such as ampicillin, tetracycline or cephalosporin) may be prescribed for infections caused by these organisms. Many types of antimicrobials are available, some specifically for the gram positive or negative organisms and the penicillin resisitant organisms. The selection and dosage of these drugs will depend upon the severity of the disease and the type of offending organism. Sensitivity series will often be done to help determine the appropriate antibiotic. Uterine cultures are taken to gain information about the organism; in severe cases blood cultures may be taken, but if they are to be of real

TABLE 35-1
TYPES OF POSTPARTUM GENITAL TRACT INFECTIONS

Type of Infection	Etiology	Signs/Symptoms	Treatment
Perineal and vulvar lesions	Bacterial invasion of episiotomy, laceration, traumatized tissue	Fever, localized pain Edema, erythema, seropurulent discharge from lesion	Antibiotics Removal of stitches and promotion of drainage, sitz baths, perineal heat lamp, analgesics
Endometritis	Bacterial invasion of placental site or entire endometrium	Fever about 38.4°C. or 101°F., chills, rapid pulse Malaise, headache, backache, loss of appetite, cramps Relaxed, tender uterus with foul-smelling discharge, dark and/or profuse lochia	Antibiotics, ergonovine Fowler's position to promote drainage, hydration
Pelvic cellulitis or parametritis	Bacterial invasion via lymphatics to tissue surrounding uterus (often following endometritis)	Fever, chills Pain and tenderness of lower abdomen, edema Signs of endometritis may be present also	Antibiotics Hydration, blood transfusion for dropping hemoglobin Bedrest, analgesics
Femoral thrombophlebitis	Infection of thrombi and vascular endothelium	Fever, chills, malaise Stiffness, pain, swelling of affected area	Rest, elevation of leg, heat or ice to leg Anticoagulants, antibiotics, analgesics
Pelvic thrombophlebitis	Infection of thrombi and pelvic veins	Severe repeated chills and dramatic temperature swings	Anticoagulants, antibiotics, blood transfusion, bedrest
Peritonitis	Spread of infection to peritoneum, local or generalized	High fever, rapid pulse Severe abdominal pain Vomiting, restlessness Distention	Antibiotics, analgesics, sedatives Bedrest, hydration, blood transfusion, oxygen, IV infusions

diagnostic value they must be taken at the time of the chill. The infected lesions are treated the same as those of any surgical wound. Drainage must be established, and since this discharge is of a highly infectious nature, care must be taken to see that it is not spread and that all contaminated pads and dressings are wrapped and burned.

Nursing Intervention. The curative treatment is antilistic therapy, but good nursing care is essential. The patient should be kept as comfortable and quiet as possible, for sleep and rest are important. Conserving the patient's strength in every way, along with giving her nourishing food and appropriate amounts of fluids, will help to increase her powers of resistance. To promote drainage the head of the bed should be kept elevated, a measure which also contributes to the patient's comfort.

Care must be exercised to prevent the spread of the infection from one patient to another. Isolation of infected patients from others is desirable in order to protect the healthy maternity patients. Ideally,

the patient with puerperal infection should be away from the maternity divisions. If it is impossible to arrange for such complete segregation, the nurse must consider every patient with puerperal infection as "in isolation" and follow scrupulous technique accordingly.

Regardless of the situation, the nurse who is caring for a patient with puerperal infection (or any infection, for that matter) should not attend other maternity patients. The hands of all attendants need special attention and should be scrubbed thoroughly after caring for a mother who has an infection. In certain cases strict isolation technique, with special gowns, masks and rubber gloves, is essential. Clean isolation gowns, masks and gloves should be available for all persons who attend the isolated patient and after being used should be left in the room and disposed of in special hampers or containers. This apparel should not be worn outside the patient's room. Nurses who care for these patients must be fully acquainted with principles of good isolation technique.

Genital Tract Infection Following Cesarean Section

The incidence of genital tract infection is significantly increased when delivery is by cesarean section. This is frequently related to several factors, such as duration of ruptured membranes, number of vaginal examinations, length of labor, various complications and the need for invasive procedures. However, the operative trauma itself increases infectious morbidity, generally caused by a mixed anaerobic/aerobic infection by organisms present in the genital tract at the time of labor and delivery. Surgical trauma, with devitalization of tissue and collection of blood and serum in the myometrium or endometrium, which have become infected with organisms that have ascended from the lower genital tract to the amniotic fluid, plays a key role in the development of postpartal endometritis, myometritis, incisional wound abscesses and pelvic abscesses.[3]

Treatment is by antimicrobial therapy and drainage of abscesses; the antibiotics commonly used include penicillin, tetracycline, kanamycin and clindamycin. The organisms most frequently causing infections following cesarean section are anaerobic streptococci, aerobic streptococci, Bacteroides species, *E. coli,* and less often Clostridium species and staphylococci. A particularly strong relationship has been found between membranes ruptured for longer than six hours and post-cesarean section infection (myometritis).[4]

Prevention of Infection

The prevention of infection throughout the maternity cycle is an important factor in the maintenance of health and the prevention of disease. During pregnancy, complete blood counts or HCT and HGB tests are done routinely and iron is prescribed as necessary, not only for the immediate value but also because anemia predisposes to puerperal infection. Health teaching is emphasized at this time, particularly in regard to diet, rest, exercise and general hygiene. The patient is advised to avoid possible sources of infection, especially upper respiratory infections.

During labor, care should be exercised to limit bacteria from extraneous sources. In the hospital, cleanliness and good housekeeping are imperative,

but, nevertheless, individual care technique reduces the chance of contamination from other patients. Each patient should have her own equipment, which includes her own bedpan. This bedpan should be cleansed after each use and sterilized once a day. Careful hand washing on the part of all personnel after contacts with each patient will do much to prevent the transfer of infection from one patient to another.

The strictest rules should be enforced for surgical cleanliness during labor and delivery. No one with an infection of the skin or the respiratory tract should work in the maternity department. The nasopharynx of attendants is the most common exogenous source of contamination of the birth canal. Regular nasopharyngeal cultures of maternity personnel are often required. To be effective, masks worn during delivery must cover the nose and the mouth and be clean and dry; thus they must be changed frequently and should not hang around the neck when not in use.

During the puerperium the same precautions should be carried out. For many days following the delivery, the surface of the birth canal is a vulnerable area for pathogenic bacteria. The birth canal is well protected against the invasion of extraneous bacteria by the closed vulva, unless this barrier is invaded. Patients, therefore, are to be taught the principles of perineal hygiene and how to give themselves self-care, without using the fingers to separate the labia, because this permits the cleansing solution to enter the vagina.

PULMONARY EMBOLISM

Pulmonary embolism is usually due to the detachment of a small part of a thrombus, which is washed along in the blood current until it becomes lodged in the right side of the heart. In many cases the thrombus originates in a uterine or a pelvic vein, although its origin may be in some other vessel. When the embolus occludes the pulmonary artery, it obstructs the passage of blood into the lungs, either wholly or in part, and the patient may die of asphyxia within a few minutes. If the clot is small, the initial episode may not be fatal, although repeated attacks may prove so. The condition may follow infection, thrombosis, severe hemorrhage or shock, and it may occur any time during the puerperium, especially after sudden exertion.

Manifestations. The symptoms of pulmonary embolism are sudden intense pain in the chest; severe dyspnea; unusual apprehension; syncope; feeble, irregular or imperceptible pulse; pallor in some cases, cyanosis in others; and eventually air hunger. Death may occur at any time from within a few minutes to a few hours, according to the amount or degree of obstruction to the pulmonary circulation. If the patient survives for a few hours, it is likely that she may recover.

Management. The treatment consists, first of all, in preventing the accident by careful attention to all details of surgical asepsis and to the proper management of labor and delivery. Following delivery, early ambulation may be an additional prophylactic measure, since circulatory stasis is undoubtedly a causative factor. In some instances it is almost impossible to prevent a fatal attack, because the patient may be recovering without elevation of temperature and without complications and yet, on the seventh or tenth day, she suddenly cries out, and passes into coma and shock due to cor pulmonale.

When embolism occurs, rapid emergency measures to combat anoxia and shock must be carried out promptly. Oxygen is administered without delay, and anticoagulants are given. Morphine or Demerol may be helpful to relieve the patient's apprehension and pain and usually is given. Dicumarol and heparin therapy will be continued to prevent recurrent emboli, for as long as six weeks to six months depending on clinical response. During hospitalization the patient must be kept warm, quiet, comfortable and as free from worry as possible. She may be given a light, nourishing diet during early convalescence.

SUBINVOLUTION OF THE UTERUS

Subinvolution is the term used to describe the condition which exists when normal involution of the puerperal uterus is retarded. The causes contributing to this condition may be 1) lack of tone in the uterine musculature, 2) imperfect exfoliation of the decidua, 3) retained placental tissue and membranes, 4) endometritis and 5) presence of uterine fibroids.

Subinvolution is characterized by a large and flabby uterus; lochial discharge prolonged beyond the usual period, sometimes with profuse bleeding; backache and dragging sensation in the pelvis.

Treatment is aimed at correcting the cause of subinvolution. Oxytocic medication, such as methylergonovine (Methergine) or ergonovine, may be administered to maintain uterine tone and prevent the accumulation of clots in the uterine cavity. Curettage is employed to remove any retained placental tissue or secundines. Endometritis will require antimicrobial therapy. If the uterus is displaced, it may delay normal involution and is usually corrected by a suitably fitting pessary.

Early ambulation is believed to have decreased the incidence of subinvolution. And, since it is recognized that breast-feeding stimulates uterine contractions, the fact that the mother is *not* breast-feeding plus the fact that she is usually taking a lactogenic suppressing drug, may be influencing factors when subinvolution occurs.

VULVAR HEMATOMAS

Blood may escape into the connective tissue beneath the skin covering the external genitalia or beneath the vaginal mucosa to form vulvar and vaginal hematomas, respectively. The condition occurs about once in every 500 to 1,000 deliveries.

Vulvar hematomas manifest themselves by severe perineal pain and the sudden appearance of a tense, fluctuant and sensitive tumor of varying size covered by discolored skin. When the mass develops in the vagina, it may temporarily escape detection, but pain and the patient's inability to void should alert the nurse to this complication.

Since these symptoms may also be indicative of other types of complications, a careful examination of the perineum and an accurate report of its condition is important. The new parturient has great difficulty in localizing any pain that she may have. Therefore the nurse usually will have to explore with the mother the nature and location of her discomfort, gradually moving from more general statements to those which are specific and more accurate. A vaginal examination which confirms the diagnosis is usually performed.

Small hematomas are usually treated supportively and allowed to resolve of their own accord. However, if the pain is severe or the tumor enlarges, incision and evacuation of the blood, with ligation of bleeding points and packing, will be required.

Vulvar or vaginal hematomas may become infected, particularly those that must be opened and drained. Therefore, attention must be given to prevention of contamination both through careful aseptic technique of attendants and by teaching the patient perineal and bowel hygiene. Dressings or perineal pads must be changed frequently and early signs of infection such as foul-smelling discharge or temperature elevation reported at once.

MASTITIS

Mastitis, or inflammation of the breast, may vary from a "simple" inflammation of the tissues around the nipple to a suppurative process that results in abscess formation in the glandular tissue. Mastitis is always the result of an infection, usually caused by *Staphylococcus aureus* or hemolytic streptococcus organisms. The disease in most instances is preceded by fissures or erosions of the nipple or the areola, which provide a portal of entry to the subcutaneous lymphatics, although under conducive conditions organisms present in the lactiferous ducts can invade the tissues and cause mastitis.

Manifestations.   Puerperal mastitis may occur any time during lactation but usually occurs about the third or fourth week of the puerperium. There is usually marked engorgement of the breast preceding mastitis, although engorgement per se does not cause the infection. When the infection occurs, the patient complains of acute pain and tenderness in the breast and often experiences general malaise, a chilly sensation or, in fact, may have a chill followed by a marked rise of temperature (to 40.5°C or 105°F.) and an increased pulse rate. On inspection the breast appears hard and reddened. The obstetrician should be notified at once and treatment instituted promptly in the hope that resolution may take place before the infection becomes localized as an abscess.

Management.   Puerperal mastitis is preventable, for the most part, by prophylactic measures. An important measure is initiated when the expectant mother learns about breast hygiene and begins to take special care of her breasts during the latter months of pregnancy (see Chapter 20).

After delivery, appropriate breast care will further help to prevent the development of lesions, but if they do occur, proper treatment must be given promptly. Any time the mother complains of sore, tender nipples, they should be inspected immediately. At this time there may be no break in the surface, but if the condition is neglected, the nipple may become raw and cracked. The alert nurse often can detect even a very small crack in the surface of the nipple if it is inspected carefully. Once a break in the skin occurs, the chances of infection mount, because pathogenic organisms are frequently brought to the breast by the hands or may reach the breast from the patient's nightgown or bedclothes.

With early treatment by antibiotics, the inflammatory process may be brought under control before suppuration occurs. A broad spectrum antibiotic is effective in treating acute puerperal mastitis if the therapy is started promptly, and often symptoms subside within 24 to 48 hours. The breasts should be well supported with a firm breast binder or well fitted brassiere. While the breasts are very painful, small side pillows used for support may give the mother some measure of comfort. Icecaps may be applied over the affected part, but if in time it becomes apparent that suppuration is inevitable, heat applications may be ordered to hasten the localization of the abscess. It is usually advised that breast-feeding be discontinued immediately in cases of mastitis.

If the treatment described above is unsuccessful, measures will have to be taken to remove the pus when abscess formation occurs. In some cases it may be preferable to aspirate the pus rather than resort to incision and drainage. When incision and drainage are done, the incision is made radially, extending from near the areolar margin toward the periphery of the gland, in order to avoid injury to the lactiferous ducts. After the pus is evacuated, a gauze drain is inserted. Following the operation the care of the patient is essentially the same as for a surgical patient. Complete recovery is usually prompt.

Another possible route for transmission of organisms to the mother's breasts is from the nasopharynx of her infant, who has become colonized by staphylococci in the hospital nursery. There need be no break in continuity of the skin of the breast or nipple. Once these organisms are introduced into the mother's breast, milk provides a superb culture medium for them. Efforts to prevent puerperal mastitis cannot be limited to the care of the mother's breasts but must extend to the hospital nursery, where the infant may acquire this penicillin-resistant strain. In the nursery such equipment as soap-solution containers, cribs, mattresses, blankets, and linens, as well as floors, can harbor the organisms. Some methods to help control the spread of infection at its source include careful nursery aseptic technique on the part of all personnel, measures to prevent the spread of organisms from infant to infant, such as proper spacing of cribs, and the exclusion of carriers from the maternity divisions as soon as they are identified.

It should be remembered that in maternity hospitals the nasopharynx of newborn infants tends to become readily infected with *Staphylococcus aureus,* and, moreover, the infection may persist for some weeks after the infant leaves the hospital. Where intensive studies have been carried out and puerperal mastitis or breast abscess appeared after discharge from the hospital, the cultures of the mothers' nares on admission to the hospital did not show evidence of the resistant strain of the organism. In these cases the infants were the source of infection, because the offending organism was cultured from the nose, the throat and the skin of the infants.

When such infections occur, in either the mother or the infant, the nurse should emphasize health teaching in care of the mother, not only concerning hygienic measures for the prevention of skin infections but also the urgency for prompt treatment of any member of the family if carbuncles, boils, burns or other skin lesions develop.

URINARY TRACT INFECTION

Postpartum urinary retention is a common occurrence, because of increased bladder capacity, decreased tonus and decreased perception of the urge to void due to perineal trauma. If the patient is unable to fully empty the bladder, the urine which is retained serves as a culture medium for bacterial growth, often leading to cystitis or pyelonephritis. Urinary tract infections occur in about 5 percent of postpartum patients and are usually caused by coliform bacteria.[5]

The increased circulatory volume of the mother that was necessary for the growth and development of the fetus during pregnancy diminishes rapidly after delivery. The two main avenues for the diminution of the circulating blood volume are the skin and the kidneys. Consequently, the newly delivered mother perspires copiously and excretes large quantities of urine within 24 to 48 hours of delivery. As much as *500 cc. to 1,000 cc.* may be voided at *each* urination; that is, as we know, two to three times what is usual in the nonparturient. The nurse will want to be particularly careful of bladder hygiene at this time because of the increase in urinary production and the danger of overdistention. Thus, one should not wait for any designated time to elapse to indicate when the bladder should be emptied; rather the nurse should observe for evidence indicating the degree of bladder distention, because the bladder may fill in a relatively short span of time. If the patient is unable to void, a catheterization order will be needed.

Retention of urine due to the inability to void is more frequently seen after operative delivery. It often lasts five or six days but may persist longer. The main cause is probably edema of the trigone muscle, which may be so pronounced that it obstructs the urethra. Very temporary urinary retention may be due to the effects of analgesia and anesthesia received in labor. As already stressed, the nurse should make every effort to have the patient void within six hours after delivery (see Chapter 28). If the patient has not done so within eight hours, or depending upon the degree of distention, catheterization is necessary.

Because of the trauma of labor and/or operative delivery, the bladder usually is not as sensitive to distention as it was prior to pregnancy and delivery. Overdistention and incomplete emptying may occur; thus, the problem of residual urine frequently results. Repeated catheterization may be necessary for several days although in these persistent cases an indwelling catheter will need to be inserted to provide constant drainage.

When the mother continues to void small amounts of urine at frequent intervals, the nurse may suspect that these voidings are merely an overflow of a distended bladder and that there is residual urine there. Catheterization for residual urine, to be completely accurate, must be done within five minutes after the patient voids. If 60 cc. or more of urine still remains in the bladder after the patient has voided, it is usually considered that the voiding has been incomplete. It is not uncommon for the catheterization to yield 800 cc. or more of residual urine.

Large amounts of urine (from 60 to 1,500 cc., as shown by catheterization) may remain in the bladder, even though the patient may feel she has completely emptied the bladder when she voided. The condition is due primarily to lack of tone in the bladder wall and is more likely to occur when the mother's bladder has been allowed to become overdistended during labor. A distended bladder requires prompt attention because of the resultant trauma; moreover, it may be a predisposing cause of postpartal hemorrhage.

In many cases of residual urine the patient is without symptoms other than frequent, scanty urination, but in others there may also be suprapubic or perineal discomfort. The treatment of this condition is usually confined to catheterization after each voiding until the residual urine becomes less than 30 cc.; in severe cases constant drainage by means of an indwelling catheter may be employed.

Cystitis.   The normal bladder is very resistant to infection, but when stagnant urine remains in a traumatized bladder, and infectious organisms are present, there is danger of cystitis. When cystitis occurs, the patient often has a low-grade fever, frequent and painful urination and marked tenderness and discomfort over the area of the bladder. A catheterized specimen of urine for microscopic examination is collected, and if pus cells are present in association with residual urine, the diagnosis of cystitis is confirmed. Since it is important in the presence of bladder infection to avoid accumulations of stagnant urine in the bladder, an indwelling bladder catheter may be inserted. In addition, antimicrobial agents are prescribed, and fluids should be forced.

If the infection spreads and involves the ureters and kidneys, the patient has a high fever and chills and a good deal of pain over the affected kidney(s). Diagnosis and treatment for pyelonephritis are essentially the same as for cystitis.

Collection of Urine Specimens.   It will be the nurse's responsibility to obtain the urine specimens which are used for the microscopic examinations and occasionally cultures. The technique of catheterization already has been discussed in Chapter 28.

However, it may be preferable to avoid catheterization, especially if the mother is having no particular difficulties in voiding. This procedure only enhances the possibility of promoting more infection. Therefore a ''clean catch'' specimen may be indicated. Different terminology for this procedure exists in various parts of the country; but the procedure is essentially the same. It consists of the collection of a ''clean'' urine specimen that is uncontaminated by lochia.

One method for this type of collection is as follows:

1. The patient is requested not to void for at least two hours and to drink as much fluid as she can in the meantime.
2. Then she is taken to the bathroom (or placed in a sitting position on a bedpan if she cannot ambulate) and the vulva and introitus are cleansed.
3. A large sterile cotton ball is placed over the introitus.
4. The mother is then requested to void a little urine forcefully into the toilet or bedpan; but *not to empty her bladder.*
5. Next, voiding is restarted and a sterile urine container or sterile basin is used to obtain the urine midstream and the specimen is sent to the laboratory for examination.

This method yields very good results with respect to uncontaminated specimens, if done carefully under the continued supervision of the nurse. It avoids the possibility of introducing bacteria into the bladder at the time of catheterization.

Management.   Diagnosis of urinary tract infection is confirmed by urine culture. Sensitivity studies are usually performed to identify the appropriate antibiotic for the causative organism. Medication is usually administered orally, except in acute febrile pyelonephritis in which intravenous antibiotics are often used. Symptoms are usually relieved within 24 to 48 hours, and treatment continued for ten days to two weeks. Repeat urine cultures are performed following the course of therapy to be certain the urine is free of organisms.

When indwelling catheters are necessary because of inability to void and residual urine which persists, it has been found that patients with catheters in place for longer than four days have a significantly higher incidence of bacteriuria than those whose catheters are removed before this time. Almost all such infections are caused by *E. coli.* Therefore, it is recommended that patients with indwelling catheters for longer than 24 hours be treated with

POSTPARTAL COMPLICATIONS: NURSING CARE

Assessment	Intervention	Evaluation

Physiological assessment
  Vital signs
  Patterns of temperature elevation
  Condition of perineum and uterus
  Character of lochia
  Tenderness and pain
  Condition of legs
  Condition of breasts
  Status of bladder and voiding
	Record and report signs and symptoms
	Administer medications and treatments
	Monitor vital signs
	Monitor fluids and hydration
	Collect specimens
		Vital signs remain stable
		Afebrile
		Able to void completely
		No symptoms of pain, dysuria, malaise, loss of appetite
		Uterus and lochia normal for stage of involution
		Breasts normal

Physical comfort
  Rest and sleep
  Appetite, nutrition and hydration
  Pain or discomfort
	Provide physical care to promote comfort (bath, backrub, clean and dry linens, positioning, etc.)
	Enhance fluid and food intake (relaxed atmosphere, preferences)
	Carry out treatments promptly and efficiently (sitz baths, medications, dressings, etc.)
		Able to rest and sleep well
		Intake of fluids and food adequate
		Reports relief of pain and discomfort

Psychosocial assessment
  Relation to infant
  Response to complication
  Response of partner
	Encourage maximum mother-infant contact, provide continuous information on infant
	Explain and discuss complication, expected course, treatment, etc.
	Involve partner in education about complication, relating to infant, understanding mother's emotional needs, providing support
	Respond to needs for support and encouragement, working through grief and fear
		Assumes as much caretaking of infant as condition permits
		Maintains interest in infant
		Understands treatment and expected course of complication
		Partner understands above, is able to provide support
		Able to express grief and fear

suppressive antimicrobial therapy, usually with such antimicrobial drugs as nitrofurantoin, sulfamethoxazole or ampicillin.[6]

OTHER COMPLICATIONS

Sheehan's Syndrome

This uncommon complication, also called postpartum anterior pituitary necrosis, occurs in about 15 percent of women who survive severe hypovolemic shock associated with postpartum hemorrhage. There is loss of function of the pituitary gland, resulting in deficiency in thyroid, adrenocortical, and ovarian functions. Symptoms include failure of lactation, decreased breast size, loss of pubic and axillary hair, genital atrophy, and myxedema in severe cases. Most women never menstruate again, although in less severe cases, there may be occasional ovulation and scanty menses.

Treatment consists of hormone replacement, usually thyroid, cortisone and estrogen. A high protein diet with ample carbohydrates is prescribed to counteract the typical cachexia. The prognosis depends on the degree of pituitary deficiency, and infertility is usual. Reasonable health can often be maintained with proper hormone replacement, but premature aging frequently results.

Chiari-Frommel Syndrome

This rare condition is characterized by prolonged lactation (galactorrhea) which can occur following normal delivery, whether or not the mother is breast-feeding. There is profuse leakage of fluid from the breasts, with headaches, hearing or visual loss, and genital atrophy. The cause is often unknown, but may be due to pituitary tumor or prolonged phenothiazine therapy. Gonadotropin and urinary estrogen excretion are reduced or absent. There is no effective treatment, although clomiphene citrate may induce ovulation and menstruation, and abnormal lactation can be suppressed by 2-bromergocryptine. Estrogen therapy or oral contraceptives may also control galactorrhea, but symptoms usually recur following discontinuation of medication.

Postpartum Vulvar Edema

An unusual syndrome which is frequently fatal, involves massive perineal edema. In the instances reported, following normal pregnancy, labor and delivery, in which local or regional anesthesia and episiotomy were used, unilateral perineal edema and induration developed beginning about the second postpartum day. This progressed to generalized vulvar, vaginal, perineal, and gluteal edema and induration. Over two or three days, the edema gradually spread to the other side and into the inner pelvis. Fever and marked leukocytosis also occurred, and in those patients who died, there was also vascular collapse. No definite etiology has been found, and while infections were present in some cases, this was not always true. Treatment consisted of various antibiotics, local heat, heparin, steroids and crystalloids, but none was particularly effective. Early recognition of asymmetric vulvar edema, associated with low-grade fever and an elevated white blood count, is recommended as possibly preventing maternal death by aggressive treatment with antibiotics and steroids.[7]

REFERENCES

1. R. C. Benson: *Current Obstetric and Gynecologic Diagnosis and Treatment.* Los Altos, Calif., Lange Medical Publishers, 1978, p. 764.

2. R. Filker and G. R. G. Monif: "The significance of temperature during the first 24 hours postpartum." *Obstet. & Gynecol.* 53, 3:358–361, March 1979.

3. L. C. Gilstrap and F. G. Cunningham: "The bacterial pathogenesis of infection following cesarean section." *Obstet. & Gynecol.* 53, 5:545—549, May 1979.

4. Ibid.

5. Benson, op. cit., p. 765.

6. R. E. Harris: "Postpartum urinary retention: Role of antimicrobial therapy." *Amer. J. Obstet. Gynecol.* 133, 2:174–175, January 15, 1979.

7. T. L. Ewing, L. E. Smale and F. A. Elliott: "Maternal deaths associated with postpartum vulvar edema." *Amer. J. Obstet. Gynecol.* 134, 2:173–179, May 15, 1979.

Assessment and Management of Perinatal Disorders

Fetal Diagnosis and Treatment

Electronic Fetal Monitoring and Fetal Intensive Care

The High Risk Infant: Disorders of Gestational Age and Birth Weight

The High Risk Infant: Developmental and Environmental Disorders

Thirty-Six

Fetal Diagnosis and Treatment

Determination of Fetal Age | Evaluation of Fetal Well-Being | Specific Fetal Problems | Fetal Treatment

Prior to the middle of the twentieth century the fetus was generally regarded as a passive participant in the entire reproductive process and fetal evaluation was limited to gross observation of growth and auscultation of the fetal heart. X-rays were used to assess fetal position and major bony abnormalities, but all of these methods clearly fell well short of determining precisely fetal age and well being. In the last few decades, however, a series of rapidly evolving developments have opened the way to increasingly accurate approaches. These developments include safer use of amniocentesis which has allowed for greater access to amniotic fluid, along with cytogenetic, biochemical, cytologic and biophysical assessment of the fluid, B mode and real time ultrasound techniques, and electronic and biochemical fetal monitoring.

In addition to these technical advances which permit evaluation of the fetus, there have been advances in understanding which permit significant albeit limited treatment of the fetus beyond simply converting the fetus to a newborn. The proliferation of this technology has been accompanied by a parallel proliferation in professional and supportive personnel in the broad area of perinatology. Subspecialties have evolved for both maternal and fetal medical specialists and neonatologists. Obstetrical anesthesia has emerged as a growing and well-defined area of study, training programs have been developed for perinatal nurse clinicians and the concept of the perinatal team has been well established; such a team includes the obstetrician, neonatologist, anesthesiologist, nurse specialist, nutritionists, social workers and adequate supporting consultants.

Regionalization of Perinatal Care

Facilities are also a concern since it is impractical and illogical for every hospital regardless of size and population served to have all the personnel and equipment necessary to deliver the most sophisticated levels of care. The concept of regionalization or centralization of perinatal care, in which three levels of care can be identified, has evolved. The basic level of care would provide for the management of only normal maternity patients and newborns. Mothers or newborns with complications would have to be transferred to either level 2 or 3 institutions. These two levels of care could not be justified in areas of high population density except under most unusual circumstances. A second level of care would be provided in most institutions with a significant maternity practice. These institutions should have the equipment and personnel to handle all but the most sophisticated and unusual problems.

These facilities should provide care for premature infants as well as most high risk mothers. Level 3 institutions would serve larger populations providing the most specialized types of care for unusual problems.

Implicit in this concept is the identification of the high risk mother and/or newborn and the transfer of that patient as required to a hospital with the appropriate level of care. Scoring systems and computerized and problem oriented record systems have been developed to aid in identifying these patients, but the key is early recognition of problems by the health care provider in order that transport may be carried out at the earliest, most optimal time. Whenever possible, infant transport is best accomplished in utero rather than after birth, when the newborn is already in a compromised state. There is considerable evidence that the outcome is far superior when intensive neonatal care begins at the moment of delivery. This, of course, is not always possible since occasionally high risk babies are born to low risk mothers, and even when the mother at risk is identified, delivery may be inevitable before transfer can be accomplished. Despite the obvious value of this concept of regionalization and mother and infant transport, there are significant problems generated relating to social and emotional aspects of patient care. Separation of patients from their families, familiar surroundings and physicians can create tremendous anxiety and require special sensitivity on the part of all involved in their care.

In the general area of fetal diagnosis there are two broad areas of concern: the determination of fetal age and/or maturity and the evaluation of fetal well-being. In the latter category are included assessment in early pregnancy for congenital disorders, later evaluation of well-being in pregnancy complications, and finally intrapartum monitoring by electronic or biochemical means. Genetic diagnosis and intrapartum monitoring are covered in Chapters 15 and 37, respectively.

DETERMINATION OF FETAL AGE

Although it is customary to use Naegele's rule to determine the period of gestation and estimated date of confinement from the first day of the last menstrual period, this method is fraught with error for various reasons, including failure to remember exact dates, irregular cycles, bleeding in the first trimester, and late registration for prenatal care. In the case of an uncomplicated pregnancy, not knowing the exact length of gestation may not represent a serious problem. However, in the high risk patient for whom timing of the delivery is critical, the information is vital. Thus, the degree to which the determination is pursued depends upon the clinical situation.

Means for Determining Fetal Age

Physical Measurements

Estimation of uterine size by pelvic examination in the first trimester is a helpful indicator of gestational growth, whereas determination of uterine size in the second trimester is less valid. Measuring the fundal height above the pelvic symphysis at each visit can give useful information about growth or lack of growth, but not about the exact period of gestation. Estimation of fetal weight is notoriously inaccurate, with the greatest error at the higher and lower weights. Other physical determinants include first auscultation of the fetal heart and serial examinations of the cervix to determine effacement and dilatation. As with all physical evaluations, there is considerable individual variation. Consequently such evaluations are not totally reliable unless they are all in agreement.

X-Ray Studies

Radiographic studies can be helpful in determining maturity. If both the distal femoral and proximal tibial epiphyses are calcified, one can be assured of a mature fetus (Fig. 36-1). However, if the epiphyses are not calcified one cannot assume immaturity, since there is considerable variation based on sex, race, and fetal weight, along with technical problems related to the position of the fetal knee relative to the maternal skeleton. Because of these inaccuracies along with concerns about radiation and the fetus, x-ray is no longer a preferred approach for the purpose of determining fetal age.

Ultrasound

Diagnostic ultrasound is now widely used in obstetrics for a variety of purposes including early diagnosis of pregnancy, confirming fetal viability, placental localization, confirmation of fetal death and estimation of fetal age. The most useful techniques are the B-mode scan with or without gray scale and the real-time scan. The diagnosis of early pregnancy and estimation of the period of gestation can be made by either technique, but real time offers the advantage of documenting viability as well since cardiac activity as well as fetal movement can be seen by that technique from early on (uniformly by eight weeks).

The most common approach to the determination of gestational age is to measure the biparietal diameter of the fetal head. This is especially useful if done during the linear phase of growth of the fetal head between 20 and 30 weeks and is further enhanced by making two measurements three to four weeks apart which will not only better fix the gestational age, but also confirm a normal rate of growth.

Fetal head growth generally proceeds at a normal rate despite late pregnancy problems which might retard overall fetal growth. This occurs because the brain is spared under such circumstances and brain growth is the major determinant of head size. To detect this type of growth retardation with head sparing, additional measurements must also be made, including the thoracic diameters, crown-rump lengths or calculations of the total intrauterine volume. It must be emphasized that although it is rather commonly done, a single measurement of the biparietal diameter late in the third trimester is of very little value in establishing the period of gestation.

Concerning the safety of diagnostic ultrasound, there is no available evidence to suggest any harmful fetal effects. This is not to say, however, that it should be used without restraint. Indeed for some practitioners ultrasound has become routine for all pregnancies, an approach which cannot be justified at this time.

Endocrine Studies

Of all the assays available, estriol (or total estrogens) and human placental lactogen (HPL)—also known as human chorionic somatomammotropin (HCS)—are the most popular. Both have normal curves which rise progressively during pregnancy; however, the range of normal is wide, and consequently these techniques are less valid in determining fetal age than fetal well-being. It is possible for a given

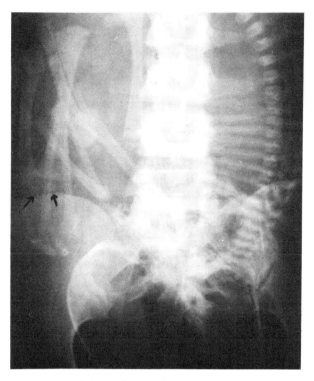

Figure 36-1. Abdominal x-ray showing a fetus with calcification of both the distal femoral and proximal tibial epiphyses *(arrows)*.

value to be in the normal range for both 35 and 40 weeks and, therefore, the age differentiation cannot be made. Both serum and 24-hour urine samples are assayed.

Amniotic Fluid Studies

Transabdominal amniocentesis has become a standard technique in modern obstetric practice (Fig. 15-8). But it must not be regarded as a totally innocuous procedure and should be undertaken only on the basis of well-founded indications. Potential complications include fetal bleeding, placental disruption, Rh sensitization, and fetal puncture. The frequency of these complications is poorly recorded and is greatly influenced by such factors as the experience of the person carrying out the procedure and the use of ultrasound to localize the placenta, but the incidence of complications is probably in the 1 percent range. Given a sample of amniotic fluid, the following determinations are useful in evaluating fetal age:

Gross Appearance. The presence of large amounts of vernix caseosa generally indicates maturity, and meconium is often present in the significantly post-date pregnancy. Neither, however, is sufficiently consistent for precise age estimation, since the meconium may be present as a sign of fetal distress in less-than-mature pregnancy.

Cytology. The cells in amniotic fluid come from both the fetus and the membranes. The bulk of fetal cells are desquamated squamous cells from the skin; cells from the respiratory, urinary, and gastrointestinal tract are also present. If amniotic fluid is mixed with a vital stain for fat (Nile blue sulfate) and a smear is made, a varying number of the squamous cells will take up the stain and appear orange on the smear. These cells normally first appear at 34 to 35 weeks gestation and increase in number as term is approached. Fifteen to 20 percent generally indicates a mature fetus, while at term the presence of 50 percent fat-containing cells and free-fat droplets is the rule. This technique has the distinct advantage of being easily done and therefore the information can be immediately available.

Creatinine. The concentration of creatinine in amniotic fluid gradually rises as the fetus' kidneys mature, increasing their ability to excrete creatinine, and also as the fetus' muscle mass increases, which causes an increase in creatine to creatinine metabolism. Values of 2 mg. per 100 ml. are indicative of fetal maturity.

Bilirubin. Although the determination of bilirubin in amniotic fluid by spectrophotometry has its greatest application in evaluating the fetus in RH sensitization, it can also be applied in evaluating the age of the fetus in nonsensitized patients. Because of the maturation of the fetal liver and the placenta, the concentration of bilirubin in amniotic fluid is progressively decreased toward term, and disappears at about 37 to 38 weeks, strongly suggesting fetal maturity. This evaluation is not sufficiently valid to be used as the sole standard but does complement the other assays.

Osmolality. Although amniotic fluid in early pregnancy is isotonic with maternal plasma, as pregnancy progresses the fluid becomes more hypotonic, presumably because of the increasing contribution of fetal urine. Values of 250 mOsm per liter per kilogram or less are generally associated with maturity, but variation is considerable.

Phospholipids. Through extensive investigation of pulmonary fluids and the genesis of the respiratory distress syndrome there have evolved what are the most important and germaine studies of fetal maturity. Because there are respiratory movements in utero, the composition of amniotic fluid does reflect the content of pulmonary fluids; consequently, several techniques measuring surfactant activity in amniotic fluid have been devised to determine fetal pulmonary maturity.

Surfactant is synthesized by the Type II cells in the lung and although present in small quantities from midpregnancy on, the mature pathway for surfactant synthesis (choline incorporation) is activated at 35 weeks in the normal pregnancy. In certain stressful circumstances, such as preeclampsia, class D and F diabetes and premature rupture of the membranes, the process is accelerated, while in others, such as class A, B, and C diabetes, it may be delayed. As will be discussed subsequently the administration of corticosteroids may under certain conditions accelerate pulmonary maturity.

There are several techniques for measuring this activity, including the "Shake" test, L/S ratio and Felma measurement. The Shake test determines the stability of foam on the surface of mixtures of ethyl alcohol and various dilutions of amniotic fluid (Fig. 36-2); maturity is indicated when the foam is stable in the presence of a 2:1 dilution.

The most widely used technique is the lecithin sphingomyelin (L/S) ratio. Since the concentration of sphingomyelin remains relatively constant, a rising L/S ratio indicates increasing surfactant production (lecithin is a major constituent of surfactant). The separation of lecithin and sphingomyelin is achieved by thin layer chromotography and the ratio determined either by visual inspection or densitometry. Pulmonary maturity is established when the L/S ratio exceeds 2:1.

With another technique, the Felma (fetal lung maturity) apparatus measures total concentrations of amniotic fluid phospholipid by an electrooptical approach. This equipment is somewhat expensive, but if the method is validated by further studies its reproducibility may make it a desirable technique. More recent studies of specific phospholipids in amniotic fluid, phospatidyl glycerol (PG) and phosphatidylinositol (PI), have proved to be valuable in borderline cases and especially in patients with class A, B, and C diabetes where pulmonary maturity is often delayed to 37 weeks or later. When PG and PI are both elevated, maturity seems assured.

EVALUATION OF FETAL WELL-BEING

There are a number of circumstances in obstetric practice in which the fetus might be in jeopardy, and it is therefore desirable to evaluate the fetal status. Such instances range from the first trimester patient with a threatened abortion, with whom there is the need to determine the viability of the pregnancy, to mid-trimester pregnancy studies to determine congenital disorders (see Chapter 15). In the third trimester, serial evaluations are necessary in chronic disorders such as diabetes and hypertension as well as in more acute problems such as preeclampsia and the postdate pregnancy. Although at the present time the application of sophisticated tests to determine fetal well-being is limited to patients with a determined fetal risk, while normal pregnancies are evaluated largely by clinical means, it is entirely possible that in the not-too-distant future some or all of these techniques may be routinely applied as a form of antenatal screening.

Antepartal Fetal Evaluation

The action to be taken by the obstetrician when the fetus at risk is in fact in jeopardy is limited and determined by the period of gestation. If in the first trimester it is determined that the pregnancy is nonviable, the uterus can evacuated. This is basically an all or none evaluation, and qualitative assessment of the first trimester pregnancy is not currently possible. As one deals with the mid-trimester and a previable fetus, evaluation of well-being is of little moment because there is generally no recourse if serious fetal problems are uncovered, given the fact that delivery is unacceptable. There are some exceptions to this in which therapy can be directed toward the fetus while allowing the pregnancy to continue. The classic example of this situation is intrauterine transfusion in the severely affected fetus with Rh hemolytic disease. In the vast majority of cases, however, these evaluations are done in the third trimester and the choice for the obstetrician

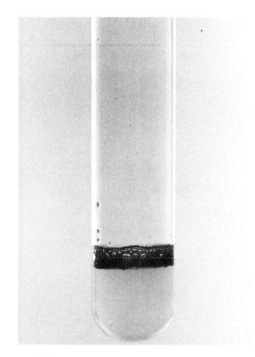

Figure 36-2. Shake test. Note bubbles on the surface maintained by surfactant in the amniotic fluid.

is between the delivery of a potentially viable premature infant or prolongation of intrauterine life with the risk of fetal death. When the indications of in utero jeopardy are severe, unfortunately the decision to deliver often results in the birth of a seriously ill newborn and a potential neonatal death. More commonly, however, the studies are reassuring and permit prolongation of the pregnancy, a much happier eventuality.

Early Pregnancy Evaluation–Threatened Abortion. A common problem in the first trimester is evaluating the significance of bleeding and deciding whether or not a pregnancy is viable and should be allowed to continue despite the persistent symptoms. Standard immunologic pregnancy tests may remain positive for some time following the point at which viability is lost. The more specific beta subunit assay is particularly reassuring if its values are appropriate for the gestational period. B-mode ultrasound scans can define a gestational sac as early as five weeks following the last menstrual period. The integrity of the sac and its appropriate dimensions are reassuring up to ten weeks. The fetus is generally visible with sac by eight weeks, and fetal activity and heart beat can be discerned by ten weeks by means of real-time equipment. These techniques have considerably more precision in assessing progress than clinical examinations evaluating uterine growth. They can therefore provide reassurance in a situation involving considerable anxiety and offer a definitive answer in situations of nonviability, thereby permitting uterine evacuation.

Late Pregnancy Evaluation

Estrogens.   Estrogen levels in maternal serum and urine rise progressively during the course of normal pregnancy, following a sigmoid curve as seen in Figure 36-3. Although estrone and estradiol also increase during pregnancy, it is estriol that is the predominant estrogen, increasing 1,000-fold and accounting for 90 percent of the total estrogen. This makes it feasible in the case of 24-hour urinary determinations to measure either estriol or total estrogens. Even more important in the clinical application of estriol measurements for problem pregnancies is the fact that at least 90 percent of the estrogen precursors are produced by the fetal zone of the fetal adrenal cortex largely as sulfates of dehydroepiandrosterone (DHEAS) and 16αOH DHEAS. Much of the DHEAS is converted to 16αOH DHEAS by the fetal liver. The conversion of these androgen precursors to estriol is a function of the placenta by processes involving splitting off of the sulfate and conjugation. Finally, estriol is excreted by the kidney largely in the conjugated form. Thus it becomes clear that, in order for there to be a normal quantity of estriol in a 24-hour urine specimen, the several parts of the cycle must be intact including the live healthy fetus with intact adrenals producing normal amounts of androgen precursors, a normally functioning placenta capable of making the conversion to estriol, and healthy maternal liver and kidneys competent to conjugate and then excrete the estriol. Consequently, estriol values that are normal for the gestational age are quite reassuring. Most commonly, measurements are made in 24-hour urine collections. Although there may be some day-to-day variation, a fall of more than 30 to 40 percent must be considered significant and the impression of fetal jeopardy pursued. Serial measurements must be done and the frequency of determination is dependent upon the seriousness and the stability of the clinical situation. In a hospitalized unstable diabetic, daily estriols may

be needed, while less frequent studies are sufficient in a less critical situation.

Because urinary estriols require a 24-hour collection, with the possibilities that it may be incomplete as well as inconvenient for the patient, and because this in effect brings about a lag in the assessment process, a number of alternatives have been suggested. Simultaneous measurement of urinary creatinine can provide a constant which then enables the clinician to utilize shorter collection periods, of 4 or 8 hours, for example, and still get meaningful information by calculating the estriol creatinine ratio. It should also be noted that there are a number of factors which can interfere with urinary estriol determinations. Obviously, in the presence of impaired maternal renal function the test loses its validity and cannot be utilized to assess the fetal status. Maternal administration of ampicillin, Mandelamine and corticosteroids all interfere with the measurement, as does a large quantity of glucose in the urine. The latter can be dealt with by diluting the specimen for the assay.

Because of these problems, a number of workers have turned to the use of plasma estriol measurements. The normal curve is similarly shaped to that for urinary measurements, although the quantities are measured in micrograms rather then milligrams. The use of plasma values does not eliminate all problems because levels vary during the day and therefore samples must be obtained at the same time each day for proper comparison. Abnormal renal function can result in false elevations of plasma levels and the technology is somewhat more difficult than urinary assays. The methodology has been improved, however, by the use of radioimmunoassay, and currently this technique when applied to unconjugated estriol is gaining in favor.

Estetrol (15αhydroxyestriol) measurements have been proposed by some as a better means of fetal evaluation. This estrogen is derived from placental estradiol and estrone with the final synthesis taking place in the fetal liver. Both serum and urinary assays have been suggested, but the current consensus, after an initial surge of enthusiasm, is that it offers no advantage over estriol.

Progesterone.   This steroid hormone is produced by the placenta in progressively increasing quantities during pregnancy. It can be measured as serum progesterone or urinary pregnanediol, but has little value in evaluating fetal well-being since progesterone does not require fetal precursors and can, in fact, persist in significant quantities even after an intrauterine fetal death has occurred.

Human Chorionic Gonadotropin (HCG).

This hormone, produced by the trophoblast, normally peaks in early pregnancy and falls off to relatively low levels in the second and third trimesters. It is the basis for most pregnancy tests, as well as for the follow-up of hydatid moles and choriocarcinoma, but is of limited value in problem pregnancies. An exception occurs in the case of severely affected erythroblastotic infants. Because of placental hypertrophy HCG values may be quite high; however, by the time these values are reached, the fetus is usually beyond salvage.

Human Placental Lactogen (HPL).

Also known as human chorionic somatomammotropin, HPL is synthesized by the syncytiotrophoblast of the placenta in progressively increasing quantities throughout pregnancy. HPL shows an incomplete immunologic cross reaction with human pituitary growth hormone. The value of this assay in monitoring fetal well-being has been a rather controversial subject and one can probably conclude that HPL is a valuable adjunct but should not be regarded as the sole end point for fetal jeopardy. It is generally concluded that those clinical situations in which fetal compromise is the direct result of impaired placental function will be heralded by falling HPL values approaching a danger zone (below 4 mg/ml after 30 weeks gestation). Thus HPL assay is most useful with hypertension disorders of pregnancy, placental insufficiency with fetal growth retardation and especially postdate pregnancies. Because placental function is not impaired in such conditions as class A and B diabetes without hypertension, congenital malformation and hemolytic disease, the study has no predictive value for such patients.

Maternal Blood Enzyme Measurement.

A number of enzymes increase in concentration in maternal serum during pregnancy, including HSAP, DAO and oxytocinase.

HEAT STABLE ALKALINE PHOSPHATASE (HSAP). This isoenzyme of alkaline phosphatase originates in the placenta and rises in concentration progressively throughout pregnancy. A sudden rapid rise in late pregnancy seems to indicate placental damage and

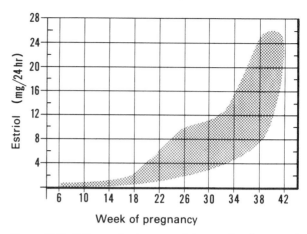

Figure 36-3. Pattern of urinary estriol excretion in normal pregnancy.

potential fetal death. In some studies this has been shown to take place prior to a drop in estriol. As with HPL, most feel this easy-to-do study is a good adjunct but not an end in itself.

PLASMA DIAMINE OXIDASE (DAO). This enzyme is probably produced by retro-placental decidua, perhaps to protect the pregnant woman against histamine produced by the fetus. It rises at a rapid linear rate in early pregnancy, but unfortunately it tends to plateau in the third trimester making it less useful for fetal evaluation.

OXYTOCINASE. Cystine aminopeptidase enzyme (oxytocinase) inactivates oxytocin during pregnancy and is synthesized by the placenta. As with HPL and HSAP it seems to be a rather pure indicator of placental function, does not reflect distress which is primary fetal, and is therefore useful as an adjunct but not for primary evaluation of well-being.

Physiologic Studies.

Since it is not feasible to measure directly the critical respiratory and nutritional function of the placenta, a number of indirect approaches have been developed. Two of these studies, the oxytocin challenge test and the nonstress test, are discussed in Chapter 37. Fetal movements and especially a change in the pattern of fetal movement are felt to be indicators of well-being. Some have suggested that patients be instructed to count the number of fetal movements in a given time period each day and record the information. Even without this formal quantitating of fetal movement, when a patient reports a reduction in fetal movements this must be evaluated further, especially if there is an underlying reason to suspect fetal jeopardy.

With the advent of real-time ultrasound, which enables one to observe fetal activity, it is possible to observe cardiac activity and respiratory movements. The latter, it has been suggested, is a good index of fetal well-being; however, the approach has not yet achieved practical clinical application, especially since long periods of observation may be needed for proper information.

Amniotic Fluid Studies. Most amniotic fluid studies are directed toward the determination of fetal maturity or genetic diagnosis, which is discussed in Chapter 15. A major exception is the quantitation of bilirubin in amniotic fluid as a means of judging the severity of hemolytic disease (see p. 607).

When chorioamnionitis is suspected, but the diagnosis is not clear, examination of amniotic fluid for the presence of polymorphonuclear leukocytes and gram-stained bacteria may be helpful. Although there are some conflicting reports concerning the importance of the white blood cells, clearly the presence of bacteria is significant.

The presence of meconium in amniotic fluid is an indication that there has been an episode of fetal stress at some time prior to the observation, but not necessarily as an ongoing situation. Indeed the presence of meconium does not indicate a fetus in distress unless there are other indicators, such as a significant alteration in the fetal heart rate. The mechanism of passage of meconium is presumably hyperperistalsis secondary to the hypoxic insult. In most cases the observation of meconium-stained fluid is made intrapartum after rupture of the membranes, although transabdominal amniocentesis or transvaginal amnioscopy may also be utilized. The latter procedure is limited to late pregnancy when the cervix is open enough to admit the lighted speculum. An advantage is that the procedure can be done repeatedly to monitor well-being in certain cases, such as the postdate pregnancy. Disadvantages of the technique are that fluid samples cannot be obtained for analysis and that occasionally the membranes may be inadvertently ruptured.

SPECIFIC FETAL PROBLEMS

Acute fetal distress will be covered in Chapter 37 in relation to intrapartum fetal monitoring, although many of the chronic fetal problems that will be discussed here can produce acute distress as well. In addition, some of these problems, such as preeclampsia, have significant maternal implications that are covered elsewhere.

Hemolytic Disease—Rh Factor

This is one of the complications of pregnancy in which there may be devastating fetal effects with virtually no maternal risk. Although the fetal pathology of severe hemolytic disease had been described before the turn of the century, the exact nature of the problem was not known until after the discovery of the Rh factor in 1940. The disease is most unusual in that within 30 years the cause, treatment, and methods for prevention have been worked out. Most of the attention has been focused on the Rh factor as a cause, but the ABO blood groups may also cause a form of hemolytic disease, as do other lesser blood groups.

The incidence of hemolytic disease is related to the occurrence of blood groups. In the Caucasian population 15 percent are Rh negative while in blacks, orientals and American Indians this figure is only 5 percent; therefore the frequency of Rh hemolytic disease is much less in these groups. Approximately 13 percent of American marriages have the setup for Rh problems (Rh negative wife, Rh positive husband) and 22 percent have the combinations for ABO disease. Ninety-eight percent of all hemolytic disease is related to either Rh or ABO incompatibilities. Fetal involvement with hemolytic disease formerly occurred with a frequency of approximately 1 in 100 deliveries; however, this incidence has been markedly reduced by the introduction of prevention by Rh immunoglobulin.

Anti-D Globulin. The ability to prevent Rh sensitization has been an established fact since Rh (anti-D) globulin became commercially available in 1969. This substance which was initially obtained from the plasma of sensitized women is now obtained by deliberately sensitizing Rh negative male volunteers. It prevents sensitization by clearing the fetal cells from the material circulating and perhaps also by depressing the patient's immune response. A single dose (300 micrograms) is capable of clearing up to 15 ml. of fetal erythrocytes. Lower doses (50 micrograms) have been made available for use in situations where only small fetomaternal transfusions are likely, such as first trimester abortion and ectopic pregnancy.

Candidates for Rh immunoglobulin are unsensitized Rh negative patients who 1) have delivered Rh positive babies, 2) and untypable pregnancies such as stillborns, ectopic pregnancies, or spontaneous or induced abortions, or 3) received ABO compatible Rh positive blood. It is of no value in the patient who is already sensitized, and although the recommendation is that it should be administered within three days of delivery this should not preclude administration at a later time if for some reason the 72-hour deadline has been missed.

Although many failures to prevent sensitization are due to failure to administer Rh immunoglobulin or inadequacy of the dose to cover the size of the fetomaternal bleed, there is a small risk (1 to 2 percent) of sensitization even when proper technique is followed. The inadequate dose problem can be dealt with by doing appropriate follow-up studies 48 hours after the anti-D globulin. This involves doing either a Kleibauer Betki Smear to demonstrate that fetal cells are no longer present, or, even more simply, doing an indirect Coombs' test to show that there is excess antibody present. If the indirect Coombs' test is negative at 48 hours, an additional dose of immunoglobulin should be given. The remainder of the failures are probably related to fetomaternal bleeding episodes which occurred long enough prior to delivery that the postpartum administration of anti-D globulin will not protect. Several projects are underway to reduce this problem by evaluating the administration of immunoglobulin antepartum in the third trimester either routinely or when there are predisposing occurrences such as third trimester bleeding.

With all of these developments, Rh hemolytic disease is becoming increasingly uncommon, but there does seem to be an irreducible group of patients who are sensitized for the reasons mentioned above. Because the problem is becoming more rare it is important that the care of the severely sensitized patient be delegated to a perinatal center.

Pathophysiology. The pathogenesis of Rh hemolytic disease is based on the fact that, even though the maternal and fetal circulations are normally completely separated, breaks in this barrier permit the entry of fetal red cells into the maternal circulation during the second and third trimesters and at delivery in up to 50 percent of pregnancies. Such breaks also occur with abortions beyond six to eight weeks of pregnancy. If these cells are Rh positive (containing the Rh + or D antigen), the mother may react to this mismatched "mini-transfusion" by forming protective antibodies. Since the formation of antibodies takes time, and since the unsensitized woman probably does not react until after she delivers, there is rarely a problem in the first pregnancy unless the patient has received a mismatched transfusion in the past. Antibodies formed as the result of the first exposure persist for life. When the woman becomes pregnant again, and the fetus is Rh positive, she will respond with rapid antibody formation as soon as she is exposed to Rh positive cells. Thus, once antibodies have been formed, all subsequent pregnancies with Rh positive infants will be a problem.

There are two types of Rh antibodies. The larger type (gamma M, or 19S) does not cross the placenta as readily as the smaller (gamma g or 7S). In the case of ABO disease where the mother who lacks the antigen has the antibody (e.g., type O has neither A nor B antigen, but has both anti-A and anti-B antibodies: type A has A antigen and anti-B antibody, and so on), these naturally occurring antibodies are the large 19S variety. Also, since these antibodies require a break in the placental barrier to get into the fetal circulation, and since this is most likely to occur at the time of delivery of the placenta, ABO disease is almost always more mild than Rh and rarely is the child stillborn or severely affected at birth. In addition, because the AB antigens are present in all body cells, this tends to absorb excess antibody and reduce the effect on the red cells. However, in Rh disease, there are both 19S and 7S antibodies (the result of sensitization). The 7S antibodies cross readily into the fetal circulation by a facilitated transport mechanism and are responsible for the destruction of the fetal red blood cells. This produces anemia, and if it is severe enough, heart failure results in an edematous hydropic infant, and possibly a stillbirth.

While the fetus is in utero, the mother is able to remove the breakdown products of the red cells (bilirubin) and handle them in her own liver; therefore, the baby is not born jaundiced. However, once separated from the mother, the baby must handle the continuing breakdown of red cells, and its liver, especially in prematures, lacks the necessary enzymes to do this efficiently. The affected newborn rapidly develops jaundice and, if untreated, brain damage may result from the deposition of the bile pigments in vital areas of the brain (kernicterus).

This is the most severe form of pathology, but it must be kept in mind that it is not only possible but likely that an Rh negative woman may have one, two or even more pregnancies without significant difficulty.

Genetic Determination. The inheritance of Rh blood type follows the simple dominant recessive rules, with Rh+ being a dominant. Each individual receives two genes (one from each parent) to determine Rh blood type. It is necessary to receive two Rh negative genes to be negative, whereas one can be Rh positive with one Rh positive and one Rh negative gene (heterozygous) or two Rh positive genes (homozygous). Thus, if the husband is heterozygous, there is a 50-50 chance of having an Rh negative child, and therefore, an unaffected one (Fig. 36-4). If the father is homozygous, all offspring will be Rh positive and subject to hemolytic disease.

In the ABO system, an individual may have genes for A, B, AB, or no antigens. Thus, the contribution to the offspring may be either A or B or none. For example: Type O individuals receive neither A nor B from the parents; a type A individual may receive an A gene from each (AA) or an A from one and none from the other (AO). The same is true for the type B individual (BB or BO). The AB individual receives an A from one parent and a B from the other.

All pregnant patients should have a blood group determination, at least with the first pregnancy. If adequate records are available, this need not be repeated with subsequent pregnancies. If the patient is Rh negative or Type O (the most common maternal type for ABO disease), the husband's blood should also be typed. If he is Rh positive, a genotype may be done to determine whether he is homozygous or heterozygous. Also, the Rh negative woman's blood should be examined for the presence of antibodies to the Rh factor (D). This is accomplished by the indirect Coomb's test and is reported in dilutions (e.g., positive 1:2, 1:4, 1:8, and so on). If the initial screening or titer is negative (i.e., shows no antibodies), this should be repeated at approximately 30 and 36 weeks of pregnancy. If both of those titers are negative, it is safe to assume that there will be no significant problem and to permit the pregnancy to run its normal course. If the titer is positive, it becomes necessary to decide how seriously the fetus is affected (i.e., how anemic it is). Since it is not possible to approach the fetus

directly and do a hemoglobin or hematocrit, less direct means must be used. In the past, the physician merely repeated the antibody titer, watching for a rise, and combining with this the patients' past history, arrived at a plan of management.

Bilirubin Levels in Fetal Diagnosis. It has now been well established that the severity of the hemolytic anemia in the fetus can best be determined by the quantity of *bilirubin* in the amniotic fluid, that is, the higher the bilirubin level, the lower the fetal hemoglobin. Thus, amniocentesis with analysis of the bilirubin in the fluid is the best basis for making therapeutic decisions in the sensitized patient. Because the quantity of bilirubin is small in the mildly sensitized or unsensitized patient, standard techniques for measuring bilirubin cannot be used and therefore a spectrophotometric approach is used. Bilirubin produces an optical density peak at 450 and it is the height of this peak (or the ΔOD_{450}) which is used to evaluate fetal involvement

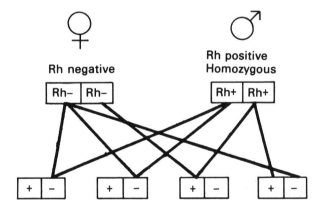

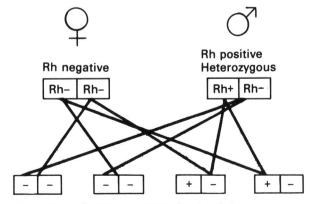

Figure 36-4. Inheritance patterns for the Rh factor.

Example Graph

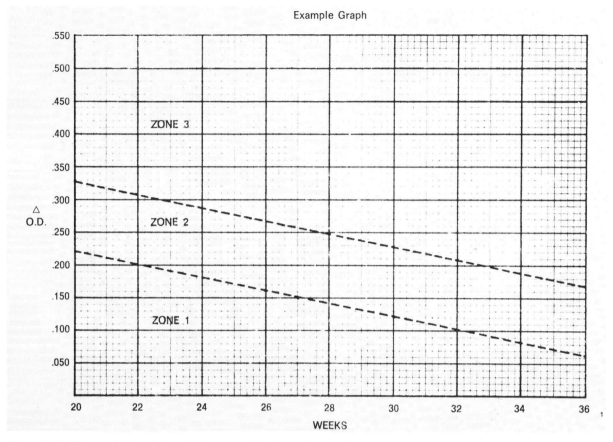

Figure 36-5. Liley graph for relating ΔOD_{450} to weeks of gestation in determining severity of hemolytic disease.

(Fig. 36-5). Amniocentesis is used to evaluate the fetus in all patients with significant sensitization. In most laboratories, a significant antibody titer below which fetal morbidity is unlikely can be determined. Although this varies from institution to institution, titers above 1:8 to 1:16 are generally considered significant. Amniocentesis is usually instituted at from 24 to 25 weeks, since intrauterine transfusion is impractical before that, although in instances with previous early stillbirths the procedure may be instituted as early as 20 weeks. The frequency of repeated amniocentesis is determined by the level of the ΔOD_{450}, weekly taps being indicated if values are high.

The common method for evaluating the ΔOD_{450} is the Liley chart illustrated in Figure 36-5. Values in the lower zone for the particular gestation indicate a mildly or even unaffected fetus, while those in the middle zone indicate an affected fetus, but one not in immediate danger of death. Values in the upper zone suggest the fetus will not survive 10 to 14 days without intervention. Management decisions are not based on single values but rather the trend. If the ΔOD_{450} remains in the lower zone, no interference is indicated and the pregnancy can be allowed to proceed to term. If the values remain in the middle zone, the fetus is best delivered as soon as there is evidence of maturity, especially of the lung, by using the L/S ratio. Upper zone values indicate immediate intervention by delivery if beyond 33 to 34 weeks or by intrauterine transfusion if before that gestational age.

This dramatic procedure was first described in 1963 by Liley and involves the instillation under fluoroscopic and/or ultrasound control of Rh negative red cells into the peritoneal cavity of the fetus in utero. The fetus is able to absorb these intact cells. If the procedure is repeated successfully every 10 to 14 days until the point of maturity (approximately 34 to 35 weeks) a stillbirth may be avoided. Only 40 to 50 percent of treated fetuses can be salvaged because the procedure is rather gross, especially in the smaller fetus, and often the fetus is very sick when the procedure is initiated. Of course, these results are far better than no survivors, which could be anticipated without the procedure.

Treatment of Newborn. The pediatric management of the newborn involves the use of exchange transfusion to correct anemia and to reduce the bilirubin concentration, thus obviating the brain damage of kernicterus. Exchange transfusion is often supplemented by administering albumin to provide more binding sites for bilirubin and the use of light or phototherapy which controls the rate of increase of bilirubin by converting it to other apparently innocuous pigments. The management of the newborn may be enhanced by the administration of drugs, such as phenobarbitol, to the mother prenatally. This drug in relatively small doses can induce in the fetus the synthesis of enzymes necessary to conjugate bilirubin and thereby make the newborn better able to deal with the jaundice.

Diabetes Mellitus

The total problem of diabetes and pregnancy is considered in Chapter 32. However, it is important to recognize the specific impact of the disease on the fetus, which is best indicated by the increase in perinatal mortality. Despite the fact that there have been marked improvements in perinatal mortality in general and in diabetic pregnancy specifically, the overall perinatal mortality in diabetic pregnancies is approximately three times that in the nondiabetic. The rate is a direct function of the severity (White classification) of the diabetes with the rate for the class A diabetic being only slightly above that for the general population while the class F/R diabetic may have not more than a 50-50 chance of having a surviving infant. It has long been known that if all diabetic pregnancies were allowed to go to term there would be a small but significant number of stillbirths based on the impact of diabetes on the blood vessels of the uterus and placenta, producing premature aging. In order to avoid these stillbirths, routine early delivery became the pattern of management. This unfortunately resulted in an increase in neonatal deaths because of the propensity of diabetic offspring to respiratory distress syndrome. Current improved survival is related to selective early delivery and antepartum testing for fetal pulmonary maturity.

The increased susceptibility of the diabetic off-spring to the respiratory distress syndrome is felt to be at least sevenfold and is related to a delay in the onset of surfactant production by the type II cells in the lung. This occurs in class A, B and C diabetics, while in class D and F diabetics, whose vascular disease predominates, pulmonary maturity is accelerated. In addition to pulmonary problems, there are several metabolic problems which are increased in the infant of a diabetic mother. Because glucose crosses the placenta readily by supple diffusion, the fetal glucose level reflects the level in the mother. Insulin, on the other hand, does not cross and consequently the fetus must deal with its hyperglycemia by hypertrophy of pancreatic islet cells and the production of insulin. The combination of high levels of insulin and glucose along with the growth hormonelike substance, HPL, is responsible for the increased size of fetuses in class A, B and C diabetic pregnancies. The magnitude of the increase in fetal size is related inversely to the adequacy of maternal blood sugar control. Macrosomia increases the likelihood of mechanical problems and fetal injury at delivery and is in part responsible for a higher cesarean section rate in diabetes. This same mechanism (fetal hyperinsulinism) is responsible for neonatal hypoglycemia when the maternal source of glucose is eliminated after delivery. These babies are also more prone to hyperbilirubinemia and hypocalcemia.

Another major problem of the diabetic newborn is birth defects. Congenital malformations are increased three times in babies born to diabetic women and lethal defects are six times as likely. Although many kinds of defects are observed, skeletal defects involving the caudal portion of the skelton (caudal regression) and ventricular septal defects are the most characteristic.

Finally, there is the question of development of diabetes in the child. The genetics of diabetes is not well understood and there may be several mechanisms involved. The suggestion that the disease is inherited as an autosomal recessive is refuted by the fact that the concordance rate is not nearly 100 percent in identical twins and also that diabetic matings do not always result in diabetic children. There is also with diabetes the question of expression, which means that an individual who has the genetic determinants for diabetes may not express the disease unless confronted with stresses such as pregnancy, obesity or infection. The best advice to be given the diabetic patient concerning these considerations is that there is an increased chance that the child may develop diabetes and that the magnitude of this increase is related to the amount of diabetes present in the pedigrees of both father and mother.

It is quite apparent then that the overall outlook for the diabetic woman producing a healthy normal infant is restricted, more severely in long-standing severe diabetes, and therefore the cost in dollars, time and emotional investment is high. Ideally, the diabetic and her family should be apprised of this information prior to undertaking a pregnancy so that the decision can be a conscious, well considered one.

Prolonged Pregnancy

The average duration of pregnancy is 280 days from the first day of the last menstrual period, or 267 days from the time of conception if the menstrual cycle is of average length. Only 5 percent of women deliver on the actual due date, although most will deliver within 10 to 14 days in either direction from the date. Since the placenta has a normal life span equal to the duration of pregnancy, one may justifiably be concerned that if the due date is exceeded by more than two weeks, the aging placenta may no longer be able to support the fetus adequately. Fortunately, in most instances the placenta is capable of such support. In fact, in a great number of patients who are postdates, the date has been miscalculated or based on faulty memory. In addition to those postmature pregnancies in which there is placental insufficiency, there is another group of late pregnancies in which the placenta functions well and the fetus becomes oversized, creating potential mechanical problems in labor and delivery.

If the circumstances including the status of the cervix, the size and position of the baby and the size of the maternal pelvis are all favorable, induction of labor should be carried out when a pregnancy exceeds the due date by 10 to 14 days. If there is any question about the dates, efforts should be made to verify the gestational age by techniques already discussed. It is important to recognize, however, that a single determination in late pregnancy has a rather significant inherent error. This is especially true of ultrasound measurements of the biparietal diameter since linear growth stops after 30 weeks. When a pregnancy is 10 to 14 days postdate and conditions are not favorable for induction of labor,

the well-being of the fetus must be established in order to permit the continuation of the pregnancy. Urinary or serum estriols may be utilized and this clinical circumstance is one of few in which HPL determinations seem helpful. The frequency of these studies is critical. Since the adequacy of placental function is not necessarily static under such circumstances these studies can provide only limited assurance and must be repeated two or three times weekly.

The oxytocin challenge test (OCT) and nonstress test are also valuable in evaluating the postdate pregnancy, and again because of the possibility of a rapid progressive decline in placental function the OCT cannot provide the usually accepted promise of seven days of well-being for the fetus.

In addition to establishing maturity in the case of uncertain gestational age, the examination of amniotic fluid for meconium may be helpful in such cases. Clear fluid is reassuring although it does not rule out fetal jeopardy. Meconium staining and scant fluid both suggest an affected fetus, and, although they are not sufficient alone to indicate aggressive action, they are confirmatory in the presence of other signs of fetal compromise. Aspiratory and severe pulmonary consequences for the newborn always exist when meconium is present. However, prevention is a dilemma. Even prompt delivery by cesarean section does not necessarily obviate aspiration, since respiratory movements can occur in utero.

The affected postmature (sometimes called dysmature) newborn has a typical appearance. It is long for its weight, which makes it appear to have lost weight. The finger and toenails are long and stained with meconium, as are the cord and membranes. These infants are especially prone to distress during labor and to respiratory problems in the neonatal period.

On the surface, it would seem simple to determine the due date and the probability that the pregnancy has gone beyond that point, but there are a number of pitfalls. Many patients do not record or cannot recall when they had their last period. Others have long cycles, with ovulation and conception occurring later than the fourteenth day. This is especially true in patients discontinuing oral contraceptive therapy, in whom the first ovulation may not occur until four to six weeks after the last withdrawal flow. One must assess these factors carefully before overtreating a patient for supposed postmaturity.

Preeclampsia-Eclampsia

Although the manifestations of preeclampsia (hypertension, edema and proteinuria) and eclampsia (convulsions in addition) are primarily maternal (see Chapter 31), the fetal impact cannot be ignored. Progressive placental insufficiency is an inherent part of the syndrome, and in fact intrauterine fetal growth is frequently retarded prior to the development of maternal manifestations. With the appearance of clinically evident preeclampsia, placental function continues to decline and fetal death may result if the pregnancy is allowed to continue. Occasionally a patient with moderate or severe preeclampsia may appear to respond so favorably to therapy that there is the temptation to allow the pregnancy to continue to permit further fetal maturity. Such a decision is fraught with the risk to failure of the fetus to prosper and the possibility of a stillbirth; and in most cases it is unwise. Should such a course be considered, amniocentesis for detection of pulmonary maturity (L/S ratio) should be done first because pulmonary maturity is often markedly accelerated in such circumstances. To attempt to prolong a pregnancy in the face of significant preeclampsia is not appropriate if the fetal lungs are already mature. If the L/S ratio is immature and a conservative course is to be followed, fetal well-being must be carefully assessed. This is not a simple matter since urinary estriol excretion may be reduced by impaired renal function, while serum levels may be falsely elevated. Interpretation of OCT's and nonstress tests is also difficult in the immature fetus.

The perinatal wastage in preeclampsia is largely a function of the stage of pregnancy at which the process develops and therefore the degree of maturity of the infant delivered. If preeclampsia does not develop until after the thirty-sixth week of gestation, the perinatal loss should be quite low. Perinatal mortality is high when convulsions (eclampsia) occur. Recent reviews indicate a rate of approximately 20 percent.

Chronic Hypertension

Approximately 75 percent of women with benign essential hypertension go through pregnancy with no problems, either maternal or fetal. Unfortunately, some 15 percent develop preeclampsia. When this happens, the fetal prognosis is very poor, especially if preeclampsia occurs at a time when the fetus is significantly premature (at the end of the second trimester, for example). The perinatal mortality rate in this group is approximately 20 percent.

In the case of the hypertensive mother without superimposed preeclampsia, the fetal risk is not great, but it is greater than that for women with normal blood pressure. Because of this, it is recommended that all hypertensive patients be followed with estriol determinations in the third trimester, in order to identify the occasional benign hypertensive patient whose fetus is in jeopardy and for whom preterm delivery is indicated. There is, in addition, an increased frequency of abruptio placentae in these hypertensive patients, with the added perinatal wastage of that problem.

TORCH Infections Affecting the Fetus

There is an increasing number of infections with recognized detrimental effects upon the fetus. These may be direct effects on fetus or indirect effects by precipitating abortion or premature labor. The term TORCH (T-toxoplasmosis, O-other, R-rubella, C-cytomegalovirus, H-herpes) has been applied to these infections, and although it does account for the majority of significant perinatal infections there are many others.

Toxoplasmosis. This disease is caused by the protozoan organism *Toxoplasma gondii* which is contracted from oocytes in cat feces or by eating uncooked meat. Only cats which are unconfined and eat infected rodents are a hazard. When primary infection, which is generally asymptomatic, occurs just before or during early pregnancy, congenital infection may result, which can lead to the birth of a child who is mentally and physically retarded with chorioretinitis and microcephaly. Approximately 10 to 15 percent of these babies die, and most of the survivors are severely compromised. If the disease is recognized clinically or by seroconversion in early pregnancy, abortion is recommended. If abortion is not accepted or the infection occurs later in pregnancy, treatment with triple sulfa may reduce the fetal impact.

Others. Many infections, such as syphilis and varicella, can be included in this category. But group B beta hemolytic streptococcus is probably most deserving of mention. This organism is not a major pathogen in the mother, but when it causes early neonatal sepsis, it produces a fulminant pneumonia with a very high mortality (greater than 40 percent). The organism is sexually transmitted and is carried asymptomatically in the cervix and vagina in a significant number (over 20 percent) of pregnant women. The route of infection is thought to be contact during the birth process and is especially prone to occur when predisposing factors such as prematurity, prolonged labor, and premature rupture of the membranes exist. The rate of newborn colonization is high; however, the attack (infection) rate is low (1 to 2 percent of colonized babies become infected). Screening of all gravidae and treatment of carriers had been recommended, but the practicality of the approach is open to serious question.

A second clinical picture, the late onset, occurs after seven to ten days, with a picture of meningitis; the source is not necessarily the cervix or vagina or even the mother. Mortality in late onset infection is considerably less.

Rubella. Although the most well-established concerns are for infection in the first trimester, serious problems are known to occur when the infection happens as late as the fifth month of gestation, and later infections may be responsible for more subtle problems. Infections in the first trimester may result in abortion in more than 33 percent of cases. Congenital rubella (the expanded rubella syndrome) may be difficult to differentiate clinically from the other TORCH infections, although culture of the virus or specific IgM measurements are diagnostic. It is especially important to recognize that these babies are highly infectious as are the placentas, and contact with nonimmune pregnant personnel should be avoided.

When the pregnant woman is exposed to rubella, she should have immediate serologic testing for rubella antibody. If this indicates immunity she is protected (85 to 90 percent of adults in the United States are immune). If she is not immune she should be carefully followed for development of clinical rubella or development of antibodies. If either of these developments occur abortion should be recommended in view of the high rate of fetal involvement. Gamma globulin is not recommended in rubella exposure unless abortion is unacceptable, and then it is important for the patient to realize that although the disease maybe modified, fetal effects are not necessarily obviated.

Immunization against rubella is recommended for all susceptible women in the child-bearing age group, but special care must be taken to avoid immunizing the pregnant woman. Although the exact risk is not known, the vaccine virus is known to have gained access to the fetus. One convenient time for rubella vaccination is the immediate postpartum period, since pregnancy is unlikely then. Rubella vaccination is not a contraindication to breast-feeding.

Cytomegalovirus. This is the most common of the congenital infections. Approximately two-thirds of adult women have antibodies to the virus and the virus can be cultured from the cervix or urine of 3 to 5 percent of pregnant women. Most adult infections are asymptomatic although this organism is a special problem among immunosuppressed patients— in transplant units, for example—and therefore a special hazard to nurses working in such areas. Congenital infection occurs in about 1 percent of births with approximately 10 percent of infected newborns exhibiting permanent damage. The severe forms of congenital infection produce a picture not dissimilar to other TORCH infections. The diagnosis can be established by viral culture or serology and there is no specific therapy unless the diagnosis can be established sufficiently early to provide an abortion option.

Herpes Simplex. There are two strains of this virus: Type I, which is primarily responsible for oral lesions, and Type II for genital lesions. These distinctions are not absolute but hold in the majority of cases. Antibodies to the herpesvirus , although specific to Types I and II, are cross protective so that a prior Type I infection will prevent viremia with a first infection of Type II and cause it to behave clinically as a recurrent rather than primary infection. Primary genital herpesvirus infections are characterized by multiple lesions, systemic symptoms and prolonged viral shedding. Once the primary infection has occurred, the virus is sequestered in the dorsal nerve route and there tends to be a series of recurrences at irregular intervals over a period of the next several (two to three) years.

Two problems are evident in pregnancy. Congenital infection which is extremely rare can occur when a primary infection (absent antibodies, viremia) occurs in pregnancy. Like other TORCH infections, the impact is greatest when this occurs in early pregnancy and the result is similar (mental retardation, microcephaly, cerebral calcification, chorioretinitis). The far more common concern is neonatal infection which is contracted during delivery by exposure to virus in genital lesions or in the asymptomatic carrier state. Disease in the newborn may be localized or systemic. The prognosis is good in newborns with localized disease, although 50 percent progress to systemic diseases with a mortality of 90 percent.

Treatment consists of avoiding the contact by cesarean section if lesions or positive cultures persist at term. Section should be carried out prior to rupture of the membranes or within four hours. Long delays after rupture of the membranes are accompanied by a high risk of neonatal infection. Chemotherapy of the infected newborn is under study. The drugs used are toxic but justified by the high mortality.

Infections Due to Premature Rupture of Membranes

Intrauterine infection as the result of premature rupture of the membranes is probably the most common infectious threat to the fetus. It is well recognized that the frequency of such infection parallels the length of time from the rupture of the membranes to the onset of labor. Infection of the fetus occurs by way of the amniotic fluid to the fetal tracheobronchial tree, as well as from the membranes and placenta through the cord vessels, producing fetal sepsis. The organisms most commonly involved are anaerobic streptococci and gram-negative bacilli.

Since it is difficult to achieve therapeutic levels of antibiotics in the amniotic fluid once the patient becomes febrile, the treatment is delivery either by induction or cesarean section. More important, however, is the prevention of infection. This is accomplished by delivery (most often by induction, but by section if necessary) of any patient with premature rupture of the membranes whose fetus is larger than 1,500 to 1,800 g. This weight range is selected because in most clinics the survival data for babies of that size are such that the risk of delivery and prematurity appears to be less than the risk of intrauterine infection. Recent data have suggested, however, that with premature rupture of the membranes, the fetal lung may mature within 24 to 48 hours and therefore a delay may be

indicated. This effect, along with the effect of glucocorticoids (administered to the mother), has yet to be clearly established in maturing the fetal lung.

Fetal Growth Retardation

This is one term applied to the clinical syndrome in which the fetus fails to prosper in utero. The terms dysmaturity, placental insufficiency, small-for-date babies, uteroplacental insufficiency, and stunted fetus have also been applied. The syndrome may occur with maternal diseases such as diabetes with severe vascular involvement, chronic renal disease, and chronic hypertension with renal involvement. Intrauterine infection with rubella, toxoplasmosis, and cytomegalovirus are causes. The most severe growth retardation is produced by multiple congenital malformations. In some cases the syndrome may be idiopathic and recurrent. In general, the earlier in gestation that retardation is apparent, the poorer the outlook.

At birth these babies appear to have lost subcutaneous fat, their skin is often wrinkled, and the finger- and toenails are long. The amniotic fluid, cord, and nails are heavily stained with meconium. The stillbirth rate is high and the frequency of respiratory problems in the newborn is increased. The most significant management problem from the obstetrical viewpoint is differentiating (antepartally) the growth-retarded fetus from a premature fetus of appropriate size. After delivery, this differentiation is less difficult and can be based on weight (particularly weight gain patterns), certain developmental criteria, such as ear cartilage development and plantar skin creases, and behavior patterns.

The question of erroneous menstrual dates often arises and this necessitates the use of the method described under fetal diagnosis. Once the diagnosis is suspected, some search for an etiology is indicated. Heroic approaches to the fetus are certainly not indicated if a diagnosis of congenital rubella or cytomegalovirus infection has been established. However, this may not be simple to do if, on the other hand, there appears to be no ominous diagnosis. The fetus must be evaluated and followed with an index of well-being (such as urinary estriol) and delivery timed appropriately. In the presence of uteroplacental insufficiency, fetal tolerance to labor may be reduced and the need for cesarean section increased. After birth, newborns with late pregnancy growth retardation and without infection or malformation tend to thrive and rapidly catch up in size with their peers. Those newborns with early pregnancy retardation have reduced cell numbers as well as cell size and tend to remain small.

Disproportionate Twin Development

Twins with disparity in size may be accounted for by the fact that there can be a connection between the two circulations. This is especially true in single-ovum twins. When this happens in early pregnancy and one heart pumps more strongly than the other, there may be monopolization of a larger area of the placenta by one twin and thus a disparity in size. Such twins are not only greatly different in size at birth, but the smaller one is often anemic and may require transfusion. The larger twin may be hypervolemic and require a phlebotomy to prevent heart failure and jaundice. This type of placental anastomosis, when it occurs in double-ovum twins, accounts for those rare situations known as "chimerism," in which an individual may have two populations of cells, as evidenced by blood groups or sex chromatin. The other important clinical significance of disparity in twin sizes is that difficulties may be encountered in delivery if the smaller of the twins is delivered first through a cervix that is not completely dilated.

FETAL TREATMENT

The art of fetal treatment is at this time far less developed than fetal diagnosis. The most common approach to the fetus by the obstetrician is to select an appropriate time for delivery, convert the fetus to a newborn, and then turn over the active treatment to the neonatologist. Perhaps the most important approach to the fetus is to provide appropriate support throughout the pregnancy. This includes adequate diet prenatally, as well as glucose and oxygen during labor, especially if there is fetal distress.

Treatment in the case of a positive prenatal diagnosis of congenital disease is generally limited to therapeutic abortion. However, in some instances of metabolic errors, maternal dietary modification may be effective in protecting the fetus with an enzyme defect.

Many drugs administered to the mother cross the placenta into the fetal circulation. Transplacental passage is generally a function of the molecular size of the drug, substances with molecular weights less than 500 crossing readily by simple diffusion. Although most often there is concern regarding the deleterious effects of drugs on the fetus, in some instances one can achieve a desirable therapeutic effect. In the case of the sensitized Rh negative patient, it is possible with certain drugs to induce the fetal liver to produce the enzymes required for bilirubin conjugation. This allows the newborn to cope better with the jaundice and reduces the need for exchange transfusion. The most effective drug is phenobarbital in small doses (15 mg., four times daily) for one or two weeks prior to delivery.

Another example of fetal drug therapy is the administration of glucocorticoids to the mother to induce the production of surfactant by the Type II cells of the fetal lung and thereby reduce the risk of respiratory distress syndrome. The evidence is that if this is done between 26 to 28 and 32 to 34 weeks of gestation and if delivery can be delayed for 24 to 48 hours, there will be a significant reduction in RDS. No deleterious results have been recorded in humans by the use of steroids; however, as with all innovative approaches the treatment must still be considered in an experimental stage.

Intrauterine fetal transfusion in Rh disease is the most publicized form of treatment. Hopefully, the use of RhoGAM will ultimately eliminate the need for this rather crude procedure.

The future undoubtedly holds many advances in this area—from the prenatal correction of congenital defects to the even more unbelievable unscrambling of genetic mishaps. There may well be treatments of maladies which are presently unknown in this rapidly developing area of fetal medicine.

SUGGESTED READING

Aubry, R. H., Beydoun, S., Cabalum, M. T., and Williams, M. L.: "Fetal growth retardation." In *Perinatal Medicine*. ed. Bolognese, R. J. and Schwarz, R. H. Baltimore, Williams & Wilkins, 1977.

Fernandez de Castro, A., Usatequi-Gomez,

M., and Spellacy, W. N.: "Amniotic fluid components as determinants of fetal maturity." *Obstet. Gynecol.* 46:76, 1975.

Gant, N. F. and Worley, R. J.: "Pregnancy induced hypertension. A chronic disease process." In *Perinatal Medicine*. ed., Bolognese, R. J. and Schwarz, R. H. Baltimore, Williams & Wilkins. 1977.

Gluck, L., Kulovich, M. V. and Borer, R. C.: "Estimates of fetal lung maturity." *Clin. Perinatal* 1:125, 1974.

Hallman, M., et al.: "Phosphatidylinostol and phosphatidylgycerol in amniotic fluid. Indices of lung maturity." *Am. J. Obstet. Gynecol.* 125:613, 1976.

Hobbins, J. C. and Winsberg, F.: *Ultrasonography in Obstetrics and Gynecology*. Baltimore, Williams & Wilkins, 1977.

Hobel, C. J., Hyvariuen, M. A., Okada, D. M. and Oh, W.: "Prenatal and intrapartum high risk screening." *Am. J. Obstet. Gynecol.* 117:1, 1973.

Nwosu, U. C.: "Post-term pregnancy." In *Perinatal Medicine*. ed., Bolognese, R. J. and Schwarz, R.H. Baltimore, Williams & Wilkins, 1977.

Queenan, J. T.: *Modern Management of the Rh Problem*. Hagerstown, Harper & Row, 1977.

Schwarz, R. H.: "Diabetes mellitus." In *Perinatal Medicine*. ed., Bolognese, R. J. and Schwarz, R. H. Baltimore, Williams & Wilkins, 1977.

Sever, J. L., and Fuceillo, D. A.: Perinatal infections." In *Perinatal Medicine*. ed., Bolognese, R. J. and Schwarz, R. H. Baltimore, Williams & Wilkins, 1977.

Thirty-Seven

Electronic Fetal Monitoring and Fetal Intensive Care

The Pros and Cons of Fetal Monitoring | Methods of Monitoring | Remedial Measures for Fetal Stress or Distress | Conclusion

The fetus, as a "patient," has always been relatively inaccessible to the nurse and the physician. For many years, the forces of labor and the well-being of the fetus could only be evaluated by palpation of the maternal abdomen and by periodic sampling of the fetal heart rate through auscultation. A greater understanding of fetal cardiorespiratory physiology and methods to measure certain maternal and fetal functions have developed over the past two decades. Among these methods, continuous electronic monitoring of fetal heart rate (FHR) and uterine activity (UA) has had widest clinical application. Experience with this instrumentation has resulted in an improved understanding and clinical interpretation of intrapartum events.

THE PROs AND CONs OF FETAL MONITORING

Several studies suggest that the majority of intrapartum fetal deaths should be avoidable when the fetal heart rate is monitored continuously. It is also generally considered that continuous fetal monitoring enables early detection of intrapartum fetal hypoxia (distress), and, when accompanied by appropriate therapy, results in lower neonatal morbidity and mortality, as well as improved neurologic development following birth. Most obstetricians believe that continuous fetal monitoring offers substantial benefit in this regard. Clinical studies of its value, however, have produced conflicting results, especially in relation to its use during normal labor. Although the observation of normal fetal monitoring data is predictive of a good fetal outcome, the interpretation of abnormal patterns has been fraught with difficulty and with considerable false-positive diagnoses (i.e., an apparently abnormal finding when the fetus is well). All of this has led the medical community, governmental agencies and the consumer to question the value of fetal monitoring. It is apparent that valid "cost-benefit" and "risk-benefit" analyses will require more data from long-term prospective studies.

Because methods of fetal monitoring are at times applied internally, several potential risks to the mother and the fetus have been suggested. The occurrence of complications such as uterine perforations or neonatal scalp infections are uncommon and rarely require therapy. The relationship of internal fetal monitoring to maternal infectious morbidity, although a concern, has generally not proved to be as important as other contributing factors, such as prolonged rupture of membranes and an excessive number of vaginal examinations.

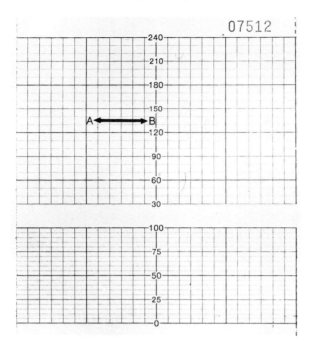

Figure 37-1. Recording paper for fetal monitor. Note FHR bpm recorded on upper channel, UA mm. Hg recorded on lower channel, and panel number at top of sheet. Distance from A to B equals one minute when paper speed is 3 cm./min.

Concerns regarding the contribution of electronic fetal monitoring to the increasing rate of cesarean sections have been raised repeatedly. Although this is difficult to evaluate, a number of investigators have suggested that the effect is not substantial. In fact, some have claimed that experience with appropriate use of monitoring can reduce the frequency of cesarean sections that are performed for fetal distress.

In spite of these controversies, the use of electronic fetal monitoring has continued to increase. Because every high risk fetus cannot be identified prior to labor, some advocate electronic monitoring of all patients during labor. On the other hand, uncertainty of the benefit in normal pregnancy and limitations of equipment and personnel frequently result in selective monitoring of high risk patients and those receiving oxytocics or conduction anesthetics. Fetal monitoring has also been extended to the evaluation of the high risk fetus prior to labor. This form of periodic evaluation, either nonstress testing (NST) or contraction stress testing (CST), is being used effectively to assess fetal well-being in a large variety of pregnancy complications.

With the development of monitoring, the role of the nurse during labor has expanded to caring for the fetus as well as for the mother. As with other diagnostic procedures, it is the nurse's responsibility to inform the patient about the purpose and the procedure of the monitoring and to screen and interpret the data initially. In many institutions nursing guidelines have been established concerning the application of fetal monitors, the interpretation of data and the institution of remedial change when abnormalities are detected. Thus, to use the fetal monitor, the nurse must be familiar with the equipment, have an understanding of the fundamental principles involved and have access to updated information concerning interpretation and management of the data.

METHODS OF MONITORING

Many different types and models of fetal monitors are available on the market. It is critically important that the nurse be thoroughly familiar with the particular model to be used, including its capabilities, limitations, and method of recording.

The Record

Fetal monitors are equipped to provide a continuous recording of fetal heart rate (FHR) and uterine activity (UA). This information is recorded on perforated paper which folds "accordion style" (Fig. 37-1). Uterine activity is generally recorded on the lower channel. The recording paper provides a vertical scale for measuring the intrauterine pressure usually in millimeters of mercury (mm. Hg). Most monitors are equipped with a zeroing and calibration device to assure that the record accurately reflects the true intrauterine pressure. The fetal heart rate in beats per minute is displayed on the upper channel. Some monitors are also equipped with a digital display of the fetal heart rate, and a small oscilloscope screen for viewing the fetal electrocardiogram.

The paper speed is usually set at 3 cm. per minute. Divisions on the horizontal scale provide a measurement of the time lapsed and are useful as markers to correlate events on both channels. Numbering on the individual sheets of the record provides a reference for rapid calculation of lapsed time for

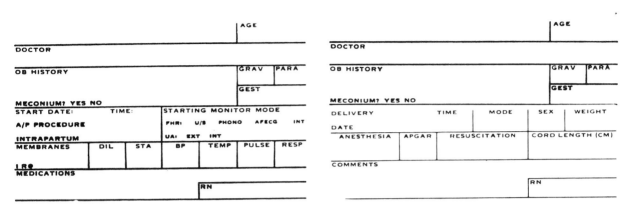

Figure 37-2. Label on left provides identification and clinical information for interpretation of tracing and is applied when monitoring is initiated. Label on right provides identification and clinical information for correlation of monitor data with neonatal condition.

longer intervals as well as for charting. For example, the nurse's record might reflect the following:

11:30 P.M. Panel #17474—Continuous external fetal monitoring initiated using ultrasound. FHR baseline 136–144 bpm. Uterine contractions every 3 min. Questionable decelerations.
11:50 P.M. Panel #17479—Dilation 6 cm. Effacement complete Station +1. Artificial rupture of membranes. Fluid clear. Internal monitor applied.
12:30 A.M. Panel #17489—FHR baseline 132–140, variability moderate. UA—baseline 10 mm Hg. Contractions g 2 min., 50 mm Hg. Periodic change—occasional mild variable decelerations to 120 bpm. with contractions, duration 30 sec., prompt recovery to baseline.

Because the data obtained become a part of the patient's permanent record, it is important that a systematic method of identification be used at the beginning and end of each fetal monitor tracing. A sample format for identification is shown in Figure 37-2. In addition, it has become common practice to record the clock time and important clinical data, such as vital signs, vaginal exams, rupture of membranes, medications (dose and route of administration), and patient activity, directly on the monitor record. This information is important for interpreting the record and is also invaluable when reviewed retrospectively for teaching purposes.

Uterine Activity (UA)

Uterine activity may be monitored by either external or internal methods. External monitoring provides a recording of the frequency and duration of uterine contractions (UC), while internal monitoring provides an accurate measurement of intrauterine pressure for assessing both baseline tone and the intensity of the contractions.

The use of an internal pressure catheter permits the most accurate assessment of UA, both quantitatively and temporally. Thus the internal method is particularly useful in evaluating patients receiving oxytocic drugs or in instances when the temporal relationship of changes in FHT to contractions is unclear. Nevertheless, the majority of labors that are monitored can be adequately assessed by the external method. The method used and any change of method should be noted directly on the fetal monitoring record as well as in the nursing record.

External Pressure Monitoring. Uterine activity is monitored by a pressure transducer called a tokodynamometer. A transducer converts one form of energy to another; this transducer converts pressure to electrical signals. The tokodynamometer is a flat disk with either a protruding or a flush plunger. It is secured to the mother's abdomen with an elastic belt. As the uterus contracts, the abdominal wall rises and presses against the transducer. The subsequent movement of the plunger is converted into an electrical signal and is recorded on the paper, giving a continuous record of the frequency and duration of contractions.

Correct placement of the tokodynamometer is necessary if interpretable data are to be gathered. The transducer is placed over the area where the greatest displacement of the uterus occurs during a contraction (i.e., the uterine fundus). Displacement of the abdominal wall by the uterus may not be adequate to record UC in patients with a small uterus (i.e., marked prematurity) or those who are extremely overweight. Because movement of the maternal abdominal wall caused by respirations, coughing, or position changes may be reflected on the fetal monitoring record, any such interfering factors should be noted as such. It may not be possible to obtain consistent data with this method from patients who are extremely restless. Occasionally patients who do not have anesthesia find that the firm elastic straps become uncomfortable or interfere with breathing techniques and effleurage. When this occurs, repositioning the tokodynamometer and straps may be useful. If this is not effective, internal pressure monitoring should be considered.

Internal method.   A soft plastic catheter filled with sterile water is passed into the uterus beyond the presenting fetal part by means of a firmer plastic introducer (Fig. 37-3). This, of course, requires that the cervix be partially dilated. Although a catheter or balloon may be placed extraamniotically, for clinical use the placement is intraamniotic and requires that the membranes be previously ruptured. The catheter is connected to a pressure transducer (strain gauge). The intrauterine pressure is transmitted from the amniotic fluid through the sterile water in the catheter to the pressure transducer. Changes in the intrauterine pressure that occur with contractions, the Valsalva maneuver, or coughing and so on are recorded on the monitor.

Because of the invasive nature of the method, the vulva should be cleansed with an antiseptic and sterile towels used to drape the patient and maintain the sterility of the catheter. The catheter is filled with sterile water prior to insertion so that air will not be introduced into the uterus. The catheter tip is protected from contamination during insertion by the plastic introducer. Before the catheter is connected, the transducer should be placed at a height which approximates that of the catheter tip (the xiphisternal junction) and "zeroed" to atmospheric pressure. If the level of the catheter tip is above the transducer, a false elevated pressure recording will result, whereas, if the catheter tip is below the transducer, a false low or negative pressure may be recorded. Calibration should be performed periodically on the record to assure accurate measurement of UA. Function of the catheter can be tested by having the patient cough. This will cause a sudden sharp positive deflection on the recording.

The internal pressure catheter provides a means of sampling amniotic fluid for meconium or bacteria during labor if this becomes clinically useful. If the catheter becomes plugged by vernix, meconium or blood, intrauterine pressure will not be transmitted to the transducer. Flushing with small amounts of sterile water will usually correct the problem. When this fails, the catheter tip should be withdrawn slightly and repositioned. The portion of the catheter in the vagina or outside the patient should not be advanced into the uterus. Not only may this result in bacterial contamination, but it is generally ineffective because the flexibility of the catheter will cause it to coil alongside the presenting fetal part. Perforation of the uterus and injury to the placenta should be considered when excessive vaginal bleeding occurs after placement of the catheter and when uterine contractions fail to be recorded.

Fetal Heart Rate (FHR)

Prior to the development of fetal monitoring, evaluation of the fetal heart rate was restricted to periodic auscultation during the interval between contractions. FHR changes occurring with the contractions or during the first 30 seconds following the contraction were usually not detected. The ability to diagnose fetal distress was limited to sustained and extreme variation in fetal heart rate, such as severe bradycardia. With auscultation, the evaluation of periodic changes, that is, those occurring over short time intervals (decelerations or accelerations), was somewhat subjective, especially when they occurred at a rate which was within the normal range.

With continuous FHR monitoring, the time interval between two successive heart beats is calculated as a rate and is recorded graphically. For example, a lapse of 375 milliseconds between beats would constitute a rate of 160 beats per minute. In order for this calculation to be made, the fetal signal obtained with a transducer is amplified and then counted by a cardiotachometer. This is converted to a rate between successive beats and recorded continuously during and in the interval between contractions.

External method. Several methods for monitoring the fetal heart rate through the maternal abdomen are available.

Phonocardiography utilizes a transducer which is essentially a microphone. With this technique the heart sounds of the fetus constitute the signal. Extraneous sounds or "noise" from within the uterus, maternal abdomen or the abdominal wall may also be detected as a signal, and thus electronic filtering is required.

Fetal electrocardiogram (FECG) is a method for obtaining the electrical signal of the fetal heart from the maternal abdominal wall. When the abdominal wall fetal ECG is used as the signal, the larger maternal ECG complex is censored or edited out by the machine. When the maternal signal coincides with a fetal signal, the machine may edit the maternal signal and insert a fetal beat automatically. This is known as compensation. Monitoring of the FECG via the maternal abdominal wall will result in clinically useful tracings in only a portion of cases in which it is attempted.

The doppler or ultrasound method is the most commonly used method of external monitoring. With this technique high frequency sound waves are transmitted from a crystal and are reflected from the moving fetal heart to a receiving crystal. The difference in frequencies of the transmitted and the reflected sound waves constitutes the signal which can be amplified for counting by the cardiotachometer and is also heard as an audible signal from the machine. Filtering is needed for other intra-abdominal motion which will constitute "noise." More recently a bidirectional doppler has been employed in fetal monitoring, which permits selection of motion either toward or away from the transducer. With this technique, whichever constitutes the better signal is selected for recording. In order to obtain clinically useful tracings with the doppler, "averaging" over two or three successive beats is performed. Some machines are also

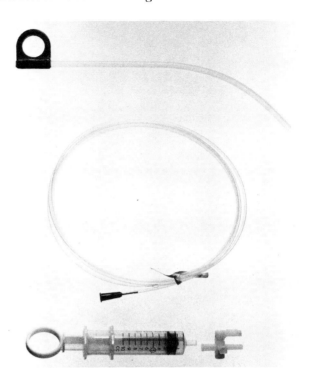

Figure 37-3. Equipment for internal pressure monitoring: plastic introducer, catheter, stopcock and syringe.

equipped with logic circuitry such that rates above a certain level (e.g., 180) will be halved on the recorder, while rates below a preset level (e.g., 90) will be doubled. Variations in equipment function such as this illustrate the importance of being familiar with the particular equipment in use.

When the doppler transducer is used, the transducer is applied to an area that will be directly over the fetal heart. This site is selected by auscultation and by palpating the fetus. By trial and error the position from which the sharpest (not necessarily the loudest) audible fetal signal can be heard is determined before securing the transducer with an elastic belt. Periodic changes of fetal or maternal position may require readjustment of the transducer to maintain high quality data.

Internal Method. Direct *fetal electrocardiography* is the most widely used method of FHR monitoring during labor. The transducer is a small electrode which is attached to the skin of the presenting part of the fetus, usually the scalp. This small silver silver-chloride electrode is commonly referred to as a "clip" because the first electrodes available were attached by two prongs to the fetal scalp. At present the most commonly used electrode is a small spiral

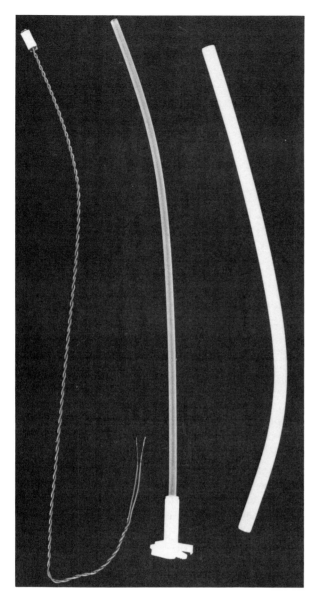

Figure 37-4. Scalp electrode and introducer for fetal heart monitoring.

wire which is advanced into the fetal skin by clockwise rotation while gentle pressure is applied (Fig. 37-4). Application of the electrode requires that the membranes be ruptured and the cervix be dilated 1 to 2 cm. or more, and that the presenting part is known and fixed in the pelvis so that the gentle pressure required will not displace the fetus.

The fetal electrocardiogram serves as the fetal signal for counting. On occasion, the maternal signal obtained by this method may produce an artifactual tracing; for example, the maternal ECG may be conducted through a dead fetus. Editing of the direct fetal ECG may result in failure to detect fetal cardiac arrhythmias. With direct fetal electrocardiography there is no need for averaging and the true beat-to-beat variation in fetal heart rate can be evaluated. Spiral electrodes are easily removed before or after delivery by counterclockwise rotation of the attached wires.

Application of the Fetal Monitor

The decision to apply the fetal monitor should be based on institutional policy and the consent of the patient. In some institutions, fetal monitoring is applied in all cases. In most programs the selection of patients to be monitored rests with the physician and the nurse. The nurse's role in selecting patients to be monitored is particularly important when the number of patients who are in labor exceeds the number of available monitors, and priorities for monitoring must be established.

In general, the decision to monitor is made on the basis of one of three primary indications:

1. *Antepartum risk factors*—these include maternal complications, such as diabetes and hypertension, or fetal problems, such as intrauterine growth retardation.
2. *Intrapartum risk factors*—such as third trimester bleeding, passage of meconium or abnormalities of FHR as indicated by auscultation.
3. *Other obstetrical factors*—such as abnormal labor, or the need to evaluate the effects of drugs, e.g., oxytocics.

Once the decision is made to monitor a patient, the method of monitoring is selected. This is contingent upon four factors: 1) status of the cervix and membranes; 2) the indication for monitoring; 3) patient acceptance; and 4) availability. When the membranes are intact or the cervix is not dilated, external methods of monitoring must be used. If adequate data cannot be obtained with the available external systems or if the belts for the transducers are unacceptable to the patient, then internal monitoring should be considered. Internal monitoring must be used in cases where the most accurate data are required, such as true beat-to-beat variation, temporal relationship of decelerations to contractions, or true intrauterine pressures.

External devices for fetal monitoring are applied by the nurse. Insertion of intrauterine catheters or

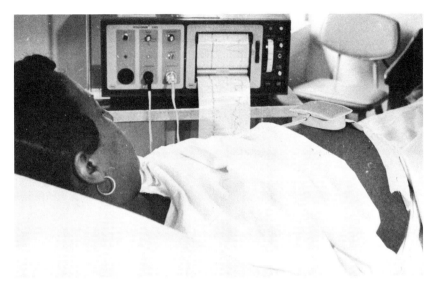

Figure 37-5. Patient with external fetal monitor applied. Note that the monitor function can be observed by the patient.

attachment of scalp electrodes is frequently performed by the obstetrician, but in some institutions nurses trained in these techniques routinely perform this function. Prior to initiating monitoring, the nurse should explain the basic concepts of monitoring and the equipment to the patient. Patients should ideally be educated about fetal monitoring during the antepartum period. Most patients readily consent to the use of monitoring when they believe that it might be of value to their fetus. The major drawback for the mother is often the need to restrict physical activity in order to maintain a consistently useful tracing. This problem as well as interference with effleurage can be circumvented somewhat by using direct methods. Newer telemetry techniques (i.e., monitoring from a distance), which may become clinically available in the near future, will reduce these restrictions on patient activity.

Since most patients wish to observe the monitor tracing (Fig. 37-5), the equipment should be placed so that it is within view of the patient, the father and the nurse. Couples often find that observing the onset and decrement (down slope) of the contractions is useful in applying breathing techniques. This is particularly true for the father. The reassurance obtained from observing or listening to the fetal heart beat during labor is often a secondary benefit to the couple. For this reason it is generally inadvisable to discontinue fetal monitoring once it has been initiated unless there is no further indication to continue and the couple wish to have the monitor disconnected.

It is important that the nurse explain the normal variation in fetal heart rate and the functions of the equipment so that patients will not become alarmed by them. When ominous patterns develop, the nurse should summon help and initiate remedial action in a calm and systematic manner. Leaving the bedside for more than a moment at such a time may cause undue panic in the patient and can be a decidedly negative feature of monitoring. Providing reassurance by orderly action is a much unrecognized benefit of protocols for remedial measures that have been established in some institutions.

Interpretation of Data

To interpret properly the data obtained from electronic fetal monitoring, a systematic approach should be used to examine the tracings and correlate them with clinical events. Interpreting monitor tracings can be learned from annotated atlases of monitor tracings (see selected reading) and clinical experience. In order to provide teaching in this area, many institutions have periodic in-service programs and, more important, conferences in which tracings are reviewed retrospectively by members of the team caring for the patients. A suggested approach for reading fetal monitor tracings is given in the Chart on page 622.

Evaluation of Uterine Activity (UA) or Uterine Contractions (UC)

External Methods. Only the frequency and duration of uterine contractions may be determined with external monitoring. The onset of the contraction is determined by the upswing of the pen and is followed by the *increment*. The peak of the contraction or highest level recorded is called the *acme*. The progressive relaxation of the uterus following the acme is referred to as the *decrement*. When the baseline is reached, the contraction is completed. The total duration of the contraction and the interval from the onset of one contraction to the onset of the next contraction may be calculated when the paper speed is known (3 cm./min.). Maternal respiratory movement may be noted as fine "saw-tooth" deflections confirmed by comparing the rate with that observed clinically. Coughing, sneezing, and so on appear as large spiking deflections. Bearing-down efforts or "pushing" cause multiple sharp spikes superimposed on the contractions. Changes of position will cause sudden sharp changes of the baseline.

Internal Method. Intrauterine pressure can be quantitated (following proper zeroing and calibration) when internal monitoring is used. Baseline tone is measured as the height of the baseline during the interval between contractions and is usually in a range of 5 to 15 mm. Hg.

Excessive baseline tone may indicate:
1. misplacement of the pressure transducer in relationship to the catheter tip;
2. excessive oxytocin administration;
3. abruptio placentae; or
4. hypertonic uterine dysfunction.

The contraction amplitude may range from 30 mm. Hg up to 60 mm. Hg. or more. Although contraction amplitudes of less than 25 to 30 mm. Hg may occur in normal active phase labor, they are most frequently associated with early labor or hypotonic uterine dysfunction.

Hypertonic labor occurs when uterine contraction amplitudes exceed normal, the frequency between onset of contractions is less than two minutes, or the resting interval between contractions is less than one minute. Coalescence of uterine contractions or a contraction of two minutes or greater duration constitutes a *tetanic contraction*. Hypertonic labor or uterine tetany are observed with administration of an excessive amount of oxytocic drugs, abruptio placentae or hypertonic uterine dysfunction. When internal pressure monitoring is applied, the geometric area beneath the contraction can be calculated. This is most easily performed by an "on-line" computer (i.e., one attached directly to the monitor). Calculation of uterine activity units or total work of the uterus by this method has proven useful for clinical studies of the forces of labor.

Evaluation of the FHR

FHR Baseline. During very early fetal development cardiac activity is initiated by the intrinsic rhythmicity of the myocardial cells. Soon after, the sinoatrial node (SA node) assumes the function of initiating the impulses which are transmitted throughout the conduction system of the heart, resulting in the mechanical events known as the heart beat.

Tachycardia and Bradycardia. The fetal heart rate decreases slightly as pregnancy advances and normally ranges between 120 to 160 beats per minute

---

APPROACH TO INTERPRETING FETAL MONITORING DATA

On the initial portion of the record (first 10 to 20 minutes):
1. Determine the clinical data which precedes the tracing and particularly identify the indication for monitoring.
2. Establish the method of monitoring used for both UA (uterine activity) and FHR (fetal heart rate)
3. Evaluate the uterine activity recording first. Determine the frequency, duration and pattern of contractions. If internal monitoring is used, determine the baseline tone and intensity of contractions.
4. Examine the fetal heart rate tracing. Determine the baseline rate. Assess the degree of variability or beat-to-beat variation. Identify any periodic changes (accelerations or decelerations) and classify them.

On subsequent portions of the tracing:
5. Note any changes in the above data.
6. Correlate these with clinical events.
7. Assess the effect of remedial measures when abnormal patterns have been noted.

(bpm). Elevation of the fetal heart rate baseline above 160 bpm is referred to as *tachycardia*. Rates between 161 and 180 bpm are classified as *mild tachycardia* and those greater than 180 bpm as *marked tachycardia*. Rates below 120 bpm are referred to as *bradycardia*. Those between 100 and 119 bpm are classified as *mild bradycardia* and those less than 100 bpm as *marked bradycardia*.

Either fetal tachycardia or bradycardia may be related to fetal hypoxia (low oxygen content of the fetal blood or inadequate delivery of oxygen to the fetal tissues). Fetal tachycardia may be an early warning sign of fetal hypoxia, while fetal bradycardia occurs somewhat later in the sequence of events. Abnormalities in baseline fetal heart rate may also be due to arrhythmias (abnormal discharge or transmission of impulses through the conduction system of the heart). These are usually benign and transient but may at times be associated with congenital heart defects or heart failure. Fetal tachycardia may also be associated with maternal fever. Because core temperature (internal body temperature) rises earlier and is higher than that measured either orally or rectally, fetal tachycardia may precede maternal fever by a short time interval. Likewise fetal bradycardia may be associated with maternal hypothermia, but this is an unusual event clinically. Abnormal fetal heart rates, either tachycardia or bradycardia, may also be caused by drugs administered to the mother.

Beat-to-beat Variation. As fetal development advances, the autonomic nervous system assumes an increasingly important role in modulating fetal heart rate. Discharge of sympathetic nerves causes an increase in rate while discharge of parasympathetic nerves causes a slowing of the heart rate. The normal continuous opposition of these two stimuli results in the beat-to-beat variation noted in the heart rate of the normal fetus and is reflected by the fine irregularity seen on the normal fetal heart rate tracing (Fig. 37-6).

It is important to note that true beat–to–beat variation can only be assessed by direct fetal electrography (i.e., internal monitoring using the spiral electrode). In the past, variability of the FHR baseline was often overlooked as an indicator of fetal status. However, recently it has assumed increasing clinical importance. When beat–to–beat variation is normal (i.e, >5 bpm) it is thought to indicate an intact nervous system with normal

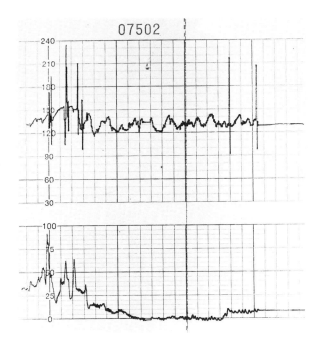

Figure 37-6. Fetal heart rate tracing. Note fine irregularity or beat-to-beat variability.

regulatory influence over the fetal heart rate. Diminished FHR variability (<5 bpm) or a flat FHR baseline in the absence of explainable causes is considered ominous and potentially indicative of hypoxia (Fig. 37-7).

Nowhere in fetal heart rate monitoring is the influence of drugs more obvious than in the assessment of FHR variability. It has become increasingly apparent that a large proportion of drugs administered to the mother will cause diminished or absent FHR-variability. For this reason it is often useful to have evaluated FHR-variability by internal monitoring before these drugs are administered.

Periodic Changes

While in utero the fetus is equipped with cardiovascular reflexes which may cause periodic or transient changes in fetal heart rate from its normal baseline. Some of these responses (e.g., accelerations with fetal movement) are indicative of normal fetal status, while other (e.g., variable deceleration with cord compression) are designed to compensate for alterations in cardiovascular dynamics. It is these periodic changes which require careful evaluation for the diagnosis of fetal stress or distress.

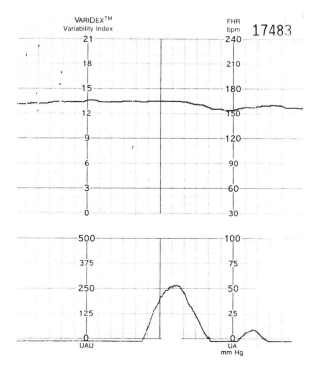

Figure 37-7. Fetal heart rate tracing with absent beat-to-beat variability. Note subtle late deceleration.

Accelerations. Transient increases of the fetal heart rate (>15 bpm for >15 sec.) have been noted during labor since fetal monitoring was first used (Fig. 37-8). At times they are associated with contractions but often are unrelated to uterine activity. The outcome of fetuses demonstrating this change has been uniformly good. It is believed that the increased FHR is due to transient discharges of the sympathetic nervous system. It has also been suggested that accelerations associated with contractions might be caused by partial compression of the cord, resulting in diminished venous return to the heart followed by a transient increase of the FHR. More recently the observation that accelerations are associated with fetal movements in the healthy fetus has led to the development of the nonstress test (NST) for antepartum evaluation of the high risk fetus (p. 630).

Early Decelerations. Transient slowing of the fetal heart rate in a pattern which is almost a mirror image of the contractions is known as an early deceleration (sometimes called a Type I dip). The occurrence of these decelerations is believed to be related to fetal head compression associated with the contraction resulting in a parasympathetic dis-

charge mediated by the vagus nerve. Parasympathetic stimulation results in slowing of the FHR. This pattern represents a normal response of the fetus to this stimulus and is associated with a uniformly good outcome.

Characteristically these decelerations have a wave form which coincides with and resembles an inverted uterine contraction (Fig. 37-9). They are uniform in shape, of short duration and of low amplitude. The fetal heart rate at the *nadir* (lowest point) of the deceleration is usually 100 bpm or greater. When slower fetal heart rates are observed with contractions, the decelerations are usually of the variable type (see below). Early decelerations do not respond to oxygen administered to the mother or to position change. They may be blocked when atropine is administered. However, because of the benign nature of this pattern, remedial action is not necessary.

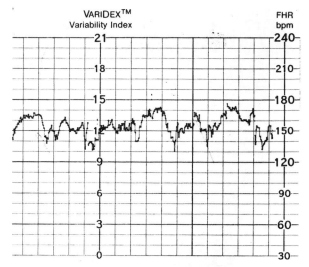

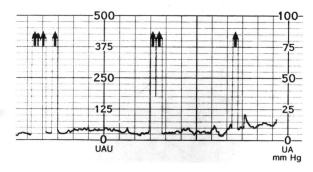

Figure 37-8. Transient accelerations of fetal heart rate noted during NST. Markers (arrows) were made by patient to indicate when fetal movements were perceived.

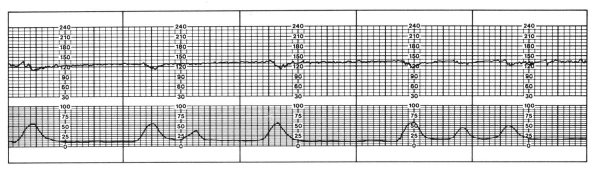

Figure 37-9. Early deceleration. The FHR baseline is the normal range, with normal variability. Uterine activity is normal with oxytocin augmentation. Early deceleration patterns are evident, approximating a mirror image of the uterine pressure curve. The nadir of the early deceleration occurs at the same time as the peak of the uterine contraction. (Parer, J. T., et al.: *A Clinical Approach to Fetal Monitoring*, San Leandro, Calif., Berkeley Bio-Engineering, Inc., 1974.)

Variable Decelerations. This type of periodic deceleration is the most commonly observed FHR change during labor. The nomenclature of this pattern is based on the fact that the relationship of these decelerations to the contractions (and, more important, the wave form) are both variable (Fig. 37-10). It is believed that these decelerations reflect a reflex response to umbilical cord compression. They are often observed in association with uterine contractions, a situation in which cord compression is more likely to occur.

Responsibility for the slowing of the fetal heart rate in variable decelerations has been attributed to a rise in systemic arterial pressure resulting from cord occlusion. This rise in pressure triggers the baroreceptor (intraarterial pressure receptor) reflex, activating a vagal impulse that causes slowing of the fetal heart rate. More recently it has been suggested that these decelerations may also be elicited by sudden hypoxia and triggering of the aortic chemoreceptor response, which also results in vagal discharge. Thus, sudden hypoxia in addition to increased arterial pressure may be important in the pathogenesis of variable decelerations.

Variable decelerations may be classified as mild, moderate, or severe (Table 37-1). Since there is a correlation between the severity of variable decelerations and fetal condition, it is important that the nurse evaluate the frequency, depth and duration of these decelerations. In addition, other indicators of hypoxia on the FHR tracing, such as abnormally low or high baseline fetal heart rate and decreased variability, should be examined. When variable decelerations are noted, remedial action should be initiated. Repetitive moderate or severe variable decelerations, especially those associated with ominous baseline change, which are not alleviated by remedial measures, may indicate that a sample of fetal scalp blood be obtained or a prompt delivery be carried out.

Late Decelerations (Type II Dips). Like early decelerations this designation indicates a uniform shape and a consistent relationship of the decelera-

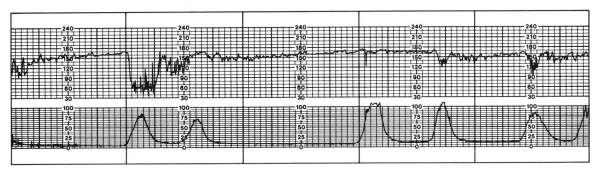

Figure 37-10. Severe variable deceleration. There is a mild fetal tachycardia, with normal baseline variability. Uterine activity is normal. The deceleration is corrected by changing the patient's position. Subsequent deceleration patterns are much less severe. (Parer, et al.: *A Clinical Approach to Fetal Monitoring.*)

TABLE 37-1
PRINCIPLES OF GRADING VARIABLE AND LATE DECELERATIONS

Criteria of grading	Mild	Moderate	Severe
Variable deceleration Level to which FHR drops and duration of deceleration	<30 sec. duration irrespective of level >80 b.p.m. irrespective of duration 70–80 b.p.m. <60 sec.	<70 b.p.m. >30<60 sec. 70–80 b.p.m. >60 sec.	<70 b.p.m. >60 sec.
Late deceleration Amplitude of drop in FHR	<15 b.p.m.	15–45 b.p.m.	>45 b.p.m.

tion to contractions. As opposed to early decelerations, the onset of the deceleration, its nadir, and its recovery do not coincide with the onset, amplitude, and recovery of the UC but rather are delayed (Fig. 37-11). In contrast to variable decelerations, late decelerations may be quite subtle, entirely within the normal FHR range, and yet be ominous. A classification of late decelerations is also given in Table 37-1.

Late decelerations are thought to reflect the effects of direct hypoxia on the fetal myocardium and cardiac conduction system. The hypoxia results from reduced oxygen exchange by the placenta due to diminished intervillous blood flow that occurs with the uterine contraction. A direct and specific relationship of hypoxia and late decelerations in monkeys has been demonstrated experimentally. Hypoxia causing late decelerations may be elicited when less oxygen is delivered to the uterus (e.g., with maternal hypoxia or hypotension), when abnormally strong uterine contractions occur, or when relative placental insufficiency exists.

Transient late decelerations associated with maternal hypotension or uterine hypertonus which responds to remedial action are thought to signal fetal stress. Removing or correcting the stress often results in fetal recovery. On the other hand, a pattern of consistent and persistent late decelerations that do not respond to remedial measures suggests fetal distress and is often associated with hypoxia, acidosis, and lower Apgar scores at birth. This latter constellation of findings, of course, indicates prompt delivery.

Sinusoidal Pattern. An unusual abnormality in fetal heart rate, in which there is a repetitive undulation of the baseline resembling a "sine wave," has been called a sinusoidal pattern (Fig. 37-12). Occasionally tracings of a normal fetal heart rate appear to have a very transient sinusoidal pattern. This has not correlated with any particular fetal abnormality. A true sinusoidal pattern occurring for longer intervals either before or during labor is almost always associated with severe fetal anemia. This is most frequently observed in fetuses suffering from hydrops fetalis due to Rhesus isoimmunization, but has also been seen with fetal anemia due to blood loss.

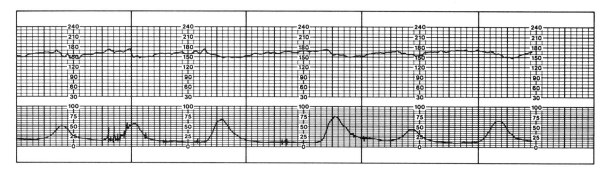

Figure 37-11. Moderate late deceleration. There is a mild fetal tachycardia, ranging between 160 and 170 beats per minute, with decreased variability. Uterine activity is normal. The nadir of late deceleration occurs when the uterine contraction is nearly over. A scalp capillary blood sample had been taken just prior to the first portion of this panel, and mild fetal acidosis was demonstrated, with scalp blood pH 7.21. (Parer, et al.: *A Clinical Approach to Fetal Monitoring.*)

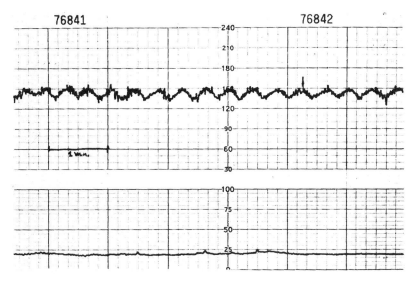

Figure 37-12. Fetal heart rate tracing demonstrating sinusoidal pattern prior to labor. Fetus was severely anemic due to Rhesus isoimmunization.

The pathophysiology of the development of a sinusoidal pattern is not understood. It has been hypothesized that this pattern may reflect an absence of central nervous system control over the fetal heart rate due to severe hypoxia. Because of the poor outcome in anemic fetuses when this pattern has been observed, the finding is considered ominous.

REMEDIAL MEASURES FOR FETAL STRESS OR DISTRESS

Fetal hypoxia may result from one or several factors which impair delivery of oxygen to the fetus. As previously discussed, alterations of FHR baseline (tachycardia, bradycardia or diminished variability) or periodic decelerations (moderate or severe variable, or late decelerations) may indicate fetal hypoxia. When mixed patterns of decelerations (i.e., early and variable, early and late, or variable and late) are observed the more ominous deceleration should be taken as the indication for action. When abnormal periodic patterns are associated with ominous baseline changes, the fetal situation should be considered more urgent.

The following etiologic factors should be considered and evaluated rapidly when fetal hypoxia is suspected: 1) impaired maternal oxygen delivery; 2) impaired placental oxygen exchange; 3) impaired fetal circulation or oxygen-carrying capacity.

Impaired Maternal Oxygen Delivery This situation may result from a number of maternal disorders. Maternal pulmonary dysfunction, associated with an acute severe asthmatic attack, amniotic fluid embolism, thromboembolism, grand mal seizure, or general anesthesia, may result in maternal hypoxia which subsequently causes fetal hypoxia. Impaired delivery of normally oxygenated maternal blood to the uterus may occur from abnormalities of cardiac function (pump failure) or decreased peripheral vascular blood flow. The latter is most often associated with hypotension and is the most frequent cause of fetal hypoxia in this category. Hypotension may be related to maternal blood loss or shock, compression of the vena cava by the gravid uterus when the patient is supine, or autonomic blockade associated with conduction anesthesia.

When maternal oxygen uptake or delivery of oxygen to the uterus is impaired, remedial measures should be taken. Oxygen should be administered by mask and the mother turned to the left lateral recumbent position. This position diminishes occlusion of the inferior vena cava by the uterus, thus promoting venous return to the heart and improved cardiovascular function. If necessary, pharmacologic correction of the respiratory or cardiovascular disorder should then be initiated.

Impaired Placental Exchange of Oxygen. The cause of this problem may be placental insufficiency (e.g., associated with intrauterine growth retardation or postmaturity) or excessively strong uterine contractions. Such contractions result in transient interruption of blood flow in the intervillous space and thus diminish oxygen exchange. When this occurs, administration of oxytocic drugs should be discontinued if they are being used. Improving maternal oxygenation and oxygen delivery by administration of oxygen and use of the left lateral position are also helpful.

Impaired Fetal Circulation or Oxygen Transport. Cord compression is the usual cause for this problem. In this situation prolapse of the cord should be determined rapidly by perineal inspection and vaginal examination. This complication requires prompt delivery, usually by cesarean section. When there is evidence of cord compression, the previously mentioned measures should be initiated: that is, maternal oxygen administration, left lateral position, and discontinuation of oxytocics. Positions other than left lateral (e.g., right lateral or knee-chest) may also be useful in alleviating variable decelerations and should be tried when the pattern does not respond to the initial remedial measures.

Fetal oxygen transport to the tissues may also be impaired when there is severe fetal anemia, as is seen in Rhesus isoimmunization associated with a sinusoidal pattern. A suggested protocol for the evaluation and treatment of fetal stress or distress is given in Table 37-2.

When fetal hypoxia is suspected on the basis of monitoring data, a single etiologic factor is often not identifiable. The combination of administering oxygen to the mother, discontinuing oxytocics, and changing the mother's position (left lateral position first) should be instituted simultaneously. Other remedial measures, such as administering tocolytics (uterine contraction inhibitors), or fetal alkali (sodium bicarbonate), are considered investigative. When nonremedial fetal distress occurs the physician may further evaluate the fetus by obtaining a sample fetal scalp blood or may proceed to prompt delivery.

Other Intrapartum Methods of Fetal Evaluation

A number of other techniques for intrapartum fetal evaluation are under investigation in the laboratory or have reached the stage of clinical trials. These include percutaneous monitoring of oxygen tension, continuous scalp pH measurement, electroencephalography and observation of fetal movements, particularly respirations, using real-time ultrasound.

pH of Fetal Blood Scalp Samples. At present, periodic measurement of the pH of fetal scalp blood has proven to be clinically useful for the diagnosis of fetal distress. For this measurement a small volume of fetal blood may be obtained by puncturing the fetal scalp and collecting the blood samples in fine glass capillary tubes. As with other invasive techniques, the membranes must be ruptured, the cervix dilated 3 to 4 cm. and the fetal presenting part fixed in the pelvis in order to perform the procedure safely. Although samples of fetal scalp blood may be obtained with the patient in bed, it is easier to carry out this procedure if the mother is in the lithotomy position in a delivery room. Transport of the patient to the delivery room may also have the secondary benefit of saving valuable time if immediate delivery becomes necessary.

A plastic or metal truncated cone known as an *amnioscope* is used to visualize the presenting part of the fetus during fetal blood sampling (Fig. 37–13). The term amnioscope was first applied because the

TABLE 37-2
IMMEDIATE CLINICAL APPROACH TO FETAL STRESS OR DISTRESS

Mechanism	Evaluation	Remedial Action
1. Equipment malfunction	Confirm monitor data by auscultation (FHR) and palpation(UC)	Substitute functional equipment
2. Impaired maternal oxygenation	Vital signs, especially skin color	Administer O_2 by mask
3. Impaired blood flow to uterus	Vital signs, especially blood pressure	Place mother in left lateral position, administer fluids, elevate legs
4. Impaired placental exchange	Uterine palpation for hypertonus	Discontinue oxytocic drugs
5. Impaired fetal circulation		
Prolapsed cord	Vaginal examination	Delivery
Cord compression	———	Maternal position change (e.g., left lateral, right lateral or knee chest)

instrument was initially designed for visualizing the fetal membranes and amniotic fluid through the partially dilated cervix. Because of the invasive nature of the procedure, sterile technique is used throughout. The amnioscope is inserted into the vagina and the dilated cervix. A light source is then attached to the amnioscope. The fetal scalp is cleansed with an antiseptic solution and dried with sterile cotton balls. A light film of petrolatum jelly or silicone spray is applied to the scalp. This will cause droplets of fetal blood to "bead," making it easier to collect the blood samples in the capillary tubes. A small metal blade attached to a long handle is used to puncture the skin. The narrow detachable blades are mounted in plastic to control the depth to which the skin is penetrated. A single brisk motion is used to penetrate the skin in a manner similar to that suggested for "sticking" the finger to draw blood. The beaded drops of fetal blood are then collected in the long, heparinized capillary tubes. A fine metal bead or short wire is added to the capillary tube prior to sealing it with wax. A magnet passed along the outside of the tube will move the metal wire and stir the sample to prevent clotting. Exposing the sample to atmospheric air can cause an exchange of oxygen and carbon dioxide which will alter the hydrogen ion concentration. Placing the capillary tube on ice will retard cellular respiration, which could also result in a change in pH.

After an adequate sample of scalp blood is obtained, the physician applies firm pressure to the puncture site for several minutes to retard bleeding. At the conclusion of the procedure the puncture site is inspected for hemostasis. Repeated scalp blood sampling may be safely performed if necessary. The risks of the procedure include continued bleeding from the puncture site, ecchymosis, hematoma and infection.

Following scalp blood sampling the nurse should observe the patient for excessive vaginal bleeding which may be fetal in origin. In addition, sustained fetal tachycardia may be observed on the monitor tracing when fetal blood loss occurs either externally or into the scalp tissues (hematoma).

The partial pressure of oxygen and carbon dioxide as well as bicarbonate ion concentration can be measured on these samples. The pH, however, has proven to be the most simple, rapid, and clinically useful measurement which can be performed on a small sample of blood. The pH of fetal scalp blood

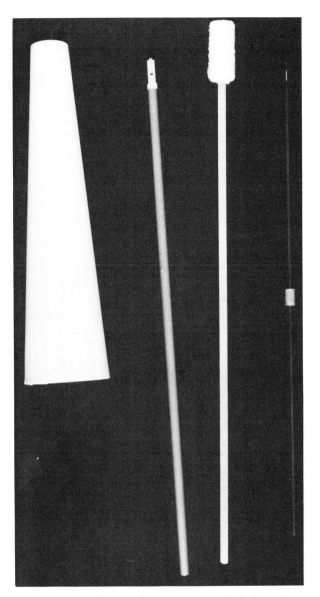

Figure 37-13. Scalp sampling equipment includes plastic amnioscope, scalpel, cotton sponge, and heparinized capillary tube.

normally ranges between 7.25 and 7.35 during labor, and correlates well with the acid-base status of the blood in the umbilical vessels. A mild progressive decline of pH within the normal range has been noted with contractions and as labor progresses. When the fetus becomes hypoxic, anaerobic glycolysis occurs, resulting in an excess production of organic acids (lactic acid) and an increase in hydrogen ion concentration. The increased hydrogen ion concentration is measured as a decrease in pH (acidosis). Thus the development of acidosis reflects the effects of hypoxia on cellular metabolism, or respiration.

Clinical studies have demonstrated a correlation between the pH of fetal scalp blood and abnormalities in fetal heart rate as well as Apgar scores. As a result of these observations, the measurement of the pH of fetal scalp blood has become an increasingly important method for diagnosing fetal distress. This measurement helps when the interpretation of fetal monitoring data is unclear and reduces the chances of false-positive diagnoses of fetal distress using fetal monitoring. Traditionally, a scalp blood pH of 7.20 or less is considered to be indicative of fetal acidosis or "fetal distress."

As with other antepartum or intrapartum methods of fetal evaluation, measurement of scalp blood pH may produce false-positive results (i.e., abnormal values when the fetus is well) or false-negative results (i.e., normal values when the fetus is hypoxic). Abnormal maternal acid-base status (e.g., maternal acidosis) may be transmitted passively to the fetus through the placenta and accounts for a portion of the false-positive cases. For this reason, obtaining a simultaneous blood sample from the mother to determine the pH of the mother's blood is of value in interpreting the fetal pH and will reduce the frequency of false-positive results. Events which occur following fetal blood sampling but before delivery (e.g., continued cord compression), may account for many of the false-negative results observed. Because these problems occur in only a small proportion of cases, they do not detract substantially from the clinical value of fetal pH measurement. In fact, it has been suggested by some that the diagnosis of fetal distress should *always* be based on the finding of fetal acidosis. However, rapid fetal deterioration, inability to obtain samples, or suspicion of false-negative results make this test as an absolute criterion in all cases impractical.

Following delivery of an infant in whom fetal blood sampling has been performed, umbilical venous and arterial blood samples should be obtained from a doubly clamped segment of cord. Measurement of blood gases and pH on these samples makes it easier to correlate the fetal monitor tracing, the scalp blood pH measurements and the neonatal condition.

When assessing the newborn, the nurse should closely inspect the scalp of the infant to identify the puncture site(s). In many institutions cleansing with an antiseptic solution and applying an antibiotic ointment are routine. Personnel in the nursery should be notified of the number and the status of scalp puncture sites at the time the infant is transferred to the nursery. In this way any complications resulting from the procedure can be detected immediately and treated.

Antepartum Fetal Heart Rate Monitoring

Periodic (usually weekly) electronic fetal monitoring during the third trimester has become a common method for evaluating the fetus in a high risk pregnancy. As with many other forms of fetal evaluation, a normal result is fairly accurate in indicating fetal well-being. On the other hand, false-positive results occur with a relatively high frequency. This has required that two or more different tests of fetal well-being be carried out before premature delivery or other remedial measures are instituted.

The observation of changes in fetal heart rate associated with spontaneous or evoked fetal movement has become known as the nonstress test or NST. Evaluation of fetal heart rate in the presence of spontaneous or oxytocin-induced contractions is termed the contraction stress test, or CST. Contraction stress testing (CST) was widely applied clinically prior to the more recent development of the NST. The ease of performing the NST and its apparent reliability as a screening tool have greatly reduced the number of CSTs performed. An example of a clinical protocol for applying these tests is given in the chart on page 631.

Contraction Stress Testing

This testing requires administration of oxytocin by intravenous infusion. For this reason it is performed in an in-patient area of a hospital, usually a labor room. Continuous external fetal monitoring is applied and oxytocin is administered in increasing dosages until uterine contractions occur. The occurrence of repeated late decelerations with contractions is classified as a positive or abnormal test, whereas, the absence of late decelerations with each of three contractions during a ten-minute interval is classified as a negative result or, commonly, a "passed test."

THE CONTRACTION STRESS TEST*

A. *Nursing Guidelines for Performing the CST:*

1. Take patient to a labor room or ante-partum testing unit.
2. Explain to the patient the testing procedure and the time involved. (The test itself requires an average of about 90 minutes but it is not uncommon for the procedure to take 3 hours.)
3. Have patient change into a gown.
4. Place patient in a semi-Fowler's position at a 30 to 45° angle with a slight left tilt.
5. Place patient on an external monitor. A phonotransducer or ultrasound transducer is used to record the fetal heart rate and a tocodynamometer to measure uterine contractions.
6. Record patient's BP initially and at 5 to 10 minute intervals.
7. Obtain at least a 10 minute baseline recording of FHR and observe for spontaneous uterine contractions.

   If spontaneous uterine contractions without late decelerations are noted at a frequency of less than three (3) in 10 minutes or no spontaneous uterine activity is observed, proceed with oxytocin infusion.
8. Prepare and begin an oxytocin infusion according to the institutional protocol or as indicated by the physician.

a. Start the oxytocin infusion (secondary line) by inserting the needle into the connector of the primary line at the connector most proximal to the primary line. Be sure to keep primary line running at a slow rate.

b. Patient is evaluated by the physician when the dosage of oxytocin reaches 10 mU/minute. If the oxytocin infusion is to be continued, the physician must write an order to increase the dosage.

B. *Guidelines for Interpretation of the CST:*

1. Test is read as:
   a. *Negative*—no late deceleration of the FHR when an adequate frequency of three contractions in 10 minutes has been established, a "negative window."
   b. *Positive*—late decelerations occurring with three contractions in 10 minutes, a "positive window."
   c. *Equivocal*—no positive or negative window.
   d. *Hyperstimulation*—excessive uterine activity is present in association with a deceleration of the FHR.
   e. *Unsatisfactory*—inadequate uterine contractions or FHR record.

---

* Courtesy of Patricia M. Graef, BSNEd.

Other terms used for classification of tests include unsatisfactory, suspicious and equivocal. Unsatisfactory tests occur when interpretable tracings cannot be obtained or the criterion of three contractions in a ten-minute interval is not met. Unsatisfactory tests are repeated within a short time interval (usually 24 hours). It has been suggested that the interpretation of the test should be based on a ten-minute testing segment known as a "testing window." The classification of equivocal and elimination of the term "suspicious tests" (occasional decelerations) has been proposed in conjunction with the concept of a "ten-minute testing window." Equivocal tests are those in which nonrepetitive late decelerations are observed (i.e., no positive or negative testing window) or in which decelerations are associated with maternal hypotension or uterine hyperstimulation. Since external methods of pressure monitoring are used, uterine hyperstimulation cannot be defined on the basis of true intrauterine

pressure (mm. Hg) but rather is defined on the basis of the frequency of contractions (greater than three contractions in ten minutes) or a tetanic contraction. It is suggested that equivocal tests be repeated in 24 hours.

Early investigators found that positive CSTs were associated with a relatively high frequency of poor outcome, such as intrauterine fetal death, fetal distress, or poor condition of the infant at birth. A normal CST gave a high degree of confidence for continued fetal survival in utero during an arbitrarily set limit of one week. Further experience has confirmed this observation. Instances of fetal death within one week of a negative CST are very infrequent. When this has occurred, the fetal deaths have often been attributed to factors (e.g., abruptio placentae or fetal malformation) other than the primary indication for testing. Some have suggested performing CSTs more frequently when there is deterioration of the maternal condition (e.g., with pregnancy-induced hypertension) or in certain very high risk disorders (e.g., diabetes with vascular disease).

Clinical studies in which patients were induced and electronically monitored following positive CST have demonstrated a high false-positive rate (25 to 40 per cent), that is, late decelerations did not recur in labor. Because of this experience it has been suggested that more than one test of fetal well-being should be carried out before a *preterm* delivery for fetal compromise is indicated. Clearly the greatest benefit of the CST lies in the reassurance which allows continuation of a high risk pregnancy when the test result is normal.

Nonstress Testing

Observation of accelerated fetal heart rate associated with fetal movements led to the development of nonstress testing. This form of testing does not require intravenous administration of drugs and thus can be safely and more quickly performed in an outpatient area. These features, coupled with the apparent reliability of the NST as a screening test,

have resulted in a marked reduction in the number of CSTs performed.

Various criteria have been applied for interpreting the NST. The occurrence of five accelerations of >15 bpm for >15 sec. in 20 minutes was initially required as a normal or reactive test. More recent studies have suggested that fewer accelerations of the same magnitude may be adequate. Because the fetus has cyclic periods of rest, external stimulation by manipulation has been used to elicit movement for this testing. Failure to demonstrate a reactive pattern due to either lack of accelerations with movement or lack of fetal movement is taken as an indication for further evaluation of the fetus by a CST (Fig. 37-14).

The NST and CST have been almost exclusively performed by nurses. Along with this function, nurses have assumed the role of educating the patients about the tests and also screening the test results. A notable secondary benefit of these functions has been the opportunity for labor and delivery nurses to establish a nurse-patient relationship with their high risk patients during the antepartum period. The benefits of this relationship in the delivery of nursing care during labor, delivery and the puerperium should be obvious.

THE NONSTRESS TEST*

A. *Nursing Guidelines for Performing the NST:*

  1. Take patient to the antepartum testing unit.
  2. Explain the procedure to the patient, including the time involved. The test requires an average of 30 minutes.
  3. Have patient change into a gown.
  4. Place patient in a semi-Fowler's position at a 30° to 45° angle with a slight left tilt.
  5. Place patient on an external monitor using ultrasound transducer or phonotransducer to record the fetal heart rate. A tocodynamometer is used to document fetal activity and spontaneous uterine activity.
  6. Record patient's BP initially and at 5 to 10 minute intervals.

  7. The patient is asked to indicate each time fetal movement occurs by pressing the record button on the monitor. A 10 to 20 minute strip is obtained.

B. *Interpretation of the NSI:*

  1. Test is read as:
    a. *Reactive*—2 FHR accelerations greater than 15 bpm above the baseline and lasting 15 seconds or more with fetal movement in 10 minute period.

    b. *Nonreactive*—none or one FHR acceleration greater than 15 bpm and lasting 15 seconds or more with fetal movement in a 10 minute period or accelerations less than 15 bpm or lasting less than 15 seconds.

---

* Courtesy of Patricia M. Graef, BSNEd.

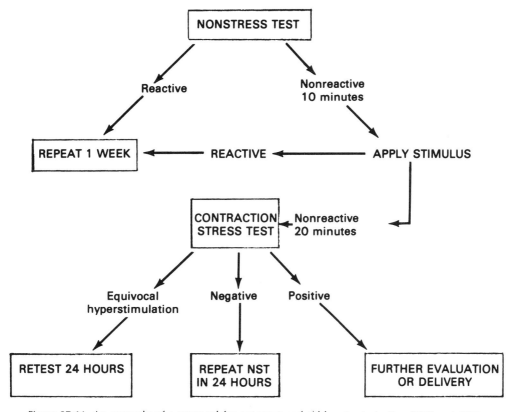

Figure 37-14. An example of a protocol for antepartum fetal heart rate testing (NST and CST).

CONCLUSION

The development and application of continuous fetal monitoring has dramatically expanded the role of the nurse in caring for the family during labor and delivery. With this expanded role have come additional responsibilities in parent education, counseling and patient care.

With consumerism becoming an increasingly important factor in the delivery of obstetrical care, the need for and the value of fetal monitoring is one of the particular aspects of clinical practice which has been questioned. The principles of fetal monitoring and the scientific basis for interpreting the data have become well understood. It seems logical to presume that the detection and alleviation of fetal stress (e.g., due to excessive uterine activity or maternal hypotension) or the detection of fetal distress (hypoxia and acidosis) should be of benefit to the patient. Nevertheless, the long-term benefits of clinically applied fetal monitoring are not as yet well sub-

stantiated. In counseling patients, the nurse should not overstate the presumed benefits of monitoring, especially during normal pregnancy; nor should the potential risks, however infrequent, be ignored. Furthermore, continuing education in interpretation of data and the use of new equipment or tests is required. It is important, therefore, that the nurse be aware of the most current information regarding the risks, benefits and applications of monitoring.

As fetal monitoring first became widely used, concerns were raised that there would develop a tendency to "nurse the machine" rather than the patients. This misgiving has not proven to be the case in most instances. On the contrary, fetal monitoring has had the beneficial result of freeing the nurse from repetitive tasks and providing an opportunity for more and better quality care for both the mother and the fetus. In applying monitoring, the nurse makes independent assessments of maternal and fetal pathophysiology and takes remedial action to correct abnormalities as they develop. These tasks have led to the concept of the nurse caring for a high risk mother and fetus as an "intensivist." As a result greater appreciation of the need for one-on-one continuous nursing care during labor and delivery has developed. Thus, rather than diminishing patient care, monitoring seems to have become an important factor in enhancing the quality of nursing care during labor and delivery.

SUGGESTED READING

General

Goodlin, R.C.: "History of fetal monitoring." *Am. J. Obstet. Gynecol.* 133:323, 1979.

Haverkamp, A. D., Thompson, H. E., McFee, J. G., and Cetrulo, C.: "The evaluation of continuous fetal heart rate monitoring in high-risk pregnancy." *Am. J. Obstet. Gynecol.* 125:310, 1976.

Haverkamp, A. D. et al.: "A controlled trial of the differential effects of intrapartum fetal monitoring." *Am. J. Obstet. Gynecol* 132:399, 1979.

Hon, E. H.: *An Introduction to Fetal Heart Rate Monitoring.* ed. 2. Los Angeles, 1975.

Johnstone, F. D., Campbell, D. M., and Hughes, G. J.: "Has continuous intrapartum monitoring made any impact on fetal outcome?" *Lancet* 1:1298, 1978.

Neutra, R. R., Feinberg, S. E., Greenland, S., and Friedman, E. A.: "Effect of fetal monitoring on neonatal death rates." *New England J. Med.* 299:324, 1978.

Paul, R. H. and Hon, E. H.: "Clinical fetal monitoring: V. Effect on perinatal outcome." *Am. J. Obstet Gynecol* 118:529, 1974.

Quilligan, E. J., and Paul, R. H.: "Fetal monitoring: Is it worth it? "*Obstet. Gynecol.* 45:96, 1975.

Renou, P., Chang, A., Anderson, I., and Wood, C.: "Controlled trial of fetal intensive care." *Am. J. Obstet. Gynecol.* 126:470, 1976.

Atlases of Fetal Monitoring

Klavan, M., Laver, A. T., and Boscola, M. A.: "Clinical concepts of fetal heart rate monitoring." Waltham, Mass., Hewlett-Packard Company, 1977.

Paul, R. H. et al.: *Fetal Intensive Care: I. An Introduction.* North Haven, Conn., William Mack Company, 1979.

Paul, R. H. et al.: *Fetal Intensive Care: II. Case Management.* North Haven, Conn., William Mack Company, 1979.

Paul, R. H. et al.: *Fetal Intensive Care: III. Case Management with Emphasis on Drug Effects.* North Haven, Conn., William Mack Company, 1979.

Fetal Scalp Blood Sampling

Saling, E.: *Fetal and Neonatal Hypoxia in Relation to Clinical Obstetric Practice.* Baltimore, Md., Williams & Wilkins, 1968.

Seeds, A. E.: "Maternal-fetal acid-base relationships and fetal scalp blood analysis." *Clinical Obstetrics and Gynecology, High Risk Obstetrics,* ed. Makowski, E. L. 21, 2, New York, Harper & Row, 1978.

Antepartum Testing

Evertson, L. R., Gauthier, R. J., Schifrin, B. S., and Paul, R. H.: "Antepartum fetal heart rate testing: I. Evolution of the nonstress test." *Am. J. Obstet. Gynecol.* 133:29, 1979.

Gauthier, R. J., Evertson, L. R., and Paul, R. H.: "Antepartum fetal heart rate testing: II. Intrapartum fetal heart rate observation and newborn outcome following a positive contraction stress test." *Am. J. Obstet. Gynecol.* 133:34, 1979.

Paul, R. H., and Miller, F. C.: "Antepartum fetal heart rate monitoring." *Clinical Obstetrics and Gynecology, High Risk Obstetrics,* ed. Makowski, E. L. 21, 2, Harper & Row, 1978.

Ray, M., Freeman, R., Pine, S., and Hesselgesser, R.: "Clinical experience with the oxytocin challenge test." *Am. J. Obstet. Gynecol.* 114:1, 1972.

Rochard, F., et al.: "Nonstressed fetal heart rate monitoring in the antepartum period." *Am. J. Obstet, Gynecol.* 126:699, 1976.

Thirty-Eight

The High Risk Infant: Disorders of Gestational Age and Birth Weight

Classification of Infants by Birth Weight and Gestational Age / Etiology / Factors which Affect Fetal Growth / Identification of the High Risk Neonate / Assessment of Gestational Age / Characteristics and Physiology of Small-for-Gestational-Age Infants / Characteristics and Physiology of the Premature Infant / Illnesses of the Premature Infant / Care of the High Risk Infant / Growth and Development / Care of the Mother and Father

The size of an infant at birth is influenced by many factors which affect the maternal and fetal environments. The relationship between low birth weight and perinatal morbidity and mortality has long been recognized, but only recently have the different implications of birth weight relative to gestational age been established. Infants of low birth weight may be of appropriate size for their gestational age but immature because they are born before pregnancy has progressed to full term. These infants are classically "premature"—born before their organ systems have matured to the point of physiological functioning. Other low birth weight infants may be undersized for the length of their gestation, whether delivered before or at term. These infants are called "small for gestational age." Often they are physiologically mature but have not attained the size and weight appropriate for gestational age for numerous reasons.

Disorders of gestational age and birth weight also include infants who are large for gestational age and who are postmature—born after pregnancy has progressed beyond full term. The associated problems and potential causes are different among these various types of altered fetal growth, requiring individualized assessment and approaches to management. The particular causes of alterations in fetal growth also determine the newborn's immediate and long-term prognosis. The challenge to effective assessment and management of fetal growth disorders begins with an understanding of the intricate and complex mechanisms which control normal fetal growth.

CLASSIFICATION OF INFANTS BY BIRTH WEIGHT AND GESTATIONAL AGE

In the past, all newborns weighing 2,500 gm. or less were termed *premature,* and those weighing more were designated *full term.* This approach assumed that intrauterine growth rates were essentially the same for all fetuses and that birth weight thus corresponded to gestational age. A considerable amount of data have now accumulated to demonstrate the inaccuracy of this assumption, and the

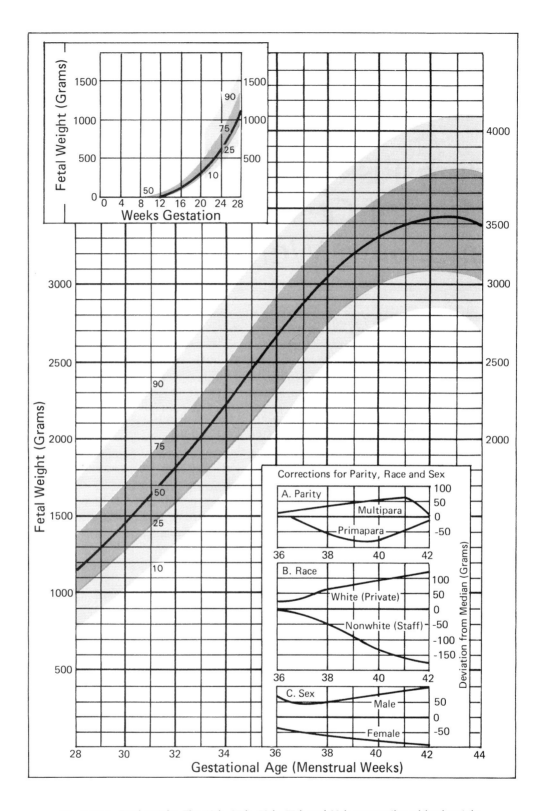

Figure 38-1. Fetal weight. The 10th, 25th, 50th, 75th and 90th percentiles of fetal weight in grams throughout pregnancy and correction factors for parity, race (socioeconomic status) and sex are graphed. Data obtained from 31,202 prostaglandin-induced abortions and spontaneous deliveries. (Courtesy of Brenner, W. E., et al.: Am. J. Obstet. Gynecol. 126:555–564, Nov. 1, 1976.)

two dimensions of *birth weight* and *gestational age* are now considered separately.

The World Health Organization (WHO) has designated a "term birth" as one occurring between 38 and 42 weeks gestation, with age calculated from the date of onset of the mother's last menstrual period. WHO advised that newborn infants not be classified as premature on the basis of weight alone. Gestational age must be used to assign categories of preterm, term, and postterm births. Also, it must be recognized that an infant weighing less than 2,500 gm. is not necessarily premature.

Intrauterine growth standards are used to compare an infant's weight and gestational age with population averages. While these have shortcomings in application to particular situations (for instance, differences in weight due to race, parity, sex, altitude), they are useful as guides in assessment of high risk infants. The most widely used growth chart was developed in Colorado and gives percentiles of intrauterine growth for weight, length and head circumference. However, the altitude effects made this estimate on the low side for the rest of the country. A more recent fetal growth chart has correction factors for parity, race and sex and presents average fetal weights for the 10th, 25th, 50th, 75th and 90th percentiles (Fig. 38-1). Infants are categorized generally as:

Gestational Age and Weight
Appropriate weight for gestational age (AGA)
Small weight for gestational age (SGA)
Large weight for gestational age (LGA)

Related to Term Pregnancy
Premature or preterm (less than 37 to 38 weeks gestation)
Term or fullterm (38 to 42 weeks gestation)
Postmature or postterm (more than 42 weeks gestation)

Weight serves in the assessment of growth, and gestational age in the assessment of maturity. An infant born at 40 weeks gestation and weighing less than 2,500 gm. (or below the 10th percentile for weight or length) would be mature but undergrown. This condition is called *intrauterine growth retardation,* with the infant classified as small for gestational age (SGA). An infant born at 36 weeks gestation and weighing 3,500 gm. (above the 90th percentile for weight) would be immature but overgrown. Such large-for-gestational-age infants (LGA) are typical for diabetic mothers. Although this infant has at-

tained average term weight, it is actually premature, with incomplete maturation of organ systems.

The term *premature* seems most appropriate for the *preterm,* immature infant regardless of birth weight. Preterm infants may also be small for gestational age, implying that at least two factors are involved: that causing the early delivery and that retarding the growth rate in utero.

Premature births have been further subdivided into the *immature fetus,* weighing 500 to 1,000 gm. and having completed 20 to 28 weeks of gestation; and the *premature infant* weighing 1,000 to 2,500 gm. with gestation of 28 to 38 weeks. Another term used is the *low birth weight infant,* which includes any live-born infant weighing 2,500 gm. or less. This category is less helpful because it fails to specify the relation of weight to gestational age, thus including both mature and immature infants whose needs and problems differ significantly (see Figs. 38-2 and 38-3).

ETIOLOGY

Preterm or Premature

Premature or preterm infants are born before the thirty-seventh week of gestation, regardless of birth weight. Most babies who weigh less than 2,500 gm. at birth are premature, as are almost all those weighing less than 1,500 gm. However, as previously stated, not all infants weighing less than 2,500 gm. are necessarily premature. The main criterion is gestational age. The majority of these preterm infants are of appropriate weight for gestational age, but some are small-for-dates. The causes of early delivery in most of these infants who are appropriately sized remain obscure.

Most studies of the factors associated with prematurity were based on birth weight as the sole criterion; thus their data are clouded. However, some conditions have been clearly related to premature labor, including chronic hypertensive disease, toxemia, placenta previa, abruptio placentae, and cervical incompetence. Other socioeconomic and environmental factors are harder to evaluate, and often several related factors are inseparable and generally associated with poverty. Mortality rates are highest among premature infants and increase as birth weight decreases.

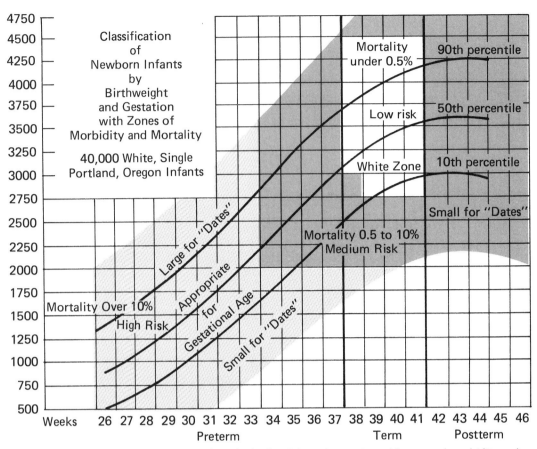

Figure 38-2. Classification of newborn infants by birthweight and gestation with areas of morbidity and mortality. (From Babson, S. G., Benson, R. C., Pernoll, M. L., and Benda, G. I.: *Management of High-Risk Pregnancy and Intensive Care of the Neonate.* St. Louis: C. V. Mosby, 1975.)

Small for Gestational Age (Growth Retardation)

Infants whose weight falls below the tenth percentile for their gestational age have experienced impairment of the normal growth process during the prenatal period. This condition may occur at any gestational age, but the majority of small-for-dates infants are born at or close to term and weigh less than 2,500 gm. Under the old classification, these would have been called "premature," although their period of intrauterine life was not significantly shortened. Though small, these infants are mature in comparison to infants of similar weight but lower gestational age.

Growth-retarded infants have increased risk of perinatal morbidity and mortality and are estimated to account for about 25 percent of the entire perinatal mortality.[1] The infant's condition is an end product of a process of intrauterine deprivation which begins many weeks before birth and is often related to abnormalities of the pregnancy or of the fetus.

There are two types of growth retardation, each of which may occur separately or simultaneously. Fetal growth involves both an increase in the number of cells (hyperplasia) and an increase in the size of cells (hypertrophy). Embryonic growth largely involves rapid increase in the number of cells as the organs and body structures are formed, and later in pregnancy these cells increase in size. If an insult to the fetus occurs early in gestation, mitosis is impaired and fewer new cells are formed, resulting in small organs of subnormal weight. The cells, however, will be of normal size. If interference with growth occurs later, the cells will be normal in number but smaller in size, again resulting in smaller organs but in this instance due to reduced amounts of cytoplasm. An intrauterine insult throughout both phases of growth results in cells that are fewer in number and smaller in size. The classic example of the latter condition is the infant with the rubella syndrome.

Fetal malnutrition and toxemia, which tend to be more prominent during later pregnancy, create the second type of growth retardation in which cell numbers are normal, but their size is reduced.

FACTORS WHICH AFFECT FETAL GROWTH

Fetal growth is influenced by a variety of factors, of maternal, placental and fetal origins. Genetic predispositions, the mother's nutritional and health status, fetal nutrition, fetal and maternal endocrine functions, developmental insults, environmental stressors, and placental function are variably involved in this process. Maturation is affected by biochemical determinants, enzymes, genes, and hor-

mones, particularly adrenal and thyroid. Development of the various organs follows a different time sequence, with hormonal action triggering a certain organ to grow and mature at a particular time during gestation. As different organs mature at different times, there are critical periods when stressors can significantly alter normal development. After that time the organ is less susceptible to damage and more capable of functioning in the extrauterine environment.

Maternal Factors

Genetic factors are important in determining fetal birth weight, but growth patterns are species specific and follow a predictable course until the last several weeks of gestation. At this time, generally after 34 to 38 weeks' gestation, fetal weights differ significantly according to parity, race and fetal sex.[2] In

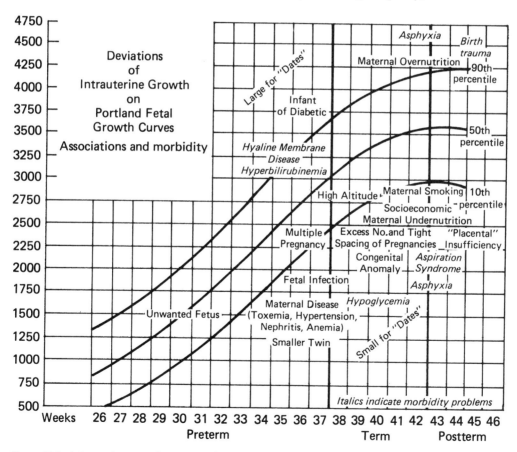

Figure 38-3. Intrauterine growth curves and associations with perinatal mortality and morbidity. (Source: Babson, S. G., Benson, R. G., Pernoll, M. L., and Benda, G. I.: *Management of High-Risk Pregnancy and Intensive Care of the Neonate.* St. Louis: C. V. Mosby, 1975.)

general, infants born to smaller parents tend to be smaller in length and weight than those infants born of larger parents. However, the greatest influence on infant birth size appears to be related to the characteristics of the maternal environment as reflected in intrauterine development. These characteristics include prepregnancy weight, weight gain during pregnancy, parity, interval between pregnancies, and age at delivery. Other factors in the mother's own environment affecting fetal growth include cigarette smoking, alcohol and drug use, infections, nutritional status, and socioeconomic conditions or changes. Finally, the occurrence of genetic defects exerts an influence on fetal growth and usually results in infants of low birth weight for their gestational age.

Nutrition

The role of nutrition in pregnancy outcome is a continuing and perplexing concern for health care providers. Although animal studies show direct causal relationships between inadequate maternal nutrition and reduced growth, altered organ function, and diminished rate of cell division in the brain and other organs in offspring, this data cannot be directly applied to humans. Malnutrition in humans is usually associated with other confounding factors, such as poverty, low socioeconomic status, wars and famines, and other types of social and psychological stress. Although birth weight has been shown to be related to maternal prepregnancy weight and weight gain during pregnancy, the latter is not a good index of nutrition and may only indicate the relative adequacy of energy intake.

The question of which nutrients are of greatest importance is under examination. Recent primate studies do not support the view that protein and calories are the major factors in favorable versus unfavorable pregnancy outcome, as measured by impaired somatic or brain growth. Reduced protein intake prolongs primate pregnancy resulting in a normal birth weight, suggesting a compensating mechanism between fetus and mother.[3] It is suggested that energy (rather than protein, carbohydrates, or combinations) is the most common nutrient affecting growth, and that primates conserve greater stores of nitrogen during pregnancy. These controlled studies could isolate the effects of protein and/or calorie restriction; observations of human populations, on the other hand, must consider multiple factors.

The adequacy of diet is difficult to assess, because of a lack of universally accepted standards of nutrition and health, imprecise determinations of needed nutrients, and limitations of study designs in doing research. In an examination of vitamin imbalance and low birth weight neonates, with mothers showing no overt signs of malnutrition, no statistically significant differences in blood levels of vitamins were found between mothers with normal and those with low birth weight infants. However, when the blood level of vitamins in the infants was tested, three vitamins were significantly lower in low birth weight infants: folate, pantothenate and vitamin B_{12}. Hematologic, neurologic and immune system dysfunctions are related to deficiencies of these vitamins. The critical questions involve the cause-effect relationships; do the low vitamin levels result from the low birth weight, are they associated with it but not directly caused by low birth weight, or are they a factor causing the impaired fetal growth.[4]

Placental Function

Under normal conditions, the size of the placenta is a major determinant of fetal size. When there is severe maternal nutritional deprivation, it appears that the maintenance needs of the placenta are met first, leading to reduction of fetal growth. In a fetus with growth retardation, however, the placenta is relatively smaller than with a normally growing fetus of the same gestational age. This is associated with higher levels of asphyxia at birth and perinatal morbidity seen among small-for-gestational-age infants. Placental mechanisms for maintaining optimal transfer of nutrients and gases between maternal and fetal blood are necessary for an adequate supply of growth-promoting substances to the fetus. The diffusion capacity of the placenta increases proportionately with fetal weight during pregnancy. Any impairment of oxygen transfer has a strikingly deleterious effect on fetal growth. Transfer of minerals, electrolytes and trace metals is also related to placental function, and these are necessary in an adequate supply for proper fetal growth.[5]

Decreased uteroplacental blood flow is believed to be a major mechanism in reduction of nutrients and oxygen to the fetus, resulting in altered growth. Maternal vascular disease is associated with the highest frequency of growth-retarded fetuses in the United States (approximately 35 percent of these cases). Hypertensive mothers with significantly reduced blood volume had infants of smaller birth weight than nonhypertensive controls. Reduction of maternal blood volume thus apparently decreases uterine blood flow.[6]

There appears to be no single placental abnormality common to infants who are small for gestational age, and placental and cord defects are present in only a small number of cases. When lesions are present, the most common include infarction, villous avascularity, fibrinosis, premature aging, and nonspecific chronic villous inflammation. Inadequate placental function is also associated with preeclampsia and diabetes.

Fetal Endocrine Influences

The hypothalamic-pituitary axis acts through the pancreas to modify fetal growth, and this is an interactional situation between mother and fetus. In the normal birth weight fetus of a normal mother, the pancreas has 2 percent endocrine tissue with 40 percent beta cells. In infants of gestational diabetic mothers, endocrine tissue is 10 percent with 60 percent beta cells, leading to significantly higher fetal insulin levels. The percentage of endocrine tissue and insulin levels are directly proportional to the excess fetal weight observed in infants of diabetic mothers. There appears to be a competitive effect between adrenal cortical hormones and insulin, related to lung maturation and formation of surfactant. Cortisol slows cell growth but enhances maturation of the fetal lung, while insulin acts as an antagonist to glucocorticoids. This effect seems related to higher incidence of respiratory distress syndrome in infants of diabetic mothers. A similar effect between insulin levels and glucocorticoids occurs with enzyme and glucose metabolism in the liver. Insulin, acting unopposed in the fetus, directly influences cytoplasmic growth and increases triglyceride concentrations in the brain, liver and lung.[7]

Thyroid and adrenal hormones are important to fetal maturation. Inadequate levels of thyroid hormone are associated with decreased fetal size, delayed skeletal ossification, delayed maturation and mental retardation. Infants of hyperthyroid mothers

may have advanced neurologic development for gestational age, greater body weight, greater placental weight, and advanced skeletal development. They appear several weeks older than gestational age. Corticosteroids are used to induce organ maturation, for instance, to promote lung maturation. They also affect maturation of the foregut (absorption of antibodies), pancreas, liver and small bowel. Liver glycogen depends on the presence of corticosteroids. It is possible that growth hormone may play a role in brain growth. Somatomedins (growth hormone ancillary factors) may be important in cell multiplication in the fetus, as high levels are found in large infants at birth and low levels in infants small for gestational age. Through an endocrine chain, hormonal regulation of fetal growth may be finely regulated by the central nervous system.[8]

Infection

Certain intrauterine infections are known to cause decreased growth of the baby, most notably cytomegalic inclusion disease and rubella. Congenital syphilis does not seem to cause growth retardation, although it has previously been identified as a cause of prematurity. Intrauterine bacterial infections usually occur just prior to or during labor but are not associated with the problem of growth retardation.

Genetic Factors

With the separation of true premature from small-for-dates infants, it became apparent that most congenital malformations occur in undergrown infants. The smaller for gestational age, the greater the frequency of congenital anomalies. Additionally, the highest incidence of severe malformations was found to occur in small-for-dates infants with the longest gestation. Congenital malformations occur 10 to 20 times more frequently in small-for-gestational-age infants than in appropriate for gestational-age infants.[9] Congenital disorders such as dwarfism often occur in infants who are small-for-dates, and in some families there are repeated births of infants who are small for age without associated abnormalities except mental retardation.

Other Factors

Various other circumstances or conditions are associated with retarded intrauterine growth. Infants born of multiple pregnancies are usually small-for-dates if born after 35 weeks gestation, presumably because the placenta can no longer supply the needs of the growing fetuses. Smoking is a significant statistical correlate to small-for-gestational-age babies, with moderate smokers having double the incidence of small birth weight babies and heavy smokers three times higher incidence than non-smokers. Mothers who smoke more than 20 cigarettes per day give birth to growth-retarded infants two to three times more often than mothers who do not smoke. Living at higher altitudes tends to be related to lower birth weight for the duration of pregnancy. Certain noxious agents such as x-ray, aminopterin and other antimetabolites result in growth impairment, malformations of the brain and cranial vault, and other anomalies depending upon timing of exposure. Infants of drug addicts, notably heroin addicts, are often small-for-dates.

IDENTIFICATION OF THE HIGH RISK NEONATE

Although the causes of prematurity and altered fetal growth are not completely understood, several associated factors have been identified which alert nurses and physicians to the possibility of these problems. Early recognition of mothers with high risk pregnancies and careful prenatal care can often contribute to a better outcome for the infant and the parents.

Many of the factors contributing to the birth of a high risk infant are not specific for a particular problem or condition but are generally related to increased morbidity and mortality. Others have specific associations with neonatal disorders or fetal abnormalities. Those related to prematurity include diabetes, placental insufficiency, multiple pregnancy, preeclampsia and hypertensive disorders, and infection. Several overlap with increased incidence of SGA (small-for-gestational-age) infants, including preeclampsia and hypertensive disorders, placental insufficiency, infections, discordant twin, and altitude. Congenital anomalies are more highly correlated to term SGA infants. (See Table 38-1 for a listing of factors associated with high risk infants.)

ASSESSMENT OF GESTATIONAL AGE

Accurate assessment of an infant's gestational age is of immediate and critical importance in the proper management of problems or anticipation of needs for care. The clinical course, outcome and problems are quite different for the preterm, immature infant and the small-for-gestational-age infant. In the first group (preterm), hyaline membrane disease, hyperbilirubinemia, apnea, and feeding problems are more common. In the second (immature), frequent problems include hypoglycemia, hypocalcemia, congenital malformations, aspiration, pneumothorax, pulmonary hemorrhage, polycythemia, and hyperviscosity.

It may be important to determine gestational age during pregnancy if fetal growth appears inappropriate for length of pregnancy, if a high risk condition exists in the mother, or if premature labor threatens. After birth, determination of gestational age may be critical in anticipating problems and planning for care when the infant is of low birth weight or experiences neonatal complications, is premature, or has high risk characteristics. A number of techniques and procedures have been developed to assess gestational age and fetal status during pregnancy and in the neonatal period.

Prenatal Assessment

Determination of the date of the *last normal menstrual period* is still an important basis for calculation of gestational age, although care must be taken in evaluating the accuracy of this date. A date may not be available if the mother was not having menstrual cycles for such reasons as a recent pregnancy or endocrine malfunctions. Postconceptional bleeding, discontinuation or omission of oral contraceptives, and simply forgetting also obscure an accurate determination of last menstrual period.

A careful obstetric history and examinations of fundal height according to *McDonald's measurements* (see Chapter 20, Antepartal Care), begun in early pregnancy and continued regularly, will enable an accurate estimation of gestational age in most pregnancies. In multiple gestations and intrauterine growth retardation, incongruent McDonald's measurements may often be a first indication that pregnancy is not progressing normally. Auscultation of *fetal heart tones* can assist in determining gestational age, as these are generally heard by fetascope about

TABLE 38-1
IDENTIFICATION OF HIGH RISK INFANT: ASSOCIATED FACTORS

Antepartal Factors

Maternal Characteristics

Age less than 15 or over 35
Lower socioeconomic status
Unmarried
Family or marital conflicts
Emotional illness or family history of
mental illness
Persistent ambivalence or conflicts
about the pregnancy
Stature under 5 feet
20 percent underweight or overweight
Inadequate diet

Reproductive History

Parity greater than 8
Two or more previous abortions
Previous stillborn or neonatal death
Previous premature labor or low birth
weight infant (2,500 gm.)
Previous excessively large infant
(>4,000 gm.)
Infant with isoimmunization or ABO
incompatibility
Infant with congenital anomaly,
genetic disorder, or birth damage
Preeclampsia or eclampsia
Uterine fibroids >5 cm. or
submucous
Abnormal Pap smear
Infertility
Prior cesarean section
Prior fetal malpresentations
Contracted pelvis
Ovarian masses
Genital tract abnormalities
(incompetent cervix, subseptate or
bicornate uterus)

Substances Abuse

Drugs
Alcohol
Heavy smoking >2 packs day

Medical Problems

Chronic hypertension
Renal disease (pyelonephritis,
glomerulonephritis, polycystic
kidney)
Diabetes mellitus
Heart disease (aortic insufficiency,
pulmonary hypertension, diastolic
murmur, cardiac enlargement, heart
failure, arrhythmia)
Sickle cell trait or disease
Anemias with hemoglobin <9 gm.
and hematocrit <32 percent

Medical Problems, cont'd
Pulmonary disease (tuberculosis,
COPD)
Endocrine disorders (hypo- or
hyperthyroidism, family history of
cretinism, adrenal or pituitary
problems)
Gastrointestinal or liver disease
Epilepsy
Malignancy (including leukemia and
Hodgkin's disease)

Complications of Present Pregnancy

Low or excessive weight gain
Hypertension (mean arterial pressure
>90, BP 140/90, increase >30 mm.
Hg systolic or >20 mm. Hg
diastolic)
Recurrent glycosuria and abnormal
FBS or glucose tolerance test
Uterine size inappropriate for
gestational age (either too large or
too small)
Recurrent urinary tract infections
Severe varicosities or
thrombophlebitis
thrombophlebitis
Recurrent vaginal bleeding
Premature rupture of membranes
Multiple pregnancy
Hydramnios with a single fetus
Rh negative with a rising titer
Late or no prenatal care
Exposure to teratogens (medications,
x-ray, radioactive isotopes)
Viral infections (rubella,
cytomegalovirus, herpes, mumps,
rubeola, chickenpox, shingles,
smallpox, vaccinia, influenza,
poliomyelitis, hepatitis, Western
equine encephalitis, Coxsackie B
virus)
Syphilis, especially late pregnancy
Bacterial infections (gonorrhea,
tuberculosis, listerosis, severe acute
infection)
Protozoan infections (toxoplasmosis,
malaria)
Postmaturity

Intrapartal Factors

Complications of Labor and Delivery
Labor longer than 24 hours in
primigravida
Labor longer than 12 hours in
multigravida
Second stage longer than 2 hours

Complications of Labor and Delivery,
cont'd
Ruptured membranes more than 24
hours
Abnormal presentation or position
Heavy sedation or injudicious
anesthesia
Maternal fever or infection
Placenta previa or abruptio placentae
Cesarean section
Meconium-stained amniotic fluid
Fetal distress by monitoring or scalp
blood sampling
Prolapsed cord
High or midforceps delivery, difficult
or operative delivery
Premature labor

Immediate Problems of Infant

Depressed, resuscitation required
Low Apgar score
Malformation or other significant
abnormality
Birth injury
Failure to begin spontaneous
respiration

Neonatal Factors

Characteristics of Infant

Preterm or premature
Small or large for gestational age
Birth weight under 5½ pounds or
over 9 pounds
Low-set ears
Enlargement of one or both kidneys
Single palmar crease
Single umbilical artery
Small head size

Clinical Problems

Sucks and takes food poorly
Anemia
Hyperbilirubinemia
Failure to maintain temperature
Respiratory distress
Hypoglycemia
Polycythemia
Infections
Rh or ABO incompatibilities

the twentieth week of gestation and by a Doppler apparatus (Dopptone) at the tenth week. *Fetal movement* (quickening) may be reported by the mother at about 16 to 18 weeks, and felt by the examiner at about 18 weeks, and can also serve as a guide to

pregnancy duration. While no one of these indicators is completely reliable alone, in combination they provide strong evidence of fetal age at a certain date, from which the estimated date of delivery can be calculated.

Diagnostic Methods

Ultrasonic scanning can be used during pregnancy to measure the biparietal diameter of the fetal skull, permitting estimation of fetal maturity and serial assessment of the rate of fetal growth. This technique is proving to be quite accurate and its use is growing as it offers the additional benefit of posing minimal danger to the fetus. Biparietal cephalometry by ultrasonography with measurements greater than 9.8 cm. indicates a term pregnancy.

X-ray examination of the fetus for ossification centers in distal femoral and proximal tibial epiphyses has been used to assess fetal growth, but the dangers of radiation appear to outweigh the benefits. The femoral epiphysis is usually seen at 36 weeks gestation and the tibial at 38 weeks. However, gestational age can be predicted accurately only to within a range of about seven weeks, and infants with intrauterine growth retardation may have absent or markedly smaller epiphyses.

A more invasive technique is injection of *radiopaque iodized lipid* into the amniotic fluid which dissolves in the vernix, thus outlining the fetal skin on x-ray. Based on the natural history of the vernix, almost all the fetal figure would be seen prior to 38 weeks' gestation, limbs and abdomen patchily outlined between 38 and 40 weeks gestation, and only the back and head visible after 40 weeks.

Laboratory Studies

Reduced excretion of *urinary estriols* by the mother during pregnancy indicate defective placental function. Serial determinations are most helpful, for a sudden drop in or disappearance of urinary estriol previously present is an ominous sign for the fetus, associated with hypoxia. Amniotic fluid obtained by amniocentesis during pregnancy provides several methods for assessing fetal status.

Rising concentrations of *creatinine* during gestation are correlated with fetal gestational age, as creatinine concentrations less than 1.8 mg. per 100 ml. occur prior to the thirty-sixth week and greater than 1.8 mg. after the thirty-sixth week. A low level or absence of *bilirubin* probably indicates fetal maturity, although this is less reliable than creatinine.

Pulmonary maturity is indicated by the sudden increase in the ratio of *lecithin to sphingomyelin* (also called the L/S ratio) which occurs in the amniotic fluid at 35 to 36 weeks' gestation. Saturated lecithins and related phospholipids arise principally from the fetal lung and are produced in greater amounts as the lungs near maturity. If the L/S ratio is 2.0 or more, hyaline membrane disease is unlikely to occur. Fetal cells probably originating from sebaceous glands can be obtained from amniotic fluid and stained with *Nile blue sulfate*. The viable, more mature cells stain orange, the immature ones stain blue. Before 34 weeks gestation, the number of orange-stained cells is less than 1 percent; between 34 and 38 weeks, 1 to 10 percent; between 38 and 40 weeks, 10 to 50 percent; and beyond 40 weeks, over 50 percent.

Oxytocin Challenge Test (OCT)

The *oxytocin challenge test* (OCT) or "stress test," while not strictly an assessment of gestational age, does provide an index to fetal status in high risk pregnancies. Information is provided about uteroplacental function and fetal response, and with diminution of placental blood flow during a contraction, a fetus with limited reserve will generally show signs of distress. Contractions are stimulated with intravenous infusion of oxytocin and compared with patterns obtained by external monitoring of fetal heart rate. If the fetus responds with a persistent pattern of late deceleration of heartrate (see Chap. 37), the test is positive and the fetus is compromised. Patients with a positive OCT have been found to have a higher incidence of growth retarded fetuses than those without a positive test. Also associated with a positive test are increased fetal distress, abnormal estriol excretion, and perinatal death.[10]

Postnatal Assessment

After the infant's birth, a number of external physical characteristics and neurologic signs can be used to assess maturity. Standardized methods using these parameters have been developed and charts and scoring systems are available to make the procedures quicker and more accurate. Nurses involved in the care of high risk infants should assess these physical characteristics and neurologic responses.

SCORING SYSTEM OF EXTERNAL PHYSICAL CHARACTERISTICS

External Sign	Score*				
	0	1	2	3	4
Edema	Obvious edema of hands and feet; pitting over tibia	No obvious edema of hands and feet; pitting over tibia	No edema		
Skin texture	Very thin, gelatinous	Thin and smooth	Smooth; medium htickness. Rash or superficial peeling	Slight thickening. Superficial cracking and peeling, especially of hands and feet	Thick and parchment like; superficial or deep cracking
Skin color	Dark red	Uniformly pink	Pale pink; variable over body	Pale; only pink over ears, lips, palms, or soles	
Skin opacity (trunk)	Numerous veins and venules clearly seen, especially over abdomen	Veins and tributaries seen	A few large vessels clearly seen over abdomen	A few large vessels seen indistinctly over abdomen	No blood vessels seen
Lanugo (over back)	No lanugo	Abundant; long and thick over whole back	Hair thinning especially over lower back	Small amount of lanugo and bald areas	At least ½ of back devoid of lanugo
Plantar creases	No skin creases	Faint red marks over anterior half of sole	Definite red marks over > anterior ½; indentations over < anterior ⅓	Indentations over > anterior ⅓	Definite deep indentations over > anterior ⅓
Nipple formation	Nipple barely visible; no areola	Nipple well defined; areola smooth and flat, diameter < 0.75 cm.	Areola stippled, edge not raised, diameter < 0.75 cm.	Areola stippled, edge raised, diameter > 0.75 cm.	
Breast size	No breast tissue palpable	Breast tissue on one or both sides, < 0.5 cm. diameter	Breast tissue both sides; one or both 0.5 to 1.0 cm.	Breast tissue both sides; one or both > 1 cm.	
Ear form	Pinna flat and shapeless, little or no incurving of edge	Incurving of part of edge of pinna	Partial incurving whole of upper pinna	Well-defined incurving whole of upper pinna	
Ear firmness	Pinna soft, easily folded, no recoil	Pinna soft, easily folded, slow recoil	Cartilage to edge of pinna, but soft in places, ready recoil	Pinna firm, cartilage to edge; instant recoil	
Genitals: Male	Neither testis in scrotum	At least one testis high in scrotum	At least one testis right down		
Genitals: Female (with hips ½ abducted)	Labia majora widely separated, labia minora protruding	Labia majora almost cover labia minora	Labia majora completely cover labia minora		

Source: Adapted by Dubowitz et al.: "Clinical assessment of gestational age in the newborn infant." *J. Pediat.* 77:1, 1970. From Farr et al.: "The definition of some external characteristics used in the assessment of gestational age of the newborn infant." *Develop. Med. Child. Neurol.* 8:507, 1966.

* If score differs on two sides, take the mean.

Physical Characteristics

During gestation, certain external physical characteristics develop and progress in an orderly fashion according to the age of the fetus. After birth, the gestational age can be determined by presence or absence of a number of these characteristics.

BREAST TISSUE AND AREOLA.   The nipples are present early in gestation, but the areola is barely visible until 34 weeks. After this time, the areola becomes raised and hair follicles become evident. Infants less than 36 weeks gestation have no breast tissue. At 36 weeks, a 1-to-2 mm. nodule of breast tissue becomes palpable. This increases with gestational age under hormonal stimulation until it reaches 7 to 10 mm. at 40 weeks.

SOLE CREASES.   The soles of the feet become wrinkled first on the anterior portion, and then in the area extending toward the heel as gestation progresses. At 32 weeks, one or two creases can be seen; they become more numerous, crisscrossed, and deeper, covering the anterior two-thirds of the sole by 37 weeks. The entire sole, including the heel, is covered at 40 weeks. In the postterm infant, creases are deeper and there may be desquamation of the soles.

EAR FORM AND CARTILAGE.   Infants of less than 33 to 34 weeks gestation have relatively flat ears. After 34 weeks, the upper pinnae begin to curve inward. By 38 weeks, the upper two-thirds of the pinnae are incurved; this extends to the earlobe by 39 to 40 weeks. An extremely premature infant's ear will remain folded over if pressed due to the absence of cartilage. Cartilage is more reliable than ear form in estimating gestational age and begins to appear at 32 weeks so that the ear slowly returns to its original position when folded over. By 36 weeks, the pinnae spring back when folded, and at term, they are firm, with the ear standing erect away from the head.

GENITALIA.   The characteristics of both male and female genitalia change with gestational age. In the female, the clitoris is prominent at 30 to 32 weeks, while the labia majora are small and widely separated. The labia majora increase in size and fullness with age, and at term they completely cover the labia minora and clitoris.

In the male, the testes are high in the inguinal canal at about 30 weeks, gradually descend to be felt high in the scrotal sac at 37 weeks and are well descended into the lower scrotal sac by 40 weeks. Rugae first appear on the scrotum anteriorly at 36 weeks and extend to cover the entire sac by 40 weeks. The postterm infant often has a pendulous scrotum covered with numerous rugae.

HAIR.   Strands of hair are very fine in early gestation and tend to mat together like wool, with small bunches sticking out from the head. The fullterm infant has silky hair which lies flat in single strands. In the postterm infant the hairline may recede. Important considerations to take into account when using hair as an assessment criterion is that hair varies in texture and characteristics with race and must be free of vernix before it is observed.

SKIN AND VERNIX.   The skin of premature infants is thin, pink, smooth, almost transparent with blood vessels visible, and thickly covered with vernix. The skin becomes thicker and more opaque with increasing age, until by 40 weeks it is pale with few vessels visible, with sparse vernix often occurring only in skin creases. In the postmature infant, there may be extensive desquamation of skin and absence of vernix.

NAILS.   At about 20 weeks the nails appear and gradually grow in subsequent weeks to cover the nailbed. At term the nails extend beyond the fingertips slightly, but long nails well beyond the fingertips are characteristic of postmature infants.

LANUGO.   This fine hair covers the infant's body at 20 weeks, and begins to disappear first from the face, then the trunk and then the extremities. At term, hair if present tends to be located only over the shoulders.

SKULL FIRMNESS.   The preterm infant has soft skull bones, particularly near the fontanels and sutures. The bones become firmer as gestation progresses, and at term the sutures are not easily displaced.

Neurologic Development

Gestational age may be assessed according to a number of neuromuscular responses of the newborn infant within the first few days of life. The infant's posture, the passive range of motion of certain parts, righting reactions, and various reflexes are evaluated.

The neurologic examination requires the infant be in a quiet, rested state, although this may not be possible immediately after delivery. Most infants can be examined during the latter part of the first day of life, but others are not ready until the second or third day. A shortened neurological examination including posture, tonicity and recoil may be done during the first few hours after birth, with the more extensive examination delayed. Charts and scoring systems are also used for these parameters (Fig. 38-4). The development of muscle tone begins in the lower extremities and progresses in a cephalad direction.

RESTING POSTURE AND EXTREMITY RECOIL. These two responses are sufficient to give a reasonable estimation of neurologic development in the first hour after birth. The remainder of the neurological examination is better carried out a day or two later to confirm the original findings. The resting posture of the premature infant is characterized by very little flexion of the upper extremities and only partial flexion of the lower. At about 30 weeks, there is slight flexion of the feet and knees. Flexion of the hips and thighs resulting in the characteristic frog position of the legs occurs at 34 weeks, but the arms are extended. At 36 to 38 weeks, the resting posture of the infant is one of complete flexion of all four extremities.

Recoil of extremities lags behind flexion by about two weeks. At 36 to 37 weeks, the extremities will remain extended but there is prompt recoil at 40 weeks.

To test recoil, flex the extremity and hold for five seconds, then extend for 30 seconds, and release. Brisk return to the flexed position indicates a fullterm infant.

HEEL TO EAR. With the infant supine and hips flat, the foot is drawn as close to the ear as possible without forcing it. In a premature infant there is very little resistance and the foot may approximate the ear, with the lag well extended. There is marked resistance in the fullterm infant, and it is impossible to draw the foot to the ear and extend the leg well.

POPLITEAL ANGLE. Passive movement of the leg reveals an inverse relationship between muscle tone and popliteal angle, with a smaller angle with greater tone. Premature infants have larger popliteal angles then term.

SCARF SIGN. In this test, the infant's arms are drawn across the neck and as far across the opposite shoulder as possible (like a scarf). In the premature infant there is less resistance and greater draping (or scarf) effect. This maneuver is best carried out by lifting the elbow across the front of the body. Note how far across the chest the elbow will go. In the premature infant, the elbow will reach near or across the midline, while in the fullterm infant it will not reach the midline (Fig. 38-5).

ANKLE AND WRIST FLEXION. Pressure is applied to the foot to push it onto the anterior aspect of the leg, and the angle between the dorsum of the foot and the leg measured. In premature infants this angle will be 45 to 90°, while in the fullterm infant the foot can be flexed until it touches the leg (Fig. 38-6). Similarly, the wrist is flexed with enough pressure to bring the hand as close to the forearm as possible. The angle between the hypothenar eminence of the wrist and the ventral aspect of the forearm is measured, with care taken not to rotate the wrist. In the premature infant this angle will be 90°, and in the fullterm infant the wrist can be flexed onto the arm.

VENTRAL SUSPENSION. The infant is suspended in the prone position with the hand of the examiner supporting it under the chest (two hands may be used for a large infant). The degree of extension of the back and head as well as the degree of flexion of the arms and legs are noted. The premature infant will hang limply with arms and legs almost straight and back rounded. The fullterm infant will extend the head, straighten the back, and flex the arms and legs.

HEAD LAG. With the infant supine, grasp the hands or arms and pull him slowly to a sitting position. Observe the position of the head in relation to the trunk. The premature infant will have no flexion of the neck. A gradual increase in flexion can be noted as gestation progresses. The fullterm infant will hold the head erect while being pulled to a sitting position.

REFLEXES. Although there are differences in reflexes *(Text continued on page 650)*

Examination First Hours

WEEKS GESTATION

PHYSICAL FINDINGS	20–25	26–30	31–34	35	36	37	38	39	40	41	42	43	44–48
Vernix	Appears → Covers body, thick layer						On back, scalp, in creases		Scant, in creases		No vernix		
Breast tissue and areola	Areola and nipple barely visible, no palpable breast tissue			Areola raised	1–2 mm nodule		3–5 mm		5–6 mm	7–10 mm			?12 mm
Ear — Form	Flat, shapeless		Beginning incurving superior		Incurving upper 2/3 pinnae		Well-defined incurving to lobe						
Ear — Cartilage	Pinna soft, stays folded		Cartilage scant, returns slowly from folding				Thin cartilage, springs back from folding		Pinna firm, remains erect from head				
Sole creases	Smooth soles without creases		1–2 anterior creases	2–3 anterior creases	Creases anterior 2/3 sole				Creases involving heel		Deeper creases over entire sole		
Skin — Thickness & appearance	Thin, translucent skin, plethoric, venules over abdomen, edema		Smooth, thicker, no edema		Pink		Few vessels		Some desquamation pale pink		Thick, pale, desquamation over entire body		
Nail plates	Appear		Nails to finger tips							Nails extend well beyond finger tips			
Hair	Appears on head	Eye brows and lashes	Fine, woolly, bunches out from head				Silky, single strands, lays flat				?Receding hairline or loss of baby hair, short, fine underneath		
Lanugo	Appears / Covers entire body			Vanishes from face			Present on shoulders				No lanugo		
Genitalia — Testes		Testes palpable in inguinal canal					In upper scrotum		In lower scrotum				
Scrotum		Few rugae			Rugae, anterior portion				Rugae cover	Pendulous			
Labia & clitoris	Prominent clitoris, labia majora small, widely separated				Labia majora larger, nearly cover clitoris				Labia minora and clitoris covered				
Skull firmness	Bones are soft	Soft to 1″ from anterior fontanelle			Spongy at edges of fontanelle, center firm		Bones hard, sutures easily displaced				Bones hard, cannot be displaced		
Posture — Resting	Hypotonic, lateral decubitus	Hypotonic	Beginning flexion, thigh	Stronger hip flexion	Frog-like	Flexion, all limbs	Hypertonic				Very hypertonic		
Recoil — leg	No recoil		Partial recoil			Prompt recoil							
Recoil — Arm	No recoil		Begin flexion, no recoil			Prompt recoil	Prompt recoil, may be inhibited				Prompt recoil after 30″ inhibition		

Confirmatory Neurologic Examination To Be Done After 24 Hours

Weeks Gestation — 20 21 22 23 24 25 26 27 28 29 30 31 32 33 34 35 36 37 38 39 40 41 42 43 44 45 46 47 48

Physical Findings		Observations (by gestational week)
Tone	Heel to ear	No resistance → Some resistance → Impossible
	Scarf sign	No resistance → Elbow passes midline → Elbow at midline → Elbow does not reach midline
	Neck flexors (head lag)	Absent → Holds head
	Neck extensors	Head begins to right itself from flexed position → Good righting cannot hold it → Holds head few seconds → Keeps head in line with trunk >40° → Turns head from side to side; Head in plane of body; Holds head
	Body extensors	Straightening of legs → Straightening of trunk → Straightening of head and trunk together
	Vertical positions	When held under arms, body slips through hands → Arms hold baby, legs extended? → Legs flexed, good support with arms
	Horizontal positions	Hypotonic, arms and legs straight → Arms and legs flexed → Head and back even, flexed extremities → Head above back
Flexion angles	Popliteal	No resistance; 150° → 110° → 100° → 90° → 80°
	Ankle	45° → 20° → 0° (A pre-term who has reached 40 weeks still has a 40° angle)
	Wrist (square window)	90° → 60° → 45° → 30° → 0°
Reflexes	Sucking	Weak, not synchronized with swallowing → Stronger, synchronized → Perfect
	Rooting	Long latency period slow, imperfect → Hand to mouth → Brisk, complete, durable → Perfect, hand to mouth → Complete
	Grasp	Finger grasp is good, strength is poor → Stronger → Can lift baby off bed, involves arms → Hands open
	Moro	Barely apparent → Weak, not elicited every time → Stronger → Complete with arm extension, open fingers, cry → Arm adduction added → ?Begins to lose Moro
	Crossed extension	Flexion and extension in a random, purposeless pattern → Extension, no adduction → Still incomplete → Extension, adduction, fanning of toes → Complete
	Automatic walk	Minimal → Begins tiptoeing, good support on sole → Fast tiptoeing → Heel-toe progression, whole sole of foot → A pre-term who has reached 40 weeks walks on toes; ?Begins to lose automatic walk
	Pupillary reflex	Absent → Appears
	Glabellar tap	Absent → Appears
	Tonic neck reflex	Absent → Appears
	Neck-righting	Absent → Appears; Present after 37 weeks

Figure 38-4. Clinical Estimation of Gestational Age (Source: Kempe, H. C., Silver, H. K., and O'Brien, D: Current Pediatric Diagnosis & Treatment. 5th Edition. Lange Medical Publishers, Palo Alto, Calif., 1978.)

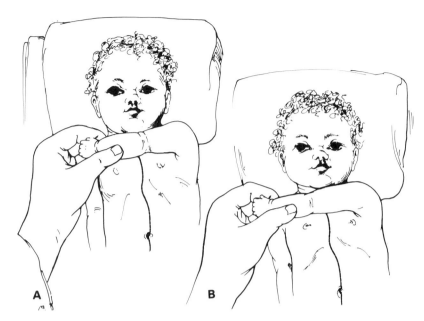

Figure 38-5. Scarf sign. In full term infant (A) the elbow will not reach midline. In premature infant (B) the elbow will reach across the midline.

with the infant's age, these are often not as pronounced as the other signs described above. The normal newborn's reflexes are discussed in Chapter 29, Care of the Newborn Infant. In the premature, the rooting reflex is less developed as evidenced by the slower response in turning the head toward the stimulus. The sucking reflex is weak or absent, depending upon prematurity and condition. The grasp reflex is weak and the infant cannot be lifted off the bed while grasping the examiner's finger. The Moro reflex is also weak, and the walking reflex often absent. The sucking reflex, which is of particular importance since it is related to the ability to take adequate nourishment with nipple feedings, occurs at about 34 weeks.

Nursing Assessment

The care of high risk infants can be individualized by determining gestational age, as well as identifying particular neonatal complications or conditions. Many of the ante- and postnatal methods described for assessment of gestational age can be done by the nurse. The non-neurological portions should optimally be performed on all infants within a few hours of birth, so that the infant's needs can be anticipated early in the neonatal course. Nurses in the delivery room or nursery are the logical ones to carry out the assessment of physical characteristics and a brief initial neurological examination (posture and recoil) to establish gestational age.

Although the examinations appear long, a few of the criteria can be selected and used regularly, providing reliable guidelines for the infant's age and related needs. For instance, observations of the breasts, ears, genitals, sole creases, posture and

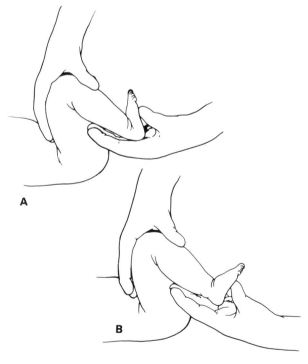

Figure 38-6. Dorsiflexion of the ankle. In full term infant (A) the foot can be flexed until it touches the leg. In the premature infant (B), the angle will be 45 to 90°.

recoil can be done rapidly and early. The correct age of the infant can usually be determined using these criteria. Recording these on a chart (Fig. 39-4) speeds the process and simplifies the procedures. Once proficiency is developed in these selected criteria, it is often easy to expand into more complete assessments. In this way, the nurse can anticipate problems and possibly prevent development of serious complications.[11]

CHARACTERISTICS AND PHYSIOLOGY OF SMALL-FOR-GESTATIONAL-AGE INFANTS

Appearance at Birth

Small-for-dates infants appear thin and wasted, with skin that is loose, often dry, and frequently scaling. Meconium staining, involving the nails, skin and umbilical cord, is common. Such infants have very little subcutaneous tissue, and the trunk and extremities do not appear to have as much musculature as would be expected. Their faces appear wizened and are not full and round, with generally sparse hair on the head. Although their weight is low, length is often normal, as is head size. Shortly after birth these infants are usually alert, active, and hungry. They frequently do not urinate during the first several hours of life, and may go as long as 24 hours without voiding if fluids are withheld. The umbilical cord tends to dry more rapidly than that of normal infants. Some small-for-dates infants appear proportionately small without wasting, meconium staining, and the other characteristics described. These babies appear old for their size and seem to have been undergrown for a long time; it is in this group that anomalies tend to occur.

Physiologic Problems

In adaptation to extrauterine life, the problems encountered by the small-for-gestational-age infant are different from those of the appropriate-for-gestational-age, preterm (premature) infant. *If the problem of poor growth in utero has been detected during pregnancy, nurses and physicians skilled in resuscitation should be present at delivery.*

Infants with intrauterine growth retardation experience three general types of complications:

1. complications related to fetal factors, including congenital malformations, congenital infections, and chromosomal malformations;
2. complications secondary to fetal distress and perinatal asphyxia including asphyxia neonatorum, meconium aspiration syndrome, persistent fetal circulation, hyperviscosity, postasphyxia encephalopathy, and renal complications; and
3. complications related to abnormalities in substrate transfer and hormonal control, including neonatal hypocalcemia, hypoglycemia, and hyperglycemia.

Another group of problems these infants encounter includes difficulties with temperature control and abnormalities in coagulation and bleeding profiles.

Asphyxia. Perinatal asphyxia is the most serious complication faced by small-for-gestational-age infants, and generally occurs in those infants whose growth retardation is due to maternal or placental factors. Limitation of substrate transfer and gas exchange across the placenta is a key factor, often leading to fetal hypoxia and acidosis which predisposes the neonate to perinatal asphyxia.

Intrauterine hypoxia can often be diagnosed during labor, through such indicators as:

1. meconium stained amniotic fluid in a cephalic presentation,
2. abnormal fetal heart rate patterns by monitoring, and
3. fetal acidosis as determined by scalp blood sampling.

Immediate resuscitation is essential for an optimal outcome for the neonate. Perinatal asphyxia is a common denominator for most of the complications occurring in infants with growth retardation, and the occurrence, severity, and outcome of complications depend upon the severity of the asphyxia.

Postasphyxia Encephalopathy. This term is used to describe various central nervous system symptoms caused by injury resulting from episodes of perinatal asphyxia. The underlying pathophysiological disorder may include cerebral edema or intracranial hemorrhage. The extent of symptoms depends on the severity of asphyxia and effectiveness of resuscitation in the delivery room.

Symptoms may include irritability, twitching, apnea, and convulsions frequently appearing during the first 6 to 12 hours of life. The prognosis is related to the underlying cause of encephalopathy, and symptoms must be differentiated from those caused by other conditions with central nervous system manifestations such as hypoglycemia and hypocalcemia.

Meconium Aspiration Syndrome.

Aspiration of meconium into the alveoli, occurring in utero or after birth, causes atelectasis and subsequent asphyxia. Meconium in the respiratory tract acts like a foreign body and blocks the flow of air into the alveoli. Increasing inflation of the alveoli distal to the obstruction can lead to their rupture and the leakage of air into the interstitial tissue. This initiates a series of complications such as pulmonary interstitial emphysema, pneumomediastinum, and pneumothorax. The asphyxia which results from these meconium effects on the lungs leads to the involvement of the central nervous system, kidney, erythropoietic system, and metabolism which are associated with the meconium aspiration syndrome. The syndrome may be prevented or minimized through appropriate obstetric management of mothers in whom there is evidence of meconium stained amniotic fluid and prompt removal of meconium from the infant's upper respiratory tract immediately after birth.

Hypoglycemia.

Neonatal hypoglycemia, or blood glucose concentration of less than 20 mg. per 100 ml., is frequent in small-for-gestational-age infants. It occurs in 50 percent of these infants who are below the third percentile for gestational age, and who are markedly wasted. Although hypoglycemia usually occurs during the first 12 hours of life, it may appear as late as 48 hours. Blood sugars of these infants must be carefully monitored and early feeding instituted.

Infants are at increased risk of hypoglycemia if their growth retardation is due to maternal undernutrition or placental insufficiency. When the placental-fetal transfer of substrates is markedly reduced, the reserve for substrates (in this case, glycogen) is also reduced. At birth, increased amounts of glucose are utilized to supply the energy required for various physiologic adaptations. Increased glucose utilization, lack of substrate reserve, inefficient gluconeogenic mechanism, and insufficient intake of glucose then result in a fall in blood glucose with consequent hypoglycemia. *Symptoms are jitteriness, twitching, convulsions, apnea, and tachypnea.* Some infants with clinically proven low levels of blood glucose are asymptomatic.

Hypocalcemia.

The most common form of this neonatal metabolic disorder is called first-day hypocalcemia and is often found in low birth weight infants (both premature and growth retarded infants weighing less than 2,000 gm.). The etiologic factor is probably not the low birth weight or status of nutrition, but the presence of asphyxia and related respiratory distress. Hypocalcemia is often found accompanying the meconium aspiration syndrome. Symptoms are nonspecific and similar to those found in hypoglycemia, and there is no correlation between symptoms and severity of hypocalcemia. Diagnosis is therefore based on clinical determinations of the serum calcium level.

Polycythemia and Hyperviscosity.

Infants with intrauterine growth retardation have been found to have increased red blood cell volume, elevated erythropoietin levels, a venous hematocrit greater than 65 percent, or hemoglobin in excess of 22 gm. per 100 ml. The cause is thought to be related to intrauterine hypoxia, as placental insufficiency leading to chronic fetal hypoxia may stimulate an increase in erythropoiesis. Hypoxia in utero can also cause redistribution of blood volume within the placental-fetal circuit with a net transfer of blood from the placenta to the fetus. In view of the high probability of increased blood volume in infants with growth retardation, the cord should be clamped or stripped quickly after birth rather than delayed, as is a common practice, to avoid the transfer of large amounts of placental blood to the infant.

Symptoms of polycythemia are related to:
1. increased destruction of red blood cells causing hyperbilirubinemia,
2. increased circulating blood volume causing congestive heart failure or pulmonary edema, and
3. the phenomenon of hyperviscosity.

Hyperviscosity frequently accompanies a venous hematocrit in excess of 65 percent. Its clinical manifestations result from sludging of blood in the microcirculation of various organs, the most commonly observed signs involving the central nervous system, cardiopulmonary system, peripheral circulation, and mesenteric vascular bed which gives rise to a high incidence of necrotizing enterocolitis.

The clinical picture varies with the system involved; in the gastrointestinal system with necrotizing enterocolitis there may be abdominal distention, ileus, bloody stools, and bilious or bloody vomiting. Cardiorespiratory signs include tachypnea, intercostal retraction, grunting, nasal flaring, tachycardia, and pleural effusion. Convulsions and other central nervous system manifestations may be present, as may scrotal edema and priapism. Treatment includes a partial exchange transfusion, replacing 10 to 15 percent of the infant's blood volume with plasma or other colloid solution.[12]

Renal Complications. The possibility of renal anomalies should always be considered in infants with growth retardation, as congenital malformations are common. The kidneys of growth retarded infants are smaller than normal infants' kidneys, but renal function tends to be adequate unless the infant suffers perinatal asphyxia. If asphyxia occurs, renal ischemia results, leading to hypotension and acute renal failure with oliguria, hyperkalemia, azotemia, water retention and dilutional hyponatremia. Treatment consists of fluid restriction and close monitoring of fluid and electrolyte status and treatment for hyperkalemia.

Thermal Regulation. Lacking subcutaneous tissue and fat, small-for-gestational-age infants have difficulty maintaining body temperature. In addition to body composition, basal metabolic rates differ from normal newborns. The temperature setting on the incubator should be determined by closely monitoring the infant's temperature, with the goal of maintaining abdominal skin temperature between 36.0 and 36.5°C. The effects of asphyxia are aggravated by stress caused by cold.

CHARACTERISTICS AND PHYSIOLOGY OF THE PREMATURE INFANT

General Description at Birth

As there are many degrees of prematurity, there are also various stages of anatomic and physiologic development. Many of the symptoms described below may vary in infants of approximately the same fetal age, depending on the factors associated with prematurity and the physical condition of the mother and the infant.

At birth the premature baby lacks the subcutaneous fat which is deposited during the last two months of intrauterine development. This gives the skin a transparent appearance so that the blood vessels are easily seen through the skin, which often is of a deep red color, sometimes with a cyanotic hue. These premature babies are prone likewise to develop icteric skin changes. Lanugo is usually abundant all over the skin surface but disappears within a few weeks.

The external ears and the nose are very soft, due to the underdeveloped cartilage. The ears lie very close to the head. The skull is round, in contrast with the long anteroposterior skull diameter of the full term infant. The fontanels are large, and the sutures prominent. The fingernails and toenails may be immature, often not reaching the ends of the fingers and the toes.

The infant may be puny and small or may approximate full term weight; yet the internal organs may be imperfectly developed, and these babies appear to be reluctant to assume the responsibility to live. The respiration is shallow and irregular, due to the lack of lung expansion and proper gaseous exchange. There are often periods of apnea.

Due to the irregular respiration and the poorly developed function of swallowing, there is danger of aspiration of milk or vomitus, causing cyanosis and predisposing to pulmonary infections. The premature baby regurgitates food readily, because the stomach is tubular and the sphincters are poorly developed. The urine is usually scanty.

The walls of the blood vessels are weak, and the tendency to hemorrhage is great. Since the central nervous system is not fully developed, the premature infant is sluggish and must be wakened to be fed, and the muscular movements are feeble. The temperature is usually subnormal and fluctuating, due to the underdeveloped heat-regulating center. The cry is monotonous, whining, "kittenlike" and effortless, showing a lack of energy. All these symptoms are evidenced in varying degrees, according to the degree of immaturity.

Physiologic Considerations

As discussed in Chapter 29, the newly born infant must make certain adaptations to extrauterine life.

For the premature infant adaptations will be even greater and more difficult due to a variety of anatomic and physiologic deficits.

Respiratory System

The development of the lungs will depend upon the degree of maturity. For instance, the lungs of an infant weighing 2 pounds (900 gm.) or less show small alveoli lined with cuboidal epithelium, surrounded by a meager supply of capillaries (which prevent efficient gaseous exchange); the lungs of an infant weighing 6 pounds (2,730 gm.), on the other hand, show large alveoli, the walls of which are virtually formed by bare capillaries. There is a great increase in the capillary network between the twenty-sixth week and the thirty-sixth week of intrauterine life, and for this reason the ability of the lungs to sustain extrauterine life increases with each week of intrauterine existence. The more immature the infant, the less blood flow there is through the lungs, the remainder being shunted through the ductus arteriosus.

As noted with the mature newborn, the most critical event in the adjustment to extrauterine life is the establishment of ventilation by the previously unused lungs. The unexpanded lungs of any fetus are not just crumpled air sacs waiting to be filled; rather they are fluid-filled organs requiring a great deal of negative intrapleural pressure (up to 60 cm. water has been used experimentally) for expansion. This great effort is necessary because of the viscosity of the fluid in the lungs, surface tension effects, and tissue resistance.

The premature baby is often not capable of this enormous task because of the previously mentioned inadequacy in the capillary anatomy which impedes appropriate gaseous exchange, and because the respiratory centers of the brain which regulate depth and rate of respiration are not fully developed. In addition, these infants are hampered by weak respiratory muscles, a yielding thoracic cage, a decreased amount of pulmonary lipoprotein (surfactant) which reduces surface tension in the lungs, and a deficient amount of fibrinolysins; hence primary and secondary atelectasis are common to these infants. The nasal passages are extremely narrow and the mucous membrane easily injured. The cough reflex is poorly developed or absent, making the danger of inhalation of regurgitated fluids very real.

In general, then, an unstable respiratory system is a result of these deficits. Respiration tends to be irregular in rhythm and depth; there are periods of apnea during which cyanosis may develop. The infant utilizes the diaphragm more than the chest in breathing, and if there is much atelectasis, the thoracic cage is dragged down with each inspiration. In severe cases, the sternum is sucked back toward the spine with inspiration, and expiration is accompanied by a short feeble grunt (Fig. 38-7). It is important to remember that with these infants, respirations must be counted for at least a minute if any accurate respiratory rate is to be determined.

Cardiovascular System

The heart is relatively large at birth and often its action is slow and feeble. Extrasystoles occur and murmurs may be present at birth or soon after, which may later disappear as the fetal openings gradually close. As previously stated there is a decrease in the density of available capillaries in vital organs to take up sufficient oxygen in babies under about 1,000 gm. The extreme capillary fragility, especially of the intracranial vessels, together with the low plasma prothrombin level leads to a bleeding tendency in these infants. This tendency is evidenced by the frequency of ecchymosis of the skin as well as intraventricular hemorrhage and other internal bleeding.

The *systolic blood pressure* at birth is lower than that of the mature infant and decreases with the birth weight. Infants weighing between 2 and 4 pounds (900 to 2270 gm.) generally have a systolic pressure of 45 to 60 mm. Hg as compared with the 80 mm. of Hg for term infants. The level rises with the age of the child, by about 20 mm. by the end of the second week, and an additional 5 mm. by the age of two months.

The *pulse rate* ranges between 100 and 160, with the average around 140. Because of the tendency to arrhythmia, the pulse rate is most accurately obtained (as with the term infant) with a stethoscope, counting the apical beat for a minute.

As with the mature baby, the premature infant has a relatively high *hemoglobin concentration* at birth, which decreases to around 7 gm. per 100 ml. of blood at four to eight weeks of age. This is due to the premature's inadequacy in manufacturing hemoglobin, together with the infant's relatively rapid rate of growth. After this time, the rate gradually

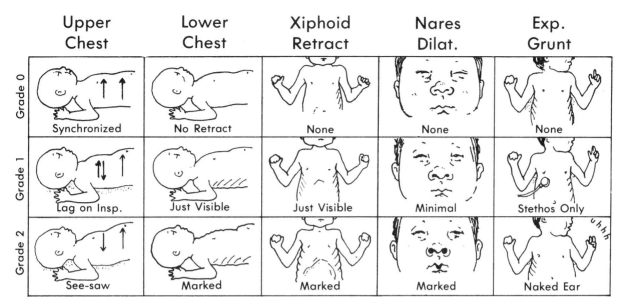

Observation of Retractions

Figure 38-7. An index of respiratory distress is determined by grading each of five arbitrary criteria; grade 0 indicates no difficulty, grade 1 moderate difficulty, and grade 2 maximum respiratory difficulty. The "retraction score" is the sum of these values; a total score of 0 indicates no dyspnea, whereas a total score of ten denotes maximal respiratory distress.

increases until about four months, when there is a second fall, characterized by hypochromia of the red cells. If a severe enough anemia develops in the first phase of hemoglobin decline, it may be treated with iron therapy. Some investigators have found for some unknown reason that *parenteral* (but not *oral*) administration of iron is useful in prevention of the first phase of anemia. However, the later phase responds well to oral iron therapy and thus it has become customary to institute the oral form of therapy from the third week onward.

White Blood Cells. The white blood cell count at birth is lower than that usually found in the term infant. There is a predominance of polymorphonuclear cells, as with the mature infant, and the same decrease occurs in the total white cell count during the first week of life. However, the change to lymphocytic predominance may occur slightly later for the mature infant.

Neurologic System

The stage of development of the nervous system at birth will depend upon the degree of maturity. As with the normal newborn, all the premature infant's neurons are present, but they are not as fully developed and remain so for months and sometimes years. The least mature infants tend to lie quietly unless disturbed, waking only at intervals for feeding. External stimulation results in weak purposeless jerky movements and perhaps a feeble cry. As the infant matures, movements tend to occur in little bursts of activity which can be quite vigorous, resulting in the infant wiggling from one end of the incubator to the other. At first the less mature infant will lie on his side in the "fetal position"; later he uncurls and after several days he lies on his back with his head rolled to one side, his hips flexed and abducted, and his knees and ankles flexed (frog position). The less mature the infant, the worse his muscle tone.

The vital centers controlling respiration and temperature are poorly developed, as are the centers controlling such important reflexes as coughing, swallowing and sucking. The Moro and tonic neck reflexes are present in normal infants of both low birth weight and early gestational age, as are the Chvostek and Babinski signs. Tendon reflexes are variable in all immature infants.

Temperature Regulation.   Even more so than the normal newborn, the premature infant's temperature regulating mechanism is poorly developed at birth. Since peripheral circulation is also poor, peripheral responses to heat and cold (i.e., sweating and shivering) are inadequate. Heat production is low and heat loss high because of the relatively greater body surface (in proportion to the weight) and the lack of subcutaneous fat.

Gastrointestinal System

Larger premature infants may have fairly good sucking and swallowing ability. The less mature infants, however, generally have feeble reflexes which, in the very immature, may be absent altogether. Because of the poorly developed mechanism for closure of the cardiac sphincter and the relatively strong pyloric sphincter, regurgitation is common.

Again the powers of digestion depend on the degree of prematurity, being rudimentary in infants of 26 to 28 weeks gestation but becoming more efficient as maturity increases. The stomach of a 2-pound (900-gm.) infant at birth shows little folding of the mucosal surface (which reduces the surface area for absorption) and poor development of the secretory glands and muscle layers, as compared with that of a term baby with deeply folded mucosal layer and relatively well-developed glands and muscle tissue.

The premature infant appears to digest and absorb carbohydrates easily, proteins less well and fats badly, even though fat-splitting enzymes are present at birth. This inability to manage fat leads to the often seen greasy and foul-smelling steatorrheic stools. When the premature newborn uses glycogen stores, he depends as usual on body fat for energy; when food becomes available, more calories are used from the carbohydrates and less from the fats than in the term baby; thus, the premature infant resembles the fetus more in this respect since the fetus also depends on carbohydrates for its main source of energy.

The musculature of the bowel is weak and easily distended, so that there may be a tendency to constipation. Because of the thin abdominal wall, gastric peristalsis is seen; if distension is present, intestinal peristalsis also becomes visible.

Urinary System

In comparison with the normal newborn, the premature infant's renal function is impaired. Since the kidney tubules continue to be formed until term, kidneys in the premature infant are poorly developed. Thus, urine cannot be concentrated well (which becomes important when conditions involving an excessive loss such as diarrhea or vomiting occur) and sodium and chloride cannot be excreted well, with resultant early water retention and edema. It is believed by many that the tendency to a more marked and prolonged acidosis in the newly born premature infant and the inability to excrete many drugs is probably due to the relatively poor development of the kidneys.

Low pH levels (normal is 7.42) are regularly found in apparently healthy immature infants and are not considered dangerous unless accompanied by conditions such as respiratory distress, vomiting or diarrhea.

Urination is scanty and infrequent for a few days after birth, due to the small amount of fluid that is usually administered. Urates are commonly present in some excess, thus giving a false positive for albumin by heat, acetic acid or trichloracetic acid tests.

Hepatic System

The liver is relatively large but its function is poorly developed in smaller infants. This immaturity of the liver predisposes to jaundice (see p. 666) because of the inability of the liver to conjugate and excrete bilirubin. It has also been suggested that the low blood sugar found in the premature is hepatogenic, due to small liver glycogen stores. Lower serum protein levels, deficiency of blood clotting factors, and the deficient conjugation and detoxification of certain drugs are all attributed to liver immaturity.

Jaundice.   The majority of premature infants become jaundiced around the second or third day of life. As is the case with term infants, the jaundice intensifies from the fourth to sixth day and generally disappears by the second week. As far as we know, the mechanism responsible for this condition is approximately the same as that described for mature infants (see Chap. 30). Weight and degree of development appear to be related to the serum bilirubin value. The smaller the infant, the higher the peak of bilirubin value; 13 mg. per 100 ml. of blood is beyond the physiologic limit. In the very small premature infant, a value of 15 to 20 mg. per 100 ml. is often found, because of the inability of the immature liver to dispose of the bilirubin which is liberated by the breakdown of the red blood cells.

When hyperbilirubinemia occurs (serum bilirubin in excess of 18 to 20 mg. per 100 ml. of blood), kernicterus may occur, and when the infant is particularly stressed (e.g., respiratory distress, difficult delivery) even lower concentrations of bilirubin can produce kernicterus. Other conditions which predispose to this condition before the second day of life are 1) erythroblastosis, concomitant with the immature liver function, and 2) early gestational age of the infant.

ILLNESSES OF THE PREMATURE INFANT

The premature infant is particularly susceptible to certain pathophysiological conditions as a consequence of organ system immaturity, asphyxia during the perinatal period, and respiratory insult often associated with the need for resuscitation and ventilation. The most common conditions seen in the premature infant include respiratory distress syndrome (hyaline membrane disease), bronchopulmonary dysplasia, pulmonary dysmaturity, and retrolental fibroplasia.

Respiratory Distress Syndrome (RDS)

Also known as *hyaline membrane disease* (*HMD*), this condition is primarily a disease of premature infants and rarely occurs in infants born at term. It is a leading cause of death among premature infants, with incidence and severity increasing with lower birth weight. It is estimated that greater than 25,000 infants are affected annually in the United States.

The greatest incidence of RDS occurs in preterm infants weighing between 1,000 and 1,500 gm., and it is observed in about 10 percent of all premature infants. It also occurs in about 50 percent of all infants of diabetic mothers and also in infants whose mothers experienced antepartal vaginal bleeding. The condition has also been noted in infants born by cesarean section; however, cesarean section in otherwise *uncomplicated* full term deliveries is probably not associated with any increased incidence of the disease. This disease is not found in stillborn infants.

Pathophysiology. In this syndrome of neonatal respiratory distress, the alveoli and the alveolar ducts are filled with a sticky exudate, a hyaline material, which prevents aeration. Although it is known that the hyaline material is a protein, the cause of hyaline membrane formation is not definitely known.

Three main theories have been postulated. The first proposes an alteration in the fibrinolytic enzyme system in the lung or blood which leads to the proliferation of the protein (fibrin) exudate. The second suggests an absence or alterations of the pulmonary surfactant which reduces alveolar ventilation and promotes atelectasis. The third indicates pulmonary hypofusion rather than surfactant deficiency. This hypofusion begins with intrauterine asphyxia and also results in reduced alveolar ventilation and atelectasis. Whatever the exact causes and mechanisms, surfactant activity is indeed deficient, and, as a result, there is incomplete expansion of the lung and failure to establish normal functional residual capacity (absence of alveolar stability). Thus, the lungs are atelectatic, and this is a hallmark of the disease.

Lecithin is thought to be the surface-active (surfactant) phospholipid responsible for maintaining alveolar stability. The production of lecithin normally begins around the thirty-second to thirty-sixth week of gestation, with the initial functioning of enzyme systems producing this phospholipid. The high glucocorticoid levels found in the fetus after the thirty-fourth week of gestation accelerate production and synthesis of surfactant and lead to lung maturation. It has been found that conditions increasing cortisol levels, such as intrauterine infections, premature rupture of the membranes, maternal hypertensive disorders, and partial abruptio placentae, are associated with lower incidence of RDS as these stressors lead to stimulation of earlier lung maturation. The use of the synthetic steroidal hormone, betamethasone, in pregnant women a few days before anticipated premature delivery stimulates maturation of the fetal lungs and holds promise of improving the outlook of RDS in the small premature.

Clinical Manifestations. Pulmonary compliance, or the capacity of the lung to increase in volume in response to a given amount of applied pressure during inspiration, is diminished in this syndrome. The stiffness of the lungs and their limited distensibility contributes significantly to the work of breathing in these sick babies. *Pulmonary vasoconstriction* is another injurious factor of major importance. This vasoconstriction results in increased resistance within the pulmonary circuit and causes hypofusion of alveolar capillaries; hence, the lungs are ischemic as well as atelectatic. Thus, the fetal circulatory state persists in varying degrees and this becomes life-threatening to the neonate. After a few breaths, continued impairment of gas exchange enhances hypoxia, hypercapnia, and acidosis. This, in turn, increases the pulmonary vasoconstriction and ischemia; surfactant activity is further diminished and atelectasis becomes more extensive. Pulmonary compliance decreases and the energy required for the simple act of breathing increases intolerably. All this leads to further impairment of gas exchange and a vicious cycle is established which soon becomes incompatible with life without intensive treatment.

It was formerly believed that a free interval existed after birth before the onset of symptoms. However, when infants are observed closely and examined carefully, symptoms can be noted immediately after birth. A chest x-ray usually confirms the diagnosis and rules out congenital cardiovascular disease.

Expiratory grunting or whining (observable when the infant is not crying), sternal and subcostal retractions, nasal flaring, rapid respirations (more than 60 per minute), and low body temperatures are seen early and are diagnostic clues. Grunting, which is the most important and useful clinical sign, may be the only and earliest indication of the disease. Conversely, cessation of grunting is often the first sign of improvement.

The infant may be cyanotic in room air. Infants who are badly affected may be cyanotic even with oxygen therapy yet paradoxically exhibit a normal respiratory rate. Auscultation of the chest reveals poor air entry, decreased breath sounds, and at times, fine rales. Arterial blood gases demonstrate decreased PO_2 and often metabolic and respiratory acidosis. There is reduced blood pH and increased nitrogen, phosphorus and potassium. Bowel sounds are often absent in the early hours of the illness and the urine output is low during the first two or three days of life.

If the disease progresses, respiratory rate increases, chest retractions become more marked, and see-saw respirations ensue (see Fig. 38-7, p. 655). Peripheral edema increases, and muscle tone decreases. With the increase in cyanosis, the body temperature tends to drop and short periods of apnea are noted. The heart rate is often fixed except for periods of bradycardia accompanied by severe cyanosis and grunting.

Many symptoms are related to asphyxia which depresses the respiratory center and causes apneic episodes as well as changes in the blood distribution throughout the body. This latter fact accounts for the pale gray skin color of the severely affected infant. In addition the rate of heat production is also decreased.

If treatment is instituted promptly, modern care has resulted in about a 50 to 70 percent salvage rate for these infants. If treatment is not prompt and/or the infant is small or does not respond to treatment, death may occur within 48 hours.

It is important that the nurse make careful observations and recordings about the respiratory signs and symptoms of infants who are born prematurely. The outcome for the premature infant usually depends a great deal on his birth weight: the smaller he is, the graver is the prognosis. For example, infants who weigh 1,000 gm. or less generally succumb, since their lungs are not developed enough to make the adjustment to extrauterine life.

Management.   Since the cause and complete pathophysiology of this entity are not understood, the principles of management center on alleviation of the clinical manifestations. Thus, approaches to treatment are made both directly, by treating the infant with oxygen and alkali, and indirectly, through influencing oxygen need and acid production by regulating the infant's body temperature, water balance, and caloric requirements. Treatment therefore involves:

1. regulation of body temperature,
2. intravenous feeding and base therapy,
3. oxygen therapy, and
4. assisted ventilation, if necessary.

The nurse is a key figure in all of these modalities. Accurate recording and reporting of all the data from the monitoring devices—skin, cardiac, apnea, and telethermometer—is necessary. The sites of these attachments must be watched carefully for abrasions or skin breakdown. Adequate oxygenation of the infant is imperative.

With mild RDS, 60 percent or less oxygen administered by hood is often adequate. As RDS becomes more severe, ventilatory assistance is needed and may be achieved by 1) continuous positive airway pressure via intratracheal tube, nasal prongs, mask or hood; 2) continuous negative airway pressure by exerting pressure on the infant's body with the head exposed and oxygen administered by mask or prongs; or 3) continuous end expiratory pressure with positive pressure exerted during expiration. Care must be taken in administration of oxygen and in ventilatory assistance because a number of complications can result from their injudicious use, as discussed below.

Prognosis. Infants with RDS generally show improvement within 72 hours after birth, or their condition deteriorates. If improvement occurs, slow recovery follows over a period of about two weeks. When the infant has remained stable for 12 to 24 hours, oral feedings are usually begun and advanced gradually. With the use of respiratory and metabolic interventions now available through new technology and equipment, premature infants with RDS can be sustained for longer time periods and the outcome not known for several weeks. Recovery or death may be postponed for varying lengths of time, creating both hope and longer periods of uncertainty for parents and health professionals.

Bronchopulmonary Dysplasia

This syndrome of characteristic pulmonary changes is believed to result from oxygen toxicity and is associated with the use of positive pressure ventilation. It is often preceded by severe RDS, with the infant treated for several days in a high oxygen environment (greater than 60 to 70 percent). The infants demonstrate tachypnea, subcostal retractions, rales and cyanosis, and it is often difficult to wean them from the respirator. On x-ray examination the lungs show similar changes to those of RDS and of pulmonary dysmaturity (Wilson-Mikity syndrome). Cardiac failure and pulmonary edema may also occur, with mortality rates as high as 50 percent observed. When improvement occurs it develops gradually over several weeks, with diminished need for oxygen, and some months are needed for complete recovery.

Pulmonary Dysmaturity (Wilson-Mikity)

This disease of premature infants has an insidious course beginning with mild respiratory symptoms after the first week of life. It is commonly noted at about three weeks of age and primarily affects infants weighing below 1,500 gm. Symptoms of respiratory distress and cardiac failure occur with typical lung changes including a diffuse, coarse and lacelike pattern of infiltrates and cystic areas of hyperaeration. Fatality is between 25 and 50 percent.

In surviving infants, the symptoms gradually disappear over weeks and months with a normal chest x-ray by six months to two years. The cause is thought to involve the increased distensibility and collapsibility of the premature infant's bronchial tree, with partial airway obstruction following aspiration of small amounts of milk or fluids as a result of a poorly developed gag reflex.

Retrolental Fibroplasia

Retrolental fibroplasia is an acquired disease, associated with prematurity, in which retinal pathology occurs in those infants receiving continuous oxygen therapy in high concentration. The incidence of the condition depends on 1) the concentration of oxygen given, and 2) the degree of immaturity of the eyes at the time when oxygen is given.

The disease is characterized by spasm, then obliteration, of the developing retinal vessels which is followed by neovascularization, hemorrhage, and retinal detachment. The disease has both an acute and a cicatricial phase; both eyes are affected, although different stages may be present in the two eyes; spontaneous arrest may occur at any stage.

The premature (and not the term) infant is susceptible to high oxygen concentrations because of the immaturity of retinal development. By 4 weeks gestational age, the retinal vessels have grown about 6 mm. from the optic nerve. Between 24 and 30 weeks no further growth occurs ("immature" fundus); after this time, however, growth again begins ("transitional" fundus). By about 34 weeks (weight 4 lb. 6 oz. or 2,000 gm.) the fundus is usually mature. During the "immature" and "transitional" developmental stages of the fundus, infants are liable to become victims of the disease, when injudicious concentrations of oxygen that initiate the above pathologic process are employed; hence the preponderance of this disease among the very early gestational age and very low birth weight infants.

The onset of the acute stage is usually between the ages of three weeks and three months and the smaller the birth weight, the *later* the onset. Dilatation and tortuosity of the retinal blood vessels occur, with the fundus becoming pale. Hemorrhages appear adjacent to the vessels and spread into the vitreous; separation of the retina follows.

After several weeks, the acute stages passes into the cicatricial stage, characterized by formation of the retrolental membrane. The anterior chamber becomes shallow and impairment of vision may be accompanied by squint, photophobia, and nystagmus. In severe cases, microphthalmia and secondary glaucoma may be sequelae. Because most of the damage is mechanical, one cannot determine the extent of detachment that will occur.

Management.   When the condition is detected early and proper measures are instituted promptly (i.e., reduction in concentration of oxygen administered), the condition in the infant may regress at any stage of the disease; on the other hand, partial or complete blindness may result.

Extensive research, carried on during the years since retrolental fibroplasia was first described, has established the cause and the means of prevention of the disease. It is now a fact that almost all cases of retrolental fibroplasia in the premature infant are the result of intensive oxygen therapy. Today oxygen is administered to an infant in the lowest concentration compatible with life and is discontinued as soon as feasible. The maximum oxygen concentration of the incubator housing the premature infant is kept at less than 40 percent whenever possible, and this is done only for as long as it is *absolutely* necessary (see Oxygen Therapy).

CARE OF THE HIGH RISK INFANT

Often, the first hours of the small-for-gestational-age or premature infant's life will determine the outcome. These babies need warmth, meticulous physical care, gentle handling, precise and careful feeding and protection from infection. Born either before the body systems have had enough time to develop and mature appropriately, or of a suboptimal uterine environment which has caused growth retardation, these infants must fight against almost insurmountable odds to make a viable adjustment to extrauterine life. The nurse is a key person in assisting these babies to maximize their resources in the struggle to live and grow, and in preventing the development of external complications which would further jeopardize their chances.

Resuscitation

All members of the delivery room team must be proficient at methods of ventilatory resuscitation. The necessary equipment should be readily available, including a suction apparatus for removal of mucus such as the bulb syringe and De Lee mucus trap, catheters and tubing, masks of assorted sizes, plastic airways, endotracheal tubes with obturators and adapters for bag insufflation, infant laryngoscopes with premature blades, mechanical aspiration equipment, a resuscitation surface such as a Krieselman crib or another type of overhead radiant heat, and the miscellaneous supplies and medications needed for effective resuscitation. These principles of care must be kept in mind during the treatment of depressed infants with asphyxia:

Gentleness.   These infants are often in a state of shock, and rough attempts to resuscitate them—as by vigorous spanking or other overvigorous methods of external stimulation—do more harm than good. Methods of physical stimulation should be limited to gentle rubbing of the back and, at the most, to light patting of the buttocks. When anoxia is present, oxygen is necessary to overcome it, and the use of measures which act as external irritants will not oxygenate the tissues.

Warmth.   Heated cribs and other means of maintaining body warmth, such as radiant lights and warm blankets, must be in readiness. This is particularly important to remember, because the measures employed to resuscitate infants, unless care is taken, tend to expose their completely naked bodies (accustomed to the temperature in utero) to room temperature; and this may aggravate the state of shock. The body of the infant should be kept covered as much as possible.

Posture.   Some obstetricians hold the infant up by the feet momentarily after birth in order to expedite drainage of mucus from the trachea, the larynx, and the posterior pharynx. Others cradle the baby in the arm with the hand supporting the head, which is held down. The baby is then placed on his back in a slight Trendelenburg position (head turned aside, lower than buttocks), also to favor gravity drainage of mucus.

Removal of Mucus.   Cleansing the air passages of mucus and fluid is essential, since effective respiration cannot be accomplished through obstructed air passages. The head down position will promote drainage of mucus and fluid from the respiratory passages, but postural drainage alone is often not adequate for this purpose, and suction of one type or another is frequently necessary. An ordinary catheter is used, size 12 to 14 French; in premature infants a smaller size (8 to 10) is advisable. A glass trap is inserted into the catheter to arrest mucus which otherwise might be drawn into the operator's mouth. Milking the trachea upward will help bring mucus and fluid into the posterior pharynx, where it may be aspirated by the catheter. Gentleness is essential, since the mucous membrane of the infant's mouth is delicate. Although the physician occasionally does so, the nurse should not introduce the catheter farther than the posterior pharynx. Mechanical suction devices are provided with most of the modern machines for infant resuscitation and are very convenient.

Indications for Resuscitation. Moderately depressed infants (Apgar score 4 to 6) are limp, cyanotic, or dusky and dyspneic. Respirations may be shallow, irregular, or gasping. However, the heart rate is normal, and there is at least a fair response when the sole of the foot is flicked. Management entails the same regimen described for normal infants during the first minute after birth (see Chaps. 23 and 29). If, however, effective spontaneous respiration is not established, thereafter, ventilatory support is essential, especially in the presence of continued cyanosis and flaccidity.

Any infant who has an Apgar score of 0, 1, or 2 is severely depressed and deserving of immediate treatment.

Mask and Bag Resuscitation. With the infant in a supine position, a flattened rolled towel is placed under the shoulders to extend the neck slightly. Initially, a laryngoscope is inserted. With the larynx visualized, suction is applied through a catheter attached to a De Lee trap. The trap may be operated by suction from the operator's mouth. This will assure removal of any blood clots, large-sized particles of meconium, vernix, or thick mucus. The suction catheter is then removed and a curved plastic airway is inserted between the tongue and palate to prevent the base of the tongue from falling backward over the glottic opening into the larynx.

The mask is placed over the nose and mouth to create a seal, with care taken that it does not extend over the eyes to avoid injury. Initial insufflation pressure may be 40 mm. H_2O, but as soon as the chest wall rises this is decreased to 15 to 20 mm. H_2O to prevent overexpansion and rupture of alveoli. Humidified oxygen is administered at 100 percent through the bag and mask.

The chest of the baby will rise with each squeeze of the bag if the oxygen is delivered adequately. If this procedure is effective, spontaneous respirations should begin within one minute and cyanosis and hypotonicity should disappear. Oxygen should still be supplied by mask, however, until the infant is stable. If color and respirations have not improved after one minute or the heart rate falls below 100 beats per minute at any time, endotracheal intubation is urgently indicated.

Endotracheal Intubation. With the laryngoscope in place, an endotracheal tube is introduced through the glottis and advanced until the flange of the tube meets resistance, usually about 1. to 1.5 cm. past the glottis (Fig. 38-8). The tube is held in place, while the laryngoscope is carefully removed and oxygen delivered through a bag attached to the endotracheal tube. The bag is briskly squeezed and then released at a rate of about 50 times per minute. The chest should rise and fall with insufflation and rest, and breath sounds should be heard through the stethoscope on both sides of the chest.

Generally, once the lungs are oxygenated, the response is gratifying. Immediate improvement may be noted, although intubation for ten minutes or longer is recommended. With the return of effective cardiac function, the baby becomes pink and some muscle activity can be noted. If heart activity is absent after three or four bag insufflations, external cardiac massage is mandatory. It is important to remember that *only after cardiovascular function is restored* intravenous administration of sodium bicarbonate and dextrose is essential since the hypoxia causes metabolic acidosis and may produce hypoglycemia as a result of rapid depletion of glycogen stores.

External Cardiac Massage. If the heartbeat has not returned after three or four insufflations, external cardiac massage is instituted immediately. It should be performed by an assistant, leaving the primary operator free to manage ventilation. Downward pressure is applied at the left margin of the lower sternum, thereby compressing the heart (systole). When the pressure is released, the heart is dilated (diastole).

The index and middle fingers are placed on the midthorax at the level of the sternum and the area is pressed downward and released (Fig. 38-9). The total downward displacement of the chest wall should not exceed one inch. Excessive vigor may

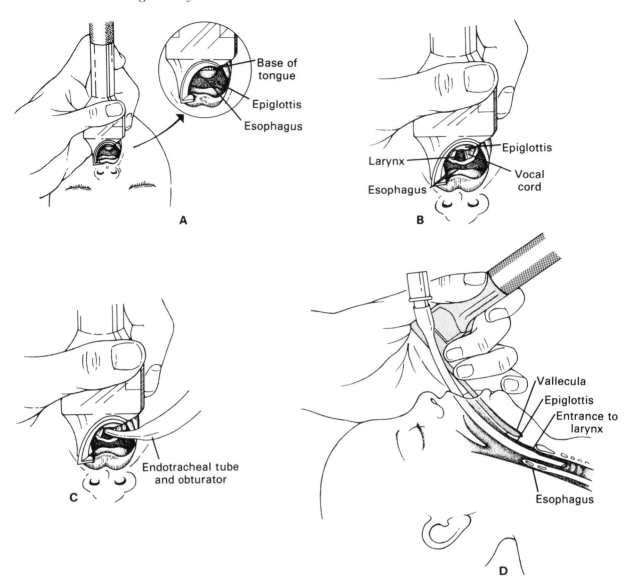

Figure 38-8. Technique of endotracheal intubation. The Miller blade should be inserted near the midline and moved to the left side of the mouth, gently deflecting the tongue. As it is advanced, the base of the tongue and epiglottis are visualized. The blade should be advanced in the same plane of movement into the vallecula (see *D*); as the blade is gently raised, the epiglottis swings anteriorly, revealing the opening of the larynx. If secretions or meconium are noted, gentle suctioning should be done before insertion of the endotracheal tube. On certain occasions when the epiglottis is not adequately raised, the blade tip may be placed posterior to the epiglottis, which can then be gently raised to expose the vocal cords. The endotracheal tube is advanced from the right corner of the mouth and inserted while maintaining direct visualization. The laryngoscope blade is then carefully withdrawn while the position of the tube is maintained by the right hand on the infant's face. Note the tip of the blade in the vallecula.

cause a laceration of the liver with severe blood loss (Fig. 38-9).

It is imperative to maintain both the cardiac massage and the ventilation. This can be accomplished by alternating the two maneuvers. The heart is compressed two or three times (approximately 120 times per minute) after which a breath of oxygen

is given. The two procedures must not be performed simultaneously because the pressure applied during cardiac massage may rupture a lung that has just been inflated by the ventilation. If the procedure is effective, the femoral or temporal artery pulses are palpable in synchrony with depression of the sternum. The procedure is to be discontinued periodically to determine the presence of spontaneous cardiac activity. When the latter occurs, cardiac compression may be discontinued.

No drugs have been found to be effective as respiratory stimulants for the infant. However, if the infant's respiratory depression is related to maternal narcosis from opiates, then the physician may administer levallorphan (Lorfan 0.25 mg.) or nalorphine (N-allylnormorphine Nalline, 0.1 mg. per kg. of body weight) into the umbilical vein. Respiration may be improved. These drugs should be used only when a specific opiate has been taken by the mother, as they otherwise will act as respiratory depressants for the baby.

Correction of Metabolic Acidosis

Prolonged hypoxia is associated with metabolic acidosis, and as part of resuscitative measures this condition must be corrected by administration of alkali, usually through an umbilical vein catheter. This procedure must not be initiated until cardiac activity has been established, even if manual ventilation is still in progress. An infusion of 10 percent glucose is started, and sodium bicarbonate administered at approximately 3 ml/kg of body weight diluted in equal amounts of glucose solution. Following alkali administration, the glucose infusion is continued with use of an infusion pump to maintain an appropriate flow rate.

General Measures

Critical observation of the infant before, during and after any procedures is especially important. The completion of necessary recording is to be accomplished quickly since early transfer of the infant is usually requested.

Because high risk babies are more susceptible to infections, asepsis is imperative. However, if the infant's condition is very labile and/or critical, the instillation of prophylactic eyedrops may have to be deferred until his condition stabilizes; in these cases, the eyes can be wiped with moist sterile gauze.

The maintenance of body temperature is essential. The high risk infant's temperature tends to fall even more precipitously than the normal infant's at birth, because of poor heat-regulating ability. Therefore the baby should be wrapped in a warmed blanket

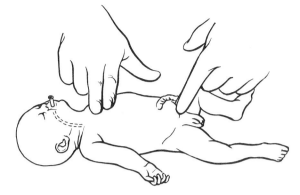

Figure 38-9. Closed-chest cardiac massage in the newborn infant. *Note:* The infant is placed on a flat surface which is tilted so that his head is on a lower level than his body, facilitating drainage of his airway. In addition, the infant's neck is extended; thus, his natural air passage is straightened.

and placed in a warm environment (90 to 92° F. or 32 to 33° C.) or under radiant overhead heat. This attention to warmth must be continued even while resuscitation is being performed.

After any immediate resuscitation efforts are concluded, the infant is generally transferred as quickly as possible to the high risk unit to ensure a proper environment. The usual weighing, temperature taking, thorough physical examination, and eye prophylaxis are generally delayed until the infant is transferred to the nursery. Obvious congenital anomalies can be noted before the infant is transferred.

Continuing Management

Because of the magnitude of the high risk problem, special nurseries and referral centers have been established for these infants in many urban areas. Space in the hospital separate from the term newborn nursery is usually allotted. In some cities, there is a large neonatal intensive care nursery (NICN) located in a medical center. When these infants must be moved from a hospital to a center or from a rural area to a hospital, effort is made whenever possible for safe transport to and from the hospital. A special transport incubator designed to maintain temperature and administer oxygen is generally used. It is strongly advised that the nurse who accompanies the infant be trained in resuscitative techniques.

As with initial management, continuing care revolves around maintaining temperature, preventing infection, and maintaining respiration and nutrition of the infant.

Neonatal Intensive Care Nursery

These special nurseries, developed to provide highly skilled nursing and medical care to high risk and sick neonates, require extensive and complicated equipment. Such life-support devices include reverse-isolation type incubators, radiant heaters, ECG-respiration-blood pressure monitors, head hoods, oxygen/air ratio controllers, oxygen analyzers, mechanical ventilators, heated nebulizers, infusion pumps, phototherapy units, and amplifying stethoscopes. The care and management of these machines are vitally important in the management of the patients. It is necessary to have technicians who can maintain this "hardware" in the intensive care nursery as well as other special units throughout the hospital. Nurses should be free from the need to "nurse the equipment" because the critical condition of their tiny patients requires constant attention and full utilization of their special skills and knowledge.

Temperature Maintenance

Many babies have subnormal temperatures, sometimes as low as 90° F. (32° C.), when they arrive at the intensive care nursery. Bringing their temperature to normal and maintaining it is extremely important, as high risk infants whose temperatures are kept between 97 and 98° F. (36 and 37° C.) from birth have significantly higher survival rates.

It is important to remember that these infants increase their heat production in cooler environments; this requires more oxygen, which places an added and at times an impossible burden on the already immature and often diseased lungs.

The body temperature of the high risk infant, as well as his respiration, is maintained in the artificial environment of the incubator, or as it is sometimes called, the Isolette. The modern air-conditioned Isolette is a miniature room in which the infant can live and be cared for under ideal conditions (i.e., desirable levels of heat, humidity and oxygen). As the infant matures, the need for all three of these elements in such exacting measured quantities will lessen. Eventually, the infant will be placed in a crib. There are several kinds of incubators currently in use, but the principle is the same, the differences being in the special construction details developed by various manufacturers.

Most incubators have controls on the outside of the unit to regulate the environment accurately and to adjust the bed from the horizontal to the tilted positions (Trendelenburg and reverse-Trendelenburg positions) to facilitate treatments and care. Some have the "Servo-Control" to automatically adjust to needed temperature and humidity settings by means of an automatic sensing device (thermistor) attached to the infant's skin. Special oxygen inlets provide adjustable oxygen concentrations (30 to 40 percent is the usual recommended "maintenance" flow). Regardless of these built-in sensors, the nurse will want to check and record the oxygen concentration with a reliable oximeter (oxygen analyzer) placed at the level of the infant's nose; a similar device can be used to ascertain the humidity level.

When oxygen therapy is no longer required, the incubator can be ventilated with fresh air from the room through a large, replaceable air filter or through an outside air attachment. Humidity can be controlled, and, by means of a nebulizer, supersaturated atmosphere can be created. Constant temperatures within the incubator can be regulated and maintained with a double-thermoswitch-controlled, sealed heating unit.

These incubators are so designed that the infant can be observed from all sides through transparent windows. Moreover, hand holes with air-tight doors and self-adjusting "sleeves" permit the nurses and the physicians to care for the infant without disturbing the atmospheric conditions (Fig. 38-10). The incubators are made of stainless steel and plastic and constructed for easy removal of all essential parts, without tools, to permit proper cleansing and sterilizing.

Prevention of Infection

Even though the incubator provides a supportive environment, maintenance of asepsis in every detail must be maintained for these fragile babies. Scrupulous hand washing and gowning technique is to be observed. Personnel are also cautioned to avoid contact with sources of infection which might be transferred to the babies. There are usually special nursery gowns which will be worn when one is assuming care of these infants. The gowning procedure will vary from institution to institution, but the underlying principle will be to keep as clean as possible anything that comes in contact with the high risk infant. Masks are infrequently used as they have been found to harbor a rich source of contam-

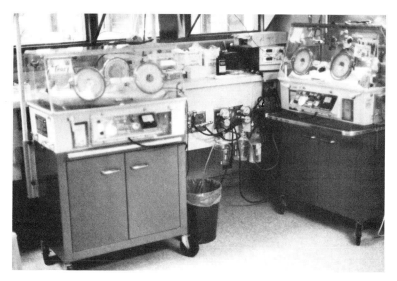

Figure 38-10. Incubators for premature infants are constructed so as to provide easy access to the infant through the hand holes so that carefully controlled environment will not be disrupted.

ination since moisture and bacteria from the nasopharynx collect in the mask folds, and even ordinary conversation distributes the infectious contents throughout the environment.

Ancillary personnel assume the task of cleaning incubators, respirators and suction equipment. All equipment is to be cultured after cleaning. Incubators that are in use are often cultured once a week and changed immediately if any bacterial growth is present. For long-term patients, it is well to change incubators once a week. For additional prophylaxis, a culture plate can be placed in each unit for two hours per day, and if any growth occurs the baby can be transferred to clean equipment.

Maintaining Respiration

As previously stated, the establishment and maintenance of respiration is of critical importance for these infants, and it is the nurse's responsibility to make careful, frequent observations and precise verbal and written recordings. It has been demonstrated that the first five minutes of life are crucial for the later successful outcome of the infant with respect to respiratory depression. Infants with unimproved respiratory function after these five minutes have a four times greater chance of dying in the first days than those infants whose condition improves or is good during this time.

Respiratory Patterns. In a quiet, larger healthy premature infant, the most common respiratory rhythm follows a steady pattern with no pause between inspiration and expiration; the next most common is the so-called adult rhythm with its inspiration, expiration, pause. Other patterns such as inspiration-pause-expiration also occur. Sighs that interrupt the regular pattern are common, and a sigh is often followed by an apneic pause. Periodic breathing, consisting of two or more periods of breathing per minute separated by an apneic pause of three seconds or more is more common among the small infants.

"Normal" respiratory rates are difficult to determine since it is difficult to define the "normal" premature and the "normal" conditions under which they prevail. Two patterns have been associated with a low mortality rate and have thus been described as "normal." In the first pattern about 40 respirations per minute occur from birth onward without any significant fluctuations. In the second pattern, rates over 60 expirations per minute occur in the first hour, with no significant increase, and subsequently decline. A significant increase is 15 or more respirations per minute above the average rate obtained in the first hour after birth.

The following patterns are always abnormal in the healthy term infant; they are also abnormal in the premature, but they are more expected because of the premature's developmental deficits.

1. *Simple retraction* may be seen, in which the chest and abdomen rise together, with a slight indentation over the sternal area. When this occurs, observations must be increased and sharpened. This pattern is a warning sign and the physician may want to be alerted.

2. *Paradoxical breathing* is considered a critical

condition; the abdomen rises while the chest sinks. There is a marked chin lag and an audible respiratory grunt, indicating respiratory distress. Since the physician should be alerted and informed of any progress in the condition, exacting observation and frequent reporting are necessary.

3. *Prolonged apnea* (which is different from the periodic apnea discussed above) often occurs in cases of respiratory distress syndrome, as well as other pathologic conditions such as infection, pneumonia and central nervous system injuries. Management usually consists of positive pressure oxygen therapy, and continuous observation since apneic spells are often repeated in these infants.

To conserve the infant's strength and prevent apnea from sheer exhaustion, other nursing measures such as bathing and weighing are scheduled with this thought in mind. Positioning the infant in a lateral Sims's position or supine position with a rolled towel under the shoulder and neck extended prevents mucus from reaching and remaining in the lungs. Changing position every two to three hours also aids in ventilating the lungs.

Oxygen Therapy

A majority of premature infants must receive oxygen initially because of respiratory depression or cyanosis or concurrent pathologic conditions such as hemorrhage or erythroblastosis. Oxygen therapy is often a life-saving measure for the infant, but it must be used judiciously and is to be administered at the lowest concentration compatible with life, since the oxygen requirements for these infants will vary according to weight, maturity and general condition of morbidity.

The administration of oxygen must be closely monitored to avoid the serious and often irreversible problems which can result from oxygen toxicity, such as bronchopulmonary dysplasia and retrolental fibroplasia. The dosage of oxygen should be adequate to relieve cyanosis, and for apneic cyanotic episodes the oxygen can be administered by mask in dosages more concentrated than 40 percent for short periods of time. Dosage is determined by laboratory blood values and may be reduced to 40 percent or less when pH is 7.35 to 7.44, arterial PO_2 is about 65 mm. Hg, and arterial hemoglobin saturation is between 85 and 90 percent.

An incubator provides a controlled source of oxygen and humidity, but it is difficult to maintain concentrations beyond 60 to 70 percent. A plastic hood is useful for oxygen levels at a constant 40 to 50 percent and can be used inside an incubator and outside during procedures (Fig. 38-11). Manual ventilatory assistance with the mask and bag is used for intermittent administration of concentrated oxygen therapy, to maintain blood gas and acid-base balance within normal ranges. Continuous positive airway pressure is generally used to improve oxygenation when the infant's respiratory efforts are inadequate, to decrease pulmonary shunting, increase residual lung capacity, and prevent atelectasis on expiration by keeping alveoli open.

Infants are weaned gradually from oxygen therapy by periodic decrements in dosage with monitoring of lab values and observations of heart rate, color, and respiratory effort.

Umbilical Catheterization

High risk neonates often require insertion of an umbilical catheter to provide a route for parenteral fluid therapy or exchange transfusions, or to obtain blood samples for gasses and metabolic studies. This is a sterile procedure in which a catheter is inserted into the umbilical artery with radiographic confirmation of placement. Antibiotic ointments and a bandage are usually applied to prevent infection, or antibiotic parenteral therapy may be used. The infant's response to the procedure is monitored and signs of complications assessed, including bleeding, emboli, infection, and blockage of the tubing.

Maintaining Nutrition

There is increasing evidence that delaying food and water in low birth weight infants lessens their chances for normal growth and development. Early feeding of these infants is associated with a reduced incidence of hyperbilirubinemia and symptomatic hypoglycemia. The nutritional requirements of low birth weight infants are higher in calories per unit of body weight than normal infants, because their growth is more comparable to that of a fetus.

During the first few days, most of these babies will need intravenous infusion of a 10 percent glucose solution with appropriate electrolytes. Caloric requirements range from 110 to 140 calories per kg. of body weight per day, depending upon maturity of the infant. Protein intake should be about 3 to 4 gm. per kg. per day, and 40 percent of the calories should be supplied by carbohydrates.

Extremely immature infants are usually given intravenous feedings. If the infant is somewhat more mature and healthy, oral feeding may start 6 to 12 hours after birth. A bottle with a soft nipple can be used if the infant is able to suck efficiently; if not, intermittent gavage is recommended. Breast-feeding may be tried for infants of 36 weeks gestational age or when a similar level of maturity is reached.

In planning the feeding schedule for the premature and low birth weight infant, it is important to establish a food tolerance, since the intestinal tract (as well as other organs) is underdeveloped. The caloric needs of the low birth weight baby are estimated according to the body weight. At first, the feeding should be in small amounts and then increased gradually to the amount that will produce a consistent gain, since vomiting and consequent aspiration, distention and diarrhea may be due to overfeeding. Early and more nearly optimal feeding in the case of the larger infant will contribute to lessening mortality and morbidity by preventing nutritive depletion and maintaining biochemical homeostasis.

Those infants in good condition (these are usually but not always the larger infants) with active peristalsis may be started on oral 5 to 10 percent glucose water 6 to 12 hours after birth. For the infant in poor condition, no matter what the cause, oral feedings are usually withheld for several days if

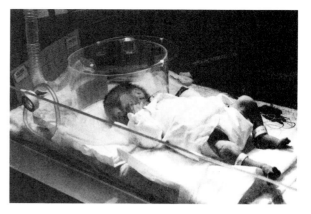

Figure 38-11. Oxygen hood maintains the level of oxygen delivered to the infant.

necessary and parenteral fluids instituted. If the infant is fed orally some physicians begin the infant on a trial of plain water; if it is retained, then glucose water or dilute modified cow's milk formula is instituted at two-hour intervals. Thus, there is a gradual replacement of water feedings by milk feedings, and a gradual increase in the amounts of milk and water at each feeding until caloric and fluid requirements are met. If an infant is taking about 180 ml. of full-strength modified cow's milk formula per kilogram of body weight per day, then he is getting about 120 calories per kilogram per day which ensures an adequate weight gain (Table 38-2).

Premature infants who weigh 1.4 kg. (3 lb.) or less may be fed every two or three hours. Infants

TABLE 38-2
DAILY FEEDING REQUIREMENTS OF LOW BIRTH WEIGHT INFANTS AND PREMATURE INFANTS

Premature, appropriate for gestational age		Low birth weight		
Item	Calories/kg/24 hr	Nutrient requirements	First week of life	Active growth period
Resting	40-50 (depending on age)	Water (ml)	80-200	130-200
Activity	10-15	Calories	50-100	110-150†
Cold stress	5-10 (depending on environmental temperature)	Protein	1-2	3-4
		Glucose } (gm)	7-12	12-15
		Fat	3-4	5-8
Specific dynamic action	8-8	Sodium	1-2	2-3
		Potassium	1-2	2-4
Fecal loss	2†-12	Chloride } (mEq)	1-2	2-3
Growth	25-25	Calcium	1-2	3-5
Total	90-120	Phosphorus	1-2	2-4
		Magnesium	—	0.5-1.0
		Iron (mg)	—	1.5-2.0

† Above 120 calories/kg. applies to infants with perinatal undergrowth.
(Source: Babson, S. G., Benson, R. C., Pernoll, M. I., and Benda, G. I.: *Management of High-Risk Pregnancy and Intensive Care of the Neonate.* St. Louis, C. V. Mosby, 1975.)

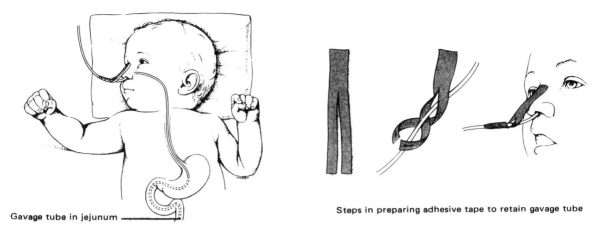

Gavage tube in jejunum _____

Steps in preparing adhesive tape to retain gavage tube

Figure 38-12. Gavage feeding. (From *The Lippincott Manual of Nursing Practice,* ed. 2. 1978.)

who weigh over 1.6 kg. (3½ lb.) may be placed on a four-hour feeding schedule. In addition to the feedings, the diets usually include vitamin and iron preparations. These additions are introduced when the feeding and schedule are fairly well established, and the infant is able to tolerate them. The stomach of the premature baby needs rest between feedings as much as that of the full-term baby; therefore, the interval should be regulated accordingly. The schedule should be as near that of a normal infant as is compatible with his progress.

Gavage Feeding.   When a very small and weak infant is on a two- to three-hour feeding schedule, gavage feeding is usually indicated (Fig. 38-12). Indwelling catheters have not been recommended because mucus is produced which can block the airway in the weak premature infant; also, purulent rhinitis and conjunctivitis may develop even with frequent tube changing; finally, the tube partially obstructs the airway.

When gavage feeding is instituted, a French catheter no. 8 is introduced through the mouth; the distance is measured from the nose to the xiphoid process and is marked on the catheter. The infant is observed for any choking or gasping, which indicates the possibility of tracheal entry.

Correct placement of the feeding catheter in the stomach is assessed by aspirating a small amount of stomach contents with a sterile syringe, injecting 5 cc. of air through the catheter into the stomach, and auscultating air bubbles over the epigastric region with a stethoscope, or placing the end of the catheter in a container of sterile water and noting if bubbles appear in conjunction with respirations.

If the tube appears to be placed in the trachea it must be removed and inserted properly. When the catheter is correctly placed, the tube is aspirated gently with a syringe; if a feeding residual of up to 1 ml. is returned, then the amount of the feeding is decreased by that amount. The residual need not be discarded; it can be fed as part of the new feeding. The nurse reports a residual of 1 ml. or more and skips that feeding. After checking the formula to determine correct temperature (tepid), the nurse will pour the formula through the barrel of the syringe; the milk is allowed to run slowly, with no pressure and minimal elevation of the syringe. During the feeding the infant is supported in a semireclining position. If the infant requires oxygen, he will be fed in the incubator. After the feeding, the infant is replaced in the incubator, and is usually positioned with the head and shoulders slightly elevated. The larger infants may be placed on the abdomen or on the right side to facilitate emptying of the stomach. These positions guard against regurgitation and aspiration.

Bottle Feeding.   Bottle-feeding requires that the infant have a good sucking and swallowing reflex which may take days or weeks to develop. The baby will indicate readiness for the bottle by consistently sucking on the gavage tubing. When bottle-feeding is instituted, the time of feeding is not to exceed 15 minutes, as this will tire the baby too much. A soft, average-sized nipple with an adequate opening is used. The infant may be helped to open his mouth to accept the nipple by applying gentle pressure on the infant's chin and touching his lips with the nipple. Again, the infant is held in the semierect position to facilitate "burping" and nursing. After the feeding the infant is positioned as described above.

There are several precautions to be aware of. The infant is not to be urged to accept more formula than is easily taken. Moreover, the bottle should be removed if the infant appears to be getting the milk too fast; in this case the infant will usually gasp,

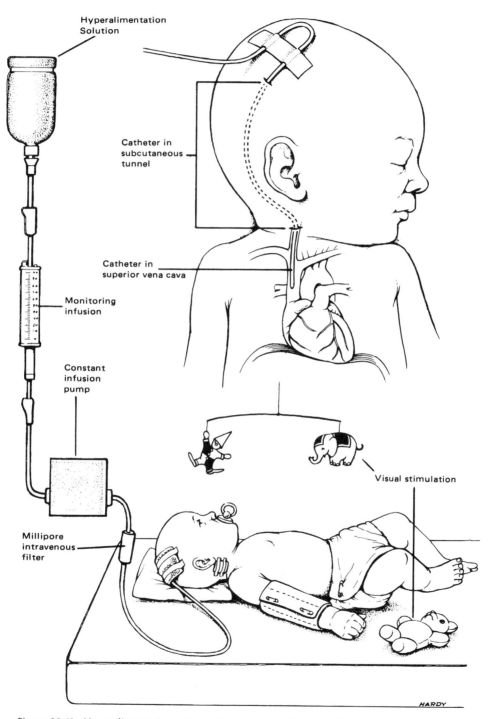

Figure 38-13. Hyperalimentation. (From *The Lippincott Manual of Nursing Practice,* ed. 2. 1978.)

choke, or swallow so quickly as to interfere with respiration. Any infant who shows reluctance to eat on two successive occasions will need critical reassessment.

Feedings are to be discontinued if the baby vomits, becomes cyanotic, overdistends or develops frequent or diarrheal stools. Feedings should also be discontinued if there is 1 ml. or more of residual; again, the infant needs reevaluation.

Finally, the bottle of the premature is never to be propped. Any change of feeding habits in these infants is critical and *may be the first sign of illness.*

Parenteral Feeding. Complete nutrition can be provided intravenously by use of hyperalimentation, and this technique can be used for substantial time periods. Hyperalimentation is generally indicated when the infant has problems of malabsorption or chronic diarrhea, requires surgery for repair of gastrointestinal abnormalities, or cannot be fed by other routes. The solution used contains glucose, electrolytes, vitamins, minerals and protein hydrolysate. An intravenous infusion using a scalp vein, or a cutdown with a catheter threaded through a scalp or arm vein, is used for administering the solution (Fig. 38-13). It is usually delivered through constant infusion pump to assure regulated flow and is monitored carefully. No other substances are generally administered through this feeding catheter. Pacifiers may be used to satisfy the infant's sucking reflex if it is present.

Other Nursing Measures

The other necessary care of the infant such as temperature taking, weighing, bathing, and dressing (if required) is usually done in conjunction with the feeding periods, so that the infant may rest without interference at the other times. The nurse will want to gather any materials needed and plan care carefully. Frequently entering the incubator is not in the interests of good aseptic technique and, of course, is very tiring to the infant.

The skin is extremely delicate and tender; and if diapers are used, they should be changed as soon as they become wet or soiled. Sometimes only a small pad is placed under the baby. Indeed, no clothing is really needed because of the controlled environment of the incubator.

Each institution will have its particular procedures for routine care in the intensive care nursery, but the principles are the same as those involved in attending the normal newborn.

GROWTH AND DEVELOPMENT

Studies of high risk infants born since the introduction of perinatal intensive care in the last two decades indicate that both mortality and morbidity have significantly decreased. Contributing to this improvement have been early identification of high risk pregnancies, maintenance of an appropriate thermal environment for the neonate, early correction of neonatal acidosis, hypoglycemia and hyperbilirubinemia, and refinement and widespread use of continuous distending pressure and ventilatory assistance methods.

In considering neurological and developmental deficiencies associated with low birth weight infants, data are confounded by the grouping together of premature (appropriate for gestational age) and small-for-gestational-age infants who also may have been born prematurely. In addition, varying criteria are used to define abnormalities, and the effects of socioeconomic status often are not included. With these limitations in mind, results of more recent studies indicate that low birth weight infants have IQ scores comparable to full-term infants at two to five years of age. Neurological studies indicate a decreased incidence of cerebral palsy, in the range of 3 to 4 percent compared to an average from previous studies of about 10 percent. Subtle neurological deficiencies vary by study design, but it appears that visual impairments and speech abnormalities are not uncommon. Studies of growth generally demonstrate a lag in low birth weight infants compared to standard growth charts, with the small-for-gestational-age infants lagging in all parameters in comparison to appropriate-for-gestational-age infants of the same birth weight.[13]

Growth and development of the premature depend primarily on the degree of immaturity at birth. Much will depend on the ability of the infant to meet the conditions attendant at birth and to adjust to the changes in the new environment. The majority (about 65 percent) of prematures weigh between 2,000 and 2,500 gm. Outcomes for these infants are good, barring complications. An additional 20 percent weigh between 1,500 to 2,000 gm. and if prompt good care is provided, they also have a chance of a good outcome. As birth weight decreases, chances of satisfactory growth and development also decrease, even though "survival" rates may be good. In general, infants who react well to prompt treatment and care make their adjustment usually by the end of the first year.

Small-for-gestational-age infants with intrauterine growth retardation have different outcomes for growth and development depending upon the cause of retardation, the severity and duration of the intrauterine insult, the extent and management of perinatal asphyxia, and early diagnosis and management of various metabolic and physiological problems. Physical growth (weight, length, head circumference) does not catch up to normal infants during the first few years of life, even with adequate caloric intake. Studies have found that IQs of small-for-gestational-age infants are generally similar to normal children, and the incidence of overt neurological handicaps is low. However, there is a high incidence of abnormal electroencephalograms, minimal brain damage, and school problems.[14]

The nurse is often asked by the parents if their premature or low birth weight baby will ever develop as well and become as strong and sturdy as a normal sized newborn. Depending upon birth weight, the infant has a good chance of doing so.

The developmental level achieved by the small premature infant during his first year generally will be lower than that expected for his chronologic age. For this reason, parents are encouraged to think of premature babies in terms of actual age since conception, which gives more realistic expectations for developmental level.

Parents of premature or low birth weight infants invariably need special guidance and support to help them develop confidence in their ability to care for their baby, particularly in anticipation of taking him home from the hospital. The nurse has a real responsibility to help them so that they are adequately prepared for the baby's homecoming.

CARE OF THE MOTHER AND FATHER

The parents of high-risk newborns often have adaptational needs or problems which necessitate sensitive and thoughtful nursing care. Not only are they making the transition to new parenthood with all its requirements, but they must cope with the unusual situation of a small, different and often sick baby. The importance of the early postpartum period for establishment of bonds between parents and the newborn and laying the groundwork for healthy attitudes toward future relationships with the child must not be underestimated.

Interactional Deprivation. Prolonged mother-infant separation, such as is routine practice in most premature and high risk nurseries, is currently under investigation for its effects on attachment. As soon as possible after the infant's birth, the mothers in the early contact group are admitted into the nursery and encouraged to touch their babies and to perform such caretaking duties as the infant's condition allows. Mothers in the late contact group are not permitted into the nursery until after their infants reach almost one month of age. Results to date reveal detectable differences in mothering performance between these two groups. In one study, high contact mothers had higher scores on an attachment interview, maternal performance, "en face" feeding and the amount of fondling of infants when tested one month after delivery.[15] In another study comparing late and early contact mothers one month after discharge of the infants, and after 200 feedings at home, the late contact mothers held their babies differently, changed positions and burped less, and were not as skillful in feeding.[16] Some mothers who were barred from interaction with their babies in the nursery resumed prior interests when they returned home, and the babies had to compete with these interests when they were discharged.

Such studies suggest that prolonged separation may adversely affect commitment or attachment between mother and infant, reduce confidence in mothering abilities, and detract from the mother's ability to develop an efficient routine of care. When mothers were allowed into the high risk nursery for early and frequent contact and caretaking of their infants, there was no increase in nursery infections or disruption of nursery routine.[17]

Modifying hospital routine to allow mothers early contact with their high risk infants appears to have a positive effect on later maternal behavior (Figs. 38-14 and 38-15). This lends support to the concept of a sensitive time for bonding to occur between the human mother and her infant. This time is probably within the first several hours of delivery. Greater maternal attentiveness and better caretaking seem related to later exploratory behavior in infants;

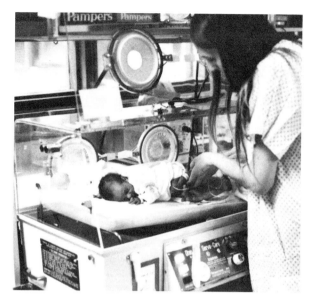

Figure 38-14. Allowing the mother to attend to the infant in the incubator enhances mother-infant bonding.

thus, removing barriers to maternal attachment during the sensitive period may have a potent influence on the later development of these babies.

Parental Reactions and Psychological Tasks

The birth of a premature or high risk infant is often experienced as an acute emotional crisis by the family. This causes a certain amount of disorganization in the parents before they are able to master their feelings and come to accept the event. Since the baby may be born before term, parents often are deprived of the last six to eight weeks in which the final psychologic (and sometimes material) preparation for the birth is made. Few of the physical and emotional signs of approaching labor (enumerated in Chapter 23) may happen. These are helpful to the mother in alerting her to the near approach of another new phase in the childbearing process, and this awareness in turn assists her in achieving psychologic preparation. The result, then may be a rather abrupt arrival of the infant, and the event may be surrounded by several anxiety-provoking features: an unattended delivery, a longer hospital stay for her baby and perhaps herself, separation from her infant, and most heartrending of all, a delicate infant who may be in danger of death.

Guilt feelings and a certain amount of grieving in both parents are an invariable accompaniment.

The parents ask themselves time and again such questions as: "What went wrong? What did we do? What made it happen? Can I really carry babies?" These guilt feelings and grief may be manifested in a variety of ways: general anger with the whole situation, self-deprecation, numerous complaints, blaming the spouse and/or attendants, insistent bids for reassurance and attention, profuse crying, or extreme quiet and immobilization.

Loneliness is also a problem, for the mother may have no opportunity to see, hold, feed and examine her child as the other mothers have. We are all familiar with the wistful figure at the nursery window, gazing longingly through the glass, while the other mothers are occupied with feeding, changing and cuddling their infants. The loneliness continues when the parents go home without their infant, and because of the continued separation, the task of integrating the new member into the household is delayed.

In addition, most mothers are concerned about whether they will be able to take adequate care of their babies when they do bring them home. The mother may still carry a picture of the frail infant

Figure 38-15. Enface contact between mother and infant should be encouraged when the infant is removed briefly from the incubator.

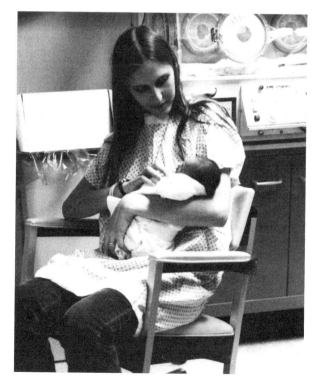

surrounded by all the nursery paraphernalia and not realize that her baby will be reasonably mature when discharged from the hospital.

To cope with this concern, she may ask many questions while she is in the hospital and demand reassurance about the baby's condition; on the other hand, she may be quiet and uncommunicative, quite overwhelmed with the anticipated enormous responsibility.

The psychologic processes the parents generally go through after the birth of a premature or high risk infant include:

shock, disbelief and denial;

anger and searching self and others for causes;

grieving over loss of perfect fantasized infant;

grieving over own inability to produce perfect infant;

anticipatory worrying over loss of infant;

initiation of contact with infant;

belief and desire that infant will live;

readiness to establish caretaking relationship.

Supportive Care

Although there is much that is specialized in the physical care activities for the premature infant, the mother's physical care remains generally the same as that for any normal postpartal course. Thus, the emphasis on care for these mothers is two-fold: 1) they need help to facilitate their emotional adjustment (this holds true for the father as well) and 2) they need help in preparing for the care of the infant when they bring him home.

The nurse can do much to strengthen the mother's ego by helping her work through her guilt feelings and grief and thus reinforce her concept of herself as an adequate, worthy person. To do this, the nurse must provide opportunities for the mother to ventilate her feelings and to question the situation. It is often difficult for the nurse to answer all the questions the mother and father ask, especially if the prognosis for the baby is guarded. Yet, to avoid the questions or problems is to deprive the parents of a valuable avenue of coping with the problem. The fears and fantasies engendered by not knowing are often worse than the facts, even though the facts are unfortunate.

As the nurse listens to the mother and the father and reflects their concerns, they are helped to arrive at a clearer notion of the reality of the situation;

thus they are able to separate fact from fancy and to work through to a more positive acceptance of their situation. The nurse can expect some negative feelings to be expressed, and the patient may go through a period of self-pity. An accepting, nonjudgmental attitude will help the patient to move to a more positive frame of mind.

Keeping the lines of communication open between the nursery staff and the patient is another useful supportive measure; the nurse on the postpartal unit can be prepared with the latest reports regarding the baby's condition, so that this information can be given to the parents. Especially when the mother cannot be taken to see her baby in the premature nursery, it is very helpful if the nurse in the premature unit can make regular visits to the mother on the ward to inform her of her infant's progress. If circumstances within the unit prevent this, contact with the mother by telephone may be substituted. This two-way communication between the floor and the nursery helps the patient to feel that everyone is "tuned in" on her situation and concerned about her. It also gives her the opportunity to know the personnel who are responsible for the care of her baby, and this is reassuring in itself.

Visiting the Nursery. When the mother is able, she can be allowed to visit the nursery at least to observe her baby for a time. Some mothers find this difficult at first, especially if the infant is very small and/or ill. It is a wise nurse who allows the mother to indicate her readiness for such visits and gives appropriate encouragement as the mother is able to face the situation and take more responsibility.

Before the mother comes to the nursery, it is best to describe all the equipment surrounding the infant and what the baby will look like. The nurse's presence beside the mother when she first sees her baby permits any questions to be answered and provides support during this difficult period. If the infant is under the bilirubin light, it is important to remove the eye patches so the mother can see the baby's eyes.

Other Sources of Support. All avenues of support are to be explored with the parents. If the mother seems to benefit from visitors or visiting with the other patients, then there need be no restriction of visiting privileges. There is no reason to isolate a mother in a room by herself (even if there has been a fetal demise) without ascertaining whether the mother needs to be alone for a time. If possible, the same nurse should be assigned to her care, for if the mother is to work through her feelings, she must have time to build a trust relationship, and this takes at least several encounters.

Other personnel, such as the social worker, may be helpful if aid is needed financially or strict budgeting is necessary. Another source of help that can prove invaluable is the public health or visiting nurse. The need for a referral for these patients and their infants should never be overlooked. Most patients are delighted to have someone to rely on during the first difficult days when they bring the baby home. Furthermore, some patients cannot make much progress in expressing their feelings and in working through the problem during their short hospital stay. Thus, they need a competent person when they return home to help them in this, as well as in making necessary arrangements in preparation for the baby's homecoming.

Instructions for Home Care.   Some hospitals encourage mothers to return to the nursery to feed and care for their babies until such time as the infant's condition permits discharge. Of particular help would be a counseling program on feeding and psychologic aspects of care, which incorporates anticipatory guidance concerning the condition and the needs of the infant on arrival home. Coping with sibling rivalry also may be included. This approach is very helpful, for it alleviates some of the separation and loneliness between mother and child and later fosters self-reliance and confidence in the mother at home.

Crisis Management.   In implementing care, the nurse will want to remember that the advent of a high risk birth is a crisis in itself; however, the parents may have to adjust to various related crises (e.g., a sudden, downward turn in the baby's condition, financial embarrassment, unexpected developments regarding other children and relatives). Nurses must be prepared to help the parents to deal with these as they arise, and to seek appropriate resources for them if the matter lies beyond their competence. Knowledge of the principles of communication and supportive care will be utilized here as they would be in any other crisis. Willingness and ability to allow the parents to ventilate and work through their feelings about the situation is of prime importance. The nurse is one of the key persons in the care of high risk infants and their parents.

REFERENCES

1. J. C. Hobbins, and R. L. Berkowitz: "Ultrasolography in the diagnosis of intrauterine growth retardation." *Amer. J. of Obstet. & Gynecol.* 129, 5: 957, Nov. 1, 1977.

2. R. M. Pilkin, and J. R. Scott: The Yearbook of Obstetrics and Gynecology, 1978. Chicago, Yearbook Medical Publishers, 1978, p. 173.

3. D. B. Cheek et al.:"Factors controlling fetal growth." *Clin. Obstet. & Gynecol.* 20, 4: 925–942, Dec. 1977.

4. H. Baker et al.: "Vitamin levels in low birth weight newborn infants and their mothers." *Amer. J. Obstet. & Gynecol.* 129, 5:521, Nov. 1, 1977.

5. Cheek, op. cit.

6. F. D. Frigoletto, and S. B. Rothchild: "Altered fetal growth: An overview." *Clin. Obstet. & Gynecol.* 20, 4:918–919, Dec. 1977.

7. Cheek, op. cit.

8. Ibid.

9. M. H. Klaus, and A. A. Fanaroff: *Care of the High Risk Neonate.* Philadelphia, W. B. Saunders, 1973.

10. C. L. Cetrulo, and R. Freeman: "Bioelectric evaluation of intrauterine growth retardation." *Clin. Obstet. & Gynecol.* 20, 4:979–989, Dec. 1977.

11. R. Sullivan, et al.: "Determining a newborn's gestational age." *MCN—J. Maternal Child Nurs.* 38-45, Jan./Feb. 1979.

12. W. Oh.: "Considerations in neonates with intrauterine growth retardaion." *Clin. Obstet. & Gynecol.* 20, 4:991–1003, Dec. 1977.

13. B. C. Dangman, and J. M. Driscoll: "Impact of perinatal intensive care on outcome." In *Perinatal Intensive Care.* S. Aladjem and A. Brown, eds. St. Louis, C. V. Mosby, 1977, pp. 396–412.

14. Oh, op. cit.

15. M. H. Klaus, et al.: "Maternal attachment: Importance of the first postpartum days. *New Eng. J. Med.* 286:460, 1972.

16. M. H. Klaus, and J. H. Kennell: "Mothers separated from their newborn infants." *Ped. Clin. North Am.* 17:1015–1037, Nov. 1970.

17. C. Barnett, et al.: "Neonatal separation: The maternal side of interactional deprivation." *Pediatrics* 45:197, 1970.

SUGGESTED READING

Black, M.: "Assessment of weight and gestational age." *Nurs. Clinics of North Amer.* 13, 1: 13-22, March 1978.

Minor, H.: "Problems and prognosis for the small-for-gestational-age and the premature infant." *MCN—Amer. J. Maternal Child Nurs.* 221–226, July/Aug. 1978.

Bliss, V. J.: "Nursing care for infants with neonatal necrotizing enterocolities." *MCN—J. Maternal Child Nurs.* 37–40, Jan./Feb. 1976.

Koch, J.: "Code pink: A system for neonatal resuscitation." *JOGN Nurs.* 49–53, Sept./Oct. 1978.

Sham, B. and Messerly, A. M.: "Apnea in the premature infant." *Nurs. Clinics of North Amer.* 13, 1:29–37, March 1978.

Pape, K. E.: "Central nervous system pathology associated with mask ventilation in the very low birth weight infant: A new etiology for intracerebellar hemorrhages." *Pediatrics* 58, 4: 473, Oct. 1976.

Dweck, H. S.: "Neonatal hypoglycemia and hypercalcemia." *Postgraduate Med.* 60, 1:92–97, July 1976.

Harris, H.: "Cardiorespiratory problems in the newborn." *Postgraduate Med.* 60, 1:92–97, July 1976.

Maherzi, M.: et al.: "Urinary tract infection in high risk newborn infants." *Pediatrics* 62, 4: 521–523, Oct. 1978.

Naeye, R.: "Neonatal apnea: Underlying disorders." *Pediatrics* 63, 1:8–11, Jan. 1979.

Fomon, S. J., and Ziegler, E. E.: "Milk of the premature infant's mother: Interpretation of data." *J. Pediatrics* 93, 1:164, July 1978.

Babson, S. G., Benson, R. C., Pernoll, M. L., and Benda, G. I.: *Management of High Risk Pregnancy and Intensive Care of the Neonate,* ed. 3. St. Louis, C. V. Mosby, 1975.

Korones, S.: *High Risk Newborn Infants—The Basis for Intensive Nursing Care,* ed. 2. St. Louis, C. V. Mosby, 1976.

Thirty-Nine

The High Risk Infant: Developmental and Environmental Disorders

Birth Trauma and Anoxia / Congenital and Genetic Anomalies / Inborn Errors of Metabolism / Neonatal Problems Secondary to Maternal Disorders / Infections / Addiction Syndromes / Musculoskeletal Defects / Parental and Staff Reactions to Defects and Disorders

During labor, delivery and the first several hours of neonatal life, many changes occur in the fetus and neonate which allow physiologic adaptation to extrauterine life. Developmental characteristics of the infant may have significant influences on this process of moving from intrauterine to extrauterine life, such as genetic or congenital abnormalities and size and gestational age (discussed in Chapter 38). Environmental factors also have an impact upon this transition, including such intrauterine influences as maternal disease and disorders, intrapartal factors such as birth trauma and anoxia, and postnatal infections and physiologic processes as affected by the newborn's environmental systems. Although the majority of neonates make this transition without difficulty, for some their later normal development and immediate survival depend in large part upon the acuity and skill of the delivery room and nursery teams in identifying and managing complications.

In some cases, high risk factors can be identified prenatally and the delivery and nursery teams alerted to a potential high risk birth. Often, however, problems may not be apparent until labor or during delivery with the occurrence of such conditions as dystocia, abnormal fetal heart rate patterns, and birth asphyxia. Other difficulties may have their onset several hours or days after birth. Perinatal teams must be constantly alert to signs of complications in the neonate, with the objectives of identifying problems early, correcting disorders quickly (or minimizing subsequent effects), preventing permanent disabilities, and promoting the parental bonding process.

BIRTH TRAUMA AND ANOXIA

Immediate observation of the newborn in the delivery room usually permits the nurse to identify injuries or anoxia resulting from the birth process. Some kinds of birth trauma require emergency intervention to save the infant's life; others can be treated later or resolve spontaneously in several days. A thorough neonatal assessment, alertness to subtle changes in the newborn's behavior and condition, efficient communication and careful recording of observations, and facility with emergency techniques enable the nurse to promote the well-being of high risk infants. Communicating with parents by providing information and support is also a major nursing responsibility (see pages 707–714).

Neonatal Asphyxia

The failure to initiate or maintain normal respiratory patterns at birth is a severe life-threatening emergency requiring immediate intervention to save the infant's life and prevent anoxic cellular damage. Usually, normal respiratory patterns are established almost immediately, and by one minute the infant is pink, crying and active with a heart rate of 120 to 160 beats per minute, normal reflexes and muscle tone, and an Apgar score of 8 to 10. If asphyxia has occurred, the infant will be apneic.

Primary apnea occurs when asphyxia has been prolonged over one to two minutes, with mild bradycardia and hypotension. The newborn is cyanotic with diminished reflexes, bradycardia of 60 to 100 per minute, and an Apgar of 3 to 5. Following gentle suctioning and the administration of oxygen, gasping respirations usually begin after about two minutes. Rapid improvement often follows, with the five-minute Apgar score reaching 8 to 10. Without other complicating conditions, these infants have an excellent immediate and long-term prognosis.

Secondary apnea occurs when there is severe bradycardia and hypotension, and death will follow shortly if there is not immediate resuscitation. The newborn is ashen, heart sounds are distant with weak pulses and bradycardia between 20 and 60 beats per minute, reflexes are absent, and the Apgar score is 1 to 3. No gasping movements are initiated with stimulation, and the infant must be resuscitated (see Chapter 38). Spontaneous respiration may not begin for 5 to 15 minutes after resuscitation is started. There is danger of irreversible effects of anoxia with long-term disabilities.[1]

The three causes of intrauterine injury of the central nervous system—narcosis, hypoxia, and brain hemorrhage—all produce a similar clinical syndrome of asphyxia, characterized by apnea. The course and prognosis of this syndrome vary with the degree of hypoxia, the location and extent of the hemorrhage, and the degree of hypercapnia and acidosis. This acidotic asphyxial state is more injurious and difficult to correct than hypoxia alone.

The normal oxygen saturation of the arterial blood of the fetus at birth is approximately 60 percent, but in severe cases may drop as low as 12 percent. In addition, the blood of these infants has a high concentration of lactic acid and a very low pH.

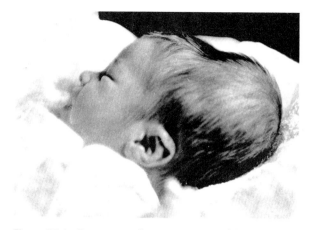

Figure 39-1. Caput succedaneum (MacDonald House, University Hospitals of Cleveland).

Management is aimed at correcting metabolic acidosis as well as maintaining tissue oxygenation. Any underlying disorder (hypoglycemia, anemia) must also be identified and corrected.

Prevention of asphyxia begins with the first antepartal visit when the pelvis is measured to make sure that it is large enough to allow passage of the infant's head without compression. Good diet and hygiene contribute greatly to the health of the infant at birth. During labor, asphyxia of the infant can be prevented through careful use of analgesic and anesthetic drugs and by avoiding as much as possible the more difficult types of operative delivery. Moreover, by monitoring the fetal heart tones, the nurse may detect early signs of impending fetal distress (slow and/or irregular rate), and, with this warning, it may be possible for the infant to be delivered before serious trouble develops. The passage of meconium-stained amniotic fluid in a cephalic presentation is another sign of fetal distress.

Caput Succedaneum

Prolonged pressure on the head during a protracted first stage of labor, when the membranes rupture before the cervix is fully dilated, causes an edematous swelling of the soft tissues of the scalp over the area where it is encircled by the cervix (Fig. 39-1). This condition is called *caput succedaneum,* and in its milder forms is very common—so common that it may be regarded as normal.

It is due to an extravasation of serum into the tissues of the scalp at the portion surrounded by the

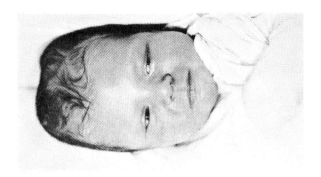

Figure 39-2. Cephalhematoma (MacDonald House, University Hospitals of Cleveland).

cervix. The term is not confined to vertex cases; the corresponding swelling which forms on any presenting part is also, for the sake of uniformity, known as caput succedaneum.

The condition always disappears within a few days without treatment. A prompt and simple explanation should be given to the parents, since this condition, although benign, can be somewhat disfiguring. Once the parents know that the caput succedaneum will disappear of its own accord, they usually are reassured and will not press for "treatment."

Cephalhematoma

Cephalhematoma is another swelling of the scalp which resembles caput succedaneum in certain respects (Fig. 39-2). It is caused by an effusion of blood between the bone and the periosteum (Fig. 39-3). This explains why the swelling appears directly over the bone. It is most common over the parietal bones. It is seldom visible when the infant

is born and may not be noticed for several hours or more after delivery, since subperiosteal bleeding occurs slowly.

The cephalhematoma increases gradually in size until about the seventh day after birth, when it remains stationary for a time and then begins to disappear. The infant usually recovers without treatment.

Cephalhematoma may be due to pressure exerted in normal labor or by forceps; but it is also seen occasionally in breech cases in which no instruments were used or prolonged pressure exerted on the aftercoming head. Such cases, however, are not common.

Sometimes an x-ray will reveal a linear skull fracture beneath the hematoma. However, there are no known pathologic sequelae, even in the presence of a fracture. Occasionally, especially if the condition is bilateral, hyperbilirubinemia may result from the breakdown of the accumulated blood. Again, the parents should receive assurance regarding the temporary nature of this condition and its spontaneous disappearance.

Intracranial Hemorrhage (Cerebral Hemorrhage, Subdural Hematoma)

In contrast to the two conditions just described, *intracranial hemorrhage* is one of the gravest complications encountered in the newborn. It may occur any place in the cranial vault, but is particularly likely to take place as the result of tears in the tentorium cerebelli with bleeding into the cerebellum, the pons, and the medulla oblongata. Since these structures contain many important centers

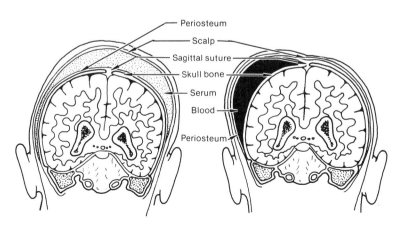

Periosteum
Scalp
Sagittal suture
Skull bone
Serum
Blood
Periosteum

Figure 39-3. Comparative diagram of the underlying pathophysiology in caput succedaneum (*Left*), and cephalhematoma (*Right*).

such as the respiratory center, hemorrhage in these areas is very often fatal.

Intracranial hemorrhage occurs most often after prolonged labor, especially in primiparae, and is particularly likely to take place in difficult forceps deliveries and in version and extractions. It is also seen more commonly in precipitate deliveries as the result of the rapid propulsion of the infant's head through the birth canal. It is due primarily to excessive or unduly prolonged pressure on the fetal skull. This causes excessive molding of the head and such overriding of the cranial bones that the delicate supporting structures of the brain (tentorium cerebelli, falx cerebri) are torn, with consequent rupture of blood vessels.

Manifestations. The development of symptoms in cerebral hemorrhage may be sudden or gradual. If the hemorrhage is severe, the infant is usually stillborn; if less marked, apnea of the newborn may result, often with fatal outcome. Many infants who are resuscitated with difficulty at birth succumb later from brain hemorrhage. On the other hand, the infant may appear normal after delivery and develop the first signs of intracranial hemorrhage several hours or several days later.

If any of the following common signs of cerebral hemorrhage occur, they should be reported immediately.

1. *Convulsions.* Convulsions may vary from mild, localized twitchings to severe pain spasms of the whole body. Twitching of the lower jaw is characteristic, particularly when associated with salivation.
2. *Cyanosis.* Cyanosis may be persistent but is more likely to occur in repeated attacks.
3. *Abnormal Respiration.* Grunting respiration is characteristic; or it may be irregular, of Cheyne-Stokes type, very rapid and shallow, or very slow. Very slow breathing, usually associated with cyanosis, suggests respiratory paralysis due to pressure on the medulla oblongata and is a grave sign.
4. *A Sharp, Shrill, Weak Cry.* This cry is similar to that seen in meningitis.
5. *Flaccidity or Spasticity.* If this condition is present, it usually portends a fatal outcome. Somnolence also may be present. In other cases there may be generalized spasticity with backward arching of the head and neck and extension of the legs (*opisthotonos*).

Management. Prevention is most important and is largely the responsibility of the provider conducting the delivery. It consists of protecting the infant from trauma, particularly in difficult or precipitate deliveries. Many obstetricians believe that the administration of vitamin K to the mother before delivery decreases the likelihood of cerebral bleeding. This is done less frequently now due to the possibility of hyperbilirubinemia. A small dose of water-soluble vitamin K_1 (1.0 mg.) may be given the infant after birth, however.

Curative treatment can be effective if damage is not too extensive.

Complete rest with the very minimum amount of handling is imperative. Infants suspected of having a cerebral hemorrhage are placed in intensive care. Supportive measures such as maintaining heat and oxygenation, and monitoring vital signs are employed along with intravenous feeding or gavage. If a subdural hematoma is suspected, a spinal tap will be done for diagnostic purposes and excess subdural bloody fluid may be removed as a therapeutic measure. Usually the physician will order some form of sedative for convulsions. Vitamin C and water-soluble vitamin K may be used to control the hemorrhage, and antibiotics may be given prophylactically. The head of the infant is kept a few inches above the level of the hips, because this position is believed to lower intracranial pressure. Moreover, the infant should *not* be placed in Trendelenburg position after delivery.

The outcome for the infant depends upon the location and extensiveness of the hemorrhage, the amount of CNS damage, and other complicating conditions such as respiratory and metabolic problems. The prognosis is guarded, and among those infants who live, there is the risk of mental retardation and cerebral palsy.

Perinatal Hemorrhage and Shock

The neonate with a hemorrhagic condition may have suffered intrauterine hemorrhage or hemolysis. As the average blood volume of a term infant is about 80 ml. per kg., rapid blood loss of as little as 50 ml. can cause shock. Intrauterine bleeding can occur from fetal to maternal circulation, from one twin to another, or from placental problems such as rupture of abnormal vessels, abruptio placentae and placenta previa.

The newborn with severe *hypovolemic shock* appears collapsed and presents a clinical picture similar to that of asphyxia, except that tachycardia is usually seen with hemorrhage and bradycardia with asphyxia. Symptoms include pallor and cyanosis, hypotonia, decreased or absent pulses and movement, gasping and retractions, tachypnea, tachycardia, and weak or absent cry.

Treatment is instituted immediately with placement of an umbilical catheter and withdrawal of blood for hemoglobin and hematocrit values, platelet count, Coombs' test, cross-matching and coagulation screen. Blood volume is then rapidly expanded by transfusion, usually with group O Rh-negative blood, or plasma (fresh or substitute) if blood is not immediately available. Subsequent management will depend upon identification of the source of hemorrhage.

Hemorrhage may also develop following birth, due to coagulation defects, internal bleeding as a result of organ laceration during traumatic delivery, and hemorrhage into the scalp due to trauma or vacuum delivery. Treatment requires careful diagnosis of the cause of bleeding. Because infants have a deficiency of most clotting factors at birth, vitamin K is administered to counteract these physiologic deficiencies. Disseminated intravascular coagulation may occur secondary to sepsis, hypoxia, acidosis and maternal eclampsia. Deficiency in the number or quality of platelets also causes hemorrhage in the newborn, characterized by cutaneous petechiae and purpuric spots.

Hemorrhage from Cord

Hemorrhage from the cord may be of two types: 1) primary, due to the umbilical clamp slipping or becoming loose, and 2) secondary, coming from the base of the cord when it separates from the body of the baby.

In the first instance, the bleeding is from the end of the cord, not from its base, and can be controlled by the proper application of a fresh clamp.

The secondary hemorrhage, from the base of the cord, occurs at about the fifth to the eighth day when separation takes place. It is often preceded by a slight jaundice; it is not an actual flow of blood but a persistent oozing which frequently resists treatment. This variety of hemorrhage, which is a rare occurrence, is usually due to one of two causes: 1) the baby may be syphilitic, or 2) the peculiar condition known as hemorrhagic diathesis may be present. In this condition, the baby's blood shows no disposition to coagulate, and bleeding from any denuded surface is persistent and often profuse.

Management. The nurse's responsibility in the treatment of secondary hemorrhage from the cord consists in applying a sterile dressing to the bleeding surface. The physician should be notified promptly. If the use of the dressing has not effectually controlled the oozing the physician will doubtless clamp the base of the umbilicus

When this form of bleeding is at all severe and persistent, recovery is doubtful; and even if the umbilical hemorrhage is controlled, bleeding may appear in the nose, the mouth, the stomach, the intestines, or the abdominal cavity; or purpuric spots may develop on various parts of the body. The prompt administration of vitamin K has greatly improved the prognosis in these cases.

Facial Paralysis

Pressure by forceps on the facial nerve may cause temporary paralysis of the muscles of one side of the face so that the mouth is drawn to the other side. This will be particularly noticeable when the infant cries. The condition is usually transitory and disappears in a few days, often in a few hours. Since the infant can look grotesque, the parents will need an explanation concerning the temporary nature of this affliction.

If the mother is allowed to feed the baby, the nurse will want to be with her more consistently during the first feedings to help her as necessary. Sucking may be difficult for the infant, and the mother will need to develop patience and skill in the feeding of her baby.

If one eye remains open because of the affected muscles, the physician will prescribe such treatment as is appropriate. Any necessary instruction regarding this continuing care after discharge should be given the mother before she leaves the hospital.

Very often parents are afraid to handle their infants when disorders occur for fear of hurting the child; this may happen even if the condition is short-term and fairly innocuous. Thus, parents should be encouraged to hold and cuddle their infants whenever the condition permits.

Arm Paralysis (Erb-Duchenne's Paralysis, Brachial Palsy)

This condition results from excessive stretching of the nerve fibers that run from the neck through the shoulder and down toward the arm (brachial plexus). It is a result of the shoulder being forcibly pulled away from the head during delivery, usually during a breech extraction.

Generally, only the muscles of the upper arm are involved, and the infant holds his arm at the side with the elbow extended and the hand rotated inward. The hand and fingers may not be involved. If the nerves are merely stretched, recovery occurs in several weeks; if they are broken within their sheaths, healing will not be complete for several months. If healing fails to occur within that time, surgery is indicated; the outcome for recovery in these cases is guarded.

To reduce tension on the brachial plexus, the physician usually will place the arm in a splint or cast in an elevated, neutral position. While the arm is healing, the physician will order gentle manipulation and massage of the muscles to prevent contractures. The mother is to be instructed in these procedures so that she may continue the care.

Fractures and Dislocations

Fracture of a long bone or dislocation of an extremity may be the result of a version; or it may occur following a breech delivery in which the arms were extended above the head and were brought down into the vagina.

Fractures of the clavicle or of the jaw, or dislocation of either of these bones, may follow forcible efforts to extract the aftercoming head in cases of breech presentation.

Fracture or dislocation of the cervical spine, usually accompanied by damage to the spinal cord, may also be the consequence of a difficult breech extraction. The vertebrae most usually affected are C5 and C6. If the cord is not completely severed, surgical repair is often effected. These babies will have a flaccid paralysis of the trunk and extremities and breathe abdominally, since the diaphragm is innervated by the nerves which have been injured in the dislocation or fracture.

Management. Fractures in the newborn baby, particularly in the long bones usually heal rapidly, but it is often difficult to keep the parts in good alignment during repair. Immobilization of the part often can be achieved by swaddling and positioning the infant on his side. Splints, slings, and other apparatus are useful. However, these devices often make handling the infant difficult and cumbersome; hence parents tend to avoid touching the infant for fear of "hurting" him. Care should be taken by the staff to encourage the parents to give their infant adequate love and attention if these apparatuses are used. This will mean that the parents will have to be shown how to manipulate the apparatus effectively to avoid traumatizing the injury.

Dislocation should be reduced at once, or there will be great danger of permanent deformity in the joint. Follow-up supervision is necessary to prevent permanent deformity. Physiotherapy under orthopedic direction is important.

Diaphragmatic Paralysis

Injury to the phrenic nerve can occur as a result of lateral hyperextension of the neck, often during a difficult breech delivery. Spinal nerve roots at C3 to C5 are involved. Paralysis of the diaphragm is usually one-sided, with irregular thoracic respirations, no abdominal movement on inspiration on the affected side, and cyanosis. The elevated diaphragm, which is displaced upward and which also displaces thoracic organs, can be demonstrated by x-ray.

Unless there is respiratory distress, in which case surgery to lower the diaphragm is necessary, the treatment consists of positioning the infant on the affected side, administering oxygen if needed, and providing nutrition by the route most appropriate for the infant's condition. Atelectasis of the involved lung should not be allowed to develop in order to prevent pneumonia. Spontaneous recovery within six weeks to one year is usual.

CONGENITAL AND GENETIC ANOMALIES

The etiology of birth defects is not completely understood, but a multifactor etiology is generally accepted and it is recognized that most of these defects have an environmental component in their causes.

Malformations may arise from

1. genetic factors such as change in the chromosome number, mutation, or structural abnormalities, and
2. environmental factors, such as irradiation, infection, and drugs.

It should be emphasized that the most frequent of the genetically influenced malformations are multifactorial. Thus, these defects result from interactions among multiple genetic and environmental factors.

There are approximately 250,000 babies born each year with abnormalities that cause a significant alteration in the structure or function of their bodies. The incidence of these disorders has not changed greatly over the decades; however, the techniques of prenatal diagnosis, repair and correction have improved immensely, thus offering a great deal of hope and consolation to the parents and the children who are afflicted with these conditions. Indeed, there is increasing specialization in *teratology*—the study of the relationship of genetic and environmental factors in the production of congenital abnormalities.

Congenital deformities may range from minor abnormalities, such as supernumerary digits to grave malformations incompatible with life, which include *anencephalia* (absence of the brain), *hydrocephalus* (excessive amount of fluid in the cerebral ventricles with tremendous enlargement of the head), and *various heart abnormalities*. These grave defects are second only to accidents as a cause of death in childhood. Moreover, these youngsters represent a serious community health problem when one considers the numerous sequential surgical procedures with the attendant expense these families must undergo. In addition, the special rehabilitation and education that many require plus the drain on the parents' time and emotional and physical reserves, can have a grave social impact.

Since these conditions are so numerous and varied, this section will present selected disorders—those more commonly seen that are apparent at birth or soon thereafter and/or those with which the maternity nurse will have to deal. The care of these infants and their parents presents a great challenge to the nurse who must give competent and, at times, complex nursing care to the babies and help the parents to convert their feelings of disappointment and often, despair to constructive efforts of habilitation of the infant. In addition, the negative feelings that are aroused in the nurse must be handled.

Congenital Heart Disease

At the time of birth and for weeks thereafter, there are great changes in the circulation of the newborn. When the cord is clamped and expansion of the lungs occurs, the pulmonary circulation increases in volume. The foramen ovale, the ductus arteriosus, and the ductus venosus are no longer needed and therefore close gradually over a period of several months. Usually the foramen ovale is closed by the third month of life and the ductus by the second; during the period of closure, signs or symptoms of patency rarely occur. When they do they may be an indication of defects in these structures or other parts of the heart.

Congenital heart disease has an incidence of about 3 per 1,000 at birth and 1 per 1,000 at the age of 10. Cardiovascular malformations account for approximately 50 percent of the deaths from congenital defects in the first year of life.

The role of heredity as an etiologic agent is not yet well understood. Congenital lesions may be recorded in as many as three generations, and siblings seem to manifest the disease more often than in the preceding or succeeding generations. *Maternal disease* during pregnancy influences the bodily structures of the developing fetus, yet the etiology and dynamics of cardiovascular lesion are not known definitively. However, there is a higher incidence of other congenital defects among infants with congenital heart disease. Thus, the infant may suffer from multiple disorders.

Assessment of Manifestations

Distress from congenital heart disease is often hard to distinguish from the distress that is secondary to pulmonary disease, such as respiratory distress syndrome. Yet accurate diagnosis is essential so that effective cardiac surgery can be instituted when indicated.

The physical signs of both the normal and the abnormal newborn infant, such as right ventricular overactivity, behavior of the second heart sound, and color, are governed largely by the pulmonary artery pressure level, the rate of constriction of the ductus arteriosus, and the amount of placental transfusion. These are important and can mask the signs of congenital heart disease.

MURMURS. The most severe of these diseases which occur in early infancy are not associated with loud murmurs, and many which eventually are associated with loud murmurs most often are not manifested immediately after birth.

HEART SOUNDS. Loud, abnormal heart sounds, however, together with a rapid rate, may constitute the first sign of serious illness. A gallop rhythm is an extremely helpful sign which indicates the presence of congestive heart failure. The presence of a single heart sound after the first 12 hours of life is almost always abnormal and should stimulate further search for cardiopulmonary disease. An ejection click is normally noted only during the first few hours of life, when it may accompany the normal hypertension which characterizes the transitional pulmonary circulation. After that time, the presence of a loud click may denote a large aorta (found in pulmonary atresia), a large pulmonary artery (found in the hypoplastic left heart syndrome), or a large single vessel (found in truncus arteriosus).

OXYGEN DEFICIENCY. It must be remembered that peripheral cyanosis occurs a great deal in the newborn period; arterial blood oxygen tensions are significantly lower shortly after birth than they will be several days later. Thus, cardiac malformations which are associated with severe arterial oxygen desaturation later in the neonatal period may be present in a relatively acyanotic form owing to the good mix of oxygenated and unoxygenated blood that results temporarily from continued patency of the ductus arteriosus or foramen ovale.

PULSES AND RESPIRATION. Reduced amplitude of arterial pulses is always an important sign in this time and implies reduced cardiac output into the aorta. Bounding pulses usually imply a large aortic run-off such as is seen with patent ductus arteriosus or truncus arteriosus.

Tachypnea is another useful sign. A respiratory rate in excess of 50 beats per minute usually means that a cardiopulmonary disorder is present. Congestive heart disease is characterized by tachypnea without much respiratory effort. In severe pulmonary disturbances, obvious labored respiration is a striking feature.

OTHER SIGNS. Close nursing observations may disclose other signs which are indicative of congenital heart disease. These include ready tiring, reluctance to feed, constant or sporadic respiratory embarrassment of varying degrees, shallow "panting" respirations, sudden periods of distress accompanied by crying suggestive of pain, changes in color characterized by pallor, grayishness, or intense cyanosis. The older infant may exhibit a failure to thrive syndrome. These symptoms can occur in any combination at any time after birth.

Diagnosis is established from the history, physical findings, roentgenographic and electrocardiographic examinations. If doubt still exists, cardiac catheterization, angiocardiography, and aortography usually supply the needed confirmatory data. These latter procedures are strenous, and, if the child is severely distressed or in danger of circulatory failure, they may very well threaten his life. Therefore, great effort is made to utilize astute observation, history findings, and the roentgen and electrocardiograph findings.

Types of Congenital Cardiac Anomalies

Transposition of the great vessels. The aorta originates from the right ventricle rather than the left, and the pulmonary artery originates from the left ventricle rather than the right. There must be an abnormal communication between these vessels to maintain life.

Atrial septal defect. An abnormal opening between the right and left atria persists after birth, with left to right shunting of blood. This may result from failure of the foramen ovale to close properly, or there may be other defects high in the ostium secundum or basally in the ostium primum.

Patent ductus arteriosus. The vascular connection between the pulmonary artery and aorta, which is functional during fetal life, persists after birth rather than closing as it normally does. When the duct remains patent after birth, the direction of blood flow through it is reversed because of the higher pressure in the aorta, thus shunting oxygenated aortic blood into the pulmonary vasculature. During fetal life, the shunt is from the pulmonary artery to the aorta.

Ventricular septal defect. There is an abnormal opening between the right and left ventricles. These vary in size and may occur in the muscular or membraneous portion of the septum. Shunting of

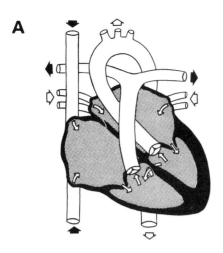

Ventricular septal defects

A ventricular septal defect is an abnormal opening between the right and left ventricle. Ventricular septal defects vary in size and may occur in either the membranous or muscular portion of the ventricular septum. Due to higher pressure in the left ventricle, a shunting of blood from the left to right ventricle occurs during systole. If pulmonary vascular resistance produces pulmonary hypertension, the shunt of blood is then reversed from the right to the left ventricle, with cyanosis resulting.

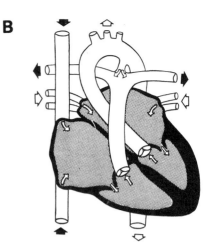

Patent ductus arteriosus

The patent ductus arteriosus is a vascular connection that, during fetal life, short circuits the pulmonary vascular bed and directs blood from the pulmonary artery to the aorta. Functional closure of the ductus normally occurs soon after birth. If the ductus remains patent after birth, the direction of blood flow in the ductus is reversed by the higher pressure in the aorta.

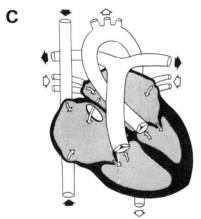

Atrial septal defects

An atrial septal defect is an abnormal opening between the right and left atria. Basically, three types of abnormalities result from incorrect development of the atrial septum. An incompetent foramen ovale is the most common defect. The high ostium secundum defect results from abnormal development of the septum secundum. Improper development of the septum primum produces a basal opening known as an ostium primum defect, frequently involving the atrio-ventricular valves. In general, left to right shunting of blood occurs in all atrial septal defects.

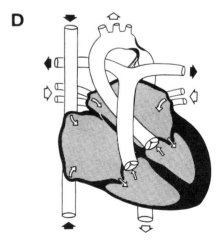

Coarctation of the aorta

Coarctation of the aorta is characterized by a narrowed aortic lumen. It exists as a preductal or postductal obstruction, depending on the position of the obstruction in relation to the ductus arteriosus. Coarctations exist with great variation in anatomical features. The lesion produces an obstruction to the flow of blood through the aorta causing an increased left ventricular pressure and work load.

Figure 39-4. Four types of congenital cardiac anomalies (Courtesy, Ross Laboratories).

blood from the left to right ventricles occurs during systole because of higher left ventricular pressure. If, however, pulmonary vascular resistance produces pulmonary hypertension, the shunt is reversed and occurs right to left, with resultant cyanosis.

Coarctation of the aorta. There is a constriction of the aorta, causing narrowing of the lumen; this partially obstructs blood flow, creating increased left ventricular pressure and work load. The coarctation may occur before or after the ductus arteriosus, and there are great variations in anatomic features of coarctations.

Tetralogy of Fallot. Four defects are combined in this anomaly, which is the most common defect causing cyanosis in children who survive beyond two years of age. There is pulmonary stenosis, ventricular septal defect, overriding aorta, and hypertrophy of the right ventricle. The severity of symptoms depends on the size of the ventricular septal defect, degree of pulmonary stenosis, and degree to which the aorta overrides the septal defect. Figure 39-4 illustrates these types of congenital cardiac anomalies.

Other Cardiac Defects. There are other types of cardiac anomalies, including tricuspid atresia, pulmonary and aortic stenosis, overriding aorta and truncus arteriosus, and anomalous venous return. Surgery can repair certain of these defects, and, in some instances, restore the infant to normal cardiac functioning. Others cannot be repaired and often are incompatible with life.

Nursing Management

Nursing care of these infants is directed at offsetting those factors which aggravate symptoms. Severely affected infants may be transferred directly to the pediatric facility; however, less distressed infants may remain on the maternity unit, especially during the time a diagnosis is being established.

The following nursing goals will be kept in mind:
1. reduction of the work of the heart
2. maintenance of nutrition
3. reduction of respiratory distress
4. prevention of respiratory and other infection
5. reduction of the parents' anxiety, and their support and teaching.

Every precaution is taken to protect the infant from exposure to infection. The principles discussed in the care of the immature infant apply here. In addition, unnecessary disturbance is to be kept at a minimum as startling or physical effort often distresses these babies.

When the infant shows signs of severe respiratory embarrassment, relief is sometimes achieved by raising the head and shoulders. When these episodes are accompanied by crying which is suggestive of pain, the baby is sometimes eased if a warm hand is applied to his abdomen and he is very gently inclined over the upper margin of the supporting hand. In the case of severe distress, the baby may lie with his head loosely retracted; this should not be corrected as the infant assumes a position most suitable for aeration.

Restlessness is often apparent, and, hence, clothes and positioning should allow for maximum freedom of movement.

Profuse disphoresis is often seen and sponge baths with tepid water can supplement the daily bath.

Oxygen is to be ready for these babies at all times, and the physician may want to prescribe digitalis if heart failure appears imminent.

Feedings are usually given more frequently and in smaller amounts than to the healthy term infant. The aim, of course, is to avoid undesirable pressure of a distended stomach on the diaphragm and heart. If the infant can suck without distress, a bottle is the feeding method of choice. If bottle feeding does result in cyanosis or impaired respiration, a spoon or gavage tube may have to be utilized. Breast-feeding is almost always discouraged because of the suddenness and capriciousness of the respiratory difficulties.

Supportive care is necessary for the parents of these babies; keeping lines of communication open between the parents and the staff (i.e., obstetrician, pediatrician, heart surgeon, nursery nurses, pediatric nurses) will do much to help alleviate anxiety and help in the adjustment (see pp. 707–714).

Cleft Lip and Cleft Palate

These deformities, which may occur separately or in combination, result from the failure of the soft and/or bony tissues of the palate and the upper jaw to unite during the fifth to tenth weeks of gestation. The defect may be unilateral or bilateral (Figure 39-5). Only the lip may be involved, or the disunion may extend into the upper jaw or the nasal cavity.

Each year about one in 700 white infants and one in 2,000 black infants are born with a cleft lip and/

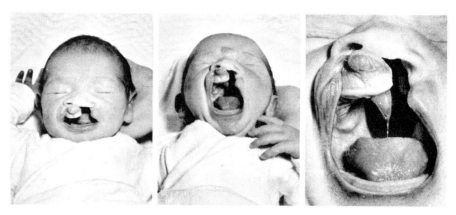

Figure 39-5. Cleft lip and complete cleft palate. In this case surgical closure of the harelip was performed less than 18 hours following birth, with excellent results. (MacDonald House, University Hospitals of Cleveland).

or cleft palate; thus, this condition is one of the most common of the birth defects. More males than females appear to be affected by the combination cleft lip and palate disorder.

A clear-cut etiologic pattern for these deformities remains obscure. Variables found to be associated with them include genetic factors, drugs (particularly corticosteroids), radiation, hypoxia in utero, maternal illness during pregnancy, and dietary influences. The hypothesis has been put forward that palatolabial defects may be due to sex-modified multifactorial inheritance.[2]

Surgical Treatment. The plan of treatment and outcome will depend on the severity of the condition. If only the lip is involved, the surgery may take place within the first few days, although some physicians prefer to wait until the child is eight to twelve weeks of age because they feel that there is more tissue available at that time to facilitate operative precision. When the palate is involved, the repair is usually done when the child is 18 to 24 months or when he reaches a weight of 9 to 10 kg. (20 to 22 lb.). Time is not the only salient variable; a child who is free from infection and nutritionally sound is perhaps even more important.

When surgery is performed later a prosthetic speech device usually is fitted so that speech development may not be hindered. Cleft palates usually involve other difficulties, frequent respiratory infections, orthodontia and speech problems, and so on; therefore, the care of these children involves the coordinated activities of the pediatrician, plastic surgeon, orthodontist, hospital and community health nurses, speech therapists and, very often, the social worker. Fortunately, modern treatment is so effective that this defect becomes a relatively minor handicap.

Nevertheless, the parents require a great deal of supportive help initially, especially since this disorder is so disfiguring. In our culture a high value is put on physical attractiveness and beauty; and when this condition occurs, particularly if the baby is a girl, it may come as a tremendous shock and burden to the parents. However, repair is generally successful, and it is very helpful if the parents know and understand this. Members of the team involved in the reconstruction process can visit the parents after a comprehensive assessment of the infant has been made, to assure them that the defect is correctable. Color transparencies are shown of an infant with a similar defect and the results of the surgery. Such visual reassurance has been found to be more effective than any verbal explanation.

The pattern of treatment is explained so parents can understand and begin to participate in the feeding and care of their child.

Nursing Management Feeding is usually one of the most immediate and difficult problems in the daily care of the infant. It can best be accomplished by placing the infant in an upright position and directing the flow of milk against the side of the mouth. This will decrease the possibility of aspiration as well as the amount of air swallowed during feeding.

Since sucking strengthens and develops the muscles needed for speech, a nipple is used for feeding whenever possible. A variety of nipples may be tried, including a regular nipple with enlarged holes, a soft rubber nipple, a presoftened "preemie" nipple, a cleft palate nipple or a duck bill nipple. The last two are more expensive. Specific instructions are necessary with their use. If the infant cannot use any of the nipples, then a spoon or a rubber-tipped asepto syringe may be tried. The flow of milk will have to be adjusted to the infant's swallowing and should not be released until the infant attempts to suck.

The feedings are given at a pace which will neither cause the infant to become unduly tired nor result in aspiration of the liquid. Thickened formulas are often used. Since these infants tend to swallow a large amount of air, they should be bubbled at frequent intervals, and the mother will need to be instructed in this technique.

The nurse will want to help the mother to attain ease in feeding her baby and should arrange to stay with her during at least several of the sessions. This is one way of assessing how well the mother is progressing.

Gavage feeding usually is unnecessary and should be used only when the other methods fail, since it does not stimulate the sucking and swallowing reflexes and promotes aspiration.

The mother may want to breast-feed her infant, and there is no contraindication as long as the milk can be given in a way that the baby can take it. This may mean that the mother may have to express her milk and offer it in a bottle.

Frenulum Linguae

The frenulum of the tongue is a sharp, thin ridge of tissue that arises in the midline from the base of the tongue and attached to its under surface for varying distances toward the top. When the attachment extends far forward, a concavity or groove is apparent at the tip of the tongue on its upper surface. This has been called tongue-tie. It never interferes with feeding nor does it produce a speech impediment as formerly thought. Therefore, incising the frenulum is not indicated, since it provides a portal of entry for infection and there is danger of severing the large vein in the area of the frenulum.

Hypospadias and Epispadias

In *male hypospadias*, the urethra opens on the under surface of the penis proximal to the usual site. Minor degrees of this condition are quite common, and no surgical intervention is necessary. If the opening is at the base of the penis or far back on the shaft, plastic surgical repair will be necessary.

In *male epispadias*, the urethral opening is on the dorsal surface of the penis. If the defect is pronounced, it also will require repair. Surgical correction is usually made by two years of age. Definitive urethroplasty should be performed before the boy enters school so that it will be possible for him to urinate in the standing position. Since the foreskin is used in the repair, boys with hypospadias are not to be circumcised.

In *female hypospadias* the urethral meatus opens into the vagina, while in *female epispadias* the upper urethral wall is absent with possible exstrophy of the bladder. The more serious types of genitourinary abnormalities often occur with numerous other anomalies.

Ambiguous Genitalia

Infants may be born with ambiguous or uncertain genitalia, or with characteristics of both male and female genitals. Abnormal sexual differentiation and fetal development can be due to genetic defects (adrenogenital syndrome, Klinefelter's syndrome, Turner's syndrome) or to the intrauterine hormonal environment (steroid sex hormone therapy given to the mother to prevent abortion). It is important for the nurse to report any instances of questionable genitalia, because establishment of genetic sex and sexual rearing are critical to later compatible psychosexual development. Chromosomal sex as well as the morphologic characteristics of internal and external sex organs are taken into consideration in sex assignment.

Often surgery to convert genitalia to one or the other sex clearly is necessary, as well as later hormonal therapy to promote the development of secondary sex characteristics. Intersex problems represent an area of specialty, and appropriate referrals to experts in this field are indicated.

Spina Bifida

Spina bifida is a rather common malformation and is due to the congenital absence of one or more vertebral arches, usually at the lower part of the

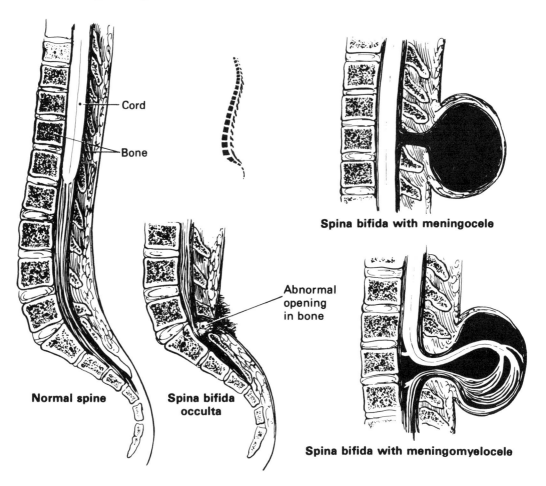

Cord

Bone

Spina bifida with meningocele

Abnormal
opening
in bone

Normal spine

**Spina bifida
occulta**

Spina bifida with meningomyelocele

Figure 39-6. Spina bifida. (From *Spina Bifida: Hope through Research.* PHS Pub. No. 1023, Health Information Series No. 103, 1970).

spine (Fig. 39-6). When the membranes covering the spinal cord bulge through the opening, the condition is known as *meningocele*. It forms a soft, fluctuating tumor filled with cerebrospinal fluid. The tumor can be diminished by pressure and enlarges when the baby cries. The extrusion of the cord along with the coverings is known as *meningomyelocele*.

When the tumor is very small and shows no signs of increasing in size, it may merely be protected from injury and infection by carefully applied dressings; but the more severe cases must be treated surgically. However, only about 60 percent of cases are operable. When the repair is massive, the outlook can be discouraging. Hydrocephalus may occur if not already present. The situation and prognosis for the infant may be guarded, and the parents will need a good deal of support and instruction about the continuing care of their infant.

Many infants with neural tube defects die or suffer from neuromuscular impairments if they survive. Permanent impairment depends upon the level of the defect and the extent of CNS tissue involvement. Prenatal diagnosis can identify neural tube defects through use of untrasound, amniography, or increased levels of α-fetoprotein in the amniotic fluid or maternal serum. Anencephaly can also be diagnosed prenatally by these techniques.

Hydrocephalus

An abnormal accumulation of fluid in the cranial vault causes enlargement of the head, atrophy of the brain, prominence of the forehead, and the typical "setting sun" appearance of the eyes due to downward pressure. These infants frequently have other anomalies, are subject to perinatal complications and have a high incidence of mental retardation, neuromuscular defects, and convulsions. The incidence is about 1 per 2,000 deliveries. The abnormal accumulation of fluid may occur between the brain and dura mater or within the ventricles of the brain. Because of the enlarged head, these infants are often breech and require delivery by cesarean section.

Surgical shunting of cerebrospinal fluid is the treatment, to reduce pressure within the cranial vault; otherwise there will be irreversible neurologic damage and death. Not all cases are operable, however, and observations over time are necessary to determine therapy.

Anencephaly

In anencephaly, there is complete or partial absence of the infant's brain and of the skull overlying the brain. The cause is not known, although there is a familial tendency in occurrences, and multiple environmental factors seem to be involved. About 70 percent of these infants are female. Often the pregnancy involves polyhydramnios. Many infants die during labor and delivery, but if they survive these, their life expectancy is quite short, usually only a few days. Supportive care is provided the infant, and the parents also need much assistance in grieving and integrating this traumatic situation.

Microcephaly

The microcephalic infant has a head which is considerably smaller than normal, with a smaller brain and accompanying mental retardation. Several causes of microcephaly have been identified, including exposure of the pregnant woman to x-ray or radiation, rubella infections during pregnancy, and cytomegalic inclusion virus infection or other prenatal infections. Many of these infants survive and need varying amounts of custodial care depending upon the extent of retardation. As with Down's syndrome, parents need assistance with decisions involving caring for the infant or child at home or seeking placement for institutional care.

Umbilical Hernia

Umbilical hernia, or rupture at the umbilicus, may appear during the first few weeks of life. The associated protrusion of intestinal contents may disappear entirely if pressure is applied, but it reappears when the pressure is removed, or when the baby cries. This is due to a weakness or an imperfect closure of the umbilical ring and is often associated with nonunion of the recti muscles. The condition usually disappears spontaneously by age one.

There is a great deal of controversy regarding the utility of strapping the abdomen to reduce the hernia. Most authorities feel that the strapping technique is useless and some feel that it may be deleterious. Surgery is usually avoided unless the hernia persists until the age of three to five years, causes symptoms, becomes strangulated or enlarges. Some mothers may need to be discouraged from placing a coin or button beneath an umbilical dressing; this practice was used for many years as a "home remedy." It has no value and prohibits adequate approximation of the margins of the abdomen.

Diaphragmatic Hernia

This neonatal emergency is caused by a defect in the development of the diaphragm which allows abdominal organs to herniate into the thoracic cavity. If the defect is small, it can be easily repaired, but must be done soon after birth as the herniated abdominal organs interfere with adequate respiration. Large defects in the diaphragm allow extensive herniation, which can prevent normal intrauterine development of pulmonary tissue, and can be incompatible with life. The outcome depends upon the size of the defect, the amount of normal pulmonary development, and the success of surgery to close the hernia.

Obstructions of the Alimentary Tract

Atresia of the Esophagus

This condition, although less common than some which have been mentioned, is quite serious, and immediate steps must be taken to prevent aspiration. The defect, which occurs during embryonic development, results in the esophagus ending in a blind pouch rather than a continuous tube to the stomach. A fistula usually occurs into the trachea near the bifurcation of the esophagus and the trachea. When

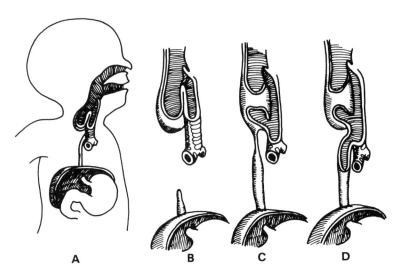

Figure 39-7. Esophageal atresia. (*A*) The most common form of esophageal atresia. (*B*) Both segments of the esophagus are blind pouches. (*C*) Esophagus is continuous, but with narrowed segment. (*D*) Upper segment of esophagus opens into trachea.

the baby attempts to swallow liquids or even normal secretions, there is an overflow into the trachea from the blind pouch (Fig. 39-7).

This malformation should be suspected whenever the infant demonstrates excessive drooling, coughing, gagging, or cyanosis during feeding. The nurse must report these symptoms immediately. Unless necessary surgery to correct the defect is prompt, the baby will contract bronchitis or pneumonia from repeated aspiration of milk and secretions.

The infant is placed in the supine position, with his head elevated 30° or more to prevent any gastric secretions from rising into the trachea through the fistula. The baby usually is placed in a heated, humidified incubator after surgery. This atmosphere is needed to liquefy the tenacious mucus that collects. Nasopharyngeal suction is necessary and the nurse should watch carefully for any cyanosis or labored respiration that indicates the need for this measure. Blood, plasma, parenteral fluids, and antibiotics are also given. The extent of the repair and the condition of the baby determine when oral feeding will be begun.

Pyloric Stenosis

This is a congenital anomaly and usually manifests its symptoms from the first week to the second or third week by the onset of vomiting which becomes projectile and occurs within 30 minutes after every feeding. The infant loses weight, the bowel elimination lessens, highly colored urine becomes scanty, and the symptoms of dehydration appear. Upon examination, gastric peristalsis is found to be pres-

ent, and the pyloric ''acornlike'' tumor may be palpated. Surgery is the treatment of choice.

Since the operation is not usually an emergency, there is sufficient time for supportive treatment to prepare the infant for surgery to correct any dehydration or electrolyte imbalance. If the hemoglobin is below 70 percent, transfusion is indicated. Gastric lavage, from one to two hours before operation, should be done until returns are clear. Maintaining body heat before and after the operation is essential. Transfusion should be given if indicated.

Four ml. of 5 percent glucose in saline is given postoperatively for four feedings. If no vomiting develops, 8 ml. are given hourly for the next four feedings, then 16 ml. hourly for four feedings. If these feedings are retained, 1 ounce of formula is given an hour after the last feeding of clear fluid and repeated two hours later. By this stepwise increment, the amount of feedings and the interval between them are increased until a full feeding program is reinstituted in about 48 hours.

Obstruction of the Duodenum and the Small Intestine

These conditions are relatively easy to diagnose. Vomiting occurs with the first feeding, and no meconium is eliminated. The vomitus may or may not be bile-stained, depending on whether the obstruction is high or low in the intestinal tract. If the obstruction is low, usually there is marked distention. A roentgenogram is used to confirm the diagnosis, and immediate surgery is indicated. However, the newborn infant should be allowed at least 12 hours for the respiration and kidney function to become stabilized.

The operation is usually accompanied by continuous parenteral fluids, and blood should be available if needed. Postoperative care includes maintaining body temperature and providing intravenous fluids until peristalsis is established (about a week), followed by feedings as given in pyloric stenosis. If distention occurs, nasoduodenal suction may be necessary. If the distention is severe, the infant is placed in an oxygen tent.

Imperforate Anus

This abnormality consists of atresia of the anus, with the rectum ending in a blind pouch. Careful examination of the infant in the delivery room usually reveals the condition. Surgical treatment is, of course, imperative. Later continence depends upon the nature of the anorectal abnormalities and effectiveness of surgery.

More males are affected by imperforate anus than females, and most females who are affected have a small fistula while this is uncommon in males. The fistulous connection may be into the vagina, bladder or urethra, or through the perineum. Male fistulas may lead into the bladder or urethra or through the perineum (Fig. 39-8). If there appears to be an anal opening, the nurse can check for patency by inserting a well-lubricated probe (thermometer, tubing, small finger), and observe physiologic func-

tioning by stroking the anus and watching for the normal "wink" response of the sphincter.

Chromosomal Abnormalities

When a particular chromosome is in triplicate rather than the usual duplicate (pair), it is called *trisomy*. Three such trisomies—trisomy 13 (D trisomy), trisomy 18 (E_1 trisomy), and trisomy 21, 22 (Down's syndrome)—have typical clinical pictures and can be recognized in the delivery room or the nursery.

As discussed in Chapter 9, in the normal person, there are 46 chromosomes in 23 pairs: one pair of sex-determining chromosomes and 22 pairs of autosomes. The extra chromosome found in trisomy results from nondisjunction (see Chap. 15) which can occur at any time in a cell's lifetime, during either meiosis or mitosis. Two different cytologic pictures emerge in trisomic cells. In the first, there is a free extra chromosome giving 47 chromosomes, or a chromosome is lacking, giving only 45. This is called nondisjunction. In the second, the extra chromosome is translocated, that is, attached to another chromosome. The total number is 46, but one of the chromosomes is the size of two chromosomes combined.

There is an increased incidence of all three types of trisomy with advanced maternal age. This phenomenon is thought to be related to the long storage of oocytes in the mother. These germ cells are laid

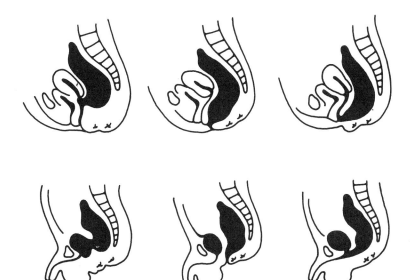

Figure 39-8. Types of imperforate anus.

down during the mother's own fetal life; they wait, however, until the time of their individual ovulation to complete their meiotic divisions. Thus, it appears that nondisjunction tends to occur in older oocytes.

Trisomy 13, or D

This trisomy is characterized by an extra chromosome in the D group which includes pairs 13 through 15 (see Chap. 15). Infants with this abnormality frequently have difficulty establishing and maintaining respiration. One of the most striking features is the abnormal cranial development. The cranium is usually small with a sloping forehead. The ears may be malformed and low-set and the eyes usually have some defect (cataracts, iris defects, unusual smallness) often bilaterally. Cleft palate and lip are commonly present. In addition, the hands and feet are often grossly deformed. Extra digits are common on both hands and feet. The thumbs may be retroflexible (double jointed) and the foot frequently has a posterior prominence of the heel sometimes accompanied by a convex sole known as "rocker bottom" foot. Other defects may include a bulbous nose, umbilical and diaphragmatic hernias, abnormal genitalia, scalp defects, and extensive capillary hemangiomata far in excess of what is usually found in the normal newborn.

Neurologic examination reveals these infants to have a weak or absent Moro reflex and little or no response to loud noises; hence they appear to be deaf. They are prone to develop myoclonic seizures and all suffer from apneic spells of unknown origin. Autopsy often reveals the complete absence of olfactory nerves and tracts. All of these infants are mentally retarded and the majority have severe cardiac defects (dextroposition of the heart, ventricular septal defects) which are the major contributors to death in these infants. The average life span for these youngsters is less than a year, although several have lived to the age of five years.

Trisomy 18, or E

This trisomy is characterized by an extra chromosome in the E group, which includes pairs 17 and 18 (see Chap. 15). These babies are usually born at term but are small, averaging about 2 kg. (5 lb.). Their placentas are often very small. The head is small with a prominent occiput but in proportion to the body size. The eyes are usually normal but the ears are generally malformed and low-set. The mouth appears small because of the short upper lip and the mandible is small, giving a receding chin.

The hands of these babies are always malformed but in a different way from the trisomy 13, and they give the best diagnostic clue to the condition. These babies keep their fists clenched most of the time with the index finger overlying the third finger.

Profuse lanugo covers the forehead, back and extremities, and the skin usually has a mottled appearance. The sternum is very short, hence the abdomen appears long. The pelvis is small with limited abduction of the hips. There also may be abnormal genitalia. Inguinal and umbilical hernias are frequent; diaphragmatic eventration (elevation of a thinned portion of the diaphragm) rather than frank hernia occurs more often in these patients.

Neurologic examination reveals abnormal muscle tone; these babies progress from a hypertonic state to frank opisthotonus. Since the sucking reflex is poor, gavage feeding is often instituted. Unlike trisomy 13, no gross brain abnormalities can be demonstrated, although cardiac abnormalities are common and either these or aspiration account for the demise of these babies.

Survival rate for these infants is less than six months on the average. During this time they become progressively undernourished and present a failure to thrive syndrome. As with trisomy 13, some infants have survived to childhood, so that death in infancy cannot be predicted.

Trisomy 21, or Down's Syndrome

In this condition an extra chromosome belonging to either pair 21 or 22 or a translocation of 15/21 is found (see Chap. 15). Although these babies are apt to have congenital defects and are more susceptible to infection, they can be expected to live much longer and have less severe mental retardation (although it can be very severe) than the other trisomies. The term "mongolism" formerly was used to refer to this syndrome, but Down's syndrome is the preferred nomenclature, because the word "mongolism" bears a negative connotation and is descriptively inaccurate for these infants.

The eyes of these infants are set close together, are slanting, and the palpebral fissures are narrow.

The nose is flat. The tongue is large, fissured, and usually is very obvious as it protrudes from the open mouth. The head is small, and posteriorly the occiput appears flat above the broad, pudgy neck. The hands are short and thick, especially the fingers (the little finger is curved), with simian creases apparent on the palmar surfaces. In addition to having defective mentality and the deformities mentioned above, these infants have underdeveloped muscles, loose joints, heart and alimentary tract abnormalities. Although these infants sometimes live past the age of puberty, the majority succumb earlier to some infection.

Incidence and Etiology. The incidence of Down's syndrome has been estimated at 1.5 in 1,000 births. However, this ratio has dropped with the lowering of maternal age. In mothers under 35 years, the incidence is about 1 per 1,500 births; in those 35 to 40 years it is 1 per 300 births; and in those over 45 years it rises to 1 per 30 to 35 births. Presently, only about 3.5 percent of pregnant women are over 35 years of age, whereas about 10 percent were this old two decades ago.[3]

Types. The most common chromosomal defect of the ovum in Down's syndrome is trisomy of the chromosome 21 or 22, resulting in a total chromosomal count of 47 instead of the normal number of 46. This type, commonly referred to as standard trisomy, usually occurs in infants born to older women and is rarely familial. The incidence of standard trisomy is 1 in 600 births.

The second type of abnormality results from a 15/21 translocation; in this type the actual chromosomal count is 46. The translocation type of Down's syndrome usually occurs in infants born to younger parents, is the familial type and is rare.

The third type of the disorder, mosaicism, is very rare. A unique factor in mosaicism is that one individual may have cells with different chromosomal counts. Laboratory tests may demonstrate that the affected person's blood cells, for example, have 47 chromosomes, whereas his skin cells may show 46 chromosomes. This is not a familial type of Down's syndrome, and, moreover, the abnormalities may be less.

Prognosis. The usual causes of death in these babies are heart defects and infectious illnesses. The average survival rate with effective antibiotic treatment has been extended to beyond nine years. Children with Down's syndrome are essentially retarded but have been found to be far more educable than was previously thought. Thus the decision to institutionalize the child is an exceedingly difficult one and should not be forced on the parents by well-meaning professionals.

Prevention and Management

The key approach to trisomy conditions lies in prevention since treatment does not alter the long-range prognosis. Education of the public regarding the effect of maternal age is the key issue in prevention. The incidence of all three trisomies goes up with increased maternal age. The later *thirties* and *forties* are less safe for childbearing (from many points of view), and childbearing is less risky when the mother is younger. Genetic counseling is another aspect of public education (see Chap. 15). Parents who have had a trisomic child (or if trisomy has appeared among their siblings) would benefit from counseling concerning the risk of having another affected child. In some families, trisomies are not the result of nondisjunction and hence have an appreciable chance of recurring, depending on the interaction of the variables of family history, maternal age, and chromosomal arrangement.

Immediate care will be supportive for the infant. Warmth, prevention of infection, fluid and electrolyte balance, and often oxygen therapy will be provided. Nursing therapy will be aimed primarily at support of the parents and helping them to work through their grief. This latter aspect is particularly important because of the grave prognosis for these babies. It is often helpful to institute community health and/or visiting nurse referrals since the parents may need technical help upon arriving home with the infant. If a fetal demise occurs, supportive help from a public health nurse is also helpful.

Phocomelia

In 1961–1962 many thousands of newborns in Germany were afflicted with an extremely pitiful type of malformation characterized either by total absence of the arms and the legs or by such stunting of the extremities that they were mere nubbins. The deformity is known as *phocomelia*. Investigation revealed that practically all the mothers who gave birth to such infants had taken a certain sedative drug, *thalidomide,* during the first part of pregnancy, and that this drug was undoubtedly the cause of the malformations.

Largely as the result of the thalidomide tragedy, the United States Food and Drug Administration, a federal agency authorized to approve new drugs, greatly tightened the regulations concerning new drug approval. But from the viewpoint of nurses and physicians, the most important lesson to be drawn from this sad experience is that *no pregnant woman should take any drug whatsoever* unless, in the opinion of her physician, it is urgently necessary for her health. This rule does not apply to the routine administration of vitamins and iron, nor to the use of stool softeners when indicated, but it does apply very strongly to most other drugs, particularly those often employed in the treatment of insomnia, nausea, and anxiety.

The child with deformed or missing limbs has special rehabilitation problems. His physical characteristics and contours are different from those of an adult, and they are constantly changing as he grows. This complicates fitting an adequate prosthesis. Furthermore, his psychosocial adjustment demands continued attention, for he does not have the chance to make his adjustment to society as a whole person, and he therefore is likely to have some feelings of inadequacy and devaluation in a culture geared to the nonhandicapped.

Even when the deformity is multiple, the child can achieve at least limited function with proper prosthetics and training. Since much of the success of the plan of treatment depends on the parents, it is particularly important that they be informed and reassured of these positive aspects in the situation. It has been demonstrated that the sooner the parents receive this knowledge, the more chance there is of an effective prosthetics program.

Management. The newborn infant with a congenital amputation will be discussed here since nurses in the maternity unit will have initial contact with these infants and will need to instruct parents on various aspects of daily care.

The usual sleeping position for the newborn is prone with the pelvis raised and the knees tucked under the abdomen. When the lower extremities are missing, the infant is unable to assume this position and, in addition, will not be able to indulge in the kicking behavior which appears to give a good deal of gratification. When the upper extremities are missing other problems occur. Prior to feeding, the infant is usually occupied with a good deal of hand to mouth contact and this, of course, will be altered. If both hands are missing the infant will be deprived of one of his major sources of sucking gratification. It is known that the need for sucking and the need for feeding often do not coincide, and, hence, the normal infant uses his fingers to complete the gratification of this need. Therefore the nurse will want to offer a pacifier to these infants. As the infant matures he tends to grasp things and bring them to his mouth, possibly for further identification. In the absence of both upper limbs, this behavior also will be altered. The nurse will also want to instruct the parents that, when the infant is older, he may not be able to life his head up (while in the prone position) since he cannot raise himself on his elbows to look around. A wedge-shaped pillow or thick folded blanket placed under the infant's chest will correct this handicap a great deal.

The development of body image begins in infancy and will play an increasingly important role in the development of these youngsters. The normally developed infant first perceives his moving arms (and legs) as part of the outside world; as he grows, he incorporates them into his body image and, hence, his self-concept. The infant amputee may not be aware that his body is different from others, but as he matures, he begins to compare himself with others and his concept about himself changes as he slowly integrates his defect into his existing body image. Obviously, the more positive attitudes he encounters with respect to his defect, the more positive his concept of himself can become.

In the parents' eyes, this defect may be catastrophic. The principles of care, as discussed on page 708, especially with regard to how the nurse actually handles the baby, are especially germane here. Guilt may be present, especially if the defect is thought to be the result of taking drugs or from contact with viral diseases. Denial also may be apparent, with the parents actually refusing to look at or admit the defect. The nurse's warm, accepting attitude in this case is very helpful since the parents' denial is often related to their apprehension regarding how others will view their infant. Once the parents have recovered from the initial shock and have worked through their grief, they can be assisted to focus on their child's rehabilitation and nurturance of his psychosocial development.

INBORN ERRORS OF METABOLISM

Numerous metabolic disorders, so-called inborn errors of metabolism, are now known to originate from mutations in the genes which alter the genetic constitution of an individual to the extent that normal function is disrupted. These biochemical disorders arise because of the disturbance (mutation) in a *molecule of the gene* itself. They *do not* stem from some mishap or alteration during the embryonic development of tissue or organs. The mode of transmission of these inborn errors usually is recessive; that is, a child, to be affected, must receive a pair of defective genes (one from the mother and one from the father). The mother and the father in these cases would be carriers of the defective genes but would not be affected by the resulting disorder per se. Fortunately, defective genes are found rather infrequently in the general population, and the chance of their joining is even rarer; hence, the diseases they produce are commensurately rare.

Some of the more familiar hereditary metabolic disorders and resulting conditions include:

1. Defects in metabolism and transport of amino acids
   a. Phenylketonuria
   b. Maple sugar urine disease
2. Defects in protein metabolism
   Agammaglobulinemia
3. Defects in metabolism and transport of carbohydrates
   a. Diabetes mellitus
   b. Gargoylism (Hurler's disease)
   c. Galactosemia
   d. Arachnodactyly (Marfan's syndrome)
4. Defects in metabolism and transport of lipids
   a. Cerebroside lipidosis (Gaucher's disease)
   b. Ganglioside lipidosis (Tay-Sachs disease)
   c. Sphingomyelin lipidosis (Niemann-Pick disease)

It is important to remember that these inborn errors of metabolism *do not produce symptoms* that are apparent at birth. Therefore, the maternity nurse

rarely will see evidence of these disorders. However, two conditions do concern us here. The one, phenylketonuria, is usually detected at an early stage by nursery personnel. The other, maternal diabetes mellitus, has a less direct effect.

Phenylketonuria

This disease, commonly known as PKU, is an inborn error of metabolism of the essential amino acid phenylalanine. It is characterized by a deficiency in the liver enzyme phenylalanine hydroxylase, which is essential in phenylalanine metabolism. High blood levels of phenylalanine occur, and phenylketone bodies are excreted in the urine. Phenylalanine makes up 5 percent of the protein factor of all foods.

Normally, phenylalanine is converted to tyrosine in the liver and then is further metabolized. The phenylketonuric child is able to digest protein and to absorb the resulting amino acids. However, there is a block in the normal metabolic pathway at this point, and the excess dietary phenylalanine, unable to be converted to tyrosine, builds up in the tissues (blood levels of this amino acid reach as high as 60 mg. per 100 ml., as compared with the normal 1 to 3 mg. per 100 ml.) and spills into the urine in the form of phenylpyruvic acid, excess phenylalanine, phenylacetic acid, and orthohydroxyphenylacetic acid. These components, excreted in the urine and the perspiration, give the child a characteristic musty odor.

Without treatment, the condition usually results in mental retardation, although the rest of the clinical picture will vary. Typically, the child with PKU is hyperactive and demonstrates unpredictable erratic behavior. Usually he does not relate well in interpersonal contacts, either within the family or with strangers, and he appears very immature and overly dependent.

The main foci of management are early detection of the condition and dietary management restricting the phenylalanine intake.

Diagnosis. This disorder may be diagnosed from both blood and urine tests. The former are more advantageous, since they can be done before the infant leaves the hospital, and they give a low rate of false positive reactions. One of the easiest and most efficient to perform is the microbiological assay (MIA), more commonly known as the Guthrie method. In this test 1 or 2 drops of blood are secured from the infant's heel from the second day to the day of discharge and are placed immediately on filter paper. The laboratory then uses a bacterial inhibition assay method on the serum phenylalanine to determine the phenylalanine level. A result of 8 mg. percent or above is considered to be diagnostic of PKU. This method is also used to monitor children on the PKU diet.

Other blood tests have been developed (LaDu-Michael, McCaman and Robins methods) which require more blood. They are as reliable as the Guthrie method and with proper laboratory facilities are often utilized.

The urine tests utilize ferric chloride as the testing agent; this solution is dropped on a freshly saturated diaper, or a prepared test-stick is pressed against a wet diaper or dipped in urine. A green reaction indicates probable phenylketonuria. The urine tests are effective only after the infant is six weeks old; they are useful in screening large populations of infants and are most often done in well-baby clinics.

Since early diagnosis is imperative, the blood tests are the tests of choice. However, since about 10 percent of newborns affected by phenylketonuria will not have high phenylalanine blood levels during the first three to four days of life, screening should be repeated in about two weeks. Diagnosis should be established and dietary treatment begun before the infant is three months old.

Management.   Restriction of phenylalanine intake is the basis of treatment, and yet enough protein must be available for growth and development; hence the child's diet becomes all-important. Commercial products (e.g., Lofenalac, a special food which is mixed with water) that provide adequate protein for growth with minimal phenylalanine content are available. The plan of dietary treatment should be reviewed carefully with both parents, so that they have an understanding of how to prepare the formula, use the meal guides and food exchange lists and prepare menus from them.

Requesting the parents to review their understanding of the problem, diet, and so on, often will elicit the areas that need clarification. The parents must be supported until they feel comfortable in discussing the problem; until this happens, they cannot be receptive to further teaching. Since this is a long-term condition and requires consistent counseling and follow-up, the need for a referral to the public health nurse becomes evident.

Care should be taken so that the parents of an affected child are not led to believe that all babies treated will have the usual pattern of growth and development (intellectual development may be slow, for instance). This cannot be guaranteed. *Early detection* and *prompt treatment* prevent mental retardation. The control of this condition demands consistent and disciplined supervision and follow-through on the part of the parents.

The Infant of the Diabetic Mother

The successful control of diabetes with insulin has led to the survival and fertility of an increasing number of diabetic women (see Chap. 32). However, despite recent advances in the management of the diabetic mother, intrauterine surveillance of the fetus and therapy during delivery and the first days of life, the infant of the diabetic mother still runs a high risk of dying. Without vascular complications, the perinatal mortality rate with modern therapy is below 10 percent, but individual risk depends upon the severity of the maternal diabetes, control of blood sugar levels during pregnancy, placental function, complications such as preeclampsia and premature labor, and the incidence of acidosis. Perinatal mortality for infants of chemical (class A) diabetic mothers is only slightly higher than normal when optimal care is provided.[4]

Infants of diabetic mothers usually have a characteristic appearance. They are usually large, often 4.5 kg. (10 lb.) or over, and present a cushingoid appearance. Their tremendous weight is not due primarily to an excess of extracellular fluid as was formerly believed, but rather to an excess of fat. The obesity is a result of fetal hyperinsulinism, originating from transformation of carbohydrates to triglycerides.[5] These infants appear bloated and tend to be "jumpy" and tremulous after the first 24 hours of life. They are also subject to cyanotic attacks, respiratory distress syndrome, hypoglycemia, hypocalcemia, and hyperbilirubinemia.

Among the many causes of death and morbidity in these babies are the higher incidences of congenital anomalies and early delivery with the resulting prematurity, respiratory distress, hypocalcemia, and hypoglycemia. Many of these problems in turn are brought about by inadequate control of the maternal diabetes. Meticulous control of maternal blood sugar, therefore, may lead to fewer problems and lower infant mortality.

Congenital anomalies are three times higher in infants of diabetic mothers, the most common including neural tube defects, cardiac malformations, and tracheoesophageal fistula. There are also increased incidences of birth trauma and asphyxia. Common types of trauma, generally related to excessive fetal size, include facial nerve paralysis, diaphragmatic paralysis, fracture of the clavicle, brachial palsy, and cephalohematoma.

Traditionally, concern has been directed toward the effect on the fetus of maternal hypoglycemia. Severe prolonged hypoglycemia will damage the fetus. However, since the newborn can tolerate a blood sugar level of as little as 20 percent with no damage, perhaps the fetus can also. Thus, loosely controlling the maternal diabetes (with one insulin injection per day and little dietary control) in an effort to provide adequate blood sugar to the fetus can instead lead to fetal death or to hypoglycemia in the newborn. The more current belief is that maternal hyperglycemia leads to the same condition in the fetus since glucose is rapidly transferred across the placenta. The fetal pancreas hypertrophies in response to repeated high "doses" of sugar and produces large amounts of insulin in an attempt to control the fetus' blood sugar and indirectly the mother's. However, since insulin in not transferred across the placenta, the fetus cannot help the mother. The excess sugar that pours across the placenta lodges in the fetal liver and other tissues, either as glycogen or fat, and produces the characteristic large, puffy infant of the diabetic mother.

It is felt that fetal hyperglycemia probably contributes to the death in utero of the fetus at 36 to 37 weeks. To combat this, most physicians wish to deliver the infant at 35 to 36 weeks. However, early delivery subjects the baby to all of the hazards associated with prematurity. If the fetus can remain in utero until 37 or 38 weeks or longer, its outlook is improved. With the newer techniques of intrauterine assessment, decisions about the fetus' ability to survive in the extrauterine environment can be made with greater certainty of a successful outcome.

When the infant is delivered and the umbilical cord cut, another problem must be faced. The baby's external supply of glucose is now cut off, yet the hypertrophied pancreas continues producing large amounts of insulin, and this cannot be readily stopped.[6] Thus, the infant rapidly becomes severely hypoglycemic and can suffer brain damage and death. Care must be taken in the administration of glucose for this condition since the hypertrophied pancreas is highly sensitized to glucose and even small quantities will trigger rebound hypoglycemia.

Management

In general, these infants are to be treated as premature infants, although their size may be deceiving. Hence, all the vital signs and blood chemistry monitoring devices are appropriate for them. Adequate temperature control and an aseptic environment are to be provided.

Intravenous Therapy. The baby's electrolyte balance is maintained with intravenous fluids until the eating pattern and sucking reflex normalize. An infusion pump should be used to ensure that fluids are given at a constant rate so that the pancreas is not stimulated to produce excess insulin in receiving more glucose one hour and less the next. Giving large quantities of glucose by vein for the maintenance of glucose levels has been found ineffective for the above reason; however, infusion of glucose for immediate *seizures* has had some effect when used in a 20-percent concentration. The use of glucagon to mobilize liver glycogen is also limited by the fact that it also stimulates insulin release and rebound hypoglycemia. Hypoglycemia can be detected by means of Dextrostix. If the infant can take fluids orally and if the blood sugar by Dextrostix is less that 45 mg. per 100 ml., the baby can be given 10-percent glucose water to bring levels to normal.

Epinephrine. 1:1,000 intramuscularly can be used to decrease the amount of insulin released since it appears to inhibit the release of insulin from the pancreas. It also stimulates the liver and muscles to release glucose, and the fat tissue to release fatty acids for glucose production. The sudden death of these infants from heart failure can be caused either directly or indirectly by a deficiency of epinephrine. Indirectly, a deficiency of this substance leads to a lack of free fatty acids, a vital part of the heart's fuel supply. Without epinephrine and fuel, the heart is overtaxed and thus cannot handle the increased stress after delivery.

When either glucagon or epinephrine are used to treat hypoglycemia, the nurse must carefully observe the infant for signs of the rebound phenomenon, because both can cause the pancreas to respond with rebound production of insulin.[7]

Hypocalcemia. The nurse will also want to be watchful of the development of hypocalcemia (serum calcium below 7 mg. per 100 ml.) which can occur with or without hypoglycemia. Symptoms are usually imperceptible and nonspecific. They include irritability, coarse tremors, twitches, and convulsions.

Two peaks of incidence occur, the first during the first 48 hours and characterized by apnea, cyanotic episodes, edema, high-pitched cry, and abdominal distention but no neuromuscular involvement. It must be noted that these manifestations have not been proved to be solely of hypocalcemic origin.

The second form occurs between the fifth and tenth days of life and is sometimes called *neonatal tetany*. It occurs when the infant is fed milk formulas (especially evaporated milk) which causes a hyperphosphatemia and depresses the activity of the parathyroid gland which, in turn, diminishes serum calcium. Here the symptoms include the neuromuscular signs—jitters, twitching, and focal or generalized convulsions.

The preventive treatment is to feed the infant a milk formula that simulates the calcium-phosphorus ratio of human milk. Actual treatment of the acute stage is intravenous instillation of 10 percent calcium gluconate 1 to 1.5 ml. per kg. of body weight, given slowly over a period of five minutes to prevent bradycardia. The heart rate is monitored constantly during the infusion and, if it drops below 100 beats per minute, the infusion is discontinued immediately. It may be restarted after the heart rate has been normal for 30 minutes.

Oxygen and Neurologic Function. The nurse will also have the responsibility to monitor the infant's blood oxygen level and neurologic function. If the infant is lethargic, frequent position change is important. Respiratory distress is managed as in any premature infant. If the baby is having respiratory difficulties, he can be positioned on his chest and neck in as straight a line as possible to reduce interference with his air passages. His shoulders can be slightly elevated and his body tilted slightly backward.

Hydration and Feeding. Hydration is also of extreme importance. It is advisable to use a urine bag connected to straight drainage to collect and measure urinary output. If the bag can be attached so that it can stay in place for 24 to 48 hours, there is less of a chance of the skin becoming excoriated from frequent bag changes. As the infant responds to treatment during the first 24 to 48 hours, oral feedings can be started. However, care must be taken to see that the baby does not aspirate formula since these infants are usually poor feeders and their size makes it difficult to handle them. It is difficult to hold up the head of such a large infant when he is in an Isolette, therefore he can be placed on his side for feeding and be bubbled by placing him on his abdomen or rotating him from side to side.

Continued Management. The infant can be placed in an open crib when his respirations, reflexes, and body temperature are stabilized and within normal ranges. However, he is still to be watched carefully since reversals can occur. Recurrence of hypoglycemia and hypocalcemia is possible and hyperbilirubinemia often occurs. Neurologically, these babies reflect their gestational age, so swallowing and evacuation may be a problem for some weeks. Parents can be taught to handle their baby as if he were premature until he is on his way to stability.

Maternal Care

Prenatally, supportive measures for the mother with diabetes should be planned with two objectives: the delivery of a normal baby and a minimum of maternal swings in blood sugar. This requires careful control of maternal blood sugar, which implies meticulous medical and nursing supervision and cooperation by the mother.

Postpartally, the parents, as part of their health education, will be alerted to the possibility that their infant may be prediabetic. If the hyperinsulinism that results from the stimulation of the fetal pancreas by maternal glucose is too prolonged or too severe, pancreatic exhaustion may ensue. This, along with genetic makeup, may lead to diabetes in the child either in the neonatal period or months or years later. Thus, parents need to receive adequate instruction about the nutritional needs of the child as well as a review of the signs and symptoms of diabetes. Parents can be encouraged to follow their child carefully following periods of stress, such as illness, injury, growth spurts, and so on. If any such symptoms occur, medical attention is indicated. Since the birth process is often traumatic for these parents and they have much to accomplish psychologically as for any trauma, a community health referral is indicated to assure follow-through on the teaching.

NEONATAL PROBLEMS SECONDARY TO MATERNAL DISORDERS

Hyperbilirubinemia of the Newborn

Hyperbilirubinemia is present when the total serum bilirubin levels reach 18 to 20 mg. per 100 ml. of blood. This may occur particularly in premature infants as an exaggeration of physiologic jaundice or as a consequence of excessive hemolysis, such as severe hemolytic disease of the newborn. Occasionally, this condition is found in term infants who have no blood group incompatibilities.

Bilirubin pigment, a product of hemoglobin breakdown, must be conjugated into a water-soluble or direct form in order to be excreted by the liver into the intestines as bile. Unconjugated or free bilirubin can escape the vascular system and become deposited in tissues, causing the yellow coloration known as *jaundice*. The liver in the full term infant is mature enough and there is adequate production of glucusyltransferase to prevent pathologic levels of bilirubin from accumulating. However, if the infant experiences cold stress, asphyxia, or hypoglycemia, or the mother has used such drugs as sulfa and aspirin shortly before delivery, the ability to excrete bilirubin is impaired.

Physiologic jaundice, occurring after the infant is 24 hours old, is common. Pathologic jaundice or hyperbilirubinemia poses a serious threat to the neonate, as accumulation of excessive bilirubin in the brain cells produces kernicterus, which can result in epilepsy, mental retardation and cerebral palsy.

The nurse can identify the risk of pathologic jaundice in the infant when jaundice appears during the first 24 hours of life, lasts more than 7 days in the full term infant and 10 days in the premature infant and when bilirubin levels increase more than 5 mg./100ml./24 hours or are above 12 mg./100 ml. in the full term and 15 mg./100 ml. in the premature infant.

Certain conditions of the mother (e.g., diabetes, as well as neonatal conditions arising from the use of certain drugs, bacteremia and prolonged cyanosis) appear to be implicated in causing this condition.

Breast Milk Jaundice. Occasionally this disorder appears among breast-fed infants during the second week of life. For some reason the mother manufactures a substance in her milk that inhibits the conjugation of bilirubin. If breast-feeding is discontinued, serum bilirubin levels return to normal within five days, and apparently no lasting damage is done to the infant.

Although high levels of bilirubin, up to 20mg./100ml., have been reported, kernicterus does not appear to occur with this condition. Breast-feeding is often continued as long as bilirubin levels remain near the upper limits of normal. Clinically jaundiced infants must be followed closely with serial serum bilirubin levels, whether breast-feeding is continued or not.

Hemolytic Disease of the Newborn. Isoimmunization due to ABO blood group incompatibility or Rh antigens can result in hemolytic anemia, hyperbilirubinemia and jaundice in the newborn. These conditions are frequently diagnosed during pregnancy so that various techniques of prenatal fetal management are employed. Depending upon the severity of the condition, intrauterine transfusions and/or early delivery may be necessary. Upon delivery, the newborn may require an exchange transfusion to promote cardiovascular function, correct anemia, remove affected red blood cells thereby reducing subsequent breakdown, and remove already formed bilirubin. The severely hydroptic (edematous) infant may also need paracentesis to alleviate ascites. As there may be pleural and pericardial effusions, positive pressure ventilation to ensure adequate oxygenation is often necessary in severe cases.

An *exchange transfusion* alternately removes a small amount of blood from the infant and replaces it with the same amount of donor blood. An infusion is started either in the umbilical stump or by cutdown into the jugular or femoral arteries. The procedure is sterile and done with minimization of cold stress to the infant. The donor blood is warmed, then after 100 ml. of the infant's blood is removed, the same amount is transfused. Following this, calcium gluconate is usually given, then the exchange transfusion procedure repeated. Usually transfusions involve replacing about twice the infant's blood volume. A 50 percent glucose solution and sodium bicarbonate should also be available for management of hypoglycemia and acidosis. Cardiac arrhythmias are also a danger, and use of warmed blood in small amounts with calcium gluconate minimizes this risk. Careful monitoring of vital signs, time, type and amount of medication and infant response is essential.

Phototherapy. The use of intense fluorescent light to reduce serum bilirubin has gained acceptance in the treatment of hyperbilirubinemia. Blue light decomposes bilirubin by photooxidatoin, which appears to take place in the skin. The chemical nature of the products formed in the breakdown of bilirubin has not been precisely determined, nor have long-term outcomes been evaluated as well as the theoretic effects of intense light upon a wide spectrum of biologic processes. For these reasons, there are some reservations about the unqualified use of this treatment for all jaundiced babies.

Phototherapy is applied by exposing the nude infant to fluorescent daylight bulbs that supply 200 to 400 foot-candles on the skin surface. Optimal intensity or duration of therapy has not been determined. The infant's eyes are shielded from the light by means of patches. The nurse will want to be sure that the lids are closed when the blindfold is applied. The bandages are to be removed at least once each shift to inspect the eyes for conjunctivitis.

INFECTIONS

Most institutions have an area designated as an isolation nursery where any infant who has or is suspected of having an infection is placed immediately. Once the infant has been tranferred to the isolation nursery, he should not be returned to the newborn nursery even though the infection has been treated and/or cured. Strict aseptic technique is used in the care of these babies, and therefore the principles of infectious disease nursing must be understood and carried out by all personnel coming in contact with the infants. Separation of the mother and the infant may be necessary, depending on the type and the severity of the infection.

Ophthalmia of the Newborn (Gonorrheal Conjunctivitis).

This is a serious condition which may result in total blindness, but if suitable treatment is adopted at the very outset of the disease and intelligently carried out, usually the sight can be saved.

State laws making the use of an antibacterial prophylaxis compulsory for all infants at birth have reduced the incidence of this infection immeasurably. Before eye prophylaxis became mandatory, however, 25 to 30 percent of all children in schools for the blind suffered impaired sight as a result of the infection. This condition is of gonorrheal origin and is characterized by a profuse, purulent discharge in the eyes due to infection, generally from the genital canal at the time of birth.

The most common reason for delay in the diagnosis is the assumption by inexperienced persons that all conjunctivitis in the first few days of life is a consequence of the prophylactic silver nitrate (or the antibiotic ointment). A degree of conjunctival inflammation with catarrhal discharge may occur with silver nitrate and to a lesser degree with the various antibiotic preparations. However, the nurse should give primary consideration to infection in the presence of purulent exudate during the first days of life or catarrhal conjunctivitis persisting longer than three days. It is well to remember also that the widely used procedure of phototherapy for neonatal hyperbilirubinemia necessitates shielding the infant's eyes during the procedure and may result in obscuring this disease—thus, the pads should be removed regularly and the eyes examined.

If the infection occurs at the time of birth, the disease appears within two or three days; but as the septic discharge may be introduced into the eye at a later period because of improper care of the infant, the onset may be later. Both eyes are usually affected; and at first they are suffused with a watery discharge and considerable inflammation of the eyelids. Within 24 hours, the lids become very much swollen, and a thick, creamy, greenish pus is discharged. Later, unless treatment has been instituted early, the swelling becomes so marked that the eyes cannot be opened, opacities of the cornea occur, the conjunctiva is ulcerated and then perforated, and the eye collapses and finally atrophies.

Preventive treatment consists of using an antibacterial agent, usually 1 percent silver nitrate, or penicillin ophthalmic ointment, which is instilled immediately after birth. However, if infection does occur, penicillin intramuscular injections may be given. The swelling and the purulent discharge usually disappear within 12 to 24 hours after treatment is begun. As gonorrheal conjunctivitis is infectious, isolation technique is essential to prevent spread to other patients and staff.

Gonorrheal Sepsis. Although the incidence is low, complications of maternal gonorrheal infection during pregnancy can include amnionitis, premature rupture of membranes, premature labor and low birth weight in the neonate. Prevention of fetal-neonatal infection is most effective, with routine gonorrheal cultures during pregnancy and treatment as needed. The newborn with mild infection usually experiences no permanent damage if antibiotic treatment is instituted. More severe infections can lead to death. Respiratory distress and pneumonia, often associated with prematurity, are also possible with significant gonorrheal infection.

Syphilis

Early congenital syphilis is apparent at birth, with skin lesions predominantly on the face, the buttocks, the palms, and the soles. Mucous patches occur in the mouth, and condylomata about the anus. These lesions are highly infectious. The eruption is usually maculopapular and not quite so generalized as in acquired syphilis. Bullae may appear on the palms and the soles, a type of lesion never found in acquired syphilis. The palms and the soles may desquamate as a result of the lesions. Less frequently seen are papular lesions or purely macular or, very rarely, vesicular or somewhat pustular ones. The nails may be deformed, and alopecia may be present. There may be destruction of the nose bridge and excoriation of the upper lip. In such cases the blood test for syphilis is usually strongly positive.

In addition to the cutaneous manifestations of syphilis, other signs and symptoms may arouse suspicion of the presence of the disease. The infant becomes restless, develops rhinitis (snuffles), and a hoarse voice and does not gain weight as it should. The lymph nodes are enlarged, especially the epitrochlear nodes. The liver and the spleen are enlarged, along with the ends of the long bones.

MANAGEMENT. Penicillin is used to treat syphilis of the newborn. If the disease was diagnosed and treated early in pregnancy, the baby seldom is born with the disease. Late congenital syphilis, if undetected, becomes apparent in the child after two years and corresponds to tertiary syphilis.

Herpesvirus Type 2

Herpesvirus type 2, usually responsible for genital herpes, can affect the fetus or neonate causing a congenital herpes infection. Fetal infection early in pregnancy is associated with increased spontaneous abortions, and later in pregnancy with prematurity, serious CNS involvement and significant risk of death. The illness may be apparent at birth, or if infection occurs during delivery may become manifest in the first week of life.

Signs and symptoms include a generalized vesiculation of the skin, progressive hepatosplenomegaly, dyspnea, jaundice, high or low temperature, signs of cardiac failure, hemorrhage, and CNS manifestations. Death often occurs in 2 to 4 days. Milder cases have a vesicular rash which may recur repeatedly during the first months of life. CNS function may be impaired, with ocular or neurologic damage frequent in survivors.

Fetal infection occurs from the infection ascending via the birth canal or from exposure during delivery, transplacental infection from maternal viremia, or contact with infected personnel.

Management. To prevent fetal infection, active genital herpes must be diagnosed during pregnancy, and the delivery done by cesarean section if the membranes are intact and maternal viremia has not occurred. There is no effective treatment for genital herpes. If lesions characteristic of herpes are observed on the mother's genitalia, these should be reported and the diagnosis established before the membranes are ruptured artificially or electrodes applied to the fetal scalp. When disease is not evident at birth, the first signs are nonspecific and include poor eating, listlessness, restlessness, and diarrhea. These symptoms become more severe and over half of the infants develop skin lesions.[8] As there is increasing incidence of genital herpes, the nurse must be alert to this possibility in newborns with the above general symptoms and a skin rash.

Bacterial Skin Infections of the Newborn

There continues to be concern about the spread of staphylococcal infection in hospitals and its increasing resistance to antibiotic therapy. The newborn nursery is one of the most vulnerable areas because of the infants' low tolerance for infections.

In studies of staphylococcal infection of the newborn, strains of the organism have been found not only in skin lesions of the infected infants, but also in the nasopharynx of a high percentage of apparently well infants. Nurseries at this time must be considered potential epidemic centers.

Many factors contribute to the large numbers of infants found to harbor these organisms. *Crowding* of infants in a nursery has always been a serious problem and a contributing factor in any epidemic disease outbreak. The usually recommended minimum of 25 square feet of space per infant may actually not be adequate to prevent spread of infection. *Hospital personnel* have been found to be carriers of staphylococcus coagulase-positive organisms. These organisms are highly resistant to most antibiotics in current use, and when they are transmitted to infants, they may result in such manifestations as skin lesions, pneumonia, septicemia, conjunctivitis, omphalitis, osteomyelitis, and other forms of infection from mild to extremely serious. In many studies, there appears to be a direct transmission of the offending organisms from hospital personnel to infant, from infant to infant, from infant to mother and to the family at home, and even into the community.

Hospital sanitation must be critically appraised, since these organisms may be airborne and can exist in many contaminated or unclean surfaces of the nurseries, wards and other hospital areas. The type of walls, floors and equipment used must be of materials which can be easily and satisfactorily cleaned. Housekeeping personnel, their equipment and methods are to be constantly evaluated and supervised. There is no substitute for cleanliness, aseptic technique and isolation of infected patients and staff in controlling the spread of infection.

Manifestations of staphylococcal infection of the newborn frequently appear as pyoderma, stuffy noses, pneumonia, and conjunctivitis. Few infants develop serious staphylococcal disease without preceding or accompanying pyoderma. Treatment usually consists of antimicrobial drugs given parenterally.

Pyoderma of the skin may occur in epidemic form in the nursery. This was formerly called "impetigo contagiosa" and the term gives some hint of its infectiousness. The condition manifests itself by the eruption of small, semiglobular vesicles or pustules. Although these may appear on any part of the body, they are most frequently encountered on moist opposing surfaces, such as the folds of the neck, the axilla and the groin. Thence they may spread rapidly by autoinoculation to any part of the body. The lesion is small and varies from the size of a pinhead to a diameter of half an inch. It contains yellow pus. The bacterium involved is usually the staphylococcus or the streptococcus.

Management.   The treatment is essentially preventive, and outbreaks rarely occur if the nursery techniques have been meticulous.

Failure to wash hands properly between handling of different infants is undoubtedly the principal mode of spread of infection by any organism. Nothing is more fundamental and important to proper nursery hygiene than handwashing.

Treatment consists of prompt isolation and local treatment of the lesions. Systemic antibiotic therapy may be required in severe outbreaks. A high nutritional level must be maintained and scratching should be controlled. If the lesion is a bleb, the fluid in it is infectious and all material coming in contact with it are to be taken care of according to isolation procedures.

Thrush

Thrush is an infection of the mouth caused by the organism *Candida albicans,* the organism which causes monilial vaginitis in the mother. The infant may acquire the infection as it passes through the birth canal of a mother so infected. However, the infection may be transferred from infant to infant on the hands of attendants and is favored by lack of cleanliness in feeding, in the care of the mother's nipples, or in the care of the bottles and the nipples. It is most likely to occur in weak, undernourished babies and in those receiving antibiotic therapy, since the use of certain antibiotics alters the oral flora making it more susceptible to this opportunistic organism.

The condition appears as small white patches (due to the fungus growth) on the tongue and in the mouth. These white plaques may be mistaken at first for small curds of milk. The infant's mouth must be kept clean, but great gentleness is required to avoid further injury to the delicate epithelium, and any attempt to wipe away the plaques will usually cause bleeding.

Management. Nystatin (Mycostatin) is the drug of choice in treating oral monilia infections, applied directly to the mucosa with cotton-tipped applicator or given as an oral instillation (100,000 units per ml.), 1 ml. four times a day at intervals of six hours. The solution is slowly and gently instilled so that there is an opportunity for it to be widely distributed throughout the oral cavity before it is swallowed.

Special care must be taken with the bottles and nipples used for infants who have thrush. These bottles and nipples must be kept separated from the the others used in the nursery. Disposable bottles and nipples are preferred for these infants. If this is impossible, both the bottles and nipples are soaked in an antiseptic solution, washed thoroughly, and sterilized before they are cared for in the routine way with bottles and nipples of other infants.

Diarrhea of the Newborn

Several bacterial agents can produce primary diarrhea. The most common and important is the enteropathic *Escherichia coli*. Serologic techniques have identified 140 groups of *E. coli*. and over a dozen have been implicated in nursery epidemics of diarrhea. Other bacteria—salmonella, shigella, and staphylococci—are infrequent causes.

Whatever the etiology, a pattern of signs and symptoms of the infection develops: refusal to feed, weight loss (as much as a pound a day), and hypoactivity. These may precede the diarrhea itself by a day or two. Blood and pus in the stool are rare, except in shigellosis. As diarrhea continues, the infant becomes toxic, dehydrated, and acidotic (metabolic acidosis). These symptoms may appear somewhat abruptly during the early phase of explosive diarrhea. Dehydration is even more rapid if vomiting is also present. An ashen gray color or pallor is indicative of impending vasomotor collapse and death. Rapid correction of the metabolic acidosis

and dehydration are therefore crucial. Milder forms of the disease are not uncommon; in these cases, there may be fewer stools, but the diarrhea is protracted and there is failure to feed.

Two of the most important predisposing factors in these outbreaks are overcrowding and faulty nursery techniques—that is, failure to scrub properly before entering the nursery, *failure to wash hands before touching a baby,* failure to maintain proper cleanliness in equipment, clothing, supplies, and so on, that come in contact with the infant. The guiding principle involved is that everything coming in contact with the baby's mouth and nose should be in a surgically aseptic condition. All nursing and medical techniques are to be planned accordingly. Various health departments have set up helpful guidelines and regulations in the hope of preventing epidemics.

Management and Prevention. When a case is discovered, immediate and absolute isolation is necessary; therefore, the infant is transferred from the newborn nursery. A culture of the stools is done to find out the causative organism and to determine specific therapy which should be instituted as soon as possible.

Neomycin or polymicin given orally have been found to be most effective against the *E. coli* organism and are instituted even before the results of the cultures are in. Often the cultures do not show either a bacterial or viral agent and to date these situations defy explanation. Drugs may be given prophylactically to exposed but uninfected infants until their discharge. Penicillin is sometimes administered to prevent or control the secondary infection that might occur in the debilitated infants.

Supportive fluid therapy by the intravenous route also may be utilized. Oral fluids—water, 5 percent glucose in water, or commercially prepared electrolyte fluid replacement for oral use—are given in small amounts. Whole blood is given by transfusion if indicated.

If necessary, the nursery is closed to new admissions until the epidemic clears up. These nurseries are washed and disinfected before being opened again for new admissions. In the prevention of this disease there seems to be nothing more effective than strict aseptic nursery technique.

Hand washing with surgical soap preparation or bacteriocidal and water after changing diapers, before feeding the infant and after handling the infant or any of its equipment is a rigid rule that should be stressed.

If an outbreak occurs, there should be a follow-up of all infants discharged in the preceding two weeks, and any infants needing treatment are readmitted to the pediatric service of the hospital. All infants exposed at the time of an outbreak are given prophylactic therapy. Complete control of this disease, which formerly led to closing of the nursery, can be gained by prompt reporting, rigid techniques, and immediate treatment.

Because of the "explosive" and virulent character of this disease and the startling debilitation of the infant, the parents usually become very anxious about their baby, and with good reason. The baby is usually not allowed to be taken to the mother, as a measure to prevent the spread of the infection and to guard against secondary infection of the infant. Thus, breast-feeding is interrupted for a time at least. The nurse can be helpful in keeping the mother and father informed about the status of the infant and helping the mother to work through her anxiety and grief positively. If it appears that breast-feeding can be resumed shortly, then the nurse can also show the mother how to empty her breast by manual expression to keep the milk supply available until nursing is resumed.

Pneumonia

This condition is the most common pulmonary cause of death in infants dying after 48 hours and is noted in as many as 20 percent of all newborn autopsies. The incidence is usually bimodal, that is, two peaks occur. One is in the first 12 hours of life and is usually secondary to maternal infection. The second peak comes after 48 hours of life, and is probably acquired in the nursery.

CONGENITAL PNEUMONIA. Infection acquired in utero is usually associated with obstetric abnormalities such as early rupture of the membranes, prolonged duration of labor, maternal infection, and uncomplicated premature delivery. The bacteria most frequently involved are *Escherichia coli* and other enteric organisms, *staphylococci* and group *B streptococci*. Symptoms may be evident at birth or within 48 hours thereafter. When these babies are affected at birth, they are flaccid, pale, or cyanotic. Resuscitation is often necessary. Once respirations

are established, they tend to be rapid and shallow with some slight retractions. When the infection is severe, repeated apneic episodes occur and these infants must be observed carefully. Temperature elevation is more likely in term, full-sized infants; the premature infants often have subnormal temperatures.

Postnatally acquired pneumonia is generally caused by *Pseudomonas aeruginosa,* penicillin-resistant staphylococci, and enteric organisms. With this infection, clinical signs usually appear after 48 hours of life. The most common presenting signs are rapid respiration, poor feeding, or aspiration during feeding. Vomiting and aspiration sometimes occur during feeding because previously unsuspected pneumonia is already present. In these instances, the chest film reveals densities that cannot be attributed with certainty to effects of aspirated formula or to preexisting pneumonia. Recovery from postnatal pneumonia is more frequent than from congenital pneumonia.

Management. Antibiotic therapy, oxygen, and supportive care together with close observation are the treatments of choice for these conditions. It is wise to place these infants on their abdomens or sides after feeding to avoid aspiration if regurgitation occurs.

Congenital Rubella

Rubella infection during pregnancy can cause various fetal manifestations, depending upon the timing of viral invasion in relation to fetal growth and development. Teratogenesis appears largely confined to rubella infections occurring in the first 16 weeks of pregnancy. Early infections also often result in spontaneous abortion. Infection which occurs later in pregnancy is associated with premature delivery and growth retardation. Deafness may also occur in later infections.

Infants with the congenital rubella syndrome exhibit varying combinations of the following problems: cardiac anomalies, eye defects, developmental ear defects, thrombocytopenia resulting in petechiae or purpura, lymphocytopenia, encephalitis and CNS disorders, immunologic defects, hepatosplenomegaly, jaundice, osteomyelitis, and pneumonitis. Many infants do not survive, but those who do can harbor the virus for up to one and one-half years after birth, and represent a source of infection to nonimmune persons, particularly pregnant women. Isolation for an extended time is thus necessary.

The potential risk to the fetus of susceptible pregnant women is great, particularly in the first three to four months of pregnancy. Inclusion of rubella testing as part of the routine prenatal laboratory panel can identify nonimmune women and precaution to avoid exposure to possible cases of rubella can be advised. Immunizing nonpregnant susceptible women is the most important preventive measure, but they should not become pregnant for three months following vaccination. The usefulness of immune globulin injections following maternal exposure to rubella has not been clearly demonstrated.[9]

ADDICTION SYNDROMES

Drug Addiction in the Newborn

This condition is being seen more frequently with the rise of drug addiction in the general population. Furthermore, it is the nurse who may be the first to discover this condition. The symptoms of the infant are due to withdrawal rather than narcosis; they may appear almost immediately after birth, or they may be delayed for several hours, depending on the time of the mother's last injection of narcotic, the dose, and the interval between the administration of the narcotic and the delivery.

The infant may manifest restlessness, tremors, shrill crying, convulsions, or twitchings of the extremities and/or face. The Moro reflex may be incomplete, and the deep tendon reflexes may be increased. Diarrhea, vomiting, anorexia, yawning, sneezing, and excessive mucus also may be present. These symptoms parallel somewhat those found in the adult undergoing withdrawal symptoms from narcotics. If the signs of withdrawal are unrecognized, the baby may die; if the infant is treated (hydration, supportive measures, and diminishing doses of sedatives), recovery and permanent cure are assured since the infant does not have a psychic dependence on narcotics.

Heroin or methadone are the narcotic drugs most commonly involved in neonatal drug addiction. Withdrawal symptoms occur in 70 to 90 percent of infants born to addict mothers. Many of these babies are also small for gestational age. In addition to CNS hyperirritability, these infants have sleep disturbances including absence of quiet sleep and inability to sleep. These problems may persist past one year of age. Abnormalities of crying (high-pitched, shrill and continuous crying) strain the mother's endurance, as do sleep disturbances. Addicted infants have a high sucking need, although sucking may be disorganized or depressed. Overfeeding because of this need to suck can compound gastrointestinal problems such as vomiting, regurgitation and diarrhea. It is advisable to provide a pacifier to meet the infant's non-nutritive sucking needs and reduce tension levels.[10] Infants of barbiturate-addicted mothers manifest the same types of symptoms, but with later onset.

Addicted babies are harder to hold, less cuddly, more difficult to console, and show depressed visual response and exaggerated auditory response. They appear to be less alert, are more irritable, have increased muscle tone, and are more labile in alternating between hyperactivity and lethargy. These characteristics make addicted infants harder to mother in a situation where every support is needed to enhance mother-infant bonding. Minimizing separation of infant and mother and assisting the mother to experience satisfying caretaking episodes are critical in promoting the relationship. An honest and open approach in discussing the effects of addiction on the baby and his needs may help the mother feel more confident in her mothering ability. She may experience guilt and anxiety, and the question of care for the infant after discharge must be discussed. A multidisciplinary approach involving drug counselors, social workers, and community health nurses is useful in providing follow-up care for both mother and baby.

Fetal Alcohol Syndrome

Maternal alcohol intake above 3 ounces of absolute alcohol or six drinks per day can result in congenital anomalies of the infant with typical craniofacial and limb defects, cardiovascular defects, intrauterine growth retardation and developmental delay. Alcohol interferes with protein synthesis and the absorption of numerous nutrients, and heavy consumption is most likely to affect fetal development during the first trimester when organogenesis is occurring. Spontaneous abortion is common among alcoholics, but improved nutrition and vitamin fortification now allows many of these pregnancies to continue. If excessive alcohol consumption occurs during the second trimester, infant weight is most affected, which leads to growth retardation.

Characteristic anomalies seen in the fetal alcohol syndrome include microcephaly, short palpebral fissures, epicanthal folds, cleft palate, maxillary hypoplasia, altered palmar creases, joint defects, cardiac defects, anomalous genitalia, fine-motor dysfunction and capillary hemangiomas. Postnatally, there often is developmental delay and growth deficiency. There may be severe mental retardation with depressed sucking and swallowing reflexes, or slight retardation which is not detected until later when developmental problems occur. The extent of immediate fetal depression at birth depends upon the time and amount of the mother's last intake of alcohol, as well as such problems as anoxia or aspiration perinatally. Difficulties in feeding and disturbances of sleep are common in the newborn with this syndrome. Prenatal detection of excessive alcohol consumption and counseling to stop or reduce drinking are the most important preventive measures.[11]

MUSCULOSKELETAL DEFECTS

Talipes Equinovarus (Clubfoot). This deformity of the foot occurs twice as often in males as in females, with an overall incidence of 1 per 1,000 births. There are three elements to this deformity; equinus or plantar flexion of the foot at the ankle, varus or inversion deformity of the heel, and forefoot adduction (Fig. 39-9). All three are present in classic talipes equinovarus. Infants with this deform-

ity should be examined for associated anomalies, especially those of the spine. There is a hereditary pattern in some families, or clubfoot may be part of a generalized neuromuscular syndrome.

Therapy begins early, often while the infant is still in the nursery, and consists of applying plaster casts after the affected foot structures have been stretched and manipulated. Casts are applied sequentially, correcting first the forefoot adduction, then inversion of the heel, and last the equinus flexion at the ankle. Serial casting is needed as the infant grows. After correction is obtained, braces are usually needed for months to years to prevent recurrences of the deformities. About half of these children require an operation to lengthen tightened foot structures.

Congenital Hip Dysplasia. There may be a disturbed relationship with partial contact or complete loss of contact between the femoral head and the acetabulum, usually with some lack of development of both acetabulum and femur and displacement of the femoral head laterally and superiorly due to muscle pull. This hereditary condition occurs more often in females because of pelvic configuration, and may be associated with breech delivery. Unless the dislocation is corrected, dysplasia becomes progressively worse and after a few years may be irreversible.

Diagnosis depends upon demonstrating instability of the joint by placing the infant on his back, flexing both hips at 90° and then slowly abducting them from the midline (Fig. 39-10). A gentle attempt is made to lift the greater trochanter forward, and slipping as the head goes into the acetabulum indicates instability. Additionally, the affected leg often appears shorter, with limited abduction (less than 60°). Assymetry of the gluteal skin folds on the dorsal thigh occurs in slightly less than half the

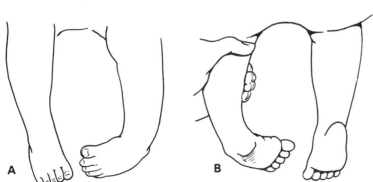

Figure 39-9. Unilateral clubfoot. (A) front view, (B) back view.

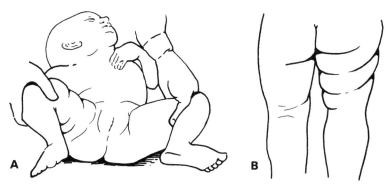

Figure 39-10. In congenital hip dislocation there is limitation of abduction of the affected leg (A) and asymmetry of skin folds of the thighs (B).

cases on the affected side, and a clicking sound may be heard during abduction of the hip.

Treatment during the first few months of life consists of thick diapers which abduct and externally rotate the leg and flex the hip, or use of a Frejka pillow often followed by a spica cast to accomplish this (Fig. 39-11). If the dislocation persists, three weeks of traction followed by six months in a plaster cast may be necessary to accomplish reduction. At an older age, operations are often required.

Parents need education and support in applying corrective measures or appliances, using adaptive feeding and holding techniques, and understanding the course of treatment and expected results. If identified and treated early, the long-term prognosis for correction is good.

Polydactyly. This hereditary condition consists of extra digits on the hands or feet. If the digits do not include bones, ligation with a silk suture during the neonatal period is often adequate to cause sloughing of the tissue, leaving only a small scar after a few days. Surgery is required if bones are present in the extra digits.

PARENTAL AND STAFF REACTIONS TO DEFECTS AND DISORDERS

The birth of an infant with congenital anomalies or developmental defects presents significant psychosocial stresses for the family and precipitates an adaptive crisis. A variety of emotional difficulties may interfere with the parents' relationship with the infant and disrupt functioning of the family. Parents often express feelings of anxiety, guilt, fear, inadequacy, helplessness, failure and anger. The way in which parents cope with crisis and work through

their feelings will influence how realistically they perceive their infant's medical condition and needs, how they are able to adapt to the infant's hospital environment, their ability to assume the primary caretaking role, their ability to assume responsibility for the infant's care after discharge, and, for some, how they will cope with the death of their infant (Fig. 39-12).[12]

Working Through a Crisis

Becoming a parent is a turning point in life, and it is particularly so for the parents of a child who has a disorder. They can emerge from this crisis less mentally and emotionally healthy than they were, or they can move on to increased maturity. If they utilize maladaptive coping mechanisms to deal with the crisis, the former no doubt will occur; if they

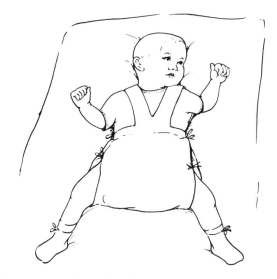

Figure 39-11. The Frejka splint is used to correct congenital dislocation of the hip.

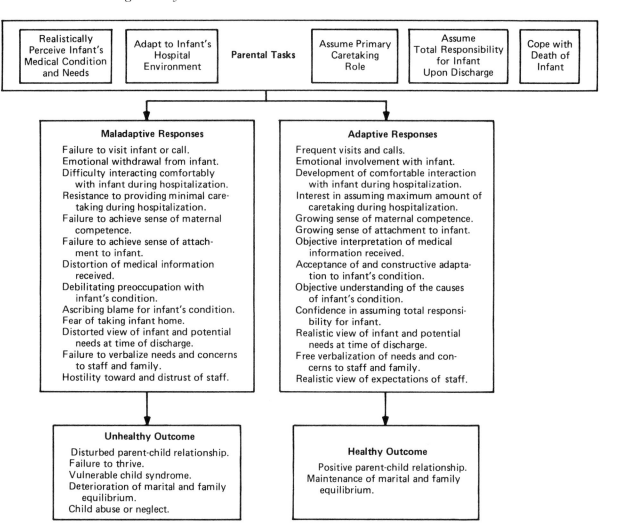

Figure 39-12. Parental response during crisis period. (Source: Grant, P.: "Psychosocial needs of families of high-risk infants." *Family & Community Health,* 1, 3, Nov. 1978, p. 93. An Aspen Publication. Article code 0160-6379/78/0013-0091.)

can be helped to work through positively, this experience will stand them in good stead for future stressful situations.

It is the responsibility of the members of the health team to help them cope with this situation adequately. However, staff members, too, are only human, and at times they are hampered by their own anxieties, feelings, and fantasies, Thus, it is especially important for the staff to understand the psychodynamics occurring in both the parents and themselves so that they may choose a therapeutic course of action to help the parents.

During pregnancy, all women wish for and fantasize about a perfect child, and they also fear that their babies might be abnormal. Their fantasies of the expected child are a composite of the images of

the people who are important to or admired by them. Thus, when the infant deviates drastically from the anticipated child, the simultaneous occurrence of the sudden loss of the idealized child and the necessity of accepting a deviant child can be overwhelming. The greater the deviation from normal, the greater can be the impact of the experience.

It is important to remember that the parents have to grieve for the lost "perfect" child before they can form an attachment to the imperfect one. The process of grief involves anger which can be directed toward anyone involved in the situation—including the infant. Mourning also impairs the capacity to recognize, evaluate, and adapt to reality appropriately. Thus, whenever possible, *long-range* planning for the infant should be delayed until the parents, particularly the mother, can participate in them; otherwise the mourning and depression may persist for an undue length of time.

Anxiety is another dominant reaction. It is thought that the sources of the most serious anxiety are the threats to the parents' sense of adequacy, self-esteem, and social status. One of the earliest questions expressed, "What caused this?" is charged with feelings of biologic inadequacy. Indeed, what the parents are really asking is, "What's the matter with us as progenitors of children?" Particularly for the mother, her failure to produce what she has so long prepared herself to create may well be a threat not only to her femininity, but to her whole unique personhood as well. Moreover, these feelings hold true even for those who have not consciously "planned" the child or who have had several children. Procreating a defective child strikes at the very core of the woman's being. This is very understandable since the child just born is still, in effect, an extension of the mother, and a defect in him is tantamount to a defect in herself. The degree of the mother's anxiety is also related to a deep narcissistic wound, since the psychologic work during pregnancy includes an increase in narcissism—the need to "take in." Hence, feelings of shame and embarrassment are the general accompaniment of personal feelings of inadequacy.

Some of the variables affecting the parents' coping behaviors include past experiences the parents have had in their own growing-up period. If their childhood experiences have fulfilled their needs for mastery, they will have gained trust, security in human relationships, feelings of optimism and the ability to cope, and freedom from crippling guilt and fear. They will also have learned tolerance for frustration. All of these will be of great help to them in their present crisis. Positive experiences with other handicapped or retarded adults and children can also affect the degree of concern and attitude the parents will have. On the other hand, if they remember hostility directed toward the defective person, or if they (or others) responded to him with guilt, pity, repugnance, or overprotectiveness, these feelings may become reactivated when they are confronted with the abnormality of their own child.

Another variable which may influence the response of the parents to their stress is the degree of energy they have at their disposal at the time of the crisis. The mother who has had a long, physically exhausting labor will have less energy for coping with stress than will the mother who has had a rapid, nonexhausting one. The father who has been at the mother's side coaching her during labor and delivery will have less reserve than one who has not performed the physical and emotional effort which accompanies coaching. In addition, having to attend to other-related life situations, such as making emergency preparations for the care of other children, making arrangements for job-related problems, and the like, also takes valuable energy away that is needed for coping.

Many other variables also may influence the responses of the parents. For example, differences in class, economic background, the physical and emotional maturity of the parents, the birth order of the child, its sex, appearance and prognosis all may have important bearing on the immediate significance which the event will have for them.[13]

Avoiding Negative Communication

In the delivery room, the physician, patient, and nurse are intensely involved with one another. Interactions are characterized by intense alertness to behavioral cues.

Whenever a disorder is apparent at birth, especially if it is of any magnitude or of a long-term nature (an anomaly, acute respiratory distress), the tension may be prolonged and intensified instead of being released in the more customary ways. The physician and the nurse will know about the disorder immediately or shortly thereafter. Both their verbal and nonverbal behavior are apt to convey their shock and disappointment to the mother. Their posture may become rigid or they may use their bodies to shield the baby from the mother; their conversation may dwindle or cease; or if an emergency ensues, their actions quicken and conversation is directed to each other and away from the mother and is of a technical nature. The mother may sense this heightened tension and become increasingly aware and terrified that all is not well.

It is not always possible for the staff to stop their activities and to respond to the mother's questions; not only are their efforts often going into lifesaving measures for the infant, but they are having to cope with their own emotional reactions. For instance, it is not unnatural for the staff (and the parents later) to have, and perhaps to express, death wishes for a severely defective child. They feel frustrated and resentful toward a situation that they can neither control nor, in many cases, change. It may be an extremely difficult time for the physician, who may have a sense of failure because the patient cannot be "healed." The mother, in turn, may sense the attendants' frustration and misinterpret it as hostility or resentment toward her—that she also has "failed." This negative communication only intensifies the trauma that is experienced by all concerned. In addition, the new mother feels sadness, a completely different emotion from the joy she had anticipated; furthermore, it comes at a time when she may be physically and emotionally exhausted.

Telling the Parents

Most professionals agree that the mother and father should be informed as soon as possible (preferably immediately) of the disorder. However, some tend to seek or develop strategies for delaying the announcement of "bad" news. If this occurs, it can mean significant and far-reaching consequences for the mother and father. Since the mother expects to see or at the very least be told about her infant, if this does not happen, she will become suspicious and alarmed and eventually mistrustful. The important immediate establishment of a "trust" relationship will be impeded.

Sometimes, however, the abnormality makes the condition of the infant so critical that he must be transferred immediately to the intensive care nursery, and the mother may not see her baby. Therefore, *what* the parents are told about the condition and *how* they are told become critical issues. All too often one hears parents complain bitterly about the "bluntness," "coldness," and "unconcern" that the staff demonstrated. Worse still is the "conspiracy of silence" that tortures the already overwrought pair, in which each professional avoids saying anything, pretending or assuming that the other will handle the matter, or that it is better left alone. It is important to recognize that the apparent coldness, avoidance, and so on, are not really manifestations of the staff members' true feelings, but rather are unsuccessful coping mechanisms on their part to allay their feelings of helplessness, anxiety, and inadequacy. However, it is part of the nurse's professional responsibility to explore these feelings and to develop more effective ways of handling them.

Cues to the best type of intervention are obtained by observing the parents' behavior at this time. The mother cannot invest feeling in the defective child until she can feel and talk about her disappointment, sense of failure, helplessness, and/or fears regarding the infant's health and future. The process of grieving is facilitated through repeated discussions before reality can be faced. Interpretations of the baby's condition must be synchronized with this mourning process so that the parents can assimilate facts and reality as they move through the process. When anger or guilt is not expressed, tremendous energy is utilized to contain it, and this energy can be better used in forming a viable relationship later with the child. Moreover, the lack of opportunity to discuss their feelings will hinder the parents' ability to test reality. Therefore, it is necessary that each fear be clarified as the parents are able to bring it into consciousness. In this way, distortions of thinking, feeling, and perception are reduced.

To accomplish this, nurses and other professional personnel will want to encourage parents to react as fully as they desire in an emotional climate and physical environment where they are assured their behavior and feelings are accepted. An attitude of warmth and acceptance which is communicated by actions (physical care, comfort measures, simply sitting with the couple), as well as words, help the couple regain self-esteem. It may be difficult for the professional personnel, since our culture frowns on frank expression of deep feeling. Yet it is much easier for the parents to accept their own feelings if they are accepted by the professionals around them. A mother will feel understood if the nurse conveys that her feelings and behavior are natural.

The nurse will want to be particularly cognizant about maintaining communication regarding the parents' responses to their situation, the condition of the infant, and any other factors that have bearing on the situation. In this way, a coordinated effort can be made by all members of the health team for comprehensive care.

Realistic Appraisal and Reassurance. In order to give the parents a realistic appraisal of the situation, many authorities feel that the parents should be informed immediately of the disorder and the prognosis, especially if repair or long-term care is involved. This information, of course, must be explained in terms that the couple can understand, and reinforcement over the days probably will be necessary.

Whatever specifics are told, it is important that two aspects of realistic reassurance be given the mother and father: first, that they and their child are acceptable and, second, that the hospital and personnel are there to render any assistance possible. Particularly in the cases of some defects and deformities (e.g., phocomelia or myelomeningocele) the parents must understand that although their child may not be made whole, he usually can be helped to some degree. This kind of reassurance demonstrates an attitude of understanding and sharing of the parents' feelings of hurt and loss, and at the same time it does not minimize the gravity of the situation.

Acceptance of the Infant by the Staff

The parents' first encounter with their infant is another crucial time. Particularly in cases in which there is an obvious anomaly, it is vitally important that the physician or the nurse who is showing the baby demonstrate an attitude of warmth and acceptance of the infant; if revulsion or rejection is manifested, the parents' own feelings of despair and ostracism will be intensified.

One way the staff can demonstrate to the parents that their child is valuable and important is to hold him close, cuddle him, and call him by name. At this time, if it seems to be indicated, the positive points in the prognosis can be reiterated or reinforced. This may be a difficult time for all concerned, since staff members are also trying to cope with their own possible feelings of rejection. Therefore, an attempt should be made to avoid a common kind of destructive behavior that tends to be demonstrated unconsciously, that of isolating the infant under the guise of "protecting" the mother.

Grieving

Grief can be considered a response to loss. It is most often known to us as a response to a loss through death or separation of a loved person, but it can occur following the loss of anything, tangible or intangible, which is highly valued. Grief is a universal, normal, developmentally evolved adaptive process. It progresses through predictable phases, and this progress enables the individual to deal adaptively with the disturbance of his psychologic equilibrium which is inevitably caused by loss. The parents can be expected to show signs of grieving when a substantial defect in their infant (or death) occurs. The couple must come to terms with a difficult and perhaps unexpected situation, one in which the prognosis may be poor. Both parents will demonstrate grief, and the father's needs, as well as the mother's, should be kept in mind.

Several phases are encountered in the grief reaction, and how intensely the parents experience these will vary according to the nature and the gravity of the disorder and their capacity for grieving.

Shock and Withdrawal

The first phase involves shock and difficulty in believing that their baby has a malformation or disorder. There is often a great urge to flee, and fathers may literally leave the situation. The parents may appear stunned or immobilized, or may try to carry on ordinary activities; intermittent flashes of anguish and despair occur as reality penetrates. Occasionally, there is an overtly intellectual response to the reality of the situation: the mother or father may try to comfort the other, make any necessary arrangements, and the like. This type of response takes place only if the full emotional impact is not allowed to reach the consciousness. The loss is recognized, but its painful character is muted. This phase may last from minutes to days; the longings for a "perfect child" may be recalled, felt intensely, and discharged gradually. This process serves to free the parents' feelings so that they may proceed to the next phase.

During the shock phase, the parents may withdraw initially. This is a strategy to escape the painful reality of the situation; hence, at times they want only silence and solitude. It is important not to label this behavior as "rejection of the child," for if criticism of this kind is manifested or implied, the parents' anger may be directed toward the child so that they continue to not wish to see him. These parents are experiencing great psychic pain and their concerns naturally center on their own feelings. They are trying to sort out what this defect or illness means to them personally. Nurses can be of great assistance, if they can respond to withdrawal with understanding and a great deal of giving, even in the face of seeming disinterest and apathy. This demonstration of giving will help relieve the mother's feelings of guilt about her lack of motherliness if the nurse helps her to understand that such feelings always develop gradually as a mother cares for and handles her child.

On the other hand, however, if the mother appears to indicate an *initial* overprotectiveness toward the infant, this behavior should also be respected since it is a defense against the mother's anxiety and disorganization. Self-pity may become displaced as pity for the child and, if the nurse is critical of this attitude, the defense will only be deepened. Thus, the mother is not to be made to feel that others are trying to intrude between her and her infant. Those appropriate aspects of nurturance and care that she attempts to give can be reinforced and praised and gradually she can be helped to realize the limits of her assistance.

Denial and Disbelief

The second phase is one of denial or disbelief that this could have happened to them. The parents wish to believe that their baby does not have a problem. This phase is affected by many factors, a significant one being the visibility of the malformation. The denial period may be longer with such conditions as Down's syndrome or other types of mental retardation which might not become clearly apparent for some time. The more obvious defects demand more immediate recognition and admission that the problem does exist. The birth of a defective child may have grave implications for the marital bond. After the immediate shock of the birth, the parents, in this second stage of grieving, begin to reflect on the many problems facing them because of the defect. Often one of them becomes very concerned about imparting information about the deviation to the other, and sometimes to close family or friends as well. This concern will be especially evident if the parent feels responsible in some way because of a family history of congenital defects, irresponsibility, or the like. This concern is manifested irrespective of whether or not the marriage is stable. Submergence of one's own feelings in deference to the partner's may occur in more stable unions, while blame may be attributed in less happy marriages. This latter response, particularly, only adds another source of stress. If either partner was afraid of what the birth of the baby might do to their relationship, the fears will only be intensified with the birth of a defective or ill child.

Anger and Sadness

The third phase involves anger and sadness, and often interweaves with the second period of denial. With developing awareness, there is often a *feeling* of loss and disappointment, accompanied at times by affective and physical symptoms (i.e., emptiness in the epigastric or chest regions, sadness, and the like). Now the painful feelings are allowed to become conscious. The parents (particularly the mother) may cry, express anger toward a variety of persons and things, talk about the situation, or be unable to express any verbal emotions, although they want to.

A relationship between the nurse and the parents that is based on helping is most effective at this time; the nurse's approach should be dictated by the parents' reactions. By accepting and encouraging the expression of feelings (and providing privacy for their expression), the nurse helps to prepare the way for the next phase. Developing awareness may take a long time—days or months. The nurse in the hospital usually will see its beginning, but very infrequently sees its termination.

During the grieving process, the mother needs more physical rest than the usual postpartum patient since she needs increased energy to cope with the tragedy. Regression is natural at this time and dependency needs are increased in the presence of anxiety.

By responding to the mother's increased need for personal care, the nurse demonstrates acceptance of both the mother and the child. By caring for the baby and showing affection and interest in him, the nurse demonstrates a realistic investment in him. This reassures the mother that the child is worthwhile and others can love and accept him—this allays her feelings of inadequacy over time. The nurse will want to be alert to the times when the mother shows signs of wanting to learn to care for the infant. Fortunately, now, mothers are given more opportunities to care for and feed their infants, even when the infants may be in a special nursery.

Balance and Equilibrium

The *fourth phase* is a period of relative equilibrium, during which some of the intense reactions have lessened. There may be little emotional resiliency at this time, however. Additional stresses can disrupt this tenuous balance, for example, the development of a new complication such as pneumonia in an infant with a congenital anomaly. With new stresses, the parents may lapse into the previous phase or begin the process over. Progression in the equilibrium phase is assisted by positive caretaking experiences.

The feeding experience is extremely significant for the mother. When she can feed her infant and sense some response in him, she will begin to have some tangible, positive reinforcement that she can perform a crucial nurturing activity for her baby. Thus, her self-esteem is increased. It must be remembered, however, that every time the mother does feed (or performs any other care-giving activity for) her infant, she must face the baby's defect or illness, and her initial feelings of anxiety, frustration, and guilt are apt to be reactivated. Over time, these initial feelings gradually diminish with successful trials of feeding or care giving. However, if the mother refuses to feed her infant or prefers to "skip" one or two feedings, it is wise to be unblaming, since nothing is to be gained by pushing the mother into prematurely caring for the infant. As the mother learns to feed her infant and do other specific activities for the infant, she channels some of her own dependency feelings into the activities and gradually gains confidence in her competence as a mother.

The arrival of a defective or ill child makes great demands on the father, and this fact is often overlooked; attention is more frequently directed toward the mother since she is hospitalized. Often the father's responsibilities are so overwhelming that he cannot perceive or provide the support his partner so earnestly needs. Unless he too receives assistance in coping with his feelings about the birth, he may have difficulty assuming his caretaking relationship. He needs to know that his feelings are important also—that he is being considered as a person, not just as an expeditor. As he realizes that his grief is acceptable and the professionals care about what he is experiencing, he will be able to cope with his feelings better and be able to offer more support to the mother.

Reorganization and Restitution

The *fifth and final phase* is that of reorganization, which may over months and years allow the parents to reach a better state of emotional organization than before they experienced this tragedy. Self-esteem can often be improved, and such parents may be more able to tolerate other stresses and tragic events and be helpful to other parents and children.[14]

During restitution mourning occurs, in which mutual grief and loss are expressed by the parents and sympathetic friends and relatives. At this stage religious beliefs and rituals are helpful in clarifying the ambiguity about suffering, eternity, and death. In this, the final phase of grief, resolution of the problem gradually occurs; this phase may take from six months to a year.

Stillbirth or Neonatal Death

Occasionally, parents and staff will be faced with the unfortunate circumstance of a stillbirth or a neonatal death. All of the responses of both personnel and parents that have just been described may be apparent in these cases. Grief and mourning will be noted particularly, and it will become the nurse's responsibility to provide an environment in which the mother and father can express their feelings. Nursing care is essentially the same as that just described.

It appears that the length and intensity of mourning after the death of an infant is proportionate to the closeness of the relationship prior to death. Moreover, it has been found that caring for an infant who subsequently dies or touching or fondling a dead infant is not unduly upsetting to an emotionally healthy mother (one who does not have a history of psychiatric problems). All too often the reason given for not allowing the mother and father contact with their dying or dead infant is that it will be "too upsetting." Fortunately, it is now known that affectional bonding is enhanced (as with all babies) with tactile stimulation and caretaking and that this type of contact does not result in pathologic grieving. It appears that affectional bonding is necessary in order that the parents may relinquish the dead child and work through the symbiotic relationship that existed before birth. Thus, a high degree of mourning appears to be a normal phenomenon of the grieving process and should not be considered pathologic or abnormal.

One of the most frequent complaints of parents, and especially mothers, is that the staff, including nurses, do not "know what to do with me." That is, the mothers are treated as if nothing had happened and no mention is made of the tragedy; this is part of the "conspiracy of silence" that we mentioned previously. It is difficult to outline specific nursing measures as the ability and depth in interaction will depend to a great extent on the nurse's own feelings about death (and deformities) and personal experience in dealing with death and dying.

One approach is for the nurse to express sympathy or sorrow that the *tragedy* had to happen to the mother. This may start the mother crying, but this emotional demonstration need not be feared. The nurse can then put an arm around the mother and encourage her to continue, assuring her that this and other grieving behavior is acceptable. If the mother continues to cry, the nurse can gently reassure her. If the mother begins to talk about the tragedy, the nurse will be able to pick up cues which may call for further reassurance that she was not "guilty" of anything or perhaps the need for factual information. It may be that, initially, the nurse will only be able to express sadness and to ask if the mother would like to talk about it. The general goal is to meet the parents' spoken and unspoken cries for compassion, understanding, and factual information.[15]

The nurse must be careful not to offer the mother unhelpful platitudes, such as, "Please don't feel so bad. You have such lovely children at home." Or "You can always have another baby." Statements of this kind are not only unhelpful but are detrimental to the situation, since they convey to the patient the nurse's great lack of understanding and appreciation of the situation. The parents will trust the nurse to the degree that they perceive an understanding and empathetic manner. To this same degree will they trust and permit the nurse to help them arrive at a positive solution of their problem.

NURSING CARE: THE HIGH RISK INFANT

Assessment	Intervention	Evaluation
Physiological Status of Newborn: Immediate care		
Respiration and oxygenation Respiratory characteristics Skin color, heart rate, cry, muscle tone Birth injury and trauma Signs of depression from CNS injury Symmetry of reflexes, facies Neuromuscular tone Symmetry of limbs Condition of skin (edema, hematoma, ecchymosis) Hemorrhage or shock Overt bleeding, source Depression, tachycardia, respiratory distress Congenital anomalies Type and characteristics Disease or illness Signs present at birth Gestational age Initial exam (posture, tonicity, recoil)	Assist ventilation (intubation, resuscitation, oxygen). Assist suctioning. Assist drawing specimens for blood gasses and electrolytes. Assist maintenance of circulation (IVs, transfusions, umbilical cath). Assist or administer emergency medications (cardiac, bicarbonate). Assist cardiac massage. Record signs of birth injury. Record congenital anomalies. Record signs of disease or illness, hemorrhage or shock. When anomaly present, examine infant carefully for other less obvious defects. Report anomalies, signs of injury or disease to members of neonatal team. Record indications of gestational age. Monitor vital signs. Conserve warmth during procedures.	Respiration maintained, spontaneous or assisted Skin color, heart rate, muscle tone, cry improve Condition stabilizes (control of hemorrhage, tremors, seizures, depression, etc.)
Continuing care		
Respiratory exchange (apnea) Later manifestations of trauma (irritability, convulsions) Signs and symptoms of disease Hypoglycemia, hypocalcemia, polycythemia, jaundice	Maintain assisted ventilation. Monitor oxygen levels. Monitor vital signs. Report and record signs and symptoms of disease, behavior indicating CNS trauma, or neurological damage.	Adequate ventilation maintained, assisted or spontaneous Vital signs stable Behavior and functions within normal limits for gestational age Treatments restore to greater physiological equilibrium

NURSING CARE: THE HIGH RISK INFANT (*Continued*)

Assessment	Intervention	Evaluation

Gestational age (thorough exam)
  Sleep patterns, restlessness, irritability
  Feeding needs and response
  Temperature regulation
  Hematologic problems
    Hemorrhage, polycythemia, anemia
  Renal and bowel function
  Signs of infection
  CNS problems
  Musculoskeletal and soft tissue trauma
	Administer treatments (medications, positioning, exchange transfusion, phototherapy, intravenous feeding or hydration, gavage feeding, etc.).
	Record and report variations in sleep patterns.
	Provide and record type, route, and amounts of feedings, responses.
	Record and report elimination.
	Report signs of infection, CNS, MS, and soft tissue problems.
	Maintain warmth in isolette, prevent heat loss during procedures.
		Sleep patterns normal for gestational age
		Takes adequate nourishment and retains feedings
		Temperature remains within normal limits
		Infant gains weight
		Elimination normal

Development Needs:
 	
  Stimulation
  Nurturance
  Activity
	According to developmental status of infant, provide balance of stimulation and rest.
	Hold and handle during feedings when condition permits.
		Infant attains expected developmental landmarks for age, both neuromuscular and interactional

Parent-Infant Bonding
 	
  Contact
  Caretaking
	Encourage bonding process through providing parents with information about status and characteristics of their infant, maximize parent-infant contact, support in caretaking activities, maintain telephone or written contact after mother is discharged, encourage visits to ICN for caretaking and holding.	Parents take active interest in progress and caretaking of their infant
		Visit regularly after mother's discharge
		Provide caretaking effectively

Parental Psychosocial Needs:
 	
  Information and support
  Grief, reactions to anomalies
  Family adaptations
	Provide information, discuss its meanings, encourage expression of feelings and reactions.
	Facilitate grieving process.
	Refer to other sources of support (parents groups, counseling, etc.).
	Discuss family responses, needs of siblings, community resources.
		Parents feel well informed and understand their infant's condition.
		Feelings of loss and grief are expressed as appropriate for the individual and family.
		Parents able to interact and care for infant, or make decisions about alternate types of care.
		Family accepts and relates to infant, plans made for special care needs.

REFERENCES

1. M. G. MacDonald and H. M. Risenberg: "Neonatal emergencies: Fetal neonatal transition, acute intensive care." In *Perinatal Medicine: Management of the High Risk Fetus and Neonate.* R. J. Bolognese and R. H. Schwartz, eds. Baltimore, Williams & Wilkins, 1977, p. 282.

2. R. L. Walton: "A study of etiological variables in palatolabial malformations." *J. Kansas Med. Soc.* 73:370–377, Aug. 1972.

3. H. C. Kempe, H. K. Silver and D. O'Brien: *Current Pediatric Diagnosis and Treatment.* Los Altos, Calif., Lange Medical Publications, 1978, p. 942.

4. R. C. Benson: *Current Obstetric and Gynecologic Diagnosis and Treatment.* Los Altos, Calif., Lange Medical Publications, 1978, p. 806.

5. F. J. Picaud et al.: "The newborn of diabetic mothers." *Biol. Neonate* 24:1–30, 1974.

6. D. W. Guthrie and R. A. Guthrie: "The infant of the diabetic mother." *Am. J. Nurs.* 11: 2008–2009, Nov. 1974.

7. M. Vogel: "When the pregnant woman is

diabetic: Care of the newborn." *Amer. J. Nurs.* 79, 3:458–460, March 1979.

8. J. E., Bahr: "Herpesvirus hominis type 2 in women and newborns." *MCN—Maternal Child Nurs.* Jan./Feb. 1978, 16–24.

9. D. W. Reynolds: "Perinatal infection—Diagnosis, treatment and prevention." *Postgrad. Medicine* 60, 1:101–106, July 1976.

10. G. K. Kantor: "Addicted mother, addicted baby—A challenge to health care providers." MCN—*Amer. J. Maternal Child Nurs.* Sept./Oct. 1978, 281–289.

11. B. Luke: "Maternal alcoholism and fetal alcohol syndrome." *Amer. J. Nurs.* 77, 12: 1924–1926, December 1977.

12. P. Grant: "Psychosocial needs of families of high-risk infants." *Fam. & Community Health* 1, 3:91–102, November 1978.

13. E. H. Waechter: "Bonding problems of infants with congenital anomalies." *Nurs. Forum* 16, 3,4:298–318, 1977.

14. J. H. Kennell: "Birth of a malformed baby: Helping the family." *Birth and Fam. J.* 5, 4: 219–222, Winter 1978.

15. H. Schuman: "Thoughts and comment." *JOGN Nursing* 48–49, May/June 1974.

SUGGESTED READING

Wyatt, D. S.: "Phenylketonuria: The problems vary during different developmental stages." *MCN—Amer. J. Maternal Child Nurs.* Sept./Oct. 1978, 296–302.

Kennell, J. H.: "Parenting in the intensive care unit." *Birth and Fam. J.* 5, 4:223–226, Winter 1978.

Arney, W. R., et al.: "Caring for parents of sick newborns." *Obstet. and Gynecol. Survey* 33, 9:603, Sept. 1978.

Bortolussi, R., et al.: "Early-onset pneumococcal sepsis in newborn infants." *Pediatrics* 60, 3:352–355, Sept. 1977.

Bresadola, C.: "One infant/one nurse/one objective: quality care." *MCN—Amer. J. Maternal Child Nurs.* Sept./Oct. 1977, 287–290.

Erdman, D.: "Parent-to-parent support: The best for those with sick newborns." *MCN—Amer. J. Maternal Child Nurs.* Sept./Oct. 1977, 291–292.

Eager, M.: "Long-distance nurturing of the family bond." *MCN—Amer. J. Maternal Child Nurs.* Sept./Oct. 1977, 293–294.

Korones, S. B., et al.: *High-Risk Newborn Infants, The Basis for Intensive Nursing Care.* St. Louis, C. V. Mosby, 1978.

Special Considerations in Maternity Nursing

Alternatives in Maternity Care

Evolution of Maternity Nursing

Forty

Alternatives in Maternity Care

History of Family-Centered Maternity Care | Resurgence of Home Births | Alternative Birthing Centers | Options Available for Cesarean Births | Options in Maternity Nursing

The purpose of this chapter is to present some of the options in maternity care which have developed during the past decade in the United States. Before presenting some of these options, it is important to reflect on some of the reasons why these alternatives have evolved.

Prior to the 1950s and 1960s a woman was generally "in the dark" regarding her pregnancy, labor and delivery. There was usually little or no exchange of educational information between the physician and the pregnant woman, and most of the decisions made about the pregnancy were made by the physician. Much of the education that a woman might obtain about childbearing and childbirth was provided by family members and friends who would share their experiences, and old wive's tales, with the woman. Often these stories would emphasize the "pain" and "suffering" women had to endure to give birth—information which only increased the pregnant woman's feelings of anxiety and apprehension about her forthcoming labor and delivery.

When a woman's labor started, she was usually taken to the hospital. Home births were less commonplace during this time because of sociological and medical pressure against this practice.[1] Once the woman was admitted to the hospital she was usually separated from the father. Except for short visiting periods during the labor, the labor and delivery rooms were "off-limits" to the father and other relatives and friends of the woman for the duration of the intrapartum period. With little knowledge about the usual course of labor and birth, and having been isolated from the father (and other support persons), the laboring woman relied heavily on the advice of the obstetrical staff to help her cope with the discomfort and apprehension she was experiencing. Analgesics and anesthetics which were administered by the well-meaning obstetrical staff to relieve the woman's pain, also relieved her of her sense of control and her sense of self-esteem. More often than not a woman would awaken after childbirth unaware that she had, in fact, given birth. It was not uncommon for the father, not the mother, to be the first to become acquainted with the newborn infant, though usually only through the nursery room window.

During the postpartum period, the mother would bathe and feed her infant according to the hospital schedule. When these tasks were completed, the infant was usually returned to the nursery where the father, mother, and the other children could gather to view the newborn infant. In some hospitals, fathers were not allowed to touch their infants until the infant was discharged and on the way home. The importance of efficiency and competency at specific medical tasks was often emphasized in the nurse's role during this period, and patient advocacy and education had little or nothing to do with maternity nursing. It is not difficult to understand why consumers became dissatisfied with this kind of maternity care. They began to question health care professionals about the rationales for some of these practices; and gradually their demands for more involvement in pregnancy and childbirth began to make a significant impact on maternity care in this country.

HISTORY OF FAMILY-CENTERED MATERNITY CARE

Family-Centered Care. The concept of *family-centered maternity care* began to gain support among nursing circles during the 1960s. This approach advocated consideration of other members of the family, particularly the fathers, during pre- and postdelivery care. The pregnant woman, who had been viewed largely in isolation as a medical problem, was recognized as having social and emotional needs which deserved the nurse's attention as did her physical needs. It seems strange now that nurses had to be reminded that pregnant women had families, with psychologic needs for some involvement in this most momentous event, as well as very real practical problems and social concerns which often could be helped by nursing attention. But this indeed had been the outcome of years of emphasis on efficiency and routinization on the one hand and influence of the medical model on the other.

Prepared Childbirth. Contributing to family-centered maternity care was the *participant childbirth movement* which brought about significant changes in the practice of obstetrics through consumer pressure. Its purposes closely paralleled the family-centered approach, but even greater involvement of the father was advocated. As the ideas and techniques of Dick-Read, Lamaze, and Bradley caught on in the United States, childbearing women and their partners began to seek knowledge and demand a right to make choices in the conduct of their own pregnancies, labors, and deliveries. Women wanted to be aware and awake, to feel a central part of the

process, to become equipped to cope with the stress of labor without heavy medication, and to have their partners by their side to share the experience. Prepared childbirth usually involved education about the processes of parturition and instruction in techniques to reduce pain perception and enhance the sense of control over the process (see Chapter 24).

Fathers frequently served as labor coaches, and through this type of involvement pressure was brought to bear on hospitals to allow their presence in the labor room. It seemed ludicrous to allow fathers to assist their partners all during labor, only to dismiss them just at the climax of the entire process. This gain was not achieved easily, and took a period of some years before reluctant physicians and nurses accepted the fact that prepared fathers were not going to faint or become irate over necessary procedures or during unexpected complications.

Mother-Baby Couple Care. Following increased concern about family involvement in the childbearing process, *mother-baby couple care* was instituted in many postpartum units to facilitate development of the early mother-infant relationship. The forerunner of this practice was *rooming-in,* when mothers who elected to do so (and could afford a private room or could be placed with a roommate who also wanted rooming-in) would have their babies placed in the room with them during the hospitalization period. Rooming-in had a varying course over the years, with persistent professional resistance which mothers had to overcome, often only to be left largely on their own with their new babies.

Mother-baby couple care represents a commitment on the part of the postpartum and nursery staff to restructure the hospital units so mothers and babies may be together the greater part of the day and night. Usually satellite nurseries are developed to serve each wing of the maternity unit, and postpartum and nursery nurses move back and forth within the wing or area. Babies are out with their mothers except for specified times when they are in the nursery for physical examinations, tests or procedures, or if the mother or baby are temporarily sick.

Although the logistics of mother-baby couple care require some working out, and nurses need some retraining in the area of their lesser experience, the benefits of each mother-baby couple having the same nurse responsible for their care are enormous. In this way, the same nurse knows the condition and needs of both mother and baby, enhancing the development of the mother-infant relationship through intimacy and close contact, immediate response to needs or problems, and elimination of the communication gap.

Breast-Feeding. The *back-to-nature* movement which was an expected reaction to the increasing use of artificial substances and chemical additives in a wide variety of material and products served as an impetus to the rediscovery of *breast-feeding*. Organizations were formed to assist mothers relearn the art of breast-feeding and encourage success through information and support, such as LaLeche League. In response to maternal need, postpartum nurses began to learn how to help mothers initiate satisfactory breast-feeding patterns during their first days of nursing their babies in the hospital.

RESURGENCE OF HOME BIRTHS

Family-centered maternity care has evolved over several years; and to some consumers the changes which have occurred are conservative. Today, routine maternity care in some areas of the country includes expensive and sophisticated tests and procedures which many women, and their partners, regard as invasive and interfering manuevers on the part of health care professionals. The increasing reliance of obstetricians on such procedures as "routine" fetal monitoring, amniotomy, administration of intravenous fluids, and oxytoxic drugs during the course of uncomplicated labors and births illustrates the still prevalent belief that pregnancy and childbirth are pathologic, not normal, processes.[2,3] Furthermore, the increasing cost of maternity and obstetrical services, especially when unnecessary tests and procedures are used routinely, is a very real concern of expectant families. As a result, there has been a gradual increase in the number of home births occurring in this country during the past decade.[4]

This current trend concerns both the consumers and providers of maternity care. The primary concern of both these groups is the potential complications which can occur during any normal birth; but which can be even more life-threatening to either the mother or the fetus when the birth occurs at home without adequate medical back-up or quick access to emergency equipment. Although some physicians and nurses are proponents of home births that utilize good medical and emergency back-up systems, most health care professionals regard this practice as exposing the mother and the fetus to unnecessary danger.[5,6] Fortunately, the dichotomy between demands for more family involvement in maternity care by consumers and the rejection of home births as a safe alternative by many health care professionals is beginning to narrow due to the development of some feasible and acceptable options in maternity care within the hospital setting.

ALTERNATIVE BIRTHING CENTERS

In 1978, a joint statement entitled "The Development of Family-Centered Maternity/Newborn Care in Hospitals" was issued by the Interprofessional Task Force on Health Care of Women and Children.[7] This task force was composed of representatives from the American College of Nurse-Midwives, the American Nurses' Association, the Nurses' Association of the American College of Obstetricians and Gynecologists, the American College of Obstetricians, and the American Academy of Pediatrics. The representatives from these grolps collaborated and agreed upon the following definition of family-centered maternity/newborn care:

> Family-centered maternity/newborn care can be defined as the delivery of safe, quality health care while recognizing, focusing on, and adapting to both the physical and psychological needs of the client-patient, the family, and the newly born. The emphasis is on the provision of maternity/newborn health care which fosters family unity while maintaining physical safety.[8]

The joint statement prepared and issued by this group of professionals also provided guidelines for implementing family-centered maternity/newborn care in hospitals interested in incorporating such programs in their obstetrical units. The statement advocated the establishment of such services as childbirth classes for the *family* taught by qualified health professionals (ideally with input from both physicians and nurses); continuing education classes for the maternity staff, which includes information on current childbirth trends and techniques; a more liberal definition of "family" to include a "significant" or other "supporting person important to the mother; the development of "Birthing Rooms" as options to the standard labor and delivery room approach to childbirth; and the option for early discharge of the mother and newborn with appropriate follow-up nursing and/or medical visits to assess their health and progress during the early postpartum period.[9] The use of professionally developed guidelines, such as those presented in this statement, combined with consumer input regarding the desires of childbearing families for a more homelike childbirth within the hospital setting, are contributing to the establishment of alternative birthing centers (or ABCs as they are often called) throughout the country. For many expectant families, birthing centers provide an acceptable option to the traditional medical "delivery" of an infant in the hospital, as well as a safe alternative to giving birth at home.

Physical Set-Up and Selection. An alternative birthing center (ABC) usually consists of one or more private birthing rooms where a woman labors and gives birth to her infant. The woman can be accompanied by the father and, in some ABCs, by her children and other family members and/or friends. The physical set-up of the birthing room is quite different from the standard labor and delivery rooms used in traditional obstetrical units. Usually there is a bed which is large enough for the mother, father, and their newborn to recline comfortably. Chairs and a dresser are included in the furnishings, as are plants and pictures. In some ABCs parents are encouraged to bring their own pictures and wall hangings to decorate the room so that the room will be similar to their own home environment. Often a stereo is provided in the room for the laboring woman to listen to her favorite music as a means of relaxing and maintaining inner calm during the labor and birth. Private bathroom facilities are incorporated into each birthing room for the convenience and comfort of the mother. The standard equipment used during childbirth is usually stored in cabinets in the room until it is needed. Also, emergency equipment which might be needed during the intrapartum period is readily available to the staff and is similarly stored.

Most ABCs are located within hospitals, and are designed for use by women who have had normal pregnancies and who are experiencing uncomplicated intrapartal periods. Strict criteria are used by physicians, nurse-midwives, and nurse practitioners during the prenatal and intrapartal periods to evaluate women who desire to give birth in an ABC. If a woman is considered to be in a high risk category during her pregnancy, she is usually not eligible for an ABC. When a woman with a normal prenatal course is initially admitted to an ABC but develops a complication during her labor, she is usually transferred to the regular obstetrical unit of the hospital.

Supportive Atmosphere. In an ABC, a woman is free to move about during her labor. She is allowed to drink fluids, and is often encouraged to bring beverages to the ABC from her home so she will have the type of fluids she desires. Analgesics are available in some ABCs; however, most couples are required to attend childbirth classes during the pregnancy so that the women will learn some breathing techniques to decrease or eliminate entirely her need for analgesics during her labor. Athough one-to-one nursing care is provided for the woman, active participaion of the father (or coach) is encouraged and supported by the nurse. In some ABCs, children are allowed to be present during the birth, but a responsible adult (other than the parents or nursing staff) must accompany the child or children to closely observe them and attend to their needs throughout this event.

The atmosphere in an ABC is usually relaxing and congenial as a woman labors and gives birth surrounded by her family and a supportive, sensitive, obstetrical staff. Since nuring care is provided on a one-to-one basis, the opportunity for establishing rapport between the expectant family and the nurse is excellent. Often a nurse will meet the family during the prenatal period and contract with that family to be their obstetric nurse throughout the labor and birth of their child. This is an ideal situation, as the nurse will become familiar with the members of the family prior to the birth and will be better able to assess their special needs and intervene appropriately to meet these needs during the intrapartum period.

Goals. In an ABC, the goal of the staff is to meet the individual desires and needs of the woman during a safe, normal childbirth while they carefully monitor the progress of her labor and the birth of her child. Enemas, pubic shaving, and stirrups are not routine in the majority of ABCs. Similarly, episiotomies are not routinely done; rather, attempts are made to stretch the woman's perineum naturally through gentle massaging of the vaginal introitus during the second stage of labor. The actual birth of the infant can occur in any position that is safe and comfortable for the mother. Since much of the amniotic fluid contained in the infant's lungs, trachea, and nasal passages is squeezed out as the infant passes through the birth canal, suctioning of the newborn's mouth and nose is not an automatic action after the birth, but is performed only when necessary.

With the safe emergence of the infant's head and shoulders, many birth attendants encourage the mother (and/or the father) to reach down and actually complete the birth by lifting the newborn onto the mother's abdomen. While the mother, father, and children become acquainted with the newborn infant through sight and touch, the nurse observes and assesses the newborn's transition to extrauterine life without interfering in the parent-infant bonding process. In some ABCs, the instillation of silver nitrate in the newborn's eyes is delayed for one-half to one hour so that the infant can have eye-to-eye contact with the mother and father—an important factor in the bonding process. Breast-feeding soon after the birth is encouraged because it enhances maternal attachment and increases uterine contractions, which facilitates placental separation. After the umbilical cord pulsations cease, the birth attendant clamps and cuts the umbilical cord (or allows the father to do this), and then delivers the placenta.

During the postpartum period, the mother and her newborn infant are carefully observed for several hours. If there are no complications, the mother and her infant can be discharged after the infant has been examined by a pediatrician or her family physician. Many ABC programs employ nurses who make follow-up home visits during the first week postpartum to assess the health of the mother and the infant. Samples for such tests as the P.K.U. and T4 can be obtained during one of these homes visits.

Other Factors. The positive responses of families who have utilized alternative birthing centers for their children's births, combined with the economic advantages of the lower cost for obstetrical care in this type of facility, have contributed to the feasibility of establishing such programs within the traditional setting of the hospital and in out-of-hospital settings.[10,11,12,13,14] Many obstetrical units

that are unable to establish an ABC in their hospitals, either because of physical or financial problems, are beginning to provide early postpartum discharge as an option to mothers and infants who have had a normal, uncomplicated intrapartum and early postpartum course.[15] Follow-up home visits by a nurse or early office visits to a pediatrician or family physician are also integral parts of this type of service. Even though this service is limited to the postpartum period, consumer response has been most favorable to it.

OPTIONS AVAILABLE FOR CESAREAN BIRTHS

Thus far, the information about the options available in family-centered maternity care has focused on the normal pregnant woman who gives birth vaginally without complications. However, a woman who undergoes a cesarean section is also in need of the sensitive and supportive care recommended by the Interprofessional Task Force on Health Care of Women and Children. Since 10 to 15 percent of all births in this country are cesarean births,[16] it is important to acknowledge the needs of these families, too. In many hospitals today, more liberal policies are being established regarding cesarean births so that the woman will experience as normal a birth as possible under the circumstances.

Information about the indications for cesarean births and what is entailed in this procedure is being incorporated into many childbirth/parenting classes to familiarize expectant families with this type of birth. Consequently, women, and their partners, are becoming more aware of the options available to them when a cesarean section must be performed.

Some of the alternatives available to women who must give birth in this manner include:

1. the choice of a general or a spinal (epidural) anesthetic so the mother can either be awake or asleep for the surgery;
2. the option of having the father (or support person) present during the birth;
3. when the woman is awake during the birth, the opportunity to hold and breast-feed the newborn immediately after birth;
4. the opportunity for father-infant bonding to occur immediately after the birth, regardless

5. initiation of rooming-in as soon as the mother desires this (often this begins in the recovery room after the birth);

6. extended or unlimited visiting privileges for the father (or support person) during the postpartum period so that the mother can have help with the care of the infant;

7. the utilization of medications (when necessary) that are not secreted in significant amounts in the mother's breastmilk.[17]

The psychological sequellae of cesarean section births are just being investigated. It is now known that the woman who undergoes a cesarean section, especially when it is not a planned event, will often have feelings of failure and guilt about not having a "normal" or "natural" childbirthing experience.[18] Furthermore, the physical discomfort of the mother after the surgery, combined with her feelings of disappointment and/or guilt, can interfere with her ability to bond to her infant. The long-term consequences of inadequate or delayed maternal-infant bonding can range from poor growth and development of the infant to blatant child abuse. Such complications of cesarean births are not common, but it is important to note such potential problems when the issue of family-centered maternity care is being presented.

Nursing Intervention. Labor and delivery nurses can play a very important role in helping the mothe and father integrate the events which precede and follow a cesarean section birth. Explaining the need for such procedures as surgical preps and cathetarizations to the couple before attempting to perform them will help to decrease the anxiety and apprehension they may feel about these invasive procedures. When the father is not allowed to accompany the mother to surgery, the nurse can accompany the woman and stay with her so the mother will have the support of at least one familiar person during this very stressful event. If the father is allowed to be with the mother during the surgery, the nurse's presence can still provide the couple with a sense of reassurance and familiarity in the foreign, sterile environment of an operating room. After the birth, the nurse can encourage and foster the parent-infant bonding prcess by providing both the mother (when she is awake) and the father the opportunity to touch and hold the newborn. When it is difficult for the mother to actually hold the infant herself, the nurse can hold the infant in an "en face" (face-to-face) position in order to facilitate the maternal-infant bonding process.[19]

One or two days after the birth, a visit from the labor and delivery nurse who assisted the couple during the childbirth is often beneficial and necessary for the integration of the event into their lives. The filling in of "missing pieces" is important for all women who experience gaps in their memories of the labor and births of their infants;[20] but this may be more important when the woman is attempting to understand the reasons for surgical intervention in what is often expected to be a "natural" process. Visits such as this also provide the couple with the opportunity to discuss any feelings of failure, guilt, or anger they may be experiencing. A sensitive and responsive nurse can effectively help the couple work through such feelings by remaining open to their comments and honestly addressing their concerns. If the family unit is to be strengthened through the childbearing process, and if childbirth is to be a family-centered event, then every attempt should be made by the obstetrical staff to help families incorporate this experience into their lives— regardless of whether or not the childbearing event is categorized as normal or abnormal according to medical criteria.

OPTIONS IN MATERNITY NURSING

Nurses today are in a unique position to foster family-centered maternity/newborn care both in the hospital setting and in out-patient facilities. The recognition of the need for expanded nursing roles to meet consumer demands for adequate, personalized health care has provided several choices for nurses pursuing careers in maternal-child health care. One such option which has been available to nurses for a number of years is nurse-midwifery (See Chap. 41 for more information on this subject.)

Maternity Clinical Specialist. A new specialty emerging within the last decade is the *maternity clinical specialist.* These clinicians undergo advanced study of maternity nursing at the graduate level and are able to provide in-depth intervention for many of the adaptational and physiologic problems encountered in maternity care. Frequently clinical specialists have an area of expertise within the specialty field, such as a maternity clinical specialist with special expertise in the care of pregnant diabetics, breast-feeding mothers, parents experiencing neonatal death or abnormalities, Rh sensitized mothers, and so on. These nurses with Master's degrees also serve as consultants to other maternity nursing staff, assisting them to plan care for difficult problems or special situations encountered on the unit. Although clinical specialists may also be involved in staff education, their primary function is direct patient services utilizing a high degree of knowledge, skill, and competence in their area of specialty.[21]

Nurse Practitioner. The latest new role to emerge on the nursing scene is that of the *nurse practitioner.* Beginning in about 1965, physicians and nurses started working together in several settings to "broaden the role" of the nurse in provision of care to patients in ambulatory and out-patient settings. Impetus for such changes was provided by the health manpower crisis and disillusionment of the American public with its health care nonsystem which erupted during the mid-sixties.

With an undersupply of physicians that was predicted to get worse, and underutilization of the knowledge and skills of hundreds of thousands of registered nurses, many voices cried out for an extension of the scope of nursing practice to help meet the health needs of the nation.

Some nurses had previously been identifying health problems and providing limited treatment, notably in community health and private office settings, but their effectiveness was reduced by lack of a systematic approach and a body of knowledge to enable them to carry out treatment.

As the nurse practitioner role evolved, it encompassed additional skills in the techniques of physical diagnosis which were formerly in the realm of medicine, as well as the knowledge base to diagnose and treat common problems and minor illness. Health prevention and maintenance, including examination, testing and education, as well as man-

agement of stabilized chronic illness are also included in nurse practitioner functions. The nurse practitioner combines the nurse's sensitivity to emotional needs and focus on adaptation and social aspects of patient care with the techniques and knowledge of medicine to diagnose and treat pathophysiologic problems. These nurses usually practice in a primary care setting, defined as the first contact in any given episode of illness with the health care system, and responsibility for continuance of care including maintenance of health, evaluation and management of symptoms, and appropriate referrals.[22, 23]

The Maternity Nurse Practitioner. The maternity nurse practitioner, or OB-GYN nurse practitioner, provides prenatal care for uncomplicated pregnancies with a physician consultant available. The nurse takes a health and pregnancy history, performs the physical and obstetrical examination, orders, and interprets laboratory and other diagnostic studies, plans for necessary treatments and medications in conjunction with the physician, and assesses family relationships and psychosocial needs.

Throughout the pregnancy the nurse practitioner sees the woman on antepartal visits, sometimes alternating with the physician, and evaluates the progress of the pregnancy as well as manages minor physical problems. Information and counseling related to pregnancy and childbirth and assessment of the couple's adjustments and family problems are also part of the nurse practitioner's role. Refferrals to community agencies, prepared childbirth classes, and other medical specialities may also be done. Most maternity nurse practitioners are skilled in provision of contraception, and can select appropriate methods for the patient including oral contraceptives, insertion of intrauterine devices, fitting for diaphragms, and teaching about the other methods.

Family nurse practitioners also provide care during pregnancy, as they are generalists who care for all family members similarly to family practice physicians. In addition to the functions described above for maternity nurse practitioners, family practitioners provide postdelivery care for the baby as it grows, thus providing continuity during the reproductive process except for the intrapartal phase.

REFERENCES

1. N. Devitt: "The transition from home to hospital birth in the United States, 1930–1960." *Birth and Fam. J.* 4, 2: 47–58, Summer 1974.

2. S. F. Anderson: "Childbirth as a pathological process: An American perspective." *MCN— Amer. J. Maternal Child Nurs.* 2, 4: 240–244, July/ August, 1977.

3. S. Arms: *Immaculate Deception*. Boston, Houghton-Mifflin, 1975.

4. L. D. Hazell: "A study of 300 elective home births." *Birth and Fam. J.* 2, 1: 11–15, Winter 1974/1975.

5. M. N. Estes: "A home obstetric service with expert consultation and back-up." *Birth and Fam. J.* 5, 3: 151–157, Fall 1978.

6. J. L. Epstein and M. McCartney: "A home birth service that works." *Birth and Fam. J.* 4, 2: 71–75, Summer 1977.

7. "The development of family-centered maternity/newborn care in hospitals." A Joint Position Statement Prepared by the Interprofessional Task Force on Health Care of Women and Children. The National Foundation/March of Dimes, June 1978.

8. Ibid, p. 3.

9. Ibid.

10. E. K. M. Ernst and M. P. Forde: "Maternity care: An attempt at an alternative." *Nurs. Clin. of North Amer.* 10, 2: 241–249, June 1975.

11. J. Goldschmidt and R. Mann: "Choices in childbirth—The nurse-midwifery service at San Francisco General Hospital." *Birth and Fam. J.* 4, 3: 120–122, Fall 1977.

12. J. Kerner and C. B. Ferris: "An alternative birth center in a community teaching hospital." *Obstet. and Gynecol.* 51, 3: 371–373, March 1978.

13. R. W. Lubic: "The childbearing center." *J. Nurse-Midwifery* 21, 3: 24–25, Fall 1976.

14. S. S. Rising: "A consumer-oriented nurse-midwifery service." *Nurs. Clin. of North Amer.* 10, 2: 251–262, June 1975.

15. M. J. Yanover, D. Jones and M. D. Miller: "Perinatal care of low risk mothers and infants— Early discharge with home care." *New Eng. J. Med.* 294, 13: 702–705, March 25, 1976.

16. M. W. Enkin: "Having a section is having a baby." *Birth and Fam. J.* 4, 3: 99–102, Fall 1977, p. 99.

17. Ibid.

18. J. S. Marut: "The special needs of the cesarean mother." *MCN—Amer. J. Maternal Child Nurs.* 3, 4: 202–206, July/August 1978.

19. M. H. Klaus and J. H. Kennell: *Maternal-Infant Bonding*. St. Louis, C. V. Mosby, 1976.

20. D. Affonso: " 'Missing pieces'—A study of postpartum feelings." *Birth and Fam. J.* 4, 4: 159–164, Winter 1977.

21. J. P. Riehl and J. W. McVay: *The Clinical Nurse Specialist: Interpretations*. New York, Appleton-Century-Crofts, 1973.

22. National Commission for the Study of Nursing and Nursing Education. Jerome Lysaught, Director. *An Abstract for Action*. New York, McGraw-Hill, 1970.

23. *Extending the Scope of Nursing Practice.* A Report of the Secretary's Committee to Study Extended Roles for Nurses. Washington, D.C., Department of Health, Education and Welfare, November 1971.

Forty-One

Evolution of Maternity Nursing

Obstetrics Over the Centuries / Developmental Maternal and Infant Care in the United States / The Emergence and Development of Maternity Nursing / Future Possibilities

OBSTETRICS OVER THE CENTURIES

The bearing of children is an event of enormous social significance, and has certain symbolic meanings for all peoples. Traditions, rites, and practices have been developed around this event to encourage positive outcomes for the individual and society. Roles for attendants during the reproductive process are formalized in one way or another, and differ greatly among cultures. Involvement of the sciences in childbearing grew gradually through the ages, but continued to be interwoven with folk beliefs and customs. In the less developed countries, ancient folk practices continue to prevail in the care provided during pregnancy, delivery, and postpartum.

In Western societies, there has been a reawakening of interest in childbearing practices that are more natural and minimize technical intervention. Family and friends once again are assuming a central role in attending laboring women, with new support roles emerging for health professionals (see Chap. 40, Alternatives in Maternity Care). As knowledge continues to advance, there is growing appreciation of the fine balance of natural ecosystems and the wisdom of restraint in applying technology to the reproductive process. While much of the modern history of obstetrical care has seen an increasing

assertion of science into difficulties of the natural process, a point of diminishing returns has been reached in which continued interventions frequently lead to iatrogenic problems and associated morbidity. A balance is required, in which technology is applied more discriminately in instances of complications, so that the normal reproductive process can proceed with the least amount of interference.

A brief account of the history of obstetrics follows, including an outline of the major stages in the development of medical involvement in care during the reproductive process.

Obstetrics Among Primitive Peoples

We know little about obstetrics among primitive peoples, but careful study of the customs of the aboriginal American Indians and the African peoples has shed some light on some aspects of obstetric practice of the ancients. Childbirth in primitive times was a relatively simple process. The mother retired to a place apart from the tribe and there gave birth to her child without great difficulty.

It is known that intertribal marriages were relatively rare; therefore, there was not the conglomeration of mingled races which exists today. A realization of this fact alone makes possible an understanding of the relative simplicity of childbirth under these circumstances. The fetal head and body were accommodated satisfactorily within the anatomic range of the maternal pelvis. The lack of mixed marriages prevented the resultant disproportion between passenger and pelvic passages.

It became customary for some women to attend other women in labor, and they became the primitive counterpart of our present-day midwife. The only real danger a primitive mother faced was that of abnormal presentation, which usually terminated fatally for both mother and child. Toxemias and other complications are largely the products of more advanced civilization and were rarely if ever met among primitive peoples.

Egyptian Obstetrics

In Egypt a highly organized state of society existed, and with it there arose a more complicated, if not more advanced, type of obstetrics. The priesthood in Egypt was interested in all the activities of society, and obstetrics was not neglected. They had a supervisory interest in it and took an active part in the care of abnormal or operative cases. They are known to have had obstetric forceps, to have performed cesarean sections on dead mothers and to have carried out podalic version.

Oriental Obstetrics

Hindu medicine was probably the first authentic system of medicine to be given to the world. Among the earliest Hindus of whom there is written record was Surata, one of the most prolific of Hindu writers. The exact date of his existence is still a matter of dispute, but he is variously stated to have worked and written between 600 B.C. and 500 A.D., more probably about the latter date. His knowledge of menstruation and gestation was quite modern. He knew and described intelligently the management of normal and abnormal labor. He described the use of forceps and cesarean section upon dead mothers to remove living children, and gave excellent antepartal and postpartal advice. He advised cleanliness on the part of the obstetrician: cutting the beard, the hair, and the nails closely, wearing clean gowns, and disinfecting the operating rooms prior to operation or delivery. His surgical antiseptic technique seems remarkable to modern students.

Chinese obstetrics was largely based on folk lore until the publication of a Chinese household manual of obstetrics, *Ta Sheng P'Ien,* which, according to the author's own statement, "is correct and needs no change or addition of prescription." There were monographs on obstetrics prior to this, but none so complete. Many of the statements are unfounded; in fact, the knowledge is scanty or incorrect, but the author had the saving grace of objecting to unnecessary interference and counseled patience in the treatment of labor.

Grecian Obstetrics

PRIOR TO HIPPOCRATES. The Asclepiads, or followers of Aesculapius, the father of medicine, had a slight and largely supervisory interest in obstetrics. Abortions were not illegal. There is little definite knowledge concerning this period, but it seems probable that obstetric treatment was primitive.

THE HIPPOCRATIC PERIOD. During this age normal obstetric cases were handled by midwives under the supervision of the physicians. Abnormal labor was entirely in the hands of the medical profession. To Hipprocates is accredited the Hippocratic oath, which is still a part of the exercises for all students graduating from medical school. Treatises on obstetrics attributed to Hippocrates are the oldest records available of the Western world's obstetric methods.

GRECO-ROMAN OBSTETRICS. This period was one of progress, which was due largely to the work of Celsus, Aëtius, and Soranus (second century). Soranus reintroduced podalic version and is responsible for the first authentic records of its use in the delivery of living children. He gave an excellent technical description of the procedure and the indications for its use.

Byzantine, Mohammedan, Jewish and Medieval Periods

These periods are characterized by a retrogression and loss of previously known practice. This was due in large part to the general failure of science in the medieval period and the inhibiting effects of religious institutions. The paucity of operative treatment in difficult labor may be judged from the recommendations contained in the only textbook of the day on obstetrics and gynecology, which reads as follows: "Place the patient in a sheet held at the corners by four strong men, with her head somewhat elevated. Have them shake the sheet vigorously by pulling on the opposite corners, and with God's aid she will give birth." However, hospitals and nursing services were organized in this age.

Although the ancient Jews specified little assistance to the woman during labor and delivery, they were interested in the hygiene of pregnancy and cleanliness at the time of childbirth. Hygiene and sanitation were practices integrated into religious law. At the time of difficult deliveries, the women "were comforted until they died." The stool or obstetric chair was used at this time and continued to be used until about the 19th century A.D. Reference is made to this chair in the Bible, in the first chapter of Exodus, "when you do the office of the midwife to the Hebrew women, and see them upon the stools. . . ."

The Renaissance Period

The Renaissance was characterized by advances in medicine and obstetrics commensurate with those in other fields. During this time the first English text on obstetrics, the *Byrthe of Mankynde,* was published by Raynalde. Both it and its German counterpart by Roesslin are copies of Soranus, and with their publication podalic version was reintroduced to obstetric practice. Many famous men were responsible for the progress in obstetrics—among them Leonardo da Vinci (who made the first accurate sketches of the fetus in utero) and Vesalius (who accurately described the pelvis for the first time).

To Ambrose Paré, the dean of French surgeons and obstetricians, must go the chief credit for making podalic version a useful and practicable procedure to be used in preference to cesarean section in difficult labor. Through his studies a significant part of obstetrical practice was removed from the hands of the midwives, where it had rested since the fall of the Roman Empire. Obstetrics was thereby established as an independent branch of medicine. Schools were established during this pe-

riod to train midwives, and laws passed to regulate their practice. Paré's work on version and his discouragement of cesarean section were opportune.

Sections had been practiced since antiquity upon dead mothers, but the first authentic section performed upon a living mother is credited to Trautman, of Wittenberg, in 1610. According to the records, the woman had a large ventral hernia which contained the uterus. Prior to this, Nufer, a sow gelder, is reputed to have performed the operation on his wife, after obstetricians and midwives had failed to deliver her. It has been stated that Jane Seymour was delivered by a section done by Frère, a noted surgeon of the time, at the request of Henry VIII. That she died a few days after the birth of Edward VI adds credence to the story, but no absolute confirmation is available. Due to the frightful mortality from hemorrhage, sepsis, and so on, it did not become popular in spite of the advocacy of the Church. Through the following centuries it was done occasionally, but not until the advent of the uterine sutures and aseptic technique did it become a practical procedure.

The origin of its name has been ascribed to Julius Caesar, but, as his mother lived many years after his birth, this seems improbable—considering the high mortality of all abdominal operations before the time of Lister. A more accurate explanation is that Numa Pompilius, one of the earlier Roman kings, passed a law making it compulsory to perform the operation upon all mothers who died while pregnant so that the mother and the child might be buried separately. This was known as the "Lex Regis" and with the advent of the Caesars as the "Lex Caesaris"—and subsequently "cesarean section." The name has been attributed to *cedere,* the Latin verb meaning to cut, but the former explanation seems to be more reasonable.

The 17th century was notable for many famous obstetricians. Mauriceau, of Paris, was the first to correct the view that the pelvic bones separated in normal labor. He was also the first man to refer to epidemic puerperal fever. His description of an obstetrician, or rather of the qualities an obstetrician should possess, is both interesting and amusing. He stated:

He must be healthful, strong and robust; because this is the most laborious of all the Operations of Chirurgery; for it will make one sometimes sweat, so he shall not have a dry Thread, tho' it were the coldest Day in Winter. . . . He ought to be well shaped, at least to outward appearance, but above all, to have small hands for the easier Introduction of them into the Womb when necessary; yet strong, with the Fingers long, especially the Fore-finger, the better to reach and touch the inner orifice. He must have no Rings on his Fingers, and his Nails well pared, when he goeth about the Work, for fear of hurting the Womb. He ought to have a pleasant Countenance, and to be as neat in his Clothes as in his person, that the poor women who have need of him be not affrighted at him. Some are of the opinion, that a Practitioner of this Art ought on the contrary to be slovenly, at least very carless, wearing a great Beard, to prevent the Occasion of the Husband's Jealousy that sends for him. Truly some believe this Policy augments their Practice but 'tis fit they should be disabused; for such a Posture and Dress resembles more a Butcher than a Chirurgeon, whom the woman apprehends already too much, that he needs not such as Disguise. Above all he must be sober, no Tipler, that he may at all times have his Wits about him. . . .

Van Deventer, of Holland, has been called the father of modern obstetrics and is credited with the first accurate description of the pelvis, its deformities and their effect on parturition. He also shares with Ould, of Dublin, the first description of the mechanism of labor.

As time passed, customs changed, and the term "accoucheur" replaced the objectionable "midman" and "man-midwife." Obstetric forceps were invented, probably about 1580, by Peter Chamberlen but were kept as a family secret until 1813 in an effort of the Chamberlens to monopolize the field. By the time the Chamberlen forceps were finally revealed to the profession, other types of forceps had been developed.

This century witnessed severe population losses due to plagues, wars, and the like. In England, William Pelty realized that controlling communicable diseases and saving infant lives would prevent continued diminution of the population. To this end he recommended isolation for plague patients and maternity hospitals for unmarried pregnant women. Such ideas were too far in advance of the time, however, and hence had no immediate consequences.

The Eighteenth Century

Population continued to be a great general concern to the governments of the world. Those who were concerned with general matters of health felt that governments ought to take a more active role in

overseeing health matters. Between 1779 and 1817, Johan Peter Frank in Germany wrote several volumes entitled *System einer vollstandigen medicinischen Polezey*. This work is even today considered a landmark in the history of thought on the social relations of health and disease. His recommendations concerning childbirth were many and as with Pelty, farsighted for his time. He insisted that all childbirth be attended by trained persons, and further urged that a midwife be consulted prior to the expected date of confinement. In addition, he proposed legislation to enforce a reasonable period of bedrest during the puerperium and to free the mother for several weeks from any work in or outside the house which might prevent her from giving the necessary attention to her infant. When necessary, he felt that the state should support parturients for the first six weeks after delivery. He then expanded upon the above and outlined a detailed child welfare program. Acceptance of his work and ideas spread to all countries in close cultural contact with Germany.

The eighteenth century was also marked by a succession of other famous men connected with obstetrics such as Palfyne, the Hunters, Smellie, White, and others. Palfyne is credited with the invention of a type of obstetric forceps, as he presented a copy in 1770 to the Academy of Medicine of Paris.

Smellie taught obstetrics with a manikin and made improvements on the obstetric forceps in use at that time, adding a steel lock and curved blades. He also laid down the first principles for their use and differentiated by measurement between contracted and normal pelves.

William Hunter, though a pupil of Smellie, was opposed to the use of forceps, and frequently exhibited his rusted blades as evidence of their uselessness. In conjunction with his brother he laid the foundation of modern knowledge of placental anatomy.

Charles White published an obstetric thesis advocating the scrubbing of the hands and general cleanliness on the part of the accoucheur; he was the pioneer in aseptic midwifery. John Harvie, 90 years before Credé, advocated external manual expression of the placenta, and it is known that a similar procedure was in use in Dublin at that time. One of the most active and famous English obstetricians of the time, John Clarke, had his fame commemorated in this epitaph:

Beneath this stone, shut up in the dark
Lies a learned man-midwife y'clep'd Dr. Clarke.
On earth while he lived by attending men's wives,
He increased population some thousands of lives;
Thus a gain to the nation was gain to himself,
An enlarged population, enlargement of pelf.
So he toiled late and early, from morning to night,
The squalling of children his greatest delight;
Then worn with labours, he died skin and bone
And his ladies he left all to Mansfield and Stone.

There were many famous obstetricians on the Continent in this period, chief among them being Baudelocque, who invented the pelvimeter and named and described positions and presentations. In America, prejudices against men in midwifery were carried over from Europe; as late as 1857 a demonstration before the graduating class at Buffalo roused such a storm of criticism that the American Medical Association had to intervene. Their judgment was that any physician who could not conduct labor by touch alone should not undertake midwifery.

The 18th century produced such men an Moultrie, Lloyd, and Shippen. The last was a pupil of Smellie and Hunter; in 1762, he opened a school for midwifery in Philadelphia, and, since he provided convenient lodgings for the accommodation of poor women during confinement, he may be said to have established the first lying-in hospital in America. With Morgan, he founded the School of Medicine of the University of Pennsylvania, becoming its first Professor of Anatomy, Surgery, and Midwifery.

The Nineteenth and the Twentieth Centuries

The increased knowledge, interest and ability which physicians brought to obstetrics were largely offset by the increased mortality due to puerperal fever. During the 17th, the 18th, and the 19th centuries it became a pestilence, at times wiping out whole communities of puerperal women. The mortality rates varied in the best European clinics at Paris and Vienna from 10 to 20 percent. The origin and the spread of the disease were little understood or studied. Obstetricians wasted futile hours on a study of minor alterations in instruments or technique and ignored the vast loss of life from puerperal fever. Oliver Wendell Holmes, of Harvard, first presented his views on the contagiousness of puerperal fever

in 1843, and in 1855 he reiterated them in a monograph on *Puerperal Fever as a Private Pestilence.* This was, and still remains, a medical classic on the subject. His statements aroused great controversy in America, and he received a great deal of abuse and criticism from Meigs and Hodge, two of the foremost American obstetricians of the day. One of them stated that it was ridiculous to conceive of any gentleman carrying contamination on his hands from patient to patient.

While Holmes first conceived the correct idea of the nature of the disease, it is to Ignaz Philipp Semmelweiss that the glory must go of finally proving without question the nature of its source and transmission. He was an assistant in the Viennese clinic for women, and while his associates fussed with unimportant details of technique, he was studying and mourning the tremendous death rate among puerperal women in the clinic. He observed that the death rate in Clinic I, where women were delivered by medical students or physicians, was always higher than that of Clinic II, where midwives officiated or received instruction. After fruitless study and manifold changes in technique in order to follow more closely that of Clinic II, the cause of the disease was brought home to him in a desperate and startling fashion. His friend, Kalletschka, an assistant in pathology, died after performing an autopsy upon a victim of puerperal fever, during which Kalletschka had sustained a slight cut on his finger.

At postmortem the findings were identical with those of puerperal sepsis, and Semmelweiss concluded that the disease was transmitted from the dead, by contact from the physicians and the students, who often went directly from the postmortem room to deliveries. Accordingly, he immediately instituted and enforced a ruling which made it obligatory that all physicians and students wash their hands in a solution of chloride of lime after attending autopsies and before examining or delivering mothers. In seven months he had reduced the mortality in Clinic I from 12 to 2 percent, and in the subsequent year had a mortality lower than Clinic II, a hitherto unheard-of feat. Subsequently, he observed that peurperal sepsis could be transmitted from patient to patient by contact of contaminated material, or attendants, as well as from the postmortem room, and in 1861 he published his immortal work on *The Cause, Concept, and Prophylaxis of Puerperal Fever.*

Medicine provides pitiful figures in profusion, but none, it seems, met such a cruel reception and ultimate fate as Semmelweiss. His colleagues (for the most part, but with a few notable and loyal exceptions) distorted and criticized his teachings. Had they stopped there, it might have been bad enough, but they carried their distaste for his views to the stage of persecution. He was forced to leave Vienna and go to Budapest, where a similar attitude—if possible a more malignant one—awaited him. A disappointed man, he died in 1865 from a brain abscess which may have originated in an infection similar to that of his friend Kalletschka. His work, however, has lived on; Pasteur and Lister added to it; and with a more modern and tolerant age his worth has been recognized.

The 19th and the 20th centuries were largely notable for their utilization of drugs to alleviate the pains of childbirth. The use of ether as an anesthetic was first discovered in America, but it was first utilized for childbirth by Simpson in Great Britain. He brought back the lost art of version by making it a safer procedure and eventually substituted chloroform for ether. As with almost every advance in medicine, it was opposed bitterly. The opposition was loudest and most vehement from the clergy, but, in 1853, Queen Victoria accepted it for delivery and by her action silenced most of the criticism. Nitrous oxide had been used in 1880 and has continued to be popular ever since that time.

Obstetric analgesia and anesthesia have made great strides during the 20th century (see Chap. 25, Analgesia and Anesthesia in Labor and Delivery).

The present century will be remembered largely for the development of antepartal clinics and the more concentrated care of the expectant mothers that came with them. The application of advances in general medicine, metabolism and public health to obstetrics has led to a marked decrease in mortality and morbidity from cardiac, pulmonic, metabolic, venereal and associated medical conditions complicating pregnancy. The consideration of adequate vitamin, mineral, and caloric contents in connection with the diet of pregnant and puerperal women not only has decreased the morbidity but also has enhanced the health of all mothers and children who receive adequate obstetric care.

Many other contributions have been made and are being added constantly to the science of obstetrics, not the least of which is more intensive training and study in this specialty demanded by the public as well as the medical profession. The advent of routine external expression of the placenta, antibacterial prophylaxis in the eyes of the newborn, purified ergot and pituitary preparations in hemorrhage control and prevention are but a few of the methods and medications which have marked the early 20th century.

The morphologic and anthropologic studies of Naegele, Roberts, Williams, Goodwin, Caldwell, Moloy, and others have done much to improve our understanding of the various types of pelves and some of their importance in labor. Roentgenologic pelvimetry, cephalometry, and tokodynamometry have greatly advanced our knowledge of the probable course of labor and delivery; Thoms, Caldwell and Moloy, Hanson, Jarcho, and countless others have contributed to our advances in this field.

DEVELOPMENT OF MATERNAL AND INFANT CARE IN THE UNITED STATES

As we know it today, maternal and child care developed into its present status through various avenues of investigation and many by-paths of interrelated activity and work. Individuals, both from the profession and the laity, as well as private and municipal organizations, contributed time, money and interest until, at last, government action was obtained.

1866. When a story was written concerning cruelty to a child, some thoughtful person referred the case to *The Society for the Prevention of Cruelty to Animals.* Henry Bergh, a former diplomat to Russia, was the founder and director of this association and was influential in having the judgment pronounced on the ground that a child was a human animal. This incident stimulated interest in the general treatment of children.

1873. *The New York Diet Kitchen Association,* the oldest public health organization in America, was opened at the request of doctors from "de Milt Dispensary" on the lower East Side of New York City. It was first organized as a soup kitchen, and milk, gruel, beef tea, and cooked rice were taken to the sick in their homes, with the idea of restoring health. In 1892, they began to make formulas for sick babies and still later dispensed free milk or sold it at 3 cents a quart. Maria L. Daniels, the first nurse director, contributed a great deal to public health progress. In 1926, this group was organized as *The Children's Health Service of New York.* The organization grew with the times, changing its program from curing the sick to preventive work—keeping well babies well. Although the organization devoted its major effort to work with babies and preschool children, it also included antepartal care in its program.

1876. The beginning of child-welfare legislation in the United States was the act passed by the New York State Legislature, granting to *The Society for the Prevention of Cruelty to Children* a charter that gave it wide power in the protection of child life. The inception of this legislation was based on the incident of the "child as a human animal" (1866).

1893. The first *Infant Milk Station* in the United States was established in New York City by Nathan Strauss. Through his persistence, milk was finally made "safe" through pasteurization; and many such stations were set up.

1900. *The United States Census Bureau* was made a permanent organization. Up to this time, *vital statistics* were considered to be of so little importance in the United States that, as soon as the population was tabulated and classified, the bureau was disbanded, to be reestablished and reorganized every ten years.

1906. *The United States Census Bureau* published mortality statistics which drew attention to the appalling loss of life among babies and children. Up to this time, very little thought had been given to maternity and infant protection.

1907. Due to growing interest, Mr. George H. F. Schrader gave money to *The Association for Improving Conditions of the Poor* (now the *Community Service Society*) for the salaries of two nurses to do antepartal work. This was the first consistent effort to prevent deaths of babies by caring for the mothers *before* the babies were born. Two reasons were given as to why antepartal care would be of value: 1) nurses in convalescent homes for postpartal mothers thought that if patients had better care during pregnancy, the health of mothers would be improved; 2) social workers going into the homes felt that they were not adequately prepared to advise pregnant mothers.

1907. *The New York Milk Committee* was organized. Its object was the reduction of infant mortality through the improvement of the city's milk supply. It established milk depots which proved beyond question their great value in the reduction of infant mortality by dispensing clean pasteurized milk and educating mothers.

1908. In this year the *Division of Child Hygiene* was established in New York City, the first in the United States, and it was important enough to be recognized nationally. Josephine Baker, M.D., was appointed chief. This was a pioneer achievement, and the methods that were evolved had no precedent.

1909 TO 1914. At approximately this time, Mrs. William Lowell Putnam, of Boston, promoted a demonstration of organized antepartal care. It was called *The Prenatal Care Committee* of the Women's Municipal League. The members of this committee worked in cooperation with the Boston Lying-In Hospital through Robert L. DeNormandie, M.D., of Harvard Medical School, Dr. Ruggles, of the then Homeopathic Hospital, and the Instructive District Nurses Association. The committee functioned long enough to establish the fact that good obstetric care was not possible without antepartal care.

1909. In this year *The American Association for the Study and Prevention of Infant Mortality* was organized and held its first meeting in New Haven, Connecticut. This committee was composed of both professional and lay members and devoted itself entirely to problems connected with child life, particularly to studying and trying to correct the high mortality rate. At this time there were no records of births or deaths, and the causes of deaths were unknown. The education of physicians and nurses was shamefully unsatisfactory; there was no public health in the schools, and practically no activity on the part of municipal, state, or the federal government to prevent infant mortality. The first president of this association was J. H. Mason Knox, M.D., and Gertrude B. Kipp was the first secretary. The committee consisted of the Honorable Herbert Hoover, Livingston Ferrand, M.D., L. Emmet Holt, M.D., Richard Bolt, M.D., and Philip Van Ingen, M.D. The work of this organization was of profound significance. In 1918, its expanding activities caused it to change its name to *The American Child Hygiene Association,* and in 1923 the name was changed to *The American Child Health Association.* In 1935, after having contributed to every angle of this pioneer work, the association was disbanded.

1909. *The First White House Conference,* on "The Dependent Child," was called by President Theodore Roosevelt. These investigations resulted in the establishment of the U.S. Children's Bureau in 1912. According to some authorities, this conference was called through the influence of a public health nurse.

1910. *The Census Bureau* published another report, this time on the mortality of infants under one year of age and at "special ages." As a result of this report maternity hospitals made an effort to improve the care given to infants.

1911. In New York City *the first strictly municipal baby-health stations* were organized under the jurisdiction of the Department of Health, and the full cost of the work was borne by the municipality. Soon the dispensing of milk was of minor importance, and emphasis was placed on prevention. They are now called *Child-Health Stations*.

1911. *The New York Milk Committee* (1907) made an investigation at the baby-health stations and found that 40 percent of all infant deaths (112 per 1,000) occurred within the first month of life before the mothers registered their babies at the health stations. This indicated the necessity for care *before* birth. The committee then decided to carry on an experiment in antepartal work. (See 1917.) They were convinced that much could be hoped for as a result of organized antepartal care.

1912. *The Babies' Welfare Association* (formerly *The Association of Infant Milk Stations* [1893]) represents the first comprehensive and successful attempt to coordinate the various child-welfare agencies in any community. All of the organizations of this type agreed to coordinate their activities by preventing duplication and overlapping without interfering with the organizations. In 1922, the name was changed to the *Children's Welfare Federation* of New York City. It continued to act as a clearing house and, among its other activities, managed the *Mother's Milk Bureau*.

1912. The *U.S. Children's Bureau* was established. It began in the Department of Commerce and Labor; in 1913 it was made a part of the Department of Labor and, in 1946, was transferred to the Federal Security Agency. This was created by Congress through a federal act (government sanction). This bureau was to set up special machinery to study and protect the child and to study all matters pertaining to the welfare of children and child life among all classes of our people, to assemble and accumulate factual information and to disseminate this information throughout the country. Miss Julia Lathrop was chosen as chief. Much of the success

of this bureau is credited to Miss Lathrop's vision. Fortunately, her successor, Miss Grace Abbott, continued the work with equal zeal.

1915. *The Birth Registration Area* was established as a federal act. The information is compiled in a uniform manner, giving the birth and the death statistics on which our information on mortality rates are based.

1915. Dr. Haven Emerson, Health Commissioner of New York City, appointed a special committee (Ralph W. Lobenstine, M.D., Clifton Edgar, M.D., and Philip Van Ingen, M.D.), in cooperation with the New York Milk Committee, to make an analysis of the facilities for maternity care in the city. The result of the survey showed that there was little antepartal work and no uniformity, and that only a very small number of pregnant mothers were receiving care. It showed also that hospitals took care of 30 percent of the deliveries, midwives delivered 30 percent, general practitioners delivered 30 percent, and private physicians, who might be classified as obstetricians, delivered 10 percent. Previous to this time little or nothing had been done to regulate or control the midwives.

1916. *The National Society for the Prevention of Blindness* was created after much pioneer work and investigation, locally and throughout the states, by Carolyn Van Blarcom, R.N. She was chosen to be the executive secretary. Through these investigations it was learned that by far the greatest cause of blindness was ophthalmia of the newborn. These findings led to the passing of a law compelling all physicians and midwives to use prophylaxis in newborn babies' eyes. Also, as a direct result of Miss Van Blarcom's surveys, a school for lay midwives, Belleview School for Midwives (no longer in existence), was started. Miss Van Blarcom took out a midwife's license and was the first nurse in the United States so to register. The first obstetrical nursing textbook to be written by a nurse is to Miss Van Blarcom's credit. Her later contribution to the better care of mothers and babies was to secure for Johns Hopkins Hospital the E. Bayard Halsted Fund for medical research.

1917. The Women's City Club of New York City and the New York Milk Committee opened three antepartal centers. The one sponsored by the Women's City Club was organized as the *Maternity Service Association* and, with Frances Perkins as the first executive secretary and Miss Mabel Choate as president, provided stimulating leadership. Dr. Ralph W. Lobenstine, a famous obstetrician, gave much time, labor, authority and direction as chairman of the medical board. In 1918, this organization was incorporated as the *Maternity Center Association* and carried out the first extensive piece of organized antepartal work in the United States. Miss Anne Stevens was director. Miss Annie W. Goodrich's wise counsel, as a member of the nursing committee, gave impetus to the organization's accomplishments. Louis I. Dublin, Ph.D., associated with this movement from the beginning, made an analysis of the first 4,000 records collected by the association. This revealed the startling fact that, through antepartal care, 50 percent of the lives of mothers might be saved and 60 percent of the lives of babies. Antepartal training and experience were extended to nurses throughout the world. This piece of intensive antepartal work fired increased interest in the care of mothers and babies. In 1929, the Maternity Center Association opened a school for the training of nurse midwives.

1919. *The Second White House Conference* was called by President Woodrow Wilson as a result of the activities of the U.S. Children's Bureau. It was organized in five sections. Each section was interested in a different phase of maternity and child care.

1919. *The American Committee on Maternal Welfare* was founded. The object of the committee was to stimulate interest of the medical profession in cooperating with public and private agencies to protect the lives and health of mothers and infants, and to teach principles and practice of personal hygiene and health to parents, physicians, nurses, and others dealing with the problems of maternity. The Committee was incorporated as a nonprofit organization in 1934 for the purpose of studying the maternal mortality rate in the United States and the management of obstetric problems generally. For more recent progress, see 1957 and 1964.

This organization publishes the magazine *The Bulletin of Maternal and Child Health*. It also promoted the American Congress of Obstetrics and Gynecology, which was held every three years.

1921. *The Sheppard-Towner Bill* was passed by Congress, an act for the promotion of the welfare and hygiene of maternity and infancy, to be administered by the U.S. Children's Bureau. This bill was introduced in the 65th Congress by Congresswoman Jeanette Rankin of New Jersey. It was reported out of committee favorably but failed to pass. A second bill was introduced in the 66th Congress. It passed in the Senate but, through delays, was not considered by the House. In the first session of the 67th Congress the bill was again introduced by Senator Sheppard and Congressman Towner and, after much agitation, finally passed— an epoch in child-welfare legislation. An appropriation of $1,240,000 per year was granted for five years. The Cooper Bill, passed in 1927, extended it for two more years. This law was accepted by all of the states except three. This legislation gave a tremendous impetus to the education not only of laity but also of physicians. Because of this legislation there was created at once, in the states which did not already have them, departments which now are quite uniformly labeled Divisions or Bureaus of Maternity and Child Health. In 1935, the Social Security Act was passed, following the plan of the Sheppard-Towner Bill. This Act appropriated $3,800,000. In 1939, the Social Security Act was amended, increasing the appropriation to $5,820,000. The amount has been increased gradually, and by 1952 (the 82nd Congress), $30,000,0000 was appropriated for Maternal and Child Health, Crippled Children and other Child Health Services.

1923. *The National Committee for Maternal Health* was formed with Robert L. Dickinson, M.D., as secretary and later as president. This was a clearinghouse and a center of information on certain medical aspects of human fertility. The object was to gather and analyze material, to stimulate research, to issue reports to the medical profession and to persuade it to take a leading part in the scientific investigations of these problems in preventive medicine. No other group existed for this purpose. It was dissolved in 1950.

1923. *The Margaret Sanger Research Bureau* came into being, an affiliation of the Planned Parenthood Federation of America, Inc., for research in the field of infertility, contraception and marriage counseling.

1923. Mary Breckinridge began her investigations in Kentucky, which led to the organization of the *Frontier Nursing Service*. With this concentrated effort of all phases of maternity and infant care, the striking results proved the value of prenatal care. Through her vision, determination and unfaltering energy, Mary Breckinridge has made this organization one of worldwide renown. In 1936, the

Frontier Nursing Service opened a school for the training of nurse midwives.

1925. *The Joint Committee on Maternal Welfare* was formed. This consisted of the American Gynecological Society, the American Association of Obstetrics and Gynecology and Abdominal Surgeons and the American Child Health Association (1909). Later the section of Obstetrics, Gynecology and Abdominal Surgeons of the American Medical Association was represented. The Committee issued a pamphlet entitled *An Outline of Delivery Care.* This stimulated the Children's Bureau to publish a concise pamphlet, *Standards of Prenatal Care* (1925), an outline for the use of physicians, which did much to standardize routine procedures.

1930. *The Third White House Conference* was called by President Herbert Hoover. Mr. Hoover's interest in child welfare was very evident. The conference was very comprehensive and far-reaching and was devoted to all aspects of maternity and child care. The Children's Charter was adopted and became a federal act. The 45,000,000 children were analyzed in chart form to show the paramount importance of care during pregnancy and the early years.

1938. *The Conference on Better Care for Mothers and Babies* was called by the Children's Bureau. This was the first time that representatives from the states, private and public organizations, both lay and professional people, met to pool ideas.

1939. *The Maternity Consultation Service* in New York City was organized to further antepartal education and care.

1940. *The Fourth White House Conference* on Children in a Democracy was called by President Franklin D. Roosevelt. It considered the aims of American civilization for the children in whose hands its future lies—how children can best be helped to grow into the kind of citizens who will know best how to preserve and protect our democracy. By 1940, the 48 states, the District of Columbia, Puerto Rico, Alaska, and Hawaii (then Territories) were cooperating with the Children's Bureau in its administration of child-welfare services.

1940. *The Cleveland Health Museum* was opened to the public—the first health museum in the Western hemisphere. It is significant in the maternity field because, in its workshops, it is reproducing the *Dickinson-Belskie models,* acquired in 1945. Dr. Bruno Gebhard, Director, says that, in his belief, the use of this sculptural series in professional and lay education will advance knowledge on this all-important subject more quickly and more accurately than any other visual means thus far available.

1943. *The Emergency Maternity and Infancy Care Program* was launched to care for the wives and the babies of enlisted men in the armed forces. From $17,000,000 to $45,000,000 per year was appropriated. This act also furthered interest in prenatal and child care.

1944. *The Public Health Service Act* was signed on July 3, 1944, and brought together all existing laws affecting the public health service. In addition, the act revised existing laws, provided authority for grants and authorized expansion of the federal-state cooperative public health programs which had bearing on maternal and child health programs. This act was to exert a great indirect impact on the care of mothers and infants because of its provisions funding research and education of personnel needed in these areas.

1946. The *World Health Organization*—an agency of the United Nations— became a reality. At the first meeting in Paris, 64 nations signed the constitution. The membership as of 1965 totaled 117 countries. The object of the organization is "the attainment of the highest possible level of health of all the peoples." So far, much has been accomplished toward that end.

1950. *The Fifth White House Conference,* with emphasis on children and youth, was called by President Harry S. Truman.

1950. *The Fred Lyman Adair Foundation* of the American Committee on Maternal Welfare was established. Its purpose is to collect funds from charitable sources to underwrite research and educational projects in this field.

1955. *The American College of Nurse-Midwifery* was established as an organization of nurse-midwives to study and evaluate the activities of nurse-midwives, to plan and develop educational programs meeting the requirements of the profession and to perform other related functions. In 1957, the College became a member of the International Confederation of Midwives, a midwifery organization with members from some 30 countries throughout the world.

1957. *The American Association for Maternal and Infant Health* (formerly the American Committee on Maternal Welfare) was activated at the Seventh American Congress held in July. Prompted by the spectacular improvements and advances in maternity care which have taken place since its founding, the board of directors of the committee voted unanimously to change the name, the role and the character of the organization. The new American Association for Maternal and Infant Health provides close integration of the various disciplines which participate in providing modern maternity care, and will serve as a forum for their mutual problems related to maternal and infant health.

1960. *The Sixth White House Conference,* concerned with the nation's children and youth, was called by President Dwight D. Eisenhower. The theme of this "Golden Anniversary" Conference was "Opportunities for Children and Youth to Realize Their Full Potential for Creative Life in Freedom and Dignity."

1962. *The Conference on Maternal and Child Health Teaching in Graduate Schools of Public Health* was convened in response to the dire reports of the lack of qualified personnel with any public health background in the area of maternal and child health. The conference recommended that an MCH career development program be established to offset the existing and predicted shortages of personnel. Such a program was established at the University of California at Berkeley with financial aid from the federal government (U.S. Children's Bureau) in 1965. The objectives of early recruitment of qualified physicians and the provision of specialized training in obstetrics or pediatrics with general community health maternal and child health content has been realized.

In the same year *The National Institute of Child Health and Human Development* was authorized. The goals of this Institute were support of research and training in special health problems and needs of mothers and children. This Institute also now conducts and supports research in the basic sciences relating to the processes of human growth and development, including prenatal development. Five conferences were held in 1967, which sought to find the problems involved in maternal and infant mortality and morbidity and to establish guidelines for change toward more optimal care.

1963. *The Maternal and Child Health and Mental Retardation Planning Amendments of 1963* was enacted. This law will make it possible for the Children's Bureau to carry out some of the major recommendations of the President's panel.

1964. *The American Association for Maternal and Child Health* (formerly the American Association for Maternal and Infant Health), as a multidisci-

plinary organization, is one of the most potentially valuable groups interested in matters concerning infant, child and maternal health. The board of directors of the Association altered the official title of the organization, not to imply any change in its proposed program but to present a more accurate definition of the organization's aims and objectives.

1964. *The Nurse Training Act,* one of the amendments of the Public Health Act, was an indirect aid to maternal and infant care. This act authorized grants for the expansion and improvement of nurse training, assistance to nursing students, scholarship grants to schools of nursing, and the establishment of a National Advisory Counsil on Nurse Training.

1965. *Amendments to the Social Security Act* provided for a new five-year program of special project grants for comprehensive health care and services for school and preschool children, particularly in low income family areas. These amendments also increased the authorization for money to support maternal and child health service programs. There are now 54 such projects in existence due to this legislation.

1965. *PKU testing* became mandatory for all infants in the states of Illinois and Michigan, thus setting a precedent for other states.

1966. *The Department of Health, Education, and Welfare* issued a policy statement on birth control which stated that the Department would support, on request, health programs making family planning information and services available. Due to this unique statement, federally supported family planning programs have since slowly begun to evolve.

The Federal Food, Drug and Cosmetic Act was instituted on June 14, 1966. This legislation required labeling of ingredients of food represented for special dietary use. Infant foods, particularly, were specified.

The Child Protection Act of 1966 banned the sale of toys and children's articles containing hazardous substances, regardless of labeling.

1967. *The Public Health Law 89–749* is considered by health authorities to be one of the most significant health measures passed by Congress since it provides for increasing flexibility at state and regional levels to attack special health problems which have regional or local impact.

1967. *Medicaid* programs were increasing among the states (30 in 1967) to provide health care for low-income families. Care during pregnancy and child care were included.

1968. *Head Start* programs provided educational opportunities for underprivileged children of preschool age, often associated with nutritional and health screening programs.

1968. The second report of the *President's Committee on Mental Retardation* noted that three-fourths of the country's mental retardation was found in isolated and impoverished urban and rural areas, and cited evidence of a close relationship between diet and mental and nervous disorders. It recommended federal action to improve manpower shortages and develop facilities for care of the mentally retarded.

1968. The *Citizens' Board of Inquiry into Hunger and Malnutrition in the United States* issued its report "Hunger—U.S.A." which supported the presence of widespread hunger among millions of U.S. citizens.

1969. A live virus vaccine for *rubella* (German measles) was released and the U.S. Public Health Service began immunization programs.

1969. The *National Center for Family Planning* was established under the Health Services and Mental Health Administration, Department of Health, Education and Welfare (DHEW), to serve as a clearinghouse for information about contraception.

1969. *Neighborhood Health Centers* pilot projects began in many Southern states and Northern urban slums to provide medical care to the poor.

1969. *Pediatric Assistants* consisting of nurses and physician's assistants were being trained in several university pediatrics departments.

1969. *Amniocentesis* was used to diagnose hereditary disease in the fetus.

1969. *The White House Conference on Food, Nutrition and Health* was charged to formulate a national nutritional program, based on reports of malnutrition among the lower income population and the consequences of nutritional deficiency for the growth and development of infants.

1970. A nationwide drive was spearheaded by the *Center for Disease Control* in Atlanta, Georgia, to vaccinate children against rubella.

1970. *The Seventh White House Conference on Children and Youth* met, and recommended the establishment of a child advocacy agency by the federal government with full ethnic, cultural, racial, and sexual representation.

1969–1970. The *Office of Child Development* was established within DHEW to administer child development programs (Head Start, day care) and coordinate activities of governmental and private agencies involved in programs for children and youth.

1970. New York state liberalized its *abortion law* to leave the decision up to the woman during the first 24 weeks of pregnancy, permitting abortion after that time only to save the woman's life.

1971. *National Commission for the Study of Nursing and Nursing Education*, Jerome Lysaught, director, reported study of nursing roles and recommended nursing roles be expanded, educational systems repatterned, and nursing input into health care increased.

1971. The American Nurses Association and American Academy of Pediatrics jointly developed guidelines for *training pediatric nurse associates* and held a national conference to implement these. The ANA and American College of Obstetricians and Gynecologists also met to draw up guidelines for training clinical nurse specialists in obstetrics-gynecology.

1971. Funds were awarded to six innovative *child advocacy demonstration projects* by two agencies of DHEW.

1972. *Home Start* programs were inaugurated to help disadvantaged parents provide child development services in their own homes and be the primary educators of their own children.

1972. The *Office of Child Development* sponsored programs to help teenagers learn how to become good parents, and in coordinated efforts with Head Start and Community Mental Health Centers strove to improve the quality of mental health care including prevention, diagnosis and treatment for Head Start children and their families.

1972. *The Committee to Study Extended Roles for Nurses* reported to the secretary of DHEW that functions of nurses "need to be broadened" so they can "assume broader responsibility in primary care, acute care, and long-term care." The new "nurse practitioner" was functioning in expanded nursing roles in many areas including obstetrics, pediatrics, psychiatry, and medical-surgical nursing.

1972. *Professional Standards Review Organizations (PSRO)* were required by an amendment to the Social Security Act to be set up to oversee care given by physicians to Medicare and Medicaid patients in hospitals.

1973. The *U.S. Supreme Court* struck down almost all state statutes prohibiting or restricting *abortion,* leaving the abortion decision to the woman and her physician during the first three months of pregnancy; after this time the state could only regulate abortion procedures in the interest of maternal health. Essentially the decision to abort became the right of the individual woman, with the state unable to interfere in her choice except to assure that the abortion be performed under safe conditions.

1973. The *Child and Family Resource Program* began as an experimental project designed to strengthen the role of the family by providing or making available prenatal health and nutritional education, after-school tutoring for primary grade children, and mental health services to parents about child development.

1973. Data showed that immunization of women with *anti-Rh antibodies* shortly after delivery was highly effective in preventing Rh sensitization in the Rh negative mother (Rhogam).

1973. *The National Commission for the Study of Nursing and Nursing Education,* directed by Jerome Lysaught, reported on the implementation phase of the study. To encourage the expansion of nursing practice, it conducted educational and informational acitivites aimed at nursing and the public, developed a national joint practice commission between medicine and nursing with state counterparts, and developed statewide planning committees to generate changes in patterns of education and practice.

1973. *National Center on Child Abuse and Neglect* was established in DHEW's Office of Child Development to act as clearinghouse on information about the problem, a *National Commission* formed to study the role of the federal government in this area and the adequacy of state laws, and funds made available to regional child abuse prevention and treatment demonstration programs.

1974. *Guidelines on Short-Term Education Modules for the Obstetric-Gynecologic Nurse Practitioner* were drawn up by the Interorganizational Committee of Obstetric-Gynecologic Health Personnel.

1974. Federal *child health screening program* strenghthened (Public Law 92-603), states required to inform Medicaid families about availability of child health screening services and provide these when requested.

1974. Funds made available to study *Sudden Infant Death Syndrome* from the National Institute of Child Health and Human Development.

1975. The Division on Maternal and Child Health Nursing Practice of the American Nurses' Associ-

ation issued a *guide for short-term continuing education* programs for nurse clinicians in neonatal and maternal-fetal care, an outgrowth of a joint effort among several organizations.

1975. The ANA Commission on Nursing Education offered *accreditation for nondegree granting nurse practitioner programs*, including the OB-GYN nurse practitioners.

1975. *The National Advisory Council on Maternal, Infant and Fetal Nutrition* was established. Annual report's submitted to the President and Congress make continuing recommendations for administrative and legislative changes in programs aimed at low income individuals at nutritional risk (PL 94-105).

1975. The *WIC* program (Special Supplemental Food Program for Women, Infants and Children) was intended to provide low income families with supplemental foods and nutrition education through local agencies, as an adjunct to good health during critical times of growth and development.

1975. *Title XX*, a comprehensive amendment to the Social Security Act, provided funds for family-planning services, child care services, child protective services, and foster care for children (as well as other benefits and services for adults).

1976. *The Early and Periodic Screening, Diagnostic and Treatment* program (EPSDT) provided Medicaid-eligible children with regular health screening and treatment through federal funding.

1975. Landmark legislation was passed, the *National Health Planning and Resources Act*, (PL 93-641) which set the framework for establishing a system of national health policy, planning and development. Health Service Areas were to be established throughout the United States to coordinate health care resources and services. To avoid duplication and overlapping services and to combat the rising costs of health care, regulations indicate that to justify a hospital having an obstetric section there should be 75 percent occupancy in the unit where there are more than 1,500 births per year. Exceptions to these regulations are provided for rural or geographically isolated communities, and for other special situations.

1976. The *Food and Drug Administration* (FDA) required pharmaceutical companies to withdraw the sequential oral contraceptives from the market because studies indicated there was an increased risk of endometrial cancer.

1976. The *FDA* ordered warning labels for physicians and pharmacists on the risks of oral contraceptives, including birth defects, tumors, blood clots, and heart attack in women over 40 years of age.

1976. The *FDA* recommended gonad shielding for men and women of reproductive age as a routine practice for x-rays, and issued proposed guidelines.

1977. A *national symposium on immunization* sponsored by the March of Dimes urged renewed attention to immunization, as an estimated 20 million children of the 52 million under age 15 were not immunized against one or more childhood diseases; a nationwide campaign was undertaken by the American Nurses' Association, March of Dimes and federal government to improve the level of immunization among children.

1977. The *Child Health Assessment Act* (CHAP) extended the early and periodic screening program (EPSDT) to broaden eligibility and to require that treatment be given for conditions discovered during assessment, with exceptions of mental retardation, mental health, developmental problems and dental care. This legislation also expanded and improved community health centers.

1977. *ANA and NAACOG* offered a national examination for maternal-gynecological-neonatal nurses.

1977. The *FDA* required patient labeling for estrogenic drug products, except those used for contraception, related to cancer risks.

1977. The *FDA* required manufacturers' labeling of IUDs for patients describing potential risks and side effects and requiring physicians to have patients read the brochure before insertion of the IUD.

1977. *The National Institute on Alcohol Abuse and Alcoholism* issued a warning that pregnant women who have more than two drinks per day risk deformed or retarded children (the fetal alcohol syndrome).

1977. Legislation was passed and upheld that *federal funds could not be used for abortions* except in cases where low-income women's lives would be endangered by continuing the pregnancy or birth would cause severe and long-lasting damage to the women's physical health, and for victims of rape and incest.

1978. The *Civil Rights Act* of 1974 was amended to protect working women from occupational discrimination because of pregnancy, requiring employers with medical disability plans to provide pregnancy disability payments on an equal basis with other medical conditions.

1978. The *Rural Health Clinic Services Act* (PL 95-210) provided for the reimbursement of nurse practitioners under Medicare and Medicaid without a physician being present on site, under jointly developed protocols, in clinics which qualified as rural.

1978. The *Committee on Maternal Health Care and Family Planning* of the American Public Health Association published guidelines to address the problems of quality, quantity, and cost of prenatal, postpartum and interconceptional care, family planning, adolescent pregnancy, health education, nutritional and social services, human resoruces, facilities and equipment, and evaluation.[1]

1979. The United Nations designated 1979 as the *International Year of the Child*, encouraging all nations to upgrade the care and well-being of children. Their Declaration of the Rights of the Child include:

The right to affection, love, and understanding.
The right to adequate nutrition and medical care.
The right to free education.
The right to full opportunity for play and recreation.
The right to a name and nationality.
The right to special care, if handicapped.
The right to be among the first to receive relief in times of disaster.
The right to learn to be a useful member of society and to develop individual abilities.
The right to be brought up in a spirit of peace and universal brotherhood.
The right to enjoy these rights, regardless of race, color, sex, religion, or national or social origin.[2]

THE EMERGENCE AND DEVELOPMENT OF MATERNITY NURSING

From time immemorial women have taken care of other women during pregnancy and childbirth; most cultures, both primitive and modern, have a well-developed "motherlore" which keeps alive instructions and practices to be used during the childbearing period.

Midwifery

In every primitive society, there seems to have been someone present to care for the mother and the infant. Usually this task fell to women, who in essence were the ancient forerunners of maternity nurses. Midwives no doubt have existed for centuries untold; Homer made reference to a nurse-midwife in the *Iliad*. They continued to attend the majority of deliveries in Roman and Medieval times, although the role of physicians was enlarging. During the 18th century maternity cases began to receive more attention, as many lying-in charities were formed and midwives were included in training programs in London and Paris.

As midwifery assumed a more scientific status, special lying-in hospitals increased, and the last 50 years of the eighteenth century saw a remarkable decrease in maternal and infant deaths in these hospitals due to better techniques of nursing management. The male physicians remained mostly uninvolved in parturient care unless needed for special procedures in difficult labors.[3] It was not until the 19th century that physicians participated extensively in obstetrics, and much opposition had to be overcome from both physicians and public before the "he-midwives" were widely accepted. In the United States, a school for midwifery was started in 1762 by a physician from Philadelphia. Both nurse-midwives and physician-midwives practiced during the eighteenth and nineteenth centuries, though the nurse-midwives predominated.

Emergence of Professional Maternity Nursing

A variety of factors, cultural, social, and technological, have had important roles in shaping the growth and development of maternity nursing. One of the most important and direct of these factors was the shift from home to hospital delivery. At the turn of the century, almost all women were delivered at home by a midwife or physician. At the present time, more than 90 percent of mothers deliver in the hospital. Two other factors, in turn, brought about this change to hospital delivery and helped shape the kind of care received there. An increase in the understanding of asepsis made physicians much more attentive to this aspect of care, particularly for maternity patients. A growing conviction developed that delivery in a hospital was mandatory. As more women began delivering in hospitals, provision had to be made for quick, efficient, aseptic care and certain time-saving devices

and work simplification procedures were borrowed from industry. "Assembly-line care" soon flourished. Compliance with "time-saving" techniques, performance of the somewhat ritualistic procedures called for to maintain asepsis, and the increasingly overall bureaucratic structure generated by the complex modernizing hospital all went into defining and shaping the very essence of maternity care. Hence there arose the ritualistic, rigid adherence to rules and procedures (with rather little thought to the patient) that characterizes so much of maternity care even today. It was during these early times that antepartal care was conceived and developed as an aspect of preventive medicine. Thus, women increasingly had longer contact with their physicians during the childbearing time and this, together with the still prevalent Victorian notion of dependency, served to cement the obstetric relationship. In order to do justice to this relationship, physicians even more strongly began to insist on hospital deliveries.

Maternity nursing developed as obstetrics developed and, not surprisingly, was based on the medical model of obstetrics in which pathology was the main focus. Thus, the nursing student's experiences were oriented to the physical care of her patients, with emphasis on technical competence. Moreover, a good deal of the student's "patient experiences" was in reality service to the hospital. The early hospitals were, in fact, staffed largely by students. This type of service-to-the-institution, technical competence orientation produced a nurse who was efficient in organizing care for many patients. However, because of the great numbers, no in-depth nursing therapy was either attempted or possible. Little or no public health experience was offered and the nurse gradually became more "institution (i.e., hospital) oriented" and the physician's veritable right arm.

Nursing Roles and Women's Status. Undoubtedly part of the reason why nursing was so subjugated by medicine was due to the powerless status of women and the distaste with which working women were viewed. It is unfortunate that maternity nursing split so completely with nurse-midwifery that two different fields were eventually formed. Midwives were also suppressed by medicine, however, to the point that their practice became illegal in some states, and was generally discredited and maligned. Maternity nurses have conducted, with more or less vigor, the long struggle toward more responsibility and autonomy that parallels the women's movement for full and equal status.

Compartmentalization and Routinization.

In the third and fourth decades of this century, hospitals themselves became larger and more complex and the nurse gradually had to assume more and more administrative and organizational duties. Similarly, medical science enlarged and with the new knowledge and progress, more functions, formerly in the province of the physician, were delegated to the nurse. These factors together with the acute hospital personnel shortage precipitated by World War II, combined to develop and promote impersonal routinized care for the mother and her infant.

As more became known about the transmission and control of pathogenic organisms, various subunits were designated for the use of the mother, the well newborn, the sick newborn, and the premature infant. Thus, restrictions and compartmentalization of nursing function (nursery nurse, postpartum nurse, and so on) proliferated in the name of "better technique" but at the expense of unity in the mother-infant relationship. Perhaps even worse was the compartmentalization of thinking and communication that also evolved. The postpartum nurse knew and cared about the progress of the particular mothers in her charge while they were on the ward. She rarely knew how they responded to their pregnancy in general. She might know something about how they had withstood their labors, but only in the physical sense, and then only in relation to their immediate postpartum course. The nursery nurse knew about the babies in her nursery, but very little about the parents who would take them home or the environment into which they would go.

The experience of childbearing, once common to all members of the social group and centered in the home with involvement of most family members, had now become a disjointed, technical, and alien process about which parents were generally ignorant. Complex and mystical, childbirth had become the province of physicians and specialized nurses, to be enacted in a strange, threatening institution in which the parents were the most powerless members. It is not hard to understand why there was widespread dissatisfaction with this state of affairs, leading to the many far-reaching and some-

times radical changes which occurred over the last 20 years.

Recent Developments.

Many factors, social, economic, political and technical, have contributed to the significant changes in maternity care which have occurred since the midcentury. Such concepts as family-centered maternity care, participant childbirth, natural childbirth, rooming-in, birth without violence, alternate birthing, and a resurgence of home births have refocused attention on childbirth as a social and family process. Less technical interference, greater humanism, a wider range of choices and options, and reaffirmation of the natural birth process have become more typical of current maternity care. More sophisticated technology has led to development of specialty centers for management of complicated pregnancy, and neonatal intensive care units along with the new field of neonatology. However, recognition of the importance of maternal-infant bonding in the first hours and days of the newborn's life has led to practices encouraging maximal mother-child contact. Many of the newer alternative approaches to maternity care are covered in Chapter 40, Alternatives in Maternity Care.

FUTURE POSSIBILITIES

In speculating about the future of maternity nursing, several significant recent developments in health care and social patterns must be taken into consideration. Perhaps the most far-reaching is the declining birthrate in the United States, with its associated slowing of the rate of population increase.

The most overt manifestation of the decrease in birthrate was the closing of maternity units in many small to moderate-sized hospitals in this country. It became economically impossible to maintain these units because of a falling census, so consolidation of obstetrical services in a few designated hospitals became common. In some of the larger cities with higher concentrations of physicians, some obstetricians and pediatricians were hard-pressed to find enough business. However, the maldistribution of health care services continued as before, with lower income and inner city or outlying rural populations still left with inadequate services.

Trends in population location show significant increases in nonmetropolitan counties, indicating the need for increased attention to health services in rural areas, and emphasis on the regional impact of health resources. Population profiles suggest that the mix of medical and health care will need to be modified during the 1980s to take into account the existence of fewer infants and more older people.[4]

Regionalized Perinatal Health Care. As a result of changing population profiles and the widespread concern over cost, quality and availability of health care services, and with the additional impetus of PL 93-641 (National Health Planning and Resources Act), there is a strong trend toward providing a regionalized system of perinatal care for mothers and infants. The goals of this system are to make complex care available to entire populations within constraints of geography, costs, population distribution, and availability of specialists and subspecialists.

The regionalized structure consists basically of four types of facilities: physicians' offices and clinics, local facilities for uncomplicated deliveries, larger urban facilities providing a fairly full range of obstetric and neonatal services, and perinatal centers and specialized units offering the full range of services for maternal and neonatal complications. Primary care units for mothers during pregnancy, and mothers and infants following delivery are generally physicians' offices and maternal-child health clinics. These provide primary perinatal care, including promotion and support for maintenance of health status, screening for complications of pregnancy, and treatment of intercurrent diseases and problems.

Level 1 facilities are generally community hospitals which are designed to provide care for mothers and neonates without major complications. These are local facilities which relate closely to the community. Because all complications cannot be identified in advance, Level 1 units must be able to provide emergency services of a more complex nature until the mother or infant can be transferred to a facility with greater capacity. Level 2 facilities are hospitals in larger, usually urban communities which offer a wider range of maternal and neonatal services. These serve as referral sources to local hospitals and physicians for high risk pregnancies or neonatal care. They provide an intermediate level of complex services and can manage the more common complications of childbearing and the newborn.

Level 3 facilities are the regional perinatal centers which provide the full range of services for perinatal complications of both mother and infant. These units can generally meet most maternal or neonatal needs related to high risk conditions and may contain specialized units as children's cardiac centers, units for management of pregnant diabetics, or units for intrauterine exchange transfusions in the cases of severe Rh sensitization. To make such a regionalized structure workable, it is necessary for health providers to develop and maintain a network through communication, consultation, transportation and outreach education.[5]

Directions for Maternity Nursing. To remain congruent with such changes in the health care delivery system, maternity nursing must also adapt and grow in new and diverse directions. The desires of the consumers of maternity care also signify a growing need for changes, as the routinized and standardized care organized in settings most convenient for the providers rather than consumers of care are less and less acceptable. Parents are asking for full participation in all phases of childbearing, the right to be involved in decisions affecting their bodies and health, and the right to institute practices which they believe are important for the happiness and well-being of parents and baby. (See The Pregnant Patient's Bill of Rights, p. 744.)

A growing body of literature and research is reaffirming the importance of early and continued close contact between mother and baby, a situation many of our modern hospital practices have made impossible to attain. The importance of natural practices, such as breast-feeding and avoidance of highly processed and chemically preserved foods suggests that health professionals support rather than discourage parents who wish to follow these practices.

The appropriateness of routine delivery of normal, uncomplicated maternity patients in the acute hospital with its focus on disease and illness is being questioned. New data about the importance of immediate, active intervention in delivery of high risk pregnancies and the postdelivery care of depressed, sick or anoxic infants reinforce the need for highly trained personnel and well-equipped

THE PREGNANT PATIENT'S BILL OF RIGHTS*

American parents are becoming increasingly aware that health professionals do not always have scientific data to support common American obstetrical practices and that many of these practices are carried out primarily because they are part of medical and hospital tradition. In the last forty years many artificial practices have been introduced which have changed childbirth from a physiological event to a very complicated medical procedure in which all kinds of drugs are used and procedures carried out, sometimes unnecessarily, and many of them potentially damaging for the baby and even for the mother. A growing body of research makes it alarmingly clear that every aspect of traditional American hospital care during labor and delivery must now be questioned as to its possible effect on the future well-being of both the obstetric patient and her unborn child.

One in every 35 children born in the United States today will eventually be diagnosed as retarded; one in every 10 to 17 children has been found to have some form of brain dysfunction or learning disability requiring special treatment. Such statistics are not confined to the lower socioeconomic group but cut across all segments of American society.

New concerns are being raised by childbearing women because no one knows what degree of oxygen depletion, head compression, or traction by forceps the unborn or newborn infant can tolerate before that child sustains permanent brain damage or dysfunction. The recent findings regarding the cancer-related drug diethylstilbestrol have alerted the public to the fact that neither the approval of a drug by the U.S. Food and Drug Administration nor the fact that a drug is prescribed by a physician serves as a guarantee that a drug or medication is safe for the mother or her unborn child. In fact, the American Academy of Pediatrics Committee on Drugs has recently stated that there is no drug, whether prescription or over-the-counter remedy, which has been proven safe for the unborn child.

The Pregnant Patient has the right to participate in decisions involving her well-being and that of her unborn child, unless there is a clear-cut medical emergency that prevents her participation. In addition to the rights set forth in the American Hospital Association's "Patient's Bill of Rights," (which has also been adopted by the New York City Department of Health) the Pregnant Patient, because she represents TWO patients rather than one, should be recognized as having the additional rights listed below.

1. *The Pregnant Patient has the right,* prior to the administration of any drug or procedure, to be informed by the health professional caring for her of any potential direct or indirect effects, risks or hazards to herself or her unborn or newborn infant which may result from the use of a drug or procedure prescribed for or administered to her during pregnancy, labor, birth, or lactation.

2. *The Pregnant Patient has the right,* prior to the proposed therapy, to be informed, not only of the benefits, risks, and hazards of the proposed therapy but also of known alternative therapy, such as available childbirth education classes which could help to prepare the Pregnant Patient physically and mentally to cope with the discomfort or stress of pregnancy and the experience of childbirth, thereby reducing or eliminating her need for drugs and obstetric intervention. She should be offered such information early in her pregnancy in order that she may make a reasoned decision.

3. *The Pregnant Patient has the right,* prior to the administration of any drug, to be informed by the health professional who is prescribing or administering the drug to her that any drug which she receives during pregnancy, labor and birth, no matter how or when the drug is taken or administered, may adversely affect her unborn baby, directly or indirectly, and that there is no drug or chemical which has been proven safe for the unborn child.

4. *The Pregnant Patient has the right,* if cesarean section is anticipated, to be informed prior to the administration of any drug, and preferably prior to her hospitalization, that minimizing her and, in turn, her baby's intake of nonessential pre-operative medicine will benefit her baby.

5. *The Pregnant Patient has the right,* prior to the administration of a drug or procedure, to be informed if there is NO properly controlled follow-up research which has established the safety of the drug or procedure with regard to its direct and/or indirect effects on the physiological, mental and neurological development of the child exposed, via the mother, to the drug or procedure during pregnancy, labor, birth, or lactation—(this would apply to virtually all drugs and the vast majority of obstetric procedures).

6. *The Pregnant Patient has the right,* prior to the administration of any drug, to be informed of the brand name and generic name of the drug in order that she may advise the health professional of any past adverse reaction to the drug.

7. *The Pregnant Patient has the right,* to determine for herself, without pressure from her attendant, whether she will accept the risks inherent in the proposed therapy or refuse a drug or procedure.

8. *The Pregnant Patient has the right* to know the name and qualifications of the individual administering a medication or procedure to her during labor or birth.

9. *The Pregnant Patient has the right* to be informed, prior to the administration of any procedure, whether that procedure is being administered to her for her or her baby's benefit (medically indicated) or as an elective procedure (for convenience or teaching purposes).

10. *The Pregnant Patient has the right* to be accompanied during the stress of labor and birth by someone she cares for, and to whom she looks for emotional comfort and encouragement.

11. *The Pregnant Patient has the right* after appropriate medical consultation to choose a position for labor and for birth which is least stressful to her baby and to herself.

12. *The Obstetric Patient has the right* to have her baby cared for at her bedside if her baby is normal, and to feed her baby according to her baby's needs rather than according to the hospital regimen.

13. *The Obstetric Patient has the right* to be informed in writing of the name of the person who actually delivered her baby and the professional qualifications of that person. This information should also be on the birth certificate.

14. *The Obstetric Patient has the right* to be informed if there is any known or indicated aspect of her or her baby's care or condition which may cause her or her baby later difficulty or problems.

15. *The Obstetric Patient has the right* to have her and her baby's hospital medical records complete, accurate, and legible and to have their records, including Nurses' Notes, retained by the hospital until the child reaches at least the age of majority, or, alternatively, to have the records offered to her before they are destroyed.

16. *The Obstetric Patient*, both during and after her hospital stay, *has the right* to have access to her complete hospital medical records, including Nurses' Notes, and to receive a copy upon payment of a reasonable fee and without incurring the expense of retaining an attorney.

It is the obstetric patient and her baby, not the health professional, who must sustain any trauma or injury resulting from the use of a drug or obstetric procedure. The observation of the rights listed above will not only permit the obstetric patient to participate in the decisions involving her and her baby's health care, but will help to protect the health professional and the hospital against litigation arising from resentment or misunderstanding on the part of the mother.

* Reprinted by permission of the Committee on Patient's Rights, Box 1900, New York, N.Y. 10001.

delivery rooms and intensive care nurseries, however. The situation appears paradoxical, and answers will not be easy. It is safe to say that what have come to be accepted as routine practices in the care of maternity and newborn patients are being seriously questioned by both experts and public.

Maternity nursing must enlarge its scope if it is to remain viable. Narrow concentration on the processes of childbearing and newborn care limit the services the maternity nurse can offer the patient and family. Because reproduction is basically a sexual event, both physiologically and in terms of role and identity, the most obvious areas for extension of maternity are into sexuality and contraception. To some extent, this is now occurring. Abortion care is another natural extension, as it is a variation within the process of reproduction.

Increasing expertise in early childhood development, and familiarity with the normal growth and development of children equips the nurse to provide much-needed assistance to families beyond the immediate childbearing period. Skill in counseling families and knowledge of family dynamics permit the nurse to be of service when problems or needs arise not only in integrating the new baby, but also with relationships between parents and other children and relatives.

Another area with potential for involvement of maternity nurses is that of women's search for a satisfying identity and sense of productivity and self-realization, generally thought of as the "women's movement." With an inquisitive mind and open attitudes, and a willingness to question personal and social tenets, perhaps both nurse and patient could attain more satisfying levels of existence.

It is hard to predict where the nurse practitioner role will go, for this certainly embodies an enlargement of the scope of maternity and other nursing practice. One possibility is an eventual merging of maternity nurse practitioner with the nurse-midwife, resulting in provision of the full range of childbearing services by such nurses to uncomplicated cases. Should this occur, relationships with the medical profession would have to be altered, as physicians would primarily provide care to high-risk and complicated cases, perform gynecologic surgery, and serve as consultants to the nurses providing care during normal childbearing.

Or, perhaps maternity nursing will split off into two separate specialties, one the nurse practitioner type involved in prenatal and postpartal followup, the other the acute hospital nurse involved in intrapartal and immediate postdelivery care. Nurse-midwifery undoubtedly will increase as restrictive laws change and programs develop to more equitably distribute care to all the American population.

Whatever the future portends, its hallmark will be change. Health care, medical care, and nursing care are all undergoing major upheavals. The issues of national health insurance, the role of third-party payers, problems with malpractice insurance, federal controls and peer review organizations, changing practice laws of nursing and medicine, the exorbitant costs of health care and the increasingly vociferous consumer advocacy movement, the development of health maintenance organizations and community health networks, all signify that health care in this country is experiencing radical changes. Maternity nursing must read the winds of change, and nursing leaders take initiative in shaping the new form this specialty will take in the years to come to serve the best interests and needs of families during all phases of childbearing.

REFERENCES

1. F. E. F. Barnes, ed.: *Ambulatory Maternal Health Care and Family Planning Services: Policies, Principles, Practices.* Committee on Maternal Health Care and Family Planning, Maternal and Child Health Section, American Public Health Association, 1978.

2. B. Bishop: Editorial on the rights of the child. *MCN*—Amer. J. Maternal Child Nurs., January/February 1979, p. 9.

3. V. L. Bullough and B. Bullough: *The Emerg-ence of Modern Nursing.* Toronto, Macmillan Co., Collier-Macmillan Canada, 1969, pp. 4, 17, 28-29, 76-78.

4. B. L. Green: "Rural health delivery systems of the 1980s" *Family & Comm. Health* 1, 2:95-108, July 1978.

5. S. N. Graven: "Perinatal health promotion: An overview." *Family & Comm. Health* 1, 3:1-11, November 1978.

SUGGESTED READING

American College of Obstetrics and Gynecologists. *Proceedings: Health Care for Mothers and Infants in Rural and Isolated Areas.* Chicago, 1978.

Anderson, E. M., Leonard, B. J., and Yates, J. A.: "Epigenesis of the nurse practitioner role". *Am. J. Nurs.* 74:1812-1816, Oct. 1974.

Barrett, J.: "The nurse specialist practitioner: A study." *Nurs. Outlook* 20:524-527, Aug. 1972.

"Changing patterns of obstetric care." *Am. J. Nurs.* 73:1723-1727, Oct. 1973.

Committee on Fetus and Newborn. *Standards and Recommendations for Hospital Care of Newborn Infants,* ed. 6. Evanston, Ill., American Academy of Pediatrics, 1977.

Committee on Perinatal Health. *Toward Improving the Outcome of Pregnancy: Recommendations for the Regional Development of Maternal and Perinatal Health Services.* New York, The National Foundation/March of Dimes, 1975.

Contemporary Nursing Series: "Maternal and newborn care: Nursing interventions." Compiled by M. H. Browning and E. P. Lewis. *Am. J. Nurs.* New York, 1973.

Fowler, M. M.: "The maternity nurse clinician in practice." In E. H. Anderson ed.: *Current Concepts in Clinical Nursing.* St. Louis, Mosby, 1973, pp. 210-215.

Lubic, R. W.: "Myths about nurse-midwifery." *Am. J. Nurs.* 74:268-269, Feb. 1974.

Lynaugh, J. E., and Bates, B.: "Physical diagnosis: A skill for all nurses?" *Am. J. Nurs.* 74:58-59, Jan. 1974.

Martin, L. M.: "I like being an FNP." *Am. J. Nurs.* 75:826-828, May 1975.

McCormack, G. B.: "The visiting nurse becomes a nurse practitioner." *Nurs. Outlook* 22:119-123, Feb. 1974.

National Health Planning and Resources Development Act of 1974, PL 93-641, 88 Stat. 2225, 1975.

Appendix

Glossary

Note: The pronunciations indicated below follow Webster's Second International Dictionary.

āle, châotic, câre, ădd, ȧccount, ärm, ȧsk, sofȧ; ēve, hẹre, ĕvent, ĕnd, sĭlĕnt, makēr; īce, ĭll, charĭty; ōld, ȯbey, ôrb, ŏdd, soft, cŏnnect; food, foot; out; oil, cūbe, ûnite, ûrn, ŭp, circŭs, menü; chair; go; sing; then, thin; natŭre; verdŭre; k = ch in German ich or ach; bon; yet zh = z in azure

abdominal (ăb-dŏm′ĭ-năl). Belonging to or relating to the abdomen.

  a. delivery. Delivery of the child by abdominal section. See *cesarean section.*

  a. gestation. Ectopic pregnancy occurring in the cavity of the abdomen.

  a. pregnancy. See *gestation* above.

ablatio placentae. See *abruptio placentae.*

abortion. The termination of pregnancy at any time before the fetus has attained a stage of viability, i.e., before it is capable of extrauterine existence.

abruptio placentae (ăb-rŭp′shĭ-ō plȧ-sen′tē). Premature separation of normally implanted placenta.

acromion (ȧ-krō′mĭ-ŏn). An outward extension of the spine of the scapula, used to explain presentation of the fetus.

adnexa (ăd-nĕk′sȧ). Appendages.

  a., uterine (ū′tēr-ĭn). The fallopian tubes and ovaries.

afibrinogenemia (ȧ-fĭ″brin-ō-jen-ē′mē-ă). Lack of fibrinogen in the blood.

afterbirth (ȧf′tēr-bûrth″). The structures cast off after the expulsion of the fetus, including the membranes and the placenta with the attached umbilical cord; the secundines.

afterpains (ȧf′tēr-pāns″). Those pains, more or less severe, after expulsion of the afterbirth, which result from the contractile efforts of the uterus to return to its normal condition.

agalactia (ăg′ȧ-lăk′shĭ-ȧ). Absence *or* failure of the secretion of milk.

allantois (ȧ-lăn′tȯ-ĭs). A tubular diverticulum of the posterior part of the yolk sac of the embryo; it passes into the body stalk through which it is accompanied by the allantoic (umbilical) blood vessel, thus taking part in the formation of the umbilical cord; and later, fusing with the chorion, it helps to form the placenta.

amenorrhea (ā-mĕn″ŏ-rē′ȧ). Absence or suppression of the menstrual discharge.

amnesia (ăm-nē′zhĭ-ȧ). Loss of memory.

amnion (ăm′nĭ-ŏn). The most internal of the fetal membranes, containing the waters which surround the fetus in utero.

amniotic (ăm″nĭ-ŏt-ĭk). Pertaining to the amnion.

  a. sac. The "bag of membranes" containing the fetus before delivery.

analgesia (ăn″-ăl-jē′zĭ-a). Drug which relieves pain, used during labor.

androgen (ăn′drȯ-jĕn). Any substance which possesses masculinizing activities, such as the testis hormone.

android (ăn′droid). The term adopted for the male type of pelvis.

anencephalia (ăn-ĕn″sĕ-fā′lĭ-ȧ). Form of monstrosity with absence of a brain.

anovular (ăn-ōv′ŭ-lēr). Not accompanied with the discharge of an ovum; said of cyclic uterine bleeding.

anoxia (an-ox′e-ah). Oxygen deficiency; any condition of absence of tissue oxidation.

antenatal (ăn-tē-nā′tȧl). Occurring or formed before birth.

antepartal (ăn″tĕ-pär′tal). Before labor and delivery or childbirth; prenatal.

areola (ȧ-rē′ȯ-lȧ). The ring of pigment surrounding the nipple.

  secondary a. A circle of faint color sometimes seen just outside the original areola about the fifth month of pregnancy.

articulation (är-tĭk″ŭ-lā′shŭn). The fastening together of the various bones of the skeleton in their natural situation; a joint. The articulations of the bones of the body are divided into two principal groups—*synarthroses,* immovable articulations, and *diarthroses,* movable articulations.

Aschheim-Zondek test (ăsh″hīm-tsŏn′dĕk). A test for the diagnosis of pregnancy. Repeated injections of small quantities of urine voided during the first weeks of pregnancy produce in infantile mice, within 100 hours, 1) minute intrafollicular ovarian hemorrhage and 2) the development of lutein cells.

asphyxia (ăs-fĭk′sĭ-á). Suspended animation; anoxia and carbon dioxide retention resulting from failure of respiration.

> **a. neonatorum** (nē″ō-ná-tō′rŭm). "Asphyxia of the newborn," deficient respiration in newborn babies.

attitude (ăt′ĭ-tūd). A posture or position of the body. In obstetrics, the relation of the fetal members to each other in the uterus; the position of the fetus in the uterus.

axis (ăk′sĭs). A line about which any revolving body turns.

> **pelvic a.** The curved line which passes through the centers of all the anteroposterior diameters of the pelvis.

bag of waters. The membranes which enclose the liquor amnii of the fetus.

ballottement (bá-lŏt′mĕnt). Literally means tossing. A term used in examination when the fetus can be pushed about in the pregnant uterus.

Bandl's ring (Bän′dls). A groove on the uterus at the upper level of the fully developed lower uterine segment; visible on the abdomen after hard labor as a transverse or slightly slanting depression between the umbilicus and the pubis. Shows overstretching of lower uterine segment. Resembles a full bladder.

Bartholin's glands (Bär′tŏ-lĭn). Glands situated one on each side of the vaginal canal opening into the groove between the hymen and the labia minora.

bicornate uterus (bī-kôr′năt). Having two horns which, in the embryo, failed to attain complete fusion.

bimanual (bī-măn′ŭ-ăl). Performed with or relating to both hands.

> **b. palpation.** Examination of the pelvic organs of a woman by placing one hand on the abdomen and the fingers of the other in the vagina.

blastoderm (blăs′tŏ-dûrm). Delicate germinal membrane of the ovum.

> **b. vesicle.** Hollow space within the morula formed by the rearrangement of cells, and by proliferation.

Braxton Hicks sign. Painless uterine contractions occurring periodically throughout pregnancy, thereby enlarging the uterus to accommodate the growing fetus.

> **B.H. version.** One of the types of operation designed to turn the baby from an undesirable position to a desirable one.

breech (brēch). Nates or buttocks.

> **b. delivery.** Labor and delivery marked by breech presentations.

bregma (brĕg′má). The point on the surface of the skull at the junction of the coronal and sagittal sutures.

brim (brĭm). The edge of the superior strait or inlet of the pelvis.

caked breast. See *engorgement.*

caput (kā′pŭt). 1. The head, consisting of the cranium, or skull, and the face. 2. Any prominent object, such as the head.

> **c. succedaneum** (sŭk″sē-dā′nĕ-ŭm). A dropsical swelling which sometimes appears on the presenting head of the fetus during labor.

catamenia (kăt-á-mē′nĭ-á). See *menses.*

caudal (kô′dăl). The term applied to analgesia or anesthesia resulting from the introduction of the suitable analgesic or anesthetic solution into the caudal canal (nonclosure of the laminae of the last sacral vertebra).

caul (kôl). A portion of the amniotic sac which occasionally envelops the child's head at birth.

cephalhematoma (sĕf″ál-hē″má-tō′má). A tumor or swelling between the bone and the periosteum caused by an effusion of blood.

cephalic (sĕ-făl′ĭk). Belonging to the head.

> **c. presentation.** Presentation of any part of the fetal head in labor.

cervix (sûr′vĭks). Neckline part; the lower and narrow end of the uterus, between the os and the body of the organ.

cesarean section (sĕ-zā′rĕ-ăn). Delivery of the fetus by an incision through the abdominal wall and the wall of the uterus.

Chadwick's sign (tshăd′wĭks). The violet color on the mucous membrane of the vagina just below the urethral orifice, seen after the fourth week of pregnancy.

change of life. See *climacteric.*

chloasma (klŏ-ăz′má). Pl. *chloasmata.* A cutaneous affection exhibiting spots and patches of a yellowish-brown color. The term chloasma is a vague one and is applied to various kinds of pigmentary discoloration of the skin.

> **c. gravidarum, c. uterinum.** Chloasma occurring during pregnancy.

chorioepithelioma (kō′rĭ-ō-ĕp-ĭ-thē-lĭ-ō′má). Chorionic carcinoma; a tumor formed by malignant proliferation of the epithelium of the chorionic villi.

chorion (kō-rĭ-ŏn). The outermost membrane of the growing zygote, or fertilized ovum, which serves as a protective and nutritive covering.

chromosome (kro′mo-sōm). One of several small, dark-staining and more or less rod-shaped bodies which appear in the nucleus of the cell at the time of cell division and particularly in mitosis.

circumcision (sûr″kŭm-sĭzh′ŏn). The removal of all or part of the prepuce, or foreskin of the penis.

cleft palate (klĕft păl′ĭt). Congenital fissure of the palate and the roof of the mouth.

climacteric (klī-măk-tĕr′ĭk). A particular epoch of the ordinary term of life at which the body undergoes a considerable change; especially, the menopause or "change of life."

clitoris (klī'tŏ-rĭs). A small, elongated, erectile body, situated at the anterior part of the vulva. An organ of the female homologous with the penis of the male.

coitus (kō'ĭt-ŭs). Sexual intercourse; copulation.

colostrum (kŏ-lŏs'trŭm). A substance in the first milk after delivery, giving to it a yellowish color.

    c. corpuscles. Large granular cells found in colostrum.

colporrhaphy (kŏl-pŏr'ă-fē). 1. The operation of suturing the vagina. 2. The operation of denuding and suturing the vaginal wall for the purpose of narrowing the vagina.

colpotomy (kŏl-pŏt'o-mē). Any surgical cutting operation upon the vagina.

conception (kŏn-sĕp'shŭn). The impregnation of the female ovum by the spermatozoon of the male, whence results a new being.

condyloma (con-dil-o'mah). Pl. *condylomata.* A wartlike excrescence near the anus or the vulva; the flat, moist papule of secondary syphilis.

confinement (kŏn-fīn'mĕnt). Term applied to child-birth and the lying-in period.

congenital (kŏn-jĕn'ĭ-tĕl). Born with a person; existing from or from before birth, as, for example, congenital disease, a disease originating in the fetus before birth.

conjugate (kŏn'joo-gŏt). The anteroposterior diameter of the pelvic inlet.

contraception (kŏn"tră-sĕp'shŭn). The prevention of conception or impregnation.

coronal (kŏrŏ-năl). Belonging to, or relating to, the crown of the head.

    c. suture. The suture formed by the union of the frontal bone with the two parietal bones.

corpus luteum (kôr'pŭs lū'tĕ-ŭm). The yellow mass found in the graafian follicle after the ovum has been expelled.

cotyledon (kŏt"ĭ-lē'dŭn). Any one of the subdivisions of the uterine surface of the placenta.

cul-de-sac (kool'dē-săk') **of Douglas.** A pouch between the anterior wall of the rectum and the uterus.

cyesis (sī-ē'sĭs). Pregnancy.

decrement (dĕk'rē-mĕnt). Decrease; also the stage of decline.

delivery (dĕ-lĭv'ĕr-ĭ). [French, *délivrer,* to free, to deliver.] 1. The expulsion of a child by the mother, or its extraction by the obstetric practitioner. 2. The removal of a part from the body; as *delivery* of the placenta.

dizygotic (dī"zī-gŏt'ĭk). Pertaining to or proceeding from two zygotes (ova).

Döderlein's bacillus (ded'er-līnz). The large gram-positive bacterium occurring in the normal vaginal secretion.

Douglas' cul-de-sac (kool'dē-săk'). A sac or recess formed by a fold of the peritoneum dipping down between the rectum and the uterus. Also called *pouch of Douglas* and *rectouterine pouch.*

ductus (dŭk'tŭs). A duct.

    d. arteriosus (är-tē"rĭ-ō'sŭ). "Arterial duct," a blood vessel peculiar to the fetus, communicating directly between the pulmonary artery and the aorta.

    d. venosus (vĕ-nō'sŭs). "Venous duct," a blood vessel peculiar to the fetus, establishing a direct communication between the umbilical vein and the inferior vena cava.

Duncan (dŭng'kăn) **mechanism.** The position of the placenta, with the maternal surface outermost; to be born edgewise.

dystocia (dĭs-tō'shĭ-ă). Difficult, slow or painful birth or delivery. It is distinguished as *maternal* or *fetal* according as the difficulty is due to some deformity on the part of the mother or on the part of the child.

    d., placental. Difficulty in delivering the placenta.

eclampsia (ĕk-lămp'sĭ-ă). Acute "toxemia of pregnancy" characterized by convulsions and coma which may occur during pregnancy, labor or the puerperium.

ectoderm (ĕk'tŏ-dŭrm). The outer layer of cells of the primitive embryo.

ectopic (ĕk-tŏp'ĭk). Out of place.

    e. gestation. Gestation in which the fetus is out of its normal place in the cavity of the uterus. It includes gestations in the interstitial portion of the tube, in a rudimentary horn of the uterus (cornual pregnancy) and cervical pregnancy as well as tubal, abdominal and ovarian pregnancies. See also *extrauterine pregnancy.*

    e. pregnancy. Same as *ectopic gestation.*

effacement (ĕ-fās'mĕnt). Obliteration. In obstetrics, refers to thinning and shortening of the cervix.

ejaculation (ĕ-jăk"ŭ-lā'shŭn). A sudden act of expulsion, as of semen.

embryo (ĕm'brĭ-ō). The product of conception in utero from the third through the fifth week of gestation; after that length of time it is called the fetus.

empathy (ĕm'pă-thĭ). The projection of one's own consciousness into that of another. Empathy may be distinguished from sympathy in that the former state includes relative freedom from emotional involvement.

endocervical (ĕn'dŏ-sûr'vĭ-kăl). Pertaining to the interior of the cervix of the uterus.

endometrium (ĕn"dŏ-mē'trĭ-ŭm). The mucous membrane which lines the uterus.

engagement (ĕn-gāj'mĕnt). In obstetrics, applies to the entrance of the presenting part into the superior pelvic strait and the beginning of the descent through the pelvic canal.

engorgement (ĕn-gôrj'mĕnt). Hyperemia; local congestion; excessive fullness of any organ or passage. In obstetrics, refers to an exaggeration of normal venous and lymph stasis of the breasts which occurs in relation to lactation.

entoderm (ĕn'tŏ-dûrm). The innermost layer of cells of the primitive embryo.

enzygotic (ĕn-zī-gŏt'ĭk). Developed from the same fertilized ovum.

episiotomy (ĕp"ĭs-ĭ-ot'ŏ-mĭ). Surgical incision of the vulvar orifice for obstetric purposes.

Erb's paralysis. Partial paralysis of the brachial plexus, affecting various muscles of the arm and the chest wall.

ergot (ûr′gŏt). A drug having the remarkable property of exciting powerfully the contractile force of the uterus, and chiefly used for this purpose, but its long-continued use is highly dangerous. Usually given in the fluid extract.

erythroblastosis fetalis (ĕ-rĭth″rō-blăs-tō′sĭs). A severe hemolytic disease of the newborn usually due to Rh incompatibility.

estrogen (ĕs′trŏ-jĕn). A hormone secreted by the ovary and the placenta.

extraperitoneal (ĕks″trȧ-pĕr-ĭ-tŏ-nē′ȧl). Situated or occurring outside the peritoneal cavity.

extrauterine (ĕks″trȧ-ū′tēr-ĭn). Outside of the uterus.

   e. pregnancy. Pregnancy in which the fetus is contained in some organ outside of the uterus, i.e., tubal, abdominal and ovarian pregnancies.

fallopian (fȧ-lō′pĭ-ȧn). [Relating to G. *Fallopius,* a celebrated Italian anatomist of the 16th century.]

   f. tubes. The oviducts—two canals extending from the sides of the fundus uteri.

fecundation (fē″kŭn-dā′shŭn). The act of impregnating or the state of being impregnated; the fertilization of the ovum by means of the male seminal element.

fertility (fĕr-tĭl′ĭ-tĭ). The ability to produce offspring; power of reproduction.

fertilization (fûr-tĭ-lĭ-zā′shŭn). The fusion of the spermatozoon with the ovum; it marks the beginning of pregnancy.

fetus (fē′tŭs). The baby in utero from the end of the fifth week of gestation until birth.

fimbria (fĭm′brĭ-ȧ). A fringe; especially the fringe-like end of the fallopian tube.

fontanel (fŏn″tȧ-nĕl′). The diamond-shaped space between the frontal and two parietal bones in very young infants. This is called the *anterior f.* and is the familiar "soft spot" just above a baby's forehead. A small, triangular one (*posterior f.*) is between the occipital and parietal bones.

foramen (fŏ-rā′mĕn). A hole, opening, aperture or orifice—especially one through a bone.

   f. ovale (ŏ-vā′lē). An opening situated in the partition which separates the right and left auricles of the heart in the fetus.

foreskin (fōr′skĭn). The prepuce—the fold of skin covering the glans penis.

fornix (fôr′nĭks). Pl. *fornices* (fôr′nĭ-sēz). An arch; any vaulted surface.

   f. of the vagina. The angle of reflection of the vaginal mucous membrane onto the cervix uteri.

fourchette (foor-shĕt). [French, "fork."] The posterior angle or commissure of the labia majora.

frenum (frē′nŭm). Lingual fold of integument or of mucous membrane that checks, curbs, or limits the movements of the tongue (ankyloglossia). Congenital shortening.

Friedman's test (frēd′mȧn). A modification of the Aschheim-Zondek test for pregnancy; the urine of early pregnancy is injected in 4-ml. doses intravenously twice daily for two days into an unmated mature rabbit. If, at the end of this time, the ovaries of the rabbit contain fresh corpora lutea or hemorrhagic corpora, the test is positive.

FSH. Abbreviation for follicle-stimulating hormone.

fundus (fŭn′dŭs). The upper rounded portion of the uterus between the points of insertion of the fallopian tubes.

funic souffle (fū′nĭc soo′f′l). A soft, blowing sound, synchronous with the fetal heart sounds and supposed to be produced in the umbilical cord.

funis (fū′nĭs). A cord—especially the umbilical cord.

galactagogue (gȧ-lăk′tȧ-gŏg). 1. Causing the flow of milk. 2. Any drug which causes the flow of milk to increase.

galactorrhea (gȧ-lak-tō-re′ȧ). Excessive flow of milk.

gamete (găm′ēt). A sexual cell; a mature germ cell, as an unfertilized egg or a mature sperm cell.

gastrula (găs′troo-lȧ). The early embryonic stage which follows the blastula.

gene (jēn). An hereditary germinal factor in the chromosome which carries on an hereditary transmissible character.

genitalia (jĕn-ĭtāl′ĭ-ȧ). The reproductive organs.

gestation (jĕs-tā-shŭn). The condition of pregnancy; pregnancy; gravidity.

gonad (gŏn′ăd). A gamete-producing gland; an ovary or testis.

gonadotropin (gŏn″ăd-ŏ-trō′pĭn). A substance having an affinity for or a stimulating effect on the gonads.

Goodell's sign (good′elz). Softening of the cervix, a presumptive sign of pregnancy.

graafian follices or **vesicles** (grăf′ĭ-ȧn). Small spherical bodies in the ovaries, each containing an ovum.

gravida (grăv′ĭT-ȧ). A pregnant woman.

habitus (hăb′ĭt-ŭs). Attitude, disposition or tendency; to act in a certain way; position acquired by frequent repetition.

Hegar's sign (hā′gärz). Softening of the lower uterine segment; a sign of pregnancy.

homologous (hŏ-mŏl′ŏ-gŭs). Corresponding in structure or origin; derived from the same source.

hormone (hôr′mōn). A chemical substance produced in an organ, which, being carried to an associated organ by the blood stream, excites in the latter organ a functional activity.

hydatidiform (hi″dah-tid′ĭ-form) **mole.** Cystic proliferation of chorionic villi, resembling a bunch of grapes.

hydramnios (hī-drăm′nĭ-ŏs). An excessive amount of amniotic fluid.

hymen (hī′mĕn). A membranous fold which partially or wholly occludes the external orifice of the vagina, especially in the virgin.

hypofibrinogenemia (hī″pŏ-fĭ-brĭn″ō-jen-ē′mē-ȧ). Deficiency of fibrinogen in the blood.

hypogalactia (hī″pŏ-gȧ-lăk′she-a). Deficiency in the secretion of milk.

hypoxia (hī-pŏks′ĭ-a). Insufficient oxygen to support normal metabolic requirements.

iliopectineal line (ĭl″ĭ-ŏ-pĕk-tĭn′ē-ăi). The linea terminalis.

impregnation (ĭm″prĕg-nā′shŭn). See *fertilization*.

increment (ĭn′krĕ-mĕnt). That by which anything is increased.

inertia (ĭn-ûr′shĭά). Inactivity; inability to move spontaneously. Sluggishness of uterine contractions during labor.

infant (ĭn′fănt). A baby; a child under two years of age.

infertility (ĭn-fûr-tĭl′ĭ-tĭ). The condition of being unfruitful or barren; sterility.

inlet (ĭn′lĕt). The upper limit of the pelvic cavity (brim).

introitis (ĭn-trō′ĭ-tŭs). A term applied to the opening of the vagina.

in utero. Inside the uterus.

inversion (ĭn-vûr′shŭn). A turning upside down, in side out, or end for end.
  i. of the uterus. The state of the womb being turned inside out, caused by violently drawing away the placenta before it is detached by the natural process of labor.

involution (ĭn″vŏ-lū′shŭn). 1. A rolling or pushing inward. 2. A retrograde process of change which is the reverse of evolution: particularly applied to the return of the uterus to its normal size and condition after parturition.

ischium (ĭs′kĭ-ŭm). The posterior and inferior bone of the pelvis, distinct and separate in the fetus or the infant, or the corresponding part of the innominate bone in the adult.

jelly (jĕl′ĭ). A soft substance which is coherent, tremulous, and more or less transparent.
  j. of Wharton. The soft, pulpy, connective tissue that constitutes the matrix of the umbilical cord.

labia (lā′bĭ-ά). The nominative plural of *labium.* Lips or liplike structures.
  l. majora (mά-jō′rά). The folds of skin containing fat and covered with hair which form each side of the vulva.
  l. minora (mĭ-nō′rά). The nymphae, or folds of delicate skin inside of the labia majora.

labor (lā′bĕr). Parturition; the series of processes by which the products of conception are expelled from the mother's body.

lactation (lăk-tā′shŭn). The act or period of giving milk; the secretion of milk; the time or period of secreting milk.

lambdoid (lăm′doid). Having the shape of the Greek letter λ (lambda).
  l. suture. The suture between the occipital and two parietal bones.

lanugo (lά-nū′gō). The fine hair on the body of the fetus. The fine, downy hair found on nearly all parts of the body except the palms of the hands and the soles of the feet.

leukorrhea (lū″kŏ-rē′ά). A whitish discharge from the female genital organs.

LH. Abbreviation for lutenizing hormone.

lightening (līt′n-ing). The sensation of decreased abdominal distention produced by the descent of the uterus into the pelvic cavity, which occurs from 2 to 3 weeks before the onset of labor.

linea (lĭn′ē-ά). Pl. *lineae* (lĭn′ē-ē). A line or thread.
  l. alba (ăl′bά). The central tendinous line extending from the pubic bone to the ensiform cartilage.
  l. nigra (nī′grä). A dark line appearing on the abdomen and extending from the pubis toward the umbilicus—considered one of the signs of pregnancy.
  l. terminalis. The oblique ridge on the inner surface of the ilium, continued on the pubis, which separates the true from the false pelvis. Formerly called the iliopectineal line.

lingua (lĭng′gwĭ). Tongue.
  l. frenum. Tonguetie.

liquir (lĭk′ĕr). A liquid.
  l. amnii (lĭ′kwôr ăm′nĭ-ī). The fluid contained within the amnion in which the fetus floats.

lochia (lō′kĭ-ά). The discharge from the genital canal during several days subsequent to delivery.

mask (mάsk) of pregnancy. See *chloasma*.

maturation (măt″ŭ-rā′shŭn). In biology, a process of cell division during which the nnmber of chromosomes in the germ cells is reduced to one half the number characteristic of the species.

meatus (mē-ā′tŭs). A passage; an opening leading to a canal, duct or cavity.
  m. urinarius (ū″-rĭ-nā′rĭ-ŭs). The external orifice of the urethra.

mechanism (mĕk′ά-niz′m). The manner of combinations which subserve a common function. In obstetrics refers to labor and delivery.

meconium (mē-kō′nĭ-ŭm). The dark-green or black substance found in the large intestine of the fetus or newly born infant.

menarche (mē-när′kĕ). The establishment or the beginning of the menstrual function.

menopause (mĕn′ŏ-pôz). The period at which menstruation ceases; the "change of life."

menorrhagia (mĕn″ŏ-rā′jĭ-ά). An abnormally profuse menstrual flow.

menses (mĕn′sēz). [Pl. of Latin *mensis,* month.] The periodic monthly discharge of blood from the uterus; the catamenia.

menstruation (mĕn″stroo-ā′shŭn). The cyclic, physiologic uterine bleeding which normally recurs at approximately four-week intervals, in the absence of pregnancy, during the reproductive period.

mentum (mĕn′tŭm). The chin.

mesoderm (mĕs′ŏ-dûrm). The middle layer of cells derived from the primitive embryo.

metrorrhagia (mē-trŏ-rā′jĭ-ά). Abnormal uterine bleeding.

migration (mĭ-grā′shŭn). In obstetrics refers to the passage of the ovum from the ovary to the uterus.

milia (mĭY′ē-ά). Plural of *milium.*

milium (mĭY′ē-ŭm). A small white nodule of the skin, usually caused by clogged sebaceous glands or hair follicles.

milk-leg. See *phlegmasia alba dolens.*

miscarriage (mĭ—-kăr′ij). Abortion.

molding (mōld′ing). The shaping of the baby's head so as to adjust itself to the size and shape of the birth canal.

monozygotic (mŏn″ŏ-zī-gŏ′tĭk). Pertaining to or derived from one zygote.

> **m. twins** (mŏn″ō-zī-gŏ′tĭk). Pertaining to or derived from one zygote.

mons veneris (mŏnz vĕn′ĕ-rĭs). The eminence in the upper and anterior part of the pubes of women.

Montgomery's tubercles (mŭnt-gŭm′er-ĭz). Small, nodular follicles or glands on the areolae around the nipples.

multigravida (mŭl″tĭ-grăv′ĭ-d*a*). A woman who has been pregnant several times, or many times.

multipara (mŭl-tĭp′*a*-r*a*). A woman who has borne several, or many, children.

navel (nāv′el). The umbilicus.

neonatal (nē″ō-nā′tăl). Pertaining to the newborn, usually considered the first four weeks of life.

nevus (nē′vŭs). A natural mark or blemish; a mole, a circumscribed deposit of pigmentary matter in the skin present at birth (birthmark).

nidation (nĭ-dā′sh*u*n). The implantation of the fertilized ovum in the endometrium of the pregnant uterus.

nullipara (nŭ-lĭp′*a*-r*a*). A woman who has not borne children.

occipitobregmatic (ŏk-sĭp″ĭt-ŏ-brĕg-măt′-ik). Pertaining the occiput (the back part of the head) and the bregma (junction of the coronal and sagittal sutures).

oligohydramnios (ŏl″ĭ-gŏ-hĭ-drăm′nĭ-ŏs). Deficiency of amniotic fluid.

omphalic (ŏm-făl′ĭk). Pertaining to the umbilicus.

oocyesis (ō′ŏ-sĭ-ē′sĭs). Ovarian pregnancy.

ophthalmia neonatorum (ŏf-thăl′mĭ-*a*). Acute purulent conjunctivitis of the newborn usually due to gonorrheal infection.

os (ŏs). Pl. *ora* (ō′r*a*). Mouth.

> **o. externum** (*external os*). The external opening of the canal of the cervix.

> **o. internum** (*internal os*). Internal opening of canal of cervix.

> **o. uteri.** "Mouth of the uterus."

ova. Plural of ovum.

ovary (ō′v*a*-rĭ). The sexual gland of the female in which the ova are developed. There are two ovaries, one at each side of the pelvis.

ovulation (ō-vŭ-lā′sh*u*n). The growth and discharge of an unimpregnated ovum, usually coincident with the menstrual period.

ovum (ō′v*u*m). The female reproductive cell. The human ovum is a round cell about $1/120$ of an inch in diameter, developed in the ovary.

oxytocic (ŏk″sĭ-tō′sĭk). 1. Accelerating parturition. 2. A medicine which accelerates parturition.

oxytocin (ŏk-sĭ-tō-sĭn). One of the two hormones secreted by the posterior pituitary.

palsy (pôl′zĭ). A synonym for paralysis, used in connection with certain special forms.

> **Bell's p.** Peripheral facial paralysis due to lesion of the facial nerve, resulting characteristic distortion of the face.

> **Erb's p.** The upper-arm type of brachial birth palsy.

para (pär′ä). The term used to refer to past pregnancies which have produced an infant which has been viable, whether or not the infant is dead or alive at birth.

parametrium (pär-*a*-mē′trĭ-*u*m). The fibrous subserous coat of the supravaginal portion of the uterus, extending laterally between the layers of the broad ligaments.

parity (păr′ĭ-tĭ). The condition of a woman with respect to her having borne children.

parovarian (pär-ŏ-vâr′ĭ-*a*n). Pertaining to the residual structure in the broad ligament between the ovary and the fallopian tube.

parturient (pär-tŭ′rĭ-ent). Bringing forth; pertaining to childbearing. A woman in childbirth.

parturition (pär″tŭ-rĭsh′*u*n). The act or process of giving birth to a child.

patulous (păt′*u*-l*u*s). Spreading somewhat widely apart; open.

pelvimeter (pĕl-vĭm′ĕ-tēr). An instrument for measuring the diameters and capacity of the pelvis.

pelvimetry (pĕl-vĭm′ĕ-trĭ). The measurement of the dimensions and capacity of the pelvis.

penis (pē′nis). The male organ of copulation.

perineorrhaphy (pĕr″ĭ-nē-ŏr′*a*-fi). Suture of the perineum; the operation for the repair of lacerations of the perineum.

perineotomy (pĕr″ĭ-nē-ŏt′ō-mī). A surgical incision through the perineum.

perineum (pĕr″ĭ-nē′*u*m). The area between the vagina and the rectum.

peritoneum (pĕr″ĭ-tŏ-nē′*u*m). A strong serous membrane investing the inner surface of the abdominal walls and the viscera of the abdomen.

phimosis (fī-mō′sĭs). Tightness of the foreskin.

phlegmasia alba dolens (flĕg-mā′zhĭ′*a* ăl′b*a* dō′lĕnz). Phlebitis of the femoral vein, occasionally following delivery.

Pitocin (pī-tō′sĭn). A proprietary solution of oxytocin.

placenta (pl*a*-sĕn′t*a*). The circular flat, vascular structure in the impregnated uterus forming the principal medium of communication between the mother and the fetus.

> **ablatio p.** See *abruptio placentae*.

> **abruptio p.** Premature separation of the normally implanted placenta.

> **previa p.** A placenta which is implanted in the lower uterine segment so that it adjoins or covers the internal os of the cervix.

polygalactia (pŏl″ē-g*a*-lăk′shē-*a*). Excessive secretion of milk.

polyhydramnios (pŏl″ĭ-hĭ-drăm′nĭ-ŏs). Hydramnios.

position (pŏ-zĭsh′*u*n). The situation of the fetus in the pelvis; determined by the relation of some arbitrarily chosen portion of the fetus to the right or the left side of the mother's pelvis.

postnatal (pōst-nā′t*a*l). Occurring after birth.

postpartal (pōst-pär′tal). After delivery or childbirth.

preeclampsia (prē-ĕk-lămp′sĭ-*a*). A disorder encountered during pregnancy or early in the puerperium, characterized by hypertension, edema and albuminuria.

pregnancy (prĕg′năn-sĭ). [Latin, *praeg′nans,* literally "previous to bringing forth."] The state of being with young or with child. The normal duration of pregnancy in the human female is 280 days, or 10 lunar months, or 9 calendar months.

premature infant. An infant which weighs 2,500 Gm. or less at birth.

prepuce (prē′pūs). The fold of skin which covers the glans penis in the male.

    p. of the clitoris. The fold of mucous membrane which covers the glans clitoris.

presentation (prē″zĕn-tā′shŭn). Term used to designate that part of the fetus nearest the internal os; or that part which is felt by the physician's examining finger when introduced into the cervix.

primigravida (prī″mĭ-grăv′ĭ-dȧ). Pl. *primigravidae* (prī″mĭ-grăv′ĭ-dē). A woman who is pregnant for the first time.

primipara (prī-mĭp′ȧ-rȧ). Pl. *primiparae* (prī-mĭp′ȧ-rē). A woman who has given birth to her first child.

primordial (prī-môr′dĭ-ăl). Original or primitive; or the simplest and most undeveloped character.

prodromal (prŏ-drŏ′măl). Premonitory; indicating the approach of a disease.

progesterone (prŏ-jĕs′tĕr-ōn). The pure hormone contained in the corpora lutea whose function is to prepare the endometrium for the reception and development of the fertilized ovum.

prolactin (prŏ-lăk′tĭn). A proteohormone from the anterior pituitary which stimulates lactation in the mammary glands.

prolan (prŏ′lăn). Zondek's term for the gonadotropic principle of human-pregnancy urine, responsible for the biologic pregnancy tests.

promontory (prŏm′ŭn-tō″rĭ). A small projection; a prominence.

    p. of the sacrum. The superior or projecting portion of the sacrum when in situ in the pelvis, at the junction of the sacrum and the last lumbar vertebra.

pseudocyesis (sū″dō-sī-ē′sĭs). An apparent condition of pregnancy; the woman really believes she is pregnant when, as a matter of fact, she is not.

puberty (pū′bĕr-tĭ). The age at which the generative organs become functionally active.

pubic (pū′bĭk). Belonging to the pubis.

pubiotomy (pū′bĭ-ŏt′ŏ-mĭ). The operation of cutting through the pubic bone lateral to the median line.

pubis (pū′bĭs). The os pubis or pubic bone forming the front of the pelvis.

pudendal (pū-dĕn′dăl). Relating to the pudenda.

pudendum (pū-dĕn′dŭm). [Latin, *pude′re,* to have shame or modesty.] The external genital parts of either sex, but especially of the female.

puerperium (pū″ĕr-pē′rĭ-ŭm). The period elapsing between the termination of labor and the return of the uterus to its normal condition, about six weeks.

quickening (kwĭk′ĕn-ĭng). The mother's first perception of the movements of the fetus.

rabbit test. See *Friedman's test.*

Rh. Abbreviation for *Rhesus,* a type of monkey. This term is used for a property of human blood cells,

because of its relationship to a similar property in the blood cells of *Rhesus* monkeys.

Rh factor. A term applied to an inherited antigen in the human blood.

Ritgen maneuver (rĭt′gĕn). Delivery of the infant's head by lifting the head upward and forward through the vulva, between contractions, by pressing with the tips of the fingers upon the perineum behind the anus.

Schultze's mechanism (shoolt′sĕz). The expulsion of the placenta with the fetal surfaces presenting.

secundine (sĕk′ŭn-dīn). The afterbirth; the placenta and membranes expelled after the birth of a child.

segmentation (sĕg″mĕn-tā′shŭn). The process of division by which the fertilized ovum multiplies before differentiation into layers occurs.

semen (sē′mĕn). 1. A seed. 2. The fluid secreted by the male reproductive organs.

show (shō). 1. Popularly, the blood-tinged mucus discharged from the vagina before or during labor.

Skene's gland. Two glands just within the meatus of the female urethra; regarded as homologues of the prostate gland in the male.

smegma. A thick cheesy secretion found under the prepuce and in the region of the clitoris and the labia minora.

souffle (soof′f'l). A soft, blowing auscultatory sound.

    funic s. A hissing souffle synchronous with the fetal heart sounds and supposed to be produced in the umbilical cord.

    placental s. A souffle supposed to be produced by the blood current in the placenta.

spermatozoon (spûr″mȧ-tŏ-zō′ŏn). Pl. *spermatozoa* (spûr″mȧ-tŏ-zō′ȧ). The mobile microscopic sexual element of the male, resembling in shape an elongated tadpole. The male reproductive cell.

stillborn (stĭl′bôrn″). Born without life; born dead.

stria (strī′ȧ). Pl. *striae* (strī′ē). A Latin word signifying a "groove," "furrow" or "crease."

    striae gravidarum (grăv-ĭ-dār′ŭm). Shining, reddish lines upon the abdomen, thighs and breasts during pregnancy.

subinvolution (sŭb′ĭn-vō-lū′shŭn). Failure of a part to return to its normal size and condition after enlargement from functional activity, as subinvolution of the uterus which exists when normal involution of the puerperal uterus is retarded.

succedaneum (sŭk′sĕ-dā′nĕ-ŭm). See *caput.*

superfecundation (sū′pĕr-fē-kŭn-dā′shŭn). The fertilization at about the same time of two different ova by sperm from different males.

superfetation (sū′pĕr-fĕ-tā′shŭn). The fecundation of a woman already pregnant.

symphysis (sĭm′fĭ-sĭs). The union of bones by means of an intervening substance; a variety of synarthrosis.

    s. pubic (pū′bĭs). "Symphysis of the pubis," the pubic articulation or union of the pubic bones which are connected with each other by interarticular cartilage.

synchondrosis (sĭng″kŏn-drō′sĭs). A union of bones by means of a fibrous or elastic cartilage.

testicle (tĕs′tĭ-k'l). One of the two glands contained in the male scrotum.

thrush. An infection caused by the fungus *Candida albicans,* characterized by whitish plaques in the mouth.

tonguetie. See *lingua frenum.*

toxemia (tŏks-ē'mĭ-à). The toxemias of pregnancy are disorders encountered during gestation, or early in the puerperium, which are characterized by one or more of the following signs: hypertension, edema, albuminuria, and in severe cases, convulsions and coma.

trichomonas (trĭk-ŏm'ŏ-năs). A genus of parasitic flagellate protozoa.

  t. vaginalis. A species sometimes found in the vagina.

trophectoderm (trof-ĕk'tŏ-dûrm). The outer layer of cells of the early blastodermic vesicle; it develops the trophoderm—the feeding layer.

umbilical (ŭm-bĭl'ĭ-kăl). Pertaining to the umbilicus.

  u. arteries. The arteries which accompany and form part of the umbilical cord.

  u. cord [Latin, *funis umbilicalis*]. The cord connecting the placenta with the umbilicus of the fetus, and at the close of gestation principally made up of the two umbilical arteries and the umbilical vein, encased in a mass of gelatinous tissue called "Wharton's jelly."

  u. hernia. Hernia at or near the umbilicus.

  u. vein. Forms a part of the umbilical cord.

uterus (ū'tĕr-ŭs). The hollow muscular organ in the female designed for the lodgement and nourishment of the fetus during its development until birth.

vagina (và-jī'nà). [Latin, a sheath.] The canal in the female, extending from the vulva to the cervix of the uterus.

vernix caseosa (vûr'nĭks kā"sĕ-ō'sà). "Cheesy varnish." The layer of fatty matter which covers the skin of the fetus.

version (vûr'shŭn). The act of turning; specifically, a turning of the fetus in the uterus so as to change the presenting part and bring it into more favorable position for delivery.

vertex (vûr'tĕks). The summit or top of anything. In anatomy, the top or crown of the head.

  v. presentation. Presentation of the vertex of the fetus in labor.

vestibule (vĕs'tĭ-būl). A triangular space between the labia minora; the urinary meatus and the vagina open into it.

viable (vī'à-b'l). A term in medical jurisprudence signifying "able or likely to live"; applied to the condition of the child at birth.

villus (vĭl'ŭs). A small vascular process or protrusion growing on a mucous surface, such as the chorionic villi seen in tufts on the chorion of the early embryo.

vulva (vŭl'và). The external genitals of the female.

Wharton's jelly (hwôr'tŭnz). [Thomas *Wharton,* English anatomist, died 1673.] The jellylike mucous tissue composing the bulk of the umbilical cord.

witches' milk (wĭch'ĕz). A milky fluid secreted from the breast of the newly born.

worm (woom). See *uterus.*

zona pellucida (zō'nà pĕll-ū'sĭd-ä). A transparent belt; translucent or shining through.

zygote (zī'gōt). A cell resulting from the fusion of two gametes.

Conversion Table for Weights of Newborn

(Gram equivalents for pounds and ounces)

For example, to find weight in pounds and ounces of baby weighing 3315 grams, glance down columns to figure nearest 3315 = 3317. Refer to number at top of column for pounds and number to far left for ounces = 7 pounds, 5 ounces.

Pounds→ Ounces↓	3	4	5	6	7	8	9	10
0	1361	1814	2268	2722	3175	3629	4082	4536
1	1389	1843	2296	2750	3203	3657	4111	4564
2	1417	1871	2325	2778	3232	3685	4139	4593
3	1446	1899	2353	2807	3260	3714	4167	4621
4	1474	1928	2381	2835	3289	3742	4196	4649
5	1503	1956	2410	2863	3317	3770	4224	4678
6	1531	1984	2438	2892	3345	3799	4252	4706
7	1559	2013	2466	2920	3374	3827	4281	4734
8	1588	2041	2495	2948	3402	3856	4309	4763
9	1616	2070	2523	2977	3430	3884	4338	4791
10	1644	2098	2551	3005	3459	3912	4366	4819
11	1673	2126	2580	3033	3487	3941	4394	4848
12	1701	2155	2608	3062	3515	3969	4423	4876
13	1729	2183	2637	3090	3544	3997	4451	4904
14	1758	2211	2665	3118	3572	4026	4479	4933
15	1786	2240	2693	3147	3600	4054	4508	4961

Or, to convert grams into pounds and *decimals* of a pound, multiply weight in grams by .0022. Thus, 3317 × .0022 = 7.2974, i.e., 7.3 pounds, or 7 pounds, 5 ounces.

To convert pounds and ounces into grams, multiply the pounds by 453.6 and the ounces by 28.4 and add the two products. Thus, to convert 7 pounds, 5 ounces, 7 × 453.6 = 3175; 5 × 28.4 = 142; 3175 + 142 = 3317 grams.

Aid for Visualization

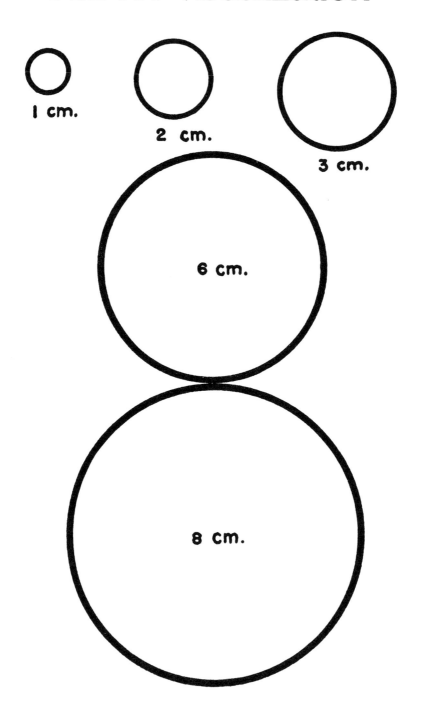

1 cm.

2 cm.

3 cm.

6 cm.

8 cm.

# of Cervical Dilatation

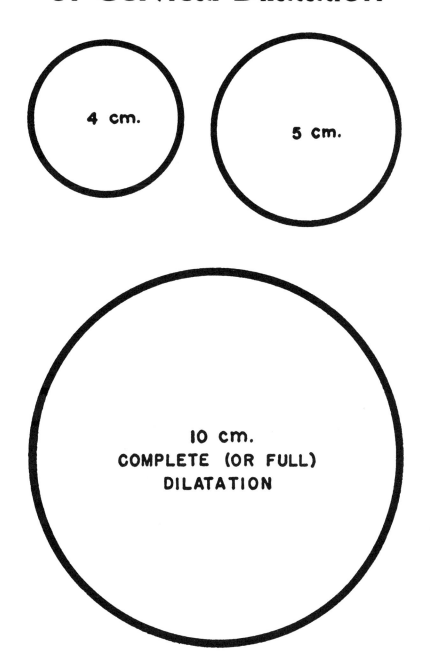

4 cm.

5 cm.

10 cm.
COMPLETE (OR FULL)
DILATATION

Index